Hensley's Practical Approach to Cardiothoracic Anesthesia

T0176444

Hensley's Practical Approach to Cardiothoracic Anesthesia

Sixth Edition

Editors

GLENN P. GRAVLEE, MD
Professor and Vice Chair for Faculty Affairs
Department of Anesthesiology
University of Colorado School of Medicine
Aurora, Colorado

ANDREW D. SHAW, MB, FRCA
Professor and Chair, Department of Anesthesiology and Pain Medicine
Faculty of Medicine and Dentistry
University of Alberta
Edmonton, Alberta, Canada

KARSTEN BARTELS, MD, MS
Assistant Professor of Anesthesiology, Medicine, and Surgery
Department of Anesthesiology
University of Colorado School of Medicine
Aurora, Colorado

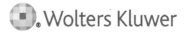. Wolters Kluwer

Philadelphia • Baltimore • New York • London
Buenos Aires • Hong Kong • Sydney • Tokyo

Acquisitions Editor: Keith Donnellan
Editorial Coordinator: Lauren Pecarich
Marketing Manager: Julie Sikora
Senior Production Project Manager: Alicia Jackson
Design Coordinator: Terry Mallon
Senior Manufacturing Coordinator: Beth Welsh
Prepress Vendor: Aptara, Inc.

6th edition

9 8 7 6 5 4

Printed in The United States of America

978-1-4963-7266-6
1-4963-7266-2
Library of Congress Cataloging-in-Publication Data
available upon request

---

shop.lww.com

Dedication

Frederick Allen Hensley, Jr., MD
(1953–2013)

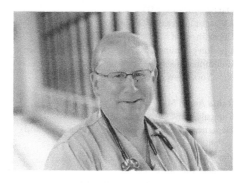

We dedicate this book to the memory of Frederick Allen Hensley, Jr., MD, who most knew simply as "Rick." As a young academician at Penn State Hershey Medical Center in the late 1980s, Rick developed a cardiac anesthesia teaching manual for local residents, fellows, and perfusionists. While preparing this manual, he recognized the wider need for a point-of-care reference book on cardiac anesthesia. He then sought to address this deficiency by compressing a readable, comprehensive cardiac anesthesia textbook into a pocket-sized paperback package. Its mission would be to provide clinical recommendations supported by their briefly-explained underlying scientific principles. Practical clinical relevance and conciseness were deemed more important than lengthy narratives and prodigious reference lists. Hensley recruited his Hershey friend and colleague, Donald E. Martin, MD, to co-edit this book. Together they envisioned a multi-author text representing multiple teaching hospitals, so they recruited chapter authors who were recognized for clinical expertise and experience. To achieve thoroughness without sacrificing readability, Rick and Don thought that the chapters should be formatted as outlines. As editors, they delicately pursued practical clinical advice while avoiding parochial institutional practices.

Their vision flew in the face of the prevailing approach to both medical textbooks and handbooks. At the time, comprehensive medical textbooks predominantly were lengthy tomes with thousands of references. Much shorter paperback handbooks typically presented single-institution "how-we-do-it" guidelines without scientific foundation or expert consensus. Hardly anything existed between those extremes. Undaunted, Hensley and Martin advanced their proposal to Little, Brown and Company, which accepted it, and *The Practice of Cardiac Anesthesia* was born in 1990. The book was warmly received by busy residents and fellows. Residency and fellowship program directors embraced it for its unique blend of quality, thoroughness, and conciseness. Part-time practitioners of cardiac anesthesiology also found it useful, in part because hardwired computers, cell phones with endless "apps," and wireless internet access had not reached anesthesia work stations. The book's success brought another edition and a new name in 1995: *A Practical Approach to Cardiac Anesthesia*. And so on through five editions and to a series of paperback subspecialty books carrying the rubric "*A Practical Approach to …*," all using Rick's visionary approach. Accordingly, the current editors have named this sixth edition *Hensley's Practical Approach to Cardiothoracic Anesthesia* in honor of Rick Hensley.

Chronology of Frederick A. Hensley's postdoctoral education and primary career appointments and positions:

1979–1983: Milton S. Hershey Medical Center, Penn State University College of Medicine: Internship, Anesthesiology Residency and Cardiac Anesthesia Fellowship

1984–1995: Penn State University College of Medicine, Assistant Professor, Associate Professor, and Professor and Director of Cardiac Anesthesia, Department of Anesthesiology

1995–2000: Sinai Hospital of Baltimore, Anesthesiologist-in-Chief and Medical Director of Perioperative Services; Associate Professor, Department of Anesthesiology and Critical Care Medicine, The Johns Hopkins University School of Medicine

2001–2009: Imogene Bassett Healthcare (Cooperstown, New York), Anesthesiologist in Chief, and Chief of Perioperative Services; Clinical Professor of Anesthesiology, College of Physicians and Surgeons of Columbia University

2009–2013: University of Alabama at Birmingham, Benjamin Monroe Carraway Endowed Professor of Anesthesiology, Department of Anesthesiology, Director, Division of Cardiothoracic Anesthesiology (2009–2011), Vice Chair of Clinical Anesthesia (2011–2013)

Contributors

Darryl Abrams, MD
Assistant Professor
Department of Medicine
Division of Pulmonary, Allergy, and Critical Care
Columbia University Medical Center
New York, New York

Rabia Amir, MD
Clinical Fellow
Department of Anesthesiology, Critical Care and
  Pain Medicine
Harvard Medical School
Resident Physician
Beth Israel Deaconess Medical Center
Boston, Massachusetts

James M. Anton, MD
Clinical Associate Professor
Department of Anesthesiology
Baylor College of Medicine
Chief
Division of Cardiovascular Anesthesiology
Texas Heart Institute, Baylor St. Luke's
  Medical Center
Houston, Texas

Yanick Baribeau
Undergraduate Research Student
Department of Anesthesia, Critical Care and Pain
  Medicine
Beth Israel Deaconess Medical Center
Boston, Massachusetts

Brandi A. Bottiger, MD
Adult Cardiothoracic Anesthesia Fellowship Director
Assistant Professor
Department of Anesthesiology
Duke University
Durham, North Carolina

Daniel Brodie, MD
Associate Professor
Department of Medicine
Columbia University Medical Center
New York, New York

John F. Butterworth, IV, MD
Professor and Chairman
Department of Anesthesiology
Virginia Commonwealth University
Chief of Anesthesiology
Virginia Commonwealth University Health System
Richmond, Virginia

Javier H. Campos, MD
Professor
Department of Anesthesia
University of Iowa Health Care
Executive Medical Director
Perioperative Services
Director of Cardiothoracic Anesthesia
University of Iowa Hospitals and Clinics
Iowa City, Iowa

Pedro Catarino, MD
Consultant Cardiothoracic Surgeon
Papworth Hospital
Cambridge, United Kingdom

Joseph C. Cleveland, Jr., MD
Professor
Department of Surgery, Division of Cardiothoracic Surgery
University of Colorado Anschutz Medical Campus
Cardiothoracic Surgeon
University of Colorado Hospital
Aurora, Colorado

Charles D. Collard, MD
Clinical Professor of Anesthesiology
Baylor College of Medicine
Attending Anesthesiologist
Division of Cardiovascular Anesthesiology
Texas Heart Institute, Baylor St. Luke's Medical Center
Houston, Texas

John R. Cooper, Jr., MD
Clinical Professor of Anesthesiology
Baylor College of Medicine
Attending Anesthesiologist
Division of Cardiovascular Anesthesiology
Texas Heart Institute, Baylor St. Luke's Medical Center
Houston, Texas

Laurie K. Davies, MD
Associate Professor
Department of Anesthesiology and Surgery
University of Florida
Medical Director
University of Florida Health
Gainesville, Florida

Ronak G. Desai, DO
Assistant Professor of Anesthesiology
Cooper Medical School of Rowan University
Division Head, Regional Anesthesia
Department of Anesthesiology
Cooper University Hospital
Camden, New Jersey

Alan Finley, MD
Associate Professor of Anesthesiology and
   Perioperative Medicine
Medical University of South Carolina
Charleston, South Carolina

Amanda A. Fox, MD, MPH
Division Chief of Cardiovascular and Thoracic
   Anesthesiology
Department of Anesthesiology and Pain Management
University of Texas Southwestern Medical School
Dallas, Texas

Steven M. Frank, MD
Professor
Department of Anesthesiology and Critical Care Medicine
Johns Hopkins School of Medicine
Baltimore, Maryland

Satoru Fujii, MD
Clinical Fellow
Department of Anesthesia
London Health Sciences Centre
London, Ontario, Canada

Chandrika R. Garner, MD, FASE
Assistant Professor
Department of Anesthesiology
Wake Forest School of Medicine
Winston-Salem, North Carolina

Thomas E. J. Gayeski, MD, PhD
Professor
Department of Anesthesiology and Perioperative
   Medicine
University of Alabama at Birmingham School of Medicine
Birmingham, Alabama

Mark A. Gerhardt, MD, PhD
Associate Professor
Department of Anesthesiology
The Ohio State University College of Medicine
The Ohio State University Wexner Medical
   Center
Columbus, Ohio

Neville M. Gibbs, MBBS, MD, FANZCA
Clinical Professor
The University of Western Australia
Perth, Australia
Specialist Anaesthetist
Department of Anaesthesia
Sir Charles Gairdner Hospital
Nedlands, WA, Australia

Glenn P. Gravlee, MD
Professor and Vice Chair for Faculty Affairs
Department of Anesthesiology
University of Colorado School of Medicine
Aurora, Colorado

Michael S. Green, DO, MBA
Chair and Program Director
Department of Anesthesiology and Perioperative
   Medicine
Drexel University College of Medicine
Hahnemann University Hospital
Philadelphia, Pennsylvania

Jonathan Hastie, MD
Assistant Professor
Department of Anesthesiology
Columbia University Medical Center
New York, New York

Nadia B. Hensley, MD
Assistant Professor
Department of Anesthesiology and Critical Care Medicine
Johns Hopkins University School of Medicine
Baltimore, Maryland

Eugene A. Hessel, II, MD
Professor of Anesthesiology and Surgery
   (Cardio-thoracic)
University of Kentucky College of Medicine
Attending Physician
Anesthesiology
Chandler Medical Center
Lexington, Kentucky

Jordan R. H. Hoffman, MD, MPH
Cardiothoracic Surgery Fellow
Department of Surgery
Division of Cardiothoracic Surgery
University of Colorado School of Medicine
Aurora, Colorado

Jay C. Horrow, MD, MS, FACC
Professor
Department of Anesthesiology and Perioperative Medicine
Drexel University College of Medicine
Philadelphia, Pennsylvania

Matthew S. Hull, MD
Adult Cardiothoracic Anesthesiology Fellow
Department of Anesthesiology and Perioperative
   Medicine
University of Alabama at Birmingham School of Medicine
Birmingham, Alabama

S. Adil Husain, MD
Professor of Surgery and Pediatrics
Chief, Section of Pediatric Cardiothoracic Surgery
University of Utah School of Medicine
Primary Children's Hospital
Salt Lake City, Utah

David Philip Jenkins, MB, BS
Consultant Cardiothoracic Surgeon
Papworth Hospital
Cambridge, United Kingdom

Rebecca Y. Klinger, MD, MS
Assistant Professor
Department of Anesthesiology
Duke University
Durham, North Carolina

Colleen G. Koch, MD, MS, MBA, FACC
Professor and Chair
Department of Anesthesiology and Critical Care Medicine
Johns Hopkins School of Medicine
Baltimore, Maryland

Megan P. Kostibas, MD
Instructor
Department of Anesthesiology and Critical Care Medicine
Johns Hopkins School of Medicine
Baltimore, Maryland

David R. Larach, MD, PhD
Chief (retired)
Division of Cardiac Anesthesiology
The Heart Institute
St. Joseph Medical Center
Towson, Maryland

Michael G. Licina, MD
Professor of Anesthesiology
Anesthesia Institute
Cleveland Clinic Lerner College of Medicine
Case Western Reserve University
Vice Chair
Department of Cardiothoracic Anesthesia
Cleveland Clinic
Cleveland, Ohio

Jerry C. Luck, Jr., MD[†]
Professor of Medicine
Department of Medicine
Penn State College of Medicine
Heart and Vascular Institute
Penn State Health Milton S. Hershey Medical Center
Hershey, Pennsylvania

Feroze U. Mahmood, MD
Professor
Department of Anesthesiology, Critical Care and
   Pain Medicine
Harvard Medical School
Director of Cardiovascular Anesthesia
Beth Israel Deaconess Medical Center
Boston, Massachusetts

S. Nini Malayaman, MD
Assistant Professor
Department of Anesthesiology
Drexel University College of Medicine
Attending Anesthesiologist
Hahnemann University Hospital
Philadelphia, Pennsylvania

Donald E. Martin, MD
Professor Emeritus
Department of Anesthesiology and Perioperative
   Medicine
Penn State College of Medicine
Hershey, Pennsylvania

Shannon J. Matzelle, MBBS, FANZCA
Specialist Anaesthetist
Department of Anaesthesia
Sir Charles Gairdner Hospital
Nedlands, WA, Australia

Thomas M. McLoughlin, Jr., MD
Chair, Department of Anesthesiology
Lehigh Valley Health Network
Allentown, Pennsylvania
Professor of Surgery, Division of Surgical Anesthesiology
University of South Florida Morsani College of Medicine
Tampa, Florida

Anand R. Mehta, MBBS
Assistant Professor of Cardiothoracic
   Anesthesia
Cleveland Clinic Lerner College of Medicine
Case Western Reserve University
Staff Physician
Department of Cardiothoracic Anesthesia
Cleveland Clinic
Cleveland, Ohio

Benjamin N. Morris, MD
Assistant Professor
Department of Anesthesiology
Wake Forest School of Medicine
Medical Director
Cardiovascular Intensive Care Unit
Wake Forest Baptist Medical Center
Winston-Salem, North Carolina

John M. Murkin, MD, FRCPC
Senate Professor
Department of Anesthesia and Perioperative Medicine
Schulich School of Medicine and Dentistry
University of Western Ontario
London, Ontario, Canada

Gary Okum, MD
Professor of Clinical Anesthesiology and Perioperative
   Medicine and Surgery
Department of Anesthesiology and Perioperative
   Medicine and Surgery
Drexel University College of Medicine
Attending Anesthesiologist
Hahnemann University Hospital
Philadelphia, Pennsylvania

[†]Deceased.

Jay D. Pal, MD, PhD
Associate Professor
Department of Surgery
Division of Cardiothoracic Surgery
University of Colorado Anschutz Medical Campus
Surgical Director, Mechanical Circulatory Support
University of Colorado Hospital
Aurora, Colorado

Nirvik Pal, MBBS, MD
Assistant Professor
Department of Anesthesiology
Cardiothoracic Division
Virginia Commonwealth University
Richmond, Virginia

Kinjal M. Patel, MD
Assistant Professor of Anesthesiology
Cooper Medical School of Rowan University
Division Head, Vascular Anesthesia
Department of Anesthesiology
Cooper University Hospital
Camden, New Jersey

Ferenc Puskas, MD, PhD
Professor
Department of Anesthesiology
University of Colorado Denver School of Medicine
Aurora, Colorado

James G. Ramsay, MD
Professor of Anesthesiology and Perioperative Care
University of California San Francisco
San Francisco, California
Medical Director
Cardiovascular Intensive Care Unit
Anesthesiology and Perioperative Care
Moffitt Hospital
San Francisco, California

Jacob Raphael, MD
Professor of Anesthesiology
University of Virginia
Charlottesville, Virginia

Anne L. Rother, MBBS, FANZCA
Staff Anesthesiologist
Department of Anesthesia
Monash Medical Centre
Clayton, VIC, Australia

Roger L. Royster, MD
Professor and Executive Vice Chair
Department of Anesthesiology
Wake Forest School of Medicine
Winston-Salem, North Carolina

Soraya M. Samii, MD, PhD
Associate Professor
Department of Medicine
Associate Program Director, Division of Cardiac
    Electrophysiology
Penn State Health Heart and Vascular Institute
Milton S. Hershey Medical Center
Hershey, Pennsylvania

Jack S. Shanewise, MD, FASE
Professor
Department of Anesthesiology
Columbia University
Chief of Cardiothoracic Anesthesiology
Columbia University Medical Center
New York, New York

Linda Shore-Lesserson, MD, FAHA, FASE
Professor of Anesthesiology
Zucker School of Medicine at Hofstra/Northwell
Vice Chair, Academic Affairs
Department of Anesthesiology
North Shore University Hospital
Northwell Health
Manhasset, New York

Peter Slinger, MD, FRCPC
Professor
Department of Anesthesia
University of Toronto
Staff Anesthesiologist
Department of Anesthesia
Toronto General Hospital
Toronto, Ontario, Canada

Alann Solina, MD
Professor and Chair
Department of Anesthesiology
Cooper Medical School of Rowan University
Chief of Anesthesia and Medical Director of Operating
    Room Services
Cooper University Health Care
Camden, New Jersey

Andrew N. Springer, MD
Assistant Professor, Clinical Anesthesiology
The Ohio State University College of Medicine
Department of Anesthesiology
The Ohio State University Wexner Medical Center
Columbus, Ohio

Mark Stafford-Smith, MD, CM, FRCP, FASE
Vice Chair of Education
Professor
Department of Anesthesiology
Duke University
Durham, North Carolina

Breandan L. Sullivan, MD
Assistant Professor
Department of Anesthesiology and Critical Care Medicine
University of Colorado School of Medicine
Medical Director, CTICU
University of Colorado Hospital
Aurora, Colorado

Erin A. Sullivan, MD, FASA
Associate Professor
Department of Anesthesiology
Program Director, Adult Cardiothoracic
    Anesthesiology Fellowship
University of Pittsburgh School of Medicine
Chief, Division of Cardiothoracic Anesthesiology
Associate Chief Anesthesiologist
UPMC Presbyterian Hospital
Pittsburgh, Pennsylvania

Matthew M. Townsley, MD, FASE
Associate Professor
Department of Anesthesiology and Perioperative
    Medicine
University of Alabama at Birmingham School of Medicine
Birmingham, Alabama

Benjamin C. Tuck, MD
Assistant Professor
Department of Anesthesiology and Perioperative
    Medicine
University of Alabama at Birmingham School
    of Medicine
Birmingham, Alabama

Kamen Valchanov, MD, BSc
Consultant Anaesthetist
Department of Anaesthesia and Intensive Care
Papworth Hospital
Cambridge, United Kingdom

Michael H. Wall, MD, FCCM
JJ Buckley Professor and Chair
Department of Anesthesiology
University of Minnesota Medical Center
Minneapolis, Minnesota

Nathaen S. Weitzel, MD
Associate Professor
Department of Anesthesiology
University of Colorado School of Medicine
Medical Director of Inpatient Operations
University of Colorado Hospital
Aurora, Colorado

Preface

WE ARE PLEASED TO PRESENT the sixth edition of a book that now exceeds a quarter century of longevity. The subspecialty of cardiothoracic anesthesiology continues to evolve, just as this book aspires to evolve with it. As it was for the first edition in 1990, our mission is to provide an easily accessible, practical reference to help trainees and practitioners prepare for and manage anesthetics within the subspecialty. As a result of Don Martin's retirement from full-time clinical practice and of Frederick Hensley's premature passing in 2013, Glenn Gravlee welcomes co-editors Andrew Shaw and Karsten Bartels to this edition. Each new editor brings a fresh and multi-institutional perspective that includes expertise in cardiothoracic anesthesia and critical care as well as clinical experience in both North America and Europe. Dr. Bartels also offers expertise in perioperative acute and chronic pain management.

The title of the sixth edition has changed to *"Hensley's Practical Approach to Cardiothoracic Anesthesia"* to honor Rick Hensley (see Dedication) and to acknowledge the incorporation of noncardiac thoracic anesthesia topics, which was actually done in previous editions without titular recognition. This edition also adds 23 links to video clips spread across Chapters 5, 11, 12, and 19. In addition to the Key Points at the beginning of each chapter (locations marked in text margins also), all chapters now include several Clinical Pearls, which are short, key clinical concepts located in the text section where their subject matter is presented. Highlighting of key references constitutes another new feature. Although we tried to keep overlap between chapters to a minimum, we allowed it when we believed that differences in content or perspective merited retention.

The sections have been subtly reorganized to flow from basic science on to general tenets of intraoperative management, then to specific cardiothoracic disorders, and to conclude with sections on circulatory support and perioperative management. Some previous chapters have been reconfigured or merged, such as Induction of Anesthesia and Precardiopulmonary Bypass Management (Chapter 6) and Anesthetic Management of Cardiac and Pulmonary Transplantation (Chapter 17). A chapter on blood management supersedes one on blood transfusion. The growth of minimally invasive valve procedures inspired the creation of a separate chapter for aortic valve procedures as well as one for those involving the mitral and tricuspid valves, each with the addition of video clips emphasizing echocardiography. Rapid development of extracorporeal membrane oxygenation in adults now merits a full chapter. Robotic surgical techniques for cardiac and thoracic surgery earn expanded coverage in Chapter 13. We decided to concede the huge topic of congenital heart disease in children to other textbooks, while retaining and updating the one on adult congenital heart disease.

We hope that learners enjoy this book's content as much as we enjoyed planning, reviewing, and editing it.

Glenn P. Gravlee, MD
Andrew D. Shaw, MB, FRCA
Karsten Bartels, MD, MS

Acknowledgments

Each edition of this book has involved a broad team effort of authors, physician editors, development editors, copy editors, typesetters, and publishing and graphics experts. The editors thank the 69 authors representing 37 institutions for their timely and tireless efforts. On the publishing side, we thank Wolters Kluwer for their continued support of this book. In particular, Keith Donellan gets warm thanks and appreciation for his dedication, experience, and wisdom. Special thanks go to Louise Bierig, whose expertise, persistence, and detail orientation during developmental editing proved indispensable.

Contents

SECTION IV: CIRCULATORY SUPPORT

SECTION V: PERIOPERATIVE MANAGEMENT

Cardiovascular Physiology and Pharmacology

1

Cardiovascular Physiology: A Primer

Thomas E. J. Gayeski

KEY POINTS

1. The heart has a fibrous skeleton that provides an insertion site at each valvular ring. This fibrous structure also connects cardiac myocytes so that "stretch" or preload results in sarcomeres lengthening and not cells sliding past each other.
2. Contractility changes as a result of myoplasmic Ca^{2+} concentration change during systole.
3. Relaxation following contraction is an active process requiring ATP consumption to pump Ca^{2+} into the sarcoplasmic reticulum (SR) as well as across the sarcolemma.
4. The fundamental unit of tension development is the sarcomere.
5. The endocardium receives blood flow only during systole while the epicardium receives blood flow throughout the cardiac cycle. The endocardium is more susceptible to infarction.
6. Oxygen or ATP consumption occurs during release of actin–myosin bonds during relaxation of this bond. The main determinants of myocardial oxygen consumption are heart rate (HR), contractility, and wall tension.
7. The external stroke volume (SV) work the ventricle does is to raise the pressure of a SV from ventricular end-diastolic pressure (VEDP, right or left) to mean arterial pressure (pulmonary or systemic, respectively).
8. The cardiovascular system regulates blood pressure (BP) and exemplifies a negative feedback loop control system. Sensors throughout the cardiovascular system detect pressure through stretch. Hence, compliance changes impact pressure sensors.
9. Physiologic reserves are expansion factors allowing the cardiovascular system to maintain BP. These reserves are HR (3-fold range), contractility (complex but significant range), systemic vascular resistance (SVR; 15-fold range), and venous capacitance (~1.3-fold range).
10. Venous capacitance reserve is approximately 1,500 mL in a 70-kg adult.

I. Introduction

As a physiologic primer for cardiac anesthesiology, this chapter requires compromise and choices! The studies of cardiac anatomy, physiology, pathology, and genomics are decades to centuries old, continue to evolve, and have a vast literature. Our focus is on presenting physiologic principles important to adult clinical management in the operating room (OR). The first compromise is that I will barely touch embryology and I chose not to discuss pediatric cardiac physiology. To complement our view, a detailed description and discussion of adult cardiac physiology can be found in Ref. [1]. A thorough understanding of the physiologic concepts contained herein will facilitate the anesthetic care of both healthy patients and those with cardiovascular disease.

II. Embryologic development of the heart

A. The cardiovascular system begins to develop during week 3 of gestation as the primitive vascular system is formed from mesodermally derived endothelial tubes. At week 4, bilateral cardiogenic cords from paired endocardial heart tubes fuse into a single heart tube (primitive heart). This fusion initiates forward flow and begins the heart's transport function.

B. The primitive heart evolves into four chambers: Bulbus cordis, ventricle, primordial atrium, and sinus venosus, eventually forming a bulboventricular loop with initial contraction commencing at 21 to 22 days. These contractions result in unidirectional blood flow in week 4.

C. From weeks 4 to 7, heart development enters a critical period, as it divides into the fetal circulation and the four chambers of the adult heart.

D. A fibrous skeleton composed of fibrin and elastin forms the framework of four rings encircling the four heart valves as well as intermyocyte connections.

E. The fibrous skeleton
  1. Serves as an anchor for the insertion into the valve cusps
  2. Resists overdistention of the annuli of the valves (resisting incompetence)
  3. Provides a fixed insertion point for the muscular bundles of the ventricles
  4. Minimizes intermyocyte sliding during ventricular filling and contraction

III. Electrical conduction

A. Purkinje fibers are made up of specialized cardiac myocytes that conduct electrical signals faster (2 m/sec) than normal myocytes (0.3 m/sec). This speed difference results in coordinated chamber contraction.

B. Purkinje fibers exist in the atrium and ventricles in the subendocardium. Hence, they can be accessed from within the respective chambers.

C. The fibrous skeleton slows the direct spread of electrical conduction between myocytes as well as between atrium and ventricles.

D. Coordinated chamber contraction depends on Purkinje signal conduction, not on intermyocyte conduction. This sequence consists of a coordinated contraction in the atrium followed by a delay as the Purkinje signal passes through AV node, which is in turn followed by coordinated contraction of ventricles.

E. Action potential
  1. A membrane potential is the difference in voltage between the inside of the cell and the outside.
  2. In a cell this membrane potential is a consequence of the ions and proteins inside and outside the cell.
  3. There is a predominance of potassium (K^+) and negatively charged proteins (anions, A^-) inside the cell and sodium (Na^+) and chloride (Cl^-) outside the cell (Fig. 1.1).
  4. At rest, potassium ions can cross the membrane readily while sodium and chloride ions have a greater difficulty in doing so.
  5. Ion channels regulate the ability of Na, K, and calcium (Ca^{2+}) to cross the membrane. They open or close in response to a stimulus, most frequently a chemical stimulus.
  6. Membrane differences in ion channel concentrations and characteristics are cell-type specific.
  7. At rest, the negative ions within the cell predominate, resulting in a negative transmembrane voltage. The resting voltage is referred to as the resting membrane potential.

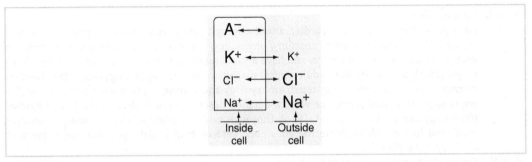

FIGURE 1.1 Major ionic content inside and outside a cell. A⁻ represents negatively charged proteins within the cell. Under normal conditions at rest, membrane potentials are negative, meaning that the voltage is more negative within the cell than outside of it.

8. Stimulation of a cell results in a change in membrane potential characteristic for that cell type because of a choreographed sequence of ion channels opening and closing. The plot of this sequence is referred to as an action potential.

F. Excitation–contraction coupling in the heart

1. The intricacies of ion channel opening due to a Purkinje action potential are beyond the scope of this chapter. However, these intricacies are important for anesthesiologists, because clinicians prescribe and administer drugs that directly affect their characteristics.

2. Excitation–contraction coupling starts when a Purkinje cell action potential triggers Ca^{2+} ion channels to open resulting in the diffusion of Ca^{2+} ions (flux) across the sarcolemma principally within the T-tubule system (Fig. 1.2).

3. The flux of Ca^{2+} across the sarcolemma is only about 1% of the Ca^{2+} needed for contraction. However, this Ca^{2+} serves as a trigger for sarcoplasmic reticulum (SR) Ca^{2+} ion channel opening and causes a graded release of Ca^{2+} to create the Ca^{2+} concentration needed for tension development. Graded release refers to the fact that the internal SR release of Ca^{2+} is dependent on the initial cytoplasmic Ca^{2+} concentration resulting from the external Ca^{2+} influx. This graded response is very different than the all-or-none response of skeletal muscle.

4. Three very important proteins within the SR are responsible for controlling calcium flux: The Ca^{2+} release channel, the sarco-endoplasmic reticulum calcium ATPase (SERCA-2), and the regulatory protein of SERCA-2 (phospholamban).

5. From relaxation to contraction, cytosolic Ca^{2+} concentration varies approximately 100-fold.

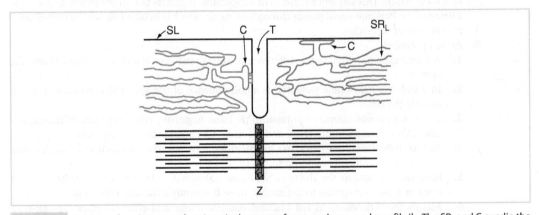

FIGURE 1.2 Relation of cardiac sarcoplasmic reticulum to surface membrane and myofibrils. The SR$_L$ and C overlie the myofilaments; they are shown separately for illustrative purposes. SL, sarcolemma; C, cisterna; T, transverse tubule; SR$_L$, longitudinal sarcoplasmic reticulum; Z, Z disc.

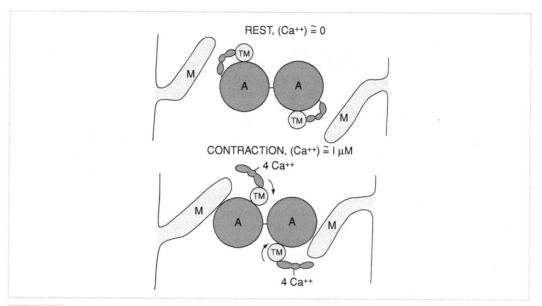

FIGURE 1.3 Schematic representation of actin–myosin dependence on Ca^{2+}–troponin binding for tension development to occur. A, actin; M, myosin; TM, tropomyosin; Ca^{++}, ionized calcium. (From Honig C. *Modern Cardiovascular Physiology*. Boston/Toronto: Little, Brown and Company; 1981.)

6. The myoplasmic (intracellular) Ca^{2+} concentration principally depends on the external Ca^{2+} concentration, the sympathetic tone (sarcolemma Ca^{2+} ion channel conductance), and the amount of Ca^{2+} stored in the SR.

7. Any increase in contractility via any drug results from increased myoplasmic Ca^{2+} concentration during systole! During systole, Ca^{2+} binds to troponin and results in a conformational change of tropomyosin. This change allows actin and myosin to interact, resulting in shortening of a sarcomere (Fig. 1.3) and oxygen consumption (see later).

> **CLINICAL PEARL**   Intracellular calcium flux is critical to the initiation of myocardial sarcomere contraction, and many anesthetic drugs impair this flux.

8. Myoplasmic Ca^{2+}, and hence contractility, is affected by all inhalational agents and some intravenous anesthetic induction drugs.

9. Intracellular acidosis presents a common physiologic reason for decreased Ca^{2+}–troponin affinity. As compared to extracellular pH, intracellular pH is greatly buffered because of intracellular proteins. Intracellular pH is normally less than extracellular pH. When either intracellular or extracellular pH changes, transmembrane reequilibration occurs. Because of the greater intracellular buffering capacity, the rate of intracellular pH change is delayed relative to extracellular pH changes.

10. Finally, for contraction to cease, Ca^{2+} must be unbound from troponin and removed from the myoplasm. Ca^{2+} is actively pumped into the SR as well as across the sarcolemma. Normally, approximately 99% of calcium is pumped back into the SR at a price of about 20% of total myocyte oxygen consumption.

IV. Cardiac myocyte

A. Sarcomere

1. The fundamental unit of tension development is the sarcomere, which is composed of myosin, actin, troponin, and tropomyosin (Fig. 1.3).

2. Actin molecules link to form a chain and two chains intertwine to form a helix. Within each groove of this helix, tropomyosin sits with troponin bound to it intermittently along its length. This complex is known as a thin filament. The length of the thin filament is

approximately 2 μm. In the absence of calcium, the actin sites of the thin filament are not available for binding to myosin.

3. About midway along the thin filament, the Z disc anchors the thin filaments in place in a regular pattern as schematized below. The Z disc is a strong meshwork of filaments that forms a band to anchor the interdigitated thin filaments.

4. Myosin molecules aggregate spontaneously, thereby forming the thick filaments. These filaments are approximately 1.6 μm long. These thick filaments are held in place by M filaments and are interdigitated among the thin filaments. At the center of each thick filament is a zone that has no myosin "heads." Each myosin head contains an actin-binding site and ATPase.

5. Together, troponin and tropomyosin and intramyocyte Ca^{2+} concentration regulate the percentage of possible actin and myosin interactions that participate in the shortening strength of the sarcomere.

6. As long as Ca^{++} is bound to troponin, actin and myosin remain adjacent to each other. During exposure of unbound actin to myosin, they bind together to shorten a sarcomere. After this binding, uncoupling occurs because of the ATPase bound to myosin. This energy-dependent step, requiring oxygen consumption, occurs multiple times within each sarcomere during a cardiac cycle. As long as actin and myosin continue to bind and unbind, the actin–myosin complex continues to shorten the sarcomere as the ventricular chamber contracts in systole.

7. Depending on preload (pre-existing "stretch" prior to contraction), the sarcomere length, or the distance between Z discs, physiologically ranges from 1.8 to 2.2 μm.

8. Intracellular calcium concentration establishes how many actin–myosin sites interact at any instant. The sarcomere length (Z-disc separation length) establishes the maximum number of actin and myosin heads that could potentially interact at any instant. Increasing the number of heads that do interact results in an increase in contractility (see below).

V. Organization of myocytes

A. A cardiac myocyte is approximately 12 μm long. Hence, each myocyte only has about 6 sarcomeres in series from end to end. Each cardiac capillary is approximately 1 mm in length, hence it serves about 80 cardiac myocytes along its length.

B. As mentioned under embryology, collagen fibers link cardiac myocytes together. In a given layer, myocytes are approximately in parallel. These collagen fiber links connect adjacent, parallel myocytes and form a skeleton. Coupled with the Purkinje system's coordinated stimulation of myocytes, this skeleton allows for a summation of the simultaneous shortening of each myocyte into a concerted shortening of the ventricle.

C. This collagen structure also limits the cardiac myocyte from being overstretched, thereby minimizing the risk of destroying a cell or reducing actin–myosin exposure through overstretching [Ref. 1, p. 9].

D. To add complexity, longitudinal alignment of the cardiac myocytes differs in overlapping layers from epicardium to endocardium. Hence, shortening in each layer results in distortion between the layers.

E. Given that blood supply comes from the surface of the heart, this distortion results in partial occlusion of penetrating arteries supplying blood to the inner layers of the myocardium.

F. Consequently, the endocardium is more vulnerable to ischemia than the epicardium. Blood flow to the endocardium occurs primarily during systole while that to the epicardium occurs during the entire cardiac cycle.

CLINICAL PEARL Systolic contraction impairs coronary arterial blood flow penetrating from epicardium to endocardium, which potentially places the endocardium at risk for ischemia.

VI. Length–tension relationship

A. Consider this thought experiment. There is an idealized, single cardiac myocyte that is 12 μm long with 6 sarcomeres in series. All distances between Z discs (sarcomere lengths) are equal for each of the 6 sarcomeres (12 μm = 6 × 2 μm). As the cardiac myocyte length

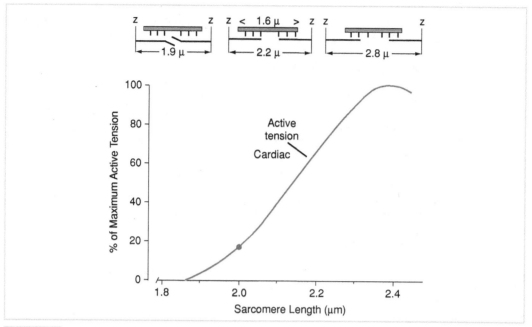

FIGURE 1.4 Top three schematic diagrams represent actin (thick filaments penetrating Z disc) and myosin (thin filaments forming sheaf between Z disc) filaments at three sarcomere lengths 1.9, 2.2, and 2.8 μm. Bottom graph represents percent of maximum tension development versus sarcomere length for strips of cardiac muscle. Note that the fibrous cardiac skeleton inhibits sarcomere stretch from approaching a sarcomere length of 2.8 μm. (Modified from Honig C. *Modern Cardiovascular Physiology*. Boston/Toronto: Little, Brown and Company; 1981.)

changes, the length of each sarcomere changes proportionately. This single myocyte is suspended so that a strain gauge measures the tension that the myocyte generates at rest and during contraction.

1. The idealized myocyte is stretched between two fixed points.
2. The tension caused by the force of stretching the muscle at rest and created by the muscle during contraction is measured.
3. The muscle is stretched at rest over a range of 10.8 to 16.2 μm. Consequently, the sarcomere lengths vary between 1.8 and 2.7 μm as this myocyte contracts.
4. At each sarcomere length, two fixed myoplasmic Ca^{2+} concentrations are set within the cell: Zero concentration (rest) and a known value (contraction).
5. Myocyte tension is measured for both Ca^{2+} concentrations.
6. Plotting resting tension as a function of length results in a resting length–(passive) tension plot.
7. Recording peak tension as a function of myocyte length, a length–(active) tension curve can be plotted for the given Ca^{2+} concentration as depicted in Figure 1.4.

B. Compliance
1. In our idealized myocyte model, a measured amount of tension resulted when the sarcomere was stretched between 1.8 and 2.7 μm. In plotting this passive tension resulting from passive stretch of the sarcomeres, note that there is very little passive tension required to stretch the sarcomeres until the compliance of the cell membrane started to play a role.
2. As the sarcomeres become stretched beyond 2.2 μm in intact cardiac muscle, the fibrous skeleton restricts further stretching. The fibrous skeleton resistance to stretch results in a rapid change in tension with very little change in length (very low compliance).
3. The slope of the line of this resting relationship between length and tension is the equivalent of ventricular compliance as will be discussed below.

C. Contractility

1. At a given Ca^{2+} concentration, a fraction of troponin molecules will bind Ca^{2+} molecules.
2. This Ca^{2+} binding to each troponin results in a conformational change in its corresponding tropomyosin that allows opposing actin and myosin head pairs, their exposure regulated by these tropomyosin molecules, to interact.
3. For this conformational change at the given Ca^{2+} concentration, the percentage of the actin and myocytes heads opposed to each other is determined.
4. If one repeats the above mental experiment with a different known Ca^{2+} concentration, a new contracting length–(active) tension curve is plotted.
5. For a range of Ca^{2+} concentrations in cardiac myocytes, a family of length–tension curves results.
6. For a given length, only through a change in myoplasmic Ca^{2+} concentration can active tension change.
7. In considering the family of curves in the context of ventricular contractility, the contractility is higher when for any given length the developed tension is greater. In vivo, determining contractility of the ventricle is complicated by the interactions of preload and afterload on any measurements.

D. Intracellular Ca^{2+} concentration

1. The range of myoplasmic Ca^{2+} concentrations during contraction varies depending upon Ca^{2+} fluxes across the sarcolemma at the initiation of contraction and the Ca^{2+} released from the SR.
2. The transmembrane flux of Ca^{2+} across the sarcolemma is only about 1% of Ca^{2+} present during contraction. However, small changes in this transmembrane flux impressively alter the amount of Ca^{2+} released from the SR.
3. The SR response is graded. The more Ca^{2+} that crosses the sarcolemma, the more Ca^{2+} is released from the SR.
4. Examples of increasing sarcolemmal Ca^{2+} flux include increasing epinephrine levels and increasing external Ca^{2+} concentration (a $CaCl_2$ bolus).
5. Increased acute SR Ca^{2+} stores result from increased Ca^{2+} flux across the sarcolemma and increased heart rate (HR)—Treppe effect.

E. Oxygen consumption

1. As described above, each interaction of actin and myosin results in a submicron shortening of the sarcomere.
2. Physiologic (15%) shortening requires multiple submicron shortenings.
3. For the sarcomere to shorten 15%, many actin–myosin interactions take place.
4. Each submicron interaction requires ATP for release of the actin–myosin head. It is relaxation of the actin–myosin interaction that requires energy and consumes oxygen.
5. Remember that the more actin–myosin cycles in a unit of time, the greater the oxygen consumption!
6. The three main determinants of myocardial oxygen consumption are:
   a. HR: more beats at the same number of actin–myosin interactions
   b. Contractility: more interactions per beat
   c. Wall tension: more interaction for a given sarcomere length change

CLINICAL PEARL   The main determinants of myocardial oxygen consumption are HR contractility, and wall tension.

VII. A heart chamber and external work

A. The chamber wall

1. To form a ventricular chamber, individual myocytes are joined together via collagen fibrin strands. This joining of myocytes, along a general orientation but not end to end, results in a sheet of muscle with myocytes oriented along a similar axis.
2. Several such layers form the ventricular wall. These layers insert on the valvular annuli.

3. Because of the rapid electrical distribution of the signal through the Purkinje system, the layers contract synchronously resulting in shortening of the muscle layers and a reduction in the volume of the chamber itself.

B. Atria

1. Atrial contraction contributes approximately 20% of the ventricular filling volume in a normal heart and may contribute even more when left ventricular end-diastolic pressure (LVEDP) is increased. In addition to the volume itself, the rate of ventricular volume addition resulting from atrial contraction may play a role in ventricular sarcomere lengthening.

C. Ventricle

1. For a given state of contractility (myoplasmic Ca^{2+} concentration), sarcomere length determines the wall tension the ventricle can achieve as discussed above. The aggregate shortening of the sarcomeres in the layers of cardiac myocytes results in wall tension that leads to ejection of blood into the aorta and pulmonary artery (PA).

2. The active range of sarcomere length is only 1.8 to 2.2 μm or ~15% of its length. Falling below 1.8 μm results from an empty ventricle and an empty heart cannot pump blood. The collagen fiber network inhibits the stretching of sarcomeres much above 2.2 μm. This integration of structure and function is important in permitting survival. If there were no skeleton, overstretch would lead to reduced emptying that would lead to more overstretch and no cardiac output (CO).

D. Preload and compliance

1. Preload

    a. Where clinicians speak of preload, muscle physiologists think of sarcomere length. The clinician's surrogate for initial sarcomere length should be end-diastolic ventricular volume, and not ventricular pressure. Compliance, a variable that can be dynamic, relates pressure and length.

    b. As discussed above, the sarcomere length determines how many actin–myosin heads interact for a given myoplasmic Ca^{2+} concentration at any instant.

    c. Measuring sarcomere length is essentially impossible clinically. As a surrogate indirect estimate of sarcomere length, clinicians measure a chamber pressure during chamber diastole. This pressure measurement is the equivalent of the myocyte resting tension measurement above.

    d. A more direct surrogate estimate of sarcomere length is chamber volume. As echocardiography is commonly available, estimates of volumes serve as direct estimates of preload (e.g., chamber pressure at the end of filling cycle) and remove some assumptions about chamber compliance that are necessary when using a pressure estimate.

    e. A plot of the relationship between resting chamber pressure and resting chamber volume results in a curve similar to the resting length–tension curve for the myocyte.

    f. The slope of this curve at any point (change in volume over the change in pressure at that point) is the compliance of the chamber at that point. The pressure–volume curve is nonlinear, and its slope varies depending on ventricular volume (Figs. 1.5 and 1.6). Ventricles become much less compliant as sarcomere length surpasses 2.2 μm because of the collagen fiber skeleton.

    g. Nonischemic changes in compliance generally occur over long time periods. However, ischemia can change ventricular compliance very quickly. Thick ventricles, ventricles with scar formation, or ischemic ventricles have a lower compliance than normal ventricles. Less compliant ventricles require a higher pressure within them to contain equal volume (sarcomere length) as compared to a more compliant ventricle.

    h. While preload is most commonly considered in the left ventricle, it is important in all four chambers. Both congenital heart disease and cardiac tamponade can make that very apparent.

E. Ventricular work

1. For a sarcomere length between approximately 1.8 and 2.2 μm (preload) with a given systolic myoplasmic Ca^{2+} concentration (contractility), the cardiac myocyte will shorten,

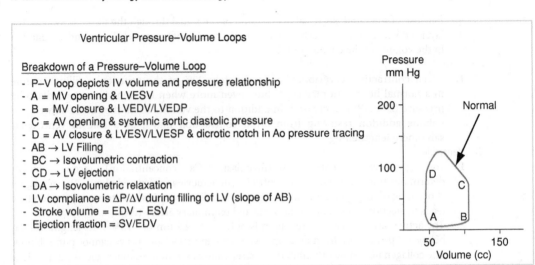

Ventricular Pressure–Volume Loops

Breakdown of a Pressure–Volume Loop
- P–V loop depicts IV volume and pressure relationship
- A = MV opening & LVESV
- B = MV closure & LVEDV/LVEDP
- C = AV opening & systemic aortic diastolic pressure
- D = AV closure & LVESV/LVESP & dicrotic notch in Ao pressure tracing
- AB → LV Filling
- BC → Isovolumetric contraction
- CD → LV ejection
- DA → Isovolumetric relaxation
- LV compliance is $\Delta P/\Delta V$ during filling of LV (slope of AB)
- Stroke volume = EDV – ESV
- Ejection fraction = SV/EDV

FIGURE 1.5 Idealized pressure–volume loop. Area within the loop represents LVSW. Dividing SV (Point B minus Point A volumes) by BSA results in SVI. The area within this indexed loop is the LVSWI. P-V, pressure-volume; IV, intraventricular; MV, mitral valve; LVESV, left ventricular end-systolic volume; LVEDP, left ventricular end-diastolic pressure; AV, aortic valve; LVESP, left ventricular end-systolic pressure; LV, left ventricle; P, pressure; V, volume; EDV, end-diastolic volume; ESV, end-systolic volume; SV, stroke volume.

develop tension that increases with increased sarcomere length, and eject blood from the ventricle to create a stroke volume (SV).

7   2. In ejecting this SV, the ventricle performs external work. This work comprises raising intraventricular pressure from end-diastolic pressure to peak systolic pressure. In the absence of valvular heart disease, the systolic left and right ventricular pressures closely match those in the aorta and PA, respectively.

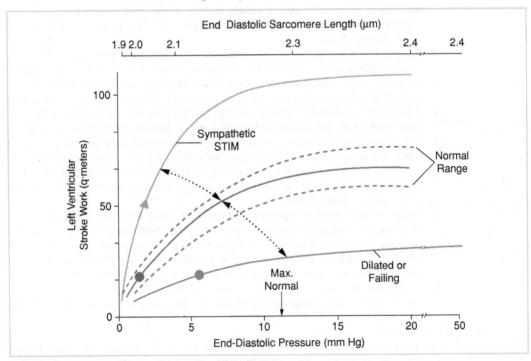

FIGURE 1.6 The Starling curve. STIM, stimulation; Max., maximum.

3. Normal blood pressures (BPs) in the aorta and PA are not dependent on body size and vary little among normal subjects. By normalizing SV to stroke volume index (SVI) (SV divided by body surface area [BSA]), the variability of SVI among subjects becomes relatively small.

4. Hydrodynamically, the external work of a ventricle is the area within the pressure volume loop seen in Figure 1.5. The definitions of various points and intervals are defined in the legend. This indexed work for the left ventricle (LVSWI) is derived by multiplying the SVI in milliliters times the difference in arterial mean pressure and ventricular pressure at the end of diastole (commonly estimated as atrial pressure or PA wedge pressure) times a constant (0.0136) to convert to clinical units:

$$LVSWI = SVI * (SBP\ mean - LVEDP) * 0.0136\ (g\ m/m^2)$$

5. The normal resting values for SVI and LVSWI are approximately 50 mL/m^2 and 50 g m/m^2, hence they are relatively easy to remember.

6. In performing this work, the efficiency of the ventricle (ratio of external work done to energy consumed to do it) approaches that of a gasoline engine, which is only 10%. This is an astonishingly inefficient process given that our lives depend on it!

7. Since external work is the product of pressure difference and SV, work does not distinguish between these two variables. Evidence suggests that the ventricles can do volume work somewhat more efficiently (require less oxygen) than pressure work. The reasoning may relate to how many actin–myosin cycles are required to shorten a sarcomere to a given distance. The hypothesis is that it takes fewer actin–myosin cycles to shorten the same distance for volume work compared to pressure work. This principle may explain an underlying reason for success using vasodilators to treat heart failure.

F. Starling curve

1. For a given myoplasmic Ca^{2+} concentration (contractile state), varying the sarcomere length between 1.9 and 2.2 μm increases the amount of external work done. For a ventricle with a normal compliance, a sarcomere length of 2.2 μm corresponds to one with an LVEDP of 10 mm Hg.

2. By plotting the relationship of LVEDP with LVSWI, a Starling curve is generated.

3. By changing the contractile state and replotting the same relationship, a new curve develops, resulting in a family of Starling curves idealized in Figure 1.6.

G. Myocardial oxygen consumption

1. Except for very unusual circumstances, substrate for ATP and phosphocreatine (PCr) production is readily available. Without external oxygen delivery, the intracellular oxygen content is capable of keeping the heart contracting for seconds. Carbohydrate and lipid stores can fuel the heart for almost an hour, albeit very inefficiently and unsustainably. Hence, capillary blood flow is crucial to maintain oxidative metabolism.

2. Myoglobin is an intracellular oxygen store. Its affinity for oxygen falls between those for hemoglobin and cytochrome aa3. The maximum oxygen concentration required in mitochondria for maximal ATP production is just 0.1 mm Hg (Torr)! Myoglobin oxygen concentration is high enough to buffer interruptions in capillary flow only for seconds. Compared to high-energy phosphate buffers, this myoglobin buffer is small relative to their ATP consumption rates.

3. Nevertheless, myoglobin's intermediate oxygen affinity enhances unloading of oxygen from the red cell into the myocyte and also serves to distribute oxygen within the cell.

4. Commonly atherosclerotic disease limits blood flow to regions of the heart, reducing oxygen delivery and cell oxygen tension. When this PO$_2$ falls below 0.1 Torr, ATP production decreases along with myocardial wall motion.

5. Capillaries are approximately 1 mm (1,000 μm) in length, apparently regardless of the organ system in which they are located. In the heart a cardiac myocyte is ~12 μm in length, so each capillary supplies multiple cardiac myocytes (~1,000/12). In contrast, a skeletal muscle fiber (cell) is perhaps 150 mm long. Since capillary length is the same (1 mm), each skeletal muscle capillary supplies a very small fraction of any given muscle cell (1/150 or 0.7%).

6. There are multiple levels of arteriolar structure. The lower-order, or initial, arterioles contribute to systemic vascular resistance (SVR) and the higher-order, or distal, arterioles regulate regional blood flow distribution at the local level. The intricacies are beyond the scope of this chapter.

7. Capillary perfusion is organized so that several capillaries are supplied from a single higher-order arteriole.

8. This structure yields regions of perfusion on the scale of mm^3 for the regional blood flow unit. Hence, the smallest volumes for "small vessel infarcts" should be this order of magnitude. As the vessel occlusions become more proximal, the infarct size grows.

9. Because length of cardiac myocytes is small relative to the capillary length, infarction due to small vessel disease only affects local zones. If the cardiac myocyte had a 15 cm length like a skeletal myocyte, the consequences of a local infarct would affect the whole length and have a much larger impact.

10. Adequate production of ATP is dependent on mitochondrial function. Approximately 30% of cardiac cell volume is occupied by mitochondria. Given the substrate distribution and the ability to produce ATP within this volume, oxygen availability is the limiting factor for maintaining ATP availability. Mitochondria can maximally produce ATP when their cell PO_2 is 0.1 Torr!

11. Before ATP production is compromised, the entire oxygen difference from ambient air—~150 Torr—to 0.1 Torr—has already happened!

12. Phosphocreatine (PCr) is an intracellular buffer for ATP concentration. The cell readily converts ATP into PCr and vice versa. PCr is an important energy reserve and also serves to transport ATP between mitochondria and myosin ATPase.

13. Myosin ATPase activity is responsible for 75% of myocardial ATP consumption. The remaining 25% is consumed by Ca^{2+} transport into the SR and across the sarcolemma.

14. The mitochondrion's role in determining the response to ischemia is evolving. Intracellular signaling pathways in response to hypoxia may direct the cell to necrosis or even apoptosis.

VIII. Control systems

A. The space program put man in space. As importantly, it brought many technical advances. In the world of systems development, control systems were central. These systems allowed us to perform tasks in unexplored environments under unimagined conditions. In simplest concept, they permitted real-time sensing of system variables that resulted in regulation of system output. In the jargon, **a feedback loop** is that portion of the system that takes signal from within the system and returns that signal to a system input that in turn affects system output.

B. Circulating levels of Ca^{2+}, thyroid hormones, antidiuretic hormone, and BP are only a few of the system variables and/or outputs that utilize a feedback loop to maintain a "normal blood level." A feedback loop is referred to as a **negative feedback loop** if a deviation of the system output from the desired output, called set point, is returned toward that set point through the system response to that deviation. Blood levels of all of the above protein moieties are controlled through negative feedback loop systems. In contrast, **positive feedback loops** increase the deviation from the normal level in response to deviation. Outside the physiology of the immune system, physiologic systems with positive feedback loops are generally pathologic. As considered below, perhaps the most studied biologic negative feedback loop is the cardiovascular system.

C. A simple example

1. A simple, manual system consists of a voltage source, a wall switch, and a light bulb. The system turns electrical energy into light through manually turning a light switch. Automation of this output would include a light detector (**sensor**) that senses light level. If the ambient light level gets below a defined level, the sensor sends a signal to a **controller** that turns the light bulb on and vice versa for high light levels. A further refinement of this automated system is one that keeps the light level constant at a defined light level (set point). In this negative feedback system, light level is referred to as a **regulated variable**. If the light level is above the set point, the constant light-level system (CLLS) does not turn on the light and adjusts the blinds to reduce the amount of light. However, when the

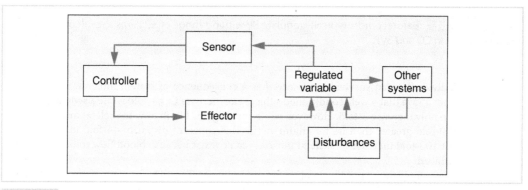

FIGURE 1.7 Diagram of a control system with a feedback loop. If the system response to a disturbance is to return the regulated variable back to the original set point, the system is a negative feedback system. Many physiologic systems are negative feedback systems.

light level gets below this set point, the CLLS **controls** the amount of light coming from the blinds and would add a light bulb if needed such that the light level at the light sensor remains constant. This control requires that the output from the light bulb must vary. One way to vary the light output is to **control** the voltage (input) to the light bulb. This new variable light bulb intensity is referred to as an **effector** because it changes the response to meet system requirements. The component of the system that regulates the voltage is called the regulator. This CLLS system has a negative feedback loop because CLLS increases light output if natural (or artificial) light decreases and vice versa.

2. The components of this CLLS consist of **inputs** to a light source (voltage), **effectors** that can vary light levels (blinds, light bulb), a **sensor** that detects the amount of light (a light detector), and a **comparator** that compares the signal from the sensor to a set point (the light level at which the system turns on or off). Finally, a **controller**, based on sensor input, varies the voltage to vary blind openness and/or light bulb output. The **controller** is the combination of the comparator and the regulator. Finally, the disturbances to the regulated variable as well as other systems impacting that variable are schematized (Fig. 1.7).

3. To be complete, there are **positive feedback systems** as well. In a positive feedback system, the response of the system increases the difference between the regulated variable and a set point. When positive feedback occurs, the system frequently becomes unstable and usually leads to system failure. In physiology, typically pathology causes positive feedback. An example of this pathology is the response of the cardiovascular system to hypotension in the presence of coronary artery disease. Hypotension leads to a demand for an increase in HR, SVR, and contractility. If the resulting increase in oxygen consumption leads to ischemia, contractility will decrease, leading to further demands that eventually result in system failure.

IX. **The cardiovascular control system**

A. The simple control system model can be used to develop a model of the cardiovascular system. This model is useful if it predicts the system response to system disturbances. Modified from Honig [Ref. 1, p. 249], components in Figure 1.6 can be broken down into sensor, controller, and effector functions. The following discussion will summarize concepts for each function.

B. For the sensor functions, the two best-characterized sensors—the baroreceptors in the carotid sinus and the volume and HR sensors in the right atrium—will be outlined in detail.

C. **Regulation** of a variable is defined as the variable remaining fixed despite changes in its determinants. The primary regulated variable in the cardiovascular system is BP, the regulation of which occurs via a negative feedback loop.

D. Our survival requires a wide range of CO and SVR. Since BP changes only by perhaps ±25% from our being asleep to maximal exercising, CO increasing is offset by SVR decreasing and vice versa. The physiologic range for each is approximately 4- to 6-fold.

E. Individual organ survival is preserved as a consequence of system integration. It is noted from above that a well-conditioned subject can increase CO 4-fold while a sedentary person can only increase 2-fold. However, while running, his blood flow to skeletal muscle must be 100-fold greater than its minimum value. This apparent disparity—4-fold increase in CO but 100-fold increase to skeletal muscle—can coexist because blood flow to other organs is reduced.

F. The brain is the site of the comparator and regulator. Together the comparator and the regulator make up the controller. While anatomic sites for individual comparator and regulator functions are known, the specifics of interaction of these sites and regulation of control balance (what effector is utilized and how much) are largely unknown.

G. For this review, details of the sympathetic and parasympathetic outputs will not receive focus. As outputs from the controller, the nervous system signals recruitment and derecruitment of the effectors in a predictable fashion through release of norepinephrine (NOR) and acetylcholine (ACH) as indicated in Figure 1.8.

H. The **effectors of the cardiovascular system—heart, venous system, and arterial system—** respond to changes in system demand. Fundamentally, the cardiovascular system must maintain BP in a normal range despite a wide range of demand, for example, exercise, eating or limitations of effector reserves such as dehydration and ischemic and valvular heart disease. To adapt, the effectors have a range over which they can expand their capacities. Globally, each effector has an expandable range known to physiologists as **physiologic reserve**.

I. Effective feedback control requires functioning sensors, a controller, and effectors to have the desired effect—in this case regulation of BP. The understanding of complexities and capacities of the sensors, comparators, and effectors as well as system integration provides a clinical basis for reducing surgical and anesthetic risk.

X. **Stretch receptors: Pressure sensors**

A. The simplified view of BP regulation presented herein is useful for organizing priorities in maintaining BP. Integration of BP regulation is more complex and requires meeting the demands of competing organs.

B. Excepting the splanchnic circulation, organs are organized in parallel with either the aorta or PA as their source of BP and the respective veins as the collecting system and reservoir.

C. As a consequence, blood flow to the individual organs can be locally adjusted and/or centrally integrated. This organization allows for individual independent organ perfusion while, or as long as, aortic or PA BP is maintained.

D. Additional sensor sites and variables sensed include systemic and pulmonary veins, heart chambers with venous blood volumes, HR, SVR, and ventricular volumes being sensed. Experiments looking at cardiovascular system responses to isolated disturbance in these locations have demonstrated their existence.

E. All known pressure-sensitive sensors in the cardiovascular system are stretch receptors. They respond to wall stretch and not container pressure. Hence, compliance of the receptor site impacts receptor signal. Compliance pathology becomes central to understanding disease of this aspect.

F. In addition to the volume of a chamber, the rate of change of that volume is sensed and commensurate afferent signals are sent to the brain.

G. Consequently, depending on the sensor location, sensor signals provide data that reflect BP, venous capacitance, SVR, ventricular contractility, SV, HR, and other parameters. Most of the knowledge of these sensor sites is inferred from indirect experiments.

XI. **Atrial baroreceptors**

A. Within the right atrium, there are receptors at the junction of the superior and inferior venae cavae with the atrium (B fibers) and in the body of this atrium (A fibers, Fig. 1.9). The corresponding impulses from the respective nerves are seen on the left.

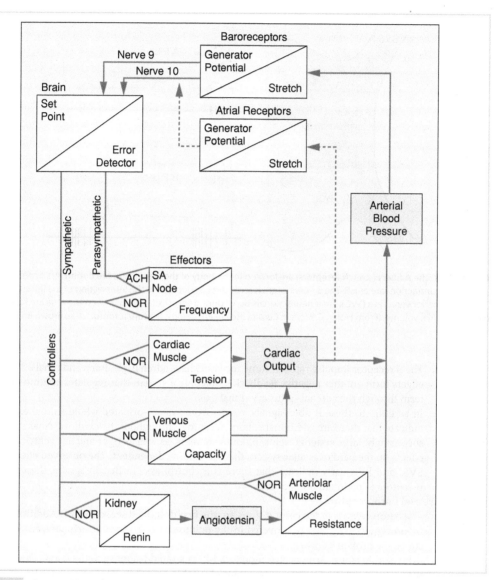

FIGURE 1.8 This simplified representation omits input to the brain from sensors throughout the vascular tree and the ventricular chambers. As discussed in the text, there are multiple inputs to the brain not represented in this simplified view. Input to the brain includes signals from sensors (receptors) that monitor blood volume, CO, SVR, and HR. Input to the effectors occurs through the sympathetic and parasympathetic systems with neural transmitters indicated. NOR, norepinephrine; ACH, acetylcholine; SA, sinoatrial. (Modified from Honig C. *Modern Cardiovascular Physiology*. Boston/Toronto: Little, Brown and Company; 1981.)

B. **A fibers**, seen in both atria, generate impulses during atrial contraction, indicating that they **detect** HR (Fig. 1.9).

C. B fibers are located only in the right atrium and impulses occur during systole when the atrium is filling. Minimum frequency occurs as filling of the atrium begins at the end of systole. Maximum frequency of B fiber impulses occurs just prior to AV valve opening and this frequency is linearly proportional to right atrial volume. **B fibers detect atrial volume filling.** When combined with A fiber information, CO can be derived potentially.

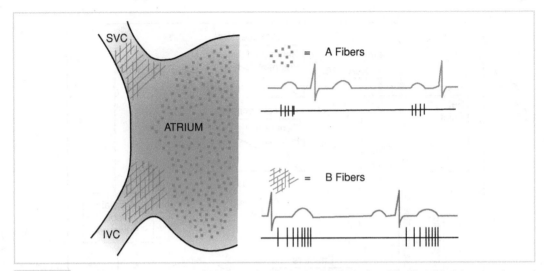

FIGURE 1.9 The A fibers (stretch receptors) are located in the body of the atrium and fire during atrial contraction and sense atrial contraction rate or HR. The B fibers (stretch receptors) are located at the intersection of the inferior vena cava (IVC) and superior vena cava (SVC). Their neural signals occur during ventricular systole when the atria are filling. Hence, they sense atrial volume. (From Honig C. *Modern Cardiovascular Physiology*. Boston/Toronto: Little, Brown and Company; 1981.)

    D. The B receptor impulse rates (volume receptor) have adrenal, pituitary, and renal effects. These effects form another negative feedback loop control system that regulates volume in the long term through the adrenal–pituitary–renal axis.

    E. In addition to these B fiber signals, results from system-oriented whole animal experiments indicate that there are additional volume receptors throughout the cardiovascular system. Not surprisingly, large systemic veins, pulmonary veins, as well as right and left ventricles all have effects on the cardiovascular system that are volume dependent. The observed effects on CO, SVR, and BP clearly indicate that there is a control system that integrates these additional receptors to maintain homeostasis.

XII. Arterial baroreceptors

    A. The baroreceptors in the carotid sinus are the first described sensors of BP. Additional arterial baroreceptors have been discovered in the pulmonary and systemic arterial trees including a site in the proximal aorta.

    B. "The carotid sinus baroreceptor monitors BP" is a rapid response to the common question of where BP is sensed. However, the details of what is sensed in this location are less frequently known [Ref. 1, p. 246].

    C. Figure 1.10 shows signals from a single neural fiber emanating from the baroreceptor. A step change in mean BP from 50 to 330 mm Hg is plotted along with the neural discharge of the carotid sinus fiber. There is a change in the neural frequency reflecting the step change in BP and then a leveling to a new steady-state discharge rate, indicating a signal correlating with mean BP.

    D. In Figure 1.11, the single neural fiber signal from a carotid sinus nerve can be seen for a pulsatile "BP waveform."

    E. Different neural firing rates are present during the upstroke of BP (possibly related to contractility), the dicrotic notch (possibly related to SVR in the peripheral circulation), and down slope following the notch (possibly related to SVR). Hence, the oscillatory shape of the BP waveform results in signals that may contain more information than simply a BP.

    F. The aortic baroreceptor is located near or in the aortic arch. Infrequently, cardiac anesthesiologists can become acutely aware of its presence. When distorted secondary to the placement of any aortic clamp, the resulting aortic baroreceptor signal results in an acute and dramatic

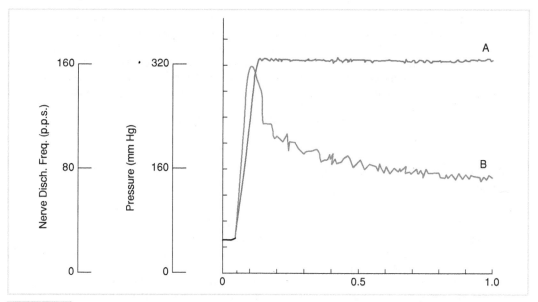

FIGURE 1.10 The nerve discharge frequency (shown in *blue*) from the baroreceptor recording changed from ~30 pulses/sec to 160 pulses/sec within 1 second after the response reached a steady state. Note that there was a transient change during the rapid response phase as well.

increase in BP. The presumed mechanism is that the clamp distorts the aortic baroreceptor. This distortion results in a signal that BP has precipitously fallen. Despite the fact that the carotid baroreceptor has no such indication, hypertension ensues, thus representing imperfect system integration. Immediately releasing a partial-occlusion clamp (when possible) usually promptly returns the BP to a more normal level. When release is not feasible, short, rapid-acting intervention—pharmacologic vasodilation or reverse Trendelenburg positioning—is required.

   G. Cardiovascular effectors

     1. BP is the product of CO, or HR times SV, times SVR plus right atrial pressure (RA):

$$BP = (CO * SVR) + RA = (SV * HR * SVR) + RA \tag{1}$$

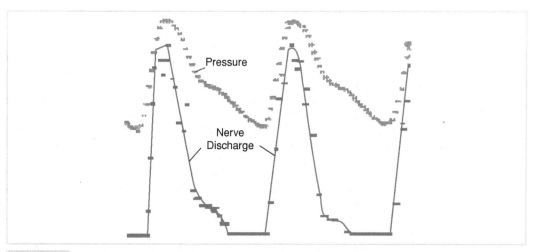

FIGURE 1.11 Note the relationship between the upslope of arterial pressure (dP/dt), the downslope (SVR), and the notch (SVR) and the action potential characteristics.

2. Organ perfusion is dependent on the difference between arterial pressure and RA and organ resistance. For homeostasis, a focus on perfusion is important in our view of BP.

3. The organs in the body are in parallel and the SVR is dependent on the individual resistance in a simple way ($1/SVR = \Sigma 1/Ri$ where Ri is the value of each individual organ in the systemic circulation). Clinicians seldom consider the resistance of individual organs.

4. SV is dependent upon contractility, preload, and afterload [Eq. (1)]. Sympathetic tone sets contractility, preload, and SVR. The myoplasmic Ca^{2+} concentration, the fraction of blood inside the thorax versus total blood volume, and the SVR are all functions of sympathetic tone.

CLINICAL PEARL SV for both the right and left ventricles depends upon contractility, preload, and afterload.

5. HR is dependent on the sympathetic tone as well.

XIII. Effectors and physiologic reserves for the healthy individual

A. The range that each of the effectors can contribute to maintaining BP through increasing CO, changing SVR or shifting venous blood into or out of the thorax in the face of everyday life requirements (sleeping to climbing a mountain) is referred to as physiologic reserve.

B. Knowing the physiologic range for each effector gives a framework to consider which reserves can be utilized to support BP in the OR.

C. Clinical situations in which additional physiologic reserves are not available (because of pathology or exceeding a range) may increase risk and jeopardize outcome.

D. Heart rate

1. A normal resting HR is perhaps 60 beats per minute (bpm). A maximum attainable HR in a 25 year old would be 220, as compared to 170 in a 55 year old. Hence, an average expansion factor is ~2.5- to 3.5-fold.

2. The clinician must keep in mind that of the three main determinants of oxygen demand—HR, contractility, and wall tension—HR correlated best with ischemia in patients under anesthesia.

E. Systemic Vascular Resistance

1. Within the systemic vascular tree, the organs in our body emanate from the aorta or the PA (recognizing the lung and liver as more complex circulations). This arrangement is referred to as organs in parallel.

2. Because of the large diameters of the normal aorta and PA, there is no physiologically important decrease in mean BP along either of their lengths. Consequently, each organ experiences the same mean BP. Through its own resistance, the organ determines its blood flow.

3. In normal life, organ blood flow requirements are met without compromising BP. Metabolic requirements (substrate supply, oxygen supply, and demand, waste removal) are met through local adjustment of each organ's own blood flow.

4. The cardiovascular system maintains BP through its effectors via central nervous system (CNS) control responding to the impact of local organ resistance.

5. Looking at Equation (1), if BP is regulated, when SVR is high then CO must be proportionately lower and vice versa. What is the observed range of SVR? For a severely dehydrated person or one with a very bad left ventricle (have cared for both), the cardiac index might be 33% of normal (1.2 LPM/M^2 [Eq. (1)]). The corresponding SVR would be three times the normal value (3,600 dyne sec/cm^5 [Eq. (1)]). For a well-trained athlete who, during maximal exercise, would increase CO 7-fold, the SVR would be ~15% of normal (~200 dyne sec/cm^5 [Eq. (1)]).

F. Contractility

1. Contractility is not a commonly measured clinical variable because of the difficulty in direct measurement due to the impact of afterload and preload on its estimate. The clinician is left to estimate any changes.

2. A consequence of an increase in contractility is the ability to increase wall tension in the left ventricle. This increased tension will lead to an increase in ejection rate of blood from the ventricle and ejection fraction (EF) under normal conditions. While there are differences in how trained and untrained healthy subjects achieve the increase, both can increase LVEF from a value of approximately 0.60 to one of approximately 0.80. This 33% increase in EF contributes to a modest but important increase in CO.

G. Intravascular volume: Venous capacitance

1. Total blood volume can be estimated from body weight. In the ideal 70-kg person, an estimate of blood volume is 70 mL/kg or about 5 L. This blood volume is considered euvolemia.

2. The distribution of that volume between intrathoracic and extrathoracic (or systemic) circulations is roughly 30% and 70%, respectively.

3. In each of these two compartments, approximately one-third of the blood is in the arteries and capillaries and two-thirds are in the venous system.

4. The pulmonary veins hold 1,100 mL and the systemic veins hold 2,400 mL (totaling about two-thirds of the blood volume).

5. Relaxation of venous tone increases venous capacity for blood. If there is no change in blood volume, this decreases right atrial volume, which leads in turn to decreases in volume in the other cardiac chambers.

6. Since atrial pressure equals ventricular end-diastolic pressure (VEDP), returning those pressures to their original values requires infusion of volume. When venous capacitance is at its largest, the amount of intravascular volume required to return these volumes to their original values is referred to as the venous capacitance reserve.

7. In addition to the blood volume defined as euvolemia, the intrathoracic and extrathoracic compartments can expand by 30%, or approximately 300 and 1,200 mL, respectively.

8. Thus, 1,500 mL of intravascular volume is a quantitative estimate of this venous capacitance reserve for this 70-kg person.

9. This reserve intravascular volume, when added to a euvolemic blood volume (5 L in a 70-kg subject), and the total intravascular volume would be 6.5 L.

10. While sustaining (i.e., "defending") BP as the primary regulated variable, maintaining CO in the face of any reduction in total blood volume, for example, standing or hemorrhage, is another important task of the cardiovascular system. Through shifting blood into the thoracic circulation from the systemic veins, the sympathetic nervous system attempts to maintain pulmonary blood volume at the expense of systemic volume. In the setting of reduced circulating blood volume, protection of pulmonary blood volume coupled with increasing HR and contractility defends BP maintenance.

11. Recognize that anesthetics, both regional and general, alter the ability of the sympathetic nervous system to defend BP. In the presence of pathology, understanding how individual anesthetics interfere with each of the reserves may reduce the anesthetic risk through choosing the anesthetic approach that preserves the most physiologic reserves.

12. In pathologic states that chronically elevate right- or left-sided atrial pressures, venous dilation results in an increase in "euvolemic" blood volume.

13. Particularly in the systemic venous system, this increase in capacity can be large. While there is no experimental data, anecdotal observations of mitral valve patients going on cardiopulmonary bypass clearly demonstrate this fact. However, the extent to which increased volumes can be recruited to maintain intrathoracic volume in normal life, which is the key to maintaining preload, remains unknown. For any patient, a portion of that additional volume is available in circulatory emergencies (e.g., hemorrhage), but the intravascular volume at the time of the emergency critically impacts this response.

14. Like hemorrhage, chronic diuresis leads to a contracted venous bed. Hence, caring for patients who are chronically or acutely hypovolemic secondary to diuresis must include understanding the state of their venous volume status (capacitance).

15. Of note, chronic diuretic administration leads to venoconstriction. However, an acute dose of furosemide will venodilate the patient with heart failure and actually lower intrathoracic blood volume by shifting blood into the dilated systemic veins.

H. Lymphatic circulation: A final reserve?

1. Interstitial space lies between the capillaries and intracellular space. Clinically this system is rarely discussed except as part of the so-called "third spacing," but physiologically it plays a vital role. For our purposes, the lymphatic system protects organs from edema. Its role in recruitment of volume in times of high sympathetic tone—for example, severe hemorrhage—will be discussed.

2. The characteristics of this space help prevent fluid accumulation in two ways—its low compliance and transport of fluid through the lymphatic conduits [2].

3. The collagen matrix is a gel and this structure results in the interstitial space having a low compliance. Consequently, fluid entering the interstitial space raises interstitial pressure rapidly (low compliance) and this increase in interstitial pressure opposes further transudation of fluid across capillaries.

4. The lymphatics are tented open by a collagen matrix. Because of this tenting, lymphatics are not compressed when the interstitium is edematous. On the contrary, lymphatic diameter and drainage increase during edematous states.

5. This increased interstitial pressure also increases lymphatic drainage as the higher interstitial pressure increases the pressure gradient between interstitial space and right atrial pressure (the lymphatics drain into the systemic venous system).

6. Consequently, more fluid leaves the interstitium via lymphatic drainage when more fluid enters the lymphatics across the capillary.

7. Proteins pass across the capillary membrane although at markedly reduced rates compared to water and solutes. With normal capillary integrity (e.g., no inflammatory response), approximately 4% of intravascular proteins cross the capillary membrane each hour.

8. Interstitial fluid exchange between capillary blood and interstitial space is dynamic during the convective transport of blood down a capillary. Exchange occurs as fluid leaves the capillary at the arteriole end and returns at the venous end. The expansion factor for this exchange is approximately 8-fold. Hence, crystalloid administration equilibrates across the vascular and interstitial volumes rapidly (minutes). Colloid, if capillary integrity is intact, remains longer (hours).

9. Remember that the time constant for colloids remaining intravascular can be markedly reduced in the presence of the inflammatory response. The inflammatory response is part of every surgical procedure.

10. With **severe hemorrhage** accompanied by maximal sympathetic stimulation, interstitial and intracellular fluid may contribute up to 2.5 L of fluid to ***intravascular volume*** [3]. While this recruitment of intracellular and interstitial fluid compensates for intravascular depletion acutely, this depletion, particularly of *intracellular volume*, does so at the expense of cell function. This eventually induces cellular acidosis, which compromises cell function.

11. All three of these compartments—intracellular, interstitial, and intravascular—have a dynamic relationship with equilibrium being reached in minutes after volume administration, change in sympathetic tone, or administration of vasoactive drugs.

12. Physiologists define the interstitial space as a fluid space outside the intracellular and intravascular spaces that contains protein and solutes. Its structural composition causes it to be a markedly noncompliant space. This space equilibrates with the intracellular and intravascular spaces by dynamically exchanging fluid, electrolytes, and proteins with both. This results in a so-called "third space" volume that is very difficult to measure. The clinical impact of this third space appears minimal in the average surgical case. However, in severe hemorrhage as described above in H.10, failure to account for its contribution to intravascular replenishment may lead to volume underresuscitation. Since the inflammatory response during surgery affects the integrity of all membranes, the normal equilibrium among intracellular, intravascular, and interstitial fluid spaces changes. Most often, the noncompliant nature of interstitial space likely minimizes its effects on fluid homeostasis.

13. Under normal conditions minimal fluid accumulation occurs in space outside of organs, referred to here as potential space. However, when fluid leaks out into this potential

space (a body cavity) due to reduced oncotic pressure or capillary integrity, pathologic accumulations such as pleural effusions and/or ascites can ensue. If fluid is removed from these spaces during surgery (e.g., opening the chest or abdomen), fluid from the adjacent organs will rapidly replace this extra-organ fluid and subsequently reduce intravascular volume and potentially induce hypotension.

14. In summary, for major hemorrhage, consideration of volume resuscitation requirements must include intracellular, interstitial, intravascular, and potential space compartments. Particularly when sympathetic tone is abruptly altered (as can happen with induction of anesthesia), the extent of circulatory collapse may be greater than anticipated as fluid within these compartments equilibrates at the new level of sympathetic tone.

I. Brain: The controller

1. It is beyond the scope of this chapter, and to an extent of our knowledge, to detail the neural pathways, interactive signaling, and psychological influences on the cardiovascular system response. Accordingly, our brain as the controller is considered a black box. In this view, this controller is designed to maintain BP assuming that all the effectors are recruitable.

2. Making the controller a black box may be justifiable on another level. Although system integration can be characterized for a given patient at the moment, the pharmacology clinicians utilize affects system integration through direct and indirect effects on effectors and perhaps on the controller and sensors as well. Other medications affect the ability of the CNS to stimulate responses through receptor or ganglion blockade. **For anesthesiologists, in many situations, our clinical management must replace system integration.** By understanding the pharmacology present and its effect on the cardiovascular system, clinical judgment dictates a plan to control BP regulation. This control responsibility must include temporizing and maintaining BP variability. Unable to rely on the cardiovascular system alone, the clinician physiologist manipulates the effector responses to maintain BP while remaining cognizant of the state (presence or absence) of physiologic reserves in the face of upcoming disturbances.

3. Understanding the impact of patient comorbidities anticipates the limitations in physiologic reserves and their availability for recruitment during stress. Through goal-directed therapy, recognition of necessary compromises for adjustment of anesthetic approach can reduce the risk of morbidity and mortality.

4. One aspect of goal-directed therapy is fluid management. Per Gan et al., the "cornerstone of Goal-directed Fluid Therapy is the use of an algorithm...based on physiology and medical evidence..."

XIV. **The cardiovascular system integration**

A. In normal, healthy subjects (no disease or anesthetics present), the cardiovascular system response to physiologic stress is predictable and reproducible. In its simplest form, if BP is altered, the integrated system response—sensors, controller, and effectors—senses the alteration and returns BP toward the original set point. This negative feedback permits us to lead our lives without considering the consequences or preparing for the disturbances to this system. As each effector is recruited to regulate BP, it can contribute less to compensating for an additional stress. It is easy to take the range and automaticity of this system response for granted.

B. In healthy subjects, the utilization of reserves depends on training levels, hydration status, and psychological state, among others. The compensatory limits of healthy humans are set through a complex physio–psycho state that ends with not being able to go on, that is, hitting the wall.

C. For patients, the response of effectors may be limited by effector pathology. The most common limiting factor is ischemic heart disease.

D. To maintain BP **in the face of hypotension** the cardiovascular system responses are predictable.

1. HR and contractility increase resulting in increased myocardial oxygen consumption. Wall tension may be increased or decreased. Since HR is a primary determinant of the onset of myocardial ischemia under anesthesia, its elevation is of particular concern.

2. Oxygen supply response is complex. Assuming no blood loss or alteration of oxygenation, increased HR leads to a reduction of diastolic time. Hence, endocardial perfusion time will be reduced. A decrease in diastolic systemic pressure may decrease the capillary perfusion pressure gradient (systemic diastolic pressure minus LVEDP) depending on the impact of hypotension on LVEDP.

3. Intervention: The anesthesiologist will most likely administer phenylephrine in response to patient hypotension. SVR will increase, and blood volume will shift from the systemic veins into the thoracic veins, increasing preload and leading to an increase in SV. BP will rise, HR will fall, contractility will be reduced, diastolic time will lengthen, and perhaps coronary perfusion pressure will rise as well. However, remember that phenylephrine has a finite half-life and that the BP response to it not only consumes physiologic reserves but also may initiate renal compromise through reduced renal blood flow leading to renal insufficiency. Consider using this half-life time to mitigate the cause of the hypotension so that continued use of phenylephrine is unnecessary.

   a. Response time required

      (1) Responding to hypotension is an everyday occurrence for an anesthesia provider. Defining hypotension is somewhat difficult. For normal subjects, physiologists would arrive at a value of around a mean BP of 50 to 60 mm Hg for preservation of organ function. Induced (i.e., intentional) hypotensive anesthesia challenges that value, and data indicate that a sitting position is different from a supine one. A prevalent clinical definition of hypotension is "±25% of the preoperative value." Given patient anxiety in the immediate preoperative period, determining that value is not always easy. Clinicians face this dilemma and must resolve it intraoperatively.

      (2) If a neuron goes without oxygen, it has a lifespan of minutes. Given that reality, sacrificing all other organ functions to maintain BP is essential on the time scale of minutes.

      (3) For the kidney, even renal insufficiency created during surgery can recover. Consequently, temporarily sacrificing renal perfusion may be acceptable to protect the neuron. However, postoperative creatinine increases of 0.3 mg/dL have been associated with increased mortality for the next year. It remains unclear how long the kidneys can tolerate a phenylephrine infusion without increasing creatinine concentration.

      (4) For a cardiac myocyte, the time constant falls somewhere between several minutes and several hours. The exact time constant is unclear for an individual myocyte, but normally it certainly approaches an hour. After 4 hours, the magic window for thrombolysis to be effective, 50% of myocytes will survive. Therefore, compromising myocardial oxygen supply and demand to preserve neurons is acceptable as a temporizing measure.

      (5) As an aside, cardiac anesthesiologists in the postbypass period are confronted with BP management in the patient who frequently has a history of hypertension, renal insufficiency, peripheral vascular disease, and whose aorta has been recently cannulated (potentially increasing the risk of rupture with even modest hypertension). Systolic pressures are often kept under 100 mm Hg in this setting.

4. If 100 mm Hg should be lower than the magic 25%, how long will it take at that pressure to cause damage? The answer is unclear, but such pressures are routinely maintained way beyond a few minutes.

5. As outlined above, phenylephrine administration elicits a potentially adverse physiologic impact **if sustained**. As the new controller of the sympathetic system, the anesthesia provider needs to consider why the hypotension occurred, if that reason is going to continue or get worse, how long the remaining physiologic reserves can maintain homeostasis in the face of further challenges, and finally the extent to which the ongoing management will negatively affect renal function.

6. These considerations are crucial in determining the likelihood of sustained—that is, through the course of the operation and the early postoperative period—hemodynamic stability of the patient.

7. Frequently, volume management is critical to this decision. Consider that if, instead of administering phenylephrine above, a volume challenge was administered and the BP response was an increase, the oxygen demand and supply benefits would remain. However, instead of consuming physiologic reserves through phenylephrine use, the controller would be providing physiologic reserves through increased venous capacitance and decreased SVR, and perhaps improving renal blood flow to reduce the chance of renal injury. The glycocalyx notwithstanding, sufficient fluid administration remains a crucial part of anesthetic care. "Masking" hypovolemia with vasopressors can lead to adversity!

> **CLINICAL PEARL**   Masking hypovolemia with vasopressors is potentially more harmful than excessive fluid administration.

   a. Achieving the balance between the need for short-term intervention and long-term stability is the responsibility of the controller, i.e., the provider's brain, during anesthesia.

XV. **Effect of anesthesia providers and our pharmacology on the cardiovascular system**

   A. The surgical patient
   1. White-coat hypertension is common. Some attribute this hypertension to the fight-or-flight response necessary for survival! The perioperative period is certainly a time of increased anxiety for many patients. In the context of their cardiovascular system, the anxiety represents an input that most likely alters the response at the controller level. Since non-white-coat hypertension may contribute to cardiac-related complications perioperatively, a patient who is hypertensive in the preoperative area will be given an anxiolytic as the first step to determine if the elevated BP is chronic or not.
   2. If the anxiolysis reduces the BP to the normal range, clinicians attribute the hypertension to anxiety and proceed. If it does not, the hypertension is attributed to an altered set point for BP and one must consider the risks and benefits, as ill defined as they are, before proceeding.

   B. The anesthetic choice
   1. For a healthy patient, for low-risk surgery, numerous retrospective studies suggest that, barring severe anesthetic overdose, in the presence of today's monitoring standards, anesthetic technique has little bearing on adverse patient outcomes [4]. Low surgical risk in the setting of normal physiologic reserves (HR, SVR, and venous volume) protects homeostasis to the extent that the margin for error is great. Provocative statement? Perhaps, but the American Society of Anesthesiologists closed claims database supports this view.
   2. For the high-risk patient with comorbidities related to diabetes, vascular or ischemic or valvular heart disease for high-risk surgery, consideration of their physiologic cardiac reserves becomes extremely important. The entire perioperative period subjects the patient to increased risk. Understanding the consequences of the patient's pathology on their physiologic reserves and use of clinical management approaches to reduce the risk should influence the anesthetic choice through goal-directed therapy [5].
   3. In this chapter, physiologic reserves in the context of normal physiology were presented. The principles related to ventricular function, determinants of myocardial oxygen consumption, and physiologic reserves apply in the pathologic situation as well.
   4. Of all the physiologic reserves discussed, one reserve is minimally affected by pathology during surgery and is not shown to affect outcomes adversely, except perhaps for gastrointestinal (GI) surgery and major trauma. That reserve is venous capacitance. Volume management constricts, replenishes, or expands venous capacitance reserve. The principle that "An empty heart cannot pump blood!!!" is true. In my personal experience as an anesthesiologist and as a consultant to others, the number of patients resuscitated from hypovolemia far exceeds the number who have incurred congestive heart failure from too much fluid.

  5. Incorporating fluid management into goal-directed therapy is of paramount importance if we are to minimize risk for the patient with cardiovascular disease.

C. Treating the cause: Goal-directed therapy

  1. When clinical signs and symptoms do not agree with clinical judgment and their conclusions, more data are necessary. Two very useful monitors in the setting of unresponsive hypotension under general anesthesia may be the PA catheter and the transesophageal echocardiography (TEE) examination.

  2. The PA catheter has been both touted and maligned as a monitoring tool, but continues to be used in cardiac surgery. Using physiologic and clinical principles based on the PA catheter to guide management over an extended perioperative period, Rao et al. [6] demonstrated reduced myocardial reinfarction rates in patients undergoing noncardiac surgery. Many large randomized clinical trials have not shown a benefit to PA catheter–guided monitoring in critically ill patients (Sandham et al.: 1,994 patients; Warszawski et al.: 676 patients; Harvey et al.: 1,041 patients [7–9]). While such definitive randomized trial studies are still lacking in the context of cardiac surgery, observational data indicate that not all cardiac surgery patients benefit from a PA catheter [10].

  3. A national survey demonstrated that clinicians did not understand or know how to apply the physiologic principles underlying the interventions guided by PA catheter data. Certainly, the mere presence of a PA catheter could not improve outcome, in other words, "The yellow snake does no good when inserted" [11]. Its use is reserved for high-risk patients and needs to be accompanied by a thorough understanding of its principles and technology, both in the OR and the intensive care unit.

CLINICAL PEARL   Many clinicians who use PA catheters lack adequate understanding of the physiologic information provided by these catheters.

  4. The ultrasound (TEE or other) probe is the optimal tool for assessing ventricular volume status and regional wall motion abnormalities. An experienced echocardiographer can assess the volume status of the ventricle (intrathoracic blood volume) within a minute and almost as quickly can assess ventricular systolic function. These two data elements provide immediate help in clinical management of unresponsive hypotension. Particularly in a setting where ventricular compliance can change rapidly (ischemia, acidosis, and sepsis), filling pressures from the PA catheter may or may not reflect volume status (actually more physiologically: sarcomere length or end-diastolic volume) of the ventricles. TEE is an essential tool precisely because it more accurately assesses cardiac preload under all conditions. As an example, TEE can assess the state of venous capacitance through observation of the impact of Trendelenburg and reverse Trendelenburg positions on diastolic volumes. With increasing availability of three-dimensional echocardiography, real-time echocardiographic measurement of CO becomes more and more accessible. The availability of all physiologic reserves—HR, contractility, venous capacitance—can then be assessed. A drawback to TEE monitoring is its limited availability in the postoperative period (i.e., once the patient has been awakened and extubated), hence transthoracic echocardiography (TTE) skills can contribute importantly to intravascular volume assessment both before and after surgery.

  5. However, if the physiologic principles of preload, afterload, and contractility are not well understood, then their application to a circulatory problem such as hypotension will be unsound. There are two approaches to this problem: ignore it or develop goal-directed protocols. Learning the principles of goal-directed therapy can allow you to scientifically manage fluid therapy for most patients. The detailed application of goal-directed therapy is complex and varied, and it extends beyond the scope of this chapter. The studies of Walsh et al. [12] and Hamilton et al. [13] demonstrate the complexity of this topic.

REFERENCES

1. **Honig C. *Modern Cardiovascular Physiology.* Boston/Toronto: Little, Brown and Company; 1981.**
2. Mellander S, Johansson B. Control of resistance, exchange, and capacitance functions in the peripheral circulation. *Pharmacol Rev.* 1968;20:117–196.
3. Mellander S. Comparative studies on the adrenergic neuro-hormonal control of resistance and capacitance blood vessels in the cat. *Acta Physiol Scand Suppl.* 1960;50(176):1–86.
4. Neumann MD, Fleisher LA. Risk of anesthesia. In: Miller RD, Eriksson LI, Fleisher LA, et al., eds. *Miller's Anesthesia.* 8th ed, Philadelphia, PA: Elsevier Saunders; 2015:1056–1084.
5. **Gan TJ, Soppitt A, Maroof M, et al. Goal-directed intraoperative fluid administration reduces length of hospital stay after major surgery. *Anesthesiology.* 2002;97:820–826.**
6. Rao TL, Jacobs KH, El-Etr AA. Reinfarction following anesthesia in patients with myocardial infarction. *Anesthesiology.* 1983;59(6):499–505.
7. **Sandham JD, Hull RD, Brant RF, et al. A randomized, controlled trial of the use of pulmonary-artery catheters in high-risk surgical patients. *New Engl J Med.* 2003;348:5–15.**
8. Richard C, Warszowski J, Anguel N, et al. Early use of the pulmonary artery catheter and outcomes in patients with shock and acute respiratory distress syndrome: a randomized controlled trial. *JAMA.* 2003;290:2713–2720.
9. Harvey S, Harrison DA, Singer M, et al. Assessment of the clinical effectiveness of pulmonary artery catheters in management of patients in intensive care (PAC-Man): a randomized controlled trial. *Lancet.* 2005;366:472–477.
10. **Schwann NM, Hillel Z, Hoeft A, et al. Lack of effectiveness of the pulmonary artery catheter in cardiac surgery. *Anesth Analg.* 2011;113:994–1002.**
11. **Iberti TJ, Fischer EP, Leibowitz AB, et al. A multicenter study of physicians' knowledge of the pulmonary artery catheter. Pulmonary Artery Catheter Study Group. *JAMA.* 1990;264(22):2928–2932.**
12. Walsh SR, Tang TY, Farooq N, et al. Perioperative fluid restriction reduces complications after major gastrointestinal surgery. *Surgery.* 2008;143(4):466–468.
13. Hamilton MA, Mythen MG, Ackland GL. Less is not more: a lack of evidence for intraoperative fluid restriction improving outcome after major elective gastrointestinal surgery. *Anesth Analg.* 2006;102(3):970–971.

2

Cardiovascular Drugs

Nirvik Pal and John F. Butterworth

KEY POINTS

1. Drug errors are a common cause of accidental injury to patients. The authors suggest referring to drug package inserts or the *Physicians' Desk Reference* to check any unfamiliar drug before it is prescribed or administered.
2. Generic sterile, injectable drugs represent a "low margin" product line for manufacturers so these agents are subject to periodic shortages when one of the few manufacturers has production issues.
3. Patients undergoing cardiac surgery may quickly recover from the need for drug support, unlike patients with chronic heart failure (CHF) receiving the identical drug(s).
4. Hemodynamic improvement has been well established with usage of vasoactive and inotropic medications but overall survival outcomes are still a matter of much debate and research.
5. Vasoactive drugs are often combined to offset unneeded side effects (e.g., milrinone + phenylephrine) or to take advantage of sequential steps in a biochemical pathway (epinephrine + milirinone).

I. **Introduction**

Numerous potent drugs are used to control heart rate (HR) and rhythm, blood pressure (BP), and cardiac output (CO) before, during, and after surgery. Patients undergoing cardiovascular and thoracic operations are particularly likely to receive one of these agents. This chapter reviews the indications, mechanisms, dosing, drug interactions, and common adverse events for these drugs. Drug errors are common causes of accidental injury to patients, particularly in hospitalized, critically ill patients. Therefore, we suggest that the package insert or *Physicians' Desk Reference* [1] (which contains the package insert information) be consulted before any unfamiliar drug is prescribed or administered [2]. Fortunately, it has never been easier to obtain drug information. Convenient sources of drug information include numerous books and websites, some of which are provided at the end of this chapter [2,3]. Using a "smart" mobile telephone, many physicians now maintain a readily updated library of drug information in their hand or pocket at all times. Note, that generic sterile, injectable drugs represent a "low margin" product line for manufacturers so these agents are subject to periodic shortages when one of the few manufacturers has production issues.

II. **Drug dosage calculations**

1. Drugs are administered in increments of weight or units. Unfortunately, drugs are not labeled in a uniform manner. Dilution of drugs and calculations are often necessary. Fortunately, most modern infusion pumps do these calculations for the operator, limiting the opportunity for mistakes.
2. To determine the dose rate (µg/min): Calculate the desired per-minute dose. Example: A 70-kg patient who is to receive dopamine at 5 µg/kg/min needs a 350 µg/min dose rate.
3. To determine the concentration (µg/mL): Calculate how many micrograms of drug are in each milliliter of solution. To calculate concentration (µg/mL), simply multiply the number of milligrams in 250 mL by 4.
4. To determine the volume infusion rate (mL/min): Divide the dose rate by the concentration (µg/min ÷ µg/mL = mL/min). The infusion pump should be set for this volume infusion rate.

A. **Vasoactive inotrope scoring** [4–6]

Common clinical practice is to have patients receive multiple vasopressors and inotropes to achieve maximal clinical benefit while minimizing side effects from the medications. In order to achieve equivalence or "common grounds" for clinical assessment and progress vasoactive inotrope score was used which has been extended with addition of newer medications in this class.

Dopamine	Micrograms/kg/min	×1
Dobutamine	Micrograms/kg/min	×1
Epinephrine	Micrograms/kg/min	×100
Norepinephrine	Micrograms/kg/min	×100
Milrinone	Micrograms/kg/min	×10
Vasopressin	Units/kg/min	×10,000
Olprinone	Micrograms/kg/min	×25

III. **Drug receptor interactions**

A. **Receptor activation**

Can responses to a given drug dose be predicted? The short answer is: *Partially.* The more accurate answer is: *Not with complete certainty.* Many factors determine the magnitude of response produced by a given drug at a given dose.

1. **Pharmacokinetics** relates the dose to the concentrations that are achieved in plasma or at the effect site. In brief, these concentrations are affected by the drug's volume of distribution and clearance, and for drugs administered orally, by the fractional absorption [7].
2. **Pharmacodynamics** relates drug concentrations in plasma or at the effect site to the drug effect.
   a. **Concentration of drug at the effect site (receptor)** is influenced by the concentration of drug in plasma, tissue perfusion, lipid solubility, and protein binding; diffusion characteristics, including state of ionization (electrical charge); and local metabolism.

    b. **Number of receptors** per gram of end-organ tissue varies.

      (1) **Upregulation** (increased density of receptors) is seen with a chronic **decrease** in receptor stimulation. Example: Chronic administration of β-adrenergic receptor antagonists increases the number of β-adrenergic receptors.

      (2) **Downregulation** (decreased density of receptors) is caused by a chronic **increase** in receptor stimulation. Example: Chronic treatment of asthma with β-adrenergic receptor agonists reduces the number of β-adrenergic receptors.

    c. **Drug** receptor affinity and efficacy may vary.

      (1) Receptor binding and receptor activation by an agonist produces a biochemical change in the cell. Example: α-Adrenergic receptor agonists increase protein kinase C concentrations within smooth-muscle cells. β-Adrenergic receptor agonists increase intracellular concentrations of cAMP.

      (2) The biochemical change may produce a cellular response. Example: Increased intracellular protein kinase C produces an increase in intracellular $[Ca^{2+}]$, which results in smooth-muscle contraction. Conversely, increased intracellular concentrations of cAMP relax vascular smooth muscle but increase the inotropic state of cardiac muscle.

      (3) The maximal effect of a partial agonist is less than the maximal effect of a full agonist.

      (4) **Receptor desensitization** may occur when prolonged agonist exposure to receptor leads to loss of cellular responses with agonist–receptor binding. An example of this is the reduced response to β_1-adrenergic receptor agonists that occurs in patients with chronic heart failure (CHF), as a result of the increased intracellular concentrations of β-adrenergic receptor kinase, an enzyme which uncouples the receptor from its effector enzyme adenylyl cyclase.

      (5) Other factors including acidosis, hypoxia, and drug interactions can reduce cellular response to receptor activation.

IV. Pharmacogenetics and genomics

In the future, pharmacogenetics, or how drug actions or toxicities are influenced by an individual's genetic make-up, may become a tool in helping anesthesiologists select among therapeutic options. The genetic profile of an individual may impact the degree to the patients will respond to adrenergic therapies, including vasopressors. Life-threatening arrhythmias, such as long QT syndrome, may result from therapy with a number of commonly prescribed agents, and relatively common genetic sequence variations are now known to be an underlying predisposing factor. Droperidol, which is highly effective and safe at small doses for preventing or treating postoperative nausea, has been shown (at larger doses) to cause QT-interval lengthening and increase risk of *Torsades de Pointes* in a small cohort of susceptible patients. Therefore, a larger number of patients will be deprived of this useful medication because of our inability to identify a small number of patients who have the genetic predisposition for this rare but disastrous complication. Industry and academia are rapidly progressing toward simple assay-based genetic screens capable of identifying patients with these and other risks for adverse or inadequate drug responses, including heparin or warfarin resistance. Unfortunately, at the present time, commercially available screens are rare and have not been sufficiently evaluated to be considered the standard care. As such, detailed family history is the only practical means through which we can identify such genetic risks. At the same time, genetic variations may occur spontaneously or be present in a family but not be manifested with symptoms (phenotypically silent). Hence, continuous monitoring for adverse or highly variable drug responses, particularly those related to arrhythmias or BP instability, is the cornerstone of cardiovascular management in the perioperative period.

V. Guidelines for prevention and treatment of cardiovascular disease

Drug treatment and drug prevention for several common cardiovascular diseases have been described in clinical practice guidelines published by national and international organizations. We provide references for the convenience of our readers. Because these recommendations evolve from year to year, we strongly recommend that readers check whether these guidelines may have been updated since publication of this volume.

A. **Coronary artery disease**
1. Primary prevention (see Refs. [8–12])
2. Established disease (see Refs. [13–15])
3. Preoperative cardiac evaluation and prophylaxis during major surgery (see Refs. [16–20])

B. **CHF** (see Refs. [21–24])

C. **Hypertension** (see (Ref. [8])

D. **Atrial fibrillation prophylaxis** (see Ref. [25])

E. **Resuscitation of patients in cardiac arrest after cardiac surgery** (see Ref. [26])

F. **Resuscitation after cardiopulmonary arrest** (see Ref. [27])

VI. **Vasopressors**

A. **α-Adrenergic receptor pharmacology** (Fig. 2.1)
1. Postsynaptic α-adrenergic receptors mediate peripheral vasoconstriction (both arterial and venous), especially with neurally released norepinephrine (NE). Selective activation of cardiac α-adrenergic receptors increases inotropy while **decreasing** the HR. (Positive

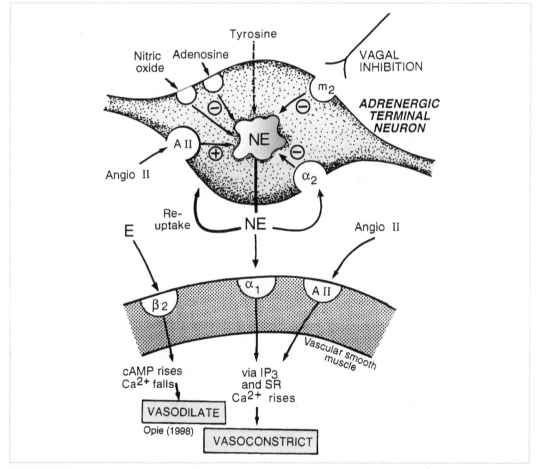

FIGURE 2.1 Schematic representation of the adrenergic receptors present on the sympathetic nerve terminal and vascular smooth-muscle cell. NE is released by electrical depolarization of the nerve terminal; however, the quantity of NE release is *increased* by neuronal (presynaptic) β_2-receptor or muscarinic–cholinergic stimulation and is *decreased* by activation of presynaptic α_2-receptors. On the *postsynaptic* membrane, stimulation of α_1- or α_2-adrenergic receptors causes vasoconstriction, whereas β_2-receptor activation causes vasodilation. Prazosin is a selective α_1-antagonist drug. Note that NE at clinical concentrations does not stimulate β_2-receptors, but epinephrine (E) does. (From Opie LH. *The Heart: Physiology from the Cell to the Circulation*. Philadelphia, PA: Lippincott Williams & Wilkins; 1998:17–41, with permission.)

inotropy from α-adrenergic agonists can only be demonstrated in vitro or by selective drug administration in coronary arteries to avoid peripheral effects that normally overwhelm the cardiac actions.)

2. α-Adrenergic receptors on presynaptic nerve terminals decrease NE release through negative feedback. Activation of brain α-adrenergic receptors (e.g., with clonidine) lowers BP by decreasing sympathetic nervous system activity and causes sedation (e.g., with dexmedetomidine). Postsynaptic α_2-adrenergic receptors mediate constriction of vascular smooth muscle.

3. **Drug interactions**
   a. **Reserpine interactions.** Reserpine depletes intraneuronal NE and chronic use induces a "denervation hypersensitivity" state. Indirect-acting sympathomimetic drugs show diminished effect because of depleted NE stores, whereas direct-acting or mixed-action drugs may produce exaggerated responses because of receptor upregulation. This is of greater laboratory than clinical interest because of the rarity with which reserpine is now prescribed to patients, but it illustrates an important concept about indirect-acting adrenergic agents.
   b. **Tricyclic (and tetracyclic) or antidepressant and cocaine interactions.** The first two categories of drugs block the reuptake of catecholamines by prejunctional neurons and increase the catecholamine concentration at receptors. Interactions between these drugs and sympathomimetic agents can be very severe and of comparable or greater danger than the widely feared monoamine oxidase (MAO) inhibitor reactions. In general, if sympathomimetic drugs are required, small dosages of direct-acting agents represent the best choice.

4. **Specific agents**
   a. **Selective agonists**
      (1) **Phenylephrine (Neo-Synephrine)** [28]
         (a) **Phenylephrine is a synthetic noncatecholamine.**
         (b) **Actions.** The drug is a selective α_1-adrenergic agonist with minimal β-adrenergic effects. It causes vasoconstriction, primarily in arterioles.

Phenylephrine	
HR	Decreased (reflex response to BP elevation)
Contractility	No direct effect with systemic administration
CO	No change or decreased
BP	Increased
Systemic vascular resistance (SVR)	Increased
Preload	Minimal

         (c) **Offset** occurs by redistribution and rapid metabolism by MAO; there is no catechol O-methyltransferase (COMT) metabolism.
         (d) **Advantages.** A direct agonist with short duration (less than 5 minutes), it increases perfusion pressure for the brain, kidney, and heart in the presence of low SVR states. When used during hypotension, phenylephrine will increase coronary perfusion pressure without altering myocardial contractility. If *hyper*tension is avoided, myocardial oxygen consumption (Mvo_2) does not increase substantially. If contractility is depressed because of ischemia, phenylephrine will sometimes produce an increased CO from an increase in coronary perfusion pressure. It is useful for correcting hypotension in patients with CAD, hypertrophic subaortic stenosis, tetralogy of Fallot, or valvular aortic stenosis.
         (e) **Disadvantages.** It may decrease stroke volume (SV) and CO secondary to increased afterload; it may increase pulmonary vascular resistance (PVR); it may decrease renal, mesenteric, and extremity perfusion. Reflex bradycardia, usually not severe, may occur but will usually respond to atropine. Phenylephrine rarely

may be associated with coronary artery spasm or spasm of an internal mammary, radial, or gastroepiploic artery bypass graft.

(f) **Indications for use**
  (i) Hypotension due to peripheral vasodilation, low SVR states (e.g., septic shock, or to counteract effects of nitroglycerin).
  (ii) For patients with supraventricular tachycardia (SVT), reflex vagal stimulation in response to increased BP may terminate the arrhythmia; phenylephrine treats both the hypotension and arrhythmia.
  (iii) It can oppose right-to-left shunting during acute cyanotic spells in tetralogy of Fallot.
  (iv) Temporary therapy of hypovolemia until blood volume is restored, although a drug with positive inotropic action (e.g., ephedrine or epinephrine) usually is a better choice in patients without CAD (or hypertrophic obstructive cardiomyopathy), and in general, vasoconstrictors should not be viewed as effective treatments for hypovolemia.

(g) **Administration.** Intravenous (IV) infusion (central line preferable) or IV bolus

(h) **Clinical use**
  (i) Phenylephrine dose
    (a) IV infusion: 0.5 to 10 μg/kg/min.
    (b) IV bolus: 1 to 10 μg/kg, increased as needed (some patients with peripheral vascular collapse may require larger bolus injections to raise SVR).
    (c) For tetralogy of Fallot spells in children: 5 to 50 μg/kg IV as a bolus dose.
  (ii) **Mixing**
    (a) IV infusion: Often mix 10 or 15 mg in 250 mL IV fluid (40 or 60 μg/mL).
    (b) IV bolus: Dilute to 40 to 100 μg/mL.
  (iii) Nitroglycerin may be administered while maintaining or increasing arterial BP with phenylephrine. This combination may serve to increase myocardial oxygen supply while minimizing increases in Mvo_2.
  (iv) Phenylephrine is the vasopressor of choice for short-term correction of excessive vasodilation in most patients with CAD or aortic stenosis.

CLINICAL PEARL Phenylephrine can be used for hypotension related to low SVR states, but only as a temporizing therapy for hypovolemia.

b. **Mixed agonists**
  (1) **Dopamine (Intropin)** [28]
    See Section VII.
  (2) **Ephedrine**
    (a) **Ephedrine is a plant-derived alkaloid with sympathomimetic effects.**
    (b) **Actions**
      (i) Mild direct α-, β_1-, and β_2-adrenergic agonists
      (ii) Indirect NE release from neurons

Ephedrine	
HR	Slightly increased
Contractility	Increased
CO	Increased
BP	Increased
SVR	Slightly increased
Preload	Increased (mobilization of blood from viscera and extremities)

(c) **Offset.** Five to 10 minutes IV; no metabolism by MAO or COMT; renal elimination

(d) **Advantages**
  (i) Easily titrated pressor and inotrope that rarely produces unexpected excessive responses
  (ii) Short duration of action with IV administration (3 to 10 minutes); lasts up to 1 hour with intramuscular (IM) administration
  (iii) Limited tendency to produce tachycardia
  (iv) Does not reduce blood flow to placenta; safe in pregnancy
  (v) Good agent to correct sympathectomy-induced relative hypovolemia and decreased SVR after spinal or epidural anesthesia

(e) **Disadvantages**
  (i) Efficacy is reduced when NE stores are depleted.
  (ii) Risk of malignant hypertension with MAO inhibitors or cocaine
  (iii) Tachyphylaxis with repeated doses (thus rarely administered by continuous infusion)

(f) **Indications**
  (i) Hypotension due to low SVR or low CO, especially if HR is low, and particularly with spinal or epidural anesthesia
  (ii) Temporary therapy of hypovolemia until circulating blood volume is restored, although, as previously noted, in general vasoconstrictors should not substitute for definitive treatment of hypovolemia

(g) **Administration.** IV, IM, subcutaneous (SC), by mouth (PO)

(h) **Clinical use**
  (i) Ephedrine dose: 5 to 10 mg IV bolus, repeated or increased as needed; 25 to 50 mg IM.
  (ii) Ephedrine is conveniently mixed in a syringe (5 to 10 mg/mL) and can be given as an IV bolus into a freely running IV line.
  (iii) Ephedrine is a useful, quick-acting, titratable IV pressor that can be administered via a peripheral vein during anesthesia.

(3) **Epinephrine (Adrenaline)**
See subsequent Section VII: Positive inotropic drugs.

(4) **NE (noradrenaline, Levophed)** [28,29]

(a) **NE is the primary physiologic postganglionic sympathetic neurotransmitter;** NE is also released by adrenal medulla and central nervous system (CNS) neurons.

(b) **Actions**
  (i) Direct α_1- and α_2-adrenergic actions and β_1-adrenergic agonist action
  (ii) Limited β_2-adrenergic effect in vivo, despite NE being a more powerful β_2-adrenergic agonist than dobutamine in vitro

	NE
HR	Variable; unchanged or may decrease if BP rises (reflex); increases if BP remains low
Contractility	Increased
CO	Increased or decreased (depends on SVR)
BP	Increased
SVR	Increased
PVR	Increased

(c) **Offset** is by redistribution, neural uptake, and metabolism by MAO and COMT.

(d) **Advantages**
   (i)   Direct adrenergic agonist. Equipotent to epinephrine at β_1-adrenergic receptors
   (ii) Redistributes blood flow to brain and heart because all other vascular beds are constricted.
   (iii) Elicits intense α_1- and α_2-adrenergic agonism; may be effective as vasoconstrictor when phenylephrine (α_1 only) lacks efficacy
(e) **Disadvantages**
   (i)   Reduced organ perfusion: Risk of ischemia of kidney, skin, liver, bowel, and extremities
   (ii) Myocardial ischemia possible; increased afterload, HR. Contractility may increase, be unchanged, or even decrease. Coronary spasm may be precipitated.
   (iii) Pulmonary vasoconstriction
   (iv) Arrhythmias
   (v)   Risk of skin necrosis with SC extravasation
(f) **Indications for use**
   (i)   Peripheral vascular collapse when it is necessary to increase SVR (e.g., septic shock or "vasoplegia" after cardiopulmonary bypass [CPB])
   (ii) Conditions in which increased SVR is desired together with cardiac stimulation
   (iii) Need for increased SVR in which phenylephrine has proved ineffective
(g) **Administration.** IV only, by central line only
(h) **Clinical use**
   (i)   Usual NE starting infusion doses: 15 to 30 ng/kg/min IV (adult); usual range, 30 to 300 ng/kg/min.
   (ii) Minimize duration of use; monitor patient for oliguria and metabolic acidosis.
   (iii) NE can be used with vasodilator (e.g., sodium nitroprusside or phentolamine) to counteract α-stimulation while leaving β_1-adrenergic stimulation intact; however, if intense vasoconstriction is not required, we recommend that a different drug be used.
   (iv) For treating severe right ventricular (RV) failure associated with cardiac surgery, the simultaneous infusion of NE into the *left atrium* (through a left atrial catheter placed intraoperatively) plus inhaled nitric oxide (NO) and/or nitroglycerin by IV infusion is useful. The left atrial NE reaches the systemic vascular bed first and it is largely metabolized peripherally before it reaches the lung where it might increase PVR (had the NE been infused through a venous line) (Table 2.1).

CLINICAL PEARL   Epinephrine is a direct α_1- and α_2- and β_1- and β_2-agonists not dependent on release of endogenous NE. In the setting of a dilated left ventricle (LV) and myocardial ischemia, epinephrine may increase coronary perfusion pressure and reduce ischemia.

(5) **Interactions with MAO inhibitors**
   (a) MAO is an enzyme that deaminates NE, dopamine, and serotonin. Thus, the MAO inhibitors treat severe depression by increasing catecholamine concentrations in the brain by inhibiting catecholamine breakdown. Administration of indirectly acting adrenergic agonists or meperidine to patients taking MAO inhibitors can produce a life-threatening hypertensive crisis. Ideally, 2 to 3 weeks should elapse between discontinuing the hydrazine MAO inhibitor phenelzine and elective surgery. Nonhydrazine MAO inhibitors (isocarboxazid, tranylcypromine) require 3 to 10 days for offset of effect. Selegiline

TABLE 2.1   Acute treatment of pulmonary hypertension and RV failure

Pulmonary hypertension	
Hyperventilation	Maintain $Paco_2$ at 25–28 mm Hg
Oxygen	Prevents hypoxic vasoconstriction
Nitric oxide (NO)	Inspired, 0.05–80 ppm
Nitroprusside	0.1–4 µg/kg/min
Nitroglycerin	0.1–7 µg/kg/min
Alprostadil	0.05–0.4 µg/kg/min
Epoprostenol	9 ng/kg/min[a]
Tolazoline	Bolus 0.5–2 mg/kg, then 0.5–10 mg/kg/hr
Phentolamine	1–20 µg/kg/min
Isoproterenol	0.02–20 µg/kg/min
Diltiazem	Effective orally; no data on IV use
Right ventricular (RV) failure	
Use therapies listed above to reduce PA pressure; in addition, the following may be utilized:	
Dobutamine	2–20 µg/kg/min
Epinephrine[b]	0.05–0.2 µg/kg/min
Inamrinone	5–20 µg/kg/min (maintenance)
Milrinone	0.5–0.75 µg/kg/min (maintenance) IV (inhaled route may be considered)
Norepinephrine (NE)[b]	0.05–0.2 µg/kg/min (maintain coronary perfusion pressure)
Right-sided mechanical assist device	Rest, unload right heart
Intra-aortic balloon counterpulsation	Unload left heart, improve coronary perfusion to left and right heart

[a]Used mainly for chronic management of primary pulmonary hypertension.
[b]May be administered via left atrial line to reduce actions on pulmonary vasculature.

at doses 10 mg or less per day should present fewer adverse drug interactions than other MAO inhibitors.

   (b) The greatest risk of inducing a hyperadrenergic state occurs with indirect-acting sympathomimetic drugs (such as ephedrine), because such agents release the intraneuronal stores of NE that were increased by the MAO inhibitor. Because dopamine releases NE, it should be initiated with caution in the MAO-inhibited patient.

   (c) In MAO-inhibited patients, preferred drugs are those with purely direct activity: epinephrine, NE, isoproterenol, phenylephrine, vasopressin, and dobutamine. All pressor drugs should be used cautiously, in small dosages with BP monitoring and observation of the electrocardiogram (ECG) for arrhythmias.

B. Vasopressin pharmacology and agonists [30–34]

   1. Actions

   a. Vasopressin is an endogenous antidiuretic hormone that in high concentrations produces a direct peripheral vasoconstriction through activation of smooth-muscle V1 receptors. Vasopressin has no actions on β-adrenergic receptors, so it may produce less tachycardia than epinephrine when used for resuscitation after cardiac arrest. Vasopressin has been administered intra-arterially in a selective fashion to control gastrointestinal bleeding.

   b. Vasopressin produces relatively more vasoconstriction of skin, skeletal muscle, intestine, and adipose tissue than of coronary or renal beds. Vasopressin causes cerebrovascular dilation.

   2. Advantages

   a. Vasopressin is a very potent agent which acts independently of adrenergic receptors.

    b. Some studies suggest that vasopressin may be effective at maintaining adequate SVR in severe acidosis, sepsis, or after CPB, even when agents such as phenylephrine or NE have proven ineffective.

    c. Vasopressin may restore coronary perfusion pressure after cardiac arrest without also producing tachycardia and arrhythmias, as is common when epinephrine is used for this purpose. However, current guidelines make vasopressin a second order choice after epinephrine for cardiac arrest.

3. Disadvantages

    a. Vasopressin produces a variety of unpleasant signs and symptoms in awake patients, including pallor of skin, nausea, abdominal cramping, bronchoconstriction, and uterine contractions.

    b. Decreases in splanchnic blood flow may be of concern in patients receiving vasopressin for more than a few hours, particularly when vasopressin is coadministered with agents such as α-adrenergic agonists and positive inotropic drugs. Increases in serum concentrations of bilirubin and of "liver" enzymes are common.

    c. Vasopressin may be associated with a decrease in platelet concentration.

    d. Lactic acidosis is common in patients receiving vasopressin infusion (but these patients are generally critically ill and already receiving other vasoactive agents).

4. Clinical use

    a. Vasopressin has been used as an alternative to epinephrine in treating countershock-refractory ventricular fibrillation (VF) in adults. The 2015 American Heart Association (AHA) Guidelines for Cardiopulmonary Resuscitation and Emergency Cardiovascular Care Science [27] states that there is no evidence that substitution of vasopressin for epinephrine during resuscitation has benefit. The typical vasopressin resuscitation dose is 40 units as an IV bolus.

    b. Vasopressin has been used in a variety of conditions associated with vasodilatory shock, including sepsis, the "vasoplegic" syndrome after CPB, and for hypotension occurring in patients receiving ACE inhibitors (or angiotensin receptor blockers [ARB]) and general anesthesia. Typical adult doses range from 4 to 6 units/hr. We have found this drug to be effective and useful, but sometimes associated with troublesome metabolic acidosis. We speculate that the latter may be the result of inadequate visceral perfusion.

    c. Vasopressin is also used for diabetes insipidus as antidiuretic hormone replacement. Oftentimes intranasal route is utilized for that.

    d. Clinical perspective [32]:
Russell in his editorial compares and contrasts the results of three trials VASST, VANISH, VANCS (see reference above). The primary end-points in VASST was 28-day mortality, VANISH was kidney failure free days, and in VANCS was mortality and severe complications. VASST and VANISH were for septic shock whereas VANCS was for cardiac surgery–related vasoplegia. Outcome benefits in primary end-points were seen in VANCS, probably attributed to "lower" serum levels of vasopressin whereas no outcome benefit in primary end-points were seen in the other two trials. Also, at the cellular level it may be hypothesized that this may be due to difference in interaction of macro-circulation versus the micro-circulation, with the macro-circulation showing improvement in hemodynamics while the micro-circulation experiencing increased oxygen debt and injury to the glycocalyx with addition of vasopressors in the presence of inflammatory cytokines.

C. Angiotensin II [35–37]

Action: Naturally occurring vasopressor as part of the renin–angiotensin–aldosterone–system (RAAS). During distributive shock, especially sepsis, it has been seen that there is synergistic downregulation of angiotensin receptor (AT-R1, AT-R2) by local release of nitric oxide (NO) and other proinflammatory cytokines. Exogenous angiotensin II acts on these receptors and plays a role in repleting and countering this effect and maintaining the vascular tone of the macro-circulation thus improving hemodynamics.

    Dose: 0.02 micrograms/kg/min to maximum of 0.04 micrograms/kg/min, titrate to effect of mean arterial pressure (MAP) between 65 and 75 mm Hg [35]

Side effects: Improves macro-circulation improving hemodynamics but may adversely affect micro-circulation at higher doses.

VII. Positive inotropic drugs

A. Treatment of low CO [28,38–41]

1. **Goals.** Increase organ perfusion and oxygen delivery to tissues.

    a. **Increase** CO by increasing SV, HR (when appropriate), or both.

    b. Maximize myocardial oxygen supply (increase diastolic arterial pressure, diastolic perfusion time, and blood O_2 content; decrease left ventricular end-diastolic pressure [LVEDP]).

    c. Provide an adequate MAP for perfusion of other organs.

    d. Minimize increases in myocardial oxygen demand by avoiding tachycardia and LV dilation.

    e. Metabolic disturbances, arrhythmias, or cardiac ischemia, if present, should be treated concurrently.

    f. Drug treatment of critically ill patients with intrinsic myocardial failure may include the following cardiac stimulants:

    (1) β_1-Adrenergic stimulation

    (2) Phosphodiesterase (PDE) inhibition

    (3) Dopaminergic stimulants

    (4) Calcium sensitizers (increase calcium sensitivity of contractile proteins)

    (5) Digoxin

2. **Monitoring.** Positive inotropic drug dosing is most effectively regulated using data from the arterial line, a monitor of CO, and/or echocardiography. In addition, monitoring of mixed venous oxygen saturation can be extremely valuable. The inotropic drug dosage can be titrated to CO and BP endpoints, together with assessment of organ perfusion, for example, urine output and concentration.

B. cAMP-dependent agents

1. **β-Adrenergic and dopaminergic receptor agonists**

    a. **Similarities among sympathomimetic drugs**

    (1) β_1-Agonist effects are primarily stimulatory.

β_1-Agonists	
HR	Increased
Contractility	Increased
Conduction velocity	Increased
Atrioventricular (AV) block	Decreased
Automaticity	Increased
Risk of arrhythmias	Increased

    (2) **β_2-Agonists** cause vasodilation and bronchodilation, and they also increase HR and contractility (albeit with less potency than β_1-agonists).

    (3) **Postsynaptic dopaminergic receptors** mediate renal and mesenteric vasodilation, increase renal salt excretion, and reduce gastrointestinal motility. Presynaptic dopaminergic receptors inhibit NE release.

    (4) **Diastolic ventricular dysfunction.** Cardiac β-receptor activation enhances diastolic ventricular relaxation by facilitating the active, energy-consuming process that pumps free intracellular Ca^{2+} into storage sites. Abnormal relaxation occurring in ischemia and other myocardial disorders leads to increased diastolic stiffness. By augmenting diastolic relaxation, β-adrenergic receptor agonists reduce LVEDP and heart size (LV end-diastolic volume [LVEDV]), improve diastolic filling, reduce left atrial pressure (LAP), and improve the myocardial oxygen supply–demand ratio.

    (5) **Systolic ventricular dysfunction.** More complete ventricular ejection during systole will reduce the LV end-systolic volume. This reduces heart size, LV systolic wall tension (by Laplace's law), and Mvo_2.

(6) **Myocardial ischemia.** The net effects of β-receptor stimulation on myocardial O_2 supply and demand are multifactorial and may be difficult to predict. Mvo_2 tends to increase as HR and contractility rise, but Mvo_2 is reduced by lowering LVEDV. β-Agonists improve O_2 supply when LVEDP is decreased, but can worsen the supply–demand ratio particularly if HR rises or diastolic BP is lowered.

(7) **Hypovolemia** is deleterious to the patient with heart failure just as it is for the patient with normal ventricular function; however, volume overload may lead to myocardial ischemia by restricting subendocardial perfusion.

(8) **There is a risk of tissue damage or sloughing when vasoactive drugs extravasate outside of a vein.** In general, catecholamine vasoconstrictors may be given through peripheral IV lines provided that

  (a) No central venous catheter is available.

  (b) The drug is injected only into a free-flowing IV line.

  (c) The IV site is observed during and after the injection for signs of infiltration or extravasation.

b. **Dobutamine (Dobutrex)** [28,42]

  (1) **Dobutamine is a synthetic catecholamine formulated as a racemic mixture.**

  (2) **Actions**

   (a) Direct $β_1$-agonist, with limited $β_2$- and $α_1$-effects. Dobutamine has no $α_2$ or dopaminergic activity.

   (b) Dobutamine increases cardiac inotropy principally via its $β_1$ (and perhaps also by $α_1$) agonism, but HR is increased only by the $β_1$-effect.

   (c) On blood vessels, dobutamine is predominantly a vasodilator drug. Mechanisms for vasodilation include the following:

    (i) $β_2$-mediated vasodilation that is only partially counteracted by (−) dobutamine's $α_1$-constrictor effects

    (ii) The (+) dobutamine enantiomer and its metabolite, (+)-3-O-methyldobutamine, are $α_1$-*antagonists*. Thus, as dobutamine is metabolized, any $α_1$-agonist actions of the drug should diminish over time.

Dobutamine	
HR	Increased
Contractility	Increased
CO	Increased
BP	Usually increases, may remain unchanged
LVEDP	Decreased
LAP	Decreased
SVR	Decreased by dilating all vascular beds; slight increase may be seen in β-blocked patients
PVR	Decreased

  (3) **Offset.** Offset of action is achieved by redistribution, metabolism by COMT, and conjugation by glucuronide in liver; an active metabolite is generated. Plasma half-life is 2 minutes.

  (4) **Advantages**

   (a) At low doses there is generally less tachycardia than with "equivalently inotropic" doses of isoproterenol or dopamine, on the other hand some studies show that "equivalently inotropic" doses of epinephrine produce LESS tachycardia than dobutamine.

   (b) Afterload reduction (SVR and PVR) may improve LV and RV systolic function, which can benefit the heart with right and/or LV failure.

   (c) Renal blood flow may increase (due to a $β_2$ effect), but not as much as with comparable (but low) doses of dopamine or dopexamine.

(5) **Disadvantages**

(a) Tachycardia and arrhythmias are dose related and can be severe.

(b) Hypotension may occur if the reduction in SVR is not fully offset by an increase in CO; dobutamine is an inotrope but is not a pressor.

(c) Coronary steal is possible.

(d) The drug is a nonselective vasodilator: Blood flow may be shunted from kidney and splanchnic bed to skeletal muscle.

(e) Tachyphylaxis has been reported when infused for more than 72 hours.

(f) Mild hypokalemia may occur.

(g) As a partial agonist, dobutamine can inhibit actions of full agonists (e.g., epinephrine) under certain circumstances.

(6) **Indications.** Low CO states, especially with increased SVR or PVR.

(7) **Administration.** IV only (central line is preferable, but dobutamine has little vasoconstrictor activity, minimizing risk of extravasation).

(8) **Clinical use**

(a) Dobutamine dose: IV infusion, 2 to 20 μg/kg/min. Some patients may respond to initial doses as low as 0.5 μg/kg/min and, at such low doses, HR usually does not increase.

(b) Dobutamine increases Mvo_2 to a lesser degree than CO. Dobutamine increases coronary blood flow to a greater degree than dopamine when either agent is given as a single drug. However, addition of nitroglycerin to dopamine may be equally effective.

(c) Dobutamine acts similar to a fixed-ratio combination of an inotropic drug and a vasodilator drug. These two components cannot be titrated separately.

(d) In patients undergoing coronary surgery, dobutamine produces more tachycardia than epinephrine when administered to produce the same increase in SV.

(e) When dobutamine is given to β-blocked patients, SVR may increase.

(f) Routine administration of dobutamine (or any other positive inotrope) is not recommended [43].

c. **Dopamine (Intropin)** [28]

(1) Dopamine is a catecholamine precursor to NE and epinephrine found in nerve terminals and the adrenal medulla.

(2) **Actions**

(a) Direct action: α_1-, β_1-, β_2-adrenergic, and dopaminergic (DA_1) agonist

(b) Indirect action: Induces release of stored neuronal NE

(c) The dose versus response relationship is often described as if "carved in stone"; however, the relationship between dose and concentration and between dose and response is highly variable from patient to patient. We provide this chart because it is expected, not because we endorse its accuracy!

Dose (μg/kg/min)	Dopamine (as commonly described)	
	Receptor activated	Effect
1–3	Dopaminergic (DA_1)	Increased renal and mesenteric blood flow
3–10	$\beta_1 + \beta_2$ (plus DA_1)	Increased HR, contractility, and CO
>10	α (plus β plus DA_1)	Increased SVR, PVR; decreased renal blood flow; increased HR, arrhythmias. Increased afterload may decrease CO

(3) **Offset** is achieved by redistribution, uptake by nerve terminals plus metabolism by MAO and COMT.

(4) **Advantages**

(a) Increased renal perfusion and urine output at low-to-moderate dosages (partially due to a specific DA_1-agonist effect)

- **(b)** Blood flow shifts from skeletal muscle to kidney and splanchnic beds.
- **(c)** BP response is easy to titrate because of its mixed inotropic and vasoconstrictor properties.

(5) Disadvantages
- **(a)** There is a significant indirect-acting component; response can diminish when neuronal NE is depleted (e.g., in patients with CHF).
- **(b)** Sinus, atrial, or ventricular tachycardia (VT) and arrhythmias may occur.
- **(c)** Maximal inotropic effect less than that of epinephrine.
- **(d)** Skin necrosis may result from extravasation.
- **(e)** Renal vasodilating effects are overridden by α-mediated vasoconstriction at dosages greater than 10 μg/kg/min with risk of renal, splanchnic, and skin necrosis. Urine output should be monitored.
- **(f)** Pulmonary vasoconstriction is possible.
- **(g)** Mvo_2 increases, and myocardial ischemia may occur if coronary flow does not increase commensurately.
- **(h)** In some patients with severe HF, the increased BP at increased doses may be detrimental. Such patients benefit from adding a vasodilator.

(6) Indications
- **(a)** Hypotension due to low CO or low SVR (although other agents are superior for the latter indication)
- **(b)** Temporary therapy of hypovolemia until circulating blood volume is restored (but vasoconstrictors should not substitute or delay primary treatment of hypovolemia)
- **(c)** "Recruiting renal blood flow" for renal failure or insufficiency (widely used for this purpose, but limited evidence basis)

(7) Administration: IV only (preferably by central venous line)

(8) Clinical use
- **(a)** Dopamine dose: 1 to 20 μg/kg/min IV.
- **(b)** Often mix 200 mg in 250 mL IV solution (800 μg/mL).
- **(c)** Good first choice for temporary treatment of hypotension until intravascular volume can be expanded or until a specific diagnosis can be made.
- **(d)** Correct hypovolemia if possible before use (as with all pressors)
- **(e)** After cardiac surgery if inotropic response is not adequate at dopamine doses of 5 to 10 μg/kg/min, we recommend a switch to a more powerful agonist such as epinephrine, or a switch to or addition of milrinone.
- **(f)** Consider adding a vasodilator (e.g., nitroprusside) when BP is adequate and afterload reduction would be beneficial (or better still, reduce the dose of dopamine).

d. Dopexamine [28]
(1) Actions
- **(a)** Dopexamine is a synthetic analog of dobutamine with vasodilator action. Its cardiac inotropic and chronotropic activity is caused by direct β_2-agonist effects and by NE actions (due to baroreceptor reflex activation and neuronal uptake-1 inhibition) that *indirectly* activate β_1-receptors. In CHF, there is selective β_1-downregulation, with relative preservation of β_2-receptor number and coupling. The latter assume greater than normal physiologic importance, making dopexamine of *theoretically* greater utility than agents with primary β_1-receptor activity. Although dopexamine has been used in Europe for nearly two decades, the drug will likely never be available in the United States.
- **(b)** Receptor activity
  α_1 and α_2: Minimal
  β_1: Little *direct* effect, some *indirect*; β_2: Direct agonist
  DA_1: Potent agonist (activation increases renal blood flow)
- **(c)** Inhibits neuronal catecholamine uptake-1, increasing NE actions

(d) Hemodynamic actions

	Dopexamine
HR	Increased
CO	Increased
SVR	Decreased
MAP	Little change or decrease
Preload	No change or slight decrease

(2) **Offset.** Half-life: 6 to 11 minutes. Clearance is by uptake into tissues (catecholamine uptake mechanisms) and by hepatic metabolism.

(3) **Advantages**
   (a) Lack of vasoconstrictor activity avoids α-mediated complications.
   (b) Decreased renovascular resistance might *theoretically* help preserve renal function after ischemic insults.

(4) **Disadvantages**
   (a) Less effective positive inotrope than other agents (e.g., epinephrine, milrinone)
   (b) Dose-dependent tachycardia may limit therapy.
   (c) Tachyphylaxis
   (d) Not approved by the U.S. Food and Drug administration for release in the United States.

(5) **Indications.** Treatment of low CO states

(6) **Administration.** IV

(7) **Clinical use**
   (a) Dopexamine dose: 0.5 to 4 μg/kg/min IV (maximum 6 μg/kg/min).
   (b) Hemodynamic and renal effects similar to the combination of variable doses of dobutamine with dopamine 1 μg/kg/min (renal dose) or fenoldopam 0.05 μg/kg/min.

e. **Epinephrine (Adrenaline)** [28]
   (1) **Epinephrine is a catecholamine produced by the adrenal medulla.**
   (2) **Actions**
      (a) Direct agonist at α_1-, α_2-, β_1-, and β_2-receptors
      (b) Dose response (adult, approximate)

Epinephrine		
Dose (ng/kg/min)	Receptors activated	SVR
10–30	β	Usually decreased
30–150	β and α	Variable
>150	α and β	Increased

   (c) Increased contractility with all dosages, but SVR may decrease, remain unchanged, or increase dramatically depending on the dosage. CO usually increased but, at extreme resuscitation dosages, α-receptor–mediated vasoconstriction may cause a lowered SV due to high afterload.

   (3) **Offset** occurs by uptake by neurons and tissue and by metabolism by MAO and COMT (rapid).

   (4) **Advantages**
      (a) This drug is direct acting; its effects are not dependent on release of endogenous NE.
      (b) Potent α- and β-adrenergic stimulation results in greater maximal effects and produce equivalent increases in SV with tachycardia after heart surgery than dopamine or dobutamine.

(c) It is a powerful inotrope with variable (and dose-dependent) α-adrenergic effect. Lusitropic effect (β_1) enhances the rate of ventricular relaxation.

(d) BP increases may blunt tachycardia due to reflex vagal stimulation.

(e) It is an effective bronchodilator and mast cell stabilizer, useful for primary therapy of severe bronchospasm, anaphylactoid, or anaphylactic reactions.

(f) With a dilated LV and myocardial ischemia, epinephrine may increase diastolic BP and decrease heart size, reducing myocardial ischemia. However, as with any inotropic drug, epinephrine may induce or worsen myocardial ischemia.

(5) **Disadvantages**

(a) Tachycardia and arrhythmias at higher doses.

(b) Organ ischemia, especially kidney, secondary to vasoconstriction, may result. Renal function must be closely monitored.

(c) Pulmonary vasoconstriction may occur, which can produce pulmonary hypertension and possibly RV failure; addition of a vasodilator may counteract this.

(d) Epinephrine may produce myocardial ischemia. Positive inotropy and tachycardia increase myocardial oxygen demand and reduce oxygen supply.

(e) Extravasation from a peripheral IV cannula can cause necrosis; thus, administration via a central venous line is preferable.

(f) As with most adrenergic agonists, increases of plasma glucose and lactate occur. This may be accentuated in diabetics.

(g) Initial increases in plasma K^+ occur due to hepatic release, followed by decreased K^+ due to skeletal muscle uptake.

(6) **Indications**

(a) Cardiac arrest (especially asystole or VF); electromechanical dissociation. Epinephrine's efficacy is believed to result from increased coronary perfusion pressure during cardiopulmonary resuscitation (CPR). Recently, the utility of high-dose (0.2 mg/kg) epinephrine was debated, the consensus as summarized in the 2015 AHA Guidelines [27] is that there is no outcome benefit to "high-dose" epinephrine.

(b) Anaphylaxis and other systemic allergic reactions; epinephrine is the agent of choice.

(c) Cardiogenic shock, especially if a vasodilator is added

(d) Bronchospasm

(e) Reduced CO after CPB

(f) Hypotension with spinal or epidural anesthesia can be treated with low-dose (1 to 4 µg/min) epinephrine infusions as conveniently and effectively as with ephedrine boluses [(12)].

(7) **Administration.** IV (preferably by central line); via endotracheal tube (rapidly absorbed by tracheal mucosa); SC

(8) **Clinical use**

(a) Epinephrine dose

(i) SC: 10 µg/kg (maximum of 400 µg or 0.4 mL, 1:1,000) for the treatment of mild-to-moderate allergic reactions or bronchospasm.

(ii) IV: Low-to-moderate dose (for shock, hypotension): 0.03 to 0.2 µg/kg bolus (IV), then infusion at 0.01 to 0.30 µg/kg/min.

High dose (for cardiac arrest, resuscitation): 0.5 to 1.0 mg IV bolus; pediatric, 5 to 15 µg/kg (may be given intratracheally in 1 to 10 mL volume). Larger doses are used when response to initial dose is inadequate.

Resuscitation doses of epinephrine may produce extreme hypertension, stroke, or myocardial infarction. A starting dose of epinephrine exceeding a 0.15 mcg/kg (10 µg in an adult) IV bolus should be given only to a patient in extremis! **Moderate doses** (0.03 to 0.06 µg/kg/min) of epinephrine are commonly used to stimulate cardiac function and facilitate separation from CPB.

(b) Watch for signs of excessive vasoconstriction. Monitor SVR, renal function, extremity perfusion.

(c) Addition of a vasodilator (e.g., nicardipine, nitroprusside, or phentolamine) to epinephrine can counteract the α-mediated vasoconstriction, leaving positive cardiac inotropic effects undiminished. Alternatively, addition of milrinone or inamrinone may permit lower doses of epinephrine to be used. We find combinations of epinephrine and milrinone particularly useful in cardiac surgical patients.

f. NE (noradrenaline, Levophed)

See the preceding Section VI: Vasopressors.

g. Isoproterenol (Isuprel)

(1) Isoproterenol is a synthetic catecholamine.

(2) Actions

    (a) Direct β_1- plus β_2-adrenergic agonist

    (b) No α-adrenergic effects

Isoproterenol	
HR	Increased
Contractility	Increased
CO	Increased
BP	Variable
SVR	Decreased; dose-related dilation of all vascular beds
PVR	Decreased

(3) Offset. Rapid (half-life, 2 minutes); uptake by liver, conjugated, 60% excreted unchanged; metabolized by MAO, COMT

(4) Advantages

    (a) Isoproterenol is a potent direct β-adrenergic receptor agonist.

    (b) It increases CO by three mechanisms:

    (c) Increased HR

    (d) Increased contractility S increased SV

    (e) Reduced afterload (SVR) S increased SV

    (f) It is a bronchodilator (IV or inhaled).

(5) Disadvantages

    (a) It is not a pressor! BP often falls (β_2-adrenergic effect) while CO rises.

    (b) Hypotension may produce organ hypoperfusion, hypotension, and ischemia.

    (c) Tachycardia limits diastolic filling time.

    (d) Proarrhythmic.

    (e) Dilates all vascular beds and is capable of shunting blood away from critical organs toward muscle and skin.

    (f) Coronary vasodilation can reduce blood flow to ischemic myocardium while increasing flow to nonischemic areas producing coronary "steal" in patients with "steal-prone" coronary anatomy.

    (g) May unmask pre-excitation in patients with an accessory AV conduction pathway (e.g., Wolff–Parkinson–White [WPW] syndrome).

(6) Indications

    (a) Bradycardia unresponsive to atropine when electrical pacing is not available.

    (b) Low CO, especially for situations in which increased inotropy is needed and tachycardia is not detrimental, such as the following:

    (c) Pediatric patients with fixed SV

    (d) After resection of ventricular aneurysm (small fixed SV)

    (e) Denervated heart (after cardiac transplantation)

    (f) Pulmonary hypertension or right heart failure

    (g) AV block: Use as temporary therapy to decrease block or increase rate of idioventricular foci. Use with caution in second-degree Mobitz type II heart block—may intensify heart block.

      (h) Status asthmaticus: IV use mandates continuous ECG and BP monitoring.

      (i) β-Blocker overdose

      (j) Isoproterenol should not be used for cardiac asystole. CPR with epinephrine or pacing is the therapy of choice because isoproterenol-induced vasodilation results in reduced carotid and coronary blood flow during CPR.

  (7) Administration. IV (safe through peripheral line, will not necrose skin); PO

  (8) Clinical use and isoproterenol dose. IV infusion is 20 to 500 ng/kg/min.

2. PDE inhibitors

  a. Inamrinone (Inocor) [28]

    (1) Inamrinone is a bipyridine derivative that inhibits the cyclic guanosine monophosphate (cGMP)–inhibited cAMP-specific PDE III, increasing cAMP concentrations in cardiac muscle (positive inotropy) and in vascular smooth muscle (vasodilation).

Inamrinone	
HR	Generally little change (tachycardia at higher doses)
MAP	Variable (the decrease in SVR may be offset by increase in CO)
CO	Increased
LAP	Decreased
SVR	Decreased
PVR	Decreased
Mvo_2	Generally little change (increase in oxygen consumption from increased CO is offset by decrease in wall tension)

    (2) Offset

      (a) The elimination half-life is 2.5 to 4 hours, increasing to 6 hours in patients with CHF.

      (b) Offset occurs by hepatic conjugation, with 30% to 35% excreted unchanged in urine.

    (3) Advantages

      (a) As a vasodilating inotrope, inamrinone increases CO by augmenting contractility *and* decreasing cardiac afterload.

      (b) Favorable effects on Mvo_2 (little increase in HR; decreases afterload, LVEDP, and wall tension)

      (c) It does not depend on activation of β-receptors and therefore retains effectiveness despite β-receptor downregulation or uncoupling (e.g., CHF) and in the presence of β-adrenergic blockade.

      (d) Low risk of tachycardia or arrhythmias

      (e) Inamrinone may act synergistically with β-adrenergic receptor agonists and dopaminergic receptor agonists.

      (f) Pulmonary vasodilator.

      (g) Positive lusitropic properties (ventricular relaxation) at even very low dosages.

    (4) Disadvantages

      (a) Thrombocytopenia after chronic (more than 24 hours) administration.

      (b) Will nearly always cause hypotension from vasodilation if given by rapid bolus administration. Hypotension is easily treated with IV fluid and α-agonists.

      (c) Increased dosages may result in tachycardia (and therefore increased Mvo_2).

      (d) Less convenient than milrinone because of photosensitivity and reduced potency

    (5) Administration. IV infusion only. Do not mix in dextrose-containing solutions.

    (6) Clinical use

      (a) Inamrinone loading dose is 0.75 to 1.5 mg/kg. When given during or after CPB, usual dosage is 1.5 mg/kg.

(b) IV infusion dose range is 5 to 20 µg/kg/min (usual dosage is 10 µg/kg/min).

(c) Used in cardiac surgical patients in a manner similar to milrinone

(d) The popularity of this agent has steadily declined since the introduction of milrinone, largely due to milrinone's lack of an adverse action on platelet function. Inamrinone is included here mostly for completeness.

b. Milrinone (Primacor) [28]

(1) Actions

(a) Milrinone has powerful cardiac inotropic and vasodilator properties. Milrinone increases intracellular concentrations of cAMP by inhibiting its breakdown. Milrinone inhibits the cGMP-inhibited, cAMP-specific PDE (commonly known by clinicians as "type III") in cardiac and vascular smooth-muscle cells. In cardiac myocytes, increased cAMP causes positive inotropy, lusitropy (enhanced diastolic myocardial relaxation), chronotropy, and dromotropy (AV conduction), as well as increased automaticity. In vascular smooth-muscle cells, increased cAMP causes vasodilation.

(b) Hemodynamic actions

Milrinone	
HR	Usually no change or slight increase
CO	Increased
BP	Variable
SVR and PVR	Decreased
Preload	Decreased
Mvo_2	Often unchanged or slight increase

(2) Onset and offset. When administered as an IV bolus, milrinone rapidly achieves its maximal effect. The elimination half-life of milrinone is considerably shorter than that of inamrinone.

(3) Advantages

(a) Used as a single agent, milrinone has favorable effects on the myocardial oxygen supply–demand balance, due to reduction of preload and afterload, and minimal tendency for tachycardia.

(b) Milrinone does not act via β-adrenergic receptors and it retains efficacy when β-adrenergic receptor coupling is impaired, as in CHF.

(c) It induces no tachyphylaxis.

(d) Milrinone has less proarrhythmic effects than β-adrenergic receptor agonists.

(e) When compared to dobutamine at equipotent doses, milrinone is associated with a greater decrease in PVR, greater augmentation of RV ejection fraction, less tachycardia, fewer arrhythmias, and lower Mvo_2.

(f) This drug may act synergistically with drugs that stimulate cAMP production, such as β-adrenergic receptor agonists.

(g) Even with chronic use, milrinone (unlike inamrinone) does not cause thrombocytopenia.

(4) Disadvantages

(a) Vasodilation and hypotension are predictable with rapid IV bolus doses.

(b) As with all other positive inotropic drugs, including epinephrine and dobutamine, independent manipulation of cardiac inotropy and SVR cannot be achieved using only milrinone.

(c) Arrhythmias may occur.

(5) Clinical use [21]:

(a) Milrinone loading dose: 25 to 75 (usual dose is 50) µg/kg given over 1 to 10 minutes. Often it is desirable to administer the loading dose before separating the patient from CPB so that hypotension can be managed more easily.

(b) Maintenance infusion: 0.375 to 0.75 µg/kg/min (usual maintenance is 0.5 µg/kg/min). Dosage should be reduced in renal failure.

(6) **Indications**

(a) Low CO syndrome, especially in the setting of increased LVEDP, pulmonary hypertension, RV failure

(b) To supplement/potentiate β-adrenergic receptor agonists

(c) Outpatient milrinone infusion has been used as a bridge to cardiac transplantation.

(d) Clinical perspective: [44–46]

No effect on mortality at 1 year or arrhythmia.

> **CLINICAL PEARL** Milrinone increases intracellular concentration of cAMP. Milrinone used as a single inotropic agent has favorable effects on myocardial supply/demand balance reducing preload and afterload and has a low tendency to produce tachycardia.

3. **Glucagon**

a. **Glucagon is a peptide hormone produced by the pancreas.**

b. **Actions.** Glucagon increases intracellular cAMP, acting via a specific receptor.

Glucagon	
Contractility	Increased
AV conduction	Increased
HR	Increased
CO	Increased, with a variable effect on SVR

c. **Offset** of action of glucagon occurs by redistribution and proteolysis by the liver, kidney, and plasma. Duration of action is 20 to 30 minutes.

d. **Advantages.** Glucagon has a positive inotropic effect even in the presence of β-blockade.

e. **Disadvantages**

(1) Consistently produces nausea and vomiting

(2) Tachycardia

(3) Hyperglycemia and hypokalemia

(4) Catecholamine release from pheochromocytomas

(5) Anaphylaxis (possible)

f. **Indications for glucagon include the following:**

(1) Severe hypoglycemia (especially if no IV access) from insulin overdosage

(2) Spasm of sphincter of Oddi

(3) β-blocker overdosage

g. **Administration.** IV, IM, SC

h. **Clinical use**

(1) Glucagon dose: 1 to 5 mg IV slowly; 0.5 to 2 mg IM or SC.

(2) Infusion: 25 to 75 µg/min.

(3) Rarely used (other than for hypoglycemia) because of gastrointestinal side effects and severe tachycardia.

C. **cAMP-independent agents**

1. **Calcium** [28]

a. **Calcium is physiologically active only as the free (unbound) calcium ion (Ca$_i$).**

(1) Normally, approximately 50% of the total plasma calcium is bound to proteins and anions and the rest remains as free calcium ions.

(2) Factors affecting ionized calcium concentration:

(a) Alkalosis (metabolic or respiratory) decreases Ca$_i$.

(b) Acidosis increases Ca$_i$.

      (c) Citrate binds (chelates) Ca_i.

      (d) Albumin binds Ca_i.

    (3) Normal plasma concentration: $[Ca_i] = 1$ to 1.3 mmol/L.

b. Actions of calcium salts

Calcium	
HR	No change or decrease (vagal effect)
Contractility	Increase (in response to Ca bolus during hypocalcemia)
BP	Increase
SVR	Usually increase
Preload	Little change
CO	Variable

c. Offset. Calcium is incorporated into muscle and bone and binds to protein, free fatty acids released by heparin, and citrate.

d. Advantages

    (1) It has rapid action with duration of approximately 10 to 15 minutes (7-mg/kg dose).

    (2) It reverses hypotension caused by the following conditions:

      (a) Halogenated anesthetic overdosage

      (b) Calcium-blocking drugs (CCBs)

      (c) Hypocalcemia

      (d) CPB, especially with dilutional or citrate-induced hypocalcemia, or when cardioplegia-induced hyperkalemia remains present (administer calcium salts only after heart has been well reperfused to avoid augmenting reperfusion injury)

      (e) β-Blockers (watch for bradycardia!)

    (3) It reverses cardiac toxicity from hyperkalemia (e.g., arrhythmias, heart block, and negative inotropy).

e. Disadvantages

    (1) Minimal evidence that calcium salts administered to patients produce even a transient increase in CO.

    (2) Calcium can provoke digitalis toxicity which can present as ventricular arrhythmias, AV block, or asystole.

    (3) Calcium potentiates the effects of hypokalemia on the heart (arrhythmias).

    (4) Severe bradycardia or heart block occurs rarely.

    (5) When extracellular calcium concentration is increased while the surrounding myocardium is being reperfused or is undergoing ongoing ischemia, increased cellular damage or cell death occurs.

    (6) Post-CPB coronary spasm may occur rarely.

    (7) Associated with pancreatitis when given in large doses to patients recovering from CPB.

    (8) Calcium may inhibit clinical responses to epinephrine and dobutamine [47].

    (9) Calcium given by bolus administration to awake patients may produce chest pain or nausea.

f. Indications for use

    (1) Hypocalcemia

    (2) Hyperkalemia (to reverse AV block or myocardial depression)

    (3) Intraoperative hypotension due to decreased myocardial contractility from hypocalcemia or CCBs

    (4) Inhaled general anesthetic overdose

    (5) Toxic hypermagnesemia

g. Administration

    (1) Calcium chloride: IV, preferably by central line (causes peripheral vein inflammation and sclerosis).

    (2) Calcium gluconate: IV, preferably by central line.

   h. Clinical use

     (1) Calcium dose

      (a) 10% calcium chloride 10 mL (contains 272 mg of elemental calcium or 13.6 mEq): adult, 200 to 1,000 mg slow IV; pediatric, 10 to 20 mg/kg slow IV

      (b) 10% calcium gluconate 10 mL (contains 93 mg of elemental calcium or 4.6 mEq): adult, 600 to 3,000 mg slow IV; pediatric, 30 to 100 mg/kg slow IV

      (c) During massive blood transfusion (more than 1 blood volume replaced with citrate-preserved blood), a patient may receive citrate, which binds calcium. In normal situations, hepatic metabolism quickly eliminates citrate from plasma, and hypocalcemia does not occur. However, hypothermia and shock may decrease citrate clearance with resultant severe hypocalcemia. Rapid infusion of albumin will transiently reduce ionized calcium levels.

      (d) Ionized calcium levels should be measured frequently to guide calcium salt therapy. Adults with an intact parathyroid gland quickly recover from mild hypocalcemia without calcium administration.

      (e) Calcium is not recommended during resuscitation (per 2015 AHA Guidelines) [27] unless hypocalcemia, hyperkalemia, or hypermagnesemia are present.

      (f) Calcium should be used with care in situations in which ongoing myocardial ischemia may be occurring or during reperfusion of ischemic tissue. "Routine" administration of large doses of calcium to all adult patients at the end of CPB is unnecessary and may be deleterious if the heart has been reperfused only minutes earlier.

      (g) Hypocalcemia is frequent in children emerging from CPB.

      (h) Digoxin **(Lanoxin)**

2. **Digoxin is a glycoside derived from the foxglove plant.**

   a. Actions

     (1) Digoxin inhibits the integral membrane protein Na–K ATPase, causing Na^+ accumulation in cells and increased intracellular Ca_i, which leads to increased Ca^{2+} release from the sarcoplasmic reticulum into the cytoplasm with each heartbeat, ultimately causing a mildly increased myocardial contractility.

     (2) Hemodynamic effects

      (a) **Digoxin**

Calcium	
Contractility	Increased
AV conduction	Decreased
Ventricular automaticity	Increased rate of phase 4 depolarization
Refractory period	Decreased (in atria and ventricles); increased in AV node

   b. Hemodynamics in CHF

Calcium	
HR	Decreased
SV	Increased
SVR	Decreased
Mvo_2	Decreased

   c. Offset. Digoxin elimination half-life is 1.7 days (renal elimination). In anephric patients, half-life is more than 4 days.

   d. Advantages

     (1) Supraventricular antiarrhythmic action

     (2) Reduced ventricular rate in atrial fibrillation or flutter

     (3) An orally active positive inotrope which is not associated with increased mortality in CHF

e. **Disadvantages**
  (1) Digoxin has an extremely low therapeutic index; 20% of patients show toxicity at some time.
  (2) Increased Mvo_2 and SVR occur in patients without CHF (angina may be precipitated).
  (3) The drug has a long half-life, and it is difficult to titrate.
  (4) There is large interindividual variation in therapeutic and toxic serum levels and dosages. The dose response is nonlinear; near-toxic levels may be needed to achieve a change in AV conduction.
  (5) Toxic manifestations may be life-threatening and difficult to diagnose. Digoxin can produce virtually any arrhythmia. For example, digitalis is useful in treating SVT, but digitalis toxicity can trigger SVT.
  (6) Digoxin may be contraindicated in patients with accessory pathway SVT. Please refer to Digoxin use for SVT in Section VIII.E.

f. **Indications for use**
  (1) Supraventricular tachyarrhythmias (see Section VIII.E)
  (2) CHF (mostly of historical interest for this condition)

g. **Administration.** IV, PO, IM

h. **Clinical use (general guidelines only)**
  (1) Digoxin dose (assuming normal renal function; decrease maintenance dosages with renal insufficiency)
    (a) Adult: Loading dose IV and IM, 0.25 to 0.50 mg increments (total 1 to 1.25 mg or 10 to 15 µg/kg); maintenance dose, 0.125 to 0.250 mg/day based on clinical effect and drug levels
    (b) **Pediatric digoxin (IV administration)**

Age	Total digitalizing dose (DD) (µg/kg)	Daily maintenance dose (divided doses, normal renal function)
Neonates	15–30	20–35% of DD
2 mos–2 yrs	30–50	25–35% of DD
2–10 yrs	15–35	25–35% of DD
>10 yrs	8–12	25–35% of DD

  (2) Digoxin has a gradual onset of action over 15 to 30 minutes or more; peak effect occurs 1 to 5 hours after IV administration.
  (3) Use with caution in the presence of β-blockers, calcium channel blockers, or calcium.
  (4) Always consider the possibility of toxic side effects.
    (a) Signs of toxicity include arrhythmias, especially with features of both increased automaticity and conduction block (e.g., junctional tachycardia with a 2:1 AV block). Premature atrial or ventricular depolarizations, AV block, accelerated junctional tachycardia, VT or VF (may be unresponsive to countershock), or gastrointestinal or neurologic toxicity may also be apparent.
  (5) Factors potentiating toxicity
    (a) Hypokalemia, hypomagnesemia, hypercalcemia, alkalosis, acidosis, renal insufficiency, quinidine therapy, and hypothyroidism may potentiate toxicity.
    (b) Beware of administering calcium salts to digitalized patients! Malignant ventricular arrhythmias (including VF) may occur, even if the patient has received no digoxin for more than 24 hours. Follow ionized calcium levels to permit use of smallest possible doses of calcium.
  (6) Therapy for digitalis toxicity
    (a) Increase serum $[K^+]$ to upper limits of normal (unless AV block is present).
    (b) Treat ventricular arrhythmias with phenytoin, lidocaine, or amiodarone.

(c) Treat atrial arrhythmias with phenytoin or amiodarone.

(d) β-Blockers are effective for digoxin-induced arrhythmias, but ventricular pacing may be required if AV block develops.

(e) Beware of cardioversion. VF refractory to countershock may be induced. Use low-energy synchronized cardioversion and slowly increase energy as needed.

(7) Serum digoxin levels

(a) Therapeutic: Approximately 0.5 to 2.5 ng/mL. Values of less than 0.5 ng/mL rule out toxicity. Values exceeding 3 ng/mL are definitely toxic.

(b) Increased serum concentrations may not produce clinical toxicity in children or hyperkalemic patients, or when digitalis is used as an atrial antiarrhythmic agent.

(c) "Therapeutic" serum concentrations may produce clinical toxicity in patients with hypokalemia, hypomagnesemia, hypercalcemia, myocardial ischemia, hypothyroidism, or those recovering from CPB.

(8) Because of its long duration of action, long latency of onset, and increased risk of toxicity, digoxin is not used to treat acute heart failure.

(9) For all indications, digoxin is much less widely used in recent years.

3. **Levosimendan** [48–53]

a. **Actions**

(1) Binds in Ca-dependent manner to cardiac troponin C, shifting the Ca^{2+} tension curve to the left. Levosimendan may stabilize Ca^{2+}-induced conformational changes in troponin C.

(2) Its effects are maximized during early systole when intracellular Ca^{2+} concentration is greatest and least during diastolic relaxation when Ca^{2+} concentration is low.

(3) Levosimendan also inhibits PDE III activity.

(4) Hemodynamic actions

Levosimendan	
HR	Increased
CO	Increased
SVR	Decreased
MAP	Unchanged
PCWP	Unchanged
Mvo_2	Unchanged

b. **Advantages**

(1) **Does** not increase intracellular Ca^{2+}

(2) Does not work via cAMP so should not interact with β-agonists or PDE inhibitors

c. **Disadvantages**

(1) Unknown potency relative to other agents

(2) Has not received regulatory approval in the United States.

d. **Indications**

Where approved, drug's indications include acute heart failure and acute exacerbations of CHF.

e. **Administration**

(1) IV

f. **Clinical use**

(1) 8 to 24 μg/kg/min

(2) Despite its biochemical actions on PDE, levosimendan is not associated with increased cAMP, so it may have reduced tendency for arrhythmias relative to sympathomimetics.

(3) Clinical perspective (see reference above):
No difference in 30-day mortality.

VIII. β-Adrenergic receptor–blocking drugs [3,54]

A. Actions

These drugs bind and antagonize β-adrenergic receptors typically producing the following cardiovascular effects:

	β-Blockers
HR	Decreased
Contractility	Decreased
BP	Decreased
SVR	Increased (unless drug has intrinsic sympathetic activity [ISA])
AV conduction	Decreased
Atrial refractory period	Increased
Automaticity	Decreased

B. Advantages of β-adrenergic-blocking drugs

1. Reduce Mvo_2 and decrease HR and contractility.
2. Increase the duration of diastole, during which majority of blood flow and oxygen are delivered to the LV.
3. Synergistic with nitroglycerin for treating myocardial ischemia; blunt reflex tachycardia and increased contractility secondary to nitroglycerin, nitroprusside, or other vasodilator drugs.
4. Have an antiarrhythmic action, especially against atrial arrhythmias.
5. Decrease LV ejection velocity (useful in patients with aortic dissection).
6. Antihypertensive, but should not be first-line agents for essential hypertension.
7. Reduce dynamic ventricular outflow tract obstruction (e.g., tetralogy of Fallot, hypertrophic cardiomyopathy).
8. Use of these agents is associated with reduced mortality after myocardial infarction, chronic angina, CHF, and hypertension.

C. Disadvantages

1. Severe bradyarrhythmias are possible.
2. Heart block (first, second, or third degree) may occur, especially if prior cardiac conduction abnormalities are present, or when IV β-blockers and certain IV calcium channel blockers are coadministered.
3. May trigger bronchospasm in patients with reactive airways.
4. CHF can occur in patients with low ejection fraction newly receiving large doses. Elevated LVEDP may induce myocardial ischemia because of elevated systolic wall tension.
5. Signs and symptoms of hypoglycemia (except sweating) are masked in diabetics.
6. SVR may increase because of inhibition of $β_2$-vasodilation; use with care in patients with severe peripheral vascular disease or in patients with pheochromocytoma without α-blockade treatment.
7. Risk of coronary artery spasm is present in rare susceptible patients.
8. Acute perioperative withdrawal of β-blockers can lead to hyperdynamic circulation and myocardial ischemia.

D. Distinguishing features of β-blockers

1. **Selectivity.** Selective β-blockers possess a greater potency for $β_1$ than for $β_2$-receptors. They are less likely to cause bronchospasm or to increase SVR than a nonselective drug. However, $β_1$-selectivity is dose-dependent (drugs lose selectivity at higher dosages). Caution must be exercised when an asthmatic patient receives any β-blocker.
2. **Intrinsic sympathomimetic activity (ISA).** These drugs possess "partial agonist" activity. Thus, drugs with ISA will block β-receptors (preventing catecholamines from binding to a receptor) but also will cause mild stimulation of the same receptors. A patient receiving a drug with ISA would be expected to have a greater resting HR and CO (which shows no change with exercise) but a lower SVR compared to a drug without ISA.

3. **Duration of action.** In general, the β-blockers with longer durations of action are eliminated by the kidneys, whereas the drugs of 4 to 6 hours duration undergo hepatic elimination. Esmolol, the ultrashort–acting β-blocker (plasma half-life, 9 minutes), is eliminated within the blood by a red blood cell esterase. After abrupt discontinuation of esmolol infusion (which under most circumstances we **do not recommend**), most drug effects are eliminated within 5 minutes. The duration of esmolol does not change when plasma pseudocholinesterase is inhibited by echothiophate or physostigmine.

E. **Clinical use**

1. **β-Blocker dosage**
2. Begin with a low dose and slowly increase until desired effect is produced.
3. For metoprolol IV dosage use 1 to 5 mg increments (for adults) as tolerated while monitoring the ECG, BP, and lung sounds. IV dosage is much smaller than oral dosage because first-pass hepatic extraction is bypassed. The usual acute IV metoprolol dose is 0.02 to 0.1 mg/kg.
4. If β-blockers must be given to a patient with bronchospastic disease, choose a selective β$_1$-blocker such as metoprolol or esmolol and consider concomitant administration of an inhalation β$_2$-agonist (such as albuterol).
5. **Treatment of toxicity.** β-agonists (e.g., isoproterenol, possibly in large doses) and cardiac pacing are the mainstays. Calcium, milrinone, inamrinone, glucagon, or liothyronine may be effective because these agents do not act via β-receptors.
6. **Assessment of β-blockade.** When β-blockade is adequate, a patient should not demonstrate an increase in HR with exercise.
7. **Use of α-agonists in β-blocked patients.** When agonist drugs with α- or both α- and β-actions are administered to patients who are β-blocked, for example, with an epinephrine-containing IV local anesthetic test dose, a greater elevation of BP can be expected owing to α-vasoconstriction unopposed by β$_2$-vasodilation. This may produce deleterious hemodynamic results (increased afterload with little increased CO).
8. Esmolol is given by IV injection (loading dose), often followed by continuous infusion. (For details on esmolol dosing for SVT, see Section VIII.E.) It is of greatest utility when the required duration of β-blockade is short (i.e., to attenuate a short-lived stimulus). Esmolol's ultrashort duration of action plus its β$_1$-selectivity and lack of ISA make it a logical choice when it is necessary to initiate a β-blocker in patients with asthma or another relative contraindication. It is also useful in critically ill patients with changing hemodynamic status.
9. Labetalol is a combined α- and β–antagonist- (α/β ratio = 1:7), which produces vasodilation without reflex tachycardia. Labetalol is useful for preoperative or postoperative control of hypertension. During anesthesia, its relatively long duration of action makes it less useful than other agents for minute-to-minute control of HR and BP. However, treatment with labetalol or another β-adrenergic receptor antagonist will reduce the needed dosage of short-acting vasodilators.
10. β-Adrenergic receptor antagonist withdrawal. Abrupt withdrawal of chronic β-blocker therapy may produce a withdrawal syndrome including tachycardia and hypertension. Myocardial ischemia or infarction may result. Thus, chronic β-blocker therapy should not be abruptly discontinued perioperatively. The authors have seen this syndrome complete with myocardial ischemia after abrupt discontinuation of esmolol when it had been infused for only 48 hours!
11. Certain β-adrenergic receptor blockers are now part of the standard therapy of patients with Class B through Class D CHF. The drugs most often used are carvedilol and metoprolol-XL, and these agents have been shown to prolong survival in heart failure. β-adrenergic receptor blocker therapy is associated with improved LV function and improved exercise tolerance over time. These agents counteract the sympathetic nervous system activation that is present with CHF. In animal studies, β-adrenergic receptor blocker therapy reduces "remodeling," which is the process by which functional myocardium is replaced by connective tissue. Importantly, not all β-adrenergic receptor blockers have been shown to

improve outcome in CHF, so reduced mortality should not be considered a "class effect" of β-adrenergic receptor blockers.

IX. **Vasodilator drugs** [28]

  A. **Comparison**

    1. **Sites of action**

Arterial (decreased SVR)	Both arterial and venous
Calcium channel blockers	Angiotensin-converting enzyme (ACE) inhibitors
Hydralazine	ARBs
Phentolamine	Nitroglycerin
	Nitroprusside
	Prazosin
	Alprostadil
	Trimethaphan
	Nesiritide

    2. **Mechanisms of action**

      a. Direct vasodilators: Calcium channel blockers, hydralazine, minoxidil, nitroglycerin, nitroprusside.

      b. α-adrenergic blockers: Labetalol, phentolamine, prazosin, terazosin, tolazoline.

      c. Ganglionic blocker: Trimethaphan.

      d. ACE inhibitor: Enalaprilat, captopril, enalapril, lisinopril.

      e. ARBs: Candesartan, irbesartan, losartan, olmesartan, valsartan, telmisartan.

      f. Central α_2-agonists (reduce sympathetic tone): Clonidine, guanabenz, guanfacine.

      g. Calcium channel blockers (see Section X).

      h. Nesiritide: Binds to natriuretic factor receptors.

    3. **Indications for use**

      a. **Hypertension, increased SVR states.** Use arterial or mixed drugs. First-line agent for long-term treatment of essential hypertension should be thiazide diuretic with ACE inhibitors, ARBs, calcium channel blockers, β-blockers, as secondary choices. Other oral agents are not associated with outcome benefit.

      b. **Controlled hypotension.** Short-acting drugs are most useful (e.g., nitroprusside, nitroglycerin, nicardipine, clevidipine, nesiritide, and volatile inhalational anesthetics).

      c. **Aortic valvular regurgitation.** Reducing SVR will tend to improve oxygen delivery to tissues.

      d. **CHF.** Vasodilation reduces Mvo_2 by lowering preload and afterload (systolic wall stress, due to reduced LV size and pressure). Vasodilation also improves ejection and compliance. More importantly, ACE inhibitors and ARBs inhibit "remodeling" and increase longevity in patients with heart failure.

      e. **Thermoregulation.** Vasodilators are often used during the cooling and rewarming phases of CPB to facilitate tissue perfusion and accelerate temperature equilibration. This is especially important during pediatric CPB procedures and others involving total circulatory arrest where an increased CBF promotes brain cooling and brain protection during circulatory arrest.

      f. **Pulmonary hypertension.** Vasodilators can improve pulmonary hypertension that is not anatomically fixed. Presently, inhaled NO is the only truly selective pulmonary vasodilator.

      g. **Myocardial ischemia.** Vasodilator therapy can improve myocardial O_2 balance by reducing Mvo_2 (decreased preload and afterload), and nitrates and calcium channel blockers can dilate conducting coronary arteries to improve the distribution of myocardial blood flow. ACE inhibitors prolong lifespan in patients who have had a myocardial infarction.

      h. **Intracardiac shunts.** Vasodilators are used in the setting of nonrestrictive cardiac shunts, especially ventricular septal defects and aortopulmonary connections, to manipulate the ratio of pulmonary artery (PA) to aortic pressures. This allows control of the direction and magnitude of shunt flow.

4. **Cautions**
   a. **Hyperdynamic reflexes.** All vasodilator drugs decrease SVR and BP and may activate baroreceptor reflexes. This cardiac sympathetic stimulation produces tachycardia and increased contractility. Myocardial ischemia resulting from increased myocardial O_2 demands can be additive to ischemia produced by reduced BP. Addition of a β-blocker can attenuate these reflexes.
   b. **Ventricular ejection rate.** Reflex sympathetic stimulation will also increase the rate of ventricular ejection of blood (dP/dt) and raise the systolic aortic wall stress. This may be detrimental with aortic dissection. Thus, addition of β-blocker (or a ganglionic blocker) is of theoretical benefit for patients with aortic dissection, aortic aneurysm, or recent aortic surgery.
   c. Stimulation of the renin–angiotensin system is implicated in the "rebound" increased SVR and PVR when some vasodilators are discontinued abruptly. Renin release can be attenuated by concomitant β-blockade, and renin's actions are attenuated by ACE inhibitors and ARBs.
   d. **Intracranial pressure (ICP).** Most vasodilators will increase ICP, except for trimethaphan and fenoldopam.
   e. Use of nesiritide for decompensated CHF was associated with increased mortality.

B. **Specific agents**
   1. **Direct vasodilators**
      a. **Hydralazine (Apresoline)**
         (1) **Actions**
             (a) This drug is a direct vasodilator.
             (b) It primarily produces an arteriolar dilatation, with little venous (preload) effect.

Hydralazine	
HR	Increased (reflex)
Contractility	Increased (reflex)
CO	May increase (reflex)
BP	Decreased
SVR and PVR	Decreased
Preload	Little change

         (2) **Offset** occurs by acetylation in the liver. Patients who are slow acetylators (up to 50% of the population) may have higher plasma hydralazine levels and may show a longer effect, especially with oral use.
         (3) **Advantages**
             (a) Selective vasodilation. Hydralazine produces more dilation of coronary, cerebral, renal, and splanchnic beds than of vessels in the muscle and skin.
             (b) Maintenance of uterine blood flow (if hypotension is avoided).
         (4) **Disadvantages**
             (a) Slow onset (5 to 15 minutes) after IV dosing; peak effect should occur by 20 minutes. Thus, at least 10 to 15 minutes should separate doses.
             (b) Reflex tachycardia or coronary steal can precipitate myocardial ischemia.
             (c) A lupus-like reaction, usually seen only with chronic PO use, may occur with chronic high doses (more than 400 mg/day) and in slow acetylators.
         (5) **Clinical use**
             (a) Hydralazine dose
                 (i) IV: 2.5 to 5 mg bolus every 15 minutes (maximum 20 to 40 mg)
                 (ii) IM: 20 to 40 mg every 4 to 6 hours

           (iii) PO: 10 to 50 mg every 6 hours

           (iv) Pediatric dose: 0.2 to 0.5 mg/kg IV every 4 to 6 hours, slowly

      (b) Slow onset limits use in acute hypertensive crises.

      (c) Doses of vasodilators can be reduced by the addition of hydralazine, decreasing the risk of cyanide toxicity from nitroprusside or prolonged ganglionic blockade from trimethaphan.

      (d) Addition of a β-blocker attenuates reflex tachycardia.

      (e) Patients with CAD should be monitored for myocardial ischemia.

      (f) Enalaprilat, nicardipine, and labetalol are replacing hydralazine for many perioperative applications, but hydralazine continues to be used for control of acute postoperative hypertension.

  b. Nitroglycerin (glyceryl trinitrate) [28]

    (1) Actions

      (a) Nitroglycerin is a direct vasodilator, producing greater venous than arterial dilation. A nitric acid–containing metabolite activates vascular cGMP production.

Nitroglycerin	
HR	Increased (reflex)
Contractility	Increased (reflex)
CO	Variable; often decreased, due to decreased preload (CO may increase when drug treats ischemia)
BP	Decreased (high dosages)
Preload	Marked decrease
SVR	Decreased (high dosages)
PVR	Decreased

      (b) Peripheral venous effects. Venodilation and peripheral pooling reduce effective blood volume, decreasing heart size and preload. This effect usually reduces Mvo_2 and increases diastolic coronary blood flow.

      (c) Coronary artery

          (i) Relieves coronary spasm.

          (ii) Flow redistribution provides more flow to ischemic myocardium and increases endocardial-to-epicardial flow ratio.

          (iii) There is increased flow to ischemic regions through collateral vessels.

      (d) Myocardial effects

          (i) Improved inotropy due to reduced ischemia

          (ii) Indirect antiarrhythmic action (VF threshold increases in ischemic myocardium because the drug makes the effective refractory period more uniform throughout the heart)

      (e) Arteriolar effects (higher dosages only)

          (i) Arteriolar dilatation decreases SVR. With reduced systolic myocardial wall stress, Mvo_2 decreases, and ejection fraction and SV may improve.

          (ii) Arteriolar dilation often requires large doses, exceeding 10 µg/kg/min in some patients, whereas much lower doses give effective venous and coronary arterial dilating effects. When reliable peripheral arteriolar dilation is needed to control a hypertensive emergency, we suggest that nicardipine, nitroprusside, or clevidipine are often better choices (and can be used together with nitroglycerin).

    (2) Offset occurs by redistribution, metabolism in smooth muscle and liver. Half-life in humans is 1 to 3 minutes.

(3) Advantages

    (a) Preload reduction (lowers LV and RV end-diastolic and LA and RA pressures)

    (b) Unlike nitroprusside, virtually no metabolic toxicity

    (c) Effective for myocardial ischemia

        (i) Decreases infarct size after coronary occlusion

        (ii) Maintains arteriolar autoregulation, so coronary steal unlikely

    (d) Useful in acute exacerbations of CHF to decrease preload and reduce pulmonary vascular congestion

    (e) Increases vascular capacity; may permit infusion of residual pump blood after CPB is terminated

    (f) Not nearly as photosensitive as nitroprusside

    (g) Dilates pulmonary vessels and can be useful in treating acute pulmonary hypertension and right heart failure

    (h) Attenuates biliary colic and esophageal spasm

(4) Disadvantages

    (a) It decreases BP as preload and SVR decrease at higher dosages. This may result in decreased coronary perfusion pressure.

    (b) Reflex tachycardia and reflex increase in myocardial contractility are dose related. Consider reducing dose or administering a β-blocker (if BP is satisfactory).

    (c) It inhibits hypoxic pulmonary vasoconstriction (but to a lesser extent than nitroprusside). Monitor PO_2 or supplement inspired gas with oxygen.

    (d) It may increase ICP.

    (e) It is adsorbed by polyvinyl chloride IV tubing. Titrate dosage to effect; increased effect may occur when tubing becomes saturated. Special infusion sets that do not adsorb drug were often used in the past, but are expensive and unnecessary.

    (f) Tolerance. Chronic continuous therapy (for longer than 24 hours) can blunt hemodynamic and antianginal effects. Tolerance during chronic therapy may be avoided by discontinuing the drug (if appropriate) for several hours daily.

    (g) Dependence. Coronary spasm and myocardial infarction have been reported after abrupt cessation of chronic industrial exposure.

    (h) Methemoglobinemia. Avoid administering doses greater than 7 μg/kg/min for prolonged periods.

(5) Clinical use

    (a) Nitroglycerin dose

        (i) IV bolus: A bolus dose of 50 to 100 μg may be superior to infusion for acute ischemia. Rapidly increasing levels in blood may cause more vasodilation than the same concentration when produced by a constant infusion (and thus may be more likely to produce hypotension).

        (ii) Infusion: Dose range, 0.1 to 7 μg/kg/min.

        (iii) Sublingual: 0.15 to 0.60 mg.

        (iv) Topical: 2% ointment (Nitropaste), 0.5 to 2 inches every 4 to 8 hours; or controlled-release transdermal nitroglycerin patch, 0.1 to 0.8 mg/hour. Nitrate-free periods of 10 to 12 hours (e.g., at night) needed to prevent tolerance.

    (b) Unless non-polyvinyl chloride tubing is used, infusion requirements may decrease after the initial 30 to 60 minutes.

    (c) Nitroglycerin is better stored in bottles than in bags if storage for more than 6 to 12 hours is anticipated.

    (d) When administered during CPB, venous pooling may cause decreases in pump reservoir volume.

> **CLINICAL PEARL** Nitroglycerin is a direct vasodilator producing greater venous pooling than arterial dilation. Venous pooling caused by dilation decreases heart size and preload reducing MvO_2 and usually lessens ongoing ischemia.

    c. Nitroprusside (Nipride) [28]

      (1) Actions

        (a) Sodium nitroprusside (SNP) is a direct-acting vasodilator. The nitrate group is converted into NO in vascular smooth muscle, which causes increased cGMP levels in cells.

        (b) It has balanced arteriolar and venous dilating effects.

	Nitroprusside
HR	Increased (reflex)
Contractility	Increased (reflex)
CO	Variable
BP	Decreased (dose-dependent)
SVR	Decreased (dose-dependent)
PVR	Decreased (dose-dependent)

      (2) Advantages

        (a) SNP has a very short duration of action (1 to 2 minutes) permitting precise titration of dose.

        (b) It has pulmonary vasodilator in addition to systemic vasodilator effects.

        (c) SNP is highly effective for virtually all causes of hypertension except high CO states.

        (d) A greater decrease in SVR (afterload) than preload is produced at low dosages.

      (3) Disadvantages

        (a) Cyanide and thiocyanate toxicity may occur.

        (b) SNP solution is unstable in light and so must be protected from light. Photo-decomposition inactivates nitroprusside over many hours but does not release cyanide ion.

        (c) Reflex tachycardia and increased inotropy (undesirable with aortic dissection because of increased shearing forces) respond to β-blockade.

        (d) Hypoxic pulmonary vasoconstriction is blunted and may produce arterial hypoxemia from increased venous admixture.

        (e) Vascular steal. All vascular regions are dilated equally. Although total organ blood flow may increase, flow may be diverted from ischemic regions (previously maximally vasodilated) to nonischemic areas that, prior to SNP exposure, were appropriately vasoconstricted. Thus, myocardial ischemia may be worsened. However, severe hypertension is clearly dangerous in ischemia, and the net effect often is beneficial. ECG monitoring is important.

        (f) Patients with chronic hypertension may experience myocardial, cerebral, or renal ischemia with abrupt lowering of BP to "normal" range.

        (g) Rebound systemic or pulmonary hypertension may occur if SNP is stopped abruptly (especially in patients with CHF). SNP should be tapered.

        (h) Mild preload reduction due to venodilation occurs (but to a lesser extent than nitroglycerin); fluids often must be infused if CO falls.

        (i) Risk of increased ICP (although ICP may decrease with control of hypertension)

        (j) Platelet function is inhibited (no known clinical consequences).

(4) Toxicity

(a) Chemical formula of SNP is $Fe(CN)_5NO$. SNP reacts with hemoglobin to release highly toxic free cyanide ion (CN^-).

(b) SNP + oxyhemoglobin S four free cyanide ions + cyanomethemoglobin (nontoxic).

(c) Cyanide ion produces inhibition of cytochrome oxidase, preventing mitochondrial oxidative phosphorylation. This produces tissue hypoxia despite adequate PO_2.

(d) Cyanide detoxification

    (i) Cyanide + thiosulfate (and rhodanase) S thiocyanate. Thiocyanate is much less toxic than cyanide ion. Availability of thiosulfate is the rate-limiting step in cyanide metabolism. Adults can typically detoxify 50 mg of SNP using existing thiosulfate stores. Thiosulfate administration is of critical importance in treating cyanide toxicity. Rhodanase is an enzyme found in liver and kidney that promotes cyanide detoxification.

    (ii) Cyanide + hydroxocobalamin S cyanocobalamin (vitamin B_{12}).

(e) Patients at increased risk of toxicity:

    (i) Those resistant to vasodilating effects at low SNP dosages (requiring dose greater than 3 μg/kg/min is necessary for effect)

    (ii) Those receiving a high-dose SNP infusion (greater than 8 μg/kg/min) for any period of time. In this setting, frequent blood gas measurements must be performed, and consideration must be given to the following:

        (a) First and foremost, decrease dosage by adding another vasodilator or a β-blocker.

        (b) Consider monitoring mixed venous oxygenation (see Chapter 4).

    (iii) Those receiving a large total dose (greater than 1 mg/kg) over 12 to 24 hours.

    (iv) Those with either severe renal or hepatic dysfunction.

(f) Signs of SNP toxicity

    (i) Tachyphylaxis occurs in response to vasodilating effects of SNP (increased renin release can be inhibited with β-blockade).

    (ii) Elevated mixed venous PO_2 (due to decreased cellular O_2 utilization) occurs in the absence of a rise in CO.

    (iii) There is metabolic acidosis.

    (iv) No cyanosis is seen with cyanide toxicity (cells cannot utilize O_2; therefore, blood O_2 saturation remains high).

    (v) Chronic SNP toxicity is due to elevated thiocyanate levels and is a consequence of long-term therapy or thiocyanate accumulation in renal failure. Thiocyanate is excreted unchanged by the kidney (elimination half-life, 1 week). Elevated thiocyanate levels (greater than 5 mg/dL) can cause fatigue, nausea, anorexia, miosis, psychosis, hyperreflexia, and seizures.

(g) Therapy of cyanide toxicity

    (i) Cyanide toxicity should be suspected when a metabolic acidosis or unexplained rise in mixed venous PO_2 appears in any patient receiving SNP.

    (ii) As soon as toxicity is suspected, SNP must be discontinued and substituted with another agent; lowering the dosage is not sufficient because clinically evident toxicity implies a marked reduction in cytochrome oxidase activity.

    (iii) Ventilate with 100% O_2.

    (iv) Mild toxicity (base deficit less than 10, stable hemodynamics when SNP stopped) can be treated by sodium thiosulfate, 150 mg/kg IV bolus (hemodynamically benign).

(v) Severe toxicity (base deficit greater than 10, or worsening hemodynamics despite discontinuation of nitroprusside):

(a) Create methemoglobin that can combine with cyanide to produce nontoxic cyanomethemoglobin, removing cyanide from cytochrome oxidase:

(1) Give 3% sodium nitrite, 4 to 6 mg/kg by slow IV infusion (repeat one-half dose 2 to 48 hours later as needed), *or*

(2) Give amyl nitrite: Break 1 ampule into breathing bag. (Flammable!)

(b) Sodium thiosulfate, 150 to 200 mg/kg IV over 15 minutes, should also be administered to facilitate metabolic disposal of the cyanide. Note that thiocyanate clearance is renal dependent.

(c) Consider hydroxocobalamin (vitamin B_{12}) 25 mg/hr.

Note: These treatments should be administered even during CPR; otherwise, O_2 cannot be utilized by body tissues.

(5) **Clinical use**

(a) SNP dose: 0.1 to 2 μg/kg/min IV infusion. Titrate dose to BP. Avoid doses greater than 2 μg/kg/min: Doses as high as 10 μg/kg/min should be infused for no more than 10 minutes.

(b) Monitor oxygenation.

(c) Solution in a bottle or bag must be protected from light by wrapping in metal foil. Solution stored in the dark retains significant potency for 12 to 24 hours. It is not necessary to cover the administration tubing with foil.

(d) Because of the potency of SNP, it is best administered by itself into a central line using an infusion pump. If other drugs are being infused through the same line, use sufficient "carrier" flow so that changes in one drug's infusion rate does not change the quantity of other drugs entering the patient per minute.

(e) Infusions should be tapered gradually to avoid rebound increases in systemic and PA pressures.

(f) Use this drug cautiously in patients with concomitant untreated hypothyroidism or severe liver or kidney dysfunction.

(g) Continuous BP monitoring with an arterial catheter is recommended.

d. **NO** [55]:

(1) **Actions**

(a) NO is a vasoactive gas naturally produced from L-arginine primarily in endothelial cells. Before its molecular identity was determined it was known as *endothelium-derived relaxing factor.* NO diffuses from endothelial cells to vascular smooth muscle, where it increases cGMP and affects vasodilation, in part by decreasing cytosolic calcium. It is an important physiologic intercellular signaling substance and NO or its absence is implicated in pathologic conditions such as reperfusion injury and coronary vasospasm.

(b) It is inhaled to treat pulmonary hypertension, particularly in respiratory distress syndrome in infancy.

NO	
PVR	Decreased
SVR	No change
RVSWI[a]	Decreased

[a]RVSWI, right ventricular stroke work index.

(2) **Offset.** NO rapidly and avidly binds to the heme moiety of hemoglobin, forming the inactive compound nitrosylhemoglobin, which in turn degrades to methemoglobin. NO's biologic half-life in blood is approximately 6 seconds.

(3) **Advantages**
   (a) Inhaled NO appears to be the long-sought "selective" pulmonary vasodilator. It is devoid of systemic actions.
   (b) Unlike parenterally administered pulmonary vasodilators, inhaled NO favorably affects lung V/Q relationships, because it vasodilates primarily those lung regions that are well ventilated.
   (c) There is low toxicity, provided safety precautions are taken.
(4) **Disadvantages**
   (a) Stringent safety precautions are required to prevent potentially severe toxicity, such as overdose or catastrophic nitrogen dioxide–induced pulmonary edema.
   (b) Methemoglobin concentrations may reach clinically important values, and blood levels must be monitored daily.
   (c) Chronic administration may cause ciliary depletion and epithelial hyperplasia in terminal bronchioles.
   (d) NO is corrosive to metal.
(5) **Clinical use**
   (a) NO is inhaled by blending dilute NO gas into the ventilator inlet gas. Therapeutic concentrations range from 0.05 to 80 parts per million (ppm). The lowest effective concentration should be used, and responses should be carefully monitored. The onset of action for reducing PVR and RVSWI is typically 1 to 2 minutes.
   (b) NO must be purchased prediluted in nitrogen in assayed tanks, and an analyzer must be used intermittently to assay the gas stream entering the patient for NO and nitrogen dioxide. NO usually is not injected between the ventilator and the patient (to avoid overdose), and it must never be allowed to contact air or oxygen until it is used (to prevent formation of toxic nitrogen dioxide).
   (c) NO has been used to treat persistent pulmonary hypertension of the newborn, other forms of pulmonary hypertension, and the adult respiratory distress syndrome with variable success and to date no effect on outcomes.
e. **Nesiritide [56–58]**
(1) **Actions**
   (a) Nesiritide binds to A and B natriuretic peptide receptors on endothelium and vascular smooth muscle, producing dilation of both arterial and venous systems from increased production of cGMP. It also has indirect vasodilating actions by suppressing the sympathetic nervous system, the RAAS, and endothelin.

Nesiritide	
HR	No direct effect
Contractility	No direct effect (reflex increase)
CO	No direct effect (reflex increase)
BP	Decreased
Preload	Decreased
Afterload	Decreased
SVR	Decreased
PVR	Decreased

   (b) Diuretic and natriuretic effects. Although nesiritide as a "cardiac natriuretic peptide" would be expected to have major diuretic and natriuretic effects, the agent seems most effective at this in healthy patients.
   (c) Nesiritide may be hydrolyzed by neutral endopeptidase. A small amount of administered drug may be eliminated via the kidneys.

(2) **Current clinical use.** Despite early studies suggesting that use of nesiritide was associated with reduced mortality in HF patients compared to the use of standard positive inotropic agents, more recent clinical trial data found that nesiritide offered no advantage over standard agents for acute decompensated HF.

    (a) Typical doses are as follows:

        (i)   2 μg/kg loading dose

        (ii) 0.01 μg/kg/min maintenance infusion

    (b) α-**Adrenergic blockers** [3,54]

2. **Labetalol (Normodyne, Trandate)**

See preceding β-adrenergic receptor blocker section in which this agent was presented. It is widely used during and after anesthesia for BP control.

a. Phentolamine (Regitine)

b. Actions

    (1) Competitive antagonist at α_1-, α_2-, and 5-hydroxytryptamine (5-HT, serotonin) receptors

        (a) Primarily arterial vasodilation with little venodilation

Phentolamine	
HR	Increased (reflex)
Contractility	Increased (reflex)
BP	Decreased
SVR	Decreased
PVR	Decreased
Preload	Little change

        (b) **Offset** occurs by hepatic metabolism, in part by renal excretion. Offset after IV bolus occurs after 10 to 30 minutes.

    (2) **Advantages**

        (a) Good for high NE states such as pheochromocytoma.

        (b) Antagonizes undesirable α-stimulation. For example, reversal of deleterious effects of NE extravasated into skin is achieved by local infiltration with phentolamine, 5 to 10 mg in 10-mL saline.

        (c) Has been combined with NE for positive inotropic support with reduced vasoconstriction after CPB.

    (3) **Disadvantages**

        (a) Tachycardia arises from two mechanisms:

            (i)   Reflex via baroreceptors

            (ii) Direct effect of α_2-blockade. Blockade of presynaptic receptors eliminates the normal feedback system controlling NE release by presynaptic nerve terminals. As α_2-stimulation decreases NE release, blockade of these receptors allows increased presynaptic release. This results in increased β_1-sympathetic effects only, as the α-receptors mediating postsynaptic α-effects are blocked by phentolamine. Myocardial ischemia or arrhythmias may result. Thus, the tachycardia and positive inotropy are β-effects that will respond to β-blockers.

        (b) Gastrointestinal motility is stimulated and gastric acid secretion increased.

        (c) Hypoglycemia may occur.

        (d) Epinephrine may cause hypotension in α-blocked patients ("epinephrine reversal") via a β_2-mechanism.

        (e) Arrhythmias occur.

        (f) There is histamine release.

        (g) It is increasingly difficult to obtain from the manufacturer.

(4) Clinical use
- **(a)** Phentolamine dose
  - **(i)** IV bolus: 1 to 5 mg (adult) or 0.1 mg/kg IV (pediatric)
  - **(ii)** IV infusion: 1 to 20 μg/kg/min
- **(b)** When administered for pheochromocytoma, β-blockade may also be instituted.
- **(c)** β-Blockade will attenuate tachycardia.
- **(d)** Phentolamine has been used to promote uniform cooling of infants during CPB prior to deep hypothermia and circulatory arrest (dose, 0.1 to 0.5 mg/kg).

c. Phenoxybenzamine (Dibenzyline)
- **(1) Actions**
  - **(a) Noncompetitive** antagonist at α_1- and α_2-receptors
  - **(b)** Primarily arterial vasodilation with little venodilation

Phentolamine	
HR	Increased (reflex)
Contractility	Increased (reflex)
BP	Decreased
SVR	Decreased
PVR	Decreased
Preload	Decreased

- **(2) Offset occurs by hepatic metabolism, in part by renal excretion. Offset after IV bolus occurs after 10 to 30 minutes.**
- **(3) Advantages**
  - **(a)** Used for high NE states such as pheochromocytoma
  - **(b)** Given PO to prepare patients for excision of pheochromocytoma
  - **(c)** Slow onset and prolonged duration of action (half-life of roughly 24 hours)
- **(4) Disadvantages**
  - **(a)** Tachycardia arises from two mechanisms:
    - **(i)** Reflex via baroreceptors
    - **(ii)** Direct effect of α_2-blockade. Blockade of presynaptic receptors eliminates the normal feedback system controlling NE release by presynaptic nerve terminals. As α_2-stimulation decreases NE release, blockade of these receptors allows increased presynaptic release. This results in increased β_1-sympathetic effects only, as the α-receptors mediating postsynaptic α-effects are blocked by phentolamine. Myocardial ischemia or arrhythmias may result. Thus, the tachycardia and positive inotropy are β-effects that will respond to β-blockers.
  - **(b)** "Stuffy" nose and headache are common.
  - **(c)** Creates marked apparent hypovolemia; adequate preoperative rehydration may result in marked postoperative edema.
  - **(d)** No IV form
- **(5) Clinical use**
  - **(a)** Phenoxybenzamine dose
  - **(b)** PO dose: 10 mg (adult) bid.
  - **(c)** Increase dose gradually up to 30 mg tid—limited by onset of side effects or by elimination of hypertension.
  - **(d)** When administered for pheochromocytoma, β-blockade should not be added until phenoxybenzamine dose has reached a steady state, unless there is exaggerated tachycardia or myocardial ischemia.
  - **(e)** Some authors advocate doxazosin or calcium channel blockers rather than phenoxybenzamine for preoperative preparation of pheochromocytoma, arguing that there are fewer side effects (preoperatively and postoperatively) with these agents.

 d. **Prazosin, doxazosin, and terazosin**
  (1) **Actions.** A selective α_1-competitive antagonist, prazosin's main cardiovascular action is vasodilation (arterial and venous) with decreased SVR and decreased preload. Reflex tachycardia is minimal.
  (2) **Offset** occurs by hepatic metabolism. The half-life is 4 to 6 hours.
  (3) **Advantages**
  (4) Virtual absence of tachycardia
  (5) The only important cardiovascular action is vasodilation.
  (6) **Disadvantages.** Postural hypotension with syncope may occur, especially after the initial dose.
  (7) **Indications.** Oral treatment of chronic hypertension (but is not a first-line agent).
  (8) **Administration.** PO
  (9) **Clinical use**
   (a) Prazosin dose: Initially 0.5 to 1 mg bid (maximum 40 mg/day).
   (b) Prazosin is closely related to two other α_1-blockers with which it shares a common mechanism of action:
    (i) Doxazosin (Cardura). Half-life: 9 to 13 hours. Dose: 1 to 4 mg/day (maximum 16 mg/day).
    (ii) Terazosin (Hytrin). Half-life: 8 to 12 hours. Dose: 1 to 5 mg/day (maximum 20 mg/day).
 3. **ACE inhibitors**
  a. **Captopril (Capoten)**
   (1) **Actions**
    (a) In common with all ACE inhibitors, captopril blocks the conversion of angiotensin I (inactive) to angiotensin II in the lung. This decrease in plasma angiotensin II levels causes vasodilation, generally without reflex increases in HR or CO.
    (b) Many tissues contain ACE (including heart, blood vessels, and kidney), and inhibition of the local production of angiotensin II may be important in the mechanism of action of ACE inhibitors.
    (c) Plasma and tissue concentrations of kinins (e.g., bradykinin) and prostaglandins increase with ACE inhibition and may be responsible for some side effects.
    (d) Captopril, enalaprilat, and lisinopril inhibit ACE directly, but benazepril, enalapril, fosinopril, quinapril, and ramipril are inactive "prodrugs" and must undergo hepatic metabolism into the active metabolites.
   (2) **Offset** occurs primarily by renal elimination with a half-life of 1.5 to 2 hours. Dosages of all ACE inhibitors (except fosinopril) should be reduced with renal dysfunction.
   (3) **Advantages** (in common with all ACE inhibitors)
    (a) Oral vasodilator that improves outcomes in chronic hypertension
    (b) No tachyphylaxis or reflex hemodynamic changes
    (c) Improved symptoms and prolonged survival in CHF, hypertension, and after MI
    (d) May retard progression of renal disease in diabetics
    (e) Antagonizes LV remodeling after myocardial infarction
   (4) **Disadvantages** (in common with all ACE inhibitors)
    (a) Reversibly decreased renal function, due to reduced renal perfusion pressure. Patients with renal artery stenosis bilaterally (or in a single functioning kidney) are at particular risk of renal failure.
    (b) Increased plasma K^+ and hyperkalemia may occur, due to reduced aldosterone secretion.
    (c) Not all angiotensin arises through the ACE pathway ("angiotensin escape").
    (d) ACE inhibition also leads to accumulation of bradykinin (which may underlie side effects of ACE inhibitors).

    (e) Allergic phenomena (including angioedema and hematologic disorders) occur rarely. Captopril may induce severe dermatologic reactions.

    (f) Many patients develop a chronic nonproductive cough.

    (g) Chronic use of ACE inhibitors (and ARBs) appears associated with exaggerated hypotension with induction of general anesthesia.

    (h) Severe fetal abnormalities and oligohydramnios may occur during second- and third-trimester exposure.

(5) Indications

    (a) Hypertension

    (b) CHF

    (c) Myocardial infarction (secondary prevention)

    (d) For all indications, outcome benefits appear to be a drug class effect; any ACE inhibitor will provide them.

    (e) Prevention of renal insufficiency (in the absence of renal artery stenosis), especially in at-risk population (diabetics)

(6) Administration. PO

(7) Clinical use

    (a) Captopril dose

        (i) Adults: 12.5 to 150 mg PO in two or three daily doses, with the lower doses being used for the treatment of heart failure

        (ii) Infants: 50 to 500 µg/kg daily in three doses

    (b) Children older than 6 mos: 0.5 to 2 mg/kg/day divided into three doses

    (c) Interactions. ACE inhibitors interact with digoxin (reduced digoxin clearance) and with lithium (Li intoxication). May predispose to exaggerated hypotension with anesthesia. Captopril interacts with allopurinol (hypersensitivity reactions), cimetidine (CNS changes), and insulin or oral hypoglycemic drugs (hypoglycemia).

b. Enalapril (Vasotec)

(1) Actions. An oral ACE inhibitor used to treat hypertension and CHF, enalapril is very similar to captopril (see Section a). The drug must first be converted to an active metabolite in the liver.

(2) Clinical use. Enalapril dose: 2.5 to 40 mg/day PO in one or two divided doses.

c. Enalaprilat (Vasotec-IV)

(1) Actions. Enalaprilat is an IV ACE inhibitor that is the active metabolite of enalapril. It is used primarily to treat severe or acute hypertension and is very similar to captopril (see Section a).

(2) Offset is by renal elimination, with a half-life of 11 hours.

(3) Advantages

    (a) This drug has a longer duration of action than nitrates, thereby avoiding the need for continuous infusion. It can help extend BP control into the postoperative period.

    (b) Unlike hydralazine, reflex increases in HR, CO, and Mvo$_2$ are absent.

(4) Disadvantages

    (a) There is a longer onset time (15 minutes) than with IV nitroprusside. Peak action may not occur until 1 to 4 hours after the initial dose.

    (b) Pregnancy. Oligohydramnios and fetal abnormalities may be induced. Use during pregnancy should be limited to life-threatening maternal conditions.

(5) Enalaprilat IV dose

    (a) Adults: 1.25 mg IV slowly every 6 hours (maximum 5 mg IV every 6 hours). In renal insufficiency (creatinine clearance less than 30 mL/min), initial dose is 0.625 mg, which may be repeated after 1 hours; then 1.25 mg.

    (b) Pediatrics: A dosage of 250 µg/kg IV every 6 hours has been reported to be effective in neonates with renovascular hypertension.

d. Other oral ACE inhibitors include: Benazepril (Lotensin), Fosinopril (monopril), Lisinopril (prinivil, zestril), Quinapril (accupril), Ramipril (altace), Aceon (perindopril), Mavik (trandolopril), Univasc (moexipril)

4. **ARBs**
    a. **Actions**
       (1) Plasma concentrations of angiotensin II and aldosterone may increase despite treatment with ACE inhibitors because of accumulation of angiotensin or because of production catalyzed via non-ACE–dependent pathways (e.g., chymase).
       (2) Selective angiotensin type-1 receptor (AT1) blockers prevent angiotensin II from directly causing the following:
           (a) Vasoconstriction
           (b) Sodium retention
           (c) Release of NE
           (d) LV hypertrophy and fibrosis
           (e) Angiotensin type-2 receptors (AT2) are not blocked: Their actions including NO release and vasodilation remain intact.
    b. **Advantages**
       (a) Oral vasodilator
       (b) No tachyphylaxis or reflex hemodynamic changes
       (c) ARBs have minimal interaction with CYP system, so few drug interactions.
       (d) Improved symptoms and survival in CHF, hypertension, and after MI
       (e) Stroke prevention in hypertension and LV dysfunction
       (f) May retard progression of renal disease (particularly in diabetics)
       (g) Antagonizes LV remodeling after myocardial infarction
       (h) Lacks common side effects of ACE inhibitors (cough, angioedema)
    c. **Disadvantages**
       (a) There is the potential for decreased renal function, due to reduced renal perfusion pressure. Patients with renal artery stenosis bilaterally (or in a single functioning kidney) are at particular risk.
       (b) Increased plasma K^+ and hyperkalemia may occur, especially when clinicians fail to recognize the consequences of reduced aldosterone secretion.
    d. **Indications**
       (a) Intolerance of ACE inhibitors—outcome benefits of ACE inhibitors in hypertension, CHF, after MI and for renal protection in diabetes appear to be largely shared by ARBs
       (b) Hypertension
       (c) CHF
       (d) Prevention of renal insufficiency (in the absence of renal artery stenosis) in at-risk population (diabetics)
       (e) Data are inconclusive as to whether there is an outcome benefit to adding ARBs to an ACE inhibitor.
    e. **Specific agents**
       (a) Available oral ACE Inhibitors include Losartan (Cozaar), Irbesartan (Avapro), Candesartan (Atacand), Eprosartan (Teveten), Telmisartan (Micardis), Valsartan (Diovan), and Olmesartan (Benicar)
5. **Direct renin inhibitor.** Aliskiren is the single member of this class. It is used for the treatment of hypertension and has the same side effects and contraindications as the ARBs. It is dosed at 150 to 300 mg in a single daily dose.
6. **Central α_2-agonists**
    a. **Clonidine (Catapres)**
       (1) **Actions**
           (a) Clonidine reduces sympathetic outflow by activating central α_2-receptors thereby reducing NE release by peripheral sympathetic nerve terminals.

(b) Clonidine is a partial agonist (activates receptor submaximally but also antagonizes effects of other α_2-agonists).

(c) There is some direct vasoconstrictor action at α_2-receptors on vascular smooth muscle, but this effect is outweighed by the vasodilation induced by these receptors.

(d) Has "local anesthetic" effect on peripheral nerve and produces analgesia by actions on spinal cord when administered via epidural or caudal route.

(e) Has been added to intermediate-duration local anesthetics (e.g., mepivacaine or lidocaine) to nearly double the duration of analgesia after peripheral nerve blocks.

(2) Offset

(a) Long duration (β half-life; 12 hours)

(b) Peak effect 1.5 to 2 hours after an oral dose

(3) Advantages

(a) α2-Agonists potentiate general anesthetics and narcotics through a central mechanism. This effect can reduce substantially doses of anesthetics and narcotics required during anesthesia.

(b) There are no reflex increases in HR or contractility.

(c) Clonidine reduces sympathetic coronary artery tone.

(d) It attenuates hemodynamic responses to stress.

(e) Prolongs duration of spinal and nerve block for regional anesthesia.

(4) Disadvantages

(a) Rebound hypertension prominent after abrupt withdrawal.

(b) Clonidine may potentiate opiate drug effects on CNS.

(c) Sedation is dose-dependent.

(5) Clinical use

(a) Clonidine dose

(i) Adult: 0.2 to 0.8 mg PO daily (maximum 2.4 mg/day). When used as anesthetic premedication, the usual dose is 5 μg/kg PO.

(ii) Pediatrics: 3 to 5 μg/kg every 6 to 8 hours.

(b) Rebound hypertension frequently follows abrupt withdrawal. Clonidine should be continued until immediately before the operation, and either it should be resumed soon postoperatively (by transdermal skin patch, nasogastric tube, or PO) or another type of antihypertensive drug should be substituted. Alternatively, clonidine can be replaced by another drug 1 to 2 weeks preoperatively.

(c) Intraoperative hypotension may occur.

(d) Transdermal clonidine patches require 2 to 3 days to achieve therapeutic plasma drug levels.

(e) Guanabenz and guanfacine are related drugs with similar effects and hazards.

(f) Use of clonidine may improve hemodynamic stability during major cardiovascular surgery.

(g) Clonidine attenuates sympathetic responses during withdrawal from alcohol or opioids in addicts.

(h) It may reduce postoperative shivering.

(i) It may be added to intermediate-duration local anesthetic solutions prior to peripheral nerve blocks to prolong the duration of action.

7. **Other vasodilators**

a. **Fenoldopam**

(1) Actions

(a) Fenoldopam is a short-acting DA-1 receptor agonist which causes peripheral vasodilation. The mechanism appears to be through stimulation of cAMP.

(b) Unlike dopamine, fenoldopam has no α- or β-adrenergic receptor activity at clinical doses and thus no direct actions on HR or cardiac contractility.

(c) Fenoldopam stimulates diuresis and natriuresis.

(2) **Advantages**

    (a) Relative to other short-acting IV vasodilators, fenoldopam has almost no systemic toxic effects.

    (b) Fenoldopam alone among vasodilators stimulates diuresis and natriuresis comparable to "renal dose" (0.5 to 2 µg/kg/min) dopamine.

    (c) Fenoldopam, unlike dopamine, reduces global and regional cerebral blood flow.

(3) **Disadvantages**

    (a) As is true for other dopaminergic agonists, fenoldopam may induce nausea in awake patients.

(4) **Clinical use**

    (a) Fenoldopam is an appropriate single agent to use whenever a combination of a vasodilator and "renal dose" dopamine is employed; for example, for hypertensive patients recovering after CPB.

    (b) Fenoldopam carries no risk of cyanide or of methemoglobinemia and may have theoretical advantages over both nitroprusside and nitroglycerin for control of acute hypertension.

    (c) For treatment of urgent or emergent hypertension in adults we initiate fenoldopam at 0.05 µg/kg/min and double the dose at 5- to 10-minute intervals until it achieves BP control. Doses of up to 1 µg/kg/min may be required.

    (d) The limited data available in pediatrics suggest that weight-adjusted doses at least as great as those used in adults are necessary.

    (e) For inducing diuresis and natriuresis, we have found that doses of 0.05 µg/kg/min are effective in adults.

b. Alprostadil (Prostaglandin E$_1$, PGE$_1$, Prostin VR)

(1) **Actions.** This drug is a direct vasodilator acting through specific prostaglandin receptors on vascular smooth-muscle cells.

(2) Offset occurs by rapid metabolism by enzymes located in most body tissues, especially the lung.

(3) **Advantages**

    (a) Alprostadil selectively dilates the ductus arteriosus (DA) in neonates and infants. It may maintain patency of an open DA for as long as 60 days of age and may open a closed DA for as long as 10 to 14 days of age.

    (b) Metabolism by lung endothelium reduces systemic vasodilation compared with its potent pulmonary vascular dilating effect.

(4) **Disadvantages**

    (a) Systemic vasodilation and hypotension

    (b) May produce apnea in infants (10% to 12%), especially if birth weight is less than 2 kg. Fever and seizures are also possible.

    (c) Expensive agent

    (d) Reversible platelet inhibition

(5) **Administration.** Infused IV or through umbilical arterial catheter

(6) **Indications for use**

    (a) Cyanotic congenital heart disease with reduced pulmonary blood flow.

    (b) Severe pulmonary hypertension with right heart failure.

(7) **Clinical use**

    (a) Alprostadil dose: Usual IV infusion starting dose is 0.05 µg/kg/min. The dose should be titrated up or down to the lowest effective value. Doses as great as 0.4 µg/kg/min may be required.

    (b) IV alprostadil is sometimes used in combination with left atrial NE infusion for treatment of severe pulmonary hypertension with right heart failure.

c. Epoprostenol (PGI$_2$) is used for the long-term treatment of primary pulmonary hypertension and pulmonary hypertension associated with scleroderma. Epoprostenol

(Veletri, Flolan) may be used for severe pulmonary arterial hypertension (WHO Class I) both in IV or inhaled form. The IV form is more common when patients are placed on a sustained infusion through a central venous access. Major harms from epoprostenol are embryonal–fetal malformations and platelet dysfunction leading to potential bleeding diathesis. In order to use it by inhaled route, patients ideally need to be intubated, which is typical in most perioperative situation. The acute treatment of pulmonary hypertension and RV failure is summarized in Table 2.1.

X. Calcium channel blockers [3,54]

A. General considerations

1. **Tissues utilizing calcium.** Calcium is required for cardiac contraction and conduction, smooth-muscle contraction, synaptic transmission, and hormone secretion.

2. **How calcium enters cells.** Calcium ions (Ca^{2+}) reach intracellular sites of action in two ways, by entering the cell from outside or by being released from intracellular storage sites. These two mechanisms are related because Ca^{2+} crossing the sarcolemma acts as a trigger (Ca-induced Ca release), releasing sequestered Ca^{2+} from the sarcoplasmic reticulum into the cytoplasm. These processes can raise intracellular free Ca^{2+} concentrations 100-fold.

3. **Myocardial effects of calcium.** The force of myocardial contraction relates to the free ionized calcium concentration in cytoplasm. Increased $[Ca^{2+}]$ causes contraction and decreased $[Ca^{2+}]$ permits relaxation. At the end of systole, energy-consuming pumps transfer Ca^{2+} from the cytoplasm back into the sarcoplasmic reticulum, decreasing free cytoplasmic $[Ca^{2+}]$. If ischemia prevents sequestration of cytoplasmic Ca^{2+}, diastolic relaxation of myocardium is incomplete. This abnormal diastolic stiffness of the heart raises LVEDP.

4. **Myocardial effects of CCBs.** CCBs owe much of their usefulness to their ability to reduce the entry of the "trigger" current of Ca^{2+}. This reduces the amount of Ca^{2+} released from intracellular stores with each heartbeat. Therefore, all CCBs in large enough doses reduce the force of cardiac contraction, although this effect often is counterbalanced by reflex actions in patients. Clinical dosages of some CCBs, such as nifedipine and nicardipine, do not produce myocardial depression in humans.

5. **Vascular smooth muscle and the cardiac conduction system are particularly sensitive to Ca^{2+} channel blockade.** All CCBs cause vasodilation.

6. **Site selectivity.** CCBs affect certain tissues more than others. Thus, verapamil in clinical dosages depresses cardiac conduction, whereas nifedipine does not.

7. **Direct versus indirect effects.** Selection of a particular CCB is based primarily on its relative potency for direct cellular effects in the target organ versus its relative potency for inducing cardiovascular reflexes.

B. Clinical effects common to all CCBs

1. **Peripheral vasodilation**

   a. **Arterial vasodilation reduces LV afterload**, and this helps offset any direct negative cardiac inotropic action.

   b. **Venous effects.** Preload usually changes little because venodilation is minimal, and negative inotropy often is offset by **reduced** afterload. However, if CCBs reduce myocardial ischemia and diastolic stiffness, filling pressures may decrease.

   c. **Regional effects.** Most vascular beds are dilated, including the cerebral, hepatic, pulmonary, splanchnic, and musculoskeletal beds. Renal blood flow autoregulation is abolished by nifedipine, making it pressure-dependent.

   d. **Coronary vasodilation is induced by all CCBs.** These drugs are all highly effective for coronary vasospasm.

   e. **CCBs versus nitrates**

      (1) Unlike nitrates, CCBs do not incite tachyphylaxis.

      (2) Unlike nitrates, several CCBs are associated with increased bleeding.

   f. **Reversal of vasodilation.** α-Agonists such as phenylephrine often restore BP during CCB-induced hypotension, but usual doses of calcium salts are often ineffective.

2. **Depression of myocardial contractility.** The degree of myocardial depression that occurs following administration of a CCB is highly variable, depending on the following factors:

   a. **Selectivity.** The relative potency of the drug for myocardial depression compared with its other actions is an important factor. Nifedipine and other dihydropyridines are much more potent as vasodilators than as myocardial depressants; clinical dosages that cause profound vasodilation have minimal direct myocardial effects. Conversely, vasodilating dosages of verapamil may be associated with significant myocardial depression in some patients.

   b. **Health of the heart.** A failing ventricle will respond to afterload reduction with improved ejection. An ischemic ventricle will pump more effectively if ischemia is reversed. As CCBs reduce afterload and ischemia, CO may rise with CCB therapy in certain situations. Direct negative inotropic effects may not be apparent.

   c. **Sympathetic reflexes** can counteract direct myocardial depression and vasodilation due to CCBs.

   d. **Reversal of myocardial depression.** Calcium salts, β-agonists, and PDE inotropes all can be used to help reverse excessive negative inotropy and heart block. Electrical pacing may be needed.

3. **Improving myocardial ischemia**

   a. **CCBs may improve oxygen supply** by the following actions:

      (1) Reversing coronary artery spasm

      (2) Vasodilating the coronary artery, increasing flow to both normal and poststenotic regions. Diltiazem and verapamil appear to preserve coronary autoregulation, but nifedipine may cause a coronary steal.

      (3) Increasing flow through coronary collateral channels

      (4) Decreasing HR (prolonging diastolic duration during which subendocardium is perfused) with verapamil and diltiazem

   b. CCBs **may improve oxygen consumption** by

      (1) Diminishing contractility

      (2) Decreasing peak LV wall stress (afterload reduction)

      (3) Decreasing HR (by verapamil and diltiazem)

4. **Electrophysiologic depression**

   a. **Spectrum of impairment of AV conduction**

      (1) Verapamil. Clinical doses usually produce significant electrophysiologic effects. Thus, verapamil has a high relative potency for prolonging AV refractoriness compared with its vasodilating potency.

      (2) Dihydropyridines. On the other hand, nifedipine and other drugs of this class in dosages that produce profound vasodilation have no effect on AV conduction.

      (3) Diltiazem is intermediate between nifedipine and verapamil.

   b. **AV node effects.** The depression of AV nodal conduction by CCBs may be beneficial for its antiarrhythmic effect.

   c. **Sinoatrial (SA) node effects.** Diltiazem and verapamil decrease sinus rate, whereas nifedipine and nicardipine often increase HR slightly.

   d. **Ventricular ectopy** due to mitral valve prolapse, atrial or AV nodal disease, and some forms of digitalis toxicity may respond to CCBs.

5. **Clinical uses**

   a. **Myocardial ischemia** mainly for symptom reduction; note that outcome benefit is not well established for CCBs.

   b. **Hypertension** (outcome benefits are better established for thiazide diuretics and ACE inhibitors; short-acting CCBs have been associated with *worsened* outcomes)

   c. **Hypertrophic cardiomyopathy** by relieving LV outflow obstruction

   d. **Cerebral vasospasm following subarachnoid hemorrhage** (nimodipine)

   e. **Possible reduction of cyclosporine nephrotoxicity with concomitant CCB therapy in transplant recipients.** Also, CCBs may potentiate the immunosuppressive action of cyclosporine.

   f. **Migraine prophylaxis**

C. **Specific IV agents**
   1. **Diltiazem (Cardizem)**
      a. **Diltiazem is a benzothiazepine calcium blocker.**
      b. **Actions.** Diltiazem has a selective coronary vasodilating action, causing a greater increase in coronary flow than in other vascular beds.

	Diltiazem
HR	Slight decrease
Contractility	No change or small decrease
BP	Decreased
Preload	No change
SVR	Decreased
AV conduction	Slowed

      c. **Offset occurs by hepatic metabolism (60%) and renal excretion (35%). Plasma elimination half-life is 3 to 5 hours. The active metabolite is desacetyldiltiazem.**
      d. **Advantages**
         (1) Diltiazem often decreases HR of patients in sinus rhythm.
         (2) It is effective in treating and preventing symptoms of classic or vasospastic myocardial ischemia. Diltiazem does *not* improve outcome in these conditions.
         (3) Used for rate control of SVT (see Section VIII.E).
         (4) Perioperative hypertension can be controlled with IV diltiazem.
      e. **Disadvantages**
         (1) Sinus bradycardia and conduction system depression are possible.
         (2) No evidence for outcome benefit in hypertension or CAD relative to other agents
      f. **Indications**
         (1) Myocardial ischemia, both classic angina and coronary artery spasm
         (2) Hypertension
         (3) SVT, including atrial fibrillation or flutter (see Section VIII.E)
         (4) Sinus tachycardia, especially intraoperative or postoperative
         (5) Diltiazem dose (adult) (see Section VIII.E)
   2. **Nicardipine (Cardene)**
      a. **Actions.** A dihydropyridine calcium blocker with actions closely resembling those of nifedipine (see Section VII), nicardipine is primarily a vasodilator without clinically important negative cardiac inotropy. It is used most commonly for treatment of hypertension.
      b. **IV nicardipine**
         (1) The IV preparation is a highly effective vasodilator that is widely used in surgical patients, causing only minimal HR increase and no increase in ICP. Nicardipine lacks the rebound hypertension that can follow nitroprusside withdrawal. Nicardipine causes less venodilation than nitroglycerin.
         (2) Offset. Metabolism occurs in the liver, with plasma α and β half-lives of 3 and 14 minutes, respectively. When IV administration is stopped, 50% offset vasodilation occurs in approximately 30 minutes.
         (3) Clinical use. Nicardipine IV is effective for control of perioperative hypertension; it also improves diastolic LV function during ischemia by acceleration of myocardial relaxation (lusitropy). Nicardipine can elevate plasma cyclosporine levels.
      c. **Nicardipine dose:** PO: 60 to 120 mg in three daily doses; IV: 1 to 4 µg/kg/min in adults, titrated to BP. The drug causes phlebitis when infused for more than 12 hours through a peripheral IV catheter.
   3. **Verapamil (Calan, Isoptin)** (see Section VIII.E).
   4. **Clevidipine** [59]: Ultra–short-acting calcium channel blocker. IV use only.
      a. **Actions:** Reducing peripheral vascular resistance, increasing CO and reducing BP. This agent is used for perioperative control of hypertension. Plasma half-life approximately

1 minute. Reduced 4.5% of systemic BP in 2 to 4 minutes (https://resources.chiesiusa.com/Cleviprex/CLEVIPREX_US_PI.pdf). Full recovery of BP can be expected in 5 to 15 minutes after infusion is stopped.

b. Metabolism: Plasma and tissue esterases. No contraindication in liver and kidney disease. Supplied as an emulsion. Potential allergic reactions to patients with egg allergy, soy allergy, abnormal lipid metabolism. The manufacturer suggests severe aortic stenosis as a contraindication, we believe that it can be used avoiding any drastic drop in BP. We have typically used it for transfemoral aortic valve replacement to control the BP after valve deployment.

c. Dose: Initiate at 1 to 2 mg/hr. Change the dose by 1 to 2 mg/hr every 5 to 10 minutes until goal is achieved. Usually maximum dose achieved is 16 mg/hr or less. Per manufacturer due to lipid load, it should be restricted to 21 mg/hr per 24-hour period.

Clevidipine	
HR	Increased (reflex)
Contractility	Increased (reflex)
CO	Increased
BP	Decreased
SVR	Markedly decreased
SV	Increased

XI. **Pharmacologic control of HR and rhythm**

A. **Overview of antiarrhythmic medications** [3,25,60]

Antiarrhythmic drugs are classified through the Vaughan Williams classification.

Class	Mechanism	Examples
Ia	Sodium channel blockers (intermediate association/dissociation)	Quinidine; Procainamide
Ib	Sodium channel blockers (fast association/dissociation)	Lidocaine; Phenytoin
Ic	Sodium channel blockers (slow association/dissociation)	Flecainide; Propafenone
II	β-blockers	Propranolol; Metoprolol
III	Potassium channel blockers	Amiodarone; Sotalol
IV	Calcium channel blockers	Verapamil; Diltiazem
V	Unknown mechanism	Adenosine; Digoxin

1. **Antiarrhythmic drugs available in IV form** [3,27,60]
   a. **Procainamide (Pronestyl, Procan-SR)**
      (1) **Class IA antiarrhythmic**
      (2) **Dosing**
         (a) **Loading dose**
            (i) IV: 10 to 50 mg/min (or 100 mg every 2 to 5 minutes) up to 17 mg/kg.
            (ii) Pediatric IV: 3 to 6 mg/kg given slowly.
         (b) **Maintenance dose**
            (i) Adult: IV infusion, 2 mg/kg/hr; PO, 250 to 1,000 mg every 3 hours
            (ii) Children: IV infusion, 20 to 50 μg/kg/min; PO, 30 to 50 mg/kg/day divided into four to six doses.
      (3) **Pharmacokinetics**
         Therapeutic plasma level is usually 4 to 10 μg/mL. With bolus administration, the duration of action is 2 to 4 hours. Metabolism is both hepatic (50%, N-acetylprocainamide) and renal. Slow acetylators are more dependent on renal elimination. Patients with reduced renal function require lower maintenance doses, and need close monitoring of serum levels and the ECG QT intervals.

(4) Adverse effects

(a) High serum levels or rapid loading may cause negative inotropic and chronotropic effects, leading to hypotension and hypoperfusion. Overdose may require pacing and/or β-agonist therapy.

(b) High serum levels of procainamide and/or its principal active metabolite (*N*-acetylprocainamide) induce QT prolongation and *Torsades de Pointes*. Discontinuation of therapy should be considered if the corrected QT interval exceeds 450 ms.

(c) CNS excitability may occur with confusion and seizures.

(d) A lupus-like syndrome may be seen with long-term therapy.

b. Amiodarone (Cordarone)

(1) Class III antiarrhythmic agent

(2) Dosing

(a) PO: 800 to 1,600 mg/day for 1 to 3 weeks, gradually reducing dosage to 400 to 600 mg/day for maintenance.

(b) IV

(i) Loading: For patients in a perfusing rhythm, 150 mg over 10 minutes in repeated boluses until sustained periods of sinus rhythm occur. For patients in pulseless VT/VF, more rapid bolus administration may be warranted. Patients often require 2 to 4 or more boluses for a sustained response.

(ii) Maintenance: 1 mg/min for 6 hours, then 0.5 mg/min thereafter, with the goal of providing approximately 1 g/day.

(3) Pharmacokinetics. The drug is metabolized hepatically, but has very high lipid solubility that results in marked tissue accumulation. The elimination half-life is 20 to 100 days. Hence, for patients treated chronically, it is usually unnecessary to "reload" amiodarone when doses are missed during surgery, and postoperatively patients usually resume their preoperative dosing.

(4) Adverse effects

(a) Amiodarone is an α- and β-receptor noncompetitive antagonist, and therefore has potent vasodilating effects, and can render negative inotropic effects. Hence, vasoconstrictors, IV fluid, and occasionally β-agonists are required for hemodynamic support, especially during the IV amiodarone loading phase.

(b) Amiodarone blocks potassium channels and typically prolongs the QT interval, but is only rarely associated with *Torsades de Pointes*. The risk of torsades on amiodarone therapy is poorly correlated with the QT interval, and QT prolongation on amiodarone, if not excessive, does not usually require cessation of therapy.

(c) Amiodarone use may cause sinus bradycardia or heart block due to β-receptor blockade, and patients requiring sustained IV amiodarone therapy sometimes require pacing or low doses of supplemental β-agonists.

(d) The side effects of long-term oral dosing (subacute pulmonary fibrosis, hepatitis, cirrhosis, photosensitivity, corneal microdeposits, hypothyroidism, or hyperthyroidism) are of little concern during short-term (days) IV therapy.

(e) This drug may increase the effect of oral anticoagulants, phenytoin, digoxin, diltiazem, quinidine, and other drugs.

c. Lidocaine (lignocaine, xylocaine)

(1) Class IB antiarrhythmic

(2) Dosing

(a) Loading dose: 1 mg/kg IV, a second dose may be given 10 to 30 minutes after first dose. Loading dose is sometimes doubled for patients on CPB who are experiencing VF prior to separation. The total dose should not exceed 3 mg/kg.

(b) Maintenance dose: 15 to 50 μg/kg/min (i.e., 1 to 4 mg/min in adults).

(3) Pharmacokinetics. Duration of action is 15 to 30 minutes after administration of a bolus dose. Metabolism is hepatic, and 95% of metabolites are inactive. However, for infusions lasting more than 24 hours, serum levels should be monitored. Many factors that reduce hepatic metabolism will increase serum levels, including CHF, α-agonists, liver disease, and advanced age.

(4) Adverse effects

(a) CNS excitation may result from mild-to-moderate overdose, producing confusion or seizures. At higher doses, CNS depression will ensue, producing sedation and respiratory depression. At still higher doses lidocaine will produce severe myocardial depression.

(b) Lidocaine, like other antiarrhythmics with sodium-channel–blocking properties (amiodarone, procainamide), slows ventricular excitation. Hence, patients with AV nodal block who are dependent upon an idioventricular rhythm may become asystolic during lidocaine therapy.

2. **Drug therapies for bradyarrhythmias** [3,27,60]

a. **Atropine**

(1) Dosing. IV bolus: In adults, use 0.4 to 1 mg (may repeat); in children, use 0.02 mg/kg (minimum 0.1 mg, maximum 0.4 mg, may repeat).

(2) Pharmacokinetics. The HR effects of IV atropine appear within seconds, and effects last as long as 15 to 30 minutes; when given IM, SC, or PO, offset occurs in approximately 4 hours. There is minimal metabolism of the drug, and 77% to 94% of it undergoes renal elimination.

(3) Adverse effects. Atropine is a competitive antagonist at muscarinic cholinergic receptors, and its adverse effects are largely systemic manifestations of this receptor activity.

(a) Tachycardia (undesirable with coronary disease)

(b) Exacerbation of bradycardia by low dosages (0.2 mg or less in an adult)

(c) Sedation (especially in pediatric and elderly patients)

(d) Urinary retention

(e) Increased intraocular pressure in patients with closed-angle glaucoma. Atropine may be safely given, however, if miotic eye drops are given concurrently.

b. **Glycopyrrolate**

(1) Dosing (adults). 0.1 mg IV, repeated at 2- to 3-minute intervals

(2) Differences from atropine. Less likely to cause sedation, but also less likely to produce tachycardia and less likely to be effective for treatment of critical bradycardia. This agent may be chosen to manage mild intraoperative bradycardia, or as an antagonist to the HR slowing effects of neostigmine when reversing neuromuscular blockade. Atropine remains the drug of choice in severe or life-threatening sinus bradycardia and glycopyrrolate should not be used for this purpose!

c. **Isoproterenol (Isuprel)**

(1) General features. Isoproterenol is a synthetic catecholamine with direct β_1- and β_2-agonist effects, and thus has both positive inotropic (through β_1-mediated enhanced contractility plus β_2-mediated vasodilation) and positive chronotropic effects. Isoproterenol is the drug of choice for drug treatment of bradycardia with complete heart block.

(2) Dosing. IV infusion is 0.02 to 0.50 μg/kg/min.

(3) Pharmacokinetics. The agent is used as a continuous infusion, and has a short half-life (2 minutes) making it titratable. It is partly metabolized in the liver (MAO, COMT) and partly excreted unchanged (60%).

(4) Adverse effects

(a) The major potential adverse effect of isoproterenol is myocardial ischemia in patients with CAD, because the combination of tachycardia, positive inotropy, and hypotension may create a myocardial oxygen supply–demand mismatch.

   (b) The agent may provoke supraventricular arrhythmias, or may unmask pre-excitation in patients with an accessory AV conduction pathway (e.g., WPW syndrome). This agent is increasingly difficult to obtain from the manufacturer in the United States.

B. Supraventricular arrhythmias [3,25,27]

  1. Therapy-based classification

    a. General. SVT often foreshadows life-threatening conditions that may be correctable in the surgical patient. Hence, the initial management of the hemodynamically stable surgical patient who suddenly develops SVT should not be on heart-directed pharmacologic therapies, but rather on potential correctable etiologies that may include hypoxemia (O_2 saturation), hypoventilation (end-tidal CO_2), hypotension (absolute or relative hypovolemia due to bleeding, anaphylaxis, etc.), light anesthesia, electrolyte abnormalities (K^+ or Mg^{2+}), or cardiac ischemia (HR, nitroglycerin).

    b. Hemodynamically unstable patients. Patients with low BP (e.g., systolic BP less than 80 mm Hg), cardiac ischemia, or other evidence of end-organ hypoperfusion require immediate *synchronous* DC cardioversion. While some patients may only respond transiently to cardioversion in this setting (or not at all), a brief period of sinus rhythm may provide valuable time for correcting the reversible causes of SVT (see earlier) and/or instituting pharmacologic therapies (see later). During cardiac or thoracic surgery, patients may experience SVT during dissection of the pericardium, placement of atrial sutures, or insertion of the venous cannulae required for CPB. If hemodynamically unstable SVT occurs during open thoracotomy, the surgeon should attempt open synchronous cardioversion. Patients with critical coronary lesions or severe aortic stenosis with SVT may be refractory to cardioversion, and thus enter a malignant cascade of ischemia and worsening arrhythmias that requires the institution of CPB. Hence, early preparation for CPB is recommended before inducing anesthesia in those cardiac surgery patients judged to be at exceptionally high risk for SVT and consequent hemodynamic deterioration.

    c. Hemodynamically stable patients

     (1) Adenosine therapy (Table 2.2)

      (a) In certain patients the SVT involves a re-entrant pathway involving the AV node. These rhythms typically have a regular R–R interval, and are common in relatively healthy patients. Adenosine administered as a 6 mg IV bolus (repeated with 12 mg if no response) may terminate the SVT.

TABLE 2.2 The response of common supraventricular tachyarrhythmias to IV adenosine

SVT	Mechanism	Adenosine response
AV nodal re-entry	Re-entry within AV node	Termination
AV reciprocating tachycardias (orthodromic and antidromic)	Re-entry involving AV node and accessory pathway (WPW)	Termination
Intra-atrial re-entry	Re-entry in the atrium	Transiently slows ventricular response
Atrial flutter/fibrillation	Re-entry in the atrium	Transiently slows ventricular response
Other atrial tachycardias	Abnormal automaticity cAMP-mediated triggered activity	Transient suppression of the tachycardia termination
AV junctional rhythms	Variable	Variable

AV, Atrioventricular.
Adapted from Balser JR. Perioperative management of arrhythmias. In: Barash PG, Fleisher LA, Prough DS, eds. *Problems in Anesthesia*. Vol. 10. Philadelphia, PA: Lippincott-Raven; 1998:201.

(b) Many of the rhythms commonly seen in the perioperative period do not involve the AV node in a re-entrant pathway, and AV nodal block by adenosine in such cases will produce only transient slowing of the ventricular rate. This may lead to "rebound" speeding of the tachycardia following the adenosine effect. Adenosine should be avoided in cases where the rhythm is recognizable and known to be refractory to adenosine (atrial fibrillation, atrial flutter). The hallmark of atrial fibrillation is an irregularly irregular R–R interval.

(c) Junctional tachycardias are common during the surgical period (particularly after surgery for congenital heart disease in children), and sometimes convert to sinus rhythm in response to adenosine, depending on the proximity of the site of origin to the AV node. Ventricular arrhythmias exhibit no response to adenosine since these rhythms originate.

2. Rate control therapy
   a. **Rationale for rate control.** In most cases, ventricular rate control is the mainstay of therapy.
      (1) Lengthening diastole serves to enhance LV filling, thus enhancing SV.
      (2) Slowing the ventricular rate reduces Mvo_2 and lowers the risk of cardiac ischemia.
   b. **Rationale for drug selection.** The most common selections are IV β-blockers or calcium channel blockers because of their rapid onset.
      (1) Among the IV β-blockers, esmolol has the shortest duration of action, rendering it titratable on a minute-to-minute basis, and allowing meaningful dose adjustments during periods of surgery that provoke changes in hemodynamic status (i.e., bleeding, abdominal traction). The drug has obligatory negative inotropic effects that are problematic for patients with severe LV dysfunction.
      (2) Both IV verapamil and IV diltiazem are calcium channel blockers that are less titratable than esmolol, but nonetheless rapidly slow the ventricular rate in SVT. Moreover, IV diltiazem has less negative inotropic action than verapamil or esmolol and is therefore preferable in patients with heart failure.
      (3) IV digoxin slows the ventricular response during SVT through its vagotonic effects at the AV node, but should be temporally supplemented with other IV agents because of its slow onset (approximately 6 hours).
   c. **Accessory pathway rhythms.** AV nodal blockade can reduce the ventricular rate in WPW, and improve hemodynamic status. However, 10% to 35% of patients with WPW eventually develop atrial fibrillation. In this case, the rapid rate of atrial excitation (greater than 300 impulses/min), normally transmitted to the ventricle after "filtering" by the AV node, is instead be transmitted to the ventricle via the accessory bundle at a rapid rate. The danger of inducing VT/VF in this scenario is exacerbated by treatment with classic AV nodal blocking agents (digoxin, calcium channel blockers, β-blockers, and adenosine) because they reduce the accessory bundle refractory period. Hence, WPW patients who experience atrial fibrillation should not receive AV nodal blockers. IV procainamide slows conduction over the accessory bundle, and is an option for treating AF in patients with accessory pathways.
   d. **Specific rate control agents** [3,27,60]
      (1) **Esmolol**
         (Please also see the earlier section on β-blockers.)
         (a) **Dosing.** During surgery and anesthesia, the standard 0.25 to 0.5 mg/kg load (package insert) may be accompanied by marked hypotension. In practice, reduced IV bolus doses of 12.5 to 25 mg are titrated to effect, followed by an infusion of 50 to 200 µg/kg/min. Transient hypotension during the loading phase may usually be managed with IV fluid or vasoconstrictors (phenylephrine).
         (b) **Pharmacokinetics.** Esmolol is rapidly eliminated by a red blood cell esterase. After discontinuation of esmolol, most drug effects are eliminated within

5 minutes. The duration of esmolol action is not affected when plasma pseudocholinesterase is inhibited by echothiophate or physostigmine.

(c) Adverse effects

(i) Esmolol is a potent, selective β_1-receptor antagonist, and may cause hypotension through both vasodilation and negative inotropic effects.

(ii) Compared to nonselective β-blockers, esmolol is less likely to elicit bronchospasm, but should still be used with caution in patients with known bronchospastic disease.

(2) Verapamil

(a) Dosing

(i) IV load (adults): 5 to 15 mg, consider administering in 1 to 2 mg increments during surgery and anesthesia, or in unstable patients. Dose may be repeated after 30 minutes.

(ii) Maintenance IV: 5 to 15 mg/hr.

(iii) PO (adults): 40 to 80 mg tid to qid (maximum 480 mg/day).

(iv) Pediatric dose: 75 to 200 µg/kg IV; may be repeated.

(b) Pharmacokinetics. Elimination occurs by hepatic metabolism, and plasma half-life is 3 to 10 hours, so lengthy intervals (hours) between dose increments for IV infusions should be utilized to avoid cumulative effects.

(c) Adverse effects

(i) Verapamil blocks L-type calcium channels and may cause hypotension because of both peripheral vasodilation and negative inotropic effects, especially during the IV loading phase. The vasodilatory effects may be mitigated by administration of IV fluid or vasoconstrictors (i.e., phenylephrine). Patients with severe LV dysfunction may not tolerate IV verapamil, and may be better candidates for IV diltiazem (see later).

(ii) Verapamil (given chronically) reduces digoxin elimination and can raise digoxin levels, producing toxicity.

(3) Diltiazem

(a) Dosing (adult)

(i) IV loading: 20 mg IV over 2 minutes. May repeat after 15 minutes with 25 mg IV if HR exceeds 110 bpm. Smaller doses or longer loading periods may be used in patients who have myocardial ischemia, hemodynamic instability, or who are anesthetized.

(ii) Maintenance: Infusion at 5 to 15 mg/hr, depending on HR control.

(iii) PO dose: 120 to 360 mg/day (sustained-release preparations are available).

(b) Pharmacokinetics. Metabolism is both hepatic (60%) and renal excretion (35%). Plasma elimination half-life is 3 to 5 hours, so lengthy intervals (hours) between dose increases for IV infusions should be utilized to avoid cumulative effects.

(c) Adverse effects

(i) Diltiazem, like all calcium channel blockers, elicits vasodilation and may evoke hypotension. At the same time, partly due to its afterload reducing properties, IV diltiazem is less likely to compromise CO in patients with reduced LV function (relative to other AV nodal blockers) and is the drug of choice for rate control in this circumstance.

(ii) Sinus bradycardia is possible, so diltiazem should be used with caution in patients with sinus node dysfunction or those also receiving digoxin or β-blockers.

(4) High-dose IV magnesium sulfate

(a) Dosing. Regimens including a 2 to 2.5 g initial bolus, followed by a 1.75 g/hr infusion, are described.

(b) **Issues with use.** High-dose magnesium is used rarely for SVT, but may nonetheless successfully provide rate control for patients with SVT. In some cases, rates of conversion to sinus rhythm exceeding placebo or antiarrhythmic agents have been noted. The use of these high magnesium doses requires close monitoring of serum levels, and should be avoided in patients with renal insufficiency. An increased requirement for temporary pacing due to the AV nodal blockade has also been noted. Magnesium potentiates neuromuscular blockers; thus, this agent can cause life-threatening hypoventilation in spontaneously breathing patients who have residual blood levels of these agents.

e. **Cardioversion of SVT**

(1) **Limitations of pharmacologic or "chemical" cardioversion**

(a) The 24-hour rate of spontaneous conversion to sinus rhythm for recent-onset perioperative SVT exceeds 50%, and many patients who develop SVT under anesthesia will remit spontaneously within hours of emergence.

(b) Most of the antiarrhythmic agents with activity against atrial arrhythmias have limited efficacy when utilized in IV form for rapid chemical conversion. Although 50% to 80% efficacy rates are cited for many IV antiarrhythmics in uncontrolled studies, these findings are an artifact of high placebo rates of conversion (approximately 60% over 24 hours). Although improved rates of chemical cardioversion are seen with high doses of IV amiodarone (approximately 2 g/day), the potential for undesirable side effects in the perioperative setting requires further study.

(c) Most agents have adverse effects, including negative inotropic effects or vasodilation (amiodarone, procainamide). In addition, these agents may provoke polymorphic ventricular arrhythmias (*Torsades de Pointes*). While less common with amiodarone, newer IV agents that exhibit high efficacy for converting atrial fibrillation (i.e., ibutilide) exhibit rates of torsades as high as 8%.

(2) **Rationale for cardioversion.** In the operating room, chemical cardioversion should be aimed mainly at patients who cannot tolerate (or do no respond to) IV rate control therapy, or who fail DC cardioversion and remain hemodynamically unstable. Intraoperative elective DC cardioversion in an otherwise stable patient with SVT also carries inherent risks (VF, asystole, and stroke). Moreover, the underlying factors provoking SVT during or shortly after surgery are likely to persist beyond the time of cardioversion, inviting recurrence. Hence, when elective DC cardioversion is considered, it may be prudent to first establish a therapeutic level of an antiarrhythmic agent that maintains sinus rhythm (i.e., procainamide, amiodarone), with a view to preventing SVT recurrence following electrical cardioversion. Guidelines for administration of IV procainamide and amiodarone are provided in an earlier section of this chapter (see Section XI.A.1.).

f. **SVT prophylaxis for postoperative patients** [27]

SVT may occur during the days following surgery, and occurs within the first 4 postoperative days in up to 40% of cardiac surgeries. Many postoperative prophylaxis regimens have been evaluated, and are discussed in recent reviews. Prophylactic administration of a number of drugs typically used to slow AV nodal conduction (particularly β-blockers and amiodarone) may reduce the incidence of postoperative atrial fibrillation (particularly after cardiothoracic surgery), but by no means eliminate the problem. Nonetheless, antiarrhythmic prophylaxis should be considered in selected patients at high risk for hemodynamic or ischemic complications from postoperative SVT.

g. Potential arrhythmogenic drugs: Table 2.3

TABLE 2.3 QT-prolonging drugs (partial listing emphasizing agents used perioperatively)

Antiarrhythmics	Quinidine, procainamide, disopyramide, sotalol, amiodarone, ibutilide, dofetilide
Antipsychotics	Haloperidol, risperidone, isoperidene, chlorpromazine, thioridazine
Antihistamines	Terfenadine, astemizole
Antifungals	Ketoconazole, fluconazole, itraconazole
Antibiotics	Trimethoprim–sulfamethoxazole, erythromycin, clarithromycin
Antidepressants	Amitriptyline, imipramine, doxepin
Opioid	Methadone
GI	Cisapride, droperidol, ondansetron

XII. Diuretics [61]
   A. Actions
   Most IV diuretics act at the loop of Henle in the kidney to block resorption of electrolytes from the tubule. Loop diuretics block the sodium–potassium–chloride transporter. Thiazide diuretics block the electroneutral sodium–chloride transporter. Amiloride and triamterene block apical (non–voltage-gated) sodium channels. Spironolactone binds and inhibits the mineralocorticoid receptor. This action increases excretion of water and electrolytes (Na, Cl, K, Ca, and Mg) from the body.
   B. Adverse effects
   1. Effect shared by all diuretics
      a. Cross-sensitivity with sulfonamides (except ethacrynic acid)
   2. Effects shared by thiazides and loop diuretics
      a. Skin reactions
      b. Interstitial nephritis
      c. Hypokalemia
      d. Hypomagnesemia (effects of thiazides and loop diuretics are diminished by potassium-sparing diuretics such as spironolactone or triamterene)
      e. Risk of hyponatremia greater with thiazides than with loop diuretics
   3. Effects specific to loop diuretics
      a. Increased serum uric acid
      b. Ototoxicity. Deafness, usually temporary, may occur with large drug doses or coadministration with an aminoglycoside antibiotic. One possible mechanism for this is drug-induced changes in endolymph electrolyte composition.
   4. Effects of thiazide diuretics
      a. Hypercalcemia
      b. Hyperuricemia
      c. Mild metabolic alkalosis ("contraction" alkalosis)
      d. Hyperglycemia, glucose intolerance
      e. Hyperlipidemia
      f. Rare pancreatitis
   5. Effects of potassium-sparing diuretics
      a. Hyperkalemia (sometimes with metabolic acidosis)
      b. Gynecomastia (with increased doses of spironolactone)
      c. Amiloride excreted by kidneys, so duration prolonged in renal failure

CLINICAL PEARL Diuretics should be used to induce diuresis, not to diagnose the characteristics or severity of acute kidney injury.

C. **Specific drugs**
  1. **Loop diuretics**
     a. **Furosemide (Lasix)**
        (1) **Pharmacokinetics.** Renal tubular secretion of unchanged drug and of glucuronide metabolite. Half-life of 1.5 hours.
        (2) **Clinical use**
           (a) **Dosing**
               (i) Adults: The usual oral dosing is 20 to 320 mg in two daily doses. The usual IV starting dose for patients not currently receiving diuretics is 2.5 to 5 mg, increasing as necessary to a 200 mg bolus. Patients already receiving diuretics usually require 20 to 40 mg initial doses to produce a diuresis. A continuous infusion (0.5 to 1 mg/kg/hr) at approximately 0.05 mg/kg/hr in adults produces a more sustained diuresis with a lower total daily dose compared with intermittent bolus dosing. Patients resistant to loop diuretics (e.g., after long-term dosing in hepatic failure) may benefit from combinations of furosemide and thiazide diuretics.
               (ii) Pediatric: 1 mg/kg (maximum, 6 mg/kg). The pediatric infusion rate is 0.2 to 0.4 mg/kg/hr.
           (b) Because furosemide is a sulfonamide, allergic reactions may occur in sulfonamide-sensitive patients (rare).
           (c) Furosemide often causes transient vasodilation of veins and arterioles, with reduced cardiac preload.
     b. **Bumetanide (Bumex)**
        (1) **Pharmacokinetics.** Combined renal and hepatic elimination. Half-life is 1 to 1.5 hours.
        (2) **Clinical use**
           (a) **Dosing:** The usual oral dosing is 25 to 100 mg in two or three daily doses. 0.5 to 1 mg IV, may be repeated every 2 to 3 hours to a maximum dose of 10 mg/day.
           (b) **Myalgias** may occur.
     c. **Ethacrynic acid (Edecrin)**
        (1) **Pharmacokinetics.** Combined renal and hepatic elimination
        (2) **Clinical use**
           (a) **Dosing:** 50 mg IV (adult dose) or 0.5 to 1 mg/kg (maximum 100 mg) titrated to effect
           (b) Usually is reserved for patients who fail to respond to furosemide or bumetanide, or who are allergic to sulfonamides (thiazides and furosemide are chemically related to sulfonamides)
  2. **Thiazide diuretics**
     a. **Mechanism/pharmacokinetics.** The mechanism of the antihypertensive effect of thiazide diuretics remains the subject of debate. All thiazides increase the urinary excretion of sodium and chloride, acting on the sodium-chloride symporter in the distal renal tubules.
  3. **Potassium-sparing diuretics**
     a. **Amiloride (Midamor)**
        (1) **Mechanism/pharmacokinetics**
            Amiloride works by inhibiting sodium channels in renal epithelium of the late distal tubule and collecting duct. This mildly increases the excretion of sodium and chloride. Amiloride decreases the lumen-negative voltage across the membrane, decreasing the excretion of K^+, H^+, Ca^{2+}, and Mg^{2+}. Amiloride has 15% to 25% oral bioavailability. It has a roughly 21-hour half-life and is predominantly eliminated by the renal excretion of the intact drug.
        (2) **Clinical use**
            Amiloride is a weak diuretic, so it is almost never used as a sole agent, but most commonly in combination with other, stronger diuretics (such as thiazides or loop

diuretics) to augment their diuretic and antihypertensive effects and reduce the risk of hypokalemia.

(a) **Dosing:** Usual dose is 5 to 10 mg/day in one or two doses added to a loop or thiazide diuretic. Doses more than 10 mg/day have rarely been given.

(b) This agent is also available as a combination product with hydrochlorothiazide (Moduretic).

b. **Eplerenone (Inspra)**

(1) **Mechanism/pharmacokinetics**

This agent has the same mechanism of action as spironolactone and it is used for the same indications. It is an effective antihypertensive. It has been shown to prolong life in patients with LV dysfunction following myocardial infarction.

(2) **Dosing:** The drug is initiated at 25 mg/day and may be increased to 100 mg/day as tolerated by the patient.

c. **Spironolactone (Aldactone)**

(1) **Mechanism/pharmacokinetics**

Spironolactone is a competitive antagonist to the mineralocorticoid receptor found in the cytoplasm of epithelial cells in the late distal tubule and collecting duct. Thus, it opposes the actions of endogenous aldosterone. After binding the receptor, the aldosterone–receptor complex migrates to the cell nucleus, regulating production of a series of "aldosterone-induced proteins." The aldosterone-induced proteins ultimately increase transepithelial sodium–chloride transport, and the lumen-negative transepithelial membrane potential, increasing the secretion of K^+ and H^+ into the tubular lumen. Spironolactone antagonizes these effects. Spironolactone has also been shown to inhibit the cardiac remodeling process and to prolong life in patients with chronic HF. The side effects of spironolactone include hyperkalemia and gynecomastia. Spironolactone has about a 65% oral bioavailability and a very short half-life. It has active metabolites with prolonged (16-hour half-life) actions.

(2) **Clinical use**

Spironolactone is a weak diuretic, so it is almost never used as a sole agent, but most commonly in combination with other, stronger diuretics (such as thiazides or loop diuretics) to augment their diuretic and antihypertensive effects and reduce the risk of hypokalemia. Spironolactone prolongs life in patients with heart failure and is now part of standard therapy for symptomatic patients with this condition.

(a) **Dosing:** The usual dose is 12.5 to 25 mg/day, but this may be increased as needed up to 100 mg/day in one or two daily doses. This agent is also available as a combination product with hydrochlorothiazide (Aldactazide).

d. **Triamterene**

(1) **Mechanism/pharmacokinetics**

This agent is believed to have the same mechanism of action as amiloride and it is used for the same indications as amiloride. It is approximately one-tenth as potent as amiloride. Triamterene has 50% oral bioavailability and a half-life of roughly 4.5 hours. It is eliminated through hepatic biotransformation to an active metabolite that is excreted in the urine.

(2) This agent is usually given in doses of 50 to 150 mg/day in one or two doses in combination with thiazide or loop diuretics. It is also found in a combination product with hydrochlorothiazide (Dyazide).

4. **Osmotic diuretics**

a. **Mannitol**

(1) **Mechanism/pharmacokinetics.** Mannitol is an osmotic diuretic that is eliminated unchanged in urine. It is also a free-radical scavenger.

(2) **Clinical use**

(a) Unlike the loop diuretics (e.g., furosemide), mannitol retains its efficacy even during low glomerular filtration states (e.g., shock).

        (b) Diuresis with this agent may have protective effects in some clinical scenarios (i.e., CPB, poor renal perfusion, hemoglobinuria, or nephrotoxins), possibly related to free-radical scavenging.

        (c) As an osmotically active agent in the bloodstream, it is sometimes used to reduce brain water content, cerebral edema and ICP. Mannitol is administered routinely (as prophylaxis) by many clinicians during anesthesia for patients with intracranial mass lesions.

    5. **Dosing**: Initial dose is 12.5 g IV to a maximum of 0.5 g/kg.

    6. **Adverse effects**

        a. It may produce hypotension if administered as a rapid IV bolus.

        b. It may induce transient pulmonary edema as intravascular volume expands before diuresis begins.

XIII. **Pulmonary hypertension** [62–64]:

For therapeutic treatment, there are essentially three established pathways that are targeted: the nitric oxide pathway, the prostacyclin pathway and endothelin receptor pathway. In perioperative settings (Table 2.1), iNO, milrinone, PGI2 (Flolan) are the most useful. For oral therapy, essentially it is the endothelin pathway–mediated drugs. Depending on their "WHO Functional Class" patients may be on multiple drug therapy. Several novel compounds are also being tried now-a-days that are still experimental (see reference above).

ACKNOWLEDGMENTS

The authors acknowledge the contributions of coauthors in previous editions: Dr. Jeffrey Balser and Dr. David Larach.

REFERENCES

1. *Physicians' Desk Reference.* 69th ed. Montvale, NJ: Medical Economics Company, Inc.; 2015.
2. Epocrates.www.epocrates.com. March 27, 2017.
3. The Medical Letter. www.medicalletter.org. March 27, 2017.
4. Gaies MG, Gurney JG, Yen AH, et al. Vasoactive-inotropic score as a predictor of morbidity and mortality in infants after cardiopulmonary bypass. *Pediatr Crit Care Med.* 2010;11(2):234–238.
5. **Maeda T, Toda K, Kamei M, et al. Impact of preoperative extracorporeal membrane oxygenation on vasoactive inotrope score after implantation of left ventricular assist device. *Springerplus.* 2015;4:821.**
6. Wernovsky G, Wypij D, Jonas RA, et al. Postoperative course and hemodynamic profile after the arterial switch operation in neonates and infants. A comparison of low-flow cardiopulmonary bypass and circulatory arrest. *Circulation.* 1995;92(8): 2226–2235.
7. LH O. *Heart Physiology from Cell to Circulation.* 4th ed. Philadelphia, PA: Lippincott Williams & Wilkins; 2004.
8. **Rosendorff C, Writing Committee. Treatment of hypertension in patients with coronary artery disease. A case-based summary of the 2015 AHA/ACC/ASH scientific statement. *Am J Med.* 2016;129(4):372–378.**
9. Rosendorff C, et al. Treatment of hypertension in patients with coronary artery disease: a scientific statement from the American Heart Association, American College of Cardiology, and American Society of Hypertension. *Circulation.* 2015;131(19):e435–e470.
10. Stone NJ, Robinson JG, Lichtenstein AH, et al. 2013 ACC/AHA guideline on the treatment of blood cholesterol to reduce atherosclerotic cardiovascular risk in adults: a report of the American College of Cardiology/American Heart Association Task Force on Practice Guidelines. *J Am Coll Cardiol.* 2014;63(25 Pt B):2889–2934.
11. Yeboah J, Sillau S, Delaney JC, et al. Implications of the new American College of Cardiology/American Heart Association cholesterol guidelines for primary atherosclerotic cardiovascular disease event prevention in a multi ethnic cohort: Multi-Ethnic Study of Atherosclerosis (MESA). *Am Heart J.* 2015;169(3):387–395.e3.
12. Jellinger PS, Handelsman Y, Rosenblit PD, et al. American Association of Clinical Endocrinologists and American College of Endocrinology Guidelines for management of dyslipidemia and prevention of cardiovascular disease. *Endocr Pract.* 2017; 23(Suppl 2):1–87.
13. Thadani U. Management of stable angina—current guidelines: a critical appraisal. *Cardiovasc Drugs Ther.* 2016;30(4):419–426.
14. **Fihn SD, Blankenship JC, Alexander KP, et al. 2014 ACC/AHA/AATS/PCNA/SCAI/STS focused update of the guideline for the diagnosis and management of patients with stable ischemic heart disease: a report of the American College of Cardiology/American Heart Association Task Force on Practice Guidelines, and the American Association for Thoracic Surgery, Preventive Cardiovascular Nurses Association, Society for Cardiovascular Angiography and Interventions, and Society of Thoracic Surgeons. *J Thorac Cardiovasc Surg.* 2015;149(3):e5–e23.**
15. Kulik A, Ruel M, Jneid H, et al. Secondary prevention after coronary artery bypass graft surgery: a scientific statement from the American Heart Association. *Circulation.* 2015;131(10):927–964.
16. **Ducceppe E, Parlow J, MacDonald P, et al. Canadian Cardiovascular Society guidelines on perioperative cardiac risk assessment and management for patients who undergo noncardiac surgery. *Can J Cardiol.* 2017;33(1):17–32.**

17. Wijeysundera DN, Duncan D, Nkonde-Price C, et al. Perioperative beta blockade in noncardiac surgery: a systematic review for the 2014 ACC/AHA guideline on perioperative cardiovascular evaluation and management of patients undergoing noncardiac surgery: a report of the American College of Cardiology/American Heart Association Task Force on practice guidelines. *J Am Coll Cardiol.* 2014;64(22):2406–2425.
18. Devereaux PJ, Mrkobrada M, Sessler DI, et al. Aspirin in patients undergoing noncardiac surgery. *N Engl J Med.* 2014; 370(16):1494–1503.
19. Devereaux PJ, POISE-2 Investigators, Rationale and design of the PeriOperative ISchemic Evaluation-2 (POISE-2) trial: an international 2 × 2 factorial randomized controlled trial of acetyl-salicylic acid vs. placebo and clonidine vs. placebo in patients undergoing noncardiac surgery. *Am Heart J.* 2014;167(6):804–809.e4.
20. Devereaux PJ, Sessler DI, Leslie K, et al. Clonidine in patients undergoing noncardiac surgery. *N Engl J Med.* 2014;370(16):1504–1513.
21. Yancy CW, Jessup M, Bozkurt B, et al. 2017 ACC/AHA/HFSA Focused Update of the 2013 ACCF/AHA Guideline for the management of heart failure: a report of the American College of Cardiology/American Heart Association Task Force on Clinical Practice Guidelines and the Heart Failure Society of America. *J Am Coll Cardiol.* 2017;23(8):628–651.
22. **Tariq S, Aronow WS. Use of Inotropic Agents in treatment of systolic heart failure. *Int J Mol Sci.* 2015;16(12): 29060–29068.**
23. **Metra M, Teerlink JR. Heart failure. *Lancet.* 2017;390(10106):1981–1995.**
24. Metra M, Ravera A, Filippatos G. Understanding worsening heart failure as a therapeutic target: another step forward? *Eur J Heart Fail.* 2017;19(8):996–1000.
25. January CT, Wann LS, Alpert JS, et al. 2014 AHA/ACC/HRS guideline for the management of patients with atrial fibrillation: a report of the American College of Cardiology/American Heart Association Task Force on Practice Guidelines and the Heart Rhythm Society. *J Am Coll Cardiol.* 2014;64(21):e1–e76.
26. Society of Thoracic Surgeons Task Force on Resuscitation After Cardiac Surgery. The Society of thoracic surgeons expert consensus for the resuscitation of patients who arrest after cardiac surgery. *Ann Thorac Surg.* 2017;103(3):1005–1020.
27. Nolan JP, Hazinski MF, Aickin R, et al. Part 1: Executive summary: 2015 International Consensus on cardiopulmonary resuscitation and emergency cardiovascular care science with treatment recommendations. *Resuscitation.* 2015;95:e1–e31.
28. Butterworth JF IV, Prielipp RC, MacGregor DA, et al. Pharmacologic cardiovascular support. In: Kvetan V, Dantzker DR, eds. *The Critically Ill Cardiac Patient: Multisystem Dysfunction and Management.* Philadelphia, PA: Lippincott-Raven; 1996:167–192.
29. Hamzaoui O, Scheeren TWL, Teboul JL., Norepinephrine in septic shock: when and how much? *Curr Opin Crit Care.* 2017;23(4):342–347.
30. Russell JA, Walley KR, Singer J, et al. Vasopressin versus norepinephrine infusion in patients with septic shock. *N Engl J Med.* 2008;358(9):877–887.
31. **Russell JA, Lee T, Singer J, et al. The Septic Shock 3.0 Definition and trials: a vasopressin and septic shock trial experience. *Crit Care Med.* 2017;45(6):940–948.**
32. **Russell JA. Vasopressin, norepinephrine, and vasodilatory shock after cardiac surgery: another "VASST" difference? *Anesthesiology.* 2017;126(1):9–11.**
33. Gordon AC, Mason AJ, Thirunavukkarasu N, et al. Effect of early vasopressin vs norepinephrine on kidney failure in patients with septic shock: the VANISH randomized clinical trial. *JAMA.* 2016;316(5):509–518.
34. Hajjar LA, Vincent JL, Barbosa Gomes Galas FR, et al. Vasopressin versus norepinephrine in patients with vasoplegic shock after cardiac surgery: the VANCS randomized controlled trial. *Anesthesiology.* 2017;126(1):85–93.
35. **Khanna A, English SW, Wang XS, et al. Angiotensin II for the treatment of vasodilatory shock. *N Engl J Med.* 2017; 377(5):419–430.**
36. Chawla LS, Russell JA, Bagshaw SM, et al. Angiotensin II for the Treatment of High-Output Shock 3 (ATHOS-3): protocol for a phase III, double-blind, randomised controlled trial. *Crit Care Resusc.* 2017;19(1):43–49.
37. Antonucci E, Gleeson PJ, Annoni F, et al. Angiotensin II in refractory septic shock. *Shock.* 2017;47(5):560–566.
38. Cerillo AG, Storti S, Kallushi E, et al. The low triiodothyronine syndrome: a strong predictor of low cardiac output and death in patients undergoing coronary artery bypass grafting. *Ann Thorac Surg.* 2014;97(6):2089–2095.
39. Hashim T, Sanam K, Revilla-Martinez M, et al. Clinical characteristics and outcomes of intravenous inotropic therapy in advanced heart failure. *Circ Heart Fail.* 2015;8(5):880–886.
40. Belletti A, Castro ML, Silvetti S, et al. The Effect of inotropes and vasopressors on mortality: a meta-analysis of randomized clinical trials. *Br J Anaesth.* 2015;115(5):656–675.
41. Baer J, Stoops S, Flynn B, Vasodilatory Shock after ventricular assist device placement: a bench to bedside review. *Semin Thorac Cardiovasc Surg.* 2016;28(2):238–244.
42. Kandasamy A, Simon HA, Murthy P, et al. Comparison of Levosimendan versus Dobutamine in patients with moderate to severe left ventricular dysfunction undergoing off-pump coronary artery bypass grafting: a randomized prospective study. *Ann Card Anaesth.* 2017;20(2):200–206.
43. Fellahi JL, Parienti JJ, Hanouz JL, et al. Perioperative use of dobutamine in cardiac surgery and adverse cardiac outcome: propensity-adjusted analyses. *Anesthesiology.* 2008;108(6):979–987.
44. Denault AY, Bussières JS, Arellano R, et al. A multicentre randomized-controlled trial of inhaled milrinone in high-risk cardiac surgical patients. *Can J Anaesth.* 2016;63(10):1140–1153.
45. Ushio M, Egi M, Wakabayashi K, et al. Impact of milrinone administration in adult cardiac surgery patients: updated meta-analysis. *J Cardiothorac Vasc Anesth.* 2016;30(6):1454–1460.
46. **Grocott HP. Updating the update: The final word on milrinone and mortality after cardiac surgery? *J Cardiothorac Vasc Anesth.* 2017;31(6):e95–e96.**
47. Patel MR, Calhoon JH, Dehmer GJ, et al. ACC/AATS/AHA/ASE/ASNC/SCAI/SCCT/STS 2017 Appropriate Use Criteria for Coronary Revascularization in Patients With Stable Ischemic Heart Disease: A Report of the American College of Cardiology Appropriate Use Criteria Task Force, American Association for Thoracic Surgery, American Heart Association,

American Society of Echocardiography, American Society of Nuclear Cardiology, Society for Cardiovascular Angiography and Interventions, Society of Cardiovascular Computed Tomography, and Society of Thoracic Surgeons. *J Am Coll Cardiol.* 2017;69(17):2212–2241.

48. Mebazaa A, Pitsis AA, Rudiger A, et al. Clinical review: practical recommendations on the management of perioperative heart failure in cardiac surgery. *Crit Care.* 2010;14(2):201.

49. Fernandez-Ruiz I. Surgery: neutral results for levosimendan in cardiac surgery. *Nat Rev Cardiol.* 2017;14(5):256.

50. Landoni G, Lomivorotov VV, Alvaro G, et al. Levosimendan for hemodynamic support after cardiac surgery. *N Engl J Med.* 2017;376(21):2021–2031.

51. Mehta RH, Leimberger JD, van Diepen S, et al. Levosimendan in patients with left ventricular dysfunction undergoing cardiac surgery. *N Engl J Med.* 2017;376(21):2032–2042.

52. Hummel J, Rücker G, Stiller B. Prophylactic levosimendan for the prevention of low cardiac output syndrome and mortality in paediatric patients undergoing surgery for congenital heart disease. *Cochrane Database Syst Rev.* 2017;3:CD011312.

53. Morelli A, Tritapepe L. Levosimendan in sepsis. *N Engl J Med.* 2017;376(8):799–800.

54. Bruton LL, Knollman BC, Hilal-Dandan R, eds. *Goodman & Gilman's: The Pharmacological Basis of Therapeutics.* 13th ed. New York: McGraw-Hill; 2017.

55. Benedetto M, Romano R, Baca G, et al. Inhaled nitric oxide in cardiac surgery: evidence or tradition? *Nitric Oxide.* 2015;49: 67–79.

56. O'Connor CM, Starling RC, Hernandez AF, et al. Effect of nesiritide in patients with acute decompensated heart failure. *N Engl J Med.* 2011;365(1):32–43.

57. Wong YW, Mentz RJ, Felker GM, et al. Nesiritide in patients hospitalized for acute heart failure: does timing matter? Implication for future acute heart failure trials. *Eur J Heart Fail.* 2016;18(6):684–692.

58. van Deursen VM, Hernandez AF, Stebbins A, et al. Nesiritide, renal function, and associated outcomes during hospitalization for acute decompensated heart failure: results from the Acute Study of Clinical Effectiveness of Nesiritide and Decompensated Heart Failure (ASCEND-HF). *Circulation.* 2014;130(12):958–965.

59. Espinosa A, Ripollés-Melchor J, Casans-Francés R, et al. Perioperative use of clevidipine: a systematic review and meta-analysis. *PLoS One.* 2016;11(3):e0150625.

60. Knollman BC, Rhoden DM. Chapter 30: Antiarrhythmic drugs. In: Brunton LL, Hilal-Dandan R, Knollman BC, eds. *Goodman & Gilman's: The Pharmacological Basis of Therapeutics.* 13th ed. New York: McGraw-Hill; 2017.

61. Hilal-Dandan R. Chapter 26. Renin and angiotensin. In: Brunton LL, Hilal-Dandan R, Knollman BC, eds. *Goodman & Gilman's: The Pharmacological Basis of Therapeutics.* 13th ed. New York: McGraw-Hill; 2017.

62. Sitbon O, Gaine S. Beyond a single pathway: combination therapy in pulmonary arterial hypertension. *Eur Respir Rev.* 2016;25(142):408–417.

63. Tsai H, Sung YK, de Jesus Perez V, et al. Recent advances in the management of pulmonary arterial hypertension. *F1000Res.* 2016;5:2755.

64. Hansmann G. Pulmonary hypertension in infants, children, and young adults. *J Am Coll Cardiol.* 2017;69(20):2551–2569.

General Approach to Cardiothoracic Anesthesia

3

The Cardiac Surgical Patient

Ronak G. Desai, Alann Solina, Donald E. Martin, and Kinjal M. Patel

KEY POINTS

1. Inability to climb two flights of stairs showed a positive predictive value of 82% for postoperative pulmonary or cardiac complications.
2. Silent ischemia is more common in the elderly and in diabetic patients, with 15% to 35% of all myocardial infarctions (MIs) occurring as silent events.
3. Isolated asymptomatic ventricular arrhythmias, even nonsustained ventricular tachycardias (VTs), have not been associated with complications following noncardiac surgery.
4. Patients with left bundle branch block (especially those right coronary artery disease) in whom a Swan–Ganz catheter is being placed are at risk of developing complete heart block during passage of the pulmonary artery catheter.
5. Preoperative hypertension at levels below 180/110 mm Hg has not been found to be an important predictor of increased perioperative cardiac risk, but may be a marker for chronic cardiovascular disease.
6. In patients undergoing cardiac surgery, the presence of carotid stenosis increases the risk of postoperative stroke from approximately 2% in patients without carotid stenosis to 10% with stenosis of greater than 50%, and to 11% to 19% with stenosis of >80%.

7. Percutaneous coronary intervention (PCI) is not therapeutically beneficial when used solely as a means to prepare a patient with coronary artery disease for noncardiac surgery.

8. Elective noncardiac surgery requiring interruption of dual antiplatelet therapy (DAPT) should not be scheduled within 1 month of bare metal stent (BMS) placement or within 6 months of drug-eluting stent (DES) placement.

9. Angiotensin-converting enzyme (ACE) inhibitors and angiotensin II receptor blockers appear to cause perioperative hypotension, so it is prudent to hold these agents the morning of surgery but restart them as soon as the patient is euvolemic postoperatively.

I. Introduction

Cardiovascular disease is our society's biggest health problem. According to Centers for Disease Control and Prevention (CDC) data from 2015, heart disease alone affects 24.8 million Americans, or about 12% of the population [1]. Of the 35 million Americans hospitalized in 2010, 3.9 million (11.1%) had heart disease [2]. Heart disease remains the leading cause of death in patients greater than age 65, with an age-adjusted death rate of 170 per 100,000 population [3]. According to the Society of Thoracic Surgeons (STS) database, 178,780 coronary artery bypass procedures were performed in 2015, which represents a 62% decrease since 2003 and is associated with an increase in the number of percutaneous coronary interventions (PCIs), including angioplasties and stents [4]. In contrast, the number of valve procedures (72,453 in 2015) has increased, with the number of valve repair procedures growing faster than the number of valve replacements [5].

The primary goal of preoperative evaluation and preparation for cardiac surgical procedures is to maximally reduce the patient's risk for morbidity and mortality during surgery and the postoperative period. The factors that are important in determining perioperative morbidity and anesthetic management must be assessed carefully for each patient.

II. Patient presentation

A. Clinical perioperative risk assessment—multifactorial risk indices

Multifactorial risk indices, which identify and assign relative importance to many potential risk factors, have become increasingly sophisticated over the last three decades. They are used to weigh multiple risk factors into a single risk estimate, to determine an individual patient's risk of morbidity and mortality following heart surgery, to guide therapy, and to "risk adjust" the surgical outcomes of populations. One of the first multifactorial risk scores was developed by Paiement, in 1983 [6], which identified eight simple clinical risk factors:

1. Poor left ventricular (LV) function
2. Congestive heart failure (CHF)
3. Unstable angina or myocardial infarction (MI) within 6 months
4. Age greater than 65 years
5. Severe obesity
6. Reoperation
7. Emergency surgery
8. Severe or uncontrolled systemic illness

Recent models still incorporate many of these eight factors.

The preoperative clinical factors that affect hospital survival following heart surgery have been studied by multiple authors from the 1990s until the present time [5,7–11]. The initial studies focused on coronary artery bypass grafting (CABG) surgery, but more recent indices have been validated for valvular surgery and combined valve and CABG surgery as well. Recent models from data collected by the STS (Table 3.1) provide odds ratios of mortality associated with a number of predictors.

In 2001, Dupuis and colleagues developed and validated the cardiac risk evaluation (CARE) score, which incorporated similar factors but viewed them more intuitively in a manner similar to the American Society of Anesthesiologists (ASA) physical status [11]. In 2004, Ouattara and colleagues [12] compared the CARE score to two other multifactorial indices, the Tu score [13] and EuroSCORE [7]. Their analysis found no difference among these scores in predicting

TABLE 3.1 Multifactorial indices of cardiovascular risk for cardiac surgical procedures: summary of risk factors in recent multifactorial indices

Risk factor	STS risk model for mortality (2009[a])	STS risk model for mortality (2009[b])	STS risk model (2009[c])
Surgical procedure(s) studied	CABG	Isolated aortic valve replacement	Valve plus CABG
Measure of risk assessment	Odds ratio	Odds ratio	Odds ratio
Age	1.36–4.7	1.43–3.34	1.29–3.95
Previous cardiac operation	3.13–4.19	2.11–2.48	2.2–2.46
Urgency of surgery	1.16–8	1.29–7.94	1.25–4.56
Left main disease or multiple vessel disease	1.17	N/A	1.12
Severity of angina	1.12	1.21	1.11
Previous MI	1.37–1.7	1.14	1.19–1.55
Cardiogenic shock	1.41–2.29	1.47–1.62	1.43–1.68
CHF	1.21–1.39	1.29–1.83	0.91–1.48
Decreased LVEF	1.19–6.0	1.09–5	1.1–5.5
Supraventricular arrhythmias	1.36	1.2	1.2
Endocarditis	N/A	1.95	2.04
Hypertension	N/A	1.12	N/A
Cerebrovascular disease (CVD)	1.14–1.31	N/A	1.0–1.22
PVD	1.42	1.25	1.29
Chronic obstructive pulmonary disease	1.22–2.35	1.27	1.19
Diabetes mellitus	1.01–1.3	1.27–1.62	1.12–1.31
Renal insufficiency	1.66–3.84	1.55–2.85	1.57–3.20
Female gender	1.31	1.23	1.36
High or low body mass index	1.6–2.2	0.98–1.75	1.04–1.58
Other factors	Immunosuppressive treatment 1.48	Immunosuppressive treatment 1.42 Co-existing mitral stenosis 1.24	Additional valve disease 1.10–1.27 Immunosuppressive therapy 1.35

[a]Shahian DM, O'Brien SM, Filardo G, et al. The Society of Thoracic Surgeons 2008 cardiac surgery risk models: part I—coronary artery bypass grafting surgery. *Ann Thorac Surg.* 2009;88:S2–S22.
[b]O'Brien SM, Shahian DM, Filardo G, et al. The Society of Thoracic Surgeons 2008 cardiac surgery risk models: part 2—isolated valve surgery. *Ann Thorac Surg.* 2009;88:S23–S42.
[c]Shahian DM, O'Brien SM, Filardo G, et al. The Society of Thoracic Surgeons 2008 cardiac surgery risk models: part 3—valve plus coronary artery bypass grafting surgery. *Ann Thorac Surg.* 2009;88:S43–S62.
CABG, coronary artery bypass grafting; CHF, congestive heart failure; LV, left ventricle; MI, myocardial infarction; LVEF, left ventricular ejection fraction; PVD, peripheral vascular disease; N/A, not applicable (either not included in this risk index or not significant); STS, Society of Thoracic Surgeons; the various studies quantify severity of each risk factor in different ways, so a range of values indicates the range of relative risk for all levels of severity.

mortality and morbidity following cardiac surgery. However, the STS continues to report more specific predictors that provide valuable risk data on CABG, valve, and combined procedures based on increasing volumes of cumulative data, making this perhaps the most robust of the risk indices.

B. **Functional status.** For patients undergoing most general and cardiac surgical procedures, perhaps the simplest and single most useful risk index is the patient's functional status, or exercise tolerance. In major noncardiac surgery, Girish and colleagues found the inability to climb two flights of stairs showed a positive predictive value of 82% for postoperative pulmonary or cardiac complications [14]. This is an easily measured and sensitive index of cardiovascular risk that accounts for a wide range of specific cardiac and noncardiac factors.

The level of exercise producing symptoms, as described classically by the New York Heart Association (NYHA) and Canadian Cardiovascular Society classifications, predicts the risk of both an ischemic event and operative mortality. During coronary revascularization procedures, operative mortality for patients with class IV symptoms (e.g., cardiac-induced dyspnea at rest) is 1.4 times that of patients without preoperative CHF [15].

CLINICAL PEARL   The patient's functional status can be a useful marker of cardiovascular risk and help determine the necessity for preoperative cardiac stress testing.

C. **Genomic contributions to cardiac risk assessment.** Genetic variations are the known basis for more than 40 cardiovascular disorders. Some of these, including familial hypercholesteremia, hypertrophic cardiomyopathy, dilated cardiomyopathy, and "channelopathies" such as the long QT syndrome, are known as monogenetic disorders, caused by alterations in one gene. These usually follow traditional Mendelian inheritance patterns, and their genetic basis is relatively easy to identify. Genetic testing is able to identify these diseases in up to 90% of patients before they become symptomatic, allowing prophylactic treatment and early therapy. For example, genetic identification of the subtype of long QT syndrome can determine an affected patient's risk of dysrhythmias associated with exercise, benefit from β-blockers, or need for implantable cardioverter defibrillator (ICD) placement [16].

   Genomic medicine's greatest recent expansion may reside in its application to chronic diseases such as coronary artery and vascular diseases. However, these disorders are multifactorial, influenced by environmental and genetic risk factors. Even when caused solely by genetic factors, it is often due to a complex interaction of many genes. Nevertheless, genetic information can be used to determine a patient's susceptibility to disease, and this information can guide prophylactic therapy. Commercial tests are currently available for susceptibility to atrial fibrillation (AF) and MI. Genetic variants have been found that help to determine susceptibility to perioperative complications, including postoperative MI and ischemia. Similarly, genetic information may be used to determine variations in patient susceptibility to drugs, as for example a single allele variation can render patients much more sensitive to warfarin. Gene therapy may also target drug delivery to specific tissues [16].

D. **Risk associated with surgical problems and procedures.** The complexity of the surgical procedure itself may be the most important predictor of perioperative morbidity for many patients. Most cardiac surgical procedures include cardiopulmonary bypass, which carries its own risks. These risks include a systemic inflammatory response and also the potential for microemboli and hypoperfusion, often involving the central nervous system (CNS), kidneys, lungs, and gastrointestinal tract. The extent of morbidity is proportional to the duration of cardiopulmonary bypass.

   Procedures on multiple heart valves or on both the aortic valve and coronary arteries carry higher morbidity and mortality rates than procedures involving only a single valve or CABG alone. The mortality rate over the last decade for each procedure, for patients in the Society of STS database, is approximately 2.3% for CABG, 3.4% for isolated valve procedures, and 6.8% for valve procedures combined with CABG [5,15,17]. Additionally, the robust STS database (accessed at http://riskcalc.sts.org/stswebriskcalc/#/) can also be used to calculate a patient's statistical likelihood of morbidity and mortality based on several individual risk factors (Table 3.1).

III. **Preoperative medical management of cardiovascular disease**

A. **Myocardial ischemia.** In patients with known coronary artery disease (CAD), the most important preoperative risk factors are: (i) the amount of myocardium at risk; (ii) the ischemic threshold, or the heart rate at which ischemia occurs; (iii) the patient's ventricular function or ejection fraction (EF); (iv) the stability of symptoms (because recent acceleration of angina may reflect a ruptured coronary plaque); and (v) adequacy of current medical therapy.

1. **Stable ischemic heart disease (SIHD).** Also known as chronic stable angina, most often results from obstruction to coronary artery blood flow by a fixed atherosclerotic coronary

lesion in at least one of the large epicardial arteries. In the absence of such a lesion, however, the myocardium may be rendered ischemic by coronary artery spasm, vasculitis, trauma, or hypertrophy of the ventricular muscle, as occurs in aortic valve disease.

Neither the location, duration, or severity of angina, nor the presence of diabetes or peripheral vascular disease (PVD), indicate the extent of myocardium at risk, or the anatomic location of the coronary artery lesions. Therefore, the clinician must depend on diagnostic studies, such as myocardial perfusion imaging (MPI), stress echocardiography, and cardiac catheterization to assist in establishing risk. Some centers use cardiac computed tomography (CT) scanning for this purpose due to its high sensitivity for detecting coronary calcification and coronary artery disease. However, the test still lacks a high enough specificity to be recommended as a definitive test.

In patients with SIHD, a reproducible amount of exercise, with its associated increases in heart rate and blood pressure (BP), often precipitates angina. This angina threshold, which can be determined on preoperative exercise testing, is an important guide to perioperative hemodynamic management. Stable angina often responds to medical therapy as well as to PCI. Patients are referred for CABG surgery when their symptoms are refractory to medical therapy and they are not candidates for PCI.

CLINICAL PEARL Preoperative stress testing can help determine the ischemic threshold, or the heart rate at which ischemic symptoms develop. This can help guide hemodynamic management during the operative procedure.

    a. Principles of the medical management of SIHD [18]
       (1) Aspirin at 75 to 162 mg daily
       (2) β-adrenergic blockade as initial therapy when not contraindicated
       (3) Calcium antagonists or long-acting nitrates as second-line therapy, or as first-line therapy when β-blockade is contraindicated
       (4) Use of angiotensin converting enzyme (ACE) inhibitors indefinitely in patients with LV EF <40%, diabetes, hypertension, or chronic renal failure
       (5) Annual influenza vaccine
       (6) Risk reduction:
          (a) Lipid management—via lifestyle modifications, dietary therapy to reduce saturated fat and trans-fat intake, and moderate- to high-dose statin therapy to reduce low-density lipoproteins.
          (b) BP control—reduce to less than 140/90 for patients with coronary disease initially treated with ACE inhibitors and/or β-blockers, with the addition of thiazide diuretics and calcium channel blockers as necessary.
          (c) Smoking cessation
          (d) Diabetes control
          (e) Weight loss
          (f) Diet and exercise

  2. Acute coronary syndrome (ACS). Sometimes called unstable angina pectoris, crescendo angina, or unstable coronary syndrome.
    a. Presentation:
       (1) Rest angina, within the first week of onset
       (2) New-onset angina markedly limiting activity, within 2 weeks of onset
       (3) Angina that is more frequent, of longer duration, or occurs with less exercise. These symptoms often indicate rapid growth, rupture, or embolus of an existing plaque. Patients in this category have a higher incidence of MI and sudden death, and increased incidence of left main coronary occlusion. The clinical factors important in determining the risk of MI or death in patients with unstable angina are shown in Table 3.2.

TABLE 3.2 Risk factors for death or MI in patients with unstable angina

	High risk	Intermediate risk	Low risk
	Any one of the following	**No high-risk factors, but any of the following**	**No high- or intermediate-risk factors, but any of the following**
History	Accelerated angina within 48 hrs	Prior MI, CVD, PVD, CABG. Aspirin use	
Angina	Prolonged rest angina (>20 min)	Prolonged (>20 min) rest pain, now resolved, with risk factors Rest angina relieved with NTG Nocturnal angina New-onset or progressive class III or IV angina within 2 wks	Increased angina frequency, severity, duration Lower angina threshold New-onset angina
Clinical findings	Pulmonary edema New or worsening MR murmur, S3, rales, hypotension, bradycardia, tachycardia, age >70 yrs	Age >70 yrs	
ECG	Angina at rest with transient >0.5 mm ST changes Bundle branch block or new sustained VT	T-wave changes Pathologic Q waves or resting ST depression less than 1 mm in multiple lead groups	Normal or unchanged ECG
Cardiac markers	Elevated cardiac TnT, TnI (>0.1 ng/mL), or CK-MB elevated	Slightly elevated cardiac TnT, TnI (>0.01 but <0.1 ng/mL) or elevated CK-MB	Normal

CABG, coronary artery bypass grafting; CK-MB, creatine kinase-MB fraction; CVD, cerebrovascular disease; ECG, electrocardiogram; MI, myocardial infarction; MR, mitral regurgitation; NTG, nitroglycerin; PVD, peripheral vascular disease; TnI, troponin I; TnT, troponin T; VT, ventricular tachycardia.
Modified from Anderson et al. ACCF/AHA UA/NSTEMI Guideline Revision. JACC Vol. 57, No. 19, 2011 May 10, 2011:e215–367, with permission.

    b. **Medical management for ACS.** Diagnostic and revascularization procedures are central to the management of most patients with ACS. Most often, medical therapy accompanies or precedes these interventions. Medical management of unstable angina or of a non-ST segment elevation MI (non-STEMI) has two parts: (i) anti-ischemic therapy and (ii) long-term dual antiplatelet therapy (DAPT). Medical anti-ischemic therapy depends largely on the presence or absence of ongoing ischemia and must be accompanied by an aggressive approach to secondary prevention or risk factor modification (Tables 3.3 and 3.4).

3. **Myocardial ischemia without angina** may be manifested by fatigue, rapid onset of pulmonary edema, cardiac arrhythmias, syncope, or an "anginal equivalent," most often characterized as indigestion or jaw pain. Silent ischemia occurs more often in elderly and in diabetic patients, for whom 15% to 35% of all MIs occur as silent events, documented only on routine electrocardiogram (ECG). Whether related to coexisting disease or delayed therapy, silent ischemia has been associated with an unfavorable prognosis.

4. **Interval between prior infarction and surgery**
In the noncardiac surgical population, the occurrence of an MI within the 30 days before surgery is a significant preoperative risk factor [19]. Bernstein [8] assigns additional risk to an MI occurring within 48 hours before surgery. Eagle et al. [20] conclude that CABG has increased risk in patients with unstable angina, early postinfarction angina (within 2 days of a non-STEMI and during an acute MI), and that risk may be reduced by delaying CABG for 3 to 7 days after MI in stable patients. Coronary revascularization procedures, however, offer improved survival in patients with unstable angina and LV dysfunction secondary to ongoing ischemia.

TABLE 3.3   Medical therapy for unstable angina: anti-ischemic therapy

Ongoing ischemia or high-risk factors[a]	Without ongoing ischemia or high-risk factors[a]
β-Blockers in the absence of contraindications[b]	β-Blockers in the absence of contraindications[b]
ACE inhibitors in any patients, especially for those with LV dysfunction (EF <40%), HF, hypertension, or diabetes mellitus	ACE inhibitors in any patients, especially for those with LV dysfunction (EF <40%), HF, hypertension or diabetes mellitus
ARB for those patients with LV dysfunction and HF intolerant to ACE inhibitors	ARB for those patients with LV dysfunction and HF intolerant to ACE inhibitors
Aldosterone receptor blockers for those patients without renal dysfunction or hyperkalemia already receiving ACE inhibitors with LV dysfunction, HF, or diabetes mellitus	Aldosterone receptor blockers for those patients without renal dysfunction or hyperkalemia already receiving ACE inhibitors with LV dysfunction, HF, or diabetes mellitus
Nitrates	
Nondihydropyridine calcium antagonists (verapamil or diltiazem) when β-blockers cannot be used	

[a]ECG changes, or ischemia associated with CHF, S_3 gallop, mitral regurgitation, hemodynamic instability, EF less than 40%, malignant ventricular arrhythmias.
[b]Contraindications to β-blocker therapy:

1. Marked first-degree AV block (ECG PR interval >0.24 sec).
2. Any second- or third-degree AV block without a pacemaker.
3. Asthma.
4. Severe LV dysfunction with CHF (may require slowly increasing doses).
5. COPD: β-Blockers may be used cautiously, beginning with low doses of β-1 selective agents.
6. Patients should not receive β-blockers during episodes of bradycardia (HR <50) or hypotension.

β-blocker, β-adrenergic blockers; LV, left ventricular; EF, ejection fraction; ACE, angiotensin-converting enzyme; ARB, angiotensin receptor blocker; AV, atrioventricular; CHF, congestive heart failure; COPD, chronic obstructive pulmonary disease; HF, heart failure. Adapted with permission from Anderson JL, Adams CD, Antman EM, et al. 2011 ACCF/AHA focused update incorporated into the ACC/AHA 2007 guidelines for the management of patients with unstable angina/non-ST-elevation myocardial infarction: a report of the American College of Cardiology Foundation/American Heart Association task force on practice guidelines. *Circulation.* 2011;123:e426–e579. Accessed August 2, 2011 at http://circ.ahajournals.org/content/123/18/e436.full.pdf

CLINICAL PEARL   Operative risk for CABG in stable postinfarction patients can be reduced by delaying surgery for 3 to 7 days. If the patient has reversible ischemia with significant myocardium at risk, early coronary revascularization offers improved survival.

B. **Congestive heart failure**
1. **Clinical assessment and medical management of heart failure.** Ventricular dysfunction can occur almost immediately in association with an ischemic event. If no infarction

TABLE 3.4   Acute coronary syndrome (ACS) and stable ischemic heart disease (SIHD): the role of dual antiplatelet therapy (DAPT)

ACS: Medical management without stenting	ACS: Medical management and PCI (BMS or DES)	SIHD: Medical management and BMS	SIHD: Medical management and DES
Aspirin—81 mg daily indefinitely	Aspirin—81 mg daily indefinitely	Aspirin—81 mg daily indefinitely	Aspirin—81 mg daily indefinitely
Clopidogrel or ticagrelor daily for 6–12 mo. May continue for longer if low bleeding risk and no overt bleeding	Clopidogrel, plasugrel, or ticagrelor daily for 6–12 mo. May continue for longer if low bleeding risk and no overt bleeding	Clopidogrel daily for at least 1 mo. May continue for longer if low bleeding risk and no overt bleeding	Clopidogrel daily for at least 1 mo. May continue for longer if low bleeding risk and no overt bleeding

BMS, bare metal stent; DES, drug-eluting stent.
Adapted from Levine GN, Bates ER, Bittl JA, et al. 2016 ACC/AHA guideline focused update on duration of dual antiplatelet therapy in patients with coronary artery disease: a report of the American College of Cardiology/American Heart Association Task Force on Clinical Practice Guidelines. *J Thorac Cardiovasc Surg.* 2016;152(5):1243–1275.

occurs and the myocardium is reperfused, the ventricle recovers function quickly. Short episodes of ischemia followed by reperfusion may actually precondition the heart, so when it is exposed to more severe ischemia, the size and severity of MI is reduced. An MI may be associated with "stunned" myocardium, which recovers function within days to weeks, or "hibernating" myocardium, which may recover months after infarction and revascularization. Ventricular dysfunction and HF have been classified into four stages, A through D, based on cardiac structural changes, symptoms of HF, and presence of serum biomarkers (e.g., B-type natriuretic peptide, N-terminal pro-B–type natriuretic peptide). Stage A refers to patients at high risk for HF without overt structural heart disease or symptoms of HF. Stage B patients have structural heart disease, but do not demonstrate signs or symptoms of HF. Patients with structural heart disease who have previously had or currently have symptoms are classified as stage C. Patients with refractory HF who require specialized interventions are classified as stage D. Management depends on the stage of the disease. Figure 3.1 details the current treatment algorithm for stages C and D HF. ACE

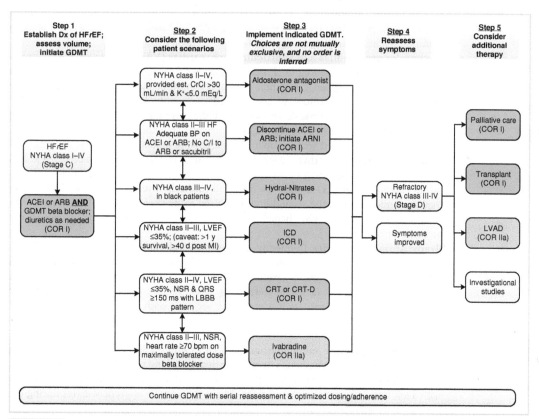

FIGURE 3.1 Treatment of HFrEF stages C and D. For all medical therapies, dosing should be optimized and serial assessment exercised. ACEI indicates angiotensin-converting enzyme inhibitor; ARB, angiotensin receptor blocker; ARNI, angiotensin receptor-neprilysin inhibitor; BP, blood pressure; bpm, beats per minute; C/I, contraindication; COR, Class of Recommendation (lower numbers and letters indicate stronger recommendation); CrCl, creatinine clearance; CRT-D, cardiac resynchronization therapy–device; Dx, diagnosis; GDMT, guideline-directed management and therapy; HF, heart failure; HFrEF, heart failure with reduced ejection fraction; ICD, implantable cardioverter-defibrillator; Hydral-Nitrates, hydralazine and/or nitrates; K+, potassium; LBBB, left bundle branch block; LVAD, left ventricular assist device; LVEF, left ventricular ejection fraction; MI, myocardial infarction; NSR, normal sinus rhythm; and NYHA, New York Heart Association. (Reprinted with permission *Circulation*. 2017;136:e137–e161 ©2017 American Heart Association, Inc.)

inhibitors and angiotensin II receptor blockers are usually used as first-line therapy, with the addition of β-blockers, aldosterone antagonists, diuretics, and implanted devices for more severely affected patients (Fig. 3.1).

2. **Perioperative morbidity.** Preoperative evidence of CHF or ventricular dysfunction is associated with increased operative mortality. Recent series summarized in Table 3.1 show a significantly increased risk of postoperative morbidity or mortality in patients with preoperative CHF and cardiogenic shock.

C. **Dysrhythmias**

1. **Incidence.** While cardiac dysrhythmias are common in patients presenting for cardiac surgery (up to 75%), life-threatening dysrhythmias occur less than 1% of the time.

2. **Supraventricular tachycardia (SVT).** Atrial fibrillation (AF) and flutter, the most common SVTs, increase in frequency with increasing age in the presence of organic heart disease. Initial management consists of heart rate control via intravenous (IV) calcium channel blockers (e.g., verapamil, diltiazem) or β-blockers. Stable reentrant tachycardias can initially be managed acutely with vagal maneuvers or adenosine to reduce heart rate and potentially convert the SVT to sinus rhythm. SVT(s) with hemodynamic instability may require urgent cardioversion. Those with AF are also managed with anticoagulation to reduce stroke risk. More recently, surgical and catheter-based ablation have become more common, especially in patients unresponsive to medical therapy.

3. **Ventricular arrhythmias and ventricular tachycardias (VTs).** Ventricular dysrhythmias have been classified according to clinical presentation (stable or unstable), type of rhythm (sustained or nonsustained VT, bundle branch reentrant or bidirectional VT, Torsades de pointes, ventricular fibrillation), or associated disease entity. Ventricular arrhythmias may lead directly to sudden cardiac death, especially if they occur in the setting of acute or recent infarction. However, isolated asymptomatic ventricular arrhythmias, even nonsustained VT, have not been associated with complications following noncardiac surgery. Patients with preoperative ventricular arrhythmias associated with LV dysfunction and an EF <30% to 35% are often managed with the prophylactic implantation of an ICD. Those not controlled with or not candidates for ICD therapy are managed medically with β-blockers as the first-line therapy. Amiodarone is the second-line drug used to prevent sudden cardiac death, with studies showing some survival benefit. Sotalol can also be effective, though it has greater proarrhythmic effects [21].

4. **Bradycardia.** Anesthetics frequently affect sinus node automaticity but rarely cause complete heart block. Asymptomatic patients with ECG-documented AV conduction disease rarely require temporary pacing perioperatively. However, symptomatic patients, or patients with Mobitz II or complete heart block, require preoperative evaluation for permanent pacing. Patients with a recent MI or with both first-degree AV block and bundle branch block may need temporary transvenous, epicardial, or transcutaneous pacing perioperatively.

Of note, patients with left bundle branch block in whom a Swan–Ganz catheter is being placed may need a transcutaneous pacemaker because of the risk of inducing right bundle branch block, and thus complete heart block. Although the risk is still quite low, patients with a left bundle branch block and right-sided CAD may be at particular risk during the passage of a Swan–Ganz catheter.

D. **Hypertension**

Systemic hypertension is one of the most common diseases of adulthood and is perhaps the most treatable cause of cardiovascular morbidity, including MI, stroke, PVD, renal failure, and HF. The contribution of hypertension to perioperative morbidity and the implications for anesthetic management depend on (i) BP level, both with stress and at rest; (ii) the etiology of hypertension; (iii) pre-existing complications of hypertension; and (iv) physiologic changes due to drug therapy.

1. **Blood pressure level.** Data summarized in the Joint National Committee on Prevention, Detection, Evaluation, and Treatment of High Blood Pressure (JNC 7) report in 2003 indicate that cardiovascular risk begins to increase at BP above 115/75 and doubles with

each increment of 20/10 [22, 22a]. Patients with blood pressures of 120 to 129/<80 are considered to have **elevated** blood pressures [22a]. Stage I hypertension is defined as SBP 130 to 139/DBP 80 to 89. Stage II hypertension is now defined as SBP ≥140/DBP ≥90. Blood pressure lowering medication should be started for patients who have the following:

- Stage I hypertension with previous cardiovascular events.
- Stage I hypertension with estimated 10 years atherosclerotic disease risk of 10% or higher.
- Stage II hypertension [22a]. Those with blood pressures >160/100 usually require combination drug therapy [22].

In contrast to the usual emphasis on the resting, unstimulated BP, the patient's preoperative BP under stress, as in the preoperative clinic or holding area, may be a better predictor of perioperative morbidity. Intraoperative cardiac morbidity in the form of dysrhythmias and ischemic ECG changes may be more frequent in stage 3 hypertensive patients with awake systolic BP greater than 180 mm Hg and diastolic BP of greater than 110 mm Hg, and this morbidity may be reduced by preoperative treatment. In these patients the benefits of improving hypertensive control preoperatively should be weighed against the risks of delaying surgery. BP lower than 180/110 has not been found to be an important predictor of increased perioperative cardiac risk, but it may be a marker for chronic cardiovascular disease [19].

2. **Etiology.** The most common "primary" or "essential" hypertension is likely caused by a combination of multiple genetic and environmental factors, with the genetic contribution (at least) being irreversible. However, it is important preoperatively to exclude the 5% to 15% of patients with treatable causes of secondary hypertension, risk factors for which are shown in Table 3.5. The most common causes of secondary hypertension are renal, endocrine, or drug related, which account for an additional 5% to 10% of hypertensive patients. Other rare disorders are found in less than 1% of patients (Table 3.6). A laboratory investigation of secondary hypertension, when indicated, should include urinalysis, creatinine, glucose, electrolytes, calcium, ECG, and chest films. More extensive testing is usually not indicated unless BP cannot be controlled or a high clinical suspicion exists [22]. Pheochromocytoma, although very rare, is particularly important because of its potential morbidity in association with anesthesia. Therefore, it should be ruled out preoperatively in patients with headache, labile or paroxysmal hypertension, abnormal pallor, or perspiration, even if delay of surgery is required.

3. **Sequelae of hypertension.** The hypertensive state can lead to sequelae most evident in the heart, CNS, and kidney. In particular, patients with established hypertension may exhibit (i) LV hypertrophy leading to decreased ventricular compliance and deleterious effects upon myocardial oxygen supply and demand; (ii) neurologic symptoms, such as headache, dizziness, tinnitus, and blurred vision that may progress to cerebral infarction; and (iii) renal vascular lesions leading to proteinuria, hematuria, and decreased glomerular filtration progressing to renal failure.

4. **Antihypertensive therapy.** Today antihypertensive medications are the most prescribed class of medications. The primary objective of antihypertensive therapy is to reduce cardiovascular morbidity by lowering the BP. However, specific classes of antihypertensive agents are effective in preventing end organ damage, especially to the heart and the kidney, and beyond that are directly associated with lowering the BP. The recommended

TABLE 3.5 Risk factors for secondary hypertension

- Blood pressure (BP) not controlled by two or more agents
- Increase in previously well-controlled BP
- Sudden onset, labile, or paroxysmal hypertension
- Hypertension with onset before age 25 or after age 50

From the sixth report of the Joint National Committee on Prevention, Detection, Evaluation, and Treatment of High Blood Pressure. *Arch Intern Med.* 1997;157:2413–2446.

TABLE 3.6 Causes of hypertension

Medical cause (incidence)	Drug-induced hypertension
Essential hypertension (85–95%)	Amphetamines
	Caffeine
Common causes of secondary hypertension	Cocaine
Renal (2–6%)	Chlorpromazine
Renal parenchymal disease	Cyclosporine
Renovascular disease	Erythropoietin
Endocrine (1–2%)	Ethanol
Pheochromocytoma	Licorice
Cushing disease	MAO inhibitors
Thyroid or parathyroid disease	Nicotine
Hyperaldosteronism	NSAIDs
Aortic coarctation (2–5%)	Oral contraceptives
Sleep apnea (1%)	Steroids
Rare causes of secondary hypertension	Sympathomimetics
Renin-producing tumors	Nasal decongestants
Adrenogenital syndrome	Weight loss regimens
Acromegaly	
Hypercalcemia	
Familial dysautonomia	
Porphyria, neuropathies	

MAO, monamine oxidase; NSAIDs, nonsteroidal anti-inflammatory drugs.
Adapted with permission from Chobanian AV, Bakris GL, Black HR, et al. The seventh report of the joint national committee on prevention, detection, evaluation, and treatment of high blood pressure. *JAMA*. 2003;289:2560–2572.

antihypertensive drug classes for patients with specific comorbid conditions are shown in Table 3.7 [22].

E. Cerebrovascular disease

    1. **The association of preoperative CVD with increased perioperative neurologic dysfunction.** Central nervous system (CNS) dysfunction of at least some degree is common after cardiopulmonary bypass, with temporary postoperative neurocognitive defects occurring in up to 80% of patients and stroke in 1% to 5% [23]. Arrowsmith et al.

TABLE 3.7 Antihypertensive therapy for patients with other systemic diseases

Medical condition	Recommended drug classes
Previous MI[a]	β-Blocker or ACEI
HF[a]	β-Blockers, diuretics, and ACEI
	Add Aldosterone antagonist, if needed
Diabetes[b]:	
Nonblack population	Thiazide-type diuretic or CCB or ACEI or ARB
Black population	Thiazide-type diuretic or CCB as necessary to maintain SBP <140, DBP <90
Recurrent stroke[c]	Diuretics and ACEI
Chronic kidney disease[b]	ACEI or ARB, add other agents as necessary to maintain SBP <140, DBP <90

[a]Aronow WS. Treatment of systemic hypertension. *Am J Cardiovasc Dis*. 2012;2:160–170.
[b]James PA, Oparil S, Carter BL, et al. 2014 evidence-based guideline for the management of high blood pressure in adults: report from the panel members appointed to the Eighth Joint National Committee (JNC 8). *JAMA*. 2014;311:507–520.
[c]Chobanian AV, Bakris GL, Black HR, et al. The seventh report of the joint national committee on prevention, detection, evaluation, and treatment of high blood pressure. *JAMA*. 2003;289:2560–2572.
ACEI, angiotensin-converting enzyme inhibitor; ARB, angiotensin II receptor blocker; CCB, calcium channel blocker; HF, heart failure; MI, myocardial infarction; SBP, systolic blood pressure; DBP, diastolic blood pressure.

found that aortic atherosclerosis is associated with the highest risk of adverse neurologic events (odds ratio 4.52) and that a history of neurologic disease ranked second, with an odds ratio of 3.19 [24]. Patients with a history of stroke are more likely to have a perioperative stroke. Even in the absence of a prior cerebral ischemic event, the presence of carotid stenosis increases the risk of postoperative stroke from approximately 2% in patients without carotid stenosis to 10% with stenosis of greater than 50%, and to 11% to 19% with stenosis of greater than 80% [25].

2. **Genetic factors.** Genetic factors may modify the risk or severity of postoperative CNS injury. Genes related to thrombotic factors and inflammatory factors such as platelet receptors, C-reactive protein, and interleukin-6 have been associated with the risk of postoperative cognitive dysfunction.

3. **Effect of the surgical procedure.** Cardiopulmonary bypass may increase the risk of postoperative cognitive dysfunction, but neurologic deficits are still seen following off pump coronary artery bypass surgery, likely because of effects such as BP lability, low cardiac output, the systemic inflammatory reaction to the procedure, or manipulation of the ascending aorta.

As may be expected, several authors have shown increased postoperative cerebral dysfunction following open aortic or mitral valve procedures compared to CABG. However, in these series, the duration of cardiopulmonary bypass was also longer for the valve procedures, making it difficult to establish a causal relationship. Even though it is apparent that carotid artery stenosis represents a risk factor for perioperative stroke, it is not nearly as clear that simultaneous carotid endarterectomy reduces this risk. Therefore, recent texts advise against combined carotid endarterectomy and CABG procedures [26]. Rather, at the present time epiaortic scanning via ultrasound to modify the surgical technique during the cardiac procedure, and possibly neurophysiologic monitoring, may offer more benefit [26].

CLINICAL PEARL Carotid stenosis is an important risk factor for perioperative stroke during cardiac surgery. However, simultaneous carotid endarterectomy with CABG does not clearly reduce stroke risk and is not routinely recommended even when carotid stenosis exceeds 50%.

IV. Noninvasive cardiac imaging

A. **Echocardiography.** Transthoracic echocardiography provides specific preoperative assessment of several types of cardiac abnormalities. Two-dimensional (2D) and Doppler echocardiography together provide quantitative assessment of the severity of valvular stenoses or insufficiency (see Chapter 12) and of pulmonary hypertension. Assessment of regional wall motion provides a more sensitive and specific assessment of the existence and extent of MI than a surface ECG. 2D echocardiography provides a quantitative assessment of global ventricular function, or EF. Echocardiography can detect even small pericardial effusions and anatomic cardiac abnormalities, including atrial septal defects (ASDs) and ventricular septal defects (VSDs), aneurysms, and mural thrombi.

Perioperative transthoracic echocardiography can predict postoperative cardiac events in noncardiac surgical patients at increased clinical cardiac risk. Decreased preoperative systolic function on echocardiography has been associated with postoperative MI, pulmonary edema, and "major cardiac events," such as ventricular fibrillation, cardiac arrest, or complete heart block. LV hypertrophy, mitral regurgitation (MR), and increased aortic valve gradient on preoperative echo also appear to predict postoperative "major cardiac events."

B. **Preoperative testing for myocardial ischemia.** Commonly used noninvasive testing modalities to evaluate for myocardial ischemic risk for both cardiac and noncardiac surgical patients are described in this section. Patients undergoing cardiac surgery will often require preoperative cardiac catheterization (Section V) to identify any correctible coronary lesions.

1. **Exercise tolerance testing.** The exercise tolerance test (ETT) is often used as a simple and inexpensive initial test to evaluate chest pain of unknown etiology. It is also used

preoperatively to determine functional capacity and identify significant ischemia or dysrhythmias for risk stratification. ETT is rarely useful as a screening test in asymptomatic patients. To better address the prognostic value of the ETT, the Duke risk score was developed [27]. This risk score equals the exercise time in minutes, minus five times the extent of the ST segment depression in millimeters, minus four times the level of angina with exercise (0—no angina, 1—typical angina, 2—typical angina requiring stopping the test). The score typically ranges from −25 to +15. These values correspond to low-risk (with a score of ≥+5), moderate-risk (with scores ranging from −10 to +4), and high-risk (with a score of <−11) categories.

a. **Limitations of ETT**
   (1) Inability to exercise because of systemic disease, particularly PVD.
   (2) Abnormal resting ECG precluding ST segment analysis (paced rhythm, left bundle branch block, LV hypertrophy, digoxin therapy).
   (3) β-Blocker therapy that prevents the patient from achieving 85% of his or her maximum permissible heart rate.

2. **Stress echocardiography.** Stress echocardiography can use exercise stress or pharmacologic stress, with dobutamine, to increase myocardial work. Abnormally contracting myocardial segments seen on stress echocardiography are classified as either *ischemic*, if their reduced contraction pattern is in response to stress, or *infarcted*, if their contractility remains consistently depressed before, during, and after stress.

   Sixteen studies evaluated in the 2007 ACC/AHA Guidelines for Perioperative Cardiovascular Evaluation for noncardiac surgery showed that 0% to 33% of open vascular surgery patients who had a positive preoperative dobutamine stress echocardiogram (DSE) subsequently suffered a postoperative MI or death. The negative predictive value was much higher—93% to 100% [19]. Wall motion abnormalities at low workloads were especially important predictors of short- and long-term outcomes. DSE has indications similar to pharmacologic perfusion imaging with comparable sensitivity, but possibly increased specificity.

   For patients with poor acoustic windows due to body habitus or severe lung disease, myocardial contrast agents (sonicated albumin microspheres) are now available to improve imaging. Still, for some patients, a difficult echocardiographic window or global poor ventricular function may preclude its use. This test may be relatively contraindicated for those patients with conditions that render them more susceptible to the deleterious effects of hypertension and tachycardia (e.g., MI, an intracranial or abdominal aneurysm, or other vascular malformation).

> **CLINICAL PEARL** Preoperative stress testing can help determine how much myocardium is "at risk" for ischemia. This information can identify which noncardiac surgical patients may benefit from a preoperative coronary evaluation and possible intervention.

3. **Radionuclide imaging.** Radionuclide stress imaging is used to assess the perfusion and the viability of areas of myocardium. This technique cannot provide an anatomic diagnosis of a cardiac lesion. It is a more sensitive and specific test than ETT and can provide an assessment of global LV function as well. Myocardial perfusion imaging (MPI) is a nuclear technique employing intravenous radioisotopes, either thallium-201 or the cardiac-specific technetium-99 perfusion agents, sestamibi (Cardiolite), or tetrofosmin (Myoview), as an indicator of the presence or absence of CAD.

   Exercise stress or pharmacologic stress is necessary to increase coronary blood flow for the test. Pharmacologic vasodilators are preferable but contraindicated in patients with severe bronchospastic lung disease, in which case dobutamine may be used. The available pharmacologic vasodilators—adenosine (Adenoscan), dipyridamole (Persantine), and regadenoson (Lexiscan)—are used to produce maximal coronary vasodilation of approximately four to five times resting values. Vessels with fixed coronary stenoses will not dilate, resulting in less isotope reaching the myocardium. Myocardium underperfused by these vessels will show up as a "defect" on stress scans when compared to surrounding myocardium supplied by nonobstructed coronaries. When compared to the images acquired at rest, any defects still present—*fixed* or *persistent defects*—are suggestive of nonviable or infarcted myocardium. Defects present on stress and not at rest, termed *reversible defects*, suggest viable myocardium at risk for ischemia when stressed. The technique used to acquire these images is single-photon emission computed tomography (SPECT).

In the studies of noncardiac surgical patients reviewed by the ACC/AHA Task Force on Perioperative Cardiovascular Evaluation, reversible defects on nuclear perfusion scanning identified 2% to 20% of patients suffering postoperative MI or cardiac death. The negative predictive value of a normal scan is much better, at approximately 99%. Fixed defects did not usually predict perioperative cardiac events. The sensitivity and specificity of nuclear perfusion imaging is similar for pharmacologic and stress-based techniques [19]. The predictive value of the test can be improved by using it in high-risk subgroups.

Contraindications to pharmacologic stress with dipyridamole, adenosine, or regadenoson are:

- unstable angina or MI within 48 hours.
- severe primary bronchospasm.
- methylxanthine ingestion within 24 hours.
- allergy to dipyridamole or aminophylline.
- for adenosine only, first-degree heart block (PR interval >0.28 seconds) and recent oral dipyridamole ingestion (<24 hours ago).

Pharmacologic vasodilators should be used in patients who cannot exercise, or who have a medical condition (e.g., cerebral aneurysm) that would contraindicate exercise. Pharmacologic stress testing with vasodilators, such as adenosine or dipyridamole, is also preferable to exercise or dobutamine in patients with left bundle branch block, because of misleading septal changes with exercise or catecholamines, which lead to false positive tests.

4. **Positron emission tomography (PET) scan.** PET scanning techniques use different radioisotopes than SPECT imaging. These isotopes decay with a higher-energy photon with a shorter half-life and can assess both regional myocardial blood flow and myocardial metabolism on a real-time basis. PET scanning techniques can be combined with CT and magnetic resonance imaging (MRI) to provide PET metabolic and anatomic information simultaneously.

5. **Magnetic resonance imaging.** MRI has been used for some time to provide both high-resolution and three-dimensional (3D) imaging of cardiac structures. It is now becoming important in perfusion imaging, atherosclerosis imaging, and coronary artery imaging. With the development of dedicated cardiovascular MRI scanning, molecular imaging techniques and biochemical markers are providing the capacity for MRI diagnosis of cardiac function. Changes in molecular composition of the myocardium can change its magnetic moment and MRI signal, allowing MRI to detect lipid accumulation, edema, fibrosis, rate of phosphate turnover, and intracellular pH in ischemic areas. Finally, MRI imaging can be gated to the cardiac cycle, allowing rapid and accurate assessment of myocardial function. Gated images are used to detect regional myocardial abnormalities that may be caused by ischemia, infarction, stunning, hibernation, and postinfarct remodeling. MRI is the diagnostic technique of choice for arrhythmogenic right ventricular (RV) dysplasia and can differentiate myocardial infiltration and diastolic dysfunction associated with sarcoidosis, hemochromatosis, amyloidosis, and endomyocardial fibrosis. Contrast-enhanced MRI has a higher sensitivity and specificity than either CT scan or TEE in aortic dissection. Dobutamine stress MRI is an accurate and rapid test for myocardial ischemia that may eventually replace dobutamine echocardiography.

MRI can be used to diagnose CAD involving the native major epicardial arteries with an accuracy of approximately 87% and is even better for assessing saphenous vein and internal mammary artery graft patency. However, it is still not commonly used clinically for this purpose.

6. **Computed tomography.** Since its introduction into clinical practice in 1973, CT has undergone significant advances. CT for calcium scoring has been utilized clinically to estimate cardiac risk, but is not effective for defining atherosclerotic disease. With the development of a higher temporal resolution scan, in conjunction with contrast injection, coronary imaging is now possible. As these imaging techniques advance in the cardiology arena, they can be used for imaging the pericardium, cardiac chambers, and great vessels. However, imaging protocols require aggressive β-blockade to achieve heart rates of 60 bpm or less in order to decrease image blurring and improve resolution.

Cardiac CT with calcium scoring is gaining widespread acceptance due to its excellent negative predictive value in determining coronary artery disease in patients without significant risk factors (advanced age, diabetes, hypertension). However, patients at higher risk for coronary artery disease should still be tested via other more established diagnostic techniques at this time.

V. Cardiac catheterization

A. **Overview.** Cardiac catheterization still is considered the gold standard for diagnosis of cardiac pathology before most open heart operations and for definition of lesions of the coronary vessels. More than 95% of all patients undergoing open heart operations have had catheterization prior to the procedure. The remaining 5% are assessed only by noninvasive techniques, such as echocardiography and Doppler flow studies. They typically have pathologic findings, such as an atrial or ventricular septal defect, that are adequately defined by noninvasive means.

As an invasive procedure, serious complications occur in approximately 0.1% of patients and include stroke, heart attack, and death. Significant access site complications occur in approximately 0.5%.

If only coronary anatomy is to be delineated, often only a systemic-arterial or left-sided catheterization will be performed. However, if any degree of LV dysfunction, valvular abnormality, pulmonary disease, or impaired RV function exists clinically, a right-sided (Swan–Ganz) catheterization usually will also be performed. A range of normal hemodynamic values obtained from right- and left-sided catheterization is included in Table 3.8.

Interpretation of catheterization data emphasizes the following areas, detailed below.

TABLE 3.8   Normal hemodynamic values obtained at cardiac catheterization

Parameter	Measurement	Value
Peripheral arterial or aortic pressure	Systolic/diastolic Mean	≤140/90 mm Hg ≤105 mm Hg
Right atrial pressure	Mean	≤6 mm Hg
Right ventricular (RV) pressure	Systolic/end diastolic	≤30/6 mm Hg
Pulmonary artery pressure	Systolic/diastolic Mean	≤30/15 mm Hg ≤22 mm Hg
Pulmonary artery wedge pressure	Mean	≤12 mm Hg
Left ventricular (LV) pressure	Systolic/end diastolic	≤140/12 mm Hg
Cardiac index		2.5–4.2 L/min/m^2
End-diastolic volume index		<100 mL/m^2
Arteriovenous O$_2$ content difference		≤5.0 mL/dL
Pulmonary vascular resistance		20–130 dynes · sec/cm^5 Or 0.25–1.6 Wood units
Systemic vascular resistance		700–1,600 dynes sec/cm^5 Or 9–20 Wood units

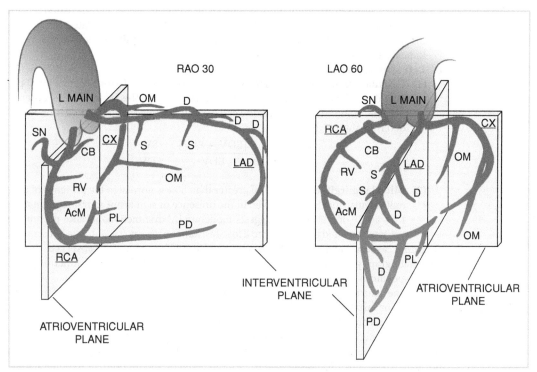

FIGURE 3.2 Representation of coronary anatomy relative to the interventricular and atrioventricular valve planes. Coronary branches are L MAIN, left main; LAD, left anterior descending; D, diagonal; S, septal; CX, circumflex; OM, obtuse marginal; RCA, right coronary artery; CB, conus branch; SN, sinus node; AcM, acute marginal; PD, posterior descending; PL, posterolateral left ventricular; RV, right ventricle; RAO 30, right anterior oblique 30 degree view; LAO 60, left anterior oblique 60 degree view. (Reproduced from Baim DS, Grossman W. Coronary angiography. In: Grossman W, ed. *Cardiac Catheterization and Angiography.* 7th ed. Philadelphia, PA: Lea & Febiger; 2005:203, with permission.)

B. **Assessment of coronary anatomy**
1. **Procedure.** Radiopaque contrast is injected through a catheter placed at the coronary ostia to delineate the anatomy of both the right and left coronary arteries. Multiple views are important to define branch lesions, decrease artifacts at points of tortuosity or vessel overlap, and determine more clearly the degree of stenosis, particularly in eccentric lesions. Two common projections of the coronary arteries are the right anterior oblique (RAO) and the left anterior oblique (LAO) views (Fig. 3.2).
2. **Interpretation.** The degree of vessel stenosis generally is assessed by the percent reduction in diameter of the vessel, which in turn correlates with the reduction in cross-sectional area of the vessel at the point of narrowing. Lesions that reduce vessel diameter by greater than 50%, reducing the cross-sectional area by greater than 70%, are considered significant. Lesions are also characterized as either focal or segmental. There is a great deal of interobserver variability in interpretation with particular concern regarding intermediate lesions (50% to 70%) and their physiologic significance. Adjunct imaging techniques include fractional flow reserve (FFR) and intravascular ultrasound (IVUS) that may assist in defining the need for revascularization of these vessels.
C. **Assessment of left ventricular function.** Both global and regional measures of ventricular function can be obtained from catheterization data.
1. **Global ventricular measurements**
   a. **Left ventricular end-diastolic pressure (LVEDP).** An elevated value above 15 mm Hg usually indicates some degree of ventricular dysfunction. LVEDP is an index that may reflect either systolic or diastolic dysfunction and is acutely affected by preload and

afterload. Without examining other indices of function, an isolated measurement of elevated LVEDP simply indicates that something is abnormal. Associated with a normal LV contractile pattern and cardiac output, an elevated LVEDP measurement may indicate a decrease in LV compliance.

b. Left ventricular EF (LVEF)

   (1) Calculation. EF is defined as the volume of blood ejected (stroke volume [SV]) per beat divided by the volume in the LV before ejection. The SV is equal to the end-diastolic volume (EDV) minus the end-systolic volume (ESV). The equation for EF determination is therefore:

$$EF = \frac{[EDV - ESV]}{EDV} = \frac{SV}{EDV}$$

   (2) Mitral regurgitation. An EF of greater than 50% is normal in the presence of normal valvular function. However, in the presence of significant mitral regurgitation MR, an EF of 50% to 55% suggests moderate LV dysfunction, because part of the volume is ejected backward into a low-resistance pathway (i.e., into the left atrium).

2. **Regional assessment of ventricular function.** LV contraction observed during ventriculography provides a qualitative assessment of overall ventricular function but is not as specific as the calculated EF.

   Routine ventriculography is less commonly performed when concerns for contrast volume, patient instability, or prior assessment of function are present. Qualitative regional differences in contraction may be evident. For examination, the heart is divided into segments. The anterior, posterior, apical, basal, inferior (diaphragmatic), and septal regions of the LV are examined (Fig. 3.3). Motion of each one of these particular regions is defined as normal, hypokinetic (decreased inward motion), akinetic (no motion), or dyskinetic (outward paradoxical motion) in relation to the other normally contracting segments. Regional wall motion abnormalities are usually secondary to prior infarction or acute ischemia. However, very infrequently myocarditis as well as rare infiltrative processes by myocardial tumors may lead to regional wall motion abnormalities.

D. Assessment of valvular function. This section will be limited to a brief discussion of the methods utilized to study lesions of the aortic and mitral valves. The specific hemodynamic patterns of acute and chronic valvular disease will be discussed in Chapters 11 and 12.

1. **Regurgitant lesions**

   a. Qualitative assessment. A relative scale of 1+ to 4+ (4+ being the most severe) is used to quantify the severity of valvular incompetence during the injection of echogenic contrast dye. Visual inspection is utilized to determine the intensity and rapidity of washout of dye from the LV after aortic root injection (aortic regurgitation) or from the left atrium after ventricular injection (MR).

   b. Pathologic V waves. In patients with mitral regurgitation MR, the pulmonary capillary wedge trace may manifest giant V waves. Normal or physiologic V waves are seen in the left atrium at the end of systole and are secondary to filling from the pulmonary veins against a closed mitral valve. With valvular incompetence, the regurgitant wave into the left atrium is superimposed on a physiologic V wave, producing a giant V wave (Fig. 3.4).

2. **Stenotic lesions.** The severity of valvular stenosis can be determined only by knowing the pressure drop across the stenotic valve *and* the simultaneous flow across the stenosis during either systolic ejection or diastolic filling. One cannot uniformly assess the severity of stenosis solely by examining the pressure gradient across the valve.

   Gorlin and Gorlin [28] described an equation for determining valve area based on these two factors in the *American Heart Journal* in 1951. A simplified version of this equation is:

$$Valve\ area = \frac{cardiac\ output\ (L/min)}{\sqrt{mean\ pressure\ gradient}}$$

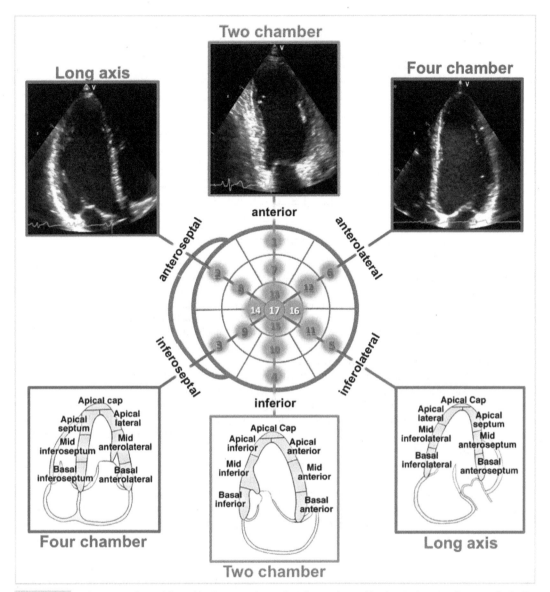

FIGURE 3.3 Orientation of apical four-chamber, apical two-chamber, and apical long-axis views in relation to the bull's-eye display of the left ventricular (LV) segments (**center**). The center diagram depicts the commonly accepted numbering system used to identify LV wall segments. Top panels show actual images, and bottom panels schematically depict the LV wall segments in each view. (Reprinted with permission from Recommendations for Cardiac Chamber Quantification by Echocardiography in Adults: An Update from the American Society of Echocardiography and the European Association of Cardiovascular Imaging. *J Am Soc Echocardiogr*. 2015;28:1–39.)

With the peak pressure gradient and cardiac output given on the catheterization report, a quick estimate of either aortic or mitral valve area can be made. For greater accuracy, the denominator of the Gorlin equation is corrected for systolic ejection time (aortic valve) or diastolic filling time (mitral valve). Values for normal and abnormal valve areas are discussed in Chapters 11 and 12.

Remember that catheterization data represent only one point in time, and medical management may have changed the hemodynamic pattern and catheterization results at the time of cardiac operation.

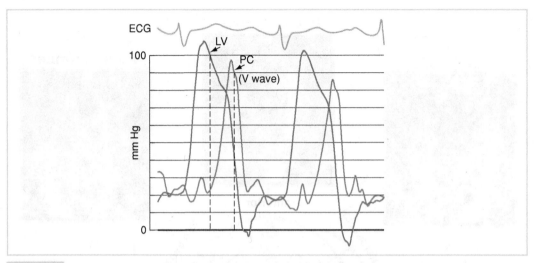

FIGURE 3.4 Left ventricular (LV) and pulmonary capillary wedge (PC) pressure tracings taken in a patient with ruptured chordae tendineae and acute mitral insufficiency. The giant V wave results from regurgitation of blood into a relatively small and noncompliant left atrium; ECG illustrates the timing of the PC V wave, whose peak follows ventricular repolarization, as manifest by the T wave of the ECG. (Reproduced from Grossman W. Profiles in valvular heart disease. In: Grossman W, Baim DS, eds. *Cardiac Catheterization, Angiography, and Intervention.* 7th ed. Philadelphia, PA: Lea & Febiger; 2005:642, with permission.)

VI. **Interventional cardiac catheterization**

A. **PCI.** In 1977, Andreas Gruentzig brought therapeutic options to cardiac catheterization practice with the first percutaneous transluminal coronary angioplasty (PTCA). Multiple technologies have been advanced since the initial balloon dilation. Current technology has evolved to include niche devices including rotational coronary atherectomy (e.g., Rotablator), various thrombectomy techniques, distal protection devices for saphenous vein grafts, vascular closure devices, and coronary stents [29].

However, post-PCI restenosis, a recurrent blockage resulting from a local vascular response to injury, occurs in one-third of balloon dilations and limits their effectiveness. Intracoronary stents were developed to provide local stabilization for PCI-induced coronary dissection and to prevent restenosis. Their widespread use has significantly reduced the need for emergent coronary bypass surgery. The original bare metal stents (BMS) reduced restenosis rates significantly, while DES covered with polymer-based antiproliferative medications have reduced restenosis rates an additional 39% to 61% [30–32].

The need for emergency coronary artery bypass graft surgery (CABG) has dramatically decreased with the use of coronary artery stents. Emergency CABG in patients undergoing PCI decreased from 2.9% before the use of stents to 0.3% with stents [33–35]. In 2009 the National Cardiovascular Data Registry (NCDR) reported the rate of emergency CABG following PCI as 0.4% [36].

Several studies have reported on the frequency of procedure-related indications for emergent CABG following PCI. These include dissection (27%), acute vessel closure (16%), perforation (8%), and failure to cross the lesion (8%). Three-vessel disease was also present in 40% of patients requiring emergency CABG [34]. The strongest predictors of the need for emergency CABG in several studies, however, are cardiogenic shock (OR = 11.4), acute MI or emergent PCI (OR = 3.2 to 3.8), multivessel or three-vessel disease (OR = 2.3 to 2.4), and complicated (type C) coronary lesion (OR = 2.6) [34]). In-hospital mortality for emergency CABG after PCI ranges from 6% to 15% [34,37,38].

When comparing CABG to PCI revascularization for patient survival, the 2011 American College of Cardiology Foundation/American Heart Association Guideline for CABG suggests improved survival in patients with greater than 50% left main coronary artery stenosis (class I evidence). In patients with three-vessel disease and greater than 70% stenosis or proximal left anterior descending disease plus additional major stenosis, CABG imparts improved survival over PCI as well (class I). Either CABG or PCI may improve survival in those who survive sudden cardiac death due to VT caused by significant coronary artery stenosis (class I) [39].

7   Though a large proportion of patients come for surgery with a history of PCI at some time in the past, it is now well established that PCI is not beneficial when used solely as a means to prepare a patient with coronary artery disease for surgery.

B. Preoperative management of patients with prior interventional procedures

1. **Postcoronary stent antiplatelet therapy and stent thrombosis**

   a. **Coronary artery stent thrombosis**

   Coronary artery stents are effective in preventing restenosis, but as foreign bodies they increase the long-term, and perhaps even permanent, risk of coronary artery thrombosis. Metal stents are associated with the greatest inflammatory response in the first 4 to 6 weeks, which then leads to reepithelialization and a decrease in the risk of subsequent thrombosis after approximately 6 weeks. In contrast, DES are designed to inhibit inflammation and so these stents remain exposed for a much longer period of time, and so are associated with a much longer risk of stent thrombosis, extending at least to (and perhaps much longer than), 1 year. Unfortunately, there is no reliable way to determine when endothelialization actually occurs.

   Because thrombosis occurs quickly, in comparison to restenosis, it is associated with a very high risk (greater than 50% in some series) of MI and death. Therefore, antiplatelet therapy is required to reduce the risk of thrombosis. Antiplatelet therapy may be particularly useful in the perioperative period, with the associated thrombotic risk during that time.

   b. **Antiplatelet agents**

   Aspirin and clopidogrel have been the mainstays of antiplatelet therapy. Since they work by different mechanisms, they have at least an additive, or perhaps superadditive effect. Ticlopidine is approximately as effective as clopidogrel in reducing the risk of thrombosis, but does have greater side effects. More recently, prasugrel, ticagrelor, and vorapaxar have been introduced, which may provide new therapeutic options preoperatively. Table 3.9 compares the properties of all of these agents except vorapaxar.

   Prasugrel and ticagrelor have both been found to have more consistent inhibition of platelet activity when compared to clopidogrel, suggesting a reduced risk of stent thrombosis, and of consequent MI and death. They are frequently used as second-line agents in patients at high risk for stent thrombosis, but there is growing evidence for their efficacy as primary agents in patients requiring DAPT. Additionally, ticagrelor appears to have a similar efficacy and a much more rapid onset and shorter duration, because of its reversible binding to $P2Y_{12}$ adenosine diphosphate (ADP) receptors.

TABLE 3.9   Antiplatelet agents commonly used to prevent coronary stent thrombosis

Drug	Drug class (mechanism)	Dosage form	Commonly used dose	Duration of action[a]
Aspirin	Salicylate (Cyclooxygenase inhibition)	Oral	325 mg loading dose 81 mg daily	7 days
Clopidogrel (Plavix)	Thienopyridine (Platelet receptor $P2Y_{12}$ ADP receptor blockade)	Oral[b]	300 mg loading dose 75 mg daily	7 days
Ticlopidine (Ticlid)	Thienopyridine (Platelet receptor $P2Y_{12}$ ADP receptor blockade)	Oral[b]	500 mg loading dose 250 mg b.i.d.	10 days
Prasugrel (Effient)	Thienopyridine (Platelet receptor $P2Y_{12}$ ADP receptor blockade)	Oral[b]	600 mg loading dose 10 mg daily	7 days
Ticagrelor[a] (Brilinta)	Nucleoside analog (Reversible platelet receptor $P2Y_{12}$ ADP receptor blockade)	Oral	180 mg loading dose 90 mg b.i.d.	2 days

[a]Information from the FDA-approved package insert.
[b]All three thienopyridines are prodrugs.
From Michelson AD. Advances in antiplatelet therapy. *Hematology Am Soc Hematol Educ Program*. 2011;62–69.

TABLE 3.10 Risk factors for coronary stent thrombosis

Clinical	Angiographic
Advanced age	Long stents
Acute coronary syndrome (ACS)	Multiple lesions
Diabetes	Overlapping stents
Low ejection fraction	Ostial or bifurcation stents
Prior brachytherapy	Small vessels
Renal failure	Suboptimal stent results

From Grines CL, Bonow RO, Casey DE Jr, et al. Prevention of premature discontinuation of dual antiplatelet therapy in patients with coronary artery stents. *Circulation.* 2007;115:813–818.

Vorapaxar blocks the action of thrombin on the platelet PAR-1 receptor, providing yet a third mechanism of inhibiting platelet activation.

c. **Prevention of coronary artery stent thrombosis**

Continuous treatment with the combination of aspirin and a $P2Y_{12}$ ADP antagonist after PCI reduces major adverse cardiac events (MACE). On the basis of randomized clinical trials, aspirin 75 to 100 mg (81 mg in the United States) daily should be given indefinitely [40].

Regarding, $P2Y_{12}$ inhibitors (thienopyridines), their duration of therapy is dependent on the indication for stent placement (SIHD vs. ACS). A SIHD indication suggests $P2Y_{12}$ inhibition after BMS placement should be continued for a minimum of 1 month, as the second part of DAPT. For DES, a SIHD indication for stent placement suggests a minimum of 6 months therapy with $P2Y_{12}$ inhibitors in all patients [40]. For patients presenting with ACS, DAPT is indicated for a minimum of 12 months (6 months if elevated bleeding risk) (see Table 3.4).

In the United States, there are currently four approved drug-eluting stents (DES): sirolimus-eluting stents (SES), paclitaxel-eluting stents (PES), zotarolimus-eluting stents (ZES), and everolimus-eluting stents (EES). Each of these stents is presumed to be associated with delayed healing and a longer period of risk for thrombosis compared with BMS, and requires a longer duration of DAPT. Current guidelines recommend at least 6 months of DAPT following any DES in order to avoid late (after 30 days) thrombosis. As of July 2016, there is also an approved bioabsorbable stent available for the treatment of coronary artery disease.

There is a growing trend among cardiologists to extend DAPT beyond 1 year (possibly indefinitely) provided the patient has not had any overt bleeding episodes and is not at a high risk for bleeding complications. Late stent thrombosis risk (after 1 year) is likely higher in DES than in BMS and has been observed at a rate of 0.2% to 0.4% per year. The greatest risk of stent thrombosis is within the first year regardless of stent type and ranges from 0.7% to 3% depending on patient and lesion complexity [41].

Risk factors for both early and late stent thrombosis are shown in Table 3.10. In addition, of course, any subsequent surgery would result in increased thrombotic risk in the perioperative period.

CLINICAL PEARL For patients with SIHD in whom coronary stent placement is required, DAPT should be continued for a minimum of 1 month after BMS placement and 6 months after DES placement. In patients requiring coronary stent placement after ACS, DAPT should be continued for at least 12 months.

d. **Perioperative antiplatelet therapy in patients with coronary artery stents**

According to current recommendations, elective noncardiac surgery requiring interruption of DAPT should not be scheduled within 1 month of BMS placement or within

6 months of DES placement [39]. Urgent or emergent surgeries require communication between the patient's cardiologist, anesthesiologist, and the surgical team. However, most guidelines recommend that, for those procedures which cannot be delayed, if the thienopyridine must be stopped, it should be stopped as close to surgery as possible, and restarted as soon as possible postoperatively, and aspirin should be continued if at all possible [40,42]. In cardiac surgery, the preoperative use of aspirin has resulted in greater blood loss and need for reoperation, but no increase in mortality, and is in fact associated with an increased saphenous vein graft patency rate [19].

VII. Management of preoperative medications

A. **β-Adrenergic blockers.** β-Adrenergic blockers are used commonly for the treatment of hypertension, stable and unstable angina, as well as for MI. These drugs can also be used to treat SVT (including that due to pre-excitation syndromes), LV systolic dysfunction (if not severe) and the manifestations of systemic disease ranging from hyperthyroidism to migraine headaches. β-Blocker therapy is beneficial in the perioperative period, and the magnitude of the benefit is directly proportional to the patient's cardiac risk [44]. Further, abrupt withdrawal of β-blockers can lead to a rebound phenomenon, manifested as nervousness, tachycardia, palpitations, hypertension, and even MI, ventricular arrhythmias, and sudden death. Many authors have found that preoperative treatment with β-blocking agents reduces perioperative tachycardia and lowers the incidence of ischemic events [19,43]. Therefore, administration of β-blockers should continue for patients on treatment chronically [44]. Continuation of preoperative β-blockade therapy intraoperatively and postoperatively is also essential to avoid rebound phenomenon.

B. **Statins (HMG-CoA inhibitors).** Statins are used chronically to reduce the levels of low-density lipoproteins. However, they have also been shown to slow coronary artery plaque formation, increase plaque stability, improve endothelial function, and exhibit antithrombogenic, anti-inflammatory, antiproliferative, and leukocyte-adhesion–limiting effects. All of these effects would be expected to reduce both short- and long-term cardiovascular morbidity. Several large recent studies have shown that preoperative statin use resulted in a significant reduction in postoperative mortality and MACE [45–47].

Currently, we are unaware of the duration of statin use needed to provide a beneficial effect or whether discontinuing statins several days preoperatively will reduce their protective effect. However, until more is known, it would be wise to continue statins preoperatively in those patients already taking the drugs, while recognizing the small incremental risks of hepatotoxicity and rhabdomyolysis.

C. **Anticoagulant and antithrombotic medication**

1. Warfarin—approaches to preoperative therapy for patients taking chronic warfarin for (a) AF, (b) mechanical prosthetic heart valve, or (c) DVT/pulmonary embolus were published by the American College of Chest Physicians in 2012 [48]. An approach to risk stratification for thromboembolism is shown in Table 3.11. Warfarin should be stopped 5 days prior to surgery and restarted within 12 to 24 hours after surgery. A suggested approach to periprocedural anticoagulation bridging with low–molecular-weight heparin is shown in Table 3.12.

2. Factor Xa inhibitors (e.g., rivaroxaban, apixaban) are a newer generation of oral medications that have been approved for stroke prevention in patients in AF. Additionally, dabigatran, a direct thrombin inhibitor, is a potent, nonpeptide small molecule that reversibly inhibits both free and clot-bound thrombin. It has also been approved for stroke prevention in patients with AF. Though peak effect occurs in 2 to 4 hours after administration, its estimated half-life is 15 hours with normal renal function. Based on the pharmacokinetics, in patients with normal renal function (eGFR >50 cc/min) discontinuation of two doses results in a decrease in the plasma level to about 25% of baseline and discontinuation of four doses will decrease the level to about 5% to 10% [49]. Restarting dabigatran for patients on chronic therapy after cardiac surgery should be delayed until 48 to 72 hours postoperatively due to the drug's quick onset of action [50].

3. **Antithrombotic and antiplatelet therapy** with agents such as clopidogrel (Plavix), cilostazol (Pletal), or combinations of agents should be stopped 1 week preoperatively, if

TABLE 3.11 Preoperative risk stratification for perioperative thromboembolism

	Indication for VKA therapy		
Risk stratum	Mechanical heart valve	Atrial fibrillation (AF)	Venous thromboembolism (VTE)
High[a]	Mitral valve prosthesis Caged ball or tilting disc aortic valve prosthesis CVA or TIA <6 mo ago	CHADS$_2$ score of 5 or 6	VTE <3 mo ago Severe thrombophilia (protein C, S, ATIII deficiency, etc.)
Moderate	Bileaflet aortic valve prosthesis and one or more of the following risk factors: atrial fibrillation AF, prior CVA or TIA, hypertension, diabetes, CHF, age >75 yrs	CHADS$_2$ score of 3 or 4	VTE 3–12 mo ago Nonsevere thrombophilia (prothrombin gene mutation, etc.) Recurrent VTE Active or recently treated cancer
Low	Bileaflet aortic valve prosthesis without atrial fibrillation AF and no other risk factors for stroke	CHADS$_2$ score of 0–2 (No prior stroke or TIAs)	VTE >12 mo ago, no other risk factors

[a]High-risk patients may also include those with a prior stroke or transient ischemic attack occurring >3 months before the planned surgery and a CHADS$_2$ score <5, those with prior thromboembolism during temporary interruption of VKAs, or those undergoing certain types of surgery associated with an increased risk for stroke or other thromboembolism (e.g., cardiac valve replacement, carotid endarterectomy, major vascular surgery).

CHADS$_2$, congestive heart failure, hypertension, age 75 years, diabetes mellitus, and stroke or transient ischemic attack; VKA, vitamin K antagonist; CVA, cerebrovascular accident; TIA, transient ischemic attack.

Reprinted with permission from Douketis JD, Spyropoulos AC, Spencer FA, et al. Perioperative management of antithrombotic therapy: antithrombotic therapy and prevention of thrombosis, 9th ed.: American College of Chest Physicians Evidence-Based Clinical Practice Guidelines. *Chest.* 2012;141(2 Suppl):e326S–e350S.

possible. Because of a concern for longer duration of action, ticlopidine (Ticlid) should be discontinued 2 weeks preoperatively, using other agents as a bridge to surgery, if needed. Glycoprotein IIb/IIIa Inhibitors (eptifibatide, tirofiban, abciximab) should be stopped approximately 48 hours preoperatively. Fondaparinux (Arixtra), a low-molecular heparin compound, should be stopped 5 days preoperatively (5 half-lives).

D. **Antihypertensives**

Preoperatively, chronic antihypertensive medications should usually be continued until the morning of surgery, and be begun again as soon as the patient is hemodynamically stable postoperatively. Continuation of β-blockers and α-2 agonists until the morning of surgery are particularly important because of the risks of rebound hypertension with sudden withdrawal of these drugs. In contrast, patients receiving ACE inhibitors and angiotensin II receptor blockers appear to be particularly prone to perioperative hypotension, so several authors recommend holding these agents the morning of surgery but restarting them as soon as the patient is euvolemic postoperatively [51].

TABLE 3.12 Suggested periprocedural anticoagulation bridging strategies

Thromboembolism risk from mechanical HV, AF, VTE	High risk		Intermediate risk		Low risk
Procedural bleeding risk	High	Low	High	Low	
Periprocedural action	Bridging[a]	Bridging[a]	No bridging[b]	Consider bridging[b]	No bridging

[a]For high-bleed risk procedures: wait a full 48 to 72 hours before reinitiating postprocedural heparin (LMWH) bridging (especially treatment dose); stepwise increase in postprocedural heparin (LMWH) dose from prophylactic dose first 24 to 48 hours to intermediate/treatment dose; no postprocedural heparin (LMWH) bridging in very high-bleed risk procedures (i.e., major neurosurgical or cardiovascular surgeries) but use of mechanical prophylaxis.

[b]Based on individual patient- and procedural-related risk factors for thrombosis and bleeding.

From Spyropoulos AC, Douketis JD. How I treat anticoagulated patients undergoing an elective procedure or surgery. *Blood.* 2012;120:2954–2962.

E. **Antidysrhythmics**
Preoperative patients may require any of a large number of oral antidysrhythmic agents, including amiodarone, or calcium channel blockers. Therapy for dysrhythmias should be continued perioperatively.

REFERENCES

1. Blackwell DL, Villarroel MA. Tables of Summary Health Statistics for U.S. Adults: 2015 National Health Interview Survey. National Center for Health Statistics. 2016. Available from https://ftp.cdc.gov/pub/Health_Statistics/NCHS/NHIS/SHS/2015_SHS_Table_A-1.pdf. Accessed July 2, 2017.
2. Number and rate of discharges by first-listed diagnostic categories: National Hospital Discharge Survey 2010. Available from https://www.cdc.gov/nchs/data/nhds/2average/2010ave2_firstlist.pdf. Accessed July 2, 2017.
3. Xu J, Murphy SL, Kochanek KD, et al. Deaths: Final data for 2013. *Natl Vital Stat Rep.* 2016;64(2):1–119.
4. Number and rate by selected surgical and nonsurgical procedure categories: National Hospital Discharge Survey 2010. Available from https://www.cdc.gov/nchs/data/nhds/4procedures/2010pro4_numberrate.pdf. Accessed July 2, 2017.
5. Shahian DM, O'Brien SM, Filardo G, et al. The Society of Thoracic Surgeons 2008 cardiac surgery risk models: part 3—valve plus coronary artery bypass grafting surgery. *Ann Thorac Surg.* 2009;88:S43–S62.
6. Paiement B, Pelletier C, Dryda I, et al. A simple classification of the risk in cardiac surgery. *Can Anaesth Soc J.* 1983;30:61–68.
7. Nashef SA, Roques F, Michael P, et al. European system for cardiac operation risk evaluation (EuroSCORE). *Eur J Cardiothorac Surg.* 1999;16:9–13.
8. Bernstein AD, Parsonnet V. Bedside estimation of risk as an aid for decision-making in cardiac surgery. *Ann Thorac Surg.* 2000;69:823–828.
9. Hannan EL, Racz MJ, Jones RH, et al. Predictors of mortality for patients undergoing cardiac valve replacements in New York state. *Ann Thorac Surg.* 2000;70:1212–1218.
10. Shroyer AL, Plomondon ME, Grover FL, et al. The 1996 coronary artery bypass risk model: the Society of Thoracic Surgeons Adult Cardiac National Database. *Ann Thorac Surg.* 1999;67:1205–1208.
11. Dupuis JY, Wang F, Nathan H, et al. The cardiac anesthesia risk evaluation score: a clinically useful predictor of mortality and morbidity after cardiac surgery. *Anesthesiology.* 2001;94:194–204.
12. Ouattara A, Niculescu M, Ghazouani S, et al. Predictive performance and variability of the cardiac anesthesia risk evaluation score. *Anesthesiology.* 2004;100:1405–1410.
13. Tu JV, Jaglal SB, Naylor D, et al. Multicenter validation of a risk index for mortality, intensive care unit stay, and overall hospital length of stay after cardiac surgery. *Circulation.* 1995;91:677–684.
14. Girish M, Trayner E, Dammann O, et al. Symptom-limited stair climbing as a predictor of postoperative cardiopulmonary complications after high-risk surgery. *Chest.* 2001;120:1147–1151.
15. Shahian DM, O'Brien SM, Filardo G, et al. The Society of Thoracic Surgeons 2008 cardiac surgery risk models: part 1—coronary artery bypass grafting surgery. *Ann Thorac Surg.* 2009;88:S2–S22.
16. Sharma S, Durieux ME. Molecular and genetic cardiovascular medicine. In: Kaplan JA, Reich DL, Savino JS, eds. *Kaplan's Cardiac Anesthesia: The Echo Era.* 6th ed. St. Louis, MO: Saunders; 2011.
17. O'Brien SM, Shahian DM, Filardo G, et al. The Society of Thoracic Surgeons 2008 cardiac surgery risk models: part 2—isolated valve surgery. *Ann Thorac Surg.* 2009;88:S23–S42.
18. **Fihn SD, Gardin JM, Abrams J, et al. 2012 ACCF/AHA/ACP/AATS/PCNA/SCAI/STS Guideline for the diagnosis and management of patients with stable ischemic heart disease: a report of the American College of Cardiology Foundation/American Heart Association Task Force on Practice Guidelines, and the American College of Physicians, American Association for Thoracic Surgery, Preventive Cardiovascular Nurses Association, Society for Cardiovascular Angiography and Interventions, and Society of Thoracic Surgeons. *J Am Coll Card.* 2012;60(24):2564–2603.**
19. Fleisher LA, Beckman JA, Brown KA, et al. 2009 ACCF/AHA focused update on perioperative beta blockade incorporated into the ACC/AHA 2007 guidelines on perioperative cardiovascular evaluation and care for noncardiac surgery: a report of the American College of Cardiology Foundation/American heart association task force on practice guidelines. *Circulation.* 2009;120:e169–e276.
20. Eagle KA, Guyton RA, Davidoff R, et al. ACC/AHA 2004 guideline update for coronary artery bypass graft surgery: a report of the American College of Cardiology/American Heart Association Task Force on practice guidelines. *Circulation.* 2004;110:e340–437.
21. Zipes DP, Camm J, Borggrefe M, et al. ACC/AHA/ESC 2006 guidelines for management of patients with ventricular arrhythmias and the prevention of sudden cardiac death—executive summary. *Circulation.* 2006;114:1088–1132.
22. Chobanian AV, Bakris GL, Black HR, et al. The seventh report of the joint national committee on prevention, detection, evaluation, and treatment of high blood pressure. *JAMA.* 2003;289:2560–2572.
22a. Whelton PK, Carey RM, Aronow WS, et al. ACC/AHA/AAPA/ABC/ACPM/AGS/APhA/ASH/ASPC/NMA/PCNA Guideline for the prevention, detection, evaluation, and management of high blood pressure in adults: a report of the American College of Cardiology/American Heart Association Task Force on Clinical Practice Guidelines. *2017 High Blood Pressure Clinical Practice Guideline.* 2017;1.
23. Newman MF, Kirchner JL, Phillips-Bute B, et al. Longitudinal assessment of neurocognitive function after coronary-artery bypass surgery. *N Engl J Med.* 2001;344:395–402.
24. Arrowsmith JE, Grocott HP, Reves JG, et al. Central nervous system complications of cardiac surgery. *Br J Anaesth.* 2000;84:378–393.
25. Ahonen J, Salmenpera M. Brain injury after adult cardiac surgery. *Acta Anaesthesiol Scand.* 2004;48:4–19.

26. Murkin JM. Central nervous system dysfunction after cardiopulmonary bypass. In: Kaplan JA, Reich DL, Savino JS, eds. *Kaplan's Cardiac Anesthesia: The Echo Era*. St. Louis, MO: Saunders; 2011.

27. Mark DB, Hlatky MA. Exercise treadmill score for predicting prognosis in coronary artery disease. *Ann Intern Med*. 1987; 106:793–800.

28. Gorlin R, Gorlin SG. Hydraulic formula for calculation of the area of the stenotic mitral valve, other cardiac valves, and central circulatory shunts. *Am Heart J*. 1951;41:1–29.

29. Kozak M, Chambers CE. Cardiac catheterization laboratory: diagnostic and therapeutic procedures in the adult patient. In: Kaplan JA, Reich DL, Savino JS, eds. *Kaplan's Cardiac Anesthesia: The Echo Era*. 6th ed. Philadelphia, PA: Elsevier; 2011:33–73.

30. Kirtane AJ, Gupta A, Iyengar S, et al. Safety and efficacy of drug-eluting and bare metal stents: comprehensive meta-analysis of randomized trials and observational studies. *Circulation*. 2009;119:3198–3206.

31. Bangalore S, Kumar S, Fusaro M, et al. Short- and long-term outcomes with drug-eluting and bare-metal coronary stents: a mixed treatment comparison analysis 117,762 patient-years of follow-up form randomized trials. *Circulation*. 2012;125(23): 2873–2891.

32. Stefanini G, Holmes D. Drug-eluting coronary-artery stents. *NEJM*. 2013;368:254–265.

33. Yang EH, Gumina RJ, Lennon RJ. Emergency coronary artery bypass surgery for percutaneous coronary interventions: changes in the incidence, clinical characteristics, and indications from 1979 to 2003. *J Am Coll Cardiol*. 2005;46:2004–2009.

34. Roy P, de Labriolle A, Hanna N, et al. Requirement for emergent coronary artery bypass surgery following percutaneous coronary intervention in the stent era. *Am J Cardiol*. 2009;103:950–953.

35. Slottosch I, Liakopoulos O, Kuhn E, et al. Outcome after coronary bypass grafting for coronary complications following coronary angiography. *J Surg Research*. 2017;210:69–77.

36. Kutcher MA, Klein LW, Ou FS, et al. Percutaneous coronary interventions in facilities without cardiac surgery on site: a report from the National Cardiovascular Data Registry (NCDR). *J Am Coll Cardiol*. 2009;54:16–24.

37. Khaladj N, Bobylev D, Peterss S, et al. Immediate surgical coronary revascularisation in patients presenting with acute myocardial infarction. *J Cardiothorac Surg*. 2013;8:167–173.

38. Seshadri N, Whitlow PL, Acharya N, et al. Emergency coronary artery bypass surgery in the contemporary percutaneous coronary intervention era. *Circulation*. 2002;106(18):2346–2350.

39. Hillis LD, Smith PK, Anderson JL, et al. 2011 ACCF/AHA guideline for coronary artery bypass graft surgery: a report of the American College of Cardiology Foundation/American Heart Association Task Force on Clinical Practice Guidelines. *Circulation*. 2011;124:e652–e735.

40. Levine GN, Bates ER, Bittl JA, et al. 2016 ACC/AHA guideline focused update on duration of dual antiplatelet therapy in patients with coronary artery disease: a report of the American College of Cardiology/American Heart Association Task Force on Clinical Practice Guidelines. *J Thorac Cardiovasc Surg*. 2016;152(5):1243–1275.

41. Levine GN, Bates ER, Blankenship JC, et al. 2011 ACCF/AHA/SCAI guidelines for percutaneous coronary intervention. A report of the American College of Cardiology Foundation/American Heart Association Task Force on Practice Guidelines and the Society for Cardiovascular Angiography and Interventions. *J Am Coll Cardiol*. 2011;58(24):e44–e122. Published online November 7, 2011.

42. American Society of Anesthesiologists Committee on Standards and Practice Parameters. Practice alert for the perioperative management of patients with coronary artery stents. *Anesthesiology*. 2009;110:22–23.

43. Lindenauer PK, Pekow P, Wang K, et al. Perioperative beta-blocker therapy and mortality after major noncardiac surgery. *N Engl J Med*. 2005;353:349–361.

44. Fleisher LA, Fleischmann KE, Auerbach AD, et al. 2014 ACC/AHA guideline on perioperative cardiovascular evaluation and management of patients undergoing noncardiac surgery: a report of the American College of Cardiology/American Heart Association Task Force on practice guidelines. *J Am Coll Cardiol*. 2014;64(22):e77–e137.

45. Lindenauer PK, Pekow P, Wang K, et al. Lipid-lowering therapy and in-hospital mortality following major noncardiac surgery. *JAMA*. 2004;291:2092–2099.

46. Liakopoulos O, Kuhn E, Slottosch I, et al. Statin therapy in patients undergoing coronary artery bypass grafting for Acute Coronary Syndrome. *Thorac Cardiovasc Surg*. 2017. doi: 10.1055/s-0037-1602257.

47. Barakat A, Saad M, Abuzaid A, et al. Perioperative statin therapy for patients undergoing coronary artery bypass grafting. *Ann Thorac Surg*. 2016;101:818–825.

48. Douketis JD, Spyropoulos AC, Spencer FA, et al. Perioperative management of antithrombotic therapy: antithrombotic therapy and prevention of thrombosis, 9th ed.: American College of Chest Physicians Evidence-Based Clinical Practice Guidelines. *Chest*. 2012;141(2 Suppl):e326S–e350S.

49. Van Ryn J, Stangier J, Haertter S, et al. Dabigatran etexilate—a novel, reversible, oral direct thrombin inhibitor: interpretation of coagulation assays and reversal of anticoagulant activity. *Thromb Haemost*. 2010;103:1116–1127.

50. Spyropoulos AC, Douketis JD. How I treat anticoagulated patients undergoing an elective procedure or surgery. *Blood*. 2012; 120:2954–2962.

51. Comfere T, Sprung J, Kumar MM, et al. Angiotensin system inhibitors in a general surgical population. *Anesth Analg*. 2005; 100:636–644.

4

Monitoring the Cardiac Surgical Patient

Mark A. Gerhardt and Andrew N. Springer

KEY POINTS

1. For cardiac anesthesia, a five-electrode surface Electrocardiogram (ECG) monitor should be used. Ischemic changes should be assessed by toggling from monitor mode to diagnostic mode.

2. After a rapid pressure change (performed by flushing the pressure line and known as the "pop test"), an underdamped system will continue to oscillate for ≥3 oscillations. Underdamped systems overestimate systolic blood pressure (sBP) and underestimate diastolic blood pressure (dBP). An overdamped system will not oscillate thus underestimating systolic and overestimating diastolic pressures. A critically damped system will settle to baseline after only one or two oscillations and will reproduce systolic pressures accurately.

3. Air within a catheter or transducer causes most pressure monitoring errors.

4. Placement of an art line ***prior to induction*** is indicated in all major cardiac procedures and most thoracic, major vascular and neurosurgical procedures.

5. The radial artery pressure may be significantly lower than the aortic pressure at the completion of cardiopulmonary bypass (CPB) and for 5 to 30 minutes following CPB.

(continued)

6. The central venous pressure (CVP) c wave *always* follows the ECG R wave and is useful for interpreting CVP waveforms.

7. The current consensus is that pulmonary artery catheter (PAC) placement benefits high-risk and complex patients. Patients with preserved left ventricular (LV) function can often be managed with CVP and TEE.

8. The PAC should be withdrawn 2 to 5 cm when initiating CPB to decrease risk of PA occlusion/infarction or rupture.

9. SvO_2 provides a global assessment of whether oxygen delivery ($\dot{D}O_2$) is meeting oxygen consumption ($\dot{V}O_2$) requirements. Normal SvO_2 is 75% with a 5% change considered significant. A decreased SvO_2 results from decreased $\dot{D}O_2$ or increased ($\dot{V}O_2$). Normal $\dot{D}O_2$ is four times the value of a normal ($\dot{V}O_2$).

10. When a pulmonary capillary wedge pressure/pulmonary artery occlusion pressure (PCWP/PAOP) waveform appears spontaneously, confirmation that the pulmonary artery catheter (PAC) balloon is deflated followed by withdrawal of the PAC until a PA waveform appears should be immediately performed.

11. Systolic pressure variation (SPV), pulse pressure variation (PPV), and stroke volume variation (SVV) depend on the interaction between intrathoracic pressure and arterial blood pressure to accurately indicate whether a patient is volume responsive. These may have some role in cardiac surgery prior to sternotomy and after chest closure, but are inaccurate while the chest is open and during CPB.

12. Monitoring temperature at one core site and one shell site is recommended. PAC temperature is recommended for core temperature, and bladder or rectal temperature for shell temperature.

13. The risk of dysrhythmia is increased following CPB. Administration of KCl and $MgSO_4$ to a goal of $K^+ \geq 4.0$ mEq/L and $Mg^{++} \geq 2.0$ mg/dL will attenuate electrolyte-mediated risk of myocardial conduction abnormalities.

14. Administration of calcium should be delayed until after reperfusion of neural tissue (15 to 20 minutes after aortic cross-clamp removal). Though low serum Ca^{++} may affect myocardial pumping function, administration of calcium during potential neural ischemia–reperfusion can result in neurotoxicity.

15. In cardiac surgical patients with ascending aortic atheroma identified by epiaortic scanning, modification of the surgical technique and neuroprotective strategies can reduce the incidence of neurologic complications from ~60% to almost 0%.

16. Splanchnic vasculature sequesters 70% of total body blood volume (TBV). The initial physiologic compensation for hypovolemia is transfer of blood from splanchnic vasculature to the central venous compartment.

17. Off-pump CABG (OPCAB) patients may be very difficult to monitor for ischemia, particularly during the most critical events of the procedure. Some cardiac anesthesiologists favor SvO_2 or $ScvO_2$ monitoring for OPCAB.

I. Introduction

Patients presenting for cardiac surgery require extensive monitoring because unstable hemodynamics and abnormal physiologic conditions associated with cardiopulmonary bypass (CPB) are the norm rather than the exception. Mechanical alterations (i.e., the surgical procedure) result in a "different patient" leaving the operating room (OR) compared to the preoperative period. Special considerations are required for minimally invasive cardiac surgery where the only two monitors that provide reliable data may be the mean arterial pressure (MAP) and mixed venous oxygen saturation (SvO_2). Current trends in hemodynamic monitoring include identification of target(s) for *goal-directed therapy*. Identification of hypovolemic patients who will have a positive response to fluid administration can be obtained with pulse pressure variation (PPV), systolic pressure variation (SPV), and stroke volume variation (SVV) for example.

Several topics remain controversial: the role of ultrasound (USN) in central line placement and pulmonary artery catheter (PAC) use in cardiac surgical patients. The American Society of Anesthesiologists (ASA) revised clinical guidelines [1] state "use real-time USN guidance for vessel localization and venipuncture when IJ selected for cannulation." This recommendation was met immediately with criticism including, within the same paper, a survey of ASA members where the

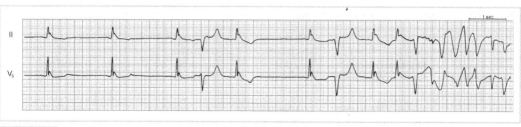

FIGURE 4.1 Cardiac monitoring during cardiopulmonary bypass (CPB). ECG changes due to hypothermia during initiation of CPB. Bradycardia progresses to frequent PVCs, followed by ventricular fibrillation. (From Mark JB. *Atlas of Cardiovascular Monitoring*. New York: Churchill Livingstone; 1998, Figure 19.1.)

majority did not agree with this recommendation. Analogous to clinical application of USN for peripheral nerve block (PNB) placement, the incidence of procedural complications and longer time for placement is only noted in *novice* anesthesia personnel. In experienced hands, success rate is not improved with USN and there is no difference in complications ± USN [2]. Reliance on technology has created anesthesiologists who are unable to place an internal jugular (IJ) catheter based on anatomical landmarks [3]. Furthermore, important critiques of this statement are that it fails to recognize the clinical experience/judgment of the anesthesiologist, particularly providing latitude to maintain anatomic-based skills for central line placement.

The PAC controversy has a long history. PAC critics cite the lack of studies demonstrating an improved outcome with PAC (see discussion in PAC section II.F.2). However, it is imperative to note: (1) most clinicians do not know how to correctly interpret PAC data [4]; (2) many studies used septic/SIRS patients with microvascular and/or mitochondrial pathology; and (3) PAC has been traditionally utilized for estimating left ventricular end-diastolic volume (LVEDV). The use of pressure in the proximal pulmonary artery (PA) as a surrogate for LVEDV simply does not work. Transesophageal echocardiography (TEE) is more consistent as a monitor for hypovolemia. However, an understanding of the nuances of waveform morphology of the arterial line, CVP and PAC can provide a wealth of information which can then be confirmed via TEE.

This chapter does not discuss TEE or point-of-care testing including coagulation monitoring (activated clotting time [ACT], thromboelastography [TEG], rotational thromboelastometry [ROTEM]). These topics are presented elsewhere. Finally, some topics (e.g., temperature monitoring) are only discussed as it relates to cardiac surgical procedures.

II. Cardiovascular monitors

    A. Electrocardiogram (ECG). The intraoperative use of the ECG facilitates the intraoperative diagnosis of dysrhythmias, myocardial ischemia, and cardiac electrical silence during cardioplegic arrest (Fig. 4.1). A five-lead system, including a V_5 lead, is preferable for cardiac surgical patients. Use of five electrodes (one lead on each extremity and one precordial lead) allows the simultaneous recording of the six standard frontal limb leads as well as one precordial unipolar lead.

        1. Indications

            a. Diagnosis of dysrhythmias

            b. Diagnosis of ischemia

            c. Diagnosis of electrolyte disturbances

            d. Monitor effect of cardioplegia during aortic cross-clamp

        2. Techniques

            a. The three-electrode system. This system utilizes electrodes only on the right arm, left arm, and left leg. The potential difference between two of the electrodes is recorded, whereas the third electrode serves as a ground. Three ECG leads (I, II, III) can be examined.

                The three-lead system has been expanded to include the augmented leads. It identifies one of the three leads as the exploring electrode and couples the remaining two at a central terminal with zero potential. This creates leads in three more axes (aVR, aVL, aVF) in the frontal plane. Leads II, III, and aVF are most useful for monitoring the inferior wall, and leads I and aVL for the lateral wall. Several additional leads have been developed for specific indications (Table 4.1).

TABLE 4.1   ECG lead placement. Bipolar and augmented leads for use with three electrodes

Lead identifier	Right arm electrode: function (location)	Left arm electrode: function (location)	Left leg electrode: function (location)	Lead select	Useful for diagnosing
■ Standard leads					
I	Negative (right arm)	Positive (left arm)	Ground (left leg)	I	Lateral ischemia
II	Negative (right arm)	Ground (left arm)	Positive (left leg)	II	Dysrhythmias (maximal P wave and QRS height); inferior ischemia
III	Ground (right arm)	Negative (left arm)	Positive (left leg)	III	Inferior ischemia
■ Augmented leads					
aVR	Positive (right arm)	Common ground (left arm)	Common ground (left leg)	aVR	
aVL	Common ground (right arm)	Positive (left arm)	Common ground (left leg)	aVL	Lateral ischemia
aVF	Common ground (right arm)	Common ground (left arm)	Positive (left leg)	aVF	Inferior ischemia
■ Special leads					
MCL_1	Ground (right arm)	Negative (underleft clavicle)	Positive (V_1 position)	III	Dysrhythmias (maximal P wave and QRS height)
CS_5	Negative (under right clavicle)	Positive (V_5 position)	Ground (left leg)	I	Anterior ischemia
CM_5	Negative (manubrium sternum)	Positive (V_5 position)	Ground (left leg)	I	Anterior ischemia
CB_5	Negative (center of right scapula)	Positive (V_5 position)	Ground (left leg)	I	Anterior ischemia; dysrhythmia (maximal P wave)
CC_5	Negative (right anterior axillary line)	Positive (V_5 position)	Ground (left leg)	I	Global ischemia

Modified from Griffin RM, Kaplan JA. ECG lead systems. In: Thys D, Kaplan J, eds. *The ECG in Anesthesia and Critical Care.* New York: Churchill Livingstone; 1987:20.

b. **The five-electrode system.** All limb leads act as a common ground for the precordial unipolar lead. The unipolar lead usually is placed in the V_5 position, along the anterior axillary line in the fifth intercostal space, to best monitor the left ventricle (LV). The precordial lead can also be placed on the right precordium to monitor the right ventricle (RV; V_{4R} lead).

(1) **Advantages.** In patients with coronary artery disease, the unipolar V_5 lead is the best single lead in diagnosing myocardial ischemia; moreover, 90% of ischemic episodes will be detected by ECG if leads II and V_5 are analyzed simultaneously. Therefore, a correctly placed V_5 and limb leads should enhance diagnosis of the vast majority of intraoperative ischemic events.

(2) **Epicardial electrodes.** Cardiac surgeons routinely place ventricular and/or atrial epicardial pacing wires at the conclusion of CPB prior to sternal closure. In addition to AV pacing, these pacing wires can be utilized to record atrial and/or ventricular epicardial ECGs.

(3) **Esophageal.** Esophageal leads can be incorporated into the esophageal stethoscope for the detection of posterior wall ischemia and atrial dysrhythmias.

(4) **Endotracheal.** ECG leads embedded into the endotracheal tube may be useful in pediatric cardiac patients for diagnosing atrial dysrhythmias.

3. **Computer-assisted ECG interpretation.** Computer programs for online analysis of dysrhythmias and ischemia are currently widely available with a 60% to 78% sensitivity in detecting ischemia compared with the Holter monitor. Typically, the current ECG signal is displayed along with a graph showing the trend (e.g., ST depression) over a recent time period, usually the past 30 minutes.

4. **ECG filters.** ECG can be analyzed via *monitor mode* or *diagnostic mode*. Diagnostic mode has a low- and high-frequency filter set at 0.05 Hz and 100 Hz, respectively. The diagnostic mode is identical to the ECG data obtained by a 12-lead ECG. Most monitors default to the monitor mode which eliminates any electrical signal below 0.5 Hz and above 40 Hz. The resulting ECG eliminates the majority of artifacts, particularly the 60-Hz interference from electrically powered devices. The ECG, in monitor mode, unfortunately distorts the ST segment. Thus ischemia monitoring is not reliable. Monitors can be toggled to diagnostic mode to assess the ECG.

5. **Myocardial ischemia detection via ECG monitoring.** ECG was the first monitor historically to be utilized to diagnose ischemia. Subendocardial ischemia results in ST segment depression whereas transmural myocardial ischemia is detected as ST segment elevation (Fig. 4.2). Myocardial blood flow anatomically originates from the epicardial

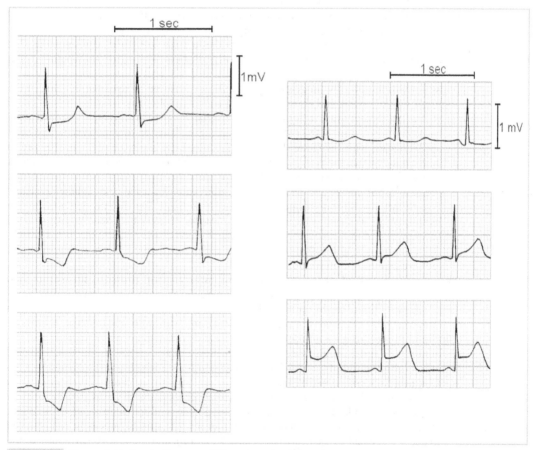

FIGURE 4.2 Myocardial ischemia. Shown are ECG tracings depicting subendocarial ischemia (**left**) and transmural ischemia (**right**). ST segment depression results from subendocardial ischemia. This patient had left main coronary disease and the ST depression worsened as her heart rate increased (63 → 75 → 86 beats/min). Transmural ischemia (full thickness) produces ST segment elevation and frequently results from proximal coronary artery occlusion. This patient underwent a redo CABG and had acute thrombosis of a saphenous vein graft. (From Mark JB. *Atlas of Cardiovascular Monitoring*. New York: Churchill Livingstone; 1998, Figures 11.1 and 11.2.)

surface of the heart and penetrates to the endocardium. Coronary perfusion transpires during both systole and diastole in the RV whereas LV perfusion is limited to diastole. Mechanically the endocardium is subjected to higher pressures than the epicardium. Thus the endocardium is typically compromised before the entire thickness of the myocardium. ST segment depression is routinely observed prior to ST segment elevation.

6. **Recommendations for ECG monitoring.** ECG is an ASA standard monitor. Five-electrode surface monitor is recommended for cardiac surgery. Correct lead placement is imperative to optimize ECG monitoring. Typically, leads V_5 and II are monitored. Automated ST segment analysis and trend history are helpful adjuncts to diagnose ischemia. Additionally ECG is the gold standard monitor to diagnose arrhythmias.

B. **Intermittent noninvasive blood pressure monitors**

1. **Indications in the cardiac patient.** Cardiac surgical patients have every indication for arterial catheter assessment and therefore preinduction arterial line placement is essential. Noninvasive cuff methods for measuring blood pressure (BP) are not adequate because BP measurement every three minutes is not practical and may cause injury. Furthermore noninvasive devices will not function when dysrhythmia alters a machine-recognized pattern, pulsatile flow is absent during CPB or when continuous-flow left ventricular assist devices (LVADs) are used.

2. **Continuous noninvasive blood pressure monitors.** Continuous noninvasive arterial pressure monitoring is a newer modality that has shown some promise in critical care settings. These systems provide a continuous arterial waveform equivalent to that provided by an arterial catheter. The majority of these devices use the volume clamp technique, in which measurements are obtained via one or more finger cuffs with integrated photoplethysmography sensors. BP is measured by dynamic inflation of the finger cuff in systole and diastole so that a constant volume is measured in the finger via the photoplethysmography sensor. An arterial waveform can then be reconstructed based on the pressure in the cuff. Monitors using applanation tonometry have also been used, typically with the radial artery. This technique measures the pressure required to flatten a segment of the artery and records this as the MAP. A proprietary algorithm then recreates the arterial waveform and systolic blood pressure (sBP) and diastolic blood pressure (dBP) are determined from this. Both methods have been validated against invasive arterial BP monitoring in critical care settings. The volume clamp technique has been evaluated with reasonable results intraoperatively with cardiac surgery patients [5]. However, during cardiac surgery, frequent blood draws (arterial blood gas [ABG], ACT, electrolytes, glucose) and periods of nonpulsatile flow (CPB) are required. Hence, invasive arterial catheterization is indicated.

C. **Physics and technical aspects for accurate intravascular pressure measurements.** Invasive monitors via intravascular catheters are required to safely administer a cardiac anesthetic. Arterial pressure can be measured by placing a catheter ("art line") in a peripheral artery or femoral artery. Central venous access is obtained to measure the central venous pressure (CVP) and to serve as a conduit for PAC placement to measure intracardiac pressures. The components of a system of intravascular pressure measurement are the intravascular catheter, fluid-filled connector tubing, a transducer, and an electronic analyzer and display system.

1. **Characteristics of a pressure waveform.** Pressure waves in the cardiovascular system can be characterized as complex periodic sine waves. These complex waves are a summation of a series of simple sine waves of differing amplitudes and frequencies, which represent the natural harmonics of a fundamental frequency. The first harmonic, or fundamental frequency, is equal to the heart rate (Fig. 4.3A and B), and the first 10 harmonics of the fundamental frequency will contribute significantly to the waveform.

2. **Properties of a monitoring system**

a. **Frequency response** (or **amplitude ratio**) is the ratio of the measured amplitude versus the input amplitude of a signal at a specific frequency. The frequency response should be constant over the desired range of input frequencies—that is, the signal is not distorted (amplified or attenuated). The ideal amplitude ratio is close to 1. The

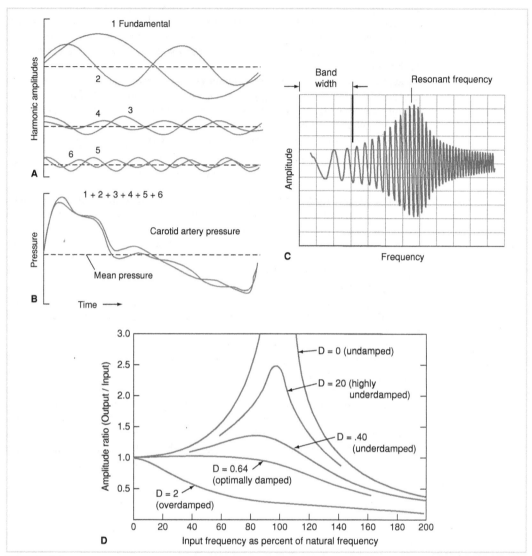

FIGURE 4.3 A: Generation of the harmonic waveforms from the fundamental frequency (heart rate) by Fourier analysis. **B:** The first six harmonics are shown. The addition of the six harmonics reproduces an actual BP wave. The first six harmonics are superimposed, showing a likeness to, but not a faithful reproduction of, the original wave. The first 10 harmonics of a pressure wave must be sensed by a catheter–transducer system, if that system is to provide an accurate reproduction of the wave. **C:** Pressure recording from a pressure generator simulator, which emits a sine wave at increasing frequencies (*horizontal axis*). The frequency response (ratio of signal amplitude$_{OUT}$ to signal amplitude$_{IN}$) is plotted on the vertical axis for a typical catheter–transducer system. The useful band width (range of frequency producing a "flat" response) and the amplification of the signal in the frequency range near the natural frequency of the system are shown. (**A–C:** From Welch JP, D'Ambra MN. Hemodynamic monitoring. In: Kofke WA, Levy JH, eds. *Postoperative Critical Care Procedures of the Massachusetts General Hospital.* Boston, MA: Little, Brown and Company; 1986:146, with permission.) **D:** Amplitude ratio (or frequency response) on the vertical axis is plotted as a function of the input frequency as a percentage of the natural frequency (rather than as absolute values). In the undamped or underdamped system, the signal output is amplified in the region of the natural frequency of the transducer system; in the overdamped system, a reduction in amplitude ratio for most input frequencies is seen. This plot exhibits several important points: (i) If a catheter–transducer system has a high natural frequency, less damping will be required to produce a flat response in the clinically relevant range of input frequencies (10 to 30 Hz); (ii) For systems with a natural frequency in the clinically relevant range (usual case), a level of "critical" (optimal) damping exists that will maintain a flat frequency response. D, damping coefficient. (From Grossman W. *Cardiac Catheterization.* 3rd ed. Philadelphia, PA: Lea & Febiger; 1985:122, with permission.)

signal frequency range of an intravascular pressure wave response is determined by the heart rate. For example, if a patient's heart rate is 120 beats/min, the fundamental frequency is 2 Hz. Because the first 10 harmonics contribute to the arterial waveform, frequencies up to 20 Hz will contribute to the morphology of an arterial waveform at this heart rate.

b. **Natural frequency** (or **resonant frequency**), a property of all matter, refers to the frequency at which a monitoring system itself resonates and amplifies the signal. The natural frequency (f_n) of a monitoring system is directly proportional to the catheter lumen diameter (D), inversely proportional to the square root of three parameters: The tubing connection length (L), the system compliance ($\Delta V/\Delta P$), and the density of fluid contained in the system (δ). This is expressed as follows:

$$f_n \propto D \cdot L^{-1/2} \cdot (\Delta V/\Delta P)^{-1/2} \cdot \delta^{-1/2}$$

To increase f_n and thereby reduce distortion, it is imperative that a pressure-sensing system be composed of short, low-compliance tubing of reasonable diameter, and filled with a low-density fluid (such as normal saline).

Ideally, the natural frequency of the measuring system should be at least 10 times the fundamental frequency to reproduce the first 10 harmonics of the pressure wave without distortion. In clinical practice, the natural frequency of most measuring systems is in the range from 10 to 20 Hz. If the input frequency is close to the system's natural frequency (which is usually the case in clinical situations), the system's response will be amplified (Fig. 4.3C). Therefore, these systems require the correct amount of **damping** to minimize distortion.

c. The **damping coefficient** reflects the rate of dissipation of the energy of a pressure wave. Figure 4.3D shows the relationship among frequency response, natural frequency, and damping coefficient.

When a pressure-monitoring system with a certain natural frequency duplicates a complex waveform with any one of the first 10 harmonics close to the natural frequency of the system, amplification will result if correct damping of the catheter–transducer unit is not performed. The problem is compounded when the heart rate is fast (as in a child or a patient with a rapid atrial rhythm), which increases the demands of the system by increasing the input frequency (Fig. 4.4).

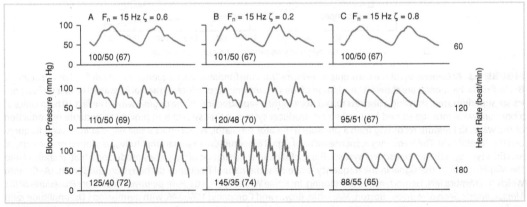

FIGURE 4.4 Comparison of three catheter–transducer systems with the same natural frequency (15 Hz) under different conditions of heart rate. Pressures are displayed as systolic–diastolic (mean). The reference BP for all panels is 100/50. **A:** A critically damped system ($\zeta = 0.6$) provides an accurate reproduction until higher heart rates (greater than 150) are reached. **B:** An underdamped system ($\zeta = 0.2$) shows distortion at lower rates, leading to overestimation of systolic and underestimation of diastolic pressures. **C:** An overdamped system ($\zeta = 0.8$) demonstrates underestimation of systolic pressure and overestimation of diastolic pressure. Also note that diastolic and mean pressures are affected less by the inadequate monitoring systems. f_n, natural frequency; ζ, damping coefficient.

Both the natural frequency and the damping coefficient of a system can be estimated using an adaptation of the square wave method known as the "pop" test. The natural frequency is estimated by measuring the time period of one oscillation as the system settles to baseline after a high-pressure flush. The damping coefficient is calculated by measuring the amplitude ratio of two successive peaks (Fig. 4.5).

After a rapid pressure change (performed by flushing the pressure line), an underdamped system will continue to oscillate for a prolonged time. In terms of pressure monitoring, this translates to an overestimation of systolic BP and an underestimation of diastolic BP. An overdamped system will not oscillate at all but will settle to baseline slowly, thus underestimating systolic and overestimating diastolic pressures. A critically damped system will settle to baseline after only one or two oscillations and will reproduce systolic pressures accurately. An optimally or *critically* damped system will exhibit a constant (or *flat*) frequency response in the range of frequencies up to the f_n of the system (Fig. 4.3D). If a given system does not meet this criterion, components should be checked, especially for air, or the system replaced. Even an optimally damped

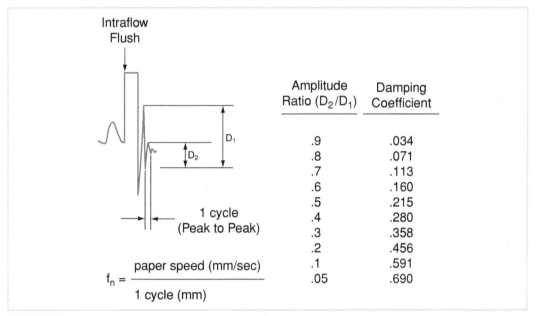

FIGURE 4.5 The "pop" test allows one to derive f_n and ζ of a catheter–transducer system. The test should be done with the catheter in situ, as all components contribute to the harmonics of the system. The test involves a rapid flush (with the high-pressure flush system used commonly), followed by a sudden release. This produces a rapid decrease from the flush bag pressure and, owing to the inertia of the system, an overshoot of the baseline. The subsequent oscillations about the baseline are used to calculate f_n and ζ. For example, the arterial pulse at the far left of the figure is followed by a fast flush and sudden release. The resulting oscillations have a definite period, or cycle, measured in millimeters. The natural frequency f_n is the paper speed divided by this period, expressed in cycles per second, or Hz. If the period were 2 mm and the paper speed 25 mm/s, $f_n = 12.5$ Hz. For determining f_n, a faster paper speed will give better reliability. The ratio of the amplitude of one induced resonant wave to the next, D_2/D_1, is used to calculate damping coefficients (**right column**). A damping coefficient of 0.2 to 0.4 describes an underdamped system, 0.4 to 0.6 an optimally damped system, and 0.6 to 0.8 an overdamped system. (From Bedford RF. Invasive blood pressure monitoring. In: Blitt CD, ed. *Monitoring in Anesthesia and Critical Care Medicine.* New York: Churchill Livingstone; 1985:59, with permission.)

system will begin to distort the waveform at higher heart rates because the 10th harmonic exceeds the system's natural frequency (Fig. 4.4).

3. **Strain gauges (transducer).** The pressure-monitoring transducer can be described as a variable-resistance transducer. A critical part of the transducer is the diaphragm, which acts to link the fluid wave to the electrical input. When the diaphragm of a transducer is distorted by a change in pressure, voltages are altered across the variable resistor of a Wheatstone bridge contained in the transducer. This in turn produces a change in current, which is electronically converted and displayed.

4. **Sources of error in intravascular pressure measurement**

   a. **Low-frequency transducer response.** Low-frequency response refers to a low-frequency range over which the ratio of output-to-input amplitude is constant (i.e., no distortion). If the natural frequency of the system is low, its frequency response will also be low. Most transducer systems used in clinical anesthesia can be described as underdamped systems with a low natural frequency. Thus, any condition that further decreases f_n response should be avoided. Air within a catheter–transducer system causes most monitoring errors. Because of its compressibility, air not only decreases the response of the system but also leads to overdamping of the system. Therefore, the myth that an air bubble placed in the pressure tubing decreases artifact by increasing the damping coefficient is incorrect. A second common cause of diminution of frequency response is the formation of a partially obstructing clot in the catheter.

   b. **Catheter whip.** Catheter "whip" is a phenomenon in which the motion of the catheter tip itself produces a noticeable pressure swing. This artifact usually is not observed with peripheral arterial catheters but is more common with PAC or LV catheters.

   c. **Resonance in peripheral vessels.** The systolic pressure measured in a radial arterial catheter may be up to 20 to 50 mm Hg higher than the aortic pressure due to decreased peripheral arterial elastance and wave summation (Fig. 4.6).

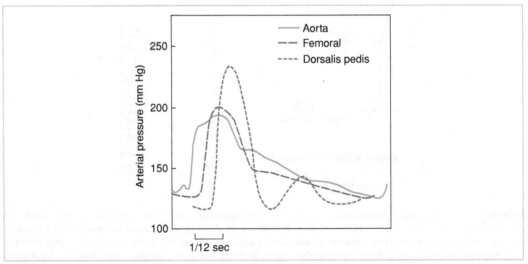

FIGURE 4.6 Change of pulse pressure waveform morphology in different arteries. Arterial waveforms do not have a single morphology. The central aortic waveform is more rounded and has a definite dicrotic notch. The dorsalis pedis and, to a lesser extent, the femoral artery show a delay in pulse transmission, sharper initial upstrokes (and thus higher systolic pressure), and slurring (femoral) and loss (dorsalis) of the dicrotic notch. The dicrotic notch is better maintained in the upper-extremity pressure wave (see Fig. 4.10). The small second "hump" in the dorsalis wave probably is due to a reflected wave from the arterial–arteriolar impedance mismatching. (From Welch JP, D'Ambra MN. Hemodynamic monitoring. In: Kofke WA, Levy JH, eds. *Postoperative Critical Care Procedures of the Massachusetts General Hospital*. Boston, MA: Little, Brown and Company; 1986:144, with permission.)

d. **Changes in electrical properties of the transducer.** *Electrical balance,* or *electrical zero,* refers to the adjustment of the Wheatstone bridge within the transducer so that zero current flows to the detector at zero pressure. Transducers should be electronically balanced periodically during a procedure because the zero point may drift, for instance, if the room temperature changes. The pressure waveform morphology may not change with baseline drift of a transducer.

e. **Transducer position errors.** By convention, the reference position for hemodynamic monitoring during cardiac surgery is the right atrium (RA). With the patient supine, the RA lies at the level of the midaxillary line. Once its zero level has been established, the transducer must be maintained at the same level as the RA. *If the transducer position changes, falsely high- or low-pressure values will result.* This can be significant especially when monitoring CVP, PA pressure, or pulmonary capillary wedge pressure (PCWP) where the observed change is a greater percentage of the measured value. For example, if a patient has a MAP of 100 mm Hg and a CVP of 10 mm Hg, a 5 mm Hg offset due to transducer position would be displayed as a 5% or 50% change in the arterial or CVP pressures, respectively.

D. **Arterial catheterization**

1. **Indications.** Arterial catheterization ("art line," or more commonly "A-line") is the gold standard in the monitoring of the cardiac surgical patient (Table 4.2). Placement of an art line *prior to induction* is imperative for a safe, smooth anesthetic induction. Note that all four indications for an art line are applicable even during routine cardiac surgery. Most thoracic, major vascular, and neurosurgical procedures will also have ≥1 indication.

2. **Sites of cannulation.** Multiple cannulation sites have been used, with radial and femoral being by far the most utilized.

   The authors typically infiltrate ≥2.5 to 3 mL of 1% lidocaine. There are issues unique to cardiac surgical procedures which may govern arterial/central line insertion site. Patients may require mechanical assistance from an intra-aortic balloon pump (IABP) which is inserted via the femoral artery. IABP is positioned in the descending thoracic aorta immediately distal to the subclavian artery. When inflation/deflation is correctly timed, the IABP improves LV cardiac output (CO) by decreasing the end-systolic aortic pressure and augmenting the LV diastolic pressure. Note that LV perfusion occurs only during diastole whereas the RV is perfused in both systole and diastole.

CLINICAL PEARL The most common mistake during radial art line insertion is infiltration of an inadequate volume of local anesthetic. Local anesthetic should eliminate discomfort during placement and attenuate arterial vasoconstriction.

a. **Radial artery.** The radial artery is the most commonly utilized site. Non-invasive blood pressure should be routinely measured in both arms prior to placement of an art line to detect differences in pressure. Usually, a *left* radial art line is preferred

TABLE 4.2 Arterial catheterization indications

Indication	Clinical application
Small/rapid changes may be harmful requiring beat-to-beat assessment	Tight control of perfusion pressure medically required; CT, major vascular, neurosurgery
Wide variation in BP or intravascular volume is anticipated	Trauma, major abdominal procedures, solid organ transplantation
Frequent blood sampling, especially arterial blood gas (ABG) analysis	Close monitoring of acid–base status, electrolytes
BP measurement cannot be performed by other methods	Dysrhythmia; marked obesity; CPB; continuous flow LVAD (nonpulsatile flow)

Arterial catheterization ("art line; A-line") is the gold standard for blood pressure monitoring of the cardiac surgical patient. Placement of an art line *prior to induction* is imperative for a safe, smooth anesthetic induction. The radial artery is the most common site.

because: (1) the primary surgeon operates on the patient's right side and can compress the right arm vasculature; (2) most patients are right dominant; and (3) improper placement of the sternal retractor can apply pressure to the brachial plexus increasing risk of neural injury. An abnormal arterial pressure wave can trigger evaluation of sternal retractor positioning.

(1) **Technique.** Ultrasound-guided radial artery cannulation is beneficial when difficulty placing the catheter via the traditional method is encountered or low flow states (shock), nonpulsatile flow during extracorporeal membrane oxygenation (ECMO), LVAD or right ventricular assist device (RVAD) or cardiac arrest.

CLINICAL PEARL   Pulse oximetry (SpO$_2$) may not be able to acquire a signal in patients with low-flow states and/or cool peripheral extremities. Performing a PNB of the SpO$_2$ digit with 1 to 2 mL of plain local anesthetic frequently restores the SpO$_2$ signal.

(2) **Complications.** Very few ischemic complications have been reported from arterial catheterization even in patients with a positive Allen test indicating limited collateral ulnar artery flow. Peripheral shunting following CPB manifesting as hypotension is occasionally observed. The difference between central arterial pressures and radial art line can exceed 25 to 30 mm Hg. This is a self-limited problem that dissipates as thermal energy is more evenly distributed in the patient. Placement of a femoral art line or passing off pressure tubing attached to the aortic cannula from the surgical field can be used to confirm this diagnosis.

(3) **Radial artery harvest.** The radial artery is an alternative option for use as a bypass conduit. Usually the radial artery to be harvested is known preoperatively, and the contralateral radial artery can be used.

b. **Femoral artery.** A femoral art line is an option that has unique considerations. The femoral artery is the site for placement of an IABP or the arterial CPB cannula when the usual placement in the ascending aorta is not possible. Aortic aneurysm and dissection are cases that may require this option.

(1) **Technique.** The femoral artery typically lies at the midpoint between the pubic tubercle and the anterior superior iliac spine. These bone landmarks can be used to guide identification of the femoral pulse in difficult cases.

(2) **Contraindications.** Cannulation of the femoral artery should be avoided in patients with prior vascular surgery involving the femoral arteries or a skin infection of the groin.

c. **Aortic root.** The surgeon can transiently assess BP by transducing the aortic cannula or aortic root while the chest is open.

d. **Axillary artery.** The axillary artery is a superficial vessel with good access to the central arterial tree.

Complications. The increased risk of cerebral embolus of air or debris must be recognized. Flushing the arterial line must be performed with caution and low pressure. Hemothorax risk is a known complication of axillary arterial lines.

e. **Brachial artery.** The brachial artery is an easily accessible artery located medially in the antecubital fossa.

Contraindications. Concern about compromised flow distal to catheter placement has limited its use at many institutions. Brachial catheterization is a secondary option or is not utilized in nonheparinized surgical procedures.

f. **Ulnar artery.** The ulnar artery is a secondary site. There is a risk of compromised perfusion if attempted placement of the ipsilateral radial artery is unsuccessful.

g. **Dorsalis pedis and posterior tibialis arteries.** In general, the distal location increases distortion of the arterial wave. The dorsalis pedis artery is technically easier to cannulate.

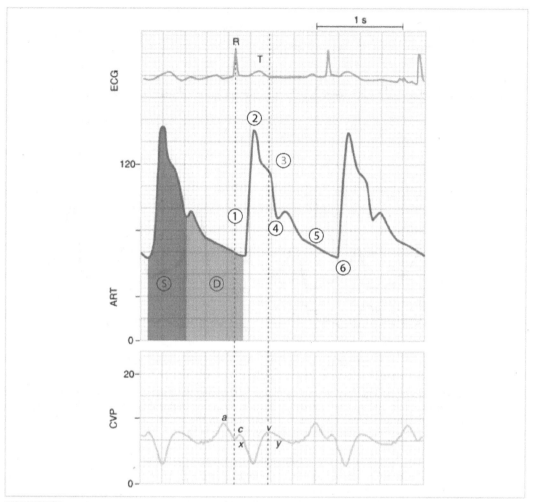

FIGURE 4.7 Normal arterial waveform morphology. Components of the normal arterial waveform include (*1*) the systolic upstroke, (*2*) systolic peak pressure, (*3*) systolic decline, (*4*) the dicrotic notch, (*5*) diastolic runoff, and (*6*) end-diastolic pressure. The area underneath the curve (shaded area on the left) divided by the beat period equals the mean arterial pressure (MAP). S, systole; D, diastole. (Modified from Mark JB. *Atlas of Cardiovascular Monitoring*. New York: Churchill Livingstone; 1998, Figures 8.1 and 8.2.)

3. **Interpretation of arterial tracings.** The arterial pressure waveform contains a great deal of hemodynamic information. Normal radial artery waveform morphology is shown in Figure 4.7. Different sites have a unique morphology although the components are identical. The dicrotic notch marks the end of systole/start of diastole. The waveform has three systolic components: systolic upstroke (a graphical representation of $\delta P/\delta t$) to a peak (sBP), then decline to the dicrotic notch, and diastolic runoff to a nadir (dBP).

    a. **Heart rate and rhythm.** The heart rate can be determined from the arterial pressure wave. This is especially helpful if the patient is being paced or if electrocautery is being used. In the presence of numerous atrial or ventricular ectopic beats, the arterial trace can provide useful information on the hemodynamic consequences of these dysrhythmias (i.e., if an ectopic beat is perfusing). The arterial waveform can also demonstrate the hemodynamic effects of ventricular versus A-V pacing (Fig. 4.8).

    b. **Pulse pressure.** The difference between the systolic and diastolic pressures provides useful information about fluid status and valvular competence. Pericardial tamponade

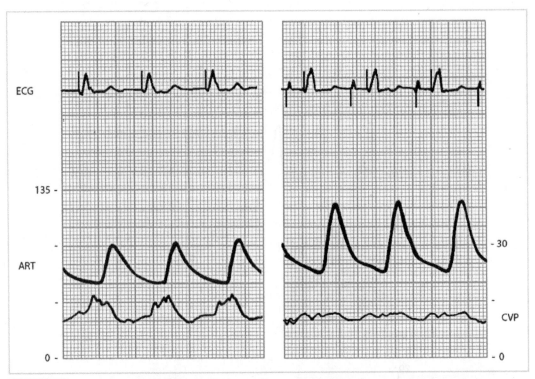

FIGURE 4.8 VOO versus AV pacing. The CVP tracing during VOO pacing (**left**) shows cannon waves due to systolic contraction of the right atrium (RA) from retrograde conduction. AV pacing (**right**) shows a normal CVP tracing and a substantial improvement in arterial blood pressure, as demonstrated by the arterial waveform. (From Mark JB. *Atlas of Cardiovascular Monitoring*. New York: Churchill Livingstone; 1998, Figure 14.16.)

and hypovolemia are accompanied by a narrow pulse pressure on the arterial waveform. An increase in pulse pressure may be a sign of worsening aortic valvular insufficiency or hypovolemia.

c. **Respiratory variation and volume status.** Hypovolemia is suggested by a decrease in arterial systolic pressure with positive-pressure ventilation (pulsus paradoxus). Positive intrathoracic pressure impedes venous return to the heart with a more pronounced effect in the hypovolemic patient. Respiratory variation of arterial sBP, stroke volume (SV), and pulse pressure can be used as goal-directed parameters to identify patients who will respond to fluid administration. This is discussed in greater depth below.

d. **Qualitative estimates of hemodynamic indices.** Inferences can be made regarding contractility, SV, and vascular resistance from the arterial waveform. sBP and dBP are the peak and nadir of the arterial waveform, respectively. Contractility can be grossly judged by $\delta P/\delta t$, the rate of pressure rise during systole keeping in mind that heart rate, preload, and afterload can affect this parameter. SV can be estimated from the area under the aortic pressure wave from the onset of systole to the dicrotic notch. Finally, the position of the dicrotic notch correlates with the systemic resistance. A notch appearing high on the downslope of the pressure trace suggests a high vascular resistance, whereas a low resistance tends to cause a dicrotic notch that is lower on the diastolic portion of the pressure trace. These elements are incorporated into the algorithms of pulse pressure analysis monitors for noninvasive CO.

e. **Intra-aortic balloon counterpulsation timing.** The arterial tracing should show a characteristic pattern when an IABP is present. A properly timed IABP should inflate the balloon starting at the dicrotic notch. The balloon remains inflated throughout diastole, and actively deflates at the start of the next systolic upstroke. Analysis of the

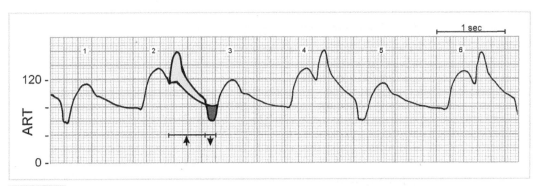

FIGURE 4.9 Arterial waveform tracing with an intra-aortic balloon pump (IABP) at 1:2. Beats 2, 4, and 6 show a properly timed inflation of the balloon at the dicrotic notch, resulting in increased diastolic arterial pressure. Deflation of the balloon just prior to the systolic upstroke results in a drop in arterial pressure at the onset of systole and a reduced peak in the following beat. (From Mark JB. *Atlas of Cardiovascular Monitoring.* New York: Churchill Livingstone; 1998, Figure 20.1.)

arterial waveform should allow appropriate adjustment of balloon inflation and deflation to optimize its function (Fig. 4.9).

4. **Complications of arterial catheterization**
   a. **Ischemia.** The incidence of ischemic complications after radial artery cannulation is low even in patients with abnormal flow patterns.
   b. **Thrombosis.** Although the incidence of thrombosis from radial artery catheterization is high, studies have not demonstrated adverse sequelae. Recanalization of the radial artery occurs in a majority of cases. Patients with increased risk include those with diabetes or severe peripheral vascular disease.
   c. **Infection.** With proper sterile technique, the risk of infection from cannulation of the radial artery should be minimal. In a series of 1,700 cases, no catheter site was overtly infected.
   d. **Bleeding.** Although transfixing the artery will put a hole in the posterior wall, the layers of the muscular media will seal the puncture. In a patient with a bleeding diathesis, however, there is a greater tendency to bleed. Unlike central venous catheters (CVCs), arterial catheters are not heparin bonded and thus have increased risk of thrombus development.

5. **Abnormal arterial waveform morphology.** Cardiac abnormalities can provide pathologic clues by altering the arterial (Fig. 4.10) waveform morphology, providing diagnostic clues which are typically underappreciated.

E. **Central venous pressure.** CVP measures RA pressure and is affected by circulating blood volume, venous tone, and RV function. Placement of a CVC (central line) is indicated in most cardiac surgical procedures to provide a large-bore conduit for rapid fluid administration and delivery of vasoactive drugs into the central vascular compartments and/or a PAC. It is very important to recognize that there are some complications that are secondary to central line placement, not PAC insertion. This is pertinent to the controversial use of a PAC in cardiac surgery. Complications of PAC insertion are much less frequent and often transient (e.g., dysrhythmia). Although CVP has severe limitations in estimating LVEDV, CVP can provide clinical clues that can trigger further therapeutic action(s). Central line placement is indicated in essentially all cardiac surgery procedures.

1. **Indications**
   a. **Monitoring.** Monitoring of CVP is indicated for all cardiac surgical patients. Anatomically, CVP is acquired at the junction of the RA, IVC, and SVC. The first step to interpretation of CVP is correctly identifying the waveform components. After eliminating all parameters that ↑ CVP (no mechanical positive pressure breaths), the end-exhalation waveform mean pressure (Fig. 4.11) is the correct value. Central venous O_2 saturation (**ScvO$_2$**) is assessed from SVC blood. ScvO$_2$ reflects venous saturation from

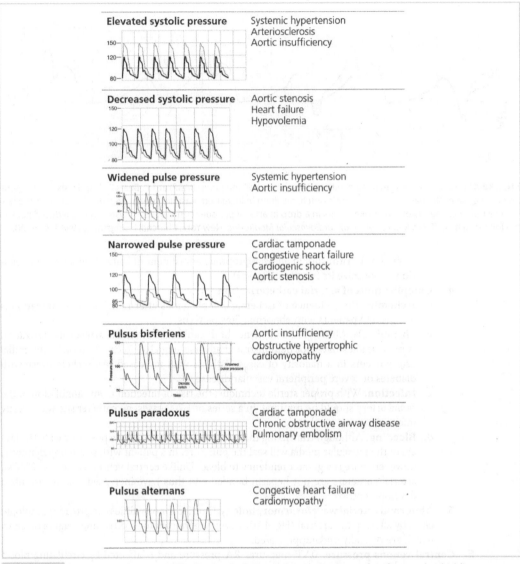

FIGURE 4.10 Arterial waveforms resulting from pathologic conditions. For the top four figures, the *thick line* represents a normal arterial waveform. (From *Quick Guide to Cardiopulmonary Care*. 3rd ed. Used with permission from Edwards Critical Care Education.)

brain and upper extremities and is typically 5% LESS than SvO_2. Oximetric CVP catheters are utilized without need to place a PAC. Normal $ScvO_2$ is 70%.

    b. Fluid and drug therapy. Central line access facilitates administration of vasoactive drugs if required. A central line also facilitates rapid fluid administration.

    c. Special issues in cardiac surgery. One may elect to place a CVP catheter, with delayed PAC placement in selected patients.

CLINICAL PEARL   Placement of a PAC can be difficult in patients with numerous congenital cardiac disorders, in those with anatomic distortion of the right-sided venous circulation, or in those requiring surgical procedures of the right heart or implantation of a right heart mechanical assist device. Insertion may need to be delayed until during the surgery.

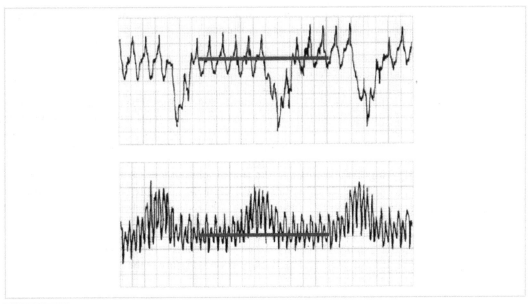

FIGURE 4.11 Central venous pressure waveforms in a spontaneously breathing patient (**top**) and a patient receiving positive-pressure ventilation (**bottom**). Note that during inspiration, the CVP decreases in the spontaneously breathing patient, whereas it increases during positive-pressure inspiration. CVP should be read at end expiration (*dark horizontal lines*) to avoid the effects of changing intrathoracic pressure. (From Pittman, JA, Ping JS, Mark JB. Arterial and central venous pressure monitoring. *Int Anesthesiol Clin.* 2004 Winter;42(1):13–30.)

    2. **Techniques.** The IJ veins, subclavian (SC) veins, and the femoral veins are the most common sites for catheter access to the central circulation (Table 4.3).

        a. **Internal jugular.** The *right* IJ (RIJ) is the most common access route for cardiac anesthesiologist because it is a straight pathway from insertion site to RA. The RSC is the most tortuous. Additionally most anesthesiologists are right handed and ergometrically the RIJ is the easier side to access.

TABLE 4.3 Central line insertion sites and complications

	IJ	SC	FEM	NOTES
IDz	+ – ++	+	+++	
Tolerability	+ – ++	+++	+	IJ posterior > middle approach
Arterial puncture	Carotid + – ++	SC or BCA (R) + – ++	Fem + – ++	Innominate art at risk via RSC lines. Experience ↓ risk
PTX	+ – ++	++ – +++	Ø	Experience ↓ risk. Low-IJ approach ↑↑↑ risk
Catheter/guidewire embolism	+	+	+	Stab wounds during attempt to place catheter. Experience ↓ risk
Thrombosis or thromboembolism	+	+	+	DVT from SC and IJ central lines are often overlooked as PE source
Nerve injury	Brachial plexus	Brachial plexus	Lumbar plexus	Difficult lines: multiple venipuncture attempts. Experience ↓ risk
Thoracic duct	LIJ	LSC	Ø	LIJ has to navigate acute angle ↑ risk
VAE	++ – +++	++ – +++	Ø	↑↑↑ NIF > fluid column → VAE. Collapse IVC ↓ Fem risk. Intermittent airway obstruction

The three primary sites for central line insertion and common complications are depicted. The relative frequency of a particular complication at a site is denoted from none (Ø) to low (+)–high (+++). Note that complication rates frequently decrease with experience. BCA, bracheocephalic artery; DVT, deep venous thrombosis; Fem, femoral; IDz, infection; IJ, internal jugular vein; IVC, inferior vena cava; L, left; PE, pulmonary embolism; PTX, pneumothorax; R, right; SC, subclavian; VAE, venous air embolism; ++, intermediate; ↑, increased; ↓, decreased.

(1) **Contraindications and recommendations.** Relative contraindications for IJ central line placement include the following:

(a) Presence of significant carotid disease

(b) Recent cannulation of the IJ (with the concomitant risk of thrombosis)

(c) Contralateral diaphragmatic dysfunction

(d) Thyromegaly or prior neck surgery

In these cases, the IJ on the contralateral side should be considered. It should be remembered that the thoracic duct lies in close proximity to the left IJ and that laceration of the left brachiocephalic vein or superior vena cava by the catheter is more likely with the left-sided approach. This risk is due to the more acute angle between the left IJ and innominate veins.

(2) **Sonographic guidance.** Ultrasound guidance of elective venous cannulation has quickly gained controversial acceptance as the preferred method for IJ catheter, particularly for inexperienced operators. Ultrasound-guided IJ cannulation requires the ability to correctly distinguish the easily compressible jugular vein from the carotid artery (Fig. 4.12).

b. **External jugular.** The external jugular vein courses superficially across the sternocleidomastoid muscle to join the subclavian vein close to the junction of the IJ and SC

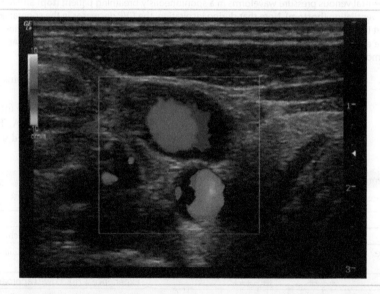

FIGURE 4.12 Ultrasound image of the internal jugular vein and carotid artery. Note that color flow visualizes blood flowing away from the transducer as blue, while blood flowing toward the transducer is *red*. So, with the probe angled caudally, blood flow in the internal jugular vein returning to the heart is *blue*, while the blood travelling up from the aortic arch into the carotid artery is *red*. (From Barash P, Cullen B, eds. *Clinical Anesthesia*. Philadelphia, PA: Lippincott Williams & Wilkins; 2009:747.)

veins. Its course is more tortuous, and the presence of valves makes central line placement more difficult. The placement of rigid central catheters (e.g., PAC introducer) via the external jugular increases the risk of vessel trauma and is not recommended. Pliable central catheters and short catheters can be used to acquire intravenous access.

   c. **Subclavian.** The subclavian vein is readily accessible and thus has been popular for use during cardiopulmonary resuscitation.

   (1) **Advantages.** The main advantage to subclavian vein cannulation is its relative ease and the stability of the catheter during long-term cannulation. Left SC insertion of a PAC introducer is the second easiest anatomical approach after the right IJ.

   (2) **Disadvantages**

   (a) Subclavian vein cannulation carries the highest rate of pneumothorax of any approach. If subclavian vein cannulation is unsuccessful on one side, an attempt on the contralateral side is contraindicated without first obtaining a chest x-ray film. Bilateral pneumothoraces can be lethal. Subclavian vein placement for cardiac surgery can be associated with compression of the central line during sternal retraction.

   (b) The subclavian artery is entered easily.

   (c) In a left-sided cannulation, the thoracic duct may be lacerated.

   (d) The right subclavian approach may make threading the PAC into the RA difficult because an acute angle must be negotiated by the catheter in order to enter the innominate vein. The left subclavian approach is recommended as the first option for PAC placement.

   d. **Arm vein**

   Techniques. Central access can be obtained through the veins of the antecubital fossa ("long-arm CVP" or "peripherally inserted central catheter—PICC"). This has a limited role in most cardiac surgical procedures.

3. **Complications.** The site-specific complications of CVP catheter insertion are listed in Table 4.3. The most severe complications of CVP insertion usually are preventable.

4. **CVP interpretation**

   a. **Normal CVP waveform morphology.** The normal CVP trace is more complex than the arterial waveform, containing three positive deflections, termed the *a*, *c*, and *v* waves, and two negative deflections termed the *x* and *y* descents. The CVP components (Table 4.4) represent mechanical events that are altered by heart function and arrhythmia (Table 4.5; Fig. 4.7, bottom). The CVP c wave *always* follows the ECG R wave and is useful for interpreting CVP waveforms.

   b. **Abnormal waves.** A common abnormality in the CVP trace is loss of the a wave secondary to atrial fibrillation (A-fib). In the presence of AV dissociation, when RA contraction occurs against a closed tricuspid valve, this produces a large "cannon A wave"

TABLE 4.4   Components of the CVP waveform

CVP waveform component	Cardiac event	S/D	Note
a wave	RA contraction	D	A-fib abolishes a wave
x descent	RA relaxation	S	Mid systolic
c wave	IVVC; TV motion	S	C wave always follows ECG R wave
v wave	Systolic RA filling	S	TR → prominent v wave
y descent	Early RV filling	D	E wave on TEE
x′	RA relaxation	S	Terminal x wave after c wave

The normal CVP waveform components are produced by distinct mechanical events. Factors which influence these events produce alterations in the CVP waveform. Note that the c wave *always* follows the ECG R wave. Aligning the ECG with the CVP assists identification of the other components and pathology. A-fib, atrial fibrillation; CVP, central venous pressure; D, diastolic; IVVC, isovolumic ventricular contraction; RA, right atrium; RV, right ventricle; S, systolic; TR, tricuspid regurgitation; TV, tricuspid valve.

TABLE 4.5   Differential diagnosis of RA-RV hemodynamic abnormalities

Abnormal waveform chart

▪ Right atrial waveforms

Decreased mean pressure	Hypovolemia
	Transducer zero level too high
Elevated mean pressure	Fluid overload states
	Right ventricular (RV) failure
	Left ventricular (LV) failure causing RV failure
	Tricuspid stenosis or regurgitation
	Pulmonic stenosis or regurgitation
	Pulmonary hypertension
Elevated "a" wave: atrial systole, increased resistance to ventricular filling	Tricuspid stenosis
	Decreased RV compliance
	RV failure
	Pulmonic stenosis
	Pulmonary hypertension
Absent "a" wave	Atrial fibrillation
	Atrial flutter
	Junctional rhythms
Elevated "v" wave: atrial filling, regurgitant flow	Tricuspid regurgitation Functional regurgitation from RV failure
Elevated "a" and "v" waves	Cardiac tamponade
	Constrictive pericardial disease
	Hypervolemia

▪ RV waveforms

Elevated systolic pressure	Pulmonary hypertension
	Pulmonic valve stenosis
	Factors that increase pulmonary vascular resistance (PVR)
Decreased systolic pressure	Hypovolemia
	Cardiogenic shock (RV failure)
	Cardiac tamponade
Increased diastolic pressure	Hypervolemia
	Congestive heart failure
	Cardiac tamponade
	Pericardial constriction
Decreased diastolic pressure	Hypervolemia

From *Quick Guide to Cardiopulmonary Care*. 3rd ed. Used with permission from Edwards Critical Care Education.

that is virtually diagnostic. These waves are also evident in VOO pacing (Fig. 4.8, left). Abnormal V waves can occur with tricuspid valve insufficiency, in which retrograde flow through the incompetent valve produces an increase in RA pressure during systole (Fig. 4.13, top).

c. **RV function.** CVP offers direct measurement of RV filling pressure.

d. **LV filling pressures.** CVP (and other PAC-obtained data) have historically been utilized as a tool to estimate LV filling pressures which in turn was dogmatically an estimate of LVEDV. Parameters that distort this estimate include LV dysfunction, decreased LV compliance (i.e., ischemia), pulmonary hypertension, or mitral valvular disease (and TR with respect to CVP). In patients with coronary artery disease but good ventricular function (ejection fraction greater than 40% and no regional wall motion abnormalities [RWMAs]), CVP correlates well with PCWP. However, because RV is a thinner-walled chamber, the compliance of the RV is higher than that of the LV. Therefore, for any given preload, CVP will be lower than either PA diastolic pressure or PCWP. Although the absolute number has not been shown to correlate with preload

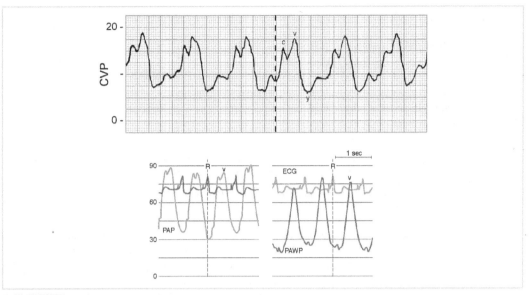

FIGURE 4.13 **Top:** CVP tracing showing a large v wave and steep y descent due to tricuspid regurgitation. The regurgitant flow during systole obscures the x descent, causing a fusion of c and v waves. RV end-diastolic pressure is best estimated from the tracing prior to the v wave, at the time of the R wave on the ECG. **Bottom:** V waves secondary to severe mitral regurgitation. The tall systolic v wave in the PA wedge pressure (PAWP) trace also distorts the PA tracing, thereby giving it a bifid appearance. LVED pressure is best estimated by measuring PAWP at the time of the ECG R wave before the onset of the regurgitant v wave. (From Mark JB. *Atlas of Cardiovascular Monitoring*. New York: Churchill Livingstone; 1998, Figures 17.1 and 17.11.)

conditions and SV, evaluating trends over time and cyclic changes during mechanical ventilation can help guide fluid therapy.

F. **Pulmonary artery catheter (PAC)**

1. **Parameters measured**

   a. **PA pressure** reflects RV function, pulmonary vascular resistance (PVR), and left atrial (LA) filling pressure.

   b. **PCWP** is a more direct estimate of LA filling pressure. With the balloon inflated and "wedged" in a distal branch PA, a valveless hydrostatic column exists between the distal port and the LA at end diastole. This measurement is often assumed to represent left ventricular end-diastolic pressure (LVEDP), and further extrapolated to reflect LVEDV; both of these assumptions, especially the latter, are fraught with potential errors.

   c. **CVP.** A sampling port of the PAC is located in the RA and allows measurement of the CVP.

   d. **CO.** A thermistor located at the tip of the PAC allows measurement of the output of the RV by the thermodilution technique. In the absence of intracardiac shunts, this measurement equals LV output.

   e. **Blood temperature.** The thermistor can provide a constant measurement of blood temperature, which is an accurate reflection of core temperature.

   f. **Derived parameters.** Advanced indices of ventricular performance and cardiovascular status can be derived from the parameters measured by PAC.

   g. **SvO_2.** Oximetric PAC can measure real-time PA venous blood oxygen saturation providing information on end-organ oxygen utilization. For standard PACs, a blood gas sample can be drawn from the distal port, which will give an intermittent SvO_2. This measurement can be repeated to trend the value.

   h. **RV performance.** New PAC technology allows for improved assessment of RV function distinct from LV dysfunction.

TABLE 4.6 PAC Indications

Assessment/management of RV failure

Assessment/management of pulmonary hypertension

Assess for adequate oxygen delivery and tissue oxygen uptake and measurement of SvO_2

Management of LV failure unresponsive to therapy, requiring escalating inotropes or IABP

Aortic surgery requiring suprarenal cross-clamping

Orthotopic heart transplantation

Myocardial protection (antegrade cardioplegia)

In cardiac surgery patients there are multiple indications for perioperative PAC utilization. Some indications may be brief but are critically important (i.e., myocardial protection during antegrade cardioplegia administration). IABP, intra-aortic balloon pump; LV, left ventricular; RV, right ventricular; SvO_2, mixed venous oxygen saturation.
Modified from Kaplan JA. Monitoring of the heart and vascular system. In: Kaplan JA, ed. *Cardiac Anesthesia, The Echo Era.* 6th ed. St. Louis, MO: Elsevier Saunders; 2011:435.

2. **Indications for PA catheterization.** There is no consensus among cardiac anesthesiologists regarding PAC use. PAC guidelines have been published [6]. In some institutions, cardiac surgery with CPB represents a universal indication for PA pressure monitoring in adults; other institutions rarely use PAC [7,8]. In the late 1990s several observational studies, randomized control trials, and meta-analyses did not show positive outcome benefits with the use of the PAC. Between 1994 and 2004, PAC use decreased 65% in medical intensive care units (ICUs) and 63% in surgical ICUs. Proponents of the PAC (Table 4.6) suggest that timing of catheter placement, patient selection, interpretation of PAC data, and early appropriate intervention are required for this monitor to meaningfully affect patient outcome. Decreased mortality has been reported in high-risk surgical patients in which PACs were inserted preoperatively and interventions were protocol driven. In elective cardiac surgical patients, Polanen reported in 2000 that PAC protocols reduce hospital and ICU length of stay [9]. Therefore, the current consensus appears to be that PACs may have benefits in high-risk patients or those with special indications. However, routine patients with preserved LV function can frequently be managed with CVP and TEE alone. Differentiation of LV versus RV function and assessment of intracardiac filling pressures during antegrade cardioplegia administration (enhanced myocardial protection) are two indications that cannot be performed with CVP alone. Discordance in right and left heart function occurs with variable frequency where pressures measured on the right side (i.e., CVP) do not adequately reflect those on the left side [10]. Knowledge of PAC waveforms and the nuances of abnormal patterns (Table 4.7) should provide a differential diagnostic list and direct examination by other monitoring modalities, particularly TEE. For example, the sudden appearance of prominent PA v waves should prompt investigation of the MV to assess MR.

   a. **Assessing volume status.** While historically PAC measurements, particularly PCWP, have been used as an indicator of a patient's volume status, several studies have demonstrated that these parameters are very poor at guiding fluid administration. Given the increase in routine usage of intraoperative TEE in cardiac surgery, we cannot advocate routine usage of PCWP for guidance of volume resuscitation.

   b. **Diagnosing RV failure.** The RV is a thin-walled, highly compliant chamber that can fail during cardiac surgery either because of a primary disease process (inferior myocardial infarction), inadequate myocardial protection, or intracoronary air (predilection for the right coronary artery) as a result of the surgical procedure. RV failure presents as an increase in CVP, a decrease in the CVP to mean PA gradient, and a low CO. The data that can be acquired from PAC can be tailored to calculating/measuring more complex hemodynamic variables (Table 4.8) to quantitate cardiac function and assess the effect of therapeutic interventions.

   c. **Diagnosing LV failure.** Knowledge of PA and wedge pressures can aid in the diagnosis of left-sided heart failure if other causes (ischemia, mitral valve disease) are eliminated. TEE can aid in correlating the clinical paradigm to PAC measurements. Simultaneous

TABLE 4.7 Differential diagnosis of PA-PCWP hemodynamic abnormalities

Pulmonary artery waveforms

Elevated systolic pressure	Pulmonary disease
	Increased blood flow, left to right shunt
	Increased pulmonary vascular resistance (PVR)
Elevated diastolic pressure	Left heart failure
	Intravascular volume overload
	Mitral stenosis or regurgitation
Reduced systolic and diastolic pressure	Hypovolemia
	Pulmonic stenosis
	Tricuspid stenosis

Pulmonary artery wedge/left atrial waveform

Decreased (mean) pressure	Hypovolemia
	Transducer level too high
Elevated (mean) pressure	Fluid overload states
	Left ventricular (LV) failure
	Mitral stenosis or regurgitation
	Aortic stenosis or regurgitation
	Myocardial infarction
Elevated "a" wave (any increased resistance to ventricular filling)	Mitral stenosis
Absent "a" wave	Atrial fibrillation
	Atrial flutter
	Junctional rhythms
Elevated "v" wave	Mitral regurgitation
	Functional regurgitation from LV failure
	Ventricular septal defect
Elevated "a" and "v" waves	Cardiac tamponade
	Constrictive pericardial disease
	LV failure

From *Quick Guide to Cardiopulmonary Care*. 3rd ed. Used with permission from Edwards Critical Care Education.

readings of high PA pressures and wedge pressure in the presence of systemic hypotension and low CO are hallmarks of LV failure.

    d. Diagnosing pulmonary hypertension. Note that with normal PVR, the PA diastolic and wedge pressure agree closely with one another. This relationship is lost with pulmonary hypertension.

    e. Assessing valvular disease

      (1) Tricuspid and pulmonary valve stenosis can be diagnosed by means of a PAC by measuring pressure gradients across these valves, although in adults TEE is the primary diagnostic modality for these lesions.

      (2) Mitral valvular disease is reflected in the PA and wedge pressure waveform morphology. Mitral insufficiency appears as an abnormal V wave and an increase in pulmonary venous pressure from the regurgitant flow into the LA. V waves can also appear in other conditions, including myocardial ischemia, ventricular pacing, and presence of a ventricular septal defect depending on the compliance of the LA. In patients with chronic mitral valve insufficiency, the LA has a high compliance and a large regurgitant volume will not always result in a dramatic V wave (Fig. 4.13, bottom).

    f. Early diagnosis of ischemia. PAC, ECG, and TEE can assist detection of myocardial ischemia. Significant ischemia (transmural or subendocardial) is often associated with a decrease in ventricular compliance, which is reflected in either an increase in PA pressure or an increase in PCWP. In addition, the development of pathologic V waves may occur secondary to ischemia of the papillary muscle.

TABLE 4.8   Hemodynamic variables and normal values

Normal hemodynamic parameters—adult

Parameter	Equation	Normal range
Arterial blood pressure (BP)	Systolic (SBP)	100–140 mm Hg
	Diastolic (DBP)	60–90 mm Hg
Mean arterial pressure (MAP)	SBP + (2 × DPB)/3	70–105 mm Hg
Right atrial pressure (RAP)		2–6 mm Hg
Right ventricular pressure (RVP)	Systolic (RVSP)	15–30 mm Hg
	Diastolic (RVDP)	0–8 mm Hg
Pulmonary artery pressure (PAP)	Systolic (PASP)	15–30 mm Hg
	Diastolic (PADP)	8–15 mm Hg
Mean pulmonary artery pressure (MPAP)	PASP + (2 × PADP)/3	9–18 mm Hg
Pulmonary artery occlusion pressure (PAOP)		6–12 mm Hg
Left atrial pressure (LAP)		4–12 mm Hg
Cardiac output (CO)	HR × SV/1,000	4.0–8.0 L/min
Cardiac index (CI)	CO/BSA	2.5–4.0 L/min/m^2
Stroke volume (SV)	CO/HR × 1,000	60–100 mL/beat
Stroke volume index (SVI)	CI/HR × 1,000	33–47 mL/m^2/beat
Stroke volume variation (SVV)	$SV_{max} - SV_{min}/SV_{mean}$ × 100	<10–15%
Systemic vascular resistance (SVR)	80 × (MAP – RAP)/CO	800–1,200 dynes·sec/cm^5
Systemic vascular resistance index (SVRI)	80 × (MAP – RAP)/CI	1,970–2,390 dynes·sec/cm^5·m^2
Pulmonary vascular resistance (PVR)	80 × (MPAP – PAOP)/CO	<250 dynes·sec/cm^5
Pulmonary vascular resistance index (PVRI)	80 × (MPAP – PAOP)/CI	255–285 dynes·sec/cm^5·m^2
Left ventricular stroke work index (LVSWI)	SVI × (MAP – PAOP) × 0.0136	50–62 g/m^2/beat
Right ventricular stroke work index (RVSWI)	SVI × (MPAP – CVP) × 0.0136	5–10 g/m^2/beat
Coronary artery perfusion pressure (CPP)	Diastolic BP – PAOP	60–80 mm Hg
Right ventricular end-diastolic volume (RVEDV)	SV/EF	100–160 mL
Right ventricular end-diastolic volume index (RVEDVI)	RVEDV/BSA	60–100 mL/m^2
Right ventricular end-systolic volume (RVESV)	EDV – SV	50–100 mL
Right ventricular ejection fraction (RVEF)	SV/EDV × 100	40–60%

From *Quick Guide to Cardiopulmonary Care*. 3rd ed. Used with permission from Edwards Critical Care Education.

    g. Monitoring intracardiac filling pressures during antegrade cardioplegia. Elevated mean PA and/or PCWPs during administration of cardioplegia into the aortic root can be a sign of aortic insufficiency leading to LV distention, indicating a need for further venting of the LV and possibly retrograde cardioplegia. It is important to remember that the PAC tip should be withdrawn 2 to 5 cm once the patient is fully on bypass to prevent collapse of the pulmonary arteries onto the catheter and cause an unintentional wedge.

3. Contraindications for PAC placement

    a. Significant tricuspid/pulmonary valvular pathology: Tricuspid/pulmonary stenosis, endocarditis, or mechanical prosthetic valve replacement.

    b. Presence of a right-sided mass (tumor/thrombosis) that would cause a pulmonary or paradoxical embolization if dislodged.

    c. Left bundle branch block (LBBB): LBBB is a relative contraindication. The incidence of transient right bundle branch block (RBBB) during PAC placement is ~5%. In a patient with LBBB, this can result in complete heart block (CHB) when floating the PAC through the RV outflow track. Therefore, external pacing should be immediately available for these patients. In addition, floating of the PAC can be delayed until the chest is open, so that CPB can be rapidly initiated should CHB occur and external pacing be ineffective.

4. **Interpretation of PA pressure data**
   a. **Effects of ventilation.** The effects of ventilation on PA pressure readings can be significant in the low-pressure system of the right-sided circulation because airway or transpleural pressure is transmitted to the pulmonary vasculature.
      (1) When a patient breathes spontaneously, the negative intrapleural pressure that results from inspiration can be transmitted to the intravascular pressure. Thus, low or even "negative" PA diastolic, wedge, and CVPs may occur with spontaneous ventilation.
      (2) Positive airway pressures are transmitted to the vasculature during positive-pressure ventilation, leading to elevations in pulmonary pressures. Mean airway pressure is the parameter which correlates most closely with the changes in PA and CVP pressure measurements.
      (3) The established convention is to evaluate pressures at **end expiration**. The digital monitor numerical readout may give incorrect information because these numbers reflect the absolute highest (systolic), lowest (diastolic), and mean (area under pressure curve) values for **several seconds**, which may include one or more breaths. Damping is not accounted for by the monitor. Thus, inspection and interpretation of the waveform data is required to correctly evaluate the clinical scenario.
   b. **Location of catheter tip.** PA pressure measurements depend on where the tip of the catheter resides in the pulmonary vascular tree. In areas of the lung that are well ventilated but poorly perfused (West zone I), the readings will be more affected by the changes in airway pressure. Likewise, even when the tip is in a good location in the middle or lower lung fields, large amounts of positive end-expiratory pressure (>10 mm Hg) will affect PA values (Fig. 4.14).
      (1) Occasionally, it may be difficult to see the transition from an RV to PA waveform while inserting a PAC. Positioning within a PA can be confirmed by observing a downward slope to the waveform in diastole, representing arterial diastolic runoff, rather than an upward slope, indicating passive RV diastolic filling.
      (2) PAC position in the PA can also be confirmed using TEE.
5. **LA pressure.** In some patients (especially pediatric), direct LA pressure can be measured after surgical insertion of an LA catheter via the LA appendage in the open chest. LA catheters are also used in corrective surgery for congenital lesions when PAC insertion is not possible. The LA pressure tracing is comparable to the CVP tracing, with A, C, and V waves occurring at identical points in the cardiac cycle. LA catheters are used to monitor valvular function (after mitral valve replacement or mitral valvuloplasty) or to monitor LV filling pressures, whether or not a PAC is available. LA pressure measured directly is more accurate than that measured with a PAC because the effects of airway pressure on the pulmonary vasculature are removed. However, LA pressure does not necessarily reflect LVEDP in the presence of mitral valvular disease. Air should be meticulously removed from LA flush systems to avoid catastrophic air emboli.
6. **Timing of placement.** Select high-risk patients may require PAC placement prior to induction. The discomfort that might be associated with placement needs to be balanced with acquisition of hemodynamic data. In appropriately sedated patients, placement of a PAC is not associated with any significant hemodynamic changes. The hemodynamic data collected in the catheterization laboratory may not accurately reflect the current hemodynamic status, especially if the patient had episodes of myocardial ischemia during the catheterization or may be experiencing ischemia when entering the operating room.
7. **Types of PACs.** A variety of PACs are currently available for clinical use. The standard thermodilution catheter has a PA port for pressure monitoring and a thermistor for CO measurements at its tip, an RA port for CVP monitoring and for injection of cold saline 30 cm from the tip, and a lumen for inflation of the balloon. In addition, PACs are available that provide the following:
   a. **Venous infusion port (VIP).** VIP PACs have a third port 1 cm proximal to the CVP (31 cm from the tip) for infusion of drugs and fluids.

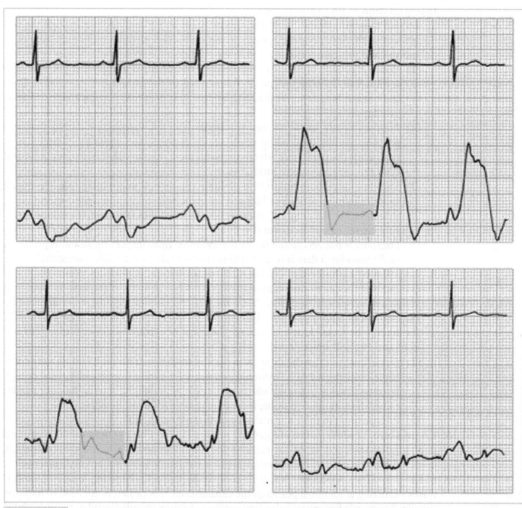

FIGURE 4.14 Pressure waveforms from the pulmonary artery catheter (PAC) tip as it passes through the right-sided heart chambers and into the pulmonary vasculature. Note that both CVP and PCWP waveforms exhibit a, c, and v waves. The shaded boxes in the RV and PA waveforms demonstrate the upward slope during diastolic filling in the RV, versus the downward sloping diastolic runoff in the PA. This is a good method for distinguishing the waveforms when inserting a PAC. (From Mark JB. *Atlas of Cardiovascular Monitoring*. New York: Churchill Livingstone; 1998, Figure 3.1.)

> **CLINICAL PEARL**   A common novice error is to forget that the VIP and CVP port are outside of the patient if the PAC has not yet been floated. Medications administered may then extravasate into the protective sheath rather than be delivered to the patient.

      b. Pacing. Pacing PACs have the capacity to provide intracardiac pacing. Pacing PACs are seldom used for cardiac procedures because usually patients already have a temporary pacing wire for symptomatic bradycardia prior to anesthetic care. Epicardial pacing wires are routinely placed by the surgeon intraoperatively for postoperative bradycardia.

      (1) Pacing PACs have a separate lumen terminating 19 cm from the catheter tip. When the catheter tip lies in the PA with a normal-sized heart, this port is positioned in the RV. A separate sterile, prepackaged pacing wire can be placed through this port to contact the RV endocardium for RV pacing.

TABLE 4.9   Invasive oximetric monitors and clinical mechanisms of SvO_2

Mechanisms which alter SvO_2, $\dot{D}O_2$ and ($\dot{V}O_2$)
  1. CO
  2. Hgb
  3. Arterial oxygen saturation
  4. ($\dot{V}O_2$)
Invasive Oximetry Monitors:
  Total body ($\dot{V}O_2$)
    SvO_2—mixed venous O_2 saturation
  Regional $\dot{V}O_2$
    $ScvO_2$—central vein O_2 saturation (SVC). Brain and upper extremities
    $ShvO_2$—hepatic vein O_2 saturation (IVC). GI and lower extremities
    $SjbO_2$—jugular bulb O_2 saturation. Neurologic monitor of cerebral hemisphere

    (2) PACs with thermodilution and atrial or AV pacing with two separate bipolar pacing probes have been shown to provide stable pacing before and after CPB.

  c. **Mixed venous oxygen saturation (SvO$_2$).** Delivery of adequate oxygen to meet the body tissue demand is best determined by SvO_2 (Table 4.9). Special fiber optic PACs can be used to monitor SvO_2 continuously. The normal SvO_2 is 75%, with a 5% to 10% increase or decrease considered significant. Decreased oxygen delivery or increased oxygen utilization result in a decreased SvO_2. Four mechanisms can result in a significant decrease in SvO_2:

    (1) Decrease in CO

    (2) Decreased hemoglobin concentration

    (3) Decrease in arterial oxygen saturation (SaO_2)

    (4) Increased O_2 utilization. These mechanisms can be understood by reviewing the oxygen consumption equation:

$$\dot{V}O_2 = CO \times Hgb \times 13.8 \times (SaO_2 - SvO_2)$$

where $\dot{V}O_2$ is oxygen consumption, CO is cardiac output in L/min, Hgb is the hemoglobin in g/dL, 13.8 is the amount of oxygen that can combine hemoglobin (1 g of Hgb can bind 1.38 mL of O_2, this factor is multiplied by 10 to convert dL to L as Hgb is measured in g/dL), SaO_2 is arterial saturation, and SvO_2 is mixed venous saturation. Based on the equation, a decrease in SvO_2 can result from a decrease in either the CO, Hgb, or SaO_2, or an increase in $\dot{V}O_2$.

CLINICAL PEARL   Changes in SvO_2 or oxygen extraction ratio (Tables 4.10 and 4.11) usually precede hemodynamic changes by a significant period of time, making this a useful clinical adjunct to other monitors. Some cardiac anesthesiologists advocate SvO_2 monitoring for off-pump coronary artery bypass (OPCAB) procedures and any patient with severe LV dysfunction and/or valve disease. Figure 4.15 presents a treatment algorithm utilizing SvO_2 to guide management.

    Attenuation of $\dot{D}O_2$ clinically is typically influenced by simultaneous changes in all three $\dot{D}O_2$ parameters. We can compare the effects of the individual mechanisms by varying them individually and comparing the results with normal CO and $\dot{D}O_2$ (Table 4.11). Note that under normal conditions $\dot{V}O_2$ consumes/requires 5.39 mL/kg O_2/min resulting in an extraction ratio of 25.5%. Thus, under normal conditions the $\dot{D}O_2$ is four times greater than required.

  d. **Ejection fraction catheter.** PACs with faster thermistor response times can be used to determine RV ejection fraction in addition to the CO. The thermistor responds rapidly enough that the exponential decay that normally results from

TABLE 4.10 Oxygen delivery variables and normal values

Parameter	Equation	Normal range
Oxygen parameters—adult		
Arterial oxygen content (CaO$_2$)	$(0.0138 \times Hgb \times SaO_2) + 0.0031 \times PaO_2$	16–22 mL/dL
Venous oxygen content (CvO$_2$)	$(0.0138 \times Hgb \times SvO_2) + 0.0031 \times PvO_2$	15 mL/dL
A-V oxygen content difference (C[a-v]O$_2$)	$CaO_2 - CvO_2$	4–6 mL/dL
Oxygen delivery (DO$_2$)	$CaO_2 \times CO \times 10$	950–1,150 mL/min
Oxygen delivery index (DO$_2$I)	$CaO_2 \times CI \times 10$	500–600 mL/min/m^2
Oxygen consumption (VO$_2$)	$C(a-v)O_2 \times CO \times 10$	200–250 mL/min
Oxygen consumption index (VO$_2$I)	$C(a-v)O_2 \times CI \times 10$	120–160 mL/min/m^2
Oxygen extraction ratio (O$_2$ER)	$(CaO_2 - CvO_2)/CaO_2 \times 100$	22–30%
Oxygen extraction index (O$_2$EI)	$(SaO_2 - SvO_2)/SaO_2 \times 100$	20–25%

Modified from *Quick Guide to Cardiopulmonary Care*. 3rd ed. Used with permission from Edwards Critical Care Education.

a thermodilution CO has end-diastolic "plateaus" with each cardiac cycle. From the differences in temperature of each succeeding plateau, the residual fraction of blood left in the RV after each contraction is calculated, as is RV stroke volume, end-diastolic volume, and end-systolic volume. Monitoring these parameters can be helpful in patients with RV dysfunction secondary to pulmonary hypertension, infarction, or reactive pulmonary disease.

  e. **Continuous CO.** PACs that use low-power thermal filaments to impart small temperature changes to RV blood have been developed (**Intellicath**, Baxter Edwards; and **Opti-Q**, Abbott Critical Care Systems, Mountain View, CA, USA). Fast-response thermistors in the PA allow for semicontinuous (every 30 to 60 seconds) CO determinations.

TABLE 4.11 Effects of hemoglobin and cardiac output (CO) on oxygen delivery

Parameter	Hgb (g/dL)	CO (L/min)	CaO$_2$ (mL O$_2$/dL)	DO$_2$ (mL O$_2$/min)
Art Blood	15	5	21.15	1057.5
SvO$_2$	15	5	15.76	
↓ Hgb	10	5	14.2	710
↓ Hgb	7	5	10.03	501.5
↓ Hgb	5	5	7.25	362.5
↓ CO 50%	15	2.5	21.15	528.75
↑ CO 50%	15	7.5	21.15	1586.25
↑ CO 100%	15	10	21.15	2,115

Effect of varying Hgb or CO on CaO$_2$ and DO$_2$. In this example, SpO$_2$ and pO$_2$ kept constant at 100% and 100 mm Hg, respectively. Changes in SvO$_2$ usually precede hemodynamic changes by a significant period of time. The top row depicts normal arterial CaO$_2$ and DO$_2$ with normal Hgb (15 g/dL), CO (5 L/min), SaO$_2$ (100%) and pO$_2$ (100 mm Hg). The normal SvO$_2$ is depicted on the second row with SvO$_2$ = 75% and PO$_2$ = 40 mm Hg. Note that under normal conditions (VO$_2$) consumes/requires 5.39 mL O$_2$/min resulting in an extraction ratio of 25.5%. Thus, under normal conditions the DO$_2$ is four times greater than required. (VO$_2$) typically does not change significantly under GA. Attenuation of DO$_2$ clinically (DO$_2$ = CO × CaO$_2$) results from change in SV, HR (CO = SV × HR) SpO$_2$ and/or Hgb abnormalities (anemia, dyshemoglobinemia). Inadequate DO$_2$ (<5.39 mL O$_2$ /min) initiate body tissues converting to anaerobic metabolism and starts oxygen debt. For example, a 50% decrease in CO results in a DO$_2$ of 5.28 mL O$_2$/min fails to meet VO$_2$ despite Hgb of 15.

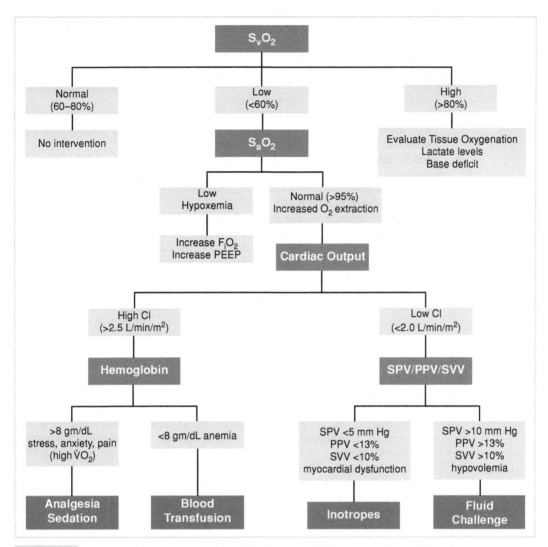

FIGURE 4.15 Treatment algorithm utilizing SvO$_2$, SaO$_2$, CO, hemoglobin concentration, and a measurement of volume status. CO, cardiac output; SvO$_2$, mixed venous oxygen saturation; SaO$_2$, arterial oxygen saturation; SPV, systolic pressure variation; PPV, pulse pressure variation; SVV, stroke volume variation. (Adapted from *Quick Guide to Cardiopulmonary Care*. 3rd ed. Used with permission from Edwards Critical Care Education.)

8. **Techniques of insertion.** The introducer is placed in a manner similar to that described for CVP insertion. However, special care should be observed with PAC placement, noting especially the following points:

    a. **Sedation.** Because the patient is under a large drape for a longer period of time, he or she should be asked questions periodically to check for oversedation. A clear drape allows visual inspection of the patient's color and may produce a less suffocating feeling.

    b. **ECG monitoring during placement.** It is essential to monitor the ECG during placement of the catheter because dysrhythmias are the most common complication associated with PAC insertion.

    c. **Pulse oximetry.** Pulse oximetry gives an audible signal of rhythm and may alert the physician to an abnormal rhythm.

d. Preferred approach. The right IJ approach offers the most direct route to the RA and thus results in the highest rate of successful PA catheterization. The left subclavian route is next most effective.

e. Balloon inflation. Air should be used for balloon inflation. If any suspicion exists about balloon competency, the PAC should be removed and the balloon inspected directly to avoid iatrogenic air embolism.

f. Waveform. A vast majority of cardiac anesthesiologists use waveform analysis to guide placement of the PAC tip. TEE or the use of fluoroscopy can aid placement in some situations. Representative waveforms are shown in Figure 4.14.

9. Complications. Complications [11] can be divided into vascular access, PAC placement/manipulation, and monitoring problems.

a. Vascular access. See Table 4.3 for complications of central venous cannulation.

b. PAC placement/manipulation

(1) Cardiac arrhythmias. Reported incidence ranges from 12.5% to 70%. PVCs are the most common arrhythmia. Fortunately, most arrhythmias resolve with either catheter withdrawal or with advancement of the catheter tip from the RV into the PA. There appears to be a higher incidence when the patient is positioned in the Trendelenburg position versus right-tilt position.

(2) Mechanical damage. Catheter knotting and entanglement of cardiac structures, although rare, can occur. Damage to intracardiac structures such as valves, chordae, and even RV perforation have been reported. The presence of IVC filters, indwelling catheters, and pacemakers can increase the risk of such complications. The incidence of knotting is estimated at 0.03% and this complication can be decreased with careful attention to depth of insertion and expected waveforms. To reduce the risk of knotting, a catheter should be withdrawn if the RV waveform is still present 20 cm after its initial appearance or when the absolute depth of 60 cm is reached without a PA tracing.

(3) PA rupture. This is a rare complication with an incidence of 0.03% to 0.2%. Risk factors include pulmonary hypertension, age greater than 60, hyperinflation of the balloon, improper (distal) catheter positioning, and coagulopathy. During CPB, distal migration of the catheter tip may occur, thus some advocate pulling the PAC back a few centimeters prior to initiating bypass.

(4) Thrombosis. Although thrombus formation on PACs has been noted at 24 hours, the incidence of thrombogenicity substantially increases by 72 hours.

(5) Pulmonary infarction. It can occur as a complication of continuous distal, wedging from catheter migration, or embolization of previously formed thrombus.

(6) Infection. The incidence of bacteremia and blood stream infection related to PAC is 1.3% to 2.3%. Additionally, the PAC can contribute to endothelial damage of the tricuspid and pulmonary valves leading to endocarditis.

(7) Other. Balloon rupture, heparin-induced thrombocytopenia (HIT) secondary to heparin-coated catheters, anaphylaxis from latex (balloon) allergy, and hepatic venous placement have all been included in PAC-related complications.

c. Monitoring complications

(1) Errors in equipment and data acquisition. Examples include inappropriate pressure transducer leveling and over/underdamping of pressure system.

(2) Misinterpretation or misapplication of data. Misinterpretation can occur when not considering ventilation modes, ventricular compliance changes, or intrinsic cardiac/pulmonary pathologies.

(3) Expense.

(4) If a PCWP/PAOP waveform appears spontaneously (indicating wedge positioning of the PAC), confirmation that the PAC balloon is deflated followed by withdrawal of the PAC until a PA waveform appears should be performed immediately.

10. Conclusions. PACs provide a wealth of information about the right and left sides of the circulation. For this reason, they are used for every cardiac surgical procedure in some institutions because their benefits are perceived to outweigh the risks. Studies that show low-morbidity rates with PAC use support this viewpoint. In other institutions, however, clinicians are more selective about which patients require PACs, because use of PA monitoring has not been demonstrated to incontrovertibly improve outcomes of cardiac surgery. The widespread application of TEE may make intraoperative PAC data less useful except for SvO_2. Additionally, noninvasive CO monitoring may also replace some uses of the PAC, although these monitors have technologic obstacles to solve prior to routine use (without invasive monitoring) during cardiac surgery. While there is increasing evidence that the risks of PA catheterization may outweigh the benefits in some clinical settings, we strongly feel that this device, especially with newer modalities such as continuous SvO_2 measurement, provides data that are not easily obtainable by any other method. The majority of studies that have failed to find a benefit for PA catheterization have typically included patients in a medical intensive care or medical cardiology setting. It is difficult to generalize these studies to the cardiothoracic surgical population, as many medical ICU patients have derangements of microvascular circulation and/or mitochondrial dysfunction, whereas surgical ICU patients, while certainly at risk for developing these microcirculatory abnormalities, tend to be earlier in the disease process. This may provide a reason why PACs tend to be more useful in a surgical population. Given the complexity of many cardiothoracic surgery cases, an anesthesia provider would be at a severe disadvantage without the data provided by a pulmonary arterial catheter. Indeed, based on data from a national registry of anesthesia outcomes, it appears that PAC use had increased in cardiac surgery cases between 2010 and 2014 [12].

G. Cardiac output (CO)
   1. Methods
      a. Thermodilution with cold injectate. This method is the most commonly utilized CO technique because of its ease of use and ability to repeat measurements over time. The indicator is an aliquot of saline (typically 10 mL, which is at a lower temperature than the temperature of blood) injected into the RA. The change in temperature produced by injection of this indicator is measured in the PA by a thermistor and is integrated over time to generate a value for RV output, which is equal to systemic CO if no intra-cardiac shunts are present. This method requires no withdrawal of blood and no arterial line, uses an inexpensive indicator, and is not greatly affected by recirculation.

CLINICAL PEARL   Thermodilution CO underestimates the CO with right-side valvular lesions, but remains accurate with mitral and aortic valve lesions (Fig. 4.16).

---

      b. Continuous thermodilution. A thermal filament in the catheter heats blood ~15 to 25 cm before its tip, thus generating a PA temperature change that is measured via a distal thermistor. The input and output signals are correlated to generate CO values.
      c. RV ejection fraction. Improved preload estimates might be obtained with this type of PAC [13].
   2. Assumptions and errors. Specific errors in CO determination are mentioned below:
      a. Thermodilution method
         (1) Volume of injectate. Because the output computer will base its calculations on a specific volume, an injectate volume less than that for which the computer is set will cause a falsely high value of CO, and vice versa.
         (2) Temperature of injectate. If the injectate temperature parameter is incorrect, errors can occur. For example, an increase of $1°C$ will cause a 3% overestimation of CO. The controversy over iced versus room-temperature injectate centers around the concept that a larger difference between the injectate temperature and blood temperature should increase the accuracy of the CO determination. Studies have not supported this hypothesis, and the extra inconvenience of keeping syringes on ice, together with the increased risk of infection (nonsterile water surrounding the Luer tip), make the iced saline method a less attractive alternative.

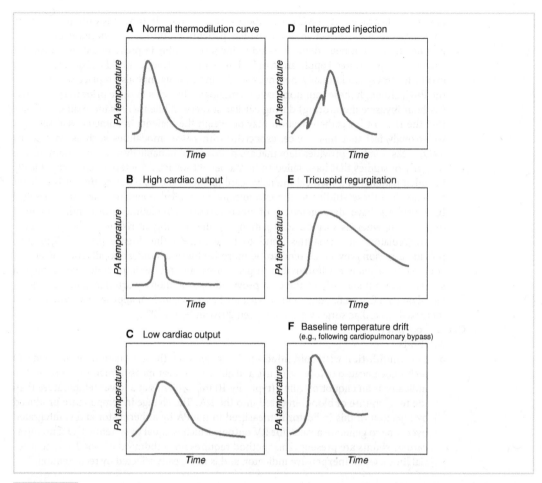

FIGURE 4.16 Thermodilution curves recorded from a pulmonary artery catheter (PAC) thermistor. Cardiac output (CO) is inversely related to the area under the curve. The curves on the left (**A, B, C**) demonstrated normal, high, and low CO, respectively. Curve **D** demonstrates an error in thermodilution technique. Curve **E** demonstrates a thermodilution curve in a patient with TR, where recirculation of the injected fluid results in distortion of the descending limb of the curve, causing an increase in the area under the curve and an underestimation of the CO. Curve **F** is representative of a patient who was recently liberated from cardiopulmonary bypass (CPB). Blood from cooled parts of the body will decrease the overall temperature of the overall circulation, leading to a drift in baseline, which will cause an overestimation of CO. (From Longnecker DE, Brown DL, Newman MF, et al. *Anesthesiology*. 2nd ed. McGraw-Hill Companies; 2012, Figure 30.14, P. 420.)

(3) **Shunts.** Intracardiac shunts will cause erroneous values for thermodilution CO values. This technique should not be used if a communication exists between the pulmonary and systemic circulations. A shunt should always be suspected when thermodilution CO values do not fit the clinical findings.

(4) **Timing with the respiratory cycle.** As much as a 10% difference in CO will result, depending on when injection occurs during the respiratory cycle. These changes are most likely due to actual changes in pulmonary blood flow during respiration.

(5) **Catheter position.** The tip of the pulmonary catheter must be in the PA and must not be "wedged"; otherwise, nonsensical curves are obtained.

3. **Minimally invasive CO monitoring.** The desire to assess cardiac function and adequate tissue perfusion in critically ill patients is traditionally accomplished using the PAC. The controversy about its invasive nature and potential harm has provoked the development of

less invasive CO monitoring devices [14,15]. Just as the PAC has its nuances, these devices have their own sets of limitations that must be considered.

a. **Accuracy and precision.** Accuracy refers to the capability of a measurement to reflect the true CO. This means that a measurement is compared to a "gold standard" method. Given the widespread use of the PAC, the thermodilution method is the practical "gold" standard to which new noninvasive CO monitors are compared. However, it is important to take into account that the inherent error for thermodilution measurements of CO are in the 10% to 20% range. *Precision* indicates the reproducibility of a measurement and refers to the variability between determinations. For the thermodilution method, studies of precision have involved probability analyses of large numbers of CO determinations. Using this approach, it was found that with two injections, there was only a 50% chance that the numbers obtained were within 5% of the true CO. If three injections yield results that are within 10% of one another, there is a 90% probability that the average value is within 10% of the true CO.

   Given that the practical gold standard carries with it some inaccuracies, new methods based on it will also hold their own similar inherent error.

b. **Methods:** Minimally invasive CO monitors can be classified into one of the four main groups: Pulse pressure analysis, pulsed Doppler technologies, applications of Fick principle using partial CO_2 rebreathing, and bioimpedance/bioreactance.

   (1) **Pulse pressure analysis:** Monitors based on that principle SV can be tracked continuously by analysis of the arterial waveform. These monitors require an optimal arterial waveform, thus arrhythmias, IABPs, LVADs, and even properties of the arterial line monitoring systems (such as over/underdamping) can alter accuracy of the CO measurement. Three common pulse contour analysis devices are compared in Table 4.12.

   (2) **Doppler devices:** CO can be measured using the change in frequency of an ultrasonic beam as it measures blood flow velocity. To achieve accurate measurements, at least three conditions must be met: (1) The cross-sectional area of the vessel must be known; (2) the ultrasound beam must be directed parallel to the flow of blood; and (3) the beam direction cannot move to any great degree between measurements. Clinical use of this technique is associated with reduced accuracy and precision.

   Two methods that use ultrasound are as follows:

   (a) **Transtracheal.** Flow in the ascending aorta is determined with a transducer bonded to the distal portion of the endotracheal tube, designed to ensure contact of the transducer with the wall of the trachea. This method is not yet fully validated in humans, and a study of cardiac patients reported poor correlation when compared to thermodilution.

   (b) **Transesophageal.** Several esophageal Doppler probes are available which are smaller than conventional TEE probes. CO is obtained by multiplying the cross-sectional area of the aorta by the blood flow velocity. Flow in the aorta is measured using a transducer placed in the esophagus. Aortic cross-sectional area is provided from a nomogram or measured by M-mode echocardiography (Fig. 4.17).

   (c) **TEE.** In addition to the Doppler technique mentioned above, TEE utilizes Simpson rule in which the LV is divided into a series of disks to estimate CO without the use of Doppler. End-diastolic and end-systolic dimensions measured by echocardiography are converted to volumes, allowing SV and CO to be determined. Given the size of the monitor and probe, this technique can provide intermittent CO, but is not ideal for continuous CO measurement desired in ICU settings.

   Summary: The PAC still remains the practical gold standard for evaluating CO. It also provides true mixed venous saturation and pulmonary pressures that cannot be obtained from noninvasive devices. Invasive hemodynamic monitoring remains the standard in the operating theater. However, select stable cardiac patients may be candidates in the ICU or stepdown units postoperatively for minimally invasive device monitoring.

TABLE 4.12 Pulse contour analysis devices

	FloTrac system	PiCCOplus system	LiDCOplus system
Requires external calibration	No	Yes	Yes
Requires central line	No	Yes	No
Type of calibration	—	Transpulmonary thermodilution via (CVL)	Pulmonary lithium indicator
Special arterial catheter	No	Yes, thermistor-tipped catheter	No
Preferred arterial site	Any site	Femoral	Any site
Alternative sites	—	Radial/brachial (require longer catheter)	—
Main advantages	Minimally invasive Operator independent Easy to use	Broad range of hemodynamic parameters More robust during hemodynamic instability (with frequent recalibration)	Minimally invasive Easy to use More robust during hemodynamic Instability (with frequent recalibration)
Main disadvantages	Reliability in vasoplegic patients low in older versions Less robust during hemodynamic instability	More invasive Requires recalibration	Disturbing factors (lithium use, neuromuscular blocking agents) Requires recalibration
Method	Concept that the area under the curve of the systolic arterial waveform is proportional to SV. Standard deviation of pulse pressure is correlated with "normal" SV based on a database of patient demographics (age, sex, weight, height). Impedance is also derived from this demographic data	Concept that the area under the curve of the systolic arterial waveform is proportional to SV. Calibration used to determine the individual aortic impedance. Recalibration recommended every 8 hrs in stable patients; increased frequency of recalibration (up to every 1 hr) needed in patients with hemodynamic instability (significant changes of vascular resistance)	Concept of conservation of mass (power). Suggests that after calibration and correction for compliance, the relationship of net power and net flow is linear. Calibration used to determine resistance of vasculature; recalibration recommended q8h. Lithium calibration negatively affected by: 1. Changes in electrolytes 2. Changes in hematocrit 3. High peak doses of muscle relaxant 4. Patient on lithium 5. Patients <40 kg
Additional assessments provided	SVV	Global end-diastolic volume; extravascular lung volume; SVV	SVV

Goal-directed assessment of fluid-responsive hypovolemia can be automatically measured by several commercially available devices. Comparison of these devices is depicted. PPV, pulse pressure variation; SPV, systolic pressure variation; SV, stroke volume; SVV, stroke volume variation.

4. **Measurements of volume responsiveness**. Fluid management is an integral part of anesthetic care. Fluid administration is regularly administered intraoperatively to improve CO. However, given frequent comorbidities associated with conditions that require cardiac surgery, including congestive heart failure and chronic kidney disease, indiscriminate administration of fluids may be contraindicated. Because of the complex physiology associated with both cardiac surgery and general anesthesia, determination of volume

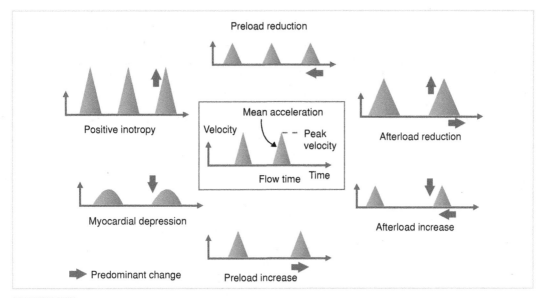

FIGURE 4.17 Doppler waveforms of aortic blood flow from esophageal Doppler monitoring. The esophageal Doppler device derives cardiac output (CO) from the measured peak velocity, mean acceleration, and systolic flow time. As illustrated in the figure, changes in contractility will affect both peak velocity and mean acceleration, while changes in preload primarily affect systolic flow time; afterload changes will alter all three variables. (From Longnecker DE, Brown DL, Newman MF, et al. *Anesthesiology*. 2nd ed. McGraw-Hill Companies; 2012, Figure 30.15, P. 422.)

responsiveness can be complex. Studies have shown that static pressure measurements that have historically been used to assess for volume responsiveness, specifically, CVP and pulmonary capillary occlusion pressure (PAOP), are unreliable [16,17]. Dynamic parameters (Table 4.13) such as SPV, PPV, and SVV have shown very promising correlations with volume responsiveness [18].

Methods

(1) **Systolic pressure variation.** Increased intrathoracic pressure generated during a positive pressure breath leads to decreased LV stroke volume, and subsequently a drop in sBP. The drop in the systolic pressure from baseline to after delivery of a fixed tidal volume the delta down (Δ down) has been shown to correlate with volume status. The advantage of this parameter is that only a standard arterial line is required (Fig. 4.18A).

(2) **Pulse pressure variation.** A similar concept to SPV, PPV compares changes in pulse pressure, that is, the difference between systolic and diastolic pressures throughout the respiratory cycle in a mechanically ventilated patient. It has been demonstrated that PPV is a more accurate surrogate of SV, most likely because SPV is influenced by both aortic transmural pressure (from the LV stroke volume) and extramural pressure from changes in pleural pressure, whereas PPV eliminates

TABLE 4.13 Measurements of fluid responsiveness

Parameter	Normal	Fluid responsive
SPV (mm Hg)	5 mm Hg	>10 mm Hg
PPV (%)	<13%	>13%
SVV (%)	<10%	>10–15%

Comparison of SPV/PPV/SVV. Goal-directed assessment of fluid responsiveness in hypovolemic patients. SPV, systolic pressure variation; PPV, pulse pressure variation; SVV, stroke volume variation.

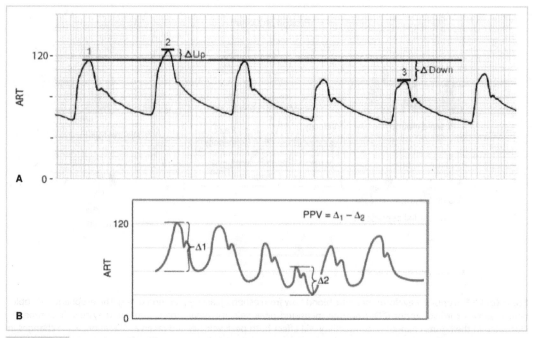

FIGURE 4.18 **A:** Arterial waveform tracing demonstrating systolic pressure variation (SPV). The first cycle is recorded during apnea, giving a baseline from which ΔUp and ΔDown are measured. In this case ΔUp is approximately 7 mm Hg, while ΔDown is 5 mm Hg, giving an SPV of 22 mm Hg, indicating that this patient would likely respond to a fluid challenge. (From Pittman JA, Ping JS, Mark JB, et al. Arterial and central venous pressure monitoring. *Int Anesthesiol Clin.* 2004 Winter;42(1):13–30.) **B:** An illustration of pulse pressure variation. In this case, the maximal pulse pressure, $\Delta1$, is approximately 60 mm Hg, and the minimal, $\Delta2$, is 35 mm Hg, giving a pulse pressure difference of $\Delta1 - \Delta2 = 25$ mm Hg. The pulse pressure difference divided by the mean of the two values (47.5 mm Hg) gives a pulse pressure variation of 53%, which is greater than 12%, indicating that this patient would also likely respond to a fluid challenge. (From Longnecker DE, Brown DL, Newman MF, et al. *Anesthesiology.* 2nd ed. McGraw-Hill Companies; 2012, Figure 30.18, P. 425.)

the effects of pleural pressure as systolic and diastolic pressures would be affected equally. While this parameter can also be measured by a standard arterial line, many of the minimally invasive CO measurement devices that rely on pulse contour analysis will automatically calculate this number (Fig. 4.18B).

(3) **Stroke volume variation.** Real-time measurement of variations in SV has been made possible using the same arterial waveform analysis used for minimally invasive continuous CO monitoring (see above). These devices determine SV using an algorithm based on the contour of the arterial pressure tracing. SVV is also measured, using the formula $SVV = (SV_{max} - SV_{min})/SV_{mean}$. SVV has been shown to very accurately predict volume responsiveness in critical care patients [19].

5. **Limitations**

CLINICAL PEARL   Generally, SPV, PPV, and SVV require a regular heart rhythm to be accurate.

Further, because all of these parameters rely on cardiopulmonary interaction, it has been noted that their utility during open heart surgery may be limited. One study demonstrated good correlation between SVV/PPV and preload surrogates before sternotomy and after sternal closure, but poor correlation while the chest was open [20]. However, it should be noted that this study did not look at fluid responsiveness, only correlation between PPV/SVV and other surrogates for preload, such as LV end-diastolic area as measured by transthoracic echocardiography and by RV end-diastolic volume measured by a PAC, both of which have their own limitations.

6. **Conclusions.** Determination of volume responsiveness via measurement of PPV and SVV is a promising newer modality that may be of some use during cardiac surgery and likely during postoperative management of volume resuscitation. These measurements are built into several of the minimally invasive CO measurement modalities, making their use increasingly available as these devices gain wider acceptance. While there are multiple limitations to utilization of PPV and SVV during cardiac surgery, these may be mitigated by future improvements in the arterial waveform analysis algorithms.

H. **Echocardiography**

TEE. TEE is discussed extensively in Chapter 5.

III. **Temperature**

Cardiac anesthesia is unique in that therapeutic hypothermia is utilized frequently and aggressively in many cases. Distribution of thermal energy can be manipulated, via CPB, more rapidly and extensively than any other anesthetic case. Unique to cardiac anesthesia are circulatory arrest procedures [21] with cooling to 17°C. Temperature monitoring for cardiac anesthesia has unique considerations. This section will introduce these topics without detailed discussion of thermal issues common to all anesthesiologists [22].

A. **Indications: CPB and hypothermia**

1. "Warm" CPB: 36° to 37°C; also known as normothermic CPB.
2. "Mild" CPB hypothermia: 32° to 34°C; occasionally termed "tepid."
3. Moderate hypothermia: 28° to 32°C. Infrequently utilized.
4. DHCA: 17° to 19°C. This unique therapeutic technique is discussed above.

Cardiac surgery utilizes the capabilities of the CPB circuit to rapidly cool or warm patients. Mild–moderate hypothermia was a common neuroprotective strategy into the 1990s. Literature comparing normothermic CPB with hypothermic CPB showed no benefit. Although hypothermic CPB is still occasionally used, the dysfunction in coagulation pathways and bleeding risk remains a major consideration. Below 32°C, the myocardium is irritable and susceptible to arrhythmias, especially during ventricular tachycardia and fibrillation. The risk of dysrhythmia is particularly high in pediatric patients. The CPB machine can exceed 37°C and the anesthesiologist should be aware of the inflow temperatures. Hyperthermia produces significant enzyme desaturation and cell damage with temperatures ≥41°C.

B. **Sites of measurement.** Numerous possible sites exist to measure temperature. These sites can be grouped into the core, brain, or the shell.

1. **Core temperature**
   a. **General considerations.** The core temperature represents the temperature of the vital organs. The term *core temperature* used here is perhaps a misnomer because gradients exist even within this vessel-rich group during rapid changes in blood temperature.
   b. **PAC thermistor.** This is the best estimate of the core temperature when pulmonary blood flow is present (i.e., before and after CPB).
   c. **Nasopharyngeal temperature.** Nasopharyngeal temperature provides an accurate reflection of brain temperature during CPB. Overinsertion is common, causing the probe to measure esophageal temperature. The probe should be inserted into the nasopharynx to a distance equivalent to the distance from the naris to the tip of the earlobe. Nasopharyngeal temperature should be monitored in all hypothermic circulatory arrest procedures and CPB cases with hypothermia requiring rewarming.
   d. **Tympanic membrane temperature.** Temperature at this site reflects brain temperature, and may provide an alternative to nasopharyngeal temperature.
   e. **Bladder temperature.** This modality has been used to measure core temperature, although it may be inaccurate in instances when renal blood flow and urine production are decreased.
   f. **Esophageal temperature.** Because the esophagus is a mediastinal structure, it will be greatly affected by the temperature of the blood returning from the extracorporeal pump and should NOT be used routinely for cases involving CPB.

    g. CPB arterial line temperature. This is the temperature of the heat exchanger (i.e., the lowest temperature during active cooling and the highest temperature during active rewarming). During either of these phases, a gradient always exists between the arterial line temperature and any other temperature.

    h. CPB venous line temperature. This is the "return" temperature to the oxygenator and probably best reflects core temperature during CPB when no active warming or cooling is occurring.

2. Shell temperature

    a. General. The shell compartment represents the majority of the body (muscle, fat, bone), which receives a smaller proportion of the blood flow, thus acting as an energy sink that can significantly affect temperature fluxes. Shell temperature lags behind core temperature during cooling and rewarming. At the point of bypass separation, the core temperature will be significantly higher than shell temperature. The final equilibrium temperature with thermal redistribution probably will be closer to the shell temperature than the core temperature measured initially.

    b. Rectal temperature. Although traditionally thought of as a core temperature, during CPB procedures the rectal temperature most accurately reflects muscle mass temperature. If the tip of the probe rests in stool, a significant lag will exist with changing temperatures.

    c. Skin temperature. Skin temperature is rarely utilized in cardiac surgery.

C. Risks of temperature monitoring. Epistaxis with nasopharyngeal temperature monitoring.

D. Recommendations for temperature monitoring. Monitoring temperature at two sites is recommended: A core site and a shell site. Arterial and venous line temperatures are available directly from the CPB apparatus. Nasal temperature monitoring is recommended for circulatory arrest cases to document brain temperature.

IV. Renal function

A. Indications for monitoring

1. Increased incidence of renal failure after CPB. Acute renal failure is a recognized complication of CPB, occurring in 2.5% to 31% of cases. Acute renal failure is related to the preoperative renal function as well as to the presence of coexisting disease. The nonpulsatile renal blood flow during CPB has been speculated as a contributing mechanism, although continuous-flow LVAD has not been associated with excessive renal failure.

2. Use of diuretics in CPB prime. Mannitol is used routinely during CPB for two reasons:

    a. Hemolysis occurs during CPB, and serum hemoglobin levels rise. Urine output should be maintained to avoid damage to renal tubules.

    b. Deliberate hemodilution is induced with the onset of hypothermic CPB. Maintenance of good urine output during and after CPB allows removal of excess free water.

B. Urinary catheter. This monitor is the single most important monitor of renal function during surgical cases involving CPB. Establishing a urinary catheter should be a priority in emergencies.

CLINICAL PEARL   Oliguria or anuria is NOT typical during CPB, as the priming fluid typically contains mannitol.

Hypothermia can be assessed with a temperature probe/Foley catheter.

C. Electrolytes. Serum electrolytes, especially potassium and magnesium, should be checked throughout the procedure including at the start of the case, prior to separation from CPB and after CPB. A therapeutic goal of $K^+ \geq 4.0$ mEq/L and $Mg^{++} \geq 2.0$ mg/dL is commonly utilized. In the vast majority of patients with adequate renal function, potassium and magnesium concentrations will decline during CPB secondary to mannitol and improved perfusion. Replacement of potassium has to account for cardioplegia which contains potassium. A low serum ionized calcium level may be the cause of diminished pump function. The timing of the calcium therapy may affect neurologic outcome, Administration of Ca^{++} during periods of neural ischemia

14

and/or reperfusion may worsen the outcome. Many cardiac anesthesiologists will not administer calcium until at least 15 to 20 minutes following acceptable perfusion (i.e., after aortic cross-clamp removal).

D. Acute kidney injury (AKI). While AKI is defined by changes in creatinine/glomerular filtration rate and urine output, novel serum markers such as neutrophil gelatinase–associated lipocalin (NGAL), may prove useful in the early detection of AKI.

V. Neurologic function

A. General considerations. Neurocognitive dysfunction is a significant complication in the cardiac surgical patient. Increased risk of poor outcomes is multifactorial. Cardiac surgical patients frequently have increased baseline susceptibility for neurocognitive insults from arterial atherosclerotic disease, diabetes, and genetic polymorphism(s) coupled. Acute neurologic injury secondary to CPB and cerebral emboli (air, atheromatous material, thrombus) are major contributing events to development of postoperative deficits. Advances in processing capability have made new devices available for neurologic assessment and risk factor modification during surgery [23–26]. Goals of monitoring include: diagnose cerebral ischemia, assess the depth of anesthesia and assess the effectiveness of medications given for brain or spinal cord protection.

B. Indications for monitoring neurologic function

1. Associated carotid disease
2. Diagnosis of embolic phenomenon
3. Diagnosis of aortic cannula malposition
4. Diagnosis of inadequate arterial flow on CPB
5. Confirmation of adequate cooling
6. Hypothermic circulatory arrest, in an adult or a child
7. Procedures with aortic cross-clamps at T5–L5 which may exclude artery of Adamkiewicz

C. Physiologic and metabolic monitoring

1. **Cerebral perfusion pressure (CPP).** Maintaining adequate CPP is the primary intervention for any neuroprotective strategy. Cerebral blood flow (CBF) undergoes autoregulation with CPP of 50 to 150 mm Hg. Hypertensive patients may have a right shift in this curve. A CPP of 60 to 70 mm Hg is a reasonable goal.

$$CPP = MAP - CVP$$

In patients with elevated intracranial pressure (ICP), the highest pressure (CVP or ICP) should be utilized. There are a number of clinical factors that can increase the CVP resulting in threatened CBF. Two therapeutic targets which can be modified are increased *CVP* and increased *mean airway pressure.*

CLINICAL PEARL Trendelenburg positioning is an often overlooked cause of increased CVP. This, along with elevated mean airway pressures, can lead to decreased cerebral perfusion pressures.

Choice of vasoactive drugs can affect CVP. Increased splanchnic resistance with low-dose α-adrenergic receptor agonists facilitates blood sequestration (↓ CVP) whereas β$_2$-adrenergic receptor activation, especially in presence of higher doses of α-adrenergic receptor agonists, results in shift of sequestered blood into central circulation from venous capacitance sites [27].

2. **End-tidal CO_2 and mean airway pressure.** Hyperventilation to a $PaCO_2$ is a core anesthesia technique to rapidly reduce CBF resulting in decreased ICP. The ventilator goal to preserve CPP is maintaining normocapnia. Ventilator settings should avoid maneuvers that increase *mean airway pressure.* PEEP/CPAP are obvious maneuvers that should be evaluated for contribution to mean airway pressure. A pressure mode of ventilation would seem most appropriate to achieve these goals.

3. **Inspired oxygen concentration (FiO_2).** Neural tissues are susceptible to ischemia/reperfusion injury including reactive oxygen species. Mannitol is an antioxidant as well as

an osmotic diuretic. Consider mannitol (0.25 to 1.0 g/kg IV) administration immediately prior to initiating CPB with a repeat dose when aortic cross-clamp removed. The lowest safe FiO_2 should be employed.

4. **Blood glucose monitoring.** Hyperglycemia markedly worsens neurologic outcomes when present during ischemia/reperfusion. An insulin continuous infusion (CI) should be immediately available in all patients with DM. It is important to note that the effects of insulin are diminished with hypothermia and increased catechol states. β-Adrenergic stimulation from the stress response to CPB increases blood glucose. Insulin CI alters K^+ and strong consideration should be given to administration of KCl and $MgSO_4$ when starting insulin CI. As a clinically applicable technical note, insulin undergoes nonspecific binding to the IV tubing. Until these nonspecific binding sites are saturated, very little insulin actually reaches the patient. The blood glucose goal has engendered controversy regarding how rigorously it should be controlled. Avoiding hypoglycemia is a critically important goal. Virtually all cardiac anesthesiologists will treat hyperglycemia exceeding 200 mg/dL.

5. **Cerebral perfusion monitoring.** Observation of the face for evenly distributed blanching and reperfusion when starting CPB is a crude method to assess cannula position. Some cardiac anesthesiologists advocate bilateral manual compression of the carotid arteries as CPB is initiated and aortic cross-clamp applied. The reasoning is that occlusion of the major vascular conduit to the brain during a high-risk period for cerebral emboli should decrease brain insult. Obviously cerebral emboli originating from the carotid arteries make this maneuver controversial.

D. Monitors of CNS electrical activity

1. **Electroencephalogram** (EEG; see Chapter 26). The EEG measures the electrical currents generated by the postsynaptic potentials in the pyramidal cell layer of the cerebral cortex. The basic principle of clinical EEG monitoring is that cerebral ischemia causes slowing (↑ latency) of the electrical activity of the brain, as well as a decrease in signal amplitude. EEG requires additional personnel (↑ cost) for monitoring and alterations of anesthetic technique. Although intriguing, there is a paucity of literature evaluating EEG in cardiac surgical patients.

2. **Processed EEG.** To increase its intraoperative utility, the EEG data are processed by fast Fourier analysis into a single power versus time **spectral array** that is more easily interpreted. Examples of power spectrum analysis include **compressed spectral array, density spectral array**, and **bispectral index (BIS)**. The BIS monitor analyzes the phase relationships between different frequency components over time. The result is reduced via a proprietary method to a single number scaled between 0 (electrical silence) and 100 (alert wakefulness). The role of BIS monitoring in cardiac surgery is in evolution [28]. The BIS may be a useful indicator of the depth of anesthesia. Studies of BIS values as a predictor of anesthetic depth during intravenous anesthesia (narcotic plus benzodiazepine) are conflicting. One study found a positive correlation between the BIS and arousal or hemodynamic responses [29], whereas another study found no such correlation between the BIS value and plasma concentrations of fentanyl and midazolam [30]. During hypothermic circulatory arrest, the BIS monitor should be isoelectric (BIS of zero). Many cardiac anesthesiologists monitor the BIS during cooling and to observe the effect of supplemental intravenous anesthetic (historically thiopental) administered for neuroprotection. Evidence supporting BIS data as a monitor of neurologic function in patients at risk for hypoxic or ischemic brain injury continues to accumulate [31]. Abnormally low BIS scores and prolonged low BIS score may be associated with poor neurologic outcomes.

3. **Evoked potentials**

   a. **Somatosensory evoked potentials (SSEPs).** SSEPs monitor the integrity of the posterior-lateral spinal cord. It is most useful in operations such as surgery for a thoracic aneurysm, in which the blood flow to the spinal cord may be compromised. A stimulus is applied to a peripheral nerve (usually the tibial nerve), and the resultant brainstem and brain activity is quantified.

    b. **Visual evoked response and brainstem audio evoked responses.** These techniques do not have routine clinical application in cardiac surgical procedures.

    c. **Motor evoked potentials (MEPs).** MEPs are useful to monitor the anterior spinal cord during surgery of the descending aorta and are discussed in more detail in Chapter 14.

E. **Monitors of regional cerebral metabolic function: Jugular bulb venous oximetry.** Measuring the oxygen saturation of the cerebral jugular bulb ($SjvVO_2$) with a fiberoptic catheter [32] is analogous to measuring the SvO_2 in the PA. The brain is the highest O_2-extracting organ in the body. If CBF decreases, oxygen extraction would increase and the jugular O_2 saturation would decrease. $SjvVO_2$ gives reliable real-time data for the ipsilateral cerebral hemisphere. Bilateral $SjvVO_2$ catheters are required to monitor the entire brain. Significant interpatient variability exists with $SjvVO_2$, trend monitoring may yield more information than individual measurements. $SjvVO_2$ catheter placement is an invasive procedure. Typically a RIJ (retrograde) $SjvVO_2$ catheter is placed as that is most common site for central line/PAC. Severe desaturation as measured by $SjvVO_2$ has been shown to correlate with poor outcome.

F. **Near-infrared spectroscopy (NIRS) and cerebral oximetry.** NIRS is a noninvasive method to monitor cerebral metabolic function [31]. A near-infrared light is emitted from a scalp sensor and penetrates the scalp, skull, cerebrospinal fluid, and brain. The light is reflected by tissue but differentially absorbed by hemoglobin-containing moieties. Cerebral oximetry, unlike $SjvVO_2$, conveniently allows for bilateral data acquisition. It is imperative that baseline cerebral oximetry measurements are acquired to allow intraoperative interpretation of the data. The actual value appears to be less important than the trend. A deviation of 20% from baseline values is considered an actionable significant difference. Currently, the role of NIRS cerebral oximetry application during cardiac surgery is controversial. Anecdotal reports have not yet transitioned to improved outcomes and the cost–benefit is unclear. A recent meta-analysis report states: "Only low-level evidence links low $rScO_2$ during cardiac surgery to postoperative neurologic complications, and data are insufficient to conclude that interventions to improve $rScO_2$ desaturation prevent stroke or POCD" [33].

G. **Monitors of CNS embolic events**

    1. **Transcranial Doppler ultrasonography (TCD).** TCD is very useful in detecting emboli in the cerebral circulation. Incorporation into clinical practice has been hindered by difficulty obtaining a reliable signal. TCD has been utilized primarily as a research tool. TCD assessment of embolic load can detect up to hundreds (sic) of discreet emboli. Embolic showers are particularly associated with aortic cross-clamp application and removal.

    2. **Epiaortic scanning.** The importance of aortic atheromas, especially in the ascending aorta and/or aortic arch, in association with poor neurologic outcomes has long been recognized. Aortic atheromas with a mobile component present the greatest risk. The introduction and use of TEE to detect aortic atheroma was a significant improvement over surgical palpation. However, TEE had significant limitations particularly in the detection of disease near the typical aortic cannulation site (distal ascending aorta, proximal aortic arch) because the airway structures interfere with the TEE signal. Epiaortic scanning is a highly sensitive and specific monitoring modality to detect atheroma in the thoracic aorta including regions where TEE evaluation is not possible. In cardiac surgical patients with identified atheroma, modification of the surgical technique and neuroprotective strategies has been reported to reduce neurologic complication from ~60% to almost 0%.

H. **Monitors of splanchnic perfusion and venous function**
   Gastric tonometry

    a. **Gastric tonometry as a hypovolemia monitor.** The management of hypovolemia is a fundamental tenet of anesthesiology. There are many causes of hypovolemia including bleeding and fluid shifts. Physiologically, the venous capacitance vessels sequester 70% of the total blood volume, which is returned to the central venous system as the initial response to hypovolemia [26]. Hypovolemia resulting in hypotension is a frequent issue in cardiac surgical procedures. Early recognition and treatment is critical as hypovolemia is a reversible problem. Multiple routine monitors directly (TEE, PAC/CVP, urine output, physical examination) or indirectly (certain labs, fluctuations in the arterial catheter waveform) assess volume status. A major clinical limitation is that loss of 10% to 25% of the total blood volume is undetectable by the typical cardiac surgery monitors whereas loss of 5% is detectable by gastric tonometry.

b. **Gastric tonometry and splanchnic hypoperfusion.** The splanchnic venous system is the key reservoir for the sequestered blood and is more responsive to sympathetic activation, especially α- and β_2-adrenergic receptor agonists, than the arterial vasculature [26]. Redistribution of splanchnic venous blood to the central circulation is the first compensatory mechanism in response to hypovolemia. Therefore, tissues that are within the splanchnic perfusion are the first to convert to anaerobic metabolism. Gastrointestinal mucosal cells produce acidic metabolites under anaerobic conditions. The tissue lining the gut neutralizes and eliminates the excess acid load by conversion to CO_2 via the HCO_3^- buffering system. The CO_2 freely diffuses across the cellular membrane and into the gut lumen. The CO_2 partial pressure can be readily detectable and quantifiable by gastric tonometry. Initially, gastric tonometry used the Henderson–Hasselbalch equation to calculate the gut mucosal intracellular pH (pHi). A pHi ≥ 7.32 was considered normal. Differences (CO_2 gap) between the pCO_2 (gut) versus $PaCO_2$ has supplanted pHi in more recent literature. In healthy human volunteers, decreased splanchnic perfusion secondary to experimental bleeding of 25% of estimated total blood volume was detected by gastric tonometry and SV, but not by other monitors of hypovolemia. Reinfusion of the blood returned all parameters to baseline [34].

c. **Clinical application of gastric tonometry.** Gastric tonometry has been studied primarily in cardiac surgery and ICU patients, where it proved to be a very sensitive predictor of poor clinical outcomes. Until recently there were no studies demonstrating that clinical interventions utilizing gastric tonometry goal-directed therapy benefitted the clinical outcome. Cardiac surgical patients receiving colloid volume expansion protocol (vs. control) had decreased major complications and length of stay (ICU and hospital) [35]. Interestingly a multicenter randomized clinical trial comparing gastric tonometry versus cardiac index goal-directed therapy failed to show a significant difference. However, "normalization of pHi within 24 hours of resuscitation is a strong signal of therapeutic success" and a "persistent low pHi despite treatment is associated with a very bad prognosis" [36]. The lack of evidence-based validation as a monitor with actionable data coupled with some initial technical issues with the manufacturer dampened enthusiasm for gastric tonometry. Reports in the literature generally agreed that a low pHi was a very sensitive marker for poor outcome but all of the studies were underpowered to determine if therapeutic normalization improved outcome. Therefore a meta-analysis was recently published that concluded that goal-directed therapy as measured by gastric tonometry does improve outcomes in critically ill patients [37].

d. **Advantages of gastric tonometry.** The diagnosis and treatment of hypovolemia is a fundamental component of anesthetic care. Due to the critically important role that the splanchnic vasculature plays with respect to hypovolemia, monitoring splanchnic function is potentially a significant clinical advancement. Gastric tonometry has several advantages compared to other monitors for hypovolemia:

(1) Monitor at organ/tissue level for regional specific function. The standard monitors for hypovolemia (art line, CVP, urine output) can only provide data at the level of the patient.

(2) Splanchnic vasculature sequesters 70% of TBV. The initial physiologic compensation for hypovolemia is transfer of blood from splanchnic vasculature to the central venous compartment.

(3) Gastric tonometry detects hypovolemia before other monitors. Loss of 10% to 12% of TBV is detected by gastric tonometry whereas some monitors (i.e., CVP) are unchanged from baseline. Bleeding of 25% TBV may not yet be reliably diagnosed by standard monitors.

(4) Minimally invasive. Gastric tonometry is measured via a nasogastric (NG) tube with a small balloon on the distal end. This is analogous to using a cuffed versus noncuffed endotracheal tube. In addition to acquiring gastric tonometry data, the NG tube is functional.

(5) Goal-directed therapy to correct splanchnic hypoperfusion may improve outcomes in critically ill patients.

(6) Gastric tonometry is a powerful predictor of poor outcome in nonresponders to goal-directed therapy.

(7) Gastric tonometry data can be collected and measured automatically.

(8) Placement is identical to any other NG tube. Although interference with acquisition of TEE images is a potential concern, clinical use without any adjustments or issues with TEE is our experience.

(9) Gastric tonometry may limit endotoxemia. Gut mucosal ischemia results in intestinal endothelial dysfunction as a barrier of translocation of bacteria/endotoxins into the systemic circulation. Gastric tonometry can detect splanchnic hypoperfusion and trigger intervention prior to endothelial dysfunction.

VI. **Cardiac surgical procedures with special monitoring considerations**

A. **OPCAB.** The standard CABG procedure is performed with CPB, which provides oxygenation and perfusion to the patient while the aortocoronary artery grafts are anastomosed. Advantageous technical aspects of CPB include a bloodless and immobile surgical field which facilitates precise placement of anastomotic sutures. Unfortunately, CPB causes neurocognitive deficits which may be exacerbated by events such as aortic cross-clamp application resulting in cerebral embolism (occasionally showering of hundreds of microemboli). This has motivated development of surgical techniques that allow cardiac revascularization without requiring CPB. Early experience had similar outcomes ± CPB. A recent meta-analysis suggests that OPCAB may improve outcomes in high-risk patients [38].

B. **OPCAB monitoring**

1. **Surgical techniques impact monitoring.** OPCAB emerged as a surgical approach that does not require CPB for revascularization. Unique components of the OPCAB procedure are placement of a myocardial stabilizer and apical suction device. The myocardial stabilizer adheres to the epicardial surface of the heart via suction and markedly restricts myocardial movement between the stabilizer arms. Inherently this results in compression of the heart and an RWMA. The apical cup attaches to, as its name implies, the apex of the heart. This allows the surgeon to manipulate the heart and the apical cup suspends the heart in the desired position. Typically, the apex is displaced anteriorly 60 to 90 degrees. Occasionally the heart is torqued to provide access to posterior and lateral targets. Additionally, a sterile pack is placed posterior to the heart to bring apex up into a position that the surgeon can quickly gain a hand grip to manually displace the heart. A "pericardial sling" is created to cradle the heart and provides another option to adjust the cardiac position while limiting manual compression.

2. **Hemodynamic monitoring during distal anastomoses.** Hemodynamic monitoring during positioning of the heart and throughout suturing of the distal anastomosis can be difficult, particularly diagnosing ischemic changes. Some cardiac anesthesiologists favor SvO$_2$ or ScvO$_2$ monitoring for OPCAB. Significant reduction of CO accompanied by hypotension and acute heart failure require immediate action. If prompt resolution of the hemodynamic instability is not achieved, conversion to (emergent) CPB is required. During the procedure, alterations commonly observed in hemodynamic monitors are:

   a. **TEE.** The posterior pericardial pack, apical displacement and pericardial sling may hinder image acquisition. Application of the epicardial stabilizer creates an obligate RWMA. Distinguishing RWMA secondary to ischemia versus mechanical impedance may not be possible.

   b. **ECG.** Low-voltage signal and distortion of the ECG tracing are very common observations. Diagnosing ischemic changes is problematic particularly when the apex is displaced because the cardiac vectors are altered in an unpredictable fashion. Dysrhythmia(s) is most likely to occur with coronary occlusion and with reperfusion. Preconditioning may attenuate ischemia/reperfusion insult.

c. **SpO$_2$.** Pulse oximetry may decrease due to low CO. Peripheral vasoconstriction from low CO may result in loss of SpO$_2$ signal. If access to the hand is available, digital nerve block with 1 to 2 mL of (plain) local anesthetic may restore the SpO$_2$ signal.

d. **Art line.** Arterial waveform may vary with impairment of CO. Systolic ejection of blood may be obstructed due to mechanical kinking of RV outflow tract or IVC/SVC. MAP of 60 to 65 mm Hg is typically utilized as a goal for perfusion pressure. Mechanical problems require mechanical solutions. Anatomic obstruction(s) due to unfavorable cardiac position can **not** be treated pharmacologically. Note that arterial pressure monitoring may indicate cardiac function without assessment of tissue $\dot{D}O_2$ to the rest of the body.

e. **SvO$_2$.** Global assessment of adequate $\dot{D}O_2$ can be inferred by determining O$_2$ consumption [$\dot{V}O_2$] from mixed venous oximetry saturation (**SvO$_2$**) of blood obtained from the PA. SvO$_2$ corresponds to CO and can be used as a surrogate CO monitor during OPCAB [39]. Furthermore, ScvO$_2$ has been shown in OPCAB patients to correspond to jugular bulb saturation (SjO$_2$) [31]. This is important because SjO$_2$ desaturation to <50 % is frequently noted during OPCAB procedures. SvO$_2$ has been advocated as the best parameter for assessment of OPCAB. A normal SvO$_2$ is 75% which corresponds to a PaO$_2$ of 40 mm Hg. SvO$_2$ ≥70% is goal for therapeutic interventions. Oximetric PACs continuously measure real-time SvO$_2$. VIP PAC can measure SvO$_2$ with a blood sample obtained from distal port. The sample must be aspirated slowly to avoid entrainment of oxygenated blood.

f. **ScvO$_2$.** It is assessed from SVC blood. ScvO$_2$ reflects from brain and upper extremities and is typically 5% LESS than SvO$_2$. Oximetric CVP catheters are utilized without need to place a PAC. Normal ScvO$_2$ is 70%. The brain extracts more oxygen than any other organ; because of this, oxygen saturation in the IVC will be greater than that in the SVC.

C. **Deep hypothermic circulatory arrest (DHCA).** DHCA is a neuroprotective technique utilizing CPB to cool the patient to 17° to 19°C. Therapeutic hypothermia incorporates modification of some monitors. DHCA is utilized more frequently in the pediatric population for correction of congenital heart defects; however there are several specialized procedures where it plays a key role, including aortic arch endarterectomy, aortic arch aneurysm, aortic dissection, giant cerebral aneurysm, ascending aortic aneurysm, and renal cell carcinoma extending into IVC and RA. Modification of anesthetic techniques is required [21].

1. **Temperature.** Temperature should be measured in at least two sites. Brain temperature determined by nasopharyngeal and/or tympanic membrane should be one of the sites. Core and/or shell temperature should be measured. Homogeneous hypothermia and normothermia should be achieved prior to DHCA and CPB separation, respectively.

2. **Brainwave electrical activity.** The goal of hypothermia is to render the brain isoelectric in order to reduce cerebral metabolic O$_2$ requirements. Prior to turning the CPB off, the temperature should be stable and at the temperature goal at all sites. The head should be packed in ice for topical cooling. The EEG/BIS should be isoelectric and stable (BIS = 0). It is not clear if pharmacologic neuroprotection adds any protection on top of hypothermia during cooling. However during rewarming, administration of pharmacologic neuroprotection should be considered as the protective effect of hypothermia is dissipating.

3. **Central line site:** The cardiovascular pathology may require alternative cannulation sites for CPB, removing those sites for central line access. For example, the surgeon may place the patient on fem-fem CPB thus eliminating the femoral artery/vein from consideration for central access.

4. **Arterial line site:** The aortic cannula and cross-clamp sites may force the surgeon to include either the innominate artery or left subclavian within the nonperfused portion of the aorta. Placement of the arterial line on the contralateral side allows continued use.

   a. Ascending aortic aneurysms require a *LEFT* radial art line.

    b. Descending aortic aneurysm or dissections require a ***RIGHT*** radial art line.

    c. Aortic arch aneurysm are repaired under DHCA thus can be either right or left.

   5. **CPB monitors:** Rapid rewarming after DHCA dramatically increases the incidence and severity of neurocognitive deficits. The temperature gradient between CPB machine venous/arterial return should be ≤4° to 5°C. Arterial inflow temperature should probably not exceed 36°C.

D. Thoracoabdominal aortic aneurysm (TAAA). TAAA are complex cases with some unique monitoring considerations. Decisions regarding which monitors will be utilized and which sites the monitors will be placed begin with a discussion with the surgeon. The surgical approach and technique will dictate monitoring decisions. Topics for discussion include:

   1. *Will the procedure be performed as an open repair or as an endovascular aortic repair (EVAR) or thoracic endovascular repair (TEVAR)?* Endovascular repair is minimally invasive, whereas open TAAA could be considered as maximally invasive. Endovascular repair options for anesthetic technique and monitors vary widely based on anatomy, experience of the surgeon/anesthesiologist and patient factors. The minimum monitoring would include an arterial catheter and two large-bore IVs (i.e., 14 g × 2). Open repair would prompt placement of an SvO_2-CCO PAC and plan for ICU postoperatively.

   2. *Which surgical technique is planned?* Partial left heart bypass versus CPB versus CPB/DHCA versus clamp and sew? Partial bypass with a centrifugal pump is managed with (right) upper and lower extremity arterial lines. Although all of the blood ejected by the RV passes through the lungs, one-lung ventilation may result in hypoxia. An SvO_2-CCO PAC is indicated for this paradigm.

   3. *What incision will be used?* A subcostal incision allowing access to both retroperitoneum and hemithorax may require ECG lead V_5 to be placed at alternative site (see Table 4.1).

   4. *What is the plan with respect to neuroprotection?* Will an intrathecal catheter be placed to drain CSF? Will full CPB ± DHCA be required with full dose of heparin? Will evoked potentials be used to monitor spinal cord hypoperfusion? If EP used which EP? Motor EP? Somatosensory EP?

VII. Additional resources

The World Wide Web provides an abundance of resources (Table 4.14) to gain further knowledge about monitoring devices.

TABLE 4.14   Internet resources

American Board of Anesthesiology	theABA.org
American Heart Association (AHA)	heart.org
American Lung Association	lung.org
American Society of Anesthesiology (ASA)	asahq.org
American Society of Echocardiography (ASE)	asecho.org
Anesthesiology	anesthesiologyonline.com
ASE/SCA Guidelines	anesthesia-analgesia.org
Anesthesia Patient Safety Foundation (APSF)	apsf.org
Canadian Society of Echocardiography (CSE)	csecho.ca
Congenital Cardiac Anaesthesiologists Society	pedsanesthesia.org/ccas
European Association of Cardiothoracic Anesthesia (EACTA)	eacta.org
Foundation for Anesthesia Education and Research (FAER)	faer.org
International Anesthesia Research Society (IARS)	iars.org
Journal of Cardiothoracic and Vascular Anesthesia (JCTVA)	jcvaonline.com
Society of Cardiovascular Anesthesiologists (SCA)	scahq.org
Society of Critical Care Medicine (SCCM)	sccm.org
Society of Thoracic Surgeons (STS)	sts.org

REFERENCES

1. **American Society of Anesthesiologists Task Force on Central Venous Access; Rupp SM, Apfelbaum JL, Blitt C, et al. Practice guidelines for central venous access: A report by the American Society of Anesthesiologists Task Force on central venous access.** *Anesthesiology.* **2012;116(3):539–573.**
2. Rando K, Castelli J, Pratt JP, et al. Ultrasound-guided internal jugular vein catheterization: a randomized controlled trial. *Heart Lung Vessels.* 2014;6(1):13–23.
3. Maizel J, Guyomarc'h L, Henon P, et al. Residents learning ultrasound-guided catheterization are not sufficiently skilled to use landmarks. *Critical Care.* 2014;18(1):R36.
4. Whitener S, Konoske R, Mark JB. Pulmonary artery catheter. *Best Pract Rec Clin Anesthesiol.* 2014;28(4):323–335.
5. Martina JR, Westerhof BE, van Goudoever J, et al. Noninvasive continuous arterial blood pressure monitoring with Nexfin®. *Anesthesiology.* 2012;116(5):1092–1103.
6. **American Society of Anesthesiologists Task Force on Pulmonary Artery Catheterization. Practice guidelines for pulmonary artery catheterization: an updated report by the American Society of Anesthesiologists Task Force on Pulmonary Artery Catheterization.** *Anesthesiology.* **2003;99(4):988–1014.**
7. Greenberg SB, Murphy GS, Vender JS. Current use of the pulmonary artery catheter. *Curr Opin Crit Care.* 2009;15(3): 249–253.
8. Leibowitz AB, Oropello JM. The pulmonary artery catheter in anesthesia practice in 2007: an historical overview with emphasis on the past 6 years. *Semin Cardiothorac Vasc Anesth.* 2007;11(3):162–176.
9. Polonen P, Hippelainen M, Takala R, et al. A prospective, randomized study of goal-oriented hemodynamic therapy in cardiac surgical patients. *Anesth Analg.* 2000;90(5):1052–1059.
10. Tuman KJ, Carroll GC, Ivankovich AD. Pitfalls in interpretation of pulmonary artery catheter data. *J Cardiothorac Anesth.* 1989;3(5):625–641.
11. Evans DC, Doraiswamy VA, Prosciak MP, et al. Complications associated with pulmonary artery catheters: a comprehensive clinical review. *Scand J Surg.* 2009;98(4):199–208.
12. **Brovman EY, Gabriel RA, Dutton RP, et al. Pulmonary artery catheter use during cardiac surgery in the United States, 2010 to 2014.** *J Cardiothorac and Vasc Anesth.* **2016;30(3):579–584.**
13. Cheatham ML, Nelson LD, Chang MC, et al. Right ventricular end-diastolic volume index as a predictor of preload status in patients on positive end-expiratory pressure. *Crit Care Med.* 1998;26(11):1801–1806.
14. **Funk DJ, Moretti EW, Gan TJ. Minimally invasive cardiac output monitoring in the perioperative setting.** *Anesth Analg.* **2009;108(3):887–897.**
15. Lee AJ, Cohn JH, Ranasinghe JS. Cardiac output assessed by invasive and minimally invasive techniques. *Anesthesiol Res Pract.* 2011;2011:475151.
16. Marik PE, Baram M, Vahid, B. Does central venous pressure predict fluid responsiveness? A systematic review of the literature and the tale of seven mares. *Chest.* 2008;134(1):172–178.
17. **Michard F, Teboul JL. Predicting fluid responsiveness in ICU patients: a critical analysis of the evidence.** *Chest.* **2002;121(6):2000–2008.**
18. Preisman S, Kogan S, Berkenstadt H, et al. Predicting fluid responsiveness in patients undergoing cardiac surgery: functional haemodynamic parameters including the respiratory systolic variation test and static preload indicators. *Br J Anaesth.* 2005; 95(6):746–755.
19. Reuter DA, Felbinger, TW, Schmidt, C, et al. Stroke volume variations for assessment of cardiac responsiveness to volume loading in mechanically ventilated patients after cardiac surgery. *Intensive Care Med.* 2002;28(4):392–398.
20. Rex S, Schälte G, Schroth S, et al. Limitations of arterial pulse pressure variation and left ventricular stroke volume variation in estimating cardiac pre-load during open heart surgery. *Acta Anaesthesiol Scand.* 2007;51(9):1258–1267.
21. Reed H, Berg KB, Janelle GM, et al. Aortic surgery and deep-hypothermic arrest: anesthetic update. *Semin Cardiothorac Vasc Anesth.* 2014;18(2):137–145.
22. Insler SR, Sessler DI. Perioperative thermoregulation and temperature monitoring. *Anesthesiol Clin.* 2006;24(4):823–837.
23. **Newman MF, Wolman R, Kanchuger M, et al. Multicenter preoperative stroke risk index for patients undergoing coronary artery bypass graft surgery. Multicenter Study of Perioperative Ischemia (McSPI) Research Group.** *Circulation.* **1996;94:(9 Suppl):II74–II80.**
24. Bhatia A, Gupta AK. Neuromonitoring in the intensive care unit I. Intracranial pressure and cerebral blood flow monitoring. *Intensive Care Med.* 2007;33(7):1263–1271.
25. Bhatia A, Gupta AK. Neuromonitoring in the intensive care unit II. Cerebral oxygenation monitoring and microdialysis. *Intensive Care Med.* 2007;33(8):1322–1328.
26. **Grocott HP, Davie S, Fedorow C. Monitoring of brain function in anesthesia and intensive care.** *Curr Opin Anesthesiol.* **2010;23(6):759–764.**
27. **Gelman S. Venous function and central venous pressure: a physiologic study.** *Anesthesiology.* **2008;108(4):735–748.**
28. Saidi N, Murkin JM. Applied neuromonitoring in cardiac surgery: patient specific management. *Semin Cardiothorac Vasc Anesth.* 2005;9(1):17–23.
29. Heck M, Kumle B, Boldt J, et al. Electroencephalogram bispectral index predicts hemodynamic and arousal reactions during induction of anesthesia in patients undergoing cardiac surgery. *J Cardiothorac Vasc Anesth.* 2000;14(6):693–697.
30. Barr G, Anderson RE, Samuelsson S, et al. Fentanyl and midazolam anaesthesia for coronary bypass surgery: a clinical study of bispectral electroencephalogram analysis, drug concentrations and recall. *Br J Anaesth.* 2000;84(6):749–752.
31. Myles PS, Daly D, Silvers A, et al. Prediction of neurological outcome using bispectral index monitoring in patients with severe ischemic-hypoxic brain injury undergoing emergency surgery. *Anesthesiology.* 2009;110(5):1106–1115.
32. Tobias JD. Cerebral oxygenation monitoring: near-infrared spectroscopy. *Expert Rev Med Devices.* 2006;3(2):235–243.

33. Zheng F, Sheinberg R, Yee MS, et al. Cerebral near-infrared spectroscopy monitoring and neurologic outcomes in adult cardiac surgery patients and neurologic outcomes: a systematic review. *Anesth Analg.* 2013;116(3):663–676.

34. Hamilton-Davies C, Mythen MG, Salmon JB, et al. Comparison of commonly used clinical indicators of hypovolaemia with gastrointestinal tonometry. *Intensive Care Med.* 1997;23(3):276–281.

35. Mythen MG, Webb AR. Perioperative plasma volume expansion reduces the incidence of gut mucosal hypoperfusion during cardiac surgery. *Arch Surg.* 1995;130(4):423–429.

36. Palizas F, Dubin A, Regueira T, et al. Gastric tonometry versus cardiac index as resuscitation goals in septic shock: a multi-center, randomized, controlled trial. *Crit Care.* 2009;13(2):R44.

37. Zhang X, Xuan W, Yin P, et al. Gastric tonometry guided therapy in critical care patients: a systematic review and meta-analysis. *Crit Care.* 2015;19:22.

38. Kowalewski M, Pawliszak W, Malvindi PG, et al. Off-pump coronary artery bypass grafting improves short-term outcomes in high-risk patients compared with on-pump coronary artery bypass grafting: meta-analysis. *J Thorac Cardiovasc Surg.* 2016; 151(1):60–77.

39. Grow, MP, Singh A, Fleming NW, et al. Cardiac output monitoring during off-pump coronary artery bypass grafting. *J Cardiothorac Vasc Anesth.* 2004;18(1):43–46.

5

Transesophageal Echocardiography

Jack S. Shanewise

KEY POINTS

1. The majority of cardiac surgical transesophageal echocardiography (TEE) imaging uses two-dimensions, which is accomplished via phased array transducers consisting of 64 to 128 small crystals activated sequentially.

2. Pulsed-wave Doppler (PWD) profiles blood flow velocity at a single point along the ultrasound beam, whereas continuous-wave Doppler (CWD) detects the maximum velocity profile along the

full length of the ultrasound beam. CWD permits measurement of higher-velocity blood flows (e.g., aortic stenosis [AS]) than PWD.

3. Color-flow Doppler (CFD) is a form of PWD that superimposes velocity information onto a two-dimensional (2D) image, which assesses blood flow direction when it is predominantly moving either toward or away from the transducer.

4. Before placing a TEE probe, significant esophageal pathology should be ruled out by asking the patient about swallowing difficulty and about known esophageal dysfunction.

5. A comprehensive TEE examination typically involves 20 standard views, which are shown in Figure 5.2.

6. Global and regional left ventricular (LV) systolic and diastolic function can be assessed qualitatively or quantitatively using TEE, as can LV preload (end-diastolic volume). Wall motion can be graded on a scale of 1 (normal) to 5 (dyskinesis).

7. Several TEE modalities can be used to assess mitral regurgitation (MR), the easiest way being CFD.

8. AS can be assessed using a variety of TEE modalities including imaging in several planes, planimetry in a short-axis (SAX) view to trace aortic valve area (AVA), and AVA assessment by continuity equation.

9. TEE is useful for interrogating the proximal ascending aorta, the aortic arch, and the descending aorta, but it has a "blind spot" for the distal ascending aorta that requires epiaortic echocardiography for diagnostic interrogation. Complete thoracic aortic interrogation is important in the presence of advanced aortic arteriosclerosis and aortic dissection.

10. TEE assessment of new LV regional wall-motion abnormalities (RWMAs) is the most sensitive bedside monitor of myocardial ischemia.

11. TEE is highly sensitive for detecting intracardiac air.

12. Intraoperative TEE is indispensable during surgery for cardiac valve repair or replacement, ventricular assist device placement, and minimally invasive cardiac surgery.

13. Real-time 3D TEE adds information to intraoperative assessment of operations for mitral valve (MV) disease and congenital heart disease.

I. Basic principles of ultrasound imaging

Medical ultrasound is produced by a piezoelectric crystal that vibrates in response to a high-frequency, alternating electrical current. The same crystal is deformed by returning echoes producing an electrical signal that is detected by the instrument. Ultrasound transmitted from the transducer into the patient interacts with the tissues in four ways: (i) Reflection, (ii) refraction, (iii) scattering, and (iv) attenuation. Ultrasound is reflected when it encounters the interface between tissues of different acoustic impedance, primarily a function of tissue density, and the timing, intensity, and phase of these echoes are processed to form the image. The velocity of transmission of ultrasound through soft tissues is relatively constant (1,540 m/sec), and the time it takes for the waves to travel to an object, be reflected, and return is determined by its distance from the transducer. Selecting the frequency of an ultrasound transducer is a trade-off between image resolution and depth of penetration. Higher frequencies have better resolution than lower frequencies, but they do not penetrate as far into tissue. The frequency of the ultrasound used in transesophageal echocardiography (TEE) typically ranges from 3.5 to 7 million cycles per second (MHz).

II. Basic principles of Doppler echocardiography

A. **Doppler echocardiography** uses ultrasound scattered from blood cells to measure the velocity and direction of blood flow. The Doppler effect increases the frequency of waves scattered from cells moving toward the transducer and decreases the frequency of waves from cells moving away. This change in the transmitted frequency (F_T) to the scattered frequency (F_S) is called Doppler shift ($F_S - F_T$) and is related to the velocity of blood flow (V) by the Doppler equation:

$$V = \frac{c(F_S - F_T)}{2F_T(\cos\theta)}$$

where c is the speed of sound in blood (1,540 m/sec) and θ is the angle between the direction of blood flow and the ultrasound beam. The 2 in the denominator corrects for the time it takes the ultrasound to travel to and from the blood cells. In order to get a reasonably accurate (less than 6% error) measurement of blood velocity with Doppler echocardiography, the angle between the flow and the ultrasound beam (θ) should be less than 20 degrees.

B. **The Bernoulli equation** describes the relationship between the flow velocity through a stenosis and the pressure gradient across the stenosis. It is a complex relationship that includes factors for convective acceleration, flow acceleration, and viscous resistance. In certain clinical applications, such as aortic and mitral stenosis, a simplified form may be used. The **simplified Bernoulli equation** is:

$$\Delta P = 4V^2$$

where ΔP is the pressure gradient in millimeters of mercury (mm Hg) and V is the velocity in meters per second (m/sec). The simplified Bernoulli equation should only be used in applications validated against another gold standard.

III. **Modes of cardiac ultrasound imaging**

A. **M-mode echocardiography** was the primary imaging mode for echocardiography for many years before the development of two-dimensional (2D) imaging in the late 1970s. It directs pulses of a single, linear beam of ultrasound into the tissues and displays the distance from the transducer of the returning echoes on the y-axis of a graph with signal strength indicated by brightness. The x-axis of the graph shows time, and motion of the structures is seen as curved lines. M-mode is useful for precisely timing events within the cardiac cycle. Its other advantage is very high temporal resolution, making thousands of images per second, which allows detection of high-frequency oscillating motion, such as vibrating vegetations.

B. **2D echocardiography** is made by very rapidly moving the ultrasound beam through a plane, creating multiple scan lines that are displayed simultaneously to construct a 2D tomographic image. Mechanical transducers accomplish this by physically rotating or oscillating the crystal. However, TEE probes usually have phased array transducers, which consist of an array of many (64 to 128) small crystals that are electrically activated in sequence to move the beam through the imaging plane. The number of 2D images that can be formed each second is called frame rate (temporal resolution), which is determined by the width (number of scan lines per image) and depth (time for each pulse to return) of the imaging sector. Typical frame rates for 2D echocardiography are 30 to 60 frames per second, which is fast enough to accurately reflect most motion in the heart.

C. **Pulsed-wave Doppler (PWD)** measures the velocity and direction of blood flow in a specific location, called sample volume, which can be placed by the user in the area of interest of a 2D image. The velocity of flow is displayed with time on the x-axis and velocity on the y-axis. Velocities going toward the transducer are above the baseline of the y-axis and velocities away from the transducer below the baseline. PWD uses one transducer to both send and receive signals, determining the depth of the sample volume from the transducer by listening at a predetermined interval after transmission. This limits the maximum rate at which pulses can be sent (pulse repetition frequency), which in turn limits the maximum Doppler shift (**Nyquist limit**) and the blood velocity that can be measured with PWD. The farther the sample volume is from the transducer, the lower the maximum velocity that can be measured. Typically, velocities more than 1.5 to 2 m/sec cannot be measured with PWD.

D. **Continuous-wave Doppler (CWD)** measures the velocity and direction of blood flow along the line of sight of the ultrasound beam. The information is displayed with time on the x-axis and velocity on the y-axis, as with PWD. CWD uses two transducers: One to continuously transmit and the other to continuously receive. As a result, all returning signals are superimposed on the display, so CWD cannot determine the depth from the transducer from which a returning signal originated (range ambiguity), only its direction. But, unlike PWD, CWD has no limit on the maximum velocity measured. CWD is used to measure blood velocity too high for PWD, such as aortic stenosis (AS), and to determine the maximum velocity of a flow profile, such as with mitral stenosis.

E. **Color-flow Doppler (CFD)** is a form of PWD that superimposes the velocity information onto the simultaneously created 2D image of the heart, allowing the location and timing of flow disturbances to be easily seen. Flow toward the transducer usually is mapped as red and away as blue. Some CFD maps, called **variance maps**, add green to indicate turbulence in the flow. Since it is a form of PWD, CFD cannot accurately measure higher flow velocities, such as mitral regurgitation (MR) and AS, and these flows appear as a mixture of red and blue, called mosaic pattern. Also, as the flow velocity passes the limit of the CFD velocity scale (Nyquist limit), the color will alias, or change from red to blue or from blue to red, depending on the direction of flow. The aliasing velocity or Nyquist limit for CFD varies with the depth of the color sector, but typically is less than 100 cm/sec. Since the instrument must develop both the 2D and Doppler images, the frame rate is lower with CFD than with 2D imaging alone, typically in the range from 12 to 24 frames per second. At frame rates below 15 frames per second, the image becomes noticeably jerky as the eye can discern the individual images. Decreasing the width and depth of the 2D image and the CFD sector within it will increase the frame rate.

F. **Tissue Doppler** is a form of PWD that measures the velocity of tissue motion at specific points in the myocardium. Its most common application is to measure the velocity of mitral annular motion to assess systolic function of the left ventricle (LV). More sophisticated analysis can be performed between two adjacent points in the myocardium to measure strain (tissue deformation over time) and strain rate (rate of deformation) to assess systolic and diastolic functions in different regions of the LV and the right ventricle (RV). Evaluation of synchrony of ventricular contraction is also possible with tissue Doppler.

IV. **Indications for TEE during cardiac surgery**
TEE can be used as a diagnostic tool during cardiac surgery to direct the surgical procedure and diagnose unanticipated problems and complications. TEE also is useful to the cardiac anesthesiologist as a monitor of cardiac function. Often, TEE is used for both purposes during heart surgery. The recently revised American Society of Anesthesiologists and the Society of Cardiovascular Anesthesiologists (ASA/SCA) Practice Guidelines for Perioperative TEE state that "For adult patients without contraindications, **TEE should be used in all open heart (e.g., valvular procedures) and thoracic aortic surgical procedures and should be considered in coronary artery bypass graft surgeries**" [1].

V. **Safety, contraindications, and risk of TEE**
A. **Preoperative screening** for esophageal disease should be completed before proceeding with TEE. The patient should be interviewed when possible and asked about a history of esophageal disease, dysphagia, and hematemesis. The medical record should be reviewed as well. Relative contraindications to TEE are listed in Table 5.1. The presence of a relative contraindication requires balancing the risk with the importance of TEE to the procedure. In patients with distal

TABLE 5.1   Relative contraindications to transesophageal echocardiography

History
Dysphagia
Odynophagia
Mediastinal radiation
Recent upper gastrointestinal surgery
Recent upper gastrointestinal bleeding
Thoracic aortic aneurysm
Esophageal pathology
Stricture
Tumor
Diverticulum
Varices
Esophagitis
Recent chest trauma

esophageal or gastric pathology, it often is possible to obtain the information needed with TEE without advancing into the distal esophagus. Preoperative esophagoscopy is another option to consider when the need for TEE is important and the risk is unclear. Another approach when facing pathology in the distal esophagus or the stomach is to confine the TEE examination to mid and upper esophageal (UE) views.

> **CLINICAL PEARL** ALWAYS think about risk factors and contraindications before inserting a TEE probe—ESPECIALLY in emergency situations.

B. **TEE probe insertion and manipulation** should be performed gently. The probe must never be forced through a resistance, and excessive force must never be applied to the control wheels.

> **CLINICAL PEARL** During probe insertion, watching or feeling the neck often allows you to tell whether the probe is going off to one side or another.

C. **Complications of TEE** are uncommon in properly screened patients, but they may be serious [2]. Complications of TEE are listed in Table 5.2. Serious injuries may not be apparent at the time of the procedure [3].

VI. Intraoperative TEE examination

A. **Probe insertion** is performed after the patient is anesthetized and the endotracheal tube is secured. An orogastric tube is inserted and the contents of the stomach and the esophagus are suctioned. As the mandible is displaced anteriorly, the probe is gently inserted into the posterior pharynx in the midline and advanced into the esophagus. A laryngoscope may be used to displace the mandible and better visualize the esophageal opening if necessary. As the probe is advanced into the thoracic esophagus (approximately 30 cm), the heart should come into view. On rare occasions, the probe cannot be placed in the esophagus, in which case the TEE is abandoned.

B. **Probe manipulation** is accomplished by advancing and withdrawing the probe within the esophagus, rotating the probe to the patient's left (counterclockwise) or right (clockwise). Assuming that the transducer is facing anteriorly (toward the heart), the tip flexes anteriorly and posteriorly with the large control wheel, and flexes to the patient's right and left (can be envisioned as "wagging," as in a dog's tail) with the small control wheel. With a multiplane TEE probe, the angle of the transducer is rotated axially from 0 degrees (horizontal plane), through 90 degrees (vertical plane), to 180 degrees (mirror image of 0-degree horizontal plane) (Fig. 5.1).

TABLE 5.2 Complications of transesophageal echocardiography
Dental and oral trauma (usually minor)
Laryngeal dysfunction
Postoperative aspiration
Endotracheal tube displacement
Bronchial compression in infants
Aortic compression in infants
Upper gastrointestinal bleeding (mucosal injury)
Pharyngeal perforation (rare)
Esophageal perforation (rare)

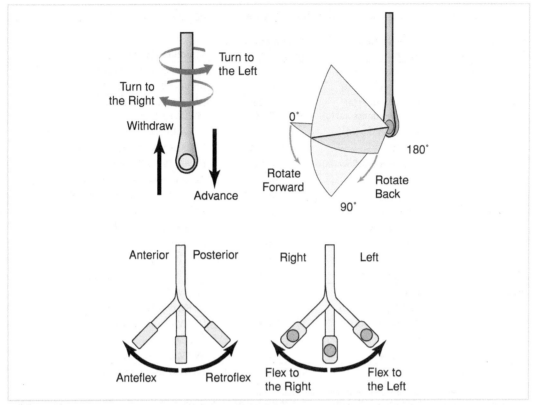

FIGURE 5.1 Terminology used to describe manipulation of the probe and transducer during image acquisition. (From Shanewise JS, Cheung AT, Aronson S, et al. ASE/SCA guidelines for performing a comprehensive intraoperative multiplane transesophageal echocardiography examination: recommendations of the American Society of Echocardiography Council for Intraoperative Echocardiography and the Society of Cardiovascular Anesthesiologists Task Force for Certification in Perioperative Transesophageal Echocardiography. *Anesth Analg.* 1999;89(4):870–884, with permission.)

  C. **Machine settings are adjusted to optimize the TEE image.** These settings are continuously adjusted by the user as the examination proceeds.

    1. **Transducer frequency** is adjusted to the highest frequency that provides adequate depth of penetration to the structure being examined.

    2. **Image depth** is adjusted to center the structure being examined in the display.

    3. **Overall image gain** and **dynamic range** (compression) are adjusted so that the blood in the chambers appears nearly black and is distinct from the shades of gray representing tissue.

    4. **Time gain compensation** controls are adjusted so that there is uniform brightness from the near field to the far field of the image.

    5. **CFD gain** is adjusted to a threshold that just eliminates any background noise within the color sector.

  D. **TEE views.** The ASE/SCA Guidelines for performing a comprehensive intraoperative multiplane TEE examination [4] define 20 views that comprise a comprehensive TEE examination (Table 5.3). These 20 views are shown in Figure 5.2. An update of these guidelines considered uses of TEE outside the perioperative arena and described a few additional views [5]. The 20 views are named for the location of the transducer (echocardiographic window), a descriptive term of the imaging plane (e.g., short axis [SAX] or long axis [LAX]), and the major anatomic structure in the view. All of these views can be developed in most patients. Additional views may be needed to completely examine a patient with a particular form of pathology. The sequence

TABLE 5.3   Recommended transesophageal echocardiographic cross section

Window (depth from incisors)	Cross section (panel in Fig. 5.2)	Multiplane angle range (degrees)	Structures imaged
UE (20–25 cm)	Aortic arch LAX (s)	0	Aortic arch, left brachiocephalic vein
	Aortic arch SAX (t)	90	Aortic arch, PA, PV, left brachiocephalic vein
Midesophageal (30–40 cm)	Four chamber (a)	0–20	LV, LA, RV, RA, MV, TV, IAS
	Mitral commissural (g)	60–70	MV, LV, LA, LAA
	Two chamber (b)	80–100	LV, LA, LAA, MV
	LAX (c)	120–160	LV, LA, AV, LVOT, MV, asc aorta
	RV inflow–outflow (m)	60–90	RV, RA, TV, RVOT, PV, PA
	AV SAX (h)	30–60	AV, IAS, coronary ostia, LVOT, PV
	AV LAX (i)	120–160	AV, LVOT, prox asc aorta, right PA
	Bicaval (l)	80–110	RA, SVC, IVC, IAS, LA, CS
	Asc aortic SAX (o)	0–60	Asc aorta, SVC, PA, right PA
	Asc aortic LAX (p)	100–150	Asc aorta, right PA
	Desc aorta SAX (q)	0	Desc thoracic aorta, left pleural space
	Desc aorta LAX (r)	90–110	Desc thoracic aorta, left pleural space
TG (40–45 cm)	Basal SAX (f)	0–20	LV, MV, RV, TV
	Mid-SAX (d)	0–20	LV, RV, papillary muscles
	Two chamber (e)	80–100	LV, MV, chordae, papillary muscles, CS, LA
	LAX (j)	0–120	LVOT, AV, MV
	RV inflow (n)	100–120	RV, TV, RA, TV chordae, papillary muscles
Deep TG (45–50 cm)	LAX (k)	0–20 (anteflexion)	LVOT, AV, asc aorta, arch

Note: Lowercase letters in parenthesis refer to views shown in Figure 4.2.
UE, upper esophageal; LAX, long axis; SAX, short axis; TG, transgastric; asc, ascending; AV, aortic valve; CS, coronary sinus; desc, descending; IAS, interatrial septum; IVC, inferior vena cava; LA, left atrium; LAA, left atrial appendage; LV, left ventricle; LVOT, left ventricular outflow tract; MV, mitral valve; PA, pulmonary artery; prox, proximal; PV, pulmonic valve; RA, right atrium; RV, right ventricle; RVOT, right ventricular outflow tract; SVC, superior vena cava; TV, tricuspid valve.
(From Shanewise JS, Cheung AT, Aronson S, et al. ASE/SCA guidelines for performing a comprehensive intraoperative multiplane transesophageal echocardiography-examination: recommendations of the American Society of Echocardiography Council for Intraoperative Echocardiography and the Society of Cardiovascular Anesthesiologists Task Force for Certification in Perioperative Transesophageal Echocardiography. *Anesth Analg.* 1999;89(4):870–884, with permission.)

in which these views are obtained will vary from examiner to examiner, but it is generally most efficient to develop the midesophageal (ME) views and then the transgastric (TG) views.

> **CLINICAL PEARL**   The goal of the TEE examination is NOT to get all 20 views, but to use the 20 views to discern the structure and function of the heart.

1. **ME views** are developed with the TEE transducer posterior to the left atrium (LA). With a multiplane TEE probe, detailed examinations of cardiac chambers and valves can be completed in most patients from this window alone.

> **CLINICAL PEARL**   Pay attention to the position of the transducer—ideally posterior to the middle of the LA. Small adjustments in or out or flexing the tip to the right can greatly improve the image.

2. **TG views** are obtained by passing the transducer into the stomach and directing the imaging plane superiorly through the diaphragm to the heart. Images of the LV and RV and the mitral valve (MV) and tricuspid valve (TV) are made from this window. Views to align the Doppler beam parallel to flow through the left ventricular outflow tract (LVOT) and aortic valve (AV) can be developed from the TG window.

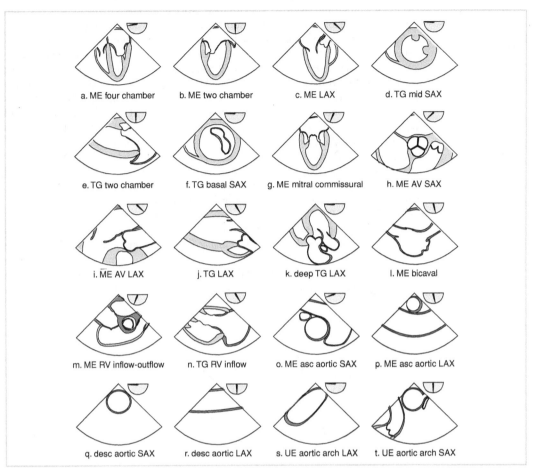

a. ME four chamber   b. ME two chamber   c. ME LAX   d. TG mid SAX

e. TG two chamber   f. TG basal SAX   g. ME mitral commissural   h. ME AV SAX

i. ME AV LAX   j. TG LAX   k. deep TG LAX   l. ME bicaval

m. ME RV inflow-outflow   n. TG RV inflow   o. ME asc aortic SAX   p. ME asc aortic LAX

q. desc aortic SAX   r. desc aortic LAX   s. UE aortic arch LAX   t. UE aortic arch SAX

FIGURE 5.2 Twenty cross-sectional views (a through t) composing the recommended comprehensive transesophageal echocardiographic examination. Approximate multiplane angle is indicated by the icon adjacent to each view. asc, ascending; AV, aortic valve; desc, descending; LAX, long axis; ME, midesophageal; RV, right ventricle; SAX, short axis; TG, transgastric; UE, upper esophageal. (From Shanewise JS, Cheung AT, Aronson S, et al. ASE/SCA guidelines for performing a comprehensive intraoperative multiplane transesophageal echocardiography-examination: recommendations of the American Society of Echocardiography Council for Intraoperative Echocardiography and the Society of Cardiovascular Anesthesiologists Task Force for Certification in Perioperative Transesophageal Echocardiography. *Anesth Analg.* 1999;89(4):870–884, with permission.)

3. **Upper esophageal views** are made with the transducer at the level of the aortic arch, which is examined in LAX and SAX. In many patients, images of the main pulmonary artery (PA) and pulmonic valve (PV) also may be developed, allowing alignment of the Doppler beam parallel to flow in these structures.

E. **Examination of specific structures**

CLINICAL PEARL   Whenever possible, at the beginning of a case perform a comprehensive examination and store the images to establish a baseline for later comparison.

1. **Left ventricle.** The LV is examined with the ME four-chamber (Video 5.1), ME two-chamber (Video 5.2), ME LAX (Video 5.3), TG mid-SAX (Video 5.4), and TG two-chamber views.
   a. **LV size** is assessed by measuring the inside diameter at the junction of the basal and mid-thirds at end diastole using the ME two- or TG two-chamber view. Normal is less than

5.4 cm for women and less than 6 cm for men. Normal thickness of the LV wall is 1.2 cm or less at end diastole and is best measured with TEE from the TG mid-SAX view [6].

b. **LV global function** may be assessed quantitatively or qualitatively. Fractional area change (FAC) is a 2D TEE equivalent of ejection fraction (EF) and is obtained by measuring the LV chamber area in the TG mid-SAX view by tracing the endocardial border to measure the end-diastolic area (EDA) and the end-systolic area (ESA) and using the formula: FAC = (EDA − ESA)/EDA. Normal FAC is greater than 0.50. This method is not as accurate when wall-motion abnormalities are present in the apex or the base of the LV. Qualitative assessment of LV function is performed by considering all views of the LV and estimating the EF (estimated ejection fraction [EEF]) as normal (EEF greater than 55%), mildly decreased (EEF 45% to 54%), moderately decreased (EEF 35% to 44%), moderately severely decreased (EEF 25% to 34%), or severely decreased (EEF less than 25%). EEF by experienced echocardiographers correlates with nonechocardiographic measures of EF as well or better than quantitative echocardiographic measurements of EF [7].

c. **Assessment of regional LV function.** The LV is divided into 17 regions or segments (Fig. 5.3). Each segment is rated qualitatively for thickening during systole using the following scale: 1 = normal (greater than 30% thickening), 2 = mild hypokinesis (10% to 30% thickening), 3 = severe hypokinesis (less than 10% thickening), 4 = akinesis (no thickening), and 5 = dyskinesis (thinning and paradoxical motion during systole). An

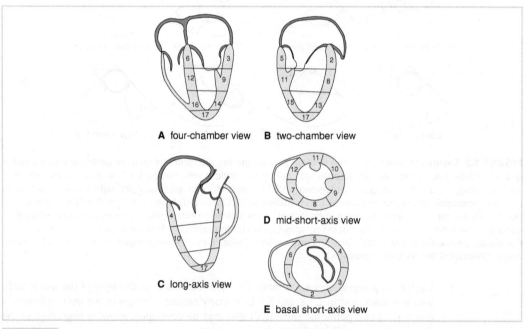

FIGURE 5.3 Seventeen-segment model of the LV. **A:** Four-chamber views show the three inferoseptal and three anterolateral segments. **B:** Two-chamber views show the three anterior and three inferior segments. **C:** Long-axis views show the two anteroseptal and two inferolateral segments. **D:** Mid–short-axis views show all six segments at the midlevel. **E:** Basal short-axis views show all six segments at the basal level. Basal segments: *1,* basal anteroseptal; *2,* basal anterior; *3,* basal anterolateral; *4,* basal inferolateral; *5,* basal inferior; *6,* basal inferoseptal. Mid-segments: *7,* mid-anteroseptal; *8,* mid-anterior; *9,* mid-anterolateral; *10,* mid-inferolateral; *11,* mid-inferior; *12,* mid-inferoseptal. Apical segments: *13,* apical anterior; *14,* apical lateral; *15,* apical inferior; *16,* apical septal; *17* apical cap or true apex. (Modified from Shanewise JS, Cheung AT, Aronson S, et al. ASE/SCA guidelines for performing a comprehensive intraoperative multiplane transesophageal echocardiography examination: recommendations of the American Society of Echocardiography Council for Intraoperative Echocardiography and the Society of Cardiovascular Anesthesiologists Task Force for Certification in Perioperative Transesophageal Echocardiography. *Anesth Analg.* 1999;89(4):870–884, with permission.)

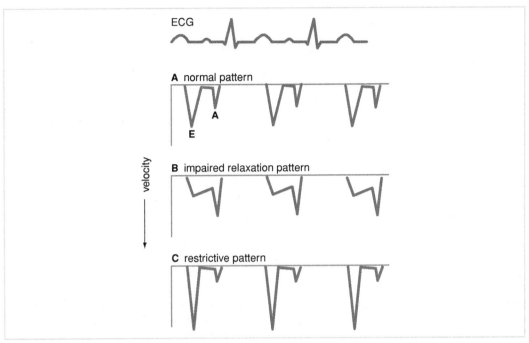

FIGURE 5.4 Transmitral inflow velocity profiles measured with PWD by placing the sample volume between the open tips of the mitral leaflets. **A:** Normal pattern. The pseudonormal pattern has a similar appearance. **B:** Impaired relaxation pattern indicative of mild diastolic dysfunction. The peak E-wave velocity is less than the A wave (E-to-A reversal) and the deceleration time of the E wave is prolonged. **C:** Restrictive pattern indicative of advanced diastolic dysfunction. The peak E-wave velocity is increased and the E-wave deceleration time is decreased. *A*, atrial filling wave; *E*, early filling wave.

increase in scale of 2 or more in a region should be considered significant and suggestive of myocardial ischemia [8].

    d. Assessment of diastolic LV function can be made by examining with PWD the transmitral inflow velocity profile during diastole. The normal pattern has an E wave corresponding to early passive filling of the LV, followed by a period of diastasis, and finally an A wave corresponding to atrial contraction in late diastole (Fig. 5.4A). Milder forms of diastolic dysfunction result in the **impaired relaxation pattern** with decreased peak E-to-A velocity ratio and prolonged E-wave deceleration time (Fig. 5.4B). Advanced diastolic dysfunction causes the **restrictive pattern** with increased peak E-to-A velocity ratio and decreased E-wave deceleration time (Fig. 5.4C). As diastolic dysfunction progresses from mild to severe over a number of years, the transmitral flow pattern may pass through a period in which it appears normal, a condition termed **pseudonormal pattern**. Normal may be distinguished from pseudonormal by examination of the pulmonary venous inflow velocity profile, which normally has positive inflow waves during systole (S wave) and diastole (D wave) and a small, negative wave corresponding to atrial contraction (A wave) (Fig. 5.5A). The pseudonormal pattern has prolongation of the A wave and attenuation of the S wave compared to the normal pattern (Fig. 5.5B). Age and preload also affect the transmitral and pulmonary venous inflow velocity patterns.

  2. Mitral valve. The MV is examined with the ME four-chamber, ME mitral commissural, ME LAX, and TG basal SAX views, with and without CFD. It consists of an anterior leaflet and a posterior leaflet joined at two commissures, the anterolateral and the posteromedial. There is a papillary muscle corresponding to each commissure. The posterior leaflet is divided into three scallops and the anterior leaflet into thirds for purposes of describing the location of lesions (Fig. 5.6). Prolapse of the MV is present when a portion of the leaflet

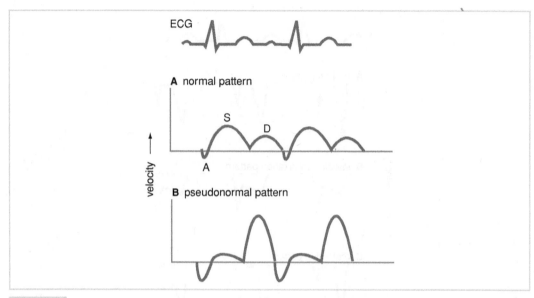

FIGURE 5.5 Pulmonary venous inflow velocity profiles measured with PWD by placing the sample volume in the left upper pulmonary vein. **A:** Profile seen with normal diastolic function and transmitral inflow. The S wave is larger than the D wave and a small A reversal is present. **B:** Pattern seen with diastolic dysfunction and pseudonormal transmitral inflow. The S wave is attenuated and smaller than the D wave and an enlarged A wave is present. *A,* atrial reversal wave; *D,* diastolic wave; *S,* systolic wave.

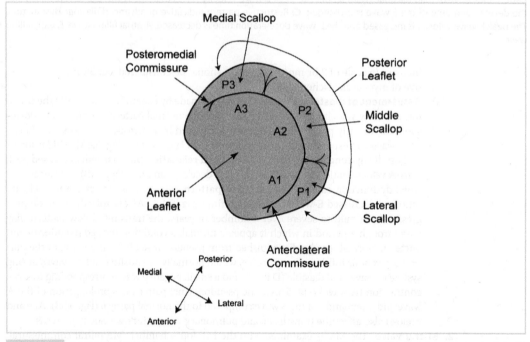

FIGURE 5.6 Anatomy of the MV. *A1,* lateral third of the anterior leaflet; *A2,* middle third of the anterior leaflet; *A3,* medial third of the anterior leaflet; *P1,* lateral scallop of the posterior leaflet; *P2,* middle scallop of the posterior leaflet; *P3,* medial scallop of the posterior leaflet. (From Shanewise JS, Cheung AT, Aronson S, et al. ASE/SCA guidelines for performing a comprehensive intraoperative multiplane transesophageal echocardiography examination: recommendations of the American Society of Echocardiography Council for Intraoperative Echocardiography and the Society of Cardiovascular Anesthesiologists Task Force for Certification in Perioperative Transesophageal Echocardiography. *Anesth Analg.* 1999;89(4):870–884, with permission.)

moves to the atrial side of the annulus during systole. Flail is said to be present when a chordae tendineae is ruptured and the corresponding segment of the valve leaflet is seen oscillating in the LA during systole.

a. **Mitral regurgitation**

(1) Judging severity of MR with TEE is based on several factors [9]. The structure of the valve leaflets is examined with 2D echocardiography, looking for defects of coaptation. CFD is used to detect retrograde flow through the valve into the LA. The width of the jet as it passes through the valve and its size in the LA are noted. Eccentric jets of MR tend to be more severe than central jets of a similar size. CFD also can detect flow convergence proximal to the regurgitant orifice, indicating more significant MR. Pulmonary venous inflow velocity profile is examined with PWD for systolic flow reversal, a specific but not very sensitive sign of severe MR. Severity is graded on a semiquantitative scale of 1+ (mild) to 4+ (severe). Most patients have at least trace amounts of MR detected with TEE.

CLINICAL PEARL Functional MR can look severe in early systole, then lessen or disappear in mid and late systole as coaptation improves.

(2) Functional **MR** is due to dilation of the MV annulus or displacement of the papillary muscles causing a decrease in the surface of coaptation of the MV leaflets. The structure of the valve leaflets is normal. Functional MR can be very dynamic and is markedly affected by loading conditions. The most common causes of functional MR are regional wall-motion abnormalities (RWMAs) from coronary artery disease and generalized dilation of the LV.

(3) Myxomatous **degeneration** of the MV is a common cause of MR requiring surgery. The leaflets are elongated and redundant, prolapsing into the LA during systole. Rupture of a chordae is common in this condition and causes a flail segment of the involved leaflet. TEE can be used to locate the portion of the MV involved and is helpful in guiding surgical therapy. Prolapse and flail of the middle scallop of the posterior leaflet is the most common form and most amenable to repair by resection of the involved portion and reinforcement of the annulus with an annuloplasty ring.

(4) Rheumatic **MR** is caused by thickening and shortening of the MV leaflets and chordae restricting motion and closure during systole. This type of MR typically is difficult to repair and usually requires prosthetic valve replacement.

(5) Proximal **isovelocity surface area** (PISA) is a method to quantify MR with echocardiography using CFD and CWD. It is most commonly applied to central MR and is probably not as accurate for eccentric MR. The flow velocity of blood increases as it converges toward the regurgitant orifice and can be seen with CFD. When the velocity reaches the limit on the CFD scale, aliasing of the signal occurs and the color mapped onto the 2D image changes from red to blue on the ventricular side of the valve. This change in color represents a hemispheric shell of blood converging toward the regurgitant orifice called PISA (Fig. 5.7). If the surface area of this hemisphere (A_{PISA}) is measured and multiplied by the aliasing velocity toward the transducer (V_{PISA}—taken from the CFD scale), the instantaneous flow at the PISA in mL/sec is obtained. A_{PISA} is calculated by measuring the radius (r) of the PISA and using the formula for the area of a hemisphere: (A_{PISA}) = $2\pi r^2 = 6.28r^2$. By the continuity principle, the instantaneous flow (mL/sec) is the same at the PISA as at the regurgitant orifice, both of which are the product of an area and a velocity: $A_{PISA} \times V_{PISA} = ROA \times V_{MR}$, where ROA is the regurgitant orifice area. The peak instantaneous velocity of the MR (V_{MR}) is measured with CWD, allowing the ROA to be calculated. Rearranging the formula,

$$ROA = \frac{(A_{PISA} \cdot V_{PISA})}{V_{MR}}$$

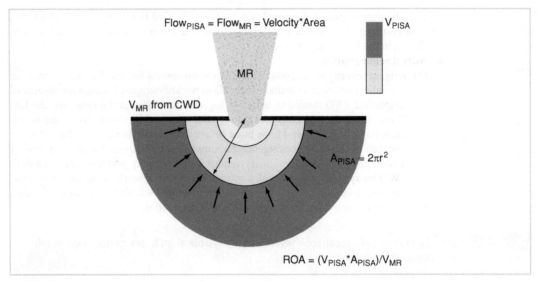

$$\text{Flow}_{\text{PISA}} = \text{Flow}_{\text{MR}} = \text{Velocity*Area} \qquad V_{\text{PISA}}$$

MR

V_{MR} from CWD

r

$A_{\text{PISA}} = 2\pi r^2$

$$\text{ROA} = (V_{\text{PISA}} * A_{\text{PISA}})/V_{\text{MR}}$$

FIGURE 5.7 Diagram of the PISA method to measure ROA in central MR. The horizontal line represents the MV with a central regurgitant orifice. As the blood flow converges on the orifice, the velocity increases and causes aliasing of the CFD signal, changing the color from red to blue creating the PISA (*small arrows*) on the ventricular side of the valve. The velocity of the blood at the PISA (V_{PISA}) is taken from the CFD scale. The size of the PISA (A_{PISA}) is calculated by measuring its radius (r, *large arrow*) and using the formula for the surface area of a hemisphere: $A_{\text{PISA}} = 2\pi r^2$. The peak velocity of the MR (V_{MR}) is measured by using CWD aimed through the orifice. $\text{Flow}_{\text{PISA}} = V_{\text{PISA}} \times A_{\text{PISA}}$ and $\text{Flow}_{\text{MR}} = V_{\text{MR}} \times \text{ROA}$. By the continuity principle, $\text{Flow}_{\text{MR}} = \text{Flow}_{\text{PISA}}$, so $\text{ROA} = (V_{\text{PISA}} \times A_{\text{PISA}})/V_{\text{MR}}$.

(6) **ROA** less than 0.2 cm² is mild MR and greater than 0.4 cm² is severe MR.

(7) **If the** CFD is adjusted so that the aliasing velocity toward the transducer is close to 40 cm/sec, and the V_{MR} is assumed to be about 500 cm/sec (most patients with reasonable hemodynamics) the formula simplifies to:

$$\text{ROA} = \frac{r^2}{2}$$

It is now possible to directly measure ROA with planimetry of three-dimensional (3D) TEE images of the MV with CFD.

b. **Mitral stenosis**

Significant mitral stenosis almost always is due to rheumatic heart disease. Severe mitral annular calcification is a rare cause of significant stenosis. 2D images show thickening of the leaflets with fusion at the commissures and restricted opening during diastole. Doppler velocity measurements of the transmitral inflow show increased peak and mean velocities, which can be used to calculate peak and mean transvalvular gradients ($\Delta P = 4V^2$).

The best gauge of severity of mitral stenosis is mitral valve area (MVA). MVA less than 1 cm² is considered severe, and from 1 to 1.5 cm² moderate.

TEE can be used to measure valve area in mitral stenosis by the following methods:

(1) **Planimetry.** Images of the stenotic orifice may be directly measured from the TG basal SAX view. The imaging plane is moved above and below the valve until the minimal orifice is seen, then the image is frozen in diastole and the orifice traced. Calcification of the annulus or leaflets may create acoustic shadowing limiting the ability to accurately image the orifice in many patients. 3D TEE imaging greatly facilitates planimetry of the stenotic MV orifice.

(2) **Pressure half-time.** The rate at which the pressure gradient decreases across a stenotic MV during diastole is directly **related** to the severity of the stenosis. A

gauge of this rate is the pressure half-time, which can be measured from the transmitral inflow velocity profile. An empirically derived formula gives the MVA in square centimeters as:

$$MVA = \frac{220}{PHT}$$

where PHT is the pressure half-time in milliseconds. This formula has been validated only for patients with rheumatic mitral stenosis. It cannot be used if there is more than mild aortic regurgitation (AR) or immediately after a mitral commissurotomy.

(3) **Proximal isovelocity surface area.** In mitral stenosis the flow velocity of blood increases as it converges toward the stenotic orifice and can be seen with CFD. When the velocity reaches the limit on the CFD scale going away from the transducer, aliasing of the signal occurs and the color mapped onto the 2D image changes from blue to red on the atrial side of the valve. This change in color represents a hemispheric shell of blood converging toward the stenotic orifice called PISA (Fig. 5.8). If the surface area of this hemisphere (A_{PISA}) is measured and multiplied by the aliasing velocity going away from the transducer (V_{PISA}—taken from the CFD scale), the instantaneous flow at the PISA in mL/sec is obtained. A_{PISA} is calculated by measuring the radius of the PISA and using the formula for the area of a hemisphere and reducing it by the ratio of the angle formed by the MV leaflets (α angle) and 180 degrees: $A_{PISA} = 2\pi r^2 \cdot (\alpha/180°) = 6.28r^2 \times (\alpha/180°)$. The CFD scale is adjusted so that the radius of the PISA is between 1 and 1.5 cm. By the continuity principle, the instantaneous flow (mL/sec) is the same at the PISA as at the stenotic orifice, both of which are the product of an area and a

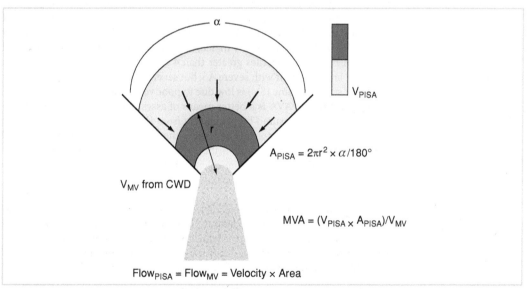

FIGURE 5.8 Diagram of the PISA method to measure MV area in mitral stenosis. The *thick lines* represent the MV with a central stenotic orifice. As the blood flow converges on the orifice, the velocity increases and causes aliasing of the CFD signal, changing the color from blue to red creating the PISA (*small arrows*) on the atrial side of the valve. The velocity of the blood at the PISA (V_{PISA}) is taken from the CFD scale. The size of the PISA (A_{PISA}) is calculated by measuring its radius (r, *large arrow*) and using the formula for the surface area of a hemisphere reduced by the ratio of the angle formed by the leaflets (α) and 180 degrees: $A_{PISA} = 2\pi r^2 \times \alpha/180°$. The peak velocity of the transmitral inflow (V_{MV}) is measured by using CWD aimed through the stenotic orifice. $Flow_{PISA} = V_{PISA} \times A_{PISA}$ and $Flow_{MV} = V_{MV} \cdot MVA$. By the continuity principle, $Flow_{MV} = Flow_{PISA}$, so $MVA = (V_{PISA} \times A_{PISA})/V_{MV}$.

velocity: $A_{PISA} \times V_{PISA} = MVA \times V_{MV}$, where MVA is the MV area and V_{MV} is the peak transmitral inflow velocity measured with CWD. Rearranging,

$$MVA = \frac{(A_{PISA} \cdot V_{PISA})}{V_{MV}}$$

3. **Aortic valve.** The AV is examined in the ME AV SAX and ME AV LAX views, with and without CFD. Doppler measurements of flow velocity through the AV are made from the TG LAX and deep TG LAX views, which allow the ultrasound beam to be directed parallel to AV flow. The AV is a semilunar valve that has three cusps: (i) The right coronary cusp, which is most anterior and adjacent to the RV outflow tract, (ii) the noncoronary cusp, which is adjacent to the atrial septum, and (iii) the left coronary cusp.

   a. **Aortic regurgitation**

   The severity of AR is assessed with TEE primarily by the size of the regurgitant jet on CFD and the depth to which it extends into the LV [8]. The valve cusps also should be examined with 2D echocardiography, looking for perforations and defects in coaptation. Other signs of severe AR include holodiastolic flow reversal in the descending thoracic aorta measured with PWD, pressure half-time of AR less than 300 msec as taken from the AR velocity profile measured with CWD from the TG LAX or deep TG LAX views, presystolic closure of the MV, and presystolic MR.

   b. **Aortic stenosis**

   Evaluation of AS with TEE is based on the appearance of the valve on 2D images and Doppler velocity measurements of the flow through the stenotic valve. In AS, the valve leaflets are thickened with markedly restricted opening during systole. Calcification of the cusps and the annulus may cause acoustic shadowing. TEE may be used to quantify the severity of AS by three methods:

   (1) **Transaortic gradients** may be calculated with the simplified Bernoulli equation ($\Delta P = 4V^2$) by using CWD to measure the flow velocity in meters per second through a stenotic AV from the TG LAX or deep TG LAX views. For example, if the peak AV outflow velocity is 5 m/sec, the peak instantaneous gradient would be 100 mm Hg. Peak velocities greater than 4 m/sec (peak gradient greater than 64 mm Hg) are consistent with severe AS, but severe AS may be present with lower velocities if stroke volume (SV) is low due to poor ventricular function.

   (2) **AVA by planimetry.** AVA is a better means of assessing severity of AS than gradients and may be measured by planimetry from the ME AV SAX view. The 2D image is frozen during systole at the level of the free edge of the leaflets, scrolled to identify the maximum systolic orifice, which is then traced using the caliper function. Acoustic shadowing from calcification may obscure the image in many patients and make planimetry difficult. AVA less than 1 cm² is considered significant.

   (3) **AVA by continuity equation.** AVA may be calculated using the continuity equation, which states that the same amount of flow passes through the AV and the LVOT with each stroke. Flow rate is equal to the velocity of the flow multiplied by the area through which the flow occurs (Flow = $V \cdot A$) and by the continuity equation is the same at the AV and the LVOT. Thus,

   $$Flow_{AV} = Flow_{LVOT}$$

   $$V_{AV} \cdot A_{AV} = V_{LVOT} \cdot A_{LVOT}$$

   rearranging, we obtain

   $$A_{AV} = \left(\frac{V_{LVOT} \cdot A_{LVOT}}{V_{AV}} \right)$$

The area of the LVOT is obtained from the ME LAX view of the AV by measuring its diameter during systole and applying the formula for the area of a circle:

$$A_{\text{CIRCLE}} = \pi r^2 = \pi \left(\frac{D}{2} \right)^2 = \left(\frac{\pi}{4} \right) \cdot D^2 = 0.785 \cdot D^2$$

V_{LVOT} is measured with PWD by placing the sample volume just proximal to the AV in the LVOT and V_{AV} by directing the CWD through the stenotic valve. It is most convenient to use units of centimeters per second and centimeters in order to obtain the AVA in units per square centimeter. Common pitfalls in using the continuity equation to measure AVA are underestimation of the LVOT diameter, an error that is squared in the calculation, and underestimating the peak AV velocity due to a large angle between the direction of the flow and the Doppler beam. It is also possible to mistake the velocity profile of MR for AS because they both are systolic and in the same general direction.

4. **Right ventricle.** The RV is examined in the ME four-chamber, ME RV inflow–outflow view, and TG RV inflow view, assessing size and global function. The RV appears to be somewhat smaller than the LV in most views and does not normally share the apex with the LV. Pressure and/or volume overload will cause RV enlargement. Global function usually is based on qualitative assessment of decrease in chamber size during systole. It is rated as normal function or as mild, moderate, or severe decrease in function.

5. **Tricuspid valve.** The TV lies between the RV and the right atrium (RA) and has three leaflets: anterior, posterior, and septal. It is examined with the ME four-chamber, ME RV inflow–outflow view, and TG RV inflow view, with and without CFD. Some tricuspid regurgitation (TR) usually is detected. Severity of TR is graded on a semiquantitative scale of 1+ (mild) to 4+ (severe) based primarily on the size of the regurgitant jet. Significant TR usually is due to annular dilation secondary to right heart failure. Tricuspid stenosis is uncommon and usually due to rheumatic heart disease. On TEE it causes high-velocity, turbulent flow across the TV detected with CFD, PWD, and CWD.

6. **Pulmonic valve.** The PV is located anterior and to the left of the AV and is examined with the ME RV inflow–outflow view and UE aortic arch SAX view, with and without CFD. PWD and CWD measurements of flow across the PV are made with the UE aortic arch SAX view because the Doppler beam is parallel to the flow in this view. Trace pulmonic regurgitation (PR) usually is seen and normal. Pulmonic stenosis usually is congenital and rare in adults. It causes high-velocity, turbulent flow across the valve seen with CFD, PWD, and CWD.

7. **Left atrium.** The LA is examined in the ME four- and ME two-chamber views for size and the presence of masses. It normally is less than 5 cm in its anteroposterior and mediolateral dimensions. Thrombus usually is associated with atrial fibrillation and LA enlargement and is most commonly in the LA appendage, seen at the superior lateral aspect of the body of the atrium.

8. **Right atrium.** The RA is examined in the ME four-chamber and ME bicaval views for size and masses. A variably sized fold of tissue at the junction of the inferior vena cava (IVC) and the RA, the **Eustachian valve**, is seen frequently. Fine, filamentous mobile strands may be seen in this region as well and are termed **Chiari network**. Both are normal structures.

9. **Interatrial septum.** The interatrial septum (IAS) is examined in the ME four-chamber, ME LAX, and ME bicaval views. Two portions usually are seen, the thinner fossa ovalis centrally and a thicker region anteriorly and posteriorly. Atrial septal defects are seen with 2D echocardiography and interatrial shunts with CFD. Atrial septal aneurysms cause redundancy and hypermobility of the IAS. Agitated saline contrast may be injected into the RA following release of positive airway pressure to look for the appearance of contrast in the LA. This indicates the presence of a patent foramen ovale (PFO), which may

predispose patients to right-to-left interatrial shunting in the presence of right heart failure causing hypoxemia and/or paradoxical systemic embolization.

CLINICAL PEARL A saline contrast injection rules out a PFO ONLY if the contrast is up against the fossa ovalis AND the atrial septum is bowing to the left (i.e., RAP > LAP).

---

10. **Thoracic aorta.** Although most of the thoracic aorta lies close to the esophagus and can be easily seen with TEE, the trachea may come between the esophagus, the distal ascending aorta, and the proximal aortic arch, obscuring TEE images of these parts of the aorta.

    a. **Ascending aorta**

    The ascending aorta is examined with the ME ascending aortic SAX and ME ascending aortic LAX views by withdrawing the TEE probe superior to the LA from the ME AV views to the level of the right PA. The distal third may be obscured by the trachea and not well seen with TEE. The inside diameter is normally less than 3.5 cm at the midlevel (anterior to the right PA). A more complete and detailed examination of the ascending aorta may be performed after sternotomy with **epiaortic echocardiography**, in which an echocardiographic transducer is covered by a sterile sheath and placed directly on the aorta in the surgical field by the surgeon.

    b. **Aortic arch**

    The aortic arch is examined with the UE aortic arch LAX and UE aortic arch SAX views. The distal arch is easily seen in most patients, but the proximal arch may be obscured by the trachea. The inside diameter normally is less than 3 cm. The great vessels often are seen coursing toward the head to the right of the image in the UE aortic arch SAX view.

    c. **Descending thoracic aorta**

    The descending thoracic aorta is examined in SAX (approximately 0-degree multiplane angle) and LAX (approximately 90-degree angle) from the arch to the diaphragm. The inside diameter normally is less than 3 cm. The proximal descending thoracic aorta is lateral to the esophagus and the distal portion is posterior, so the probe must be rotated as different levels are examined to keep the aorta centered in the image. It often is possible to see the proximal abdominal aorta by advancing the probe past the diaphragm.

    d. **Aortic diseases.** Three common abnormalities of the aorta are detected with TEE:

    (1) **Atherosclerosis**

    Atherosclerosis causes thickening and irregularity of the intimal layer of the aorta that is easily seen with TEE. The normal intima is smooth and less than 2 mm thick. Severity of atherosclerosis is graded on a five-point scale: Grade 1 for normal or minimal disease (intima less than 2 mm thick), grade 2 for mild disease (intima 2 to 3 mm thick), grade 3 for moderate or sessile disease (intima 3 to 5 mm thick), grade 4 for severe or protruding disease (intima greater than 5 mm thick), and grade 5 for mobile lesions. The location and extent of the lesions also are noted.

    (2) **Aneurysm**

    Aneurysmal dilations of the aorta are classified by their location and shape as either diffuse (sometimes termed fusiform) or saccular (a sac coming out the side of the vessel, similar in concept to a bulging hernia). They often are associated with atherosclerotic changes and/or mural thrombus, which are easily seen with TEE. Aneurysms with inside diameter 4 cm or less are considered mild and those greater than 6 cm are considered severe.

    (3) **Dissection**

    An aortic dissection is the separation through the media of the intimal layer from the rest of the aorta. With TEE, a mobile membrane is seen within the aorta dividing the vessel into a true and a false lumen. CFD is applied to the aorta to characterize the flow in the true and false lumens. Dissections are classified into type A, which involve the ascending aorta and are a surgical emergency, and type B, which do not involve the ascending aorta and usually are treated without surgery. TEE findings that may be associated with type A aortic dissections include aneurysmal dilation of the aorta, hemopericardium and tamponade, left hemothorax, AR, and RWMAs due to coronary artery ostial involvement.

VII. **Monitoring applications of TEE**

A. **Assessing preload**

The most direct measurement of preload is LV end-diastolic volume. TEE provides 2D images of the LV, so LV EDA of the TG mid-SAX view has been used as an estimation of end-diastolic volume. Studies have shown that decreases in blood volume as little as 1.5% can be detected by this technique [10] and that correlation between EDA and cardiac output is better than that between PA occlusion pressure and cardiac output [11].

B. **Measuring intracardiac pressures**

Measuring flow velocities with Doppler echocardiography and applying the modified Bernoulli equation allow calculation of gradients between chambers of the heart at various locations. If the absolute pressure of one of these chambers is known, the pressure of the other chamber can be calculated. Thus, by measuring the peak velocity of TR with CWD, one can estimate the peak RV systolic pressure as the RV to RA gradient ($\Delta P = 4V_{TR}^2$) plus the RA pressure. This equals the PA systolic pressure if there is no pulmonic stenosis. Similar logic can be used to measure LA, PA diastolic, and LV end-diastolic pressures by measuring the velocities of MR, PR, and AR jets and knowing the LV systolic (same as systolic BP), RV diastolic (same as central venous pressure [CVP]), and aortic diastolic (same as diastolic BP) pressures.

C. **Measuring cardiac output**

Calculating SV with TEE requires making two measurements: (i) The velocity profile of flow with PWD or CWD and (ii) the area through which the flow occurs with 2D echocardiography. These measurements can be made with TEE in several locations: AV, LVOT, MV, and PA. The accuracy of this technique depends on both the velocity and area measurements being made **in the same location and at the same time in the cardiac cycle**. The velocity profile of the flow is traced and integrated through time to yield a value called **velocity time integral** (VTI), which is in units of length, usually centimeters. Then the area A through which the flow passes is measured with 2D echocardiography to give a value in units of length squared, usually square centimeters. The product of VTI and A yields the SV in units of volume, usually cubic centimeters or milliliters. SV times the heart rate gives the cardiac output. The best validated technique for intraoperative TEE uses CWD across the AV from the TG LAX or deep TG LAX views [12]. The area of the valve then is calculated from the ME AV SAX view by measuring the intercommissural distance S and applying the formula for the area of an equilateral triangle: $A_\Delta = 0.433S^2$. This technique is only applicable if the AV is normal.

D. **Detecting myocardial ischemia**

Appearance of a new RWMA on TEE during surgery has been shown to be a more sensitive indicator of myocardial ischemia than electrocardiographic changes and a better predictor of progression to myocardial infarction [13]. After complete baseline examination of all LV segments is recorded for comparison, the TG mid-SAX view is monitored because it simultaneously shows regions supplied by all three major coronary arteries. An increase in the wall-motion score of two or more grades in a segment suggests acute ischemia. Severe hypovolemia also may produce wall-motion abnormalities without ischemia [14]. TEE is not a true monitor for ischemia unless it is continuously observed during surgery and is more often checked at crucial points of the operation, such as aortic cross-clamping, or when another monitor suggests ischemia, such as electrocardiographic or hemodynamic changes.

E. **Intracardiac air**

Air in the heart is easily seen with TEE as hyperdense or white areas within the chambers. In a supine patient, air in the LA accumulates along the IAS and adjacent to the right upper pulmonary vein. Air in the LV accumulates along the apical septum. Tiny white spots seen floating within the chambers are microscopic bubbles and are not of great concern. Large bubbles have air–fluid levels visible on TEE as straight lines perpendicular to the direction of gravity that wobble as the heart beats. They typically have a shimmering artifact extending from the air–fluid level away from the transducer. Large bubbles should be evacuated before discontinuing cardiopulmonary bypass (CPB).

VIII. TEE for specific types of surgery

A. Coronary artery bypass grafting (CABG)

TEE for CABG surgery focuses on global and regional LV functions. Baseline examination of all segments of the LV is performed and recorded for later comparison. A baseline RWMA may represent previously infarcted, nonviable myocardium, chronically ischemic hibernating myocardium, or acutely ischemic myocardium. Examination of the LV is repeated after grafting. The appearance of a new RWMA before or after bypass grafting should be considered acute ischemia. A new RWMA seen immediately after CPB may indicate stunned myocardium, that is, viable muscle that is perfused but transiently not functioning due to inadequate myocardial protection during CPB. RV infarction causes dilation and hypokinesis of the RV on TEE, often associated with significant TR. Complications of coronary artery disease, such as ischemic MR, LV thrombus, LV aneurysm, ruptured papillary muscle, and postinfarction ventricular septal defect, may be detected with TEE. TEE also is important in detecting atherosclerosis in the aorta, which may increase the risk of stroke during CABG surgery.

B. Valve repair surgery

Intraoperative TEE is very helpful during valve repair surgery. Detailed baseline examination of the diseased valve can provide the surgeon with information about the mechanism and etiology of the lesion, indicating the feasibility of repair and the type of repair needed. Assessment of the repair after CPB is done so that problems can be detected and immediately addressed. MV repairs are assessed with TEE for three potential problems:

1. **Residual regurgitation.** Residual MR is assessed with CFD after MV repair. Ideally there is no or only trace MR. Mild (1+) MR probably is acceptable. Moderate (2+) or more MR should lead to consideration of revision of the repair or valve replacement.

2. **Systolic anterior motion (SAM) of the MV.** Repair of myxomatous MVs with redundant leaflets can cause mitral SAM, which is easily diagnosed with TEE. There is abnormal anterior motion of the excessive leaflet tissue toward the ventricular septum during systole. This leads to dynamic LVOT obstruction and MR. SAM can be managed successfully in some cases by increasing intravascular volume, administering pure vasoconstricting drugs, and stopping positive inotropic drugs. In severe cases that do not respond to appropriate treatment, revision of the repair or valve replacement is needed.

3. **Stenosis.** Excessive narrowing of the mitral orifice by valve repair creating stenosis is possible but very uncommon. This is seen on TEE by limited opening of the leaflets and high peak transmitral inflow velocity (greater than 2 m/sec).

C. Valve replacement surgery

After valve replacement surgery, the prosthesis is evaluated with TEE. CFD is used to examine the valve annulus for paravalvular leaks. Trace paravalvular leaks often are seen after CPB and are not a cause for concern. Moderate (2+) or more regurgitation may need to be addressed surgically. Different types of prosthetic valves have characteristic normal CFD patterns of regurgitation that should not be confused with pathologic regurgitation. Bileaflet mechanical valve prostheses may have a leaflet immobilized, usually in the closed position, by impinging tissue, so TEE evaluation of these valves should document that both leaflets move freely. An immobile leaflet should be corrected immediately with surgical intervention. Stentless aortic bioprostheses and aortic homograft prostheses may develop significant AR if they are not inserted properly. This can be detected with CFD. Moderate (2+) or more AR usually warrants further surgical intervention.

D. Surgery for congenital heart disease

TEE can confirm the diagnosis before CPB and occasionally finds previously undiagnosed lesions in patients with complex congenital heart disease. Septal defect closure and adequacy of flow through prosthetic conduits and intracardiac baffles are assessed intraoperatively with TEE using CFD, PWD, and CWD, allowing immediate correction of inadequate repairs.

E. **Surgery for infective endocarditis**

TEE is helpful in confirming the location and extent of infection and assessing the severity of associated lesions such as valvular regurgitation, abscesses, and fistulae. Intraoperative TEE often detects progression of the infection since the preoperative studies guiding the surgical intervention. TEE examination after CPB confirms the adequacy of the resection of infected tissue and repair of hemodynamic lesions.

F. **Surgery for hypertrophic obstructive cardiomyopathy**

TEE is used before CPB to measure the thickness of the ventricular septum and the location of contact of the MV with the septum to guide the surgeon in sizing the myectomy. The adequacy of the myectomy is assessed with TEE after CPB by looking for residual SAM, measuring residual gradients across the LVOT, and assessing severity of residual MR. Moderate (2+) or more MR and a peak LVOT gradient greater than 50 mm Hg indicate that a more extensive myectomy is needed. Complications of the repair such as ventricular septal defect and AR are assessed with TEE after CPB. CFD often reveals a small jet of diastolic flow in the region of the myectomy from the transected septal perforator artery, which is inconsequential.

G. **Thoracic aortic surgery**

TEE is helpful in monitoring cardiac function and providing definition of thoracic aortic pathology, but it is often difficult to image the distal ascending aorta and proximal arch with TEE. Caution should be used while performing TEE in patients with thoracic aortic aneurysms, especially involving the aortic arch, as the esophagus may be deviated, increasing the risk of injury. A complete baseline examination of the LV is important to identify changes occurring during application and removal of the aortic cross-clamp during surgery on the descending thoracic aorta. When left atrial to aortic or femoral artery partial left heart bypass is used, TEE LV EDA is used to assess adequacy of LV filling to balance flow between the proximal and the distal aorta.

H. **Transplantation surgery**

1. **Heart transplantation**

Pre-transplant examination of the recipient heart focuses on identifying left heart thrombus to help prevent dislodgement with surgical manipulation. Right heart pressures are estimated and aortic cannulation sites are also assessed before CPB. Adequacy of air evacuation from the donor heart is checked with TEE before coming off CPB. Evaluation of donor heart function with TEE after CPB helps direct hemodynamic support. Stenosis of the PA anastomosis is excluded by measuring the peak velocity across it with CWD. RV dysfunction after CPB is common and is manifested on TEE by a hypocontractile, dilated RV with TR secondary to annular dilatation. After CPB, the atrial transplant suture line often creates a mass visible with TEE along the lateral aspects of the LA and RA and the midportion of the atrial septum. If the vena cavae are individually anastomosed, both the superior vena cava (SVC) and IVC anastomoses should be interrogated using the bicaval view within 1 to 3 cm of the cavoatrial junction for stenosis and CFD flow acceleration (suggesting or confirming a stenotic anastomosis).

2. **Lung transplantation**

A comprehensive baseline examination is recorded for comparison later during the procedure. For single lung transplants and bilateral sequential lung transplants, TEE is used to monitor RV function during PA clamping. RV failure causes increased size and decreased contractility seen with TEE, usually associated with increasing TR secondary to annular dilatation and may necessitate going on CPB. Cardiac function is monitored as well during reperfusion, watching for changes in volume and contractility of the ventricles. Air embolism with reperfusion is also detected with TEE. After transplantation, patency of the pulmonary vein-to-LA anastomoses is assessed using CFD and PWD to measure pulmonary venous inflow velocity.

I. **Ventricular assist device implantation**

Intraoperative TEE plays a crucial role during VAD implantation surgery. For a VAD to function properly, the native valve at the outflow of the assisted ventricle must be reasonably competent (PV for right ventricular assist device [RVAD], AV for left ventricular assist device

[LVAD]). TEE is used to assess these valves, and if significant regurgitation is present, a prosthetic valve may be inserted or the native valve sewn shut. TEE is used to detect any intracardiac shunts with TEE such as PFO, atrial septal defect, or VSD, because a properly functioning VAD will decompress the assisted side of the heart and can change the direction of an existing intracardiac shunt. TEE is used to detect thrombus within the left heart to avoid systemic embolization with manipulation or insertion of the VAD cannulae into the heart. The aorta is examined for atherosclerosis to avoid atheroembolism with aortic cannulation, clamping, or anastomosis of the outflow conduit. Before separating from CPB, TEE is used to check the orientation of the VAD cannulae to detect and correct obstruction of the inflow cannula against the wall of the ventricle. Intracardiac air is identified and removed. While weaning a VAD patient from CPB, TEE helps maintain stable hemodynamics with its ability to assess the assisted ventricle's decompression and the nonassisted ventricle's volume and function, including the detection of acute atrioventricular valve incompetence that can accompany acute ventricular failure. This is especially an issue with LVAD patients, where impaired RV function may limit LV preload, and hence the VAD's ability to deliver a normal cardiac output. Once off CPB but before decannulation, agitated saline contrast is injected into the RA to rule out right-to-left shunting not detected before CPB because of elevated left heart filling pressures. With a properly functioning LVAD, the AV typically will not open after CPB. The function of a VAD depends on an adequate filling volume, and TEE can be helpful in making decisions about fluid replacement therapy. Some LVAD patients are expected to have recovery of ventricular function and eventual explantation of the VAD. Usually, the timing of the explantation is determined by periodically decreasing the VAD flow while TEE is used to assess the function of the recovering ventricle. TEE is also very helpful in the detection of postoperative complications such as cardiac tamponade and VAD prosthetic valve dysfunction.

J. **Minimally invasive cardiac surgery**

TEE monitoring is critical to the safe conduct of cardiac surgery with CPB performed through percutaneous access and limited surgical incisions. It is used to assure the proper placement of guide wires and to position cannulae and catheters, as well as detect their displacement during the procedure. Because there is limited or no direct view of the heart during minimally invasive surgery, TEE is relied on to detect distention or inappropriate myocardial contraction during CPB. Likewise, TEE is the best way of judging cardiac volume and function while weaning from CPB. As with conventional cardiac surgery, TEE is necessary to follow deairing of the left heart and the adequacy of the surgical intervention during minimally invasive cardiac surgery.

K. **Transcatheter valve interventions**

Catheter-based techniques to repair or replace cardiac valves have undergone great advances in recent years and are being performed more often at more medical centers. Guidelines for the use of echocardiography during these procedures have been published [15].

The most widespread of these procedures is transcatheter aortic valve replacement (TAVR) for AS. TEE may be used to help size the device, but this is probably best done before the procedure, and other techniques such as CT and MRI may be more accurate. TEE can be used to help position the device during TAVR, but fluoroscopy is probably more important in most cases. TAVR complications, such as annular rupture or RV perforation, may be detected with TEE, and TEE, as with other types of cardiac interventions, can be a very useful monitor of cardiac function during the procedure. TEE is probably the best way to detect and localize AR during TAVR, but it is possible to rule out significant AR fluoroscopically with an aortic root injection. Many anesthesiologists believe that general anesthesia with endotracheal intubation is the safest way to manage the airway during TEE for TAVR, and many centers are forgoing TEE in favor of sedation techniques. In some cases, transthoracic echocardiography is employed with moderate conscious sedation, and TEE is used on an as-needed basis.

Transcatheter repair of the MV for MR is emerging as an effective procedure in selected cases considered too high risk for conventional surgery. In contrast to TAVR, where the role of TEE is diminishing, most of the transcatheter mitral procedures require TEE to properly position and deploy the device, and these patients are typically anesthetized and intubated. The use of real-time TEE imaging in three-dimensions has probably contributed to some of the success of these mitral interventions by clearly showing the position as the device is being manipulated into position. TEE is also unsurpassed in assessing the severity and mechanism of MR in real time, often guiding the conduct of the procedure.

IX. 3D echocardiography

3D reconstruction of echocardiographic images from a series of 2D images has been in clinical use for over 20 years. This technique has been most helpful in assessing complex congenital heart defects. TEE transducers that acquire echocardiographic data from a volume of space and create a 3D image in real time are now commercially available and are being used at many centers for intraoperative applications. Reports are appearing in the literature describing how 3D echocardiography adds important information to the standard 2D examination. 3D TEE is already providing new and useful information about the anatomical relationships of complex structures close to the LA, such as the MV. As this technology continues to evolve and becomes more practical, echocardiography will be transformed in the same way as was in the 1970s with the development of 2D imaging.

A. Fundamental limitations of ultrasound imaging

The ability to use ultrasound to make medical images is based on a fundamental, physical fact: The velocity of sound transmission through soft tissue is relatively constant at about 1,540 m/sec. But this fact also imposes a fundamental limitation that becomes important in 2D echocardiography and critical in 3D. Since it takes a fixed amount of time for ultrasound to leave a transducer, travel to and from the reflector in the tissues, and be detected by the transducer, there is an absolute limit to the pulses per second of ultrasound (pulse repetition frequency) a system can transmit without one pulse interfering with the reflection of the previously sent pulse. Thus, the absolute maximum pulse repetition frequency, when imaging at 15 cm depth (30 cm travel distance), is about 5,000 pulses/sec. An ultrasound system constructs the image by synthesizing information from many pulses, rapidly scanning the ultrasound beam through a plane for 2D or a volume of space in real-time 3D, and is limited in either the width and depth of the image or the speed with which it can generate a coherent image (frame rate).

There are two methods of producing 3D images with ultrasound: (i) Off-line computed rendering of a series of 2D images acquired separately within a short period of time and (ii) real-time insonation of a volume of tissue.

B. Computed rendering of 2D images into 3D

Off-line rendering has been available for over 20 years and uses the same computing algorithms developed in radiology for 3D renderings of CT and MRI images. In the past, these techniques had been limited to the radiology suite, but as the cost and size of computers dramatically fell, the technology was applied to portable ultrasound systems and currently is capable of producing a high-quality 3D image with a TEE transducer in about 2 minutes. The process begins with the positioning of the TEE probe and development of a 2D image of the structure to be examined. Then, as the probe is held perfectly still, a series of 2D images are acquired by automatically advancing the multiplane angle through 180 degrees stepwise in 3- to 5-degree increments. Image acquisition is triggered by the ECG so that each 2D image starts and ends at the same point in the cardiac cycle, and translation of the heart (changing of the heart's position within the thorax) minimized, usually by gating acquisition to end expiration or by pausing ventilation, which is easily accomplished in anesthetized patients. With TEE, acquisition takes about 1 minute. Once image acquisition is completed, the system then combines the series of 2D images into a 3D image in about 20 or 30 seconds. The main advantages of the off-line rendering are the ability to create 3D images of larger volumes at higher frame rates than real-time 3D and images that include CFD in much greater detail. Off-line rendering can be done with a conventional 2D multiplane TEE probe. The disadvantages are the time it takes to create the image and the requirement to keep the heart from translating during acquisition. Also, 3D rendering is less accurate in patients with irregular rhythms.

C. Real-time insonation of a volume of tissue

TEE probes capable of real-time 3D image acquisition have been commercially available since 2009. The 3D TEE transducer has a rectangular array of over 2,000 elements that systematically scans an ultrasound beam through a pyramidal volume of tissue with the apex at

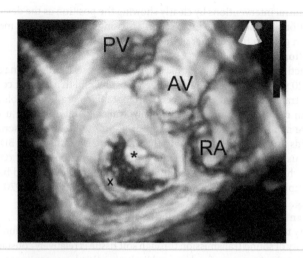

FIGURE 5.9 The MV in mid-diastole viewed from the atrial side. * indicates the anterior leaflet and × the posterior leaflet. An oblique view of the AV is seen, as well. PV, pulmonic valve; AV, aortic valve; RA, right atrium.

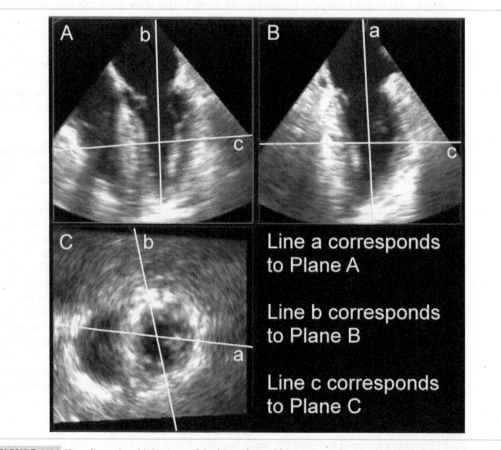

FIGURE 5.10 Two-dimensional (2D) views of the heart derived from a three-dimensional (3D) volume of data. Plane A is a four-chamber view, Plane B is a two-chamber view, and Plane C is an SAX view. The lines show how the 2D planes are aligned within the 3D volume and can be manipulated with the software to modify the 2D images displayed.

the probe. This creates a 3D image that responds to real-time probe manipulation and heart translation and requires no extended time to acquire or render. But real-time 3D is much more limited than off-line rendering in its frame rate and its displayed image width and depth, and real-time CFD is much more limited as well. Newer versions of real-time 3D systems can increase the size of the volume acquired or the quality of CFD by acquiring five to seven real-time beats and "stitching" them into a more detailed or larger image. This requires ECG and respiratory gating, but over a shorter period than conventional off-line rendering systems. The real-time 3D TEE probe is a little larger than a 2D multiplane probe, and considerably more expensive.

D. 3D image display and manipulation

Once a 3D echo image (dataset) has been acquired, it can be displayed in a number of ways. It is typically shown as a pyramidal-shaped volume that may be manipulated using the system software (Fig. 5.9). The volume can be rotated on each of three axes, allowing it to be seen from any point of view; top or bottom, front or back, left or right. The volume of data may also be cropped from any side by using an editing function that removes part of the image with an erasure plane that is gradually brought into the pyramid until the desired structure is exposed. Some systems can create a 2D image by orienting a plane through the 3D volume. Another display mode shows two or more 2D images of the structures simultaneously in synchronized motion (Fig. 5.10). The 3D volumetric displays are highly processed images that require smoothing and interpolation by computer algorithms and are thus prone to artifacts, especially dropout. It takes some time and practice to learn how to properly fine tune the settings of the system to optimize 3D image quality, but this technology is advancing rapidly, making it simpler and quicker to get high-quality 3D images. While 3D echo will provide us with new insights into the structure and function of complex structures such as the MV, for now significant findings should be confirmed and refined with 2D imaging.

REFERENCES

1. Practice guidelines for perioperative transesophageal echocardiography. A report by the American Society of Anesthesiologists and the Society of Cardiovascular Anesthesiologists Task Force on Transesophageal Echocardiography. *Anesthesiology.* 1996; 84(4):986–1006.

2. Kallmeyer IJ, Collard CD, Fox JA, et al. The safety of intraoperative transesophageal echocardiography: a case series of 7200 cardiac surgical patients. *Anesth Analg.* 2001;92(5):1126–1130.

3. Brinkman WT, Shanewise JS, Clements SD, et al. Transesophageal echocardiography: not an innocuous procedure. *Ann Thorac Surg.* 2001;72(5):1725–1726.

4. **Shanewise JS, Cheung AT, Aronson S, et al. ASE/SCA guidelines for performing a comprehensive intraoperative multiplane transesophageal echocardiography examination: recommendations of the American Society of Echocardiography Council for Intraoperative Echocardiography and the Society of Cardiovascular Anesthesiologists Task Force for Certification in Perioperative Transesophageal Echocardiography. *Anesth Analg.* 1999;89(4):870–884.**

5. **Hahn RT, Abraham T, Adams MS, et al.; American Society of Echocardiography; Society of Cardiovascular Anesthesiologists. Guidelines for performing a comprehensive transesophageal echocardiographic examination: recommendations from the American Society of Echocardiography and the Society of Cardiovascular Anesthesiologists. *Anesth Analg.* 2014;118(1):21–68.**

6. **Lang RM, Bierig M, Devereux RB, et al.; Chamber Quantification Writing Group; American Society of Echocardiography's Guidelines and Standards Committee; European Association of Echocardiography. Recommendations for chamber quantification: a report from the American Society of Echocardiography's Guidelines and Standards Committee and the Chamber Quantification Writing Group, developed in conjunction with the European Association of Echocardiography, a branch of the European Society of Cardiology. *J Am Soc Echocardiogr.* 2005;18(12):1440–1463.**

7. Stamm RB, Carabello BA, Mayers DL, et al. Two-dimensional echocardiographic measurement of left ventricular ejection fraction: prospective analysis of what constitutes an adequate determination. *Am Heart J.* 1982;104(1):136–144.

8. Smith JS, Cahalan MK, Benefiel DJ, et al. Intraoperative detection of myocardial ischemia in high-risk patients: electrocardiography versus two-dimensional transesophageal echocardiography. *Circulation.* 1985;72(5):1015–1021.

9. **Zoghbi WA, Enriquez-Sarano M, Foster E, et al.; American Society of Echocardiography. Recommendations for evaluation of the severity of native valvular regurgitation with two-dimensional and Doppler echocardiography. *J Am Soc Echocardiogr.* 2003;16(7):777–802.**

10. Cheung AT, Savino JS, Weiss SJ, et al. Echocardiographic and hemodynamic indexes of left ventricular preload in patients with normal and abnormal ventricular function. *Anesthesiology.* 1994;81(2):376–387.

11. Thys DM, Hillel Z, Goldman ME, et al. A comparison of hemodynamic indices derived by invasive monitoring and two-dimensional echocardiography. *Anesthesiology.* 1987;67(5):630–634.
12. Darmon PL, Hillel Z, Mogtader A, et al. Cardiac output by transesophageal echocardiography using continuous-wave Doppler across the aortic valve. *Anesthesiology.* 1994;80(4):796–805.
13. Leung JM, O'Kelly B, Browner WS, et al. Prognostic importance of postbypass regional wall-motion abnormalities in patients undergoing coronary artery bypass graft surgery. SPI Research Group. *Anesthesiology.* 1989;71(1):16–25.
14. Seeberger MD, Cahalan MK, Rouine-Rapp K, et al. Acute hypovolemia may cause segmental wall motion abnormalities in the absence of myocardial ischemia. *Anesth Analg.* 1997;85(6):1252–1257.
15. **Zamorano JL, Badano LP, Bruce C, et al. EAE/ASE recommendations for the use of echocardiography in new trans-catheter interventions for valvular heart disease. *J Am Soc Echocardiogr.* 2011;24(9):937–965.**

6 Induction of Anesthesia and Precardiopulmonary Bypass Management

Ferenc Puskas, Anand R. Mehta, Michael G. Licina, and Glenn P. Gravlee

KEY POINTS

1. On the day of surgery, most cardiovascular medications should be administered, with the exceptions of angiotensin-converting enzyme (ACE) inhibitors, angiotensin receptor blockers, and (selectively) diuretic agents.
2. Prior to induction of anesthesia, critical emergency drugs should be prepared for immediate administration. Practices vary, but these drugs should include a vasopressor, vasodilator, inotrope, β-adrenergic blocker, and heparin.
3. Induction of anesthesia can be achieved using many different approaches. The most important underlying principle is avoiding hypotension while also suppressing the stress response.
4. Hemodynamically tenuous patients likely will not tolerate traditional induction doses of propofol, but even drugs typically unassociated with hypotension can cause hypotension in cardiac surgical patients as a result of anesthetic-induced reduction in sympathetic tone, synergistic circulatory depression when some induction drugs are given in combination, and/or initiation of positive pressure ventilation.
5. Opioids suppress the stress response in a dose-related manner until a maximum effect is reached at an approximate dose-equivalency of 8 µg/kg of fentanyl.

(continued)

6. Etomidate offers hemodynamic stability during induction, but also suppresses adrenal cortical function for approximately 24 hours.
7. **Potent inhalational agents induce vasodilation and** some myocardial depression, but can be safely used during induction especially to complement intravenous (IV) agents such as etomidate and fentanyl.
8. The reported incidence of ischemia during the precardiopulmonary bypass (pre-CPB) period ranges from 7% to 56%.
9. The Society of Thoracic Surgeons (STS) recommends a cephalosporin as the primary prophylactic antibiotic for adult cardiac surgery. In patients considered high risk for staphylococcus infection (either presumed or known staphylococcal colonization), it is reasonable to combine cephalosporins with vancomycin.
10. During a high-dose narcotic-based anesthetic, the reported incidence of hypertension during sternotomy is as high as 88%.
11. Sinus tachycardia with heart rates (HRs) greater than 100 beats/min has been associated with a 40% incidence of ischemia. HR greater than 110 beats/min was associated with a 32% to 63% incidence of ischemia.

I. Introduction

Induction of anesthesia in a cardiac patient is more than a simple transition from an awake to a stable anesthetic state. Considering all aspects of the patient's cardiac condition allows selection of an anesthetic that best accommodates the patient's current cardiac status and medications. No single agent or technique can guarantee hemodynamic stability. Hemodynamic change with induction can be attributed to the patient's pathophysiology and to a reduction in sympathetic tone potentially causing vasodilation, cardiac depression, and relative hypovolemia. The period between anesthetic induction and the initiation of cardiopulmonary bypass (CPB) also poses numerous challenges to the anesthesia and surgical teams.

II. Premedication

A. Just as the patient's chronic medications can mostly be used to advantage, so can anesthetic premedication (e.g., intravenous [IV] midazolam, lorazepam, or fentanyl) become an integral component of the anesthetic technique.

B. **With rare exception, chronic cardiac medications should be administered orally preoperatively on the day of surgery** with as little water as possible.
   1. **Some** clinicians prefer to withhold diuretics on the morning of surgery, which seems reasonable.
   2. Angiotensin-converting enzyme (ACE) inhibitors and angiotensin receptor blockers have been associated with hypotension following induction of anesthesia (and perhaps during separation from CPB). Although somewhat controversial, we prefer to discontinue the patient's usual dose of these drugs 1 day (24 hours) before surgery in order to reduce the risk for hypotension and for acute kidney injury that has been associated with ACE inhibitor use in cardiac surgery [1].

III. Preinduction period

Unstable patients (e.g., critical aortic stenosis, congestive heart failure) probably should not be premedicated before they reach a preanesthetic holding area that permits observation by an anesthesia caregiver, and we perceive that few practitioners currently administer sedatives or opioids prior to the patient's arrival in such an area. Some examples of premedication regimens are shown in Table 6.1, but monitoring catheters, such as arterial and central venous "lines," ideally should be placed under the influence of premedication, such as IV midazolam (if not after induction of anesthesia).

A. **Basic monitors** and supplemental oxygen are important to initiate before giving supplemental sedation (if needed) and placing invasive monitors.
   1. Electrocardiogram
   2. Noninvasive blood pressure (BP)
   3. Pulse oximeter

TABLE 6.1 Anesthetic premedication for cardiac surgical patients

Poorly compensated patients	Lorazepam or midazolam 1–2 mg intravenously (approximately 15–20 µg/kg)
Compensated patients	I. Midazolam 1–5 mg (15–70 µg/kg) intravenously, titrated to effect with or without IV morphine 2–5 mg (0.03–0.07 mg/kg), hydromorphone 1–2 mg (15–30 µg/kg), sufentanil 5–10 ug (0.05–0.10 µg/kg), or fentanyl 50–100 µg (0.5–1 µg/kg) intravenously after arrival in the preinduction area or the operating room.
	II. Lorazepam 2–4 mg (30–40 µg/kg) by mouth with or without an orally (e.g., methadone 5–10 mg or 0.1 mg/kg) or intramuscularly (e.g., morphine 0.1 mg/kg) administered narcotic 30–60 min before arrival in operating room area.
	III. Benzodiazepines probably contribute to postoperative delirium in elderly patients. Alternatives include dexmedetomidine and carefully titrated propofol.

B. **Invasive monitors can be useful during induction** [2], so some clinicians choose to place central "access" catheters, such as a central venous catheter or pulmonary artery catheter (PAC), before induction of anesthesia. It appears that most anesthesiologists defer central line placement until after anesthetic induction, which is an equally acceptable approach that does not appear to affect patient outcomes. In patients with low cardiac outputs, onset time for anesthetic induction drugs and for vasoactive drugs can be noticeably delayed when this approach is chosen. It appears that most anesthesiologists prefer to place the arterial catheter before inducing anesthesia, as do we, but some prefer to await induction of anesthesia for this intervention as well.

CLINICAL PEARL Most practitioners place central venous catheters (including PACs) after induction of anesthesia, although this can also be accomplished before induction with the aid of judicious sedation.

1. In emergency situations, it may be necessary to proceed with anesthetic induction before placing invasive monitors. In these situations, if a large-bore IV catheter is already present, opening the chest is far more important than PAC or central venous pressure (CVP) catheter measurements. It is highly desirable to initiate intra-arterial BP monitoring before anesthetic induction in such cases. If the anesthesiologist is busy stabilizing the patient and preparing for induction, the surgery team can be asked to assist with radial or femoral arterial catheter (henceforth termed "line") placement under local anesthesia.

C. **Clinical tips** in preparing for cardiac anesthesia
1. Emergency drugs that may be needed can be prepared as dilute bolus doses in syringes or as IV or syringe infusion pumps attached to a peripheral IV or to the infusion port or side-port of the introducer of the pulmonary artery (PA) (or some other central venous) catheter via a manifold.
2. **The drugs selected for anesthesia depend on the patient's condition and the preferences of the anesthesiologist.**
   a. Commonly fentanyl or sufentanil, and less commonly remifentanil, are selected as opioids.
   b. Among the potent inhalational agents, isoflurane probably should be selected for economy, desflurane for rapid titratability, and sevoflurane for inhalational induction or for an airway that is suspected to be difficult (as a judgment-based alternative to awake intubation).
   c. IV amnestic agents may include benzodiazepines such as midazolam, lorazepam, or diazepam, or any of the traditional induction agents described below.
   d. For muscle relaxation, succinylcholine (or no muscle relaxant) is suggested for a suspect airway; pancuronium for low heart rates (HRs); vecuronium, rocuronium, or cisatracurium for hemodynamic blandness; and cisatracurium in the case of liver or renal failure. Note that even moderate-to-severe impairment in renal or

hepatic function need not contraindicate any muscle relaxant per se, but may instead simply merit adjustments in dosing frequency.

3. **Specific cardiovascular medications to have available** before surgery:
   a. Anticholinergic: Atropine (preferred over glycopyrrolate for faster onset)
   b. **Inotrope: Epinephrine, dobutamine, or dopamine as infusions; epinephrine also in a syringe for bolus administration**
   c. Phosphodiesterase III inhibitor: Milrinone
   d. Calcium chloride (27.2 mg/mL elemental calcium) or calcium gluconate (9.3 mg/mL elemental calcium)
   e. Ephedrine as a bolus (mixed vasopressor/inotrope)
   f. Vasopressors
      (1) **Phenylephrine as a 50- to 100-µg bolus, or as an infusion, or norepinephrine**
      (2) Vasopressin (for vascular collapse and resuscitation, especially after left ventricular (LV) assist device placement and with pulmonary hypertension)
   g. **Vasodilators: Nitroglycerin**, nicardipine, clevidipine, or nitroprusside
   h. Antiarrhythmics and antitachycardic agents
      (1) Adenosine
      (2) Esmolol, metoprolol
      (3) Diltiazem or verapamil
      (4) Lidocaine
      (5) Amiodarone
      (6) Magnesium
   i. Anticoagulation and its reversal
      (1) **Heparin**
      (2) Protamine

CLINICAL PEARL   To be most prepared, at least one inotrope, one vasopressor, and one vasodilator should be set up and connected in a pump that is preprogrammed and ready to use. Similarly, syringes should be prepared for bolus administration of at least one vasopressor, inotrope, vasodilator, and probably a β-adrenergic blocker as well.

   j. A custom-built IV pole with a built-in electrical outlet and the capability for attachment of multiple IV infusion or syringe pumps should be available. In the case of syringe pumps, battery operation is acceptable if there is a reliable mechanism for recharging the syringe pumps before each procedure.

D. **Last-minute checks.** Immediately before anesthetic induction, the following points should be considered:
   1. Reassessment of the patient's overall cardiopulmonary and airway status
   2. Integrity of breathing circuit and immediate availability of suction
   3. Availability of blood for transfusion
   4. Proximity of a surgeon or a senior resident
   5. Any special endotracheal tube (double-lumen, bronchial blocker) or intubation (video laryngoscope, intubating stylet) needs
   6. Immediate availability of emergency cardiac drugs

IV. Induction

The cardiac anesthesiologist must often induce a patient who under normal circumstances would not receive a general anesthetic. Objectives include:

A. **Attenuation of hemodynamic responses** to laryngoscopy and surgery without undue hypotension
   1. Conservative drug amounts, as the anesthetic requirement rapidly becomes relatively minor during surgical skin preparation and draping (exception: high-dose opioid induction technique, e.g., 50 µg/kg of fentanyl) (Table 6.2)

TABLE 6.2 Recommended induction doses

Drug	Induction dose
▬ **Hypnotics**	
Propofol	1–2 mg/kg
Etomidate	0.15–0.3 mg/kg
Ketamine	0.5–1.5 mg/kg
▬ **Opioids**	
Fentanyl	3–10 µg/kg
Sufentanil	0.1–1 µg/kg
Remifentanil	0.1–0.75 µg/kg/min or bolus 0.5–1 µg/kg
▬ **Muscle relaxants**	
Cisatracurium	70–100 µg/kg
Vecuronium	70–100 µg/kg
Rocuronium	0.3–1.2 mg/kg
Succinylcholine	1–2 mg/kg
▬ **Maintenance of anesthesia in critically ill patients**	
Sedative/hypnotic agent	
Propofol infusion	20–120 µg/kg/min
Lorazepam single bolus	2–4 mg (25–50 µg/kg)
Diazepam intermittent boluses	4–8 mg (50–100 µg/kg)
Midazolam infusion	0.25–0.5 µg/kg/min
Plus	
An opioid infusion (or intermittent boluses)	
Remifentanil	0.05–0.1 µg/kg/min
Fentanyl	0.03–0.1 µg/kg/min
Sufentanil	0.1–0.5 µg/kg/hr
or	
Dexmedetomidine	0.5–1 µg/kg/hr

    2. Use drug onset time and interactions to advantage.

    3. Adapt induction drug doses to physical status of patient.

B. **Guiding principles** for anesthetic induction include:

    1. Modifications of techniques as new knowledge are gained. For example, trace the history of sufentanil as used during anesthetic induction.

        a. In the 1980s, the recommended induction dose of sufentanil was as high as 25 µg/kg.

        b. In the 1990s, recommendations changed to 6 to 10 µg/kg.

        c. In the new millennium, as little as 0.1 µg/kg is used.

        d. Combinations of sufentanil or fentanyl with etomidate and muscle relaxants exemplify efficient induction techniques.

    2. Physiologic issues

        a. Hypovolemia, which is often difficult to assess, is frequently caused by diuretics and prolonged nothing by mouth (NPO) status.

            (1) This is difficult to assess because of the usual absence of preoperative urine output documentation or LV preload assessment.

            (2) Many cardiac surgical patients do not tolerate more than 10% depletion of intravascular volume without hemodynamic compromise.

            (3) Tachycardia and vasoconstriction, which are useful compensatory mechanisms in normal individuals, may be deleterious in cardiac patients or may be impaired or even precluded as a result of the patient's chronic cardiovascular drug regimen.

(4) Anesthetic drugs may impair appropriate hemodynamic responses [3].

    (a) Propofol reduces BP by inducing venodilation with peripheral pooling of blood, decreasing sympathetic tone to decrease systemic vascular resistance (SVR), and depressing myocardial contractility.

    (b) In decreasing order of circulatory depression, propofol is most depressant, midazolam is intermediate, and etomidate is the least depressant.

(5) The most physiologically efficient method of combating hypovolemia is to augment intravascular volume in the preinduction period using balanced salt solutions, being careful not to overdo this in patients with mitral valve lesions or congestive heart failure. The presence or absence of susceptibility to congestive heart failure may be subtle in patients with LV diastolic dysfunction. In general, the trend has been toward more conservative use of fluids in the pre-CPB period in order to minimize hemodilution and the need for erythrocyte (RBC) transfusion. At times, this occurs at the expense of circulatory support with vasopressors. This philosophy is sound as long as sufficient cardiac output is maintained to perfuse the vital organs and (arguably) is most safely applied if one can measure cardiac output to ensure an adequate cardiac index (under anesthesia, probably greater than or equal to 1.8 L/min/m^2). The preinduction initiation of a prophylactic inotropic infusion (e.g., low-dose epinephrine 0.01 to 0.03 mcg/kg/min or dopamine 1 to 3 mcg/kg/min) in patients with low LV ejection fractions (or with preserved LV function with documented episodes of diastolic heart failure) sometimes helps to maintain a stable perfusion pressure and cardiac output until surgical incision commences.

  3. **Pharmacodynamic issues.** With the exception of ketamine, which can stimulate the cardiovascular system, all anesthetics decrease BP by some combination of removing sympathetic tone, directly decreasing SVR, directly depressing the myocardium, increasing venous pooling (reducing venous return), or inducing bradycardia.

Important individual drug characteristics to be considered:

  a. In critically ill patients, ketamine can decrease BP because depletion of catecholamines may lead to an inability of indirect central nervous system (CNS)-mediated sympathomimetic effects to counterbalance its direct negative inotropic effects. Even in such patients, hypotension appears to be an uncommon response to ketamine.

  b. The conflict between the need to attenuate the hemodynamic response to intubation and other noxious stimuli without overdosing can be illustrated by propofol.

    (1) Propofol may induce hypotension if used for induction, yet a small dose may not suppress the hypertensive response to laryngoscopy.

    (2) In combination with other drugs: After an induction dose of propofol, systolic BP fell an average of 28 mm Hg when no fentanyl was administered, whereas it fell 53 mm Hg when 2 μg/kg of fentanyl was administered. However, the hemodynamic response to intubation was decreased in proportion to the preinduction dose of fentanyl [4].

    (3) Propofol can be given in small increments (0.5 to 1 mg/kg) judging from the patient's physical status and can be used with a small well-timed dose of opioid (e.g., 1 to 3 μg/kg of fentanyl 2 to 4 minutes preceding propofol).

CLINICAL PEARL   During induction of anesthesia, the dosing and timing of sedative–hypnotics, inhalational agents, opioids, and muscle relaxants to avoid awake paralysis and chest wall rigidity while optimizing stress response suppression, mask ventilation, and intubating conditions epitomize the "art" of cardiac anesthesia.

---

  c. The principle of using the relationship between the plasma drug concentration and the bioeffector site onset (biophase or Ke$_0$) must be considered, such that the maximal effects of both the opioid and hypnotic are used to best advantage.

(1) The mean onset time for peak effect of propofol is 2.9 minutes and for fentanyl is 6.4 minutes. Ideally, endotracheal intubation should be performed at the peak concentration of both drugs and after optimal muscle relaxation has been achieved. This may require a second dose or a continuous infusion of ultra–short-acting induction agents such as propofol, because the muscle relaxant onset time may occur after the peak effect of the bolus dose of the induction agent has dissipated from rapid redistribution.

CLINICAL PEARL Increasing the opioid dose beyond 8 µg/kg of fentanyl, 0.75 µg/kg of sufentanil, or 1.2 µg/kg/min of remifentanil does not further attenuate the stress response (increased BP and HR) to intubation.

d. Depth of anesthesia provided by propofol or other sedative–hypnotic agents does not determine the degree of stress–response suppression; rather, the CNS level of opioid analgesia tends to do so.

e. Reducing the doses of anesthetic drugs is often the safest way to induce critically ill patients.

f. For a hemodynamically stable patient, one might prefer a hemodynamically bland muscle relaxant. For patients with a baseline HR less than 50 beats/min or with valvular regurgitation, either pancuronium (if available) or a small dose of glycopyrrolate (e.g., 0.2 mg) or atropine (e.g., 0.4 mg) might be useful to increase HR to 70 to 80 beats/min.

g. Induction drugs are administered most efficiently through a central venous catheter, such as the side-port introducer, or an infusion port in a PAC. *This is one disadvantage to central venous/PA catheter placement after induction of anesthesia.*

h. Muscle relaxants are given early in the sequence. Onset time is important to consider. This can be defined for most agents in the context of ED_{95}, or the average dose required to induce 95% suppression of the twitch response. For most nondepolarizing neuromuscular blockers, the time to achieve maximum twitch suppression at a dose of $1 \times ED_{95}$ is 3 to 7 minutes. Use of $2 \times$ or $3 \times ED_{95}$ reduces onset time to 1.5 to 3 minutes, and to as low as 1 to 1.5 minutes for $3 \times ED_{95}$ with rocuronium (0.9 mg/kg).

(1) Succinylcholine (1 to 2 mg/kg) can be used to reduce onset time of neuromuscular blockade to 1 to 1.5 minutes.

CLINICAL PEARL Muscle relaxant timing is important during induction, that is, early enough to avert opioid-induced chest wall rigidity but late enough to avoid awake paralysis.

i. An example of a drug combination that combines rapid onset (intubating conditions in 1 to 2 minutes) and good suppression of the stress response to laryngoscopy is remifentanil 1 µg/kg, etomidate 0.2 mg/kg, and succinylcholine 1.5 mg/kg, all administered as a simultaneous bolus.

j. High-dose opioid induction techniques:

(1) Achieved popularity in the early 1970s with morphine (1 to 2 mg/kg) and in the late 1970s with fentanyl (50 to 100 µg/kg) because of the combination of excellent stress–response suppression and hemodynamic stability.

(2) Sufentanil (10 to 25 µg/kg) rose to popularity for the same reasons in the 1980s.

(3) This technique lost favor in the 1990s because of long postoperative intubation times, but it is still potentially useful for high-risk patients who will require overnight mechanical ventilation regardless of the anesthetic technique chosen.

(4) Because of the marked vagotonic effects of bolus high-dose opioids, pancuronium nicely complements this technique, especially if given early enough in the induction sequence to minimize chest wall rigidity.

(5) These doses of fentanyl and sufentanil can be given as a bolus or over 3 to 5 minutes. Morphine, now seldom used in cardiac anesthesia, must be given slowly (5 to 10 mg/min) to avoid hypotension. A 2009 study indicated that morphine may still have a place in cardiac anesthesia, as it reduced the degree of postoperative pain and the incidence of postoperative fever [5].

(6) Beware of hypotension if hypnotics are given simultaneously and of inadequate amnesia if they are not.

C. **Anticipated difficult intubation. The cardiac patient with a difficult airway imposes a conflict between our instincts to preserve and protect the airway and those to avoid hemodynamic stress. Concerns about loss of airway control supersede those about hemodynamic stimulation, yet both airway safety and hemodynamic stability can be achieved with awake intubation.** Suggestions for accomplishing "awake" endotracheal intubation (by any of several techniques) while still preventing potentially deleterious hemodynamics follow:

1. **Adequate airway anesthesia either** greatly attenuates or prevents the hemodynamic stress of endotracheal intubation. Specific techniques that may prove helpful include:

   a. Nebulized 4% lidocaine for 15 or more minutes prior to airway instrumentation.

   b. Topical sprays such as 2 sec of Cetacaine or 4% lidocaine, although toxicity can result from either of these agents if used to excess.

   c. Nerve blocks: Glossopharyngeal and superior laryngeal blocks can anesthetize the pharynx down to the level of the vocal cords. They should be used with caution, as subsequent anticoagulation could lead to hematoma in case of vascular puncture.

   d. Transcricoid or transtracheal injection of 4% lidocaine can suppress the cough reflex, as can injection of 4% lidocaine via the suction or injection port of a fiberoptic bronchoscope upon reaching the vocal cords and trachea.

   e. A dexmedetomidine bolus and/or infusion offers a useful adjunct to awake intubation, because it provides some analgesia and stress response suppression while preserving respiration and responsiveness to verbal commands. An IV bolus or a continuous infusion of esmolol can also assist in suppressing hypertension and tachycardia during awake intubation.

> **CLINICAL PEARL** Awake intubation is safe in cardiovascularly unstable patients as long as adequate airway anesthesia is provided.

2. **Low-to-moderate levels of sedation** can facilitate patient cooperation and may induce amnesia:

   a. Midazolam titrated to effect.

   b. Opioids in low doses (not amnestic), but beware of the combined sedative and respiratory depressant effects of opioids combined with sedative/hypnotics, such as midazolam.

   c. Conservative infusion doses of propofol (e.g., 10 to 40 µg/kg/min) can be helpful and may reduce the gag and cough reflex modestly, but can also result in dysphoria or airway obstruction.

   d. Some practitioners select dexmedetomidine for this purpose, whereas others remain unimpressed with its efficacy or desirability. Favorable aspects include sedation (without reliable amnesia!), tendency to decrease HR and BP, and possibly modest airway reflex suppression. For awake intubation, typically a bolus dose of 1 µg/kg administered is administered intravenously for awake intubation over approximately 10 minutes, followed by a regular infusion of 0.2 to 1.0 µg/kg/hr as maintenance.

3. **Adjuncts that may help prevent or treat hypertension or tachycardia:**

   a. β-Adrenergic blockers (e.g., **esmolol** bolus [0.25 to 1 mg/kg] or infusion [100 to 300 µg/kg/min])

   b. Vasodilators (e.g., nicardipine 500 to 750 µg or nitroglycerin 50- to 100-µg bolus, or continuous infusion titrated to effect)

    c. Mixed adrenergic blocker: IV labetalol titrated to effect (bolus dose typically 10 to 20 mg every 5 to 10 minutes)

  4. Be prepared to proceed with a gentle IV induction once endotracheal intubation has been achieved. If the preparations above have been successful, the patient will tolerate the presence of the endotracheal tube without coughing or distress, which reduces the urgency to proceed with induction.

V. Drugs and pharmacology applied to induction of anesthesia

A. Opioids

  1. Basic structures and opioid receptors

    a. Rigid interlocked molecules of the morphine group known as pentacyclides and flexible molecules of phenylpiperidine rings, such as fentanyl

    b. There are three opioid receptors (μ, κ, and δ) with subgroups.

      (1) Opioid receptors are γ-protein–coupled receptors.

  2. Properties of opioids. Analgesia is more than the relief of pain or of the conscious perception of a nociceptive stimulus. A noxious stimulus can affect an ostensibly unconscious (and unparalyzed) person as demonstrated by movement in the form of a withdrawal reflex. The stimulus can produce increased autonomic activity. Narcotics in general are poor hypnotics and cannot be counted upon to induce amnesia.

  3. Induction pharmacokinetics:

    a. Pharmacokinetics are similar among three modern synthetic opioids (fentanyl, sufentanil, and alfentanil) with a few differences [6].

      (1) All have a three-compartment model.

      (2) Ninety-eight percent of fentanyl is redistributed from the plasma in the first hour.

      (3) Brain levels parallel plasma levels with a lag of 5 minutes.

      (4) Fentanyl has a large volume of distribution, which can limit hepatic access. However, the liver will clear all the fentanyl it gets.

      (5) Sufentanil is 7 to 10 times more potent than fentanyl. It has a higher pKa and only 20% is ionized.

      (6) Sufentanil is half as lipid soluble as fentanyl and is more tightly bound to receptors. It has a lower volume of distribution and a faster recovery time.

      (7) Alfentanil, typically administered as a continuous infusion, is less potent than fentanyl and shorter acting than sufentanil, but has been largely superseded by remifentanil (see below).

  4. Remifentanil pharmacokinetics:

    a. Remifentanil has a unique pharmacokinetic profile, as it is subject to widespread extrahepatic hydrolysis by nonspecific tissue and blood esterases.

    b. It has an onset time of 1 minute and a recovery time of 9 to 20 minutes. These properties make it very advantageous when there is variation of surgical stimulus or a desire for early postoperative extubation. The anesthesiologist can give as much as he or she feels is needed without impeding rapid recovery.

    c. Careful provision of postoperative pain control is essential, as remifentanil-induced analgesia dissipates rapidly after the infusion is terminated.

B. Other intravenous (IV) anesthetic agents for induction

  1. Etomidate

    a. Etomidate, a very useful induction agent for cardiac patients, is 10 times more potent than propofol, with a recommended dose range of 0.15 to 0.3 mg/kg.

    b. It is reliable at achieving hypnosis, especially when combined with an opioid. Administering the primary dose just after giving an opioid may attenuate myoclonus, which sometimes occurs as a result of subcortical disinhibition.

    c. Etomidate reaches the brain in 1 minute.

    d. There may be an increased incidence of epileptiform activity in patients with known epileptic seizure disorders.

    e. An induction dose of etomidate typically produces a 10% to 15% decrease in mean arterial pressure (MAP) and SVR and a 3% to 4% increase in HR and cardiac output.

6

f. Importantly, stroke volume, left ventricular end-diastolic volume (LVEDV), and contractility remain unchanged in normovolemic patients.

g. Etomidate can be used to anesthetize heart transplant patients, because it preserves myocardial contractility better than any induction technique other than a high-dose opioid induction.

h. Although traditional induction doses of etomidate and opioids given individually most often preserve hemodynamics, when they are given together hypotension may ensue.

i. Since even a single dose of etomidate has been shown to induce significant adrenal suppression for more than 24 hours (not associated with increased vasopressor requirement), it should be used with caution in high-risk cardiac surgical patients or followed by glucocorticoid supplementation for 24 to 48 hours [7].

2. **Propofol**

a. A normal induction dose of 2 mg/kg will drop BP 15% to 40%.

b. Because propofol resets the baroreceptor reflex, lower BP does not increase HR.

c. There are significant reductions in SVR, cardiac index, stroke volume, and LV stroke work index.

d. There is direct myocardial depression at doses above 0.75 mg/kg.

e. Propofol should be titrated according to the patient's age, weight, and individual need and ideally injected into a central vein, thereby allowing the smallest dose to be used effectively and avoiding pain on injection.

f. Propofol's metabolic clearance is 10 times faster than that of thiopental.

g. There is extensive redistribution and movement from the central compartment to a peripheral one, which enables rapid recovery.

h. Because it has direct myocardial depressant effects and easily induces hypotension, propofol should be used with caution (e.g., titrated over 2 to 3 minutes) or reserved for use in hemodynamically stable cardiac patients with good ventricular function.

3. **Thiopental**

a. **Thiopental is currently not available in the United States**, but it is still used in some other countries.

b. **It has a rapid onset and can be used safely in hemodynamically stable patients.**

c. Rapid redistribution to highly perfused tissues causes cessation of thiopental's effects.

d. Cardiovascular effects
   (1) Predominantly venous pooling and resultant decreased cardiac preload.
   (2) Myocardial depressant above 2 mg/kg.
   (3) Increases HR by activating baroreceptor reflex.
   (4) In patients who have low cardiac output, a greater proportion of the drug dose goes to the brain and myocardium; thus, a smaller amount of thiopental has a larger effect.
   (5) Overall, there is a dose-related negative inotropic effect from a decrease in calcium influx.

4. **Midazolam**

a. **Midazolam is a good premedicant but is difficult to titrate to a minimum effective dose for induction because of a large variation in the hypnotic dose and a relatively slow onset time to peak CNS effect of 3 to 7 minutes. A typical induction dose is 0.1 to 0.2 mg/kg.**

b. It is an effective amnestic, and this constitutes its appeal.

c. The hypotensive effect from an induction dose is similar to or less than that for thiopental, and it is dose related.

d. In patients who have high cardiac filling pressures, midazolam seems to mimic low-dose nitroglycerin by reducing filling pressures.

e. The addition of opioids produces a supra-additive hypotensive effect.

CLINICAL PEARL   Carefully titrated boluses or infusions of midazolam have become a mainstay of cardiac anesthesia.

5. **Lorazepam and diazepam**
   a. Lorazepam is a very potent benzodiazepine (approximately 1.5 times as potent as midazolam), and diazepam is approximately half as potent as midazolam.
   b. Because of its potency, lorazepam produces anxiolytic, sedative, and amnestic effects in lower doses and with fewer side effects than midazolam. Diazepam's cardiovascular effects are comparable to those for midazolam, that is, generally modest preload and afterload reduction that appears to be enhanced in the presence of potent opioids such as fentanyl, sufentanil, and remifentanil.
   c. Lorazepam is useful in sick cardiac patients when only small amounts of drugs are desired. Both lorazepam and diazepam can complement high-dose opioid inductions as long as the slower onset times are understood and accommodated.
   d. If rapid recovery is expected, as in minimally invasive direct coronary artery bypass surgery, lorazepam is a poor choice because of its relatively long clinical action (typically several hours). Diazepam in moderate-to-high doses (greater than 0.15 mg/kg for most patients) can exhibit a prolonged action as well, and it has an active metabolite. Diazepam's clinical offset is disproportionately prolonged in elderly patients when compared to lorazepam or midazolam.
   e. Onset times are relatively slow (lorazepam peaks in 5 to 10 minutes, diazepam is slightly faster) in the context of induction of anesthesia, but are acceptable in the context of IV sedation for "line" placement before induction of anesthesia.
6. **Ketamine**
   a. Ketamine produces a unique cataleptic trance known as dissociative anesthesia.
   b. It is extensively redistributed and eliminated.
   c. Bioavailability on IV injection is 97% and 2 mg/kg produces unconsciousness in 20 to 60 seconds.
   d. **Ketamine induces significant increases in HR, MAP, and plasma epinephrine levels.** This sympathetic nervous system stimulation is centrally mediated.
   e. Ketamine may be advantageous in hypovolemia, major hemorrhage, or cardiac tamponade.
   f. It allows amnestic obtundation of the hemodynamically unstable patient, giving the surgeon an opportunity to rapidly intervene and correct a life-threatening problem (e.g., cardiac tamponade). In these situations, skin preparation should be performed before induction.
   g. **The hemodynamic stimulatory effect of ketamine depends on the presence of a robust myocardium and sympathetic reserve. In the absence of either, hypotension may ensue from myocardial depression** [8].
   h. Coronary blood flow may not be sufficient to meet the increased oxygen demands induced by sympathetic stimulation.
   i. Ketamine should be avoided in patients with elevated intracranial pressure.
   j. Ketamine is very useful for patients who have experienced severe acute blood loss.
   k. The analgesic effects of ketamine are increasingly recognized and appreciated, especially in opioid-dependent patients.
   l. Ketamine increases salivation and tracheobronchial secretions, so we advise simultaneous administration of glycopyrrolate in the absence of tachycardia.
C. **Inhalational agents**
   1. **Hemodynamic effects.** Similar but generally modest levels of myocardial depression occur with all three popular inhalational agents, **isoflurane, desflurane**, and **sevoflurane**. Serious consequences may occur in patients with congestive heart failure, however, as a narrow range of anesthetic concentrations may be tolerated by the compromised myocardium. **The predominant hemodynamic effect of these three agents is dose-dependent vasodilation**, hence reducing BP and SVR [9]. All three agents also induce a dose-dependent reflex tachycardia that can be attenuated or prevented by β-adrenergic blockers or opioids.
   2. **Desflurane** is uniquely titratable for induction of anesthesia because of its rapid onset and offset, which remarkably matches that of a remifentanil infusion. Because of its

pungent aroma, however, desflurane is poorly tolerated unless it is preceded by an IV induction.

3. **Sevoflurane** has a much more pleasant aroma, suitable for inhalational induction, offers hemodynamic stability in most induction situations, and has an onset time only slightly slower than that of desflurane.

4. **Isoflurane**, like desflurane, has a pungent aroma, and it is best introduced after an IV induction.

5. **Nitrous oxide** is seldom used during anesthetic induction in cardiac surgical patients, but it is generally safe to use for induction with the probable exception of patients with markedly increased pulmonary vascular resistance (PVR). Some find it useful in the hiatus between induction and incision, because one can achieve a minimum alveolar concentration (MAC) level (see below) proportionate to its inspired concentration with minimal reduction in BP.

6. **Clinical use.** Whereas clinically significant brain concentrations (greater than or equal to 1 × minimal alveolar concentration [MAC]) can be attained with desflurane and sevoflurane in 2 to 4 minutes, generally lower concentrations are achieved over the same time frame with isoflurane. Consequently, **desflurane and sevoflurane are more likely to reach concentrations consistent with stress–response suppression (generally 1.3 to 1.5 times MAC) during a customary induction period than isoflurane**. One potential drawback to desflurane is sympathetic stimulation when the inspired concentration is increased rapidly, perhaps owing to its airway irritant effects. Any of these inhalation agents can be used during induction as a complement to an IV induction. Desflurane can be useful in cardiac anesthesia not as much because of its rapid offset as because of its rapid onset.

D. **Muscle relaxants**

1. **A suspected difficult intubation** precludes giving the patient a neuromuscular blocker before achieving intubation unless one is highly confident that mask ventilation will succeed and that an emergency alternative airway (e.g., laryngeal mask) can also succeed.

2. **Succinylcholine** still has the fastest onset and offset of all muscle relaxants.

3. Significant β-adrenergic blockade and high-dose opioid induction are potential indications for otherwise obsolescent pancuronium, as its vagolytic effects tend to counter the vagotonia and bradycardia induced by higher doses of opioids.

4. **Intermediate-duration agents:** Cisatracurium, rocuronium, and vecuronium are hemodynamically bland.

   a. If hepatic or renal failure exists, cisatracurium appears to be the wisest choice.

5. **Timing of the administration** of the muscle relaxant is important.

   a. Laryngoscopy should await optimal relaxation (see Section I.B.3.h). Early administration obviates opioid-induced truncal rigidity, which may impair mask ventilation and result in systemic oxygen desaturation, yet one should also ensure amnesia with a sedative–hypnotic agent before administering the muscle relaxant.

E. **Applications of old drugs in sick patients**

One busy cardiac surgery center blends the principles of careful patient assessment, cautious dosing, and fiscal restraint by commonly choosing the following preinduction sequence:

1. Patient arrives in anesthetic preinduction area or operating room.

   a. A large-bore (16-gauge or larger) IV catheter is placed.

   b. Light premedication is administered, typically midazolam 1 to 2 mg IV.

   c. A 20-gauge radial or brachial arterial catheter is placed using local anesthesia.

2. IV induction of anesthesia proceeds using the following:

   a. Fentanyl 250 to 500 µg in consideration of the patient's size and hemodynamic stability.

   b. Etomidate 0.15 to 0.2 mg/kg with the same consideration.

   c. After ensuring that mask ventilation can be accomplished, succinylcholine 1 to 2 mg/kg is administered.

   d. Endotracheal intubation is accomplished.

3. After endotracheal intubation, the next steps are as follows:
   a. Placement of central venous access (e.g., double-lumen CVP or 9 French introducer with single-lumen IV catheter or a PAC placed through the introducer for hemodynamic monitoring)
   b. As hemodynamics permit, careful initiation of isoflurane is administered at 0.5 to 1 MAC with titration to BP and bispectral index (BIS).
   c. If needed, IV phenylephrine is titrated to support BP.
   d. Upon recovery from succinylcholine, transition to vecuronium (initial dose approximately 0.03 to 0.05 mg/kg, subsequent doses 0.01 to 0.02 mg/kg) or rocuronium (initial dose 0.3 to 0.6 mg/kg, subsequently 0.1 to 0.2 mg/kg) for maintenance of neuromuscular blockade.

F. **Inhalational induction in very sick patients**
This technique is a good alternative to gently induce very sick patients with low ejection fraction undergoing left ventricular assist device (LVAD) placement or heart transplantation. The technique is recommended only in patients who clearly have empty stomachs to avoid the potential for aspiration, as the induction period is prolonged:
   1. Patient is in the operating room, monitors placed.
   2. Large-bore (16-gauge or larger) IV catheter is placed.
   3. Light premedication with midazolam 1 to 2 mg IV.
   4. Twenty-gauge radial arterial catheter is placed using local anesthetic (1–2% lidocaine).
   5. An inotropic infusion (usually epinephrine or dopamine) is connected to the peripheral IV, programmed and ready to go.
   6. Start preoxygenation and 2% sevoflurane, maintain 2% during entire induction period, and decrease it only if hemodynamic instability ensues.
   7. Administer fentanyl typically 150 to 500 µg in divided doses, depending on the patient size and age.
   8. Consider administering additional midazolam boluses usually up to 5 mg total, for younger patients (age <65), or increasing the inspired concentration of sevoflurane to 3% to 4% if hemodynamics remain stable.
   9. Upon loss of consciousness, after testing the airway (e.g., oropharyngeal airway insertion), administer 0.6 to 0.9 mg/kg rocuronium to allow for rapid intubation.
   10. When mask ventilating, hyperventilate with small tidal volumes to decrease PA pressure, and to avoid intrathoracic overinflation that may increase PVR and decrease venous return. For similar reasons, avoid positive end-expiratory pressure (PEEP) and be aware of the possibility of "breath-stacking" in patients with reactive airways disease or chronic obstructive pulmonary disease (COPD). The latter patients may require prolonged expiratory time.

VI. **Immediate postinduction period**
After induction and intubation, several different techniques may be used for maintenance of anesthesia. First priorities, however, are to assess the airway (confirm endotracheal tube location via end-tidal CO_2 and auscultation), assess hemodynamic stability, and respond appropriately to any problems identified.
A. A low-dose continuous infusion of the opioid used for induction or of remifentanil (e.g., 0.1 µg/kg/min) can be implemented.
B. Consider adding an inhalational agent for maintenance of anesthesia and amnesia.
C. Continuous infusion or intermittent bolus doses of a sedative–hypnotic agent (e.g., midazolam or ketamine) can be initiated if no potent inhalational agent is used.
D. A propofol infusion may be useful in hemodynamically robust patients.
E. Some clinicians prefer a dexmedetomidine infusion for its augmentation of analgesia and tendency to avoid hypertension, although its offset time is relatively long (15 minutes or more), it can induce hypertension at onset, and bradycardia and hypotension may occur. Further, it lacks reliable amnestic effects.
F. The treatment of postinduction hypotension deserves mention. There is a tendency to administer phenylephrine boluses of 100 to 200 µg as a "knee-jerk" response to hypotension, when

at times either rapid volume infusion, an alternative vasoactive drug, or both may be more appropriate.

1. If the heart appears empty based on filling pressures, echocardiography findings, cardiac output measurement, or respiratory variation in systolic pressure, then rapid administration of crystalloid or colloid is appropriate.

2. If the induction has used drugs most likely to reduce SVR and preload without affecting myocardial contractility (e.g., midazolam or etomidate with an opioid and a muscle relaxant), then phenylephrine is appropriate. If the need appears likely to be sustained because of a lengthy interval to surgical incision, then consider a continuous phenylephrine infusion of 0.1 to 1 µg/kg/min.

3. If the HR is low or if there is a strong possibility of myocardial depression as well (e.g., propofol was used for induction or >0.5 MAC of a volatile agent is in use), then consider using a bolus of ephedrine (5 to 15 mg) or epinephrine (10 to 25 µg).

A simple technique used frequently and varied in dosage according to the physical status of the patient probably provides the most consistent results for most clinicians.

VII. **Management of events between anesthetic induction and cardiopulmonary bypass (CPB)**

   A. **General principles**

   The time between induction of anesthesia and institution of CPB is characterized by widely varying surgical stimuli. Anesthetic management during this high-risk period must strive to:

   8

   1. Optimize the myocardial O_2 supply/demand ratio and monitor for myocardial ischemia. The reported incidence of ischemia during this period varies from as low as 7% to as high as 56% [10].

   2. Hemodynamics must be optimized to maintain adequate organ perfusion. This is best achieved by optimizing the preload, afterload, contractility, HR, and rhythm depending on underlying cardiac dysfunction and its associated complications.

   3. Manage "fast-track" patients with short-acting anesthetic agents.

   4. Adverse hemodynamic changes increase the risk of developing ischemia, heart failure, hypoxemia, or dysrhythmias. These complications may alter surgical management and lead to urgent institution of CPB with failure to perform internal mammary artery (IMA) or radial artery dissection, along with an increased risk of bleeding.

   A few simple rules may assist in the management of cardiac patients before CPB:

   a. **"Keep them where they live."**

   A review of the preoperative vital signs and tests of cardiac performance (echocardiography, cardiac catheterization, and other imaging modalities) helps guide the management of hemodynamics during this period.

   b. **"The enemy of good is better."**

   If the patient's BP and HR are acceptable, does it matter if the cardiac index is 1.8 L/min/m²? When a patient is anesthetized, oxygen consumption decreases, so a lower cardiac index may be adequate. Trying to increase it to "normal" may lead to other problems, such as dysrhythmias or myocardial ischemia. Additional parameters such as mixed venous oxygen saturation (SvO_2) and presence of acidosis should be considered prior to treatment.

   c. **"Do no harm."**

   These patients are frequently very ill. If you are having problems managing the patient, ask for help.

   5. **Stages of the pre-CPB period.** The pre-CPB period can be subdivided into stages based on the level of surgical stimulation.

   a. **High levels of stimulation** include incision, sternal split, sternal spread, sympathetic nerve dissection, pericardiotomy, and aortic cannulation. Inadequate anesthesia or sympathetic activation at these times leads to increased catecholamine levels, possibly resulting in hypertension, dysrhythmias, tachycardia, ischemia, or heart failure (Table 6.3).

   b. **Low-level stimulation** occurs during preincision, radial artery or saphenous vein harvesting, internal mammary (thoracic) artery dissection, and CPB venous cannulation. Risks during these periods include hypotension, bradycardia, dysrhythmias, and ischemia (Table 6.3).

TABLE 6.3 Typical hemodynamic responses to surgical stimulation before cardiopulmonary bypass (CPB)

	Preincision	Incision	Sternotomy and sternal spread	Sympathetic dissection	IMA dissection	Cannulation
Surgical stimulation	↓	↑	↑↑	↑	↓	↓
Heart rate (HR)	↓ or —	— or ↑	↑↑	— or ↓	— or ↓	— or ↓[a]
Blood pressure (BP)	↓↓	↑	↑↑↑	↑ or ↑↑	— or ↓	↓
Preload	— or ↓	— or ↑	— or ↑	— or ↑	— or ↓	↓
Afterload	— or ↓	↑↑	↑↑ or ↑↑↑	↑ or ↑↑	— or ↓	— or ↓
Myocardial O₂ demand	↓	— or ↑	↑↑ or ↑↑↑	↑ or ↑↑	↓	↓

[a]Dysrhythmias secondary to mechanical stimulation of the heart are likely.
IMA, internal mammary artery; ↑, slightly increased; ↑↑, moderately increased; ↑↑↑, markedly increased; ↓, slightly decreased; ↓↓, moderately decreased; —, unchanged. All values are compared with control (preinduction) values.

B. Preincision

This period includes surgical preparation and draping. Several parameters should be checked during this time:

1. **Confirm bilateral breath sounds** after final patient positioning.
2. **Check pressure points.** Ischemia, secondary to compression and compounded by decreases in temperature and perfusion pressure during CPB, may cause peripheral neuropathy or damage to soft tissues.
   a. **Brachial plexus injury** can occur if the arms are hyperextended or if chest retraction is excessive (e.g., occult rib fracture using a sternal retractor) [11]. Excessive chest retraction can occur not only with the sternal spreader but also during IMA dissection even if the arms are tucked to the sides. If the arms are placed on arm boards, obtain the proper position by minimizing pectoralis major muscle tension. Do not extend arms more than 90 degrees from the body to avoid stretching the brachial plexus.
   b. **Ulnar nerve injury** can **occur** from compression of the olecranon against the metal edge of the operating room table. To obtain the proper position, provide adequate padding under the olecranon. Do not allow the arm to contact the metal edge of the operating room table.
   c. **Radial nerve injury** can occur from **compression** of the upper arm against the "ether screen" or the support post of the chest wall sternal retractors used in IMA dissection.
   d. If the fingers are **positioned** improperly, **finger injury** can result from members of the operating team leaning against the operating table. To obtain the proper position, hands should be next to the body, with fingers in a neutral position away from the metal edge of the table. One method to prevent upper extremity injury is to have the patient position himself or herself. A rolled surgical towel can be placed in each hand to ensure that the fingers are in a comfortable and protected position.
   e. **Occipital alopecia** can occur 3 weeks after the operation secondary to ischemia of the scalp, particularly during hypothermia. To obtain the proper position, pad and reposition the head frequently during the operation. A "doughnut" type of pillow protects against this injury as well.
   f. **Heel skin ischemia and tissue necrosis** are possible. Heels should be well padded in such a way as to redistribute weight away from the heel to the lower leg.
   g. **The eyes** should be closed, taped, and free from any pressure.
   h. Commercial foam dressings may be applied prophylactically to various pressure points (sacrum and heels) to prevent pressure sores.
3. **Adjust fresh gas flow**
   a. Use of 100% O₂ maximizes inspired O₂ tension. A lower inspired oxygen concentration may prevent absorption atelectasis and reduce the risk of O₂ toxicity. The inspired

oxygen concentration can be titrated based on pulse oximeter readings and arterial blood gases (ABGs).

b. Nitrous oxide can be used during the pre-CPB period in stable patients. It will, however,

(1) Decrease the concentration of inspired oxygen (Fio_2)

(2) Increase PVR

(3) Increase catecholamine release

(4) Possibly induce ventricular dysfunction

(5) Some evidence suggests that nitrous oxide should not be used in patients with an evolving myocardial infarct or in patients with ongoing ischemia because the decrease in Fio_2 and potential catecholamine release theoretically can increase the risk of ischemia and infarct size. This point remains controversial.

(6) At inspired concentrations of 50% to 60%, nitrous oxide may facilitate hemodynamic stability while augmenting amnesia in the period between induction and surgical incision.

4. Check all monitors and lines after final patient position is achieved

a. IV infusions should flow freely, and the arterial pressure waveform should be assessed for overdamping (flattening of waves) or hyperresonance (typically seen as exaggeration of systolic peak or "overshoot").

b. IV injection ports should be accessible.

c. All IV and arterial line connections (stopcocks) should be taped or secured to prevent their movement and minimize the risk of blood loss from an open connection.

d. Confirm electrical and patient reference "zero" of all transducers.

e. Nasopharyngeal temperature probes, if required, must be placed prior to heparinization to avoid excessive nasal bleeding.

5. Check hemodynamic status

a. When available through existing monitors, cardiac index, ventricular filling pressures, and SvO_2 should be evaluated after intubation, in addition to end-tidal CO_2, HR, BP, and SpO_2.

b. If transesophageal echocardiography (TEE) is used, check and document the position of the probe and the presence or absence of dental and oropharyngeal injury. The TEE probe should be placed before heparinization to avoid excessive bleeding. Make sure the TEE probe is not in a locked position, as this may lead to pressure necrosis in the gastrointestinal tract. Bite blocks are recommended in order to avert expensive probe repairs.

c. A baseline TEE examination should be performed to document the ejection fraction, wall-motion abnormalities, valve function, and the presence or absence of intracardiac shunts (see Chapter 5).

6. Check blood chemistry

a. Once a stable anesthetic level is achieved, and ventilation and Fio_2 have been constant for 10 minutes, an ABG measurement should be obtained to confirm adequate oxygenation and ventilation, and to correlate the ABG with noninvasive measurements (pulse oximetry and end-tidal CO_2 concentration). Maintain normocapnia, as hypercapnia may increase PVR. Hypocapnia may promote myocardial ischemia and cardiac dysrhythmias. Hypocapnia and resulting alkalosis shift the oxyhemoglobin curve to the left, thereby limiting unloading of oxygen to the cells.

b. Mixed venous hemoglobin O_2 saturation can be measured with a mixed venous blood gas at this time, if necessary, to calibrate a continuous mixed venous PAC.

c. Electrolytes, calcium, and glucose levels should be determined as clinically indicated. High glucose levels should be treated to minimize neurologic injury and to decrease postoperative infection rates. Intraoperative hyperglycemia is an independent risk factor for other perioperative complications, including death, after cardiac surgery [12]. Perioperative glucose management of diabetic patients must be started in the prebypass period. Glucose control may be achieved by a continuous infusion of insulin with the infusion rate depending on the patient's blood glucose level. Boluses of IV insulin may lead to large swings in blood glucose, thus, an IV infusion is preferred. It is as important to assess the trends of blood glucose as the absolute blood glucose levels, especially so to avoid intraoperative hypoglycemia. Hence, glycemic control should be based on the velocity of glucose change as well as the absolute value.

   d. A blood sample to determine a baseline activated clotting time (ACT) before heparinization may be drawn at the same time as the sample for ABG. The blood can be taken from the arterial line after withdrawal of 5 to 10 mL of blood, depending on the dead space of the arterial line tubing and avoiding residual heparin, if present, in the flush solution. The perfusionist may require a blood sample to perform a heparin dose–response curve, which in some institutions is used to determine the initial heparin dosage.

   e. Before any manipulation of the arterial line (zeroing, blood sample withdrawal), it is important to announce your intentions. This avoids alarming your colleagues, who may notice the loss of the arterial waveform.

7. **Antibiotics**

   a. Antibiotics are administered before incision and should be timed not to coincide with the administration of other medications, should an allergic reaction occur.

   b. For cardiac patients, the Surgical Care Improvement Project (SCIP) and the Society of Thoracic Surgeons (STS) Practice guidelines recommend that preoperative prophylactic antibiotics be administered within 1 hour prior to incision (2 hours for vancomycin or fluoroquinolones) and discontinued 48 hours after the end of surgery for cardiac surgical patients.

   c. The STS recommends a cephalosporin as the primary prophylactic antibiotic for adult cardiac surgery. In patients considered high risk for staphylococcus infection (either presumed or known staphylococcal colonization), it would be reasonable to combine cephalosporins with vancomycin. Loading doses of vancomycin are based on total body weight. Suggested initial dose is 10 to 15 mg/kg with a maximum dose being 1,000 mg. Administration over 1 hour is advised to avoid hypotension.

   d. Exclusive vancomycin use for cardiac surgical prophylaxis should be avoided as it provides no gram-negative coverage.

   e. In patients with a history of an immunoglobulin-E–mediated reaction to penicillin, vancomycin should be administered with additional gram-negative coverage [13,14].

8. **Antifibrinolytics**
   Excessive fibrinolysis is one of the causes of blood loss following cardiac surgery. Antifibrinolytic agents are commonly used to minimize bleeding and thereby reduce the exposure to blood products.

   a. **Aprotinin (serine protease inhibitor).** The FDA suspended the use of aprotinin after the Blood Conservation using Antifibrinolytics in a Randomized Trial (BART) trial which demonstrated that aprotinin has a worse risk–benefit profile than the lysine analogs with a trend toward increased mortality in patients receiving aprotinin [15].

   b. **Epsilon-aminocaproic acid (EACA) and tranexamic acid (lysine analogs).** With the suspended use of aprotinin, EACA and tranexamic acid are the only antifibrinolytics available. Both are effective agents in reducing **postoperative** blood loss. However, EACA at equipotent doses to tranexamic acid is associated with a higher rate of temporary renal dysfunction. Tranexamic acid is associated with seizures at higher doses [16].

9. **Preparation for saphenous vein excision** involves lifting the legs above the level of the heart. Increased venous return increases cardiac preload. This change is desirable in patients with low filling pressures and normal ventricular function but may be detrimental in patients with borderline ventricular reserve and/or pre-existing hypervolemia. Gradual elevation of the legs may be useful in attenuating the hemodynamic changes. The reverse occurs when the legs are returned to the neutral position.

10. **Endoscopic saphenectomy** for harvesting vein grafts for coronary artery bypass grafting is now common. As in a laparoscopic procedure, carbon dioxide is the insufflating gas of

choice during this procedure. Mechanical ventilation may have to be adjusted depending on the rise in CO_2 as detected by an end-tidal monitor and ABG analysis. When using carbon dioxide insufflation, CO_2 embolism has been reported. Frail, elderly patients with fragile tissue are at risk for this complication. Preventive measures include maintenance of a right atrial pressure to insufflation pressure gradient of greater than or equal to 5 mm Hg and addition of PEEP. Hemodynamic deterioration from transmission of gas through a patent foramen ovale into the left heart and coronary circulation has also been reported [17].

11. **Maintenance of body temperature** is not a concern during the pre-CPB time period with the exception of off-pump coronary artery bypass grafting (OPCAB). It is often preferable to allow the temperature to drift down slowly, as this allows for more homogeneous hypothermia at institution of CPB, and modest hypothermia is inconsequential in an anesthetized patient, especially in the presence of neuromuscular blockade. Before CPB, increasing the room temperature, humidifying anesthetic gases, warming IV solutions, and using a warming blanket are not necessary. These measures must be available for post-CPB management, however. In an anesthetized patient, the physiologic changes associated with mild hypothermia (34° to 36°C) include the following:

   a. Decrease in O_2 consumption and CO_2 production (8% to 10% for each degree Celsius)
   b. Increase in SVR and PVR
   c. Increase in blood viscosity
   d. Decrease in CNS function (amnesia, decrease in cerebral metabolic rate or O_2 consumption [$CMRO_2$] and decrease in cerebral blood flow)
   e. Decrease in anesthetic requirement (MAC decreases 5% for each degree Celsius)
   f. Decrease in renal blood flow and urine output
   g. Decrease in hepatic blood flow
   h. Minimal increase in plasma catecholamine levels

12. **Maintain other organ system function**
   a. Renal system [18]
      (1) Inadequate urine output must be addressed:
         (a) Rule out technical problems first (kinked urinary catheter tubing or disconnected tubing).
         (b) Optimize and maintain an adequate intravascular volume and cardiac output using CVP, PAC, or TEE as a measure of preload and cardiac performance.
         (c) Avoid or treat hypotension.
         (d) Maintain adequate oxygenation.
         (e) Mannitol (0.25 g/kg IV) may be used to redistribute renal blood flow to the cortex and to maintain renal tubular flow, although this has not been proven to improve renal outcomes.
         (f) Dopamine (2.5 to 5 μg/kg/min) infusion may be given to increase renal blood flow by renal vascular dilation. Currently, there is no evidence that "renal" dose dopamine will prevent perioperative renal dysfunction. Its use may increase the incidence of atrial dysrhythmias.
         (g) Diuretics (furosemide, 10 to 40 mg; bumetanide, 0.25 to 1 mg) can be given to maintain renal tubular flow if other measures are ineffective or if the patient has taken preoperative diuretics.
      (2) Patients undergoing emergent surgery may have received a large radiocontrast dye load at angiography. Avoiding dye-induced acute tubular necrosis, utilizing the techniques mentioned earlier, is crucial.
   b. Central nervous system
      (1) Adequate cerebral perfusion pressure must be maintained.
         (a) The patient's preoperative lowest and highest MAPs should be the limits accepted in the operating room to avoid cerebral ischemia. Remember, "keep them where they live."

      (b) Elderly patients have a decreased cerebral reserve and are more sensitive to changes in cerebral perfusion pressure.

    (2) Patients at risk for an adverse cerebral event include those with known carotid artery disease, peripheral vascular disease, or a known embolic focus.

  c. Lungs

    (1) Maintain normal pH, $Paco_2$, and adequate Pao_2.

    (2) Treatment of systemic hypertension with a vasodilator may induce hypoxemia secondary to inhibition of hypoxic pulmonary vasoconstriction. Fio_2 may have to be increased.

    (3) Use of an air–oxygen mixture may prevent absorption atelectasis.

13. Prepare for incision

  a. Ensure adequate depth of anesthesia using clinical signs. If available, a bispectral (BIS) monitor may be helpful. A small dose of a narcotic or hypnotic or increased concentration of inhaled agent may be necessary.

  b. Ensure adequate muscle relaxation to avoid movement with incision and sternotomy. If movement occurs, make sure the patient is sufficiently anesthetized, as you are preventing movement with neuromuscular blockade.

C. Incision

1. Adequate depth of anesthesia is necessary but may not be sufficient to avoid tachycardia and hypertension in response to the stimulus of incision. If hemodynamic changes occur, they are usually short lived, so medications with a brief duration of action are recommended.

  a. Treatment can include:

    (1) Vasodilators

      (a) Nitroglycerin (20- to 80-µg bolus) or infusion

      (b) Nicardipine infusion

    (2) β-Blockers

      (a) Esmolol (0.25 to 1 mg/kg)

2. Observe the surgical field for patient movement and blood color. Despite an abundance of monitors, the presence of bright red blood remains one of the best ways to assess oxygenation and perfusion.

3. If the patient responds clinically to the incision (tachycardia, hypertension, other signs of "light" anesthesia, or clinically significant BIS monitor value changes), then the level of anesthesia must be deepened before sternotomy. Do not allow sternal split until the patient is anesthetized adequately and hemodynamics are controlled.

D. Opening the sternum

1. A very high level of stimulation accompanies sternal "split." The incidence of hypertension has been reported to be as high as 88% even during a high-dose narcotic-based anesthetic, for example, a cumulative dose of fentanyl, 50 to 70 µg/kg [19]. Hypertension and tachycardia, if they occur, should be treated as described for skin incision.

    Bradycardia secondary to vagal discharge can occur. It is usually self-limiting, but if it is persistent and causes hemodynamic compromise, then a dose of atropine, glycopyrrolate, and/or ephedrine may be necessary.

2. A reciprocating power saw is often used to open the sternum. The lungs should be "deflated" during opening of the internal table of the sternum to avoid damage to the lung parenchyma. Forgetting to turn the ventilator back on poses a potential safety hazard.

3. The patient should have adequate muscle relaxation during sternotomy to avoid an air embolism. If the patient gasps as the right atrium is cut, air can be entrained owing to the negative intrapleural pressure.

4. This is the most common time period for awareness and recall due to the intense stimulation. The risk is greatest with "pure" high-dose opioid techniques, which are obsolete.

  a. Awareness has been reported with fentanyl dosages as large as 150 µg/kg and with lower fentanyl doses supplemented with amnestic agents. Awareness usually, but not always, is associated with other symptoms of light anesthesia (movement, sweating, increased pupil size, hypertension, or tachycardia). A BIS or other type of anesthesia depth monitor may be helpful, but recall has occurred in patients with an "adequate" BIS reading.

   b. If an amnestic agent has not been administered previously, it should be considered before sternotomy because these agents decrease the incidence of recall but will not produce retrograde amnesia. Amnestic supplements do not always protect against the hypertension and tachycardia associated with awareness. However, amnestic supplements may cause hypotension. The most common amnestic agents, their dosages, and side effects include:

   (1) Benzodiazepines (midazolam, 2.5 to 10 mg; diazepam, 5 to 15 mg; lorazepam, 1 to 4 mg) in divided doses usually are well tolerated but can decrease SVR and contractility in patients with poor ventricular function, especially when the drugs are added to a narcotic-based anesthetic.

5. Supplementation of opioids (e.g., fentanyl 1 to 3 μg/kg) in anticipation of sternotomy will attenuate the stress response somewhat.

CLINICAL PEARL   Sternotomy is the time of the highest incidence of awareness during cardiac surgery.

---

6. At this point, any potential benefit to nitrous oxide becomes questionable, as it may augment catecholamine release, cause LV dysfunction, and increase PVR and the risk of hypoxemia. Its use in the noncardiac surgery (ENIGMA) trial was associated with an increased long-term risk of myocardial infarction. Nitrous oxide–induced inactivation of methionine synthetase increases plasma homocysteine levels in the postoperative period. This can lead to endothelial dysfunction and hypercoagulability [20].

7. Inhalation agents are useful at the time of sternal spread. Primarily they decrease BP through vasodilation, but can also cause myocardial depression, bradycardia, tachycardia, or dysrhythmias. They are effective in low concentrations (e.g., 0.5 MAC) as a component of a "balanced" anesthetic including other agents such as fentanyl and midazolam, and have become a standard component of most "fast-track" techniques.

8. Propofol (10- to 50-mg bolus) can rapidly decrease BP if needed.

E. During and after sternal spreading

1. Visually confirm equal inflation of the lungs after the chest is open. Usually the right lung is visible through its parietal pleura, but the left lung might not be visible unless left IMA (LIMA) dissection is performed.

2. PAC malfunction with sternal spread has been reported. Most occurrences are with external jugular or subclavian insertion approaches and involve kinking of the PAC as it exits the introducer sheath. A reinforced introducer can decrease the incidence of kinking. If this occurs, the surgeon can often assist by slightly decreasing the amount of sternal retraction.

   Sheath withdrawal may rectify the problem but can lead to the following:

   a. Loss of the side-port IV line (distal tip of introducer may become extravascular)

   b. Bleeding

   c. Contamination of the access site

3. Innominate (brachiocephalic) vein rupture, as well as brachial plexus injury, is possible after aggressive sternal spread.

F. Concerns with cardiac reoperation ("redo heart")

1. The pericardium is usually not closed after heart surgery, and the aorta, RV, and bypass grafts may adhere to the underside of the sternum. At reoperation, these structures can be easily injured when the sternum is opened. A clue to this potential problem may be provided radiologically if there is no space between the heart and the inner sternal border. Although using an oscillating saw decreases this risk, it does not eliminate it. As this takes longer than the usual sternotomy, ventilation should not be held. Knowing the proximity of mediastinal structures to the sternum is necessary, and if preoperative imaging suggests that they may be in jeopardy, extra measures before reopening the sternum, such as peripheral cannulation and CPB (with or without deep hypothermic circulatory arrest), may be necessary to avoid catastrophe [21]. A venous cannula may be passed into the right atrium through the femoral vein. The correct positioning of this cannula may be identified on the mid-esophageal bicaval view using TEE. Axillary or subclavian cannulation may be the preferred site for peripheral arterial inflow site as compared to the femoral artery in patients with concurrent descending, thoracoabdominal, or abdominal aortic aneurysms. A discussion with the surgeon is necessary to place the arterial line for monitoring in the contralateral superior extremity in case of either subclavian or axillary cannulation. Femoral arterial cannulation may be an alternative.

2. If a pre-existing coronary artery bypass graft is cut, the patient may develop profound ischemia. Nitroglycerin may be helpful, but if significant myocardial dysfunction or hypotension occurs, the ultimate treatment is prompt institution of CPB followed by revascularization of the affected coronary artery.

3. If the right atrium, RV, or great vessels are cut, a surgeon or assistant will put a "finger in the dike" while the tear is fixed or a decision is made to go emergently onto CPB. CPB can be initiated using the following:
   a. After full heparinization, "sucker bypass" with a femoral artery cannula or aortic cannula and the cardiotomy suckers are used as the venous return line if the right atrium cannot be cannulated.
   b. Femoral vein–femoral artery bypass

4. Prolonged surgical dissection increases the risk of dysrhythmias.
   a. The availability of external defibrillator pads or sterile external paddles should be considered. Defibrillation may be necessary before complete exposure of the heart, rendering internal paddles ineffective.
   b. Some institutions use a defibrillation pad that adheres to the back and is placed before induction of anesthesia. This allows for use of an internal paddle even if the heart is not totally exposed, as current will flow in an anteroposterior fashion through the heart.

5. Volume replacement (crystalloid, colloid, blood) may be necessary to provide adequate preload if hemorrhage is brisk during the dissection.
   a. Adequate IV access for volume replacement must be available prior to the start of the surgical procedure. This may be accomplished by securing two large-bore peripheral IV lines or a large-bore multilumen central venous access catheter in a central vein.
   b. Have at least 2 units of blood available in case it is necessary to transfuse the patient.
   c. After the patient is heparinized, the surgical team should use the CPB suckers to help salvage blood.

G. **Concerns with urgent or emergent cardiac operation**
   1. Indications include:
      a. Cardiac catheterization complications (failed angioplasty with persistent chest pain, coronary artery dissection) [22]
      b. Persistent ischemia with or without chest pain that is refractory to medical therapy or an intra-aortic balloon pump (IABP)
      c. Left main coronary artery disease or left main equivalent
      d. Acute aortic dissection
      e. Fulminant infective endocarditis
      f. Ruptured chordae tendineae
      g. Acute ischemic ventricular septal defect
      h. Multiple high-grade lesions with significant myocardium at risk
      i. Emergent LVAD placement
      j. Ruptured or rupturing thoracic aneurysm
      k. Cardiac tamponade
      l. Ventricular rupture

2. Continue BP, pulse oximeter, and electrocardiographic (ECG) monitoring during transport and preparation.
3. Aggressively treat ischemia and dysrhythmias that may be present.
4. If a heparin infusion is being given, continue it until sternotomy. This will increase operative bleeding but will decrease the risk of worsening coronary thrombosis.
   a. Consider heparin resistance and increase the initial heparin dose to avoid delays in starting CPB because the ACT is too low.
5. Continue antianginal therapy, particularly the nitroglycerin infusion, during an acute myocardial ischemic event.
6. Maintain coronary perfusion pressure. Phenylephrine or norepinephrine boluses and/or infusions may be necessary. An IABP may be in use or required. Maintain IABP timing triggers (ECG or arterial pulse wave).
7. In these cases, time is of the essence. Decisions must be made regarding the risks and benefits of additional monitoring (arterial line and PAC) relative to the delay required for catheter insertion. Access to the central circulation and some form of direct BP monitoring are preferred before beginning surgery.
8. If the patient continues to have significant hemodynamic and ischemic changes, after induction, that are unresponsive to treatment, proceed to CPB urgently.
9. In a cardiac arrest situation, go directly to CPB. The surgeon can place central venous and PA lines from the surgical field before weaning the patient from CPB. TEE is a fast alternative to obtain much of the information derived from a PAC.
   a. Urgency of initiating CPB does not supersede obtaining adequate heparinization documented by ACT, or adequate anesthetic levels. In a cardiac arrest situation, consider administering twice the usual dose of heparin (e.g., 600 USP units/kg) to ensure adequate heparinization. The surgeon may give the heparin directly into the heart if access is not available.
10. If a "bailout" (coronary perfusion) catheter has been placed across a coronary dissection, it should not be disturbed. It can be withdrawn from the femoral arterial sheath just before application of the aortic cross-clamp.
11. Fibrinolytic or antiplatelet agents may have been given in the catheterization laboratory. These drugs will increase bleeding before and after CPB.

H. **Internal mammary artery (IMA) and radial artery dissection**
   1. This is a period of low-level stimulation.
   2. The chest is retracted to one side using the chest wall retractor, and the table is elevated and rotated away from the surgeon. The LIMA is most commonly grafted to the left anterior descending artery.
      a. This procedure can cause difficulties in BP measurement.
         (1) Left-sided radial arterial lines may not function during LIMA dissection owing to compression of the left subclavian artery with sternal retraction. The same may be true with a right-sided catheter and a right IMA (RIMA) dissection.
         (2) Transducers must be kept level with the right atrium.
   3. Although rare, accidental extubation is possible from thoracic wall movement during sternal retraction.
   4. Radial nerve injury due to compression by the support post of the sternal retractor is possible.
   5. **Bleeding** may be extensive but hidden from view in the chest cavity (consider volume replacement to treat hypotension), especially if the ipsilateral pleura has been opened.
   6. **Heparin**, 5,000 units, may be given during the vessel dissection process.
   7. Papaverine may be injected into the IMA for dilation and to prevent spasm. Systemic effects may include hypotension or anaphylaxis.
   8. IMA blood flow usually should be more than 100 mL/min (25 mL collected in 15 seconds) to be considered acceptable for grafting.
   9. Mechanical ventilation may need to be adjusted if the motion of the lungs interferes with the surgical dissection of the IMA. This may be achieved by reducing the tidal volume and increasing the respiratory rate to achieve constant minute ventilation.

    10. If the radial artery is being harvested as a conduit, the arterial line should be placed on the other side.

I. **Sympathetic nerve dissection**

    1. After the pericardium is opened, the postganglionic sympathetic nerves are dissected from the aorta to allow insertion of the aortic cannula.

    2. This is the most overlooked period of high-level stimulation because of sympathetic discharge. Treatment of hemodynamic changes is explained above.

J. **Perioperative stress response**

The body responds to stress with a catabolic response and an increase in substrate mobilization. This response is mediated primarily through the hypothalamic–pituitary–adrenal axis. Stimuli include intubation, surgical incision, sternotomy, and CPB. Inadequate depth of anesthesia and analgesia elevates the magnitude of this response.

    1. **Humoral mediators** and the systemic effects of the stress response (see Table 6.4)

    2. **Modification of the stress response**

        a. Systemic opioids (high dose)

            (1) Techniques using high-dose **fentanyl (50 to 150 μg/kg) or sufentanil (10 to 30 μg/kg)** became popular in the 1980s, as they blunt almost all responses except for prolactin increase and an occasional increase in myocardial lactate production before CPB. Even in astronomical doses such as these, opioids alone do not provide sufficient depth of anesthesia to prevent hypertension and possibly tachycardia for a surgical stimulus as potent as sternal division (see above under induction techniques).

        b. Inhalational anesthetics

            (1) Minimum alveolar concentration (MAC) BAR is defined as the inhalational anesthetic partial pressure that blocks adrenergic response (BAR) in 50% of patients

                (a) MAC BAR is approximately equal to 1.5 MAC.

                (b) Cortisol and growth hormone (GH) levels will increase with the depth of anesthesia.

TABLE 6.4 Stress response—mediators and systemic response

Humoral mediators	End-organ responses
Adrenocorticotropic hormone (ACTH) ↑ Cortisol ↑	Blood glucose ↑
Catecholamines ↑	Hypertension Tachycardia Dysrhythmias Myocardial O_2 demand ↑ Cerebral metabolic rate ↑ Bronchodilation and dead space ↑ Lactate levels ↑
Insulin (inappropriate ↓ for glucose level) Glucagon ↑	Blood glucose ↑ Inotropy ↑ Fatty acids ↑
Growth hormone (GH) ↑	Protein synthesis ↑
Antidiuretic hormone (ADH) ↑ Renin ↑	Blood volume (preload) ↑ SVR (afterload) ↑ Urine output ↓ Plasma K^+ ↓ Plasma Na^+ ↑ Renal blood flow ↓ Aldosterone ↑
Prolactin ↑ Endorphins ↑	MAC ↓

MAC, minimum alveolar concentration; SVR, systemic vascular resistance.

    (c) To reduce catecholamine responses in 95% of patients, 2 MAC is needed.

    (d) MAC BAR is associated with decreased BP, myocardial depression, and increased pulmonary capillary wedge pressure (PCWP).

  c. Systemic medications that decrease catecholamine effects:

    (1) β-Adrenergic blockers

      (a) β-Blockers attenuate increases in HR and myocardial O_2 demand.

      (b) Adverse effects include decreased myocardial contractility and bronchospasm.

  d. Centrally acting α_2-adrenergic agonists (clonidine, dexmedetomidine) [23]

    (1) Both agents decrease peripheral efferent sympathetic activity.

    (2) They cause a decrease in all catecholamine levels (reduced norepinephrine levels are most prominent) and enhance cardiovascular stability.

    (3) They can decrease HR, BP, and SVR in the perioperative period.

    (4) Some attenuation of adrenergic response during or after CPB is seen with preoperative dosing.

    (5) They may cause bradycardia and hypotension, especially when combined with ACE inhibitors or vasodilators. Paradoxically, high doses may cause increases in PVR, hypertension, and decreases in cardiac index.

    (6) Dexmedetomidine will produce analgesia and sedation. Infusions often are used after CPB for "fast-track" anesthesia.

  e. Vasodilators

    (1) Vasodilators are used as treatment for increases in BP (usually from increased SVR), often secondary to elevated norepinephrine levels.

    (2) Adverse effects include: reflex increase in catecholamines, reflex increase in HR, and inhibition of hypoxic pulmonary vasoconstriction.

  f. Regional (epidural or subarachnoid) anesthetic techniques [24]

    (1) Local anesthetics

      (a) These drugs decrease GH, adrenocorticotropic hormone (ACTH), antidiuretic hormone (ADH), and catecholamine responses to lower abdominal procedures.

      (b) Thoracic epidural anesthesia is inconsistent in blocking the stress response to thoracic surgery, possibly due to insufficient somatic or sympathetic blockade or from unblocked afferent fibers.

      (c) Adverse effects include decreased SVR, bradycardia, decreased inotropy from sympathectomy, and risk of epidural hemorrhage after heparinization.

      (d) In elective cardiac surgery, thoracic epidural analgesia combined with general anesthesia followed by patient-controlled thoracic epidural analgesia offers no major advantage with respect to hospital length of stay, quality of recovery, or morbidity when compared with general anesthesia alone followed by patient-controlled analgesia with IV morphine [25]. Time to extubation was shorter and consumption of anesthetics was lower in the patient-controlled thoracic epidural analgesia group. Pain relief, degree of sedation, ambulation, and lung volumes were similar in both the study groups. There was a trend toward lower incidences of pneumonia and confusion in the patient-controlled thoracic epidural analgesia group, whereas lung volumes, and cardiac, renal, and neurologic outcomes were similar between the groups [25].

    (2) Narcotics

      (a) Peridural narcotics poorly block the stress response to surgery.

      (b) They provide postoperative analgesia.

K. Treatment of hemodynamic changes

Vasopressor and vasodilator treatment of any hemodynamic change ideally should involve the use of agents with a very short half-life, for the following reasons: (i) The surgical stimuli and the patient response are usually short lived (after sternotomy, the duration of hemodynamic

TABLE 6.5 Differential diagnosis of hypotension[a]
I. Hypovolemia
II. Deep anesthetic plane for level of stimulation
III. Decreased venous return
A. Mechanical compression of the heart or great vessels
B. Increased airway pressure
C. Tension pneumothorax
IV. Impaired myocardial contractility
V. Ischemia
VI. Dysrhythmia
A. Bradycardia
B. Tachycardia (decrease in diastolic filling time)
C. Dysrhythmia leading to loss of atrial contraction and its contribution to ventricular filling
VII. Decrease in SVR
VIII. Constrictive pericarditis in reoperation cases
IX. Steroid depletion with chronic steroid administration

[a]Causes of hypotension are listed in approximate order of frequency of occurrence.
SVR, systemic vascular resistance.

response is usually limited to 5 to 15 minutes). (ii) Many agents (β-blockers, calcium channel blockers, vasodilators, ACE inhibitors, and phosphodiesterase inhibitors) will affect hemodynamic parameters for longer than 15 minutes and have half-lives of several hours. Their actions could affect weaning from CPB or postoperative management. For these reasons, the use of short-acting agents (e.g., esmolol, nitroglycerin, sodium nitroprusside, clevidipine, phenylephrine, and ephedrine) should be encouraged.

1. **Hypotension**
   a. Causes
      (1) Mechanical causes must first be ruled out before pharmacologic treatment. Among these are the following:
         (a) Surgical compression of the heart
         (b) Technical problems with invasive BP measurement (kinked catheter, wrist position, and air bubbles)
         (c) Transient dysrhythmias from surgical manipulation of the heart (see below)
      (2) The most common cause of hypotension is hypovolemia (Table 6.5).
      (3) Myocardial ischemia is another potentially treatable cause of hypotension. Treatment is outlined in Figure 6.1.

2. **Hypertension**
   a. Hypertension is less common in patients with LV dysfunction than in patients with normal contractility, but it still occurs.
   b. The most likely cause of hypertension is sympathetic discharge. This is seen most often in younger patients and in those with preoperative hypertension (Table 6.6).
   c. Treatment is outlined in Figure 6.2.

3. **Sinus bradycardia**
   a. The most common cause of sinus bradycardia is vagal stimulation, which often results from the vagotonic effects of narcotics.
   b. Treatment
      (1) Treatment is indicated for the following:
         (a) Any HR decrease associated with a significant decrease in BP.
         (b) HR less than 40 beats/min, even without decrease in BP, if it is associated with a junctional or ventricular escape rhythm.
      (2) The underlying cause should be treated.
      (3) Atropine, 0.2 to 0.4 mg IV, can cause an unpredictable response. Emergency bradycardia treatment dose is 0.4 to 1.0 mg.

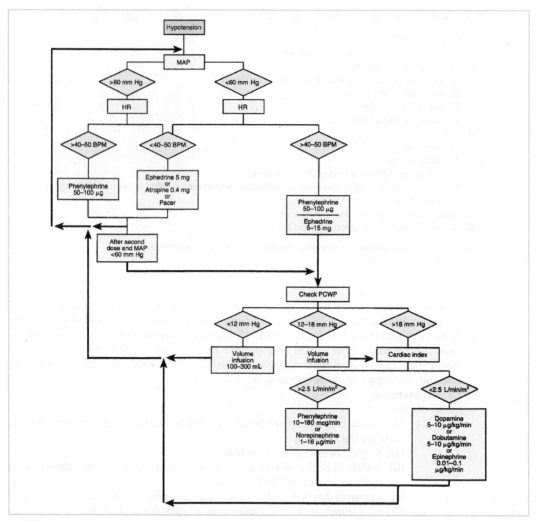

FIGURE 6.1 Treatment of hypotension in the prebypass period. Once hypotension is identified: (i) supply 100% O_2; (ii) check end-tidal carbon dioxide level (ETCO$_2$) and blood gas; (iii) decrease inhalation agent concentration; (iv) rule out dysrhythmias and technical or mechanical factors, and then treat per algorithm. Algorithm presumes presence of PCWP, for which either pulmonary artery (PA) diastolic pressure (same values assuming absence of elevated pulmonary vascular resistance [PVR]) or central venous pressure (CVP) (decrease values 2 to 4 mm Hg). HR, heart rate; MAP, mean arterial pressure; PCWP, pulmonary capillary wedge pressure (also called pulmonary artery occlusion pressure or PAOP); BPM, beats per minute.

    (a) It may cause uncontrolled tachycardia and ischemia.
    (b) It can be ineffective, but it is still indicated in the emergency treatment of bradycardia.
    (c) Glycopyrrolate (0.1 to 0.2 mg IV), another vagolytic agent, may induce less increase in HR, but it is unpredictable and has a longer half-life than atropine.
  (4) Pancuronium, 2 to 4 mg IV, is often effective owing to its sympathomimetic activity, but it can be unpredictable.
  (5) Ephedrine, 2.5 to 25 mg IV, is indicated if bradycardia is associated with hypotension. The response may be unpredictable.
  (6) PACs with pacing capabilities and esophageal atrial pacing may provide safe and predictable, although expensive, means of increasing the HR.

TABLE 6.6   Differential diagnosis of hypertension[a]

I.	Light anesthesia (increased narcotic requirements are noted in patients with chronic tobacco, alcohol, or caffeine use)
II.	Dissection of sympathetic nerves from the aorta in preparation for aortic cannulation
III.	Hypoxia
IV.	Hypercapnia
V.	Hypervolemia
VI.	Withdrawal syndromes
	A. β-Blockers
	B. Clonidine
	C. Alcohol
VII.	Thyroid storm
VIII.	Malignant hyperpyrexia
IX.	Pheochromocytoma

(Items V–IX bracketed as) Rare

[a]Causes of hypertension are listed in approximate order of frequency of occurrence.

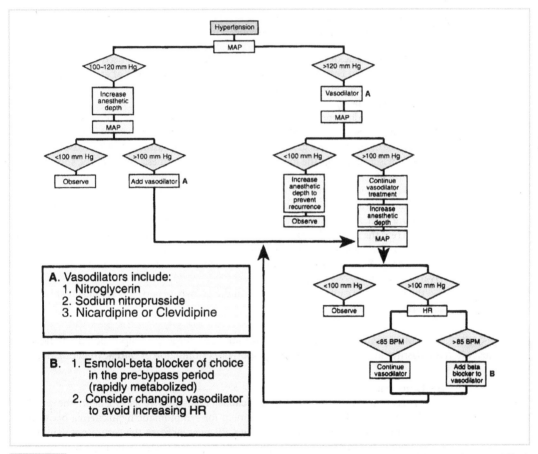

FIGURE 6.2 Treatment of hypertension in the prebypass period. First, rule out technical problems and airway difficulties. HR, heart rate; MAP, mean arterial pressure.

TABLE 6.7   Common causes of dysrhythmias[a]

   I. Mechanical stimulation of the heart (e.g., placement of purse-string sutures, cannulation, vent placement, and lifting the heart to study coronary anatomy)
  II. Pre-existing dysrhythmias
 III. Increase in catecholamine levels
     A. Light anesthesia
     B. Hypercapnia
     C. Nitrous oxide
  IV. Direct and indirect autonomic stimulants
     A. Pancuronium (now seldom used)
     B. Inotropic agents
     C. Aminophylline preparations (seldom used)
     D. β-Agonists
     E. Monoamine oxidase inhibitors and tricyclic antidepressants (rare)
   V. Electrolyte abnormalities including hypokalemia
  VI. Hypertension
 VII. Hypotension
VIII. Ischemia[b]
  IX. Hypoxemia

[a]Causes of dysrhythmias are listed in approximate order of frequency of occurrence.
[b]More frequent in patients with severe coronary disease.

---

        (7) Extrathoracic or direct epicardial ventricular pacing can be used for life-threatening bradycardia. For minimally invasive procedures, placement of external patches may be needed to provide pacing.

4. Sinus tachycardia

    a. Sinus tachycardia appears to be the most significant risk factor for intraoperative myocardial ischemia. Sinus tachycardia greater than 100 beats/min has been associated with a 40% incidence of ischemia. HR greater than 110 beats/min was associated with a 32% to 63% incidence of ischemia [26]. The most likely cause is light anesthesia (sympathetic stimulation).

    b. Treatment

        (1) Rule out ventilation abnormalities and correct them if present.

        (2) Increase anesthetic depth if other signs of light anesthesia or BIS monitor changes are seen. An empiric small dose of narcotic is often used.

        (3) Treat the underlying cause.

            (a) Give volume infusion if low preload is evident.

            (b) β-Blockade with esmolol can be used, particularly if ischemia is noted.

5. Dysrhythmias

    a. The most likely cause of dysrhythmia in the prebypass period is surgical manipulation of the heart (Table 6.7).

CLINICAL PEARL   Most prebypass dysrhythmias are caused by surgical manipulation of the heart, and most often the dysrhythmia ceases immediately upon discontinuation of cardiac manipulation.

---

    b. Treatment

        (1) Treatment of the underlying cause. Potassium replacement in the pre-CPB period should be limited to treatment for symptomatic hypokalemia because the cardioplegic solution used during CPB may increase the serum potassium level significantly. Magnesium replacement has been useful in patients who have dysrhythmias and are hypomagnesemic.

        (2) Dysrhythmias causing minor hemodynamic disturbances

            (a) Supraventricular tachycardia (including acute atrial fibrillation or flutter): Stop mechanical irritation or use vagal maneuvers, adenosine, calcium channel blockers, β-blockers (typically esmolol), phenylephrine, or edrophonium (often not available in the United States).

        (b) Premature ventricular contractions (PVCs) are mostly benign: Stop mechanical irritation.

        (c) Antiarrhythmics do not reduce PVCs caused by mechanical irritation.

        (d) If not from mechanical irritation, they can be treated with lidocaine, procainamide, β-blockers, and/or amiodarone, but this is seldom necessary in the absence of runs of ventricular tachycardia.

    (3) Dysrhythmias causing severe hemodynamic compromise

        (a) Cardioversion or defibrillation for atrial dysrhythmias, ventricular tachycardia, or ventricular fibrillation

            (i) Internal cardioversion:

                (a) Internal paddles are applied directly to the heart when the chest is open.

                (b) Low-energy levels (10 to 25 J) are needed for cardioversion (skin and chest wall impedance are bypassed).

                (c) Synchronization capabilities are desirable for atrial dysrhythmias and ventricular tachycardia. This may require additional cables or equipment to transmit ECG signal to defibrillator.

                (d) Defibrillation requires similar energy levels in a nonsynchronized mode.

            (ii) External cardioversion

                (a) Usual paddle size is used with the chest closed.

                (b) Energy levels of 50 to 300 J are needed.

                (c) Sterile external paddles are desirable if defibrillation pads were not placed prior to incision and excluded from the sterile surgical skin preparation area.

L. Preparation for cardiopulmonary bypass

  1. Anticoagulation with heparin [27]

    Unfractionated heparin is the preferred agent for anticoagulation. It is a water-soluble mucopolysaccharide with an average molecular weight of 15,000 Da.

    a. Mechanism of action: Binds to antithrombin III (AT III), a protease inhibitor, and increases the speed of the reaction between AT III and several activated clotting factors (II, IX, X, XI, XII, XIII).

    b. Onset time: Less than 1 minute if cardiac output is normal.

    c. Half-life: Approximately 2.5 hours at usual cardiac surgery dose.

    d. Metabolism: Approximately 50% by liver (heparinase) or reticuloendothelial system, approximately 50% unchanged by renal elimination.

    e. Potency of different preparations may differ markedly.

      (1) Potency is measured in units (not milligrams).

      (2) Heparin solutions usually contain 100 to 140 units/mg, depending on the lot or manufacturer.

    f. Dosage

      (1) The initial dosage of heparin for anticoagulation before CPB is 300 to 400 units/kg. This initial dose has been established by many investigators. However, some patients may remain inadequately anticoagulated using this dose, so adequate anticoagulation must be established on an individual basis according to the ACT (see Chapter 21).

      (2) Some institutions use a heparin dose–response titration to establish an initial dose.

    g. Routes of administration. Heparin must be administered directly into a central vein or into the right atrium, with documentation that heparin is being administered into the intravascular space (aspiration to confirm blood return, adequate ACT level).

  2. Cannulation (Fig. 6.3)

    a. A pericardial sling is created before cannulation to increase working space and to provide a dam for external cooling fluid and ice slush solution. The sling may lift the heart, which can decrease venous return and lead to hypotension.

    b. Purse-string sutures are used to keep the aortic and venous cannulae in place during surgery and to close the incisions after decannulation.

    c. If in use, nitrous oxide is discontinued to avoid enlargement of air emboli.

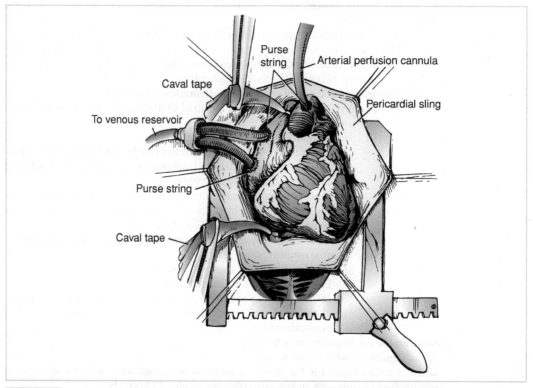

FIGURE 6.3 View of an open chest with formation of a pericardial sling (see text). Note arterial and venous cannulation sites. Caval tapes, placed around the superior and inferior vena cava, are tightened to institute complete cardiopulmonary bypass (CPB).

  d. Heparin is **always** given before cannulation.
  e. The aortic cannula is ideally inserted first to allow infusion of volume in case of hemorrhage associated with venous cannulation. Systolic BP should be decreased to 90 to 100 mm Hg to reduce the risk of aortic dissection and to facilitate cannulation. If necessary, emergency CPB can be instituted using cardiotomy suckers to deliver venous return (the so-called "sucker bypass").
  f. The surgical and anesthesia teams both should check the aortic cannula for air bubbles as it is filled with saline and connected to CPB tubing. A test transfusion of 100 mL should be performed to ensure proper placement and functioning of the cannula.
  g. If you request an infusion of volume before CPB, make sure the surgical team or the perfusionist does not have any clamps on the tubing.
  h. PEEP may be applied to increase intracardiac pressures to avoid air entrainment during cannulation of the right atrium.
  i. Complications of aortic cannulation
   (1) Embolic phenomena from air or atherosclerotic plaque dislodgment can occur. Epiaortic echocardiography is sometimes used to identify intimal plaque and to find a "safe" location for the cannula.
   (2) Hypotension
    (a) Hypotension is usually secondary to hypovolemia (blood loss).
    (b) It may result from mechanical compression of the heart.
    (c) A partial occlusion clamp used for cannulation may narrow the aortic lumen (more common in children). Check the aortic pressure immediately when the clamp is applied.
   (3) Dysrhythmias (uncommon) are most likely due to surgical manipulation.

(4) Aortic dissection can occur due to cannula misplacement. A pulsatile pressure from the aortic cannula that correlates with the radial mean arterial BP effectively rules out dissection, as can TEE.

(5) Bleeding

   (a) Minor bleeding is not uncommon with cannulation.

   (b) Major bleeding may occur if the aorta is torn.

   (c) Treatment consists of infusion of volume as needed or initiation of CPB.

(6) Rarely, air entrainment around the cannula occurs, with resultant systemic embolization.

j. Complications of venous cannulation

   (1) Hypotension

      (a) Venous cannulation may temporarily impair venous return to cause reduced cardiac output and hypotension. If a venous cannula is sufficiently large that it occludes a vena cava, then the most reasonable option to treat hypotension may be to initiate CPB.

      (b) If hypotension is due to hypovolemia, give volume in 100-mL increments for adults and 10 to 25 mL for pediatric patients through the aortic line as needed.

      (c) Mechanical compression of the heart may cause hypotension, especially during inferior vena caval cannulation.

   (2) Bleeding

      (a) Bleeding can occur from a tear of the right atrium or the superior or inferior vena cava.

      (b) Treatment is accomplished by infusing volume or initiating emergency CPB.

   (3) Dysrhythmias

      (a) Dysrhythmias usually result from surgical manipulation.

      (b) No treatment is required if they do not cause hemodynamic deterioration.

      (c) Cessation or limitation of mechanical stimulation may be all that is necessary.

   (4) Air entrainment from around the cannula with subsequent signs of pulmonary embolization is possible.

3. Autologous blood removal

a. Sequestration of platelets and clotting factors. Autologous blood may be removed to sequester platelets and clotting factors from damage during CPB, with return at the conclusion of CPB. Some practitioners believe this practice enhances coagulation after CPB and decreases the need for transfusion of homologous blood and blood products during this period. However, there is controversy about the benefits of this procedure. Sequestration of platelets and clotting factors can be accomplished in a variety of ways.

   (1) Techniques

      (a) Blood, 500 to 1,000 mL, can be withdrawn in the pre-CPB period and stored in a citrate phosphate dextrose (CPD) solution, similar to banked blood.

      (b) Before initiation of bypass, 500 to 1,000 mL of heparinized blood can be removed from the venous bypass drainage line and saved for later infusion.

      (c) Plateletpheresis cell salvage equipment can be used in the prebypass period to remove blood, if necessary, from a central venous catheter. After centrifugation, the red cells are returned to maintain hemoglobin levels and O_2 transport. The platelet-poor fraction may be returned to maintain intravascular volume or reserved along with the platelet-rich fraction for later infusion after bypass.

   (2) Risks

      (a) Hypotension from hypovolemia. Treat with vasopressors and decrease the withdrawal rate while increasing the infusion rate.

      (b) Decreased O_2-carrying capacity, as evidenced by decreased mixed venous oxygenation saturation. Treat with 100% Fio_2, halt blood removal, return red cells as needed, and begin CPB as soon as possible.

      (c) Infection. Maintain sterile technique for removal and return of blood.

(3) Relative contraindications

    (a) Left main coronary disease or equivalent

    (b) LV dysfunction

    (c) Anemia with hemoglobin less than 12 g/dL

    (d) Emergent surgery

ACKNOWLEDGMENT

The authors gratefully acknowledge the contributions of Michael Howie, M.B.Ch.B., to previous versions of this chapter. His vast clinical experience and knowledge of pharmacology form essential foundations for this chapter.

REFERENCES

1. Sun J-Z, Cao L-H, Liu H. ACE inhibitors in cardiac surgery: Current studies and controversies. *Hypertension Res.* 2011;34:15–22.
2. **Mittnacht AJC, Reich DL, Sander M, Kaplan JA. Monitoring of the heart and vascular system. In: Kaplan JA, et al., eds. *Cardiac Anesthesia*. 7th ed. Philadelphia, PA: Elsevier; 2017:390–426.**
3. **Harrison NL, Sear JW. Barbiturates, etomidate, propofol, ketamine, and steroids. In: Evers AS, Maze M, eds. *Anesthetic Pharmacology: Physiologic Principles and Clinical Practice*. Philadelphia, PA: Churchill Livingstone; 2004:395–416.**
4. Billard V, Moulla F, Bourgain JL, et al. Hemodynamic response to induction and intubation: Propofol/fentanyl interaction. *Anesthesiology.* 1994;81:1384–1393.
5. **Murphy GS, Szokil JW, Marymont JH, et al. Morphine-based cardiac anesthesia provides superior early recovery compared with fentanyl in elective cardiac surgery patients. *Anesth Analg.* 2009;109:311–319.**
6. Bovill JG. Opioids. In: Bovill JG, Howie MB, eds. *Clinical Pharmacology for Anaesthetists.* London: WB Saunders; 1999:87–102.
7. Morel J, Salard M, Castelain C, et al. Hemodynamic consequences of etomidate administration in elective cardiac surgery: A randomized double blinded study. *Br J Anesth.* 2011;107(4):503–509.
8. Schuttler J, Zsigmond EK, White PF. Ketamine and its isomers. In: White PF, ed. *Textbook of Intravenous Anesthesia.* Philadelphia, PA: Williams & Wilkins; 1997:171–188.
9. **Pagel PS, Warltier DC. Anesthetics and left ventricular function. In: Warltier DC, ed. *Ventricular Function, a Society of Cardiovascular Anesthesiologists Monograph*. Baltimore, MD: Williams & Wilkins; 1995:213–252.**
10. O'Connor JP, Ramsey JG, Wynands JE, et al. The incidence of myocardial ischemia during anesthesia for coronary artery bypass surgery in patients receiving pancuronium or vecuronium. *Anesthesiology.* 1989;70:230–236.
11. **Sharma AD, Parmley CL, Sreeram G, et al. Peripheral nerve injuries during cardiac surgery: Risk factors, diagnosis, prognosis, and prevention. *Anesth Analg.* 2000;91:1358–1369.**
12. Gandhi GY, Nuttall GA, Abel MD, et al. Intraoperative hyperglycemia and perioperative outcomes in cardiac surgery patients. *Mayo Clin Proc.* 2005;80:862–866.
13. Edwards FH, Engelman RM, Houck P, et al. The Society of Thoracic Surgeons Practice Guideline Series: Antibiotic prophylaxis in cardiac surgery, part I: Duration. *Ann Thorac Surg.* 2006;81:397–404.
14. **Engelman R, Shahian D, Shemin R, et al. The Society of Thoracic Surgeons Practice Guideline Series: Antibiotic prophylaxis in cardiac surgery, part II: Antibiotic choice. *Ann Thorac Surg.* 2007;83:1569–1576.**
15. Fergusson DA, Hebert PC, Mazer CD, et al. A comparison of aprotinin and lysine analogues in high-risk cardiac surgery. *N Engl J Med.* 2008;358:2319–2331.
16. Martin K, Knorr J, Breuer T, et al. Seizures after open heart surgery: Comparison of ε-aminocaproic acid and tranexamic acid. *J Cardiothorac Vasc Anesth.* 2011;25:20–25.
17. Perrault LP, Kollpainter R, Page R, et al. Techniques, complications, and pitfalls of endoscopic saphenectomy for coronary artery bypass grafting. *J Card Surg.* 2005;20:393–402.
18. Aronson S, Blumenthal R. Perioperative renal dysfunction and cardiovascular anesthesia: Concerns and controversies. *J Cardiothorac Vasc Anesth.* 1998;12:567–586.
19. Bovill JG, Sebel PS, Stanley TH. Opioid analgesics in anesthesia: With special reference to their use in cardiovascular anesthesia. *Anesthesiology.* 1984;61:731–755.
20. Leslie K, Myles PS, Chan MT, et al. Nitrous oxide and long-term morbidity and mortality in the ENIGMA trial. *Anesth Analg.* 2011;112:387–393.
21. Sabik JF 3rd, Blackstone EH, Houghtaling PL, et al. Is reoperation still a risk factor in coronary artery bypass surgery? *Ann Thorac Surg.* 2005;80:1719–1727.
22. Bates ER. Ischemic complications after percutaneous transluminal coronary angioplasty. *Am J Med.* 2000;108:309–316.
23. Kamibayashi T, Maze M. Clinical uses of [alpha]2-adrenergic agonists. *Anesthesiology.* 2000;93:1345–1349.
24. Liu S, Carpenter RL, Neal JM. Epidural anesthesia and analgesia: Their role in postoperative outcome. *Anesthesiology.* 1995;82:1474–1506.
25. Hansdottir V, Philip J, Olsen MF, et al. Thoracic epidural versus intravenous patient-controlled analgesia after cardiac surgery: A randomized controlled trial on length of hospital stay and patient-perceived quality of recovery. *Anesthesiology.* 2006;104:142–151.
26. **Slogoff S, Keats AS. Randomized trial of primary anesthetic agents on outcome of coronary artery bypass operations. *Anesthesiology.* 1989;70:179–188.**
27. Despotis GJ, Gravlee G, Kriton F, et al. Anticoagulation monitoring during cardiac surgery: A review of current and emerging techniques. *Anesthesiology.* 1999;91:1122–1129.

7

Management of Cardiopulmonary Bypass

Neville M. Gibbs, Shannon J. Matzelle, and David R. Larach

1. Prior to cannulation for cardiopulmonary bypass (CPB), the anesthesiologist must ensure that adequate anticoagulation has been achieved. This is typically achieved by heparin administration and confirmed by an activated clotting time (ACT) >400 seconds.

2. After commencement of CPB, once a target perfusion flow rate has been confirmed (e.g., full flow) with adequate oxygenation, the anesthesiologist should discontinue mechanical ventilation and commence monitoring of CPB variables.

3. Cardioplegic solutions have a variety of "recipes." In most cases, a cold hyperkalemic crystalloid solution is used, either alone or in combination with blood. Cardioplegia can be administered antegrade (via coronary arteries) or retrograde (via coronary sinus).

4. Anesthesia during CPB can be maintained with various combinations of volatile agents, opioids, and hypnotic agents. Anesthetic requirements are reduced during hypothermia. Maintaining neuromuscular blockade is important in order to avoid spontaneous breathing and visible or subclinical shivering.

5. Appropriate perfusion flows and pressures during CPB are controversial, but for most patients, a normothermic perfusion index (equivalent to a cardiac index) of 2.2 to 2.4 L/min/m^2 and mean arterial pressure (MAP) of 50 to 70 mm Hg suffice. Continuous monitoring of mixed venous oxygen saturation (MvO$_2$) is a guide to the adequacy of perfusion but must be supplemented by other indices, including arterial blood gas measurements to ensure optimal flows to all organs.

6. Moderate hemodilution is useful during CPB and aided by clear CPB circuit priming solutions. Minimum safe hemoglobin (Hb) concentrations during CPB are controversial and must be discussed pre-CPB. For most patients, a Hb ≥6.5 g/dL (hematocrit [Hct] ≥20%) is safe in the absence of evidence for inadequate oxygen delivery (e.g., metabolic acidosis, low MvO$_2$).

7. Hypothermia is commonly used during CPB to reduce oxygen consumption and metabolism and to confer organ protection. Often temperatures of 32° to 34°C are used in combination with alpha-stat arterial blood gas management. Rewarming should be accomplished slowly and should not proceed beyond a core temperature of 37°C.

8. During cardioplegic arrest, the anesthesiologist monitors the adequacy of left ventricular (LV) emptying via direct observation of the heart, the presence of low cardiac filling pressures, and the absence of all electrical activity on the ECG.

9. Organ protection should be promoted, especially of the brain, but also of the kidneys, lungs, and gut, by ensuring adequate oxygen delivery (e.g., flows, Hct) and perfusion pressures (arterial–venous), as well as by measures to minimize the inflammatory response to CPB.

10. CPB may be associated with catastrophic events such as aortic dissection, aortic or venous cannula malposition, venous obstruction from air lock, massive air embolism, circuit disruption, pump or oxygenator failure, and blood clots in the extracorporeal circuit. A high level of expertise and vigilance is required with mandatory safety precautions and checks.

11. Minimally invasive cardiac procedures typically require additional instrumentation and monitoring for CPB due to the limited surgical exposure, with the use of transesophageal echocardiography (TEE) to guide venous and other cannula placement and lung management to optimize surgical access.

12. Several rare conditions such as sickle cell disease, cold agglutinin disease, malignant hyperthermia (MH), and angioedema have implications for CPB and may require additional interventions or CPB modifications.

I. Preparations for cardiopulmonary bypass (CPB)

This requires close communication and coordination between surgeon, perfusionist, and anesthesiologist.

A. Assembling and checking the CPB circuit

The perfusionist assembles the CPB circuit (Fig. 7.1) before commencement of surgery, so that CPB can be instituted rapidly if necessary. The circuit components (e.g., pump [roller or

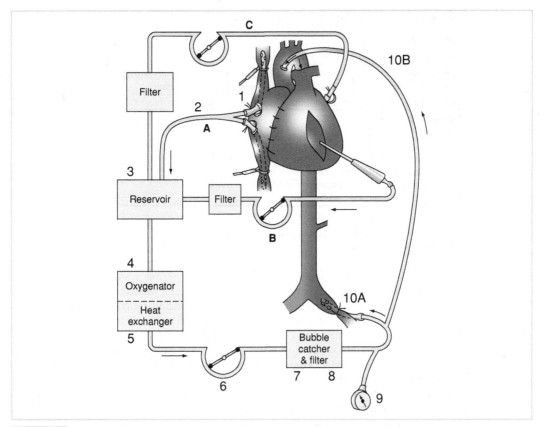

FIGURE 7.1 CPB circuit (example). Blood drains by gravity (or with vacuum assistance) (**A**) from venae cavae (**1**) through venous cannula (**2**) into venous reservoir (**3**). Blood from surgical field suction and from vent is pumped (**B, C**) into cardiotomy reservoir (not shown) and then drains into venous reservoir (**3**). Venous blood is oxygenated (**4**), temperature adjusted (**5**), raised to arterial pressure (**6**), filtered (**7, 8**), and injected into either aorta (**10B**) or femoral artery (**10A**). Arterial line pressure is monitored (**9**). Note that items **3, 4,** and **5** often are single integral units. CPB, cardiopulmonary bypass. (Modified from Nose Y. *The Oxygenator*. St. Louis, MO: Mosby; 1973:53.)

centrifugal], tubing [e.g., standard or heparin-bonded], reservoir [venous and possibly arterial], oxygenator, filters, and safety monitors) are decided by institutional preference and should comply with guidelines of professional organizations. Similarly, the type and volume of CPB prime are decided by the perfusionist, in consultation with surgeon and anesthesiologist. The perfusionist checks all components using an approved checklist. See Chapter 20 for details on CPB circuit design and use.

B. Anesthesiologist's pre-CPB checklist (Table 7.1)

A separate pre-CPB checklist is undertaken by the anesthesiologist (Table 7.1). This includes ensuring that anticoagulation is sufficient for cannulation and CPB (e.g., activated clotting time [**ACT**] **>400 seconds)**, adequate anesthesia will be provided during CPB, fluid infusions are ceased, and monitors are withdrawn to safe positions for CPB (e.g., Swan–Ganz catheter, if present, is withdrawn into the proximal pulmonary artery [PA] and a transesophageal echocardiography [TEE] probe, if present, is returned to a neutral [unflexed] position). The urinary catheter drainage bag should be emptied, and the patient's face and pupils should be checked so that any changes as a result of CPB can be recognized. If cerebral oximetry is used, the pre-CPB values should be recorded.

C. Management of arterial and venous cannulation

Prior to cannulation, adequate anticoagulation must be confirmed, and nitrous oxide, if used, must be ceased (to avoid the expansion of any air bubbles inadvertently introduced during

TABLE 7.1   Prebypass checklist
Anticoagulation—ACT >400 sec
Anesthesia—Continuous delivery ensured; nitrous oxide ceased
Cannulation—Ensure appropriate arterial line pressure and pulsatility and absence of arterial air bubbles; check cannula position with TEE where necessary
Infusions—Review drug infusions and cease fluid infusions
Monitoring Withdraw PA catheter into main PA Return TEE probe to neutral position Check correct "zero" of pressure transducers Ensure optimally placed core temperature measurement Record pre-CPB cerebral oximetry measurements (if used) Urinary catheter drainage bag emptied
Hemodilution: Discuss safe limits and transfusion trigger

ACT, activated clotting time; TEE, transesophageal echocardiography; PA, pulmonary artery; CPB, cardiopulmonary bypass.

cannulation). The anesthesiologist typically reduces the systemic systolic blood pressure to about 80 to 100 mm Hg to reduce the risk of arterial dissection while the cannula is placed. In most cases, the arterial cannulation site will be the distal ascending aorta. If so, this site should be checked for at-risk atherosclerotic plaques (mobile or >3 mm thickness) by TEE or epiaortic scanning. The perfusionist then checks that the pressure trace through the arterial cannula matches the systemic blood pressure trace (mean arterial pressure [MAP] and pulsatility). This ensures that the **arterial cannula has been placed within the aortic lumen**. Depending on the type of aortic cannula, it may be possible to check the correct position of the tip using TEE. Once the aortic cannula is in place and its correct position has been checked (and adequate anticoagulation has been confirmed), it is possible to transfuse fluid from the CPB circuit to treat transient hypotension. If a two-stage venous cannula is selected, the surgeon then inserts the venous cannula into the right atrium and guides the distal stage of the cannula into the inferior vena cava (IVC). If retrograde cardioplegia is planned, a separate smaller cannula is guided via the right atrium into the coronary sinus, which can also be checked using TEE. Femoral or arterial cannulation may be used if access to the distal ascending aorta is limited: The axillary approach avoids retrograde flow in the often atherosclerotic thoracic and abdominal aorta. The venous cannula can also be inserted peripherally through a femoral vein, if necessary, but must be advanced to the right atrium for adequate drainage. In these cases, TEE is required to confirm satisfactory venous cannula position. Management of arterial and venous cannulation for minimally invasive procedures is covered in Section VIII.

II. Commencement of CPB

A. Establishing "full flow"

Once the cannulae are in place and all other checks and observations are satisfactory, the surgeon indicates that CPB should commence. The perfusionist gradually increases the flow of oxygenated blood through the arterial cannula into the systemic circulation. At the same time, the venous clamp is gradually released, allowing an increasing proportion of systemic venous blood to drain into the CPB reservoir. Care is taken to match the arterial flow to the venous drainage. Typically, the arterial inflow is increased over about 30 to 60 seconds to provide a "normal" cardiac output (CO), based on a cardiac index of about 2.2 to 2.4 L/min/m². This is known as "full flow." At this stage, the left ventricle (LV) should have ceased to eject, and the central venous pressure (CVP) should be close to zero.

B. Initial CPB checklist (Table 7.2)

As CPB commences, the anesthesiologist should check the patient's face for asymmetry of color and the patient's pupils for asymmetry of size and can repeat the check of the arterial cannula tip position using TEE. Satisfactory oxygenator function should be confirmed by checking the color of the arterial blood, oxygen saturation monitors, and, if available, the in-line PaO_2.

TABLE 7.2 Initial cardiopulmonary bypass (CPB) checklist (see also 2-minute drill, Chapter 20)

Cannula position:
Arterial line: Pressure and pulsatility should match patient blood pressure
Face: Color and temperature should be symmetrical without plethora or edema
Eyes: Pupil sizes should be symmetrical with no conjunctival edema
Recheck with TEE if necessary

Oxygenation:
Arteriovenous color difference should be visible in pump lines
Confirm with in-line PaO_2 or SaO_2 if available; check satisfactory SvO_2

Hemodynamics:
MAP normally 30–60 mm Hg transiently
CVP <5 mm Hg
PA pressure <15 mm Hg (if used)

Heart: Should be empty, with atria and ventricles decompressed

Perfusion flow: This should increase to "full flow" (perfusion index 2.2–2.4 L/min/m²)
over 30–60 sec, with absence of cardiac ejection as the heart empties

Ventilation:
Cease ventilation when "full flow" achieved

TEE, transesophageal echocardiography; MAP, mean arterial pressure; CVP, central venous pressure; PA, pulmonary artery.

Adequate venous drainage is confirmed by the absence of pulsatility in the arterial waveform and low CVP (typically <5 mm Hg). Transient hypotension (MAP 30 to 50 mm Hg) is not uncommon following initiation of CPB, but if persistent, aortic dissection should be ruled out.

CLINICAL PEARL If there is doubt about the ability to achieve full flow or adequate oxygenation, separation from CPB should be considered, so that the cannula position and CPB equipment can be rechecked.

C. **Cessation of ventilation and lung management**
If the observations of the initial CPB checklist are satisfactory and full flow is established, ventilation of the lungs is ceased. Optimal lung management during CPB and the relative benefits of continuous positive pressure (5 to 10 cm H_2O) and lower or higher FiO_2 are not known, although the use of 100% oxygen may promote atelectasis. For some minimally invasive procedures, all positive pressure on the operative side must be avoided.

D. **Monitoring**
Patient monitoring during CPB includes continuous **ECG, MAP, CVP, core temperature (e.g., nasopharyngeal, tympanic membrane, bladder), blood temperature, and urine output.** Continuous monitoring of **venous hemoglobin (Hb) oxygen saturation** (and ideally arterial Hb oxygen saturation) is required and in-line monitoring of arterial blood gases, pH, electrolytes, and hematocrit (Hct) are recommended. Measurement errors may lead to inappropriate management with potentially disastrous consequences, so calibration and frequent checks confirming accuracy are advised. Depth of anesthesia monitoring (e.g., bispectral index, entropy) should be continued during CPB. Intermittent monitoring of **coagulation (e.g., ACT), laboratory arterial blood gases, electrolytes (including calcium, potassium, blood glucose, and lactate), and Hb** are necessary. Estimates of Hb and blood glucose can be obtained rapidly using **point-of-care devices. Cerebral oximetry** using near-infrared spectroscopy (NIRS) provides an indication of brain tissue oxygenation and is used in selected patients or for selected procedures [1] (see Sections II.E.4, IV.E.5, and VI.B).

E. **Adequacy of perfusion**
1. **Oxygen delivery** (DO_2) is the most important reason for establishing adequate perfusion ($DO_2 = CaO_2$ [blood oxygen content] × effective perfusion flow rate). The margin of error

is often reduced due to hemodilution, but oxygen utilization may also be decreased by hypothermia. Inadequate DO_2 will cause a reduction in the mixed venous O_2 saturation due to increased oxygen extraction. However, below a critical point, tissue hypoxia and lactic acidosis will also begin to occur. DO_2 can be improved by raising Hct values (by transfusion or hemoconcentration) or by increasing pump flow rates. Oxygen demand is reduced by hypothermia and muscle relaxation. Calculation of oxygen consumption may assist in ensuring that adequate oxygen is being delivered.

2. **Mixed venous oxygen saturation (MvO_2, SvO_2)** provides clues to the adequacy of oxygen delivery (DO_2) for any given oxygen demand (VO_2).

CLINICAL PEARL　The SvO_2 provides a valuable guide to the adequacy of global perfusion, but additional information is required to ensure adequate perfusion to individual organs and to exclude regional ischemia.

Normally, MvO_2 is above 75%, even at normothermia. Below this value, inadequate VO_2 should be suspected, and below 50%, tissue hypoxia is likely. Unfortunately, satisfactory MvO_2 does not exclude regional ischemia. **Thus, although a low venous oxygen saturation should always be remedied, a normal or high venous saturation does not always imply adequate perfusion to all organs.**

3. **Metabolic and lactic acidosis:** Tissue hypoxia due to inadequate DO_2 will result in metabolic acidosis, primarily due to increases in lactic acid. The reduction in pH and bicarbonate and increase in base deficit can be monitored by in-line or serial arterial blood gas measurement. An increase in lactate level suggests a metabolic cause for acidosis.

4. **Cerebral oximetry** (e.g., NIRS). In addition to its role as a monitor of the adequacy of cerebral oxygen delivery, recent studies have suggested that cerebral oximetry may be a useful surrogate to assess adequacy of total body oxygen delivery [2]. As cerebral blood flow is autoregulated more closely than other organs, decreases in cerebral oxygenation suggest that flow to other tissues is also impaired.

5. Adequacy of regional perfusion to specific organs: See Section VI.A–F.

III. **Typical CPB sequence**

A. **Typical coronary artery bypass graft (CABG) operation**

A typical CABG operation proceeds as follows. Total CPB is initiated and mild-to-moderate hypothermia is either actively induced (32° to 34°C) or permitted to occur passively (sometimes called "drifting"). The aorta is cross-clamped and cardioplegic solution is infused antegrade through the aortic root and/or retrograde cannula via the coronary sinus to arrest the heart. During antegrade cardioplegia administration, it is important to monitor for distention of the LV, and during retrograde cardioplegia infusion, it is important to monitor delivery pressures. The distal saphenous vein grafts are placed on the most severely diseased coronary arteries first, to facilitate administration of additional cardioplegic solution (via the vein graft) distal to the stenosis if necessary. The internal mammary artery anastomosis (if used) is often undertaken last because of its fragility and shorter length. Rewarming typically begins when the final distal anastomosis is started. Once the distal anastomoses are completed, the aorta is unclamped, and either an aortic side clamp is applied or an internal occlusive device is used to permit proximal vein graft anastomoses while cardioplegic solution is being washed out of the heart. In some patients, the proximal anastomoses are completed with the aortic cross clamp in place, in order to reduce instrumentation of the aorta (with the risk of dislodging atheroma). Total CPB continues until the heart is reperfused from its new blood supply. Finally, when the patient is adequately rewarmed and the coronary artery grafts are completed, the heart is defibrillated if necessary, epicardial pacing wires are placed, and separation from CPB commences.

B. **Typical aortic valve replacement (or repair) operation**

After initiation of CPB and application of the aortic cross-clamp, cardioplegia is infused as per the CABG procedure, unless the aortic valve is incompetent, in which case the aortic root is opened and cardioplegic solution is infused into both coronary artery ostia under direct vision (to prevent the cardioplegic solution entering the LV through the incompetent aortic valve instead of the coronary arteries). For this reason, cardioplegia is often administered retrograde via the coronary sinus, either instead of or in addition to antegrade cardioplegia. The valve is then either replaced or repaired. Carbon dioxide is often suffused into the thoracic cavity to displace air from open heart chambers. Rewarming commences toward the end of valve repair or replacement. The heart is irrigated to remove residual air or tissue debris, and the aortotomy is closed except for a vent. The aortic cross-clamp is removed (often with the patient in a head-down position) and the heart is defibrillated if necessary. Final deairing occurs as venous drainage to the pump is retarded, the heart fills and begins to eject (partial CPB), and residual bubbles are aspirated through the aortic vent, an LV vent, or a needle placed in the apex of the heart. During deairing, the lungs are inflated to help flush air out of pulmonary veins and the heart chambers, and TEE is viewed to monitor air evacuation and exclude residual air.

C. **Typical mitral valve replacement (or repair) operation**
This operation is similar to aortic valve surgery (see Section III.B above), except that the left atrium (or right atrium for a transatrial septal approach) is opened instead of the aorta, and the cardioplegia infusion can take place through the aortic root and the coronary sinus. If a transatrial approach is used, bicaval venous cannulation is required. The valve is replaced or repaired, and a vent tube is passed through the mitral valve into the LV to prevent ejection of blood into the aorta until deairing is completed. Before bicaval cannulation, a PA catheter, if present, should be withdrawn into the superior vena cava (SVC), and CVP measurement cephalad to the SVC cannula should be assured. If a PA catheter introducer is in place, attaching the CVP monitor to the side port of the introducer is recommended. Carbon dioxide is often suffused into the thoracic cavity to displace air from open heart chambers. After thorough irrigation of the field and closure of the atriotomy except for the LV vent, the aortic cross-clamp is removed, often with the patient in a head-down position. The heart is defibrillated, if necessary, and deairing occurs as described above. Finally, the LV vent is removed.

D. **Typical combined procedures**
For combined valve–CABG procedure, the distal vein graft anastomoses are created first to permit cardioplegia of the myocardium distal to severe coronary stenoses. Also, lifting the heart to access the posterior wall vessels can disrupt myocardium if an artificial valve has been inserted, especially in the case of mitral valve replacement. Next, the valve repair or replacement is undertaken, and the operation proceeds as described above. When combined aortic and mitral valve surgery is performed, usually the mitral valve surgery is performed first.

IV. **Maintenance of CPB**
A. **Anesthesia**
1. **Choice of agent and technique.** Just as in the pre-CPB period, anesthesia is typically provided by a **potent volatile agent** or an infusion of **intravenous (IV) anesthetic** (e.g., propofol) on a background of **opiates** (e.g., fentanyl, sufentanil) and other **sedative drugs** (e.g., benzodiazepines). Volatile agents have a more defined role in myocardial protection than other anesthetics through ischemic preconditioning and reduction of reperfusion injury [3].
2. **Potent volatile agent via pump oxygenator.** This requires a vaporizer mount in the gas inlet line to the oxygenator. A flow- and temperature-compensated vaporizer, typically containing sevoflurane or isoflurane, is then attached to the mount. The concentration of agent is typically about 1.0 MAC at normothermia but depends on the amount of supplementary opiates and sedatives and is reduced with hypothermia. With most oxygenators, uptake and elimination of the volatile agent are more rapid than through an anesthesia circuit and a patient's lungs. Volatile agent administration can be confirmed by connecting the gas analysis line from the anesthesia circuit to a side port of the oxygenator outlet during CPB [4]. If volatile agents are used, appropriate scavenging of the oxygenator outlet is required. Nitrous oxide is never used because of its propensity to enlarge gas-filled spaces, including micro and macro gas emboli.
3. **Total intravenous anesthesia.** Total intravenous anesthesia (TIVA) can be provided during CPB using a combination of opiates and sedatives, either by intermittent bolus

or by infusion. For propofol, the typical infusion rates are 3 to 6 mg/kg/hr or a target plasma concentration of 2 to 4 μg/mL, depending on the use of other IV agents and the patient's temperature. The advantages of TIVA are simplicity, less myocardial depression, and the absence of a need for oxygenator scavenging. However, as with all forms of TIVA, ensuring adequate depth is more difficult, providing greater justification for anesthesia depth monitoring (e.g., bispectral index, entropy) [5].

4. **Muscle relaxation.** Movement of the patient during CPB risks cannula dislodgement. If additional muscle relaxants are not used, adequate depth of anesthesia to prevent movement must be ensured. Similarly, spontaneous breathing must be avoided, as this risks the development of negative intravascular pressures and potential air entrainment. If spontaneous breathing occurs, adequate depth of anesthesia should be checked, and elevated $PaCO_2$, if present, should be corrected.

5. **Effect of temperature.** Anesthetic requirements fall as temperature drops. However, due to its relatively high blood supply, brain temperature changes faster than core temperature. For this reason, particular care should be taken to ensure **adequate anesthesia** as soon as **rewarming commences**, and additional opiates or sedatives may be required. When the patient is normothermic, anesthetic requirements are the same as the pre-CPB phase, although the context-sensitive half-time for most anesthetic drugs increases substantially during and after CPB.

6. **Monitoring anesthetic depth. Awareness** may be difficult to exclude clinically due to the use of high-dose opiates, cardiovascular drugs (e.g., β-adrenergic blockers), and muscle relaxants. Moreover, hemodynamic cues cannot be used during CPB. The patient should be checked for pupillary dilation and sweating, but these signs may be affected by opiate medication and rewarming. Therefore, emphasis should be placed on ensuring delivery of adequate anesthesia, preferably with the use of depth-of-anesthesia monitors [5].

7. **Altered pharmacokinetics and pharmacodynamics.** At the onset of CPB, the **circulating blood volume is increased** by the addition of the priming solution in the extracorporeal circuit, but the percentage change in the total volume of distribution of most anesthetic agents is minimal. Neuromuscular blockers are an exception; hence, supplementary doses may be required at the onset of CPB. **Hemodilution reduces the concentration of plasma proteins**, increasing the unbound active proportion of many drugs (e.g., propofol) to offset the reduced total plasma concentration induced by the increased circulating blood volume. A small proportion of some agents (e.g., fentanyl, nitroglycerin) may be **absorbed onto the foreign surfaces** of the CPB circuit. **Hypothermia** reduces the rate of drug metabolism and elimination, as does reduction in blood flow to the liver and kidneys. **Bypassing the lungs reduces pulmonary metabolism** and sequestration of certain drugs and hormones. **Reduced blood supply to vessel-poor tissues** such as muscle and fat may result in sequestration of drugs given pre-CPB. The response to drugs may also be altered by hypothermia and hemodynamic alterations associated with CPB. The combined effect of these pharmacologic changes may be difficult to predict, so the **principle of titrating drugs** to achieve a certain endpoint is particularly important during CPB.

B. **Hemodynamic management.** See also Chapter 20.

1. **Systemic perfusion flow rate.** The most fundamental hemodynamic change during CPB is the generation of the CO by the CPB pump rather than the patient's heart. The perfusionist regulates the CPB pump to deliver the desired perfusion flow rate for the patient. This is usually based on a nomogram taking into consideration the patient's height and weight and the core temperature. Typically, the perfusion flow rate is set to deliver a perfusion flow rate of **2.4 L/min/m² at 37°C and about 1.5 L/min/m² at 28°C**. The amount delivered by the CPB pump is usually set slightly higher than the target flow rate to account for any recirculation within the CPB circuit. For example, a continuous flow of about 200 mL/min from the arterial line filter may be returned to the reservoir through a purge line to provide a mechanism for purging trapped microbubbles. The **effective perfusion flow rate** is the amount delivered by the CPB pump minus the amount recirculated. An **inadequate effective perfusion flow rate** will result in a **low venous**

Hb oxygen saturation (continuously monitored in the CPB venous return) and the development of a **metabolic acidosis** due to anaerobic metabolism and the accumulation of **lactic acid**. If other causes for a low venous Hb oxygen saturation can be excluded (e.g., excessive hemodilution, inadequate anesthesia, excessive rewarming), the perfusion flow rate should be increased accordingly. Unfortunately, a normal venous oxygen saturation does not confirm adequate perfusion of all tissues. **Shunting** may occur leaving some tissue beds underperfused. An **increased metabolic rate** due to shivering, which may be subclinical during hypothermia (or much more rarely due to thyrotoxicosis or malignant hyperthermia [MH]), may also reduce venous HbO_2 saturations despite normal flow rates.

2. **MAP.** The optimum MAP during CPB is not known [6]. Systolic and diastolic pressures are generally of little concern because the vast majority of CPB is conducted using nonpulsatile flow. If an **adequate perfusion flow rate** is delivered, the actual MAP may be less important, so long as it is **above the lower limit of autoregulation**, and there is **no critical stenosis** in the arterial supply to individual organs. However, the lower limits of autoregulation vary widely between patients [7]. Therefore, in adults, a conservative approach is usually taken, maintaining the MAP between **50 and 70 mm Hg**. This assumes a CVP close to zero and should be adjusted **higher if the CVP is raised**. Higher pressures may be required in the presence of **pre-existing hypertension** or known **cerebrovascular disease**. Lower levels may be tolerated in children. The possibility of **measurement error due to inappropriate position of the pressure transducers or zero drift should be checked frequently and corrected if necessary.**

3. **Hypotension.** The most important consideration in the management of hypotension is to ensure that an **adequate effective perfusion flow rate** is being delivered. While a transient reduction of perfusion flow rate (such as may be requested by the surgeon at particular stages of the procedure) is of little consequence, sustained reductions must be avoided. Once an adequate perfusion flow rate is confirmed, the MAP may be corrected by increasing the systemic vascular resistance (SVR) with the use of vasoconstrictors such as phenylephrine (0.5 to 10 µg/kg/min or norepinephrine 0.03 to 0.3 µg/kg/min), on the basis of the following relationship:

$$SVR = (MAP - CVP)/\text{effective perfusion flow rate (L/min)}$$

where MAP is expressed in mm Hg, CVP in mm Hg, and SVR in mm Hg/L/min (to convert to dyne·s·cm^{-5}, multiply by 80). As there is substantial individual variability in response to vasoconstrictors, especially during CPB, the dose should be titrated, commencing with less potent agents (e.g., phenylephrine) or smaller doses and progressing to higher doses of more potent agents (e.g., norepinephrine), if required. Occasionally, vasopressin (e.g., 0.01 to 0.05 units/min) is required. The perfusion flow rate can be increased above normal to correct hypotension temporarily (e.g., while vasoconstrictors take effect), but this is not an appropriate strategy to correct persistent hypotension. The onset of CPB is typically associated with sudden **hemodilution**, which decreases SVR. **Cardioplegia solution** entering the circulation also reduces SVR and is a common cause of hypotension. Reperfusion of the myocardium after release of the aortic cross-clamp is another common cause of transient hypotension. For these reasons, the use of vasoconstrictors during CPB is common. Continuous infusions are preferable to intermittent boluses to avoid inadvertent periods of hypertension or "roller coaster" changes in MAP.

4. **Hypertension.** Hypertension is usually the result of an increase in SVR, which may be due to endogenous sympathetic stimulation or hypothermia. Before treating hypertension with direct vasodilators (e.g., nitroglycerin 0.1 to 10 µg/kg/min, sodium nitroprusside 0.1 to 2 µg/kg/min, nicardipine 2 to 5 mg/hr), **adequate anesthesia** should be ensured. Artifactual hypertension due to aortic cannula malposition should also be excluded (see Sections I.C and VII.A). The perfusion flow rate can be decreased below normal to correct hypertension temporarily (e.g., while vasodilators take effect), but not to correct persistent hypertension. Hypertension should be avoided during all **aortic cross-clamp manipulations**, including the application and release of side-biting clamps. Typically,

nitroglycerin is the first-line drug with more venous than arterial vasodilation. Sodium nitroprusside is more potent if nitroglycerin alone is insufficient. Nicardipine has a longer duration of action and offset.

5. **Central venous pressure.** With appropriate venous drainage, the CVP should be low (0 to 5 mm Hg). A persistently high CVP indicates poor venous drainage, which may require adjustment of the venous cannula or cannulae by the surgeon. Venous drainage can also be improved slightly by raising the operating table height, thereby increasing the hydrostatic gradient between the heart and the venous reservoir. Increasingly, in recent years, suction (vacuum-assisted venous drainage [VAVD]) is applied to the venous reservoir, especially for miniaturized circuits (see Chapter 20) or for femoral venous cannulation (see Section VIII). Excessive suction should be suspected if the CVP reading falls below −5 mm Hg. As the CVP is a low-range pressure, it is very sensitive to measurement error (e.g., hydrostatic gradient between transducer and right atrium). Care should also be taken to ensure that the catheter measuring the CVP is in a large central vein and is not snared by surgical tapes.

C. **Fluid management and hemodilution**

1. **CPB prime.** The CPB circuit is "primed" with a balanced isotonic crystalloid solution, to which colloids, mannitol, or buffers may be added, depending on perfusionist, anesthesiologist, and surgical preference (see Chapter 20). CPB prime also usually contains a small dose of heparin (e.g., 5,000 to 10,000 units). A dose of the antifibrinolytic agent being used may also be added (e.g., aminocaproic acid 5 g or tranexamic acid 1 g). The volume of the prime depends on the circuit components. It is typically about 1,400 to 2,000 mL for adults. It is lower for pediatric CPB circuits and for miniaturized CPB systems (see Chapter 20).

2. **Hemodilution.** The use of a nonsanguineous prime inevitably results in hemodilution. The degree of hemodilution on commencement of CPB can be estimated prior to CPB by multiplying the Hb concentration (or Hct) prior to CPB by the ratio of the patient's estimated blood volume to the patient's estimated blood volume *plus* the CPB prime volume. Moderate hemodilution is usually well tolerated because oxygen delivery remains adequate and oxygen requirements are often reduced during CPB, especially if hypothermia is used. Moderate hemodilution may also be beneficial because it reduces blood viscosity, which counters the increase in blood viscosity induced by hypothermia that would otherwise impede blood flow.

3. **Limits of hemodilution.** While the safe limit of hemodilution during CPB in individual patients is not known, a conservative approach is to **avoid Hb levels <6.5 g/dL (approximately an Hct of 20%)**. If the estimated degree of hemodilution on commencement of CPB is too low, allogeneic red blood cells (RBCs) can be added to the CPB prime. This is particularly important for smaller patients (due to their lower estimated blood volumes) (e.g., pediatric patients) and anemic patients. If venous oxygen saturations are low during CPB despite normal effective perfusion flow rates, excessive hemodilution as a cause should be considered and additional RBCs added if necessary. Similarly, inadequate oxygen delivery will result in anaerobic metabolism and the development of **acidosis**. Patients with **known stenoses** of cerebral or renal arteries may be **less tolerant** of hemodilution.

CLINICAL PEARL The predicted effect of CPB on the Hct, the safe limit of hemodilution, and transfusion triggers should be discussed prior to CPB.

---

4. **Time course of hemodilution.** During the course of CPB, crystalloid fluid will diffuse from the vascular to the extracellular space and also will be filtered by the kidney, gradually reducing the extent of hemodilution. However, **crystalloid cardioplegia** returning to the circulation will increase hemodilution, as will the addition of other crystalloids or colloids used to replace blood loss or redistribution of fluid into nonvascular compartments.

5. **Monitoring hemodilution.** The Hb (or Hct) should be measured at least every 30 to 60 minutes and more frequently if there is ongoing blood loss, or low mixed venous oxygen saturations. If possible, Hct should be monitored continuously.

6. **Acute normovolemic hemodilution.** In adult patients with average (or greater) body size and normal preoperative Hb, acute normovolemic hemodilution prior to, or at the time of commencement of, CPB should be considered. Typically, 1 to 2 units of anticoagulated blood are collected and replaced with colloids, crystalloids, or a combination. This blood, containing pre-CPB Hb, platelet, and clotting factor levels can be reinfused post-CPB.

7. **Allogeneic RBC transfusion trigger.** The trigger for allogeneic RBC transfusion varies between institutions and will depend on patient and surgical factors. It must take into account the balance of harmful effects of allogeneic RBC transfusion versus the harmful effects of inadequate oxygen carriage. Ideally, the transfusion trigger for the individual patient should be discussed between anesthesiologist, perfusionist, and surgeon prior to the commencement of CPB. Conservative triggers are an Hb <6.5 g/dL during the maintenance phase of CPB and <8.0 g/dL at the time of separation, although **lower levels** may be tolerated in selected patients, and **higher levels** may be required in others.

8. **Cardiotomy suction.** Shed blood may be returned to the CPB circuit using cardiotomy suction. However, shed blood often contains activated coagulation and fibrinolytic factors, especially if exposed to the pericardium. Excessive cardiotomy suction may also be associated with hemolysis, especially if there is co-aspiration of air. For this reason, some choose to return only brisk blood loss to the CPB circuit. An alternative is separate cell salvage with washing of RBCs before returning them to the CPB circuit.

9. **Fluid replacement.** Fluid may be lost from the circuit through blood loss, redistribution to other compartments, and filtration by the kidney. A reduction in the circulating blood volume will manifest as a fall in the CPB reservoir fluid level. A falling CPB reservoir fluid level is dangerous, as it reduces the margin of safety for air embolism. In many circuits, an alarm will be activated if the reservoir volume falls to unsafe levels. The replacement fluid is typically crystalloid, with colloid added depending on perfusionist, surgeon, and anesthesiologist preference.

10. **Diuresis and ultrafiltration.** Occasionally, the return of cardioplegia solution to the CPB circuit or contraction of the vascular space by vasoconstrictors or hypothermia will cause the reservoir level to increase. If high levels persist, diuresis can be encouraged by the use of diuretic agents such as furosemide or mannitol. Alternatively, an ultrafiltration device can be added to the circuit to remove water and electrolytes (see Chapter 20).

11. **Urine production** should be identified and quantified as a sign of adequate renal perfusion and to assist in appropriate fluid management. Very high urine flow rates (e.g., >300 mL/hr) may be seen during hemodilution (due to low plasma oncotic pressure), especially if mannitol is also present in the priming solution. Oliguria (less than 1 mL/kg/hr) should prompt an investigation because it may indicate inadequate renal perfusion. However, some hypothermic patients demonstrate oliguria without an apparent cause. Kinking of urinary drainage catheters may manifest as apparent oliguria, so this should be checked before initiating treatment.

D. **Management of anticoagulation** (see also Chapter 21)

1. **Monitoring anticoagulation.** The ACT or a similar rapid test of anticoagulation must periodically confirm adequate anticoagulation (e.g., ACT >400 seconds; see also Chapter 21). The ACT should be checked before and after initiating CPB and at least every 30 minutes thereafter. The ACT can be checked within 2 minutes of administering heparin [8]. As the ACT falls over time, often a higher target is chosen (e.g., >500 seconds), so that the lowest ACT remains >400 seconds. During periods of **normothermia**, heparin elimination is faster, so a requirement for heparin supplementation is more likely.

2. **Additional heparin** is usually given in 5,000- to 10,000-unit increments, and the ACT is repeated to confirm an adequate response. Use of fully heparin-coated circuits does not eliminate the need for heparin; an ACT of 400 seconds or greater is often recommended.

3. **Heparin resistance** is a term used to describe the inability to achieve adequate heparinization despite conventional doses of heparin. It may be due to a variety of causes, but it is most common in patients who have received heparin therapy for several days preoperatively. Most cases will respond to **increased doses of heparin**. However, if an ACT >400 seconds cannot be achieved despite heparin >600 units/kg, consideration should be given to administering **supplemental antithrombin III** (AT-III). A dose of 1,000 units of AT-III concentrate will increase the AT-III level in an adult by about 30%. Fresh frozen plasma, 2 to 4 units, is a less expensive alternative, but it is also less specific and carries a low risk of infectious and other complications. For a detailed discussion of heparin resistance and AT-III deficiency, see Chapter 21.

E. **Temperature management**

1. **Choice of maintenance temperature.** The optimal temperature during the maintenance phase of CPB is not known. Typically, the patient's core temperature at the onset of CPB is 35° to 36°C. Core temperature is usually measured in the **nasopharynx or tympanic membrane**, but the bladder or midesophagus may also be used. The target temperature is chosen on the basis of the type and length of surgical procedure, patient factors, and surgical preference. Often the temperature is allowed to drift lower to about 34°C without active cooling (tepid CPB). Alternatively, the heat exchanger is used to provide moderate hypothermia, which may be as low as 28°C but is more often 32°C or above. If there is a concern about the adequacy of myocardial protection, lower temperatures may be used (see also Chapter 23).

2. **Hypothermia.** Hypothermia during CPB reduces metabolic rate and oxygen requirements and provides organ protection against ischemia. However, it may promote coagulation abnormalities and may increase the risk of microbubble formation during rewarming. Hypothermia shifts the Hb oxygen saturation curve to the left, reducing peripheral oxygen delivery, but this is countered by the reduced oxygen requirements. The rewarming phase may prolong CPB duration and may also risk overheating, particularly the brain.

3. **Normothermia.** Normothermia (or mild hypothermia, >34°C) has been reported to be as safe as lower target temperatures and may improve some outcomes [9].

4. **Slow cooling.** Lack of response of the **nasopharyngeal or tympanic temperature** during the cooling phase may indicate **inadequate brain cooling** and should prompt investigation of the cause (e.g., ineffective heat exchanger, inadequate cerebral perfusion). The position and function of the temperature monitor should also be checked to exclude artifactual causes.

5. **Deep hypothermic circulatory arrest** (DHCA). For certain surgical procedures in which circulatory arrest is required (e.g., repairs of the aortic arch), deep hypothermia is used as part of a **strategy to prevent cerebral injury**. The typical target temperature prior to circulatory arrest is about 15° to 17°C, although if anterograde cerebral perfusion is planned, 22° to 24°C may suffice. Other strategies to minimize injury include limiting the period of circulatory arrest to as short a time as possible, **anterograde or retrograde cerebral perfusion** during the period of DHCA and **pharmacologic protection** using **barbiturates** (e.g., thiopental 10 mg/kg), **corticosteroids** (e.g., methylprednisolone 30 mg/kg), and **mannitol** (0.25 to 0.5 g/kg). These must be given before DHCA is commenced. Ensuring deep neuromuscular blockade prior to DHCA is advisable. Cerebral oximetry should also be used. For details of DHCA management, including monitoring, see Chapters 14 and 26.

6. **Rewarming.** Rewarming should commence early enough to ensure that the patient's core temperature has returned to 37°C by the time the surgical procedure is completed, so that separation from CPB is not delayed. The surgeon will usually advise the perfusionist when rewarming should commence, taking into account the patient's core temperature at the time, how long the patient has been at this temperature, and the patient's body size. The rate of rewarming is limited by the **maximum safe temperature gradient** between the water temperature in the heat exchanger and the blood which should be no greater than 10°C and less as normothermia is approached. Higher gradients risk the formation

of microbubbles. The arterial blood temperature should also be limited to 37°C to prevent cerebral hyperthermia [10]. Typically, patients' core temperatures rise about 0.3°C/min. Vasodilators may facilitate rewarming by improving distribution of blood and permitting higher pump flow rates.

7. **Hypothermia and arterial blood gas analysis.** Hypothermia increases the solubility of oxygen and carbon dioxide, thereby reducing their partial pressures. However, arterial blood gas measurement is performed at 37°C, so the values have to be "temperature corrected" to the patient's blood temperature if the values at the patient's blood temperature are required. The reduced PaO_2 is of limited clinical significance, so long as increased fractions of oxygen are administered ($FiO_2 >0.5$). However, the reduced $PaCO_2$ produces an apparent respiratory alkalosis when temperature-corrected values are used. To keep the pH normal **(pH stat)**, it would be necessary to add CO_2 to the oxygenator. The alternative is to avoid temperature correction of arterial blood gases on the basis that the **degree of dissociation of H^+** also varies with temperature **(alpha stat)**. With this strategy, there is no requirement to add CO_2 to maintain neutrality. These complex biochemical considerations are avoided by using **non–temperature-corrected values** and making decisions based on the values measured at 37°C, irrespective of the patient's blood temperature. See Chapter 26 for further discussion of arterial blood gas management.

8. **Shivering.** Shivering should be avoided by ensuring adequate anesthesia. Muscle relaxants will also prevent shivering.

F. **ECG management**

Isolated atrial and ventricular ectopic beats are common during cardiac manipulation and require no specific intervention. If ventricular fibrillation occurs before aortic cross-clamp placement, defibrillation may be required. Ventricular fibrillation once the aortic cross-clamp has been placed is likely to be short-lived because the delivery of cardioplegia will achieve cardiac standstill. After aortic cross-clamp, ECG complexes change shape, become less frequent, and then cease. Absence of an isoelectric ECG indicates insufficient or ineffective cardioplegia. Return of electrical activity after cardioplegic arrest suggests washout of cardioplegia solution. The surgeon should be notified, as additional cardioplegia may be required. Ventricular fibrillation may occur during the rewarming phase after the release of the aortic cross-clamp. This often resolves spontaneously but may require defibrillation, especially if the patient remains hypothermic.

G. **Myocardial protection** (see also Chapter 23)

1. **Cardioplegia.** Once the myocardial blood supply is interrupted by the placement of an aortic cross-clamp, cardioplegic arrest of the myocardium is required. The **antegrade technique** is achieved by administering cardioplegia solution into the aortic root between the aortic valve and aortic clamp. The interval between the placement of the cross-clamp and the administration of the cardioplegia is kept to a minimum (no more than a few seconds) to prevent any warm ischemia. Conventional cardioplegia solutions are high in potassium, arresting the heart in diastole. The solution is typically administered cold (8° to 12°C) to provide further protection, although warm continuous cardioplegic techniques are used in some institutions. The solution may be administered alone **(crystalloid cardioplegia)** or mixed with blood **(blood cardioplegia)**. Cardioplegia may also be administered **retrograde** through a catheter in the **coronary sinus**. In patients with aortic regurgitation, administration of cardioplegia directly into the left and right coronary ostia may be required. Cardioplegia is typically given intermittently every 20 to 30 minutes but may be given continuously by infusion. An alternative novel low-sodium crystalloid cardioplegic solution (Custodiol HTK, Franz Kohler Chemie GmbH, Benshein, Germany), which lasts up to 3 hours, is often used for minimally invasive and other complex cardiac procedures because it typically involves less disruption for repeated intermittent cardioplegia administration [11].

2. **Cold.** Most myocardial protection techniques involve cold cardioplegia, and ice may be placed around the heart to provide further protection. Systemic hypothermia, if used, contributes to keeping the myocardium cold.

3. **Venting.** During cross-clamping, vents are typically placed in the aortic root to ensure that the heart does not distend. For open-chamber procedures, vents are placed also in the left atrium or LV to remove both blood and air. Inadequate venting may result in the **development of tension** in the LV, causing potential **subendocardial ischemia.** The coronary perfusion pressure for cardioplegia is also reduced.

4. **Avoiding electrical activity.** See Section IV.F above.

H. **Arterial blood gas and acid–base management**

1. **Alpha stat or pH stat strategy?** (see Section IV.E.7 and Chapter 26)

2. The **arterial PO_2** is typically maintained between **150 and 300 mm Hg** by adjusting the percentage oxygen in the sweep (analogous to inspired) gas delivered to the oxygenator. **Arterial hypoxemia** may indicate **inadequate oxygenator sweep gas flow** (or leak) or **inadequate oxygen percentage** in the oxygenator sweep gas. Alternatively, it may indicate **oxygenator dysfunction.**

3. The **arterial PCO_2** is maintained at approximately **40 mm Hg** by adjusting the sweep gas flow rate through the oxygenator. There is an inverse relationship between the sweep gas flow rate and the arterial PCO_2. **Hypercapnea** ($PaCO_2$ >45 mm Hg) should be avoided as it is associated with sympathetic stimulation and **respiratory acidosis.** Hypercapnea may be caused by an inadequate sweep gas flow rate, absorption of CO_2 used to flood the chest cavity during open chamber procedures [12], or increased CO_2 production. Administration of bicarbonate also increases the $PaCO_2$. **Hypocapnea** ($PaCO_2$ <35 mm Hg) should also be avoided, as it is associated with **respiratory alkalosis and left shift of the HbO_2 dissociation curve** (further reducing oxygen delivery) and **cerebral vasoconstriction.**

4. **Metabolic acidosis** (e.g., lactic acidosis) is prevented where possible by ensuring adequate oxygen delivery and tissue perfusion. Severe metabolic acidosis should be corrected cautiously with the use of sodium bicarbonate. If unexplained acidosis occurs with signs of an increased metabolic rate (e.g., low mixed venous oxygen saturations, elevated $PaCO_2$), MH should be considered.

I. **Management of serum electrolytes**

1. **Hyperkalemia** may occur when cardioplegia solution (which contains high potassium concentrations) enters the circulation. This is usually mild or transient unless **large amounts of cardioplegia** are used or the patient has **renal dysfunction.** Hyperkalemia more often follows the first dose of cardioplegia than later ones because both the volume and potassium concentration are typically higher for the initial administration. Hyperkalemia can cause **heart block, negative inotropy,** and **arrhythmias.** Hyperkalemia can be treated by promoting potassium elimination by loop diuretics (e.g., **furosemide**) or by **ultrafiltration.** Potassium can also be shifted into cells by the administration of **insulin and glucose** or by creating an **alkalosis.** A **normal ionized calcium** level should also be ensured. In rare cases, **hemodialysis** is required. If the patient has severe renal dysfunction or the serum potassium remains above the normal range, the cardioplegia delivery technique should be modified to ensure that cardioplegia is vented separately and not returned to the circulation.

2. **Hypokalemia.** If a patient is hypokalemic, initiating K^+ replacement during CPB is much safer than waiting until after bypass, thus avoiding hypokalemic dysrhythmias during CPB weaning or potential cardiac arrest during rapid K^+ replacement post-CPB.

3. **Sodium.** Serum sodium should be maintained within the normal range where possible. Rapid corrections should be avoided due to the risk of acute changes in **intracranial pressure** as a result of the changes in **plasma osmolality.** The use of low-sodium cardioplegic solutions (e.g., custodial HTK) is associated with hyponatremia, but hypo-osmolality is avoided by the presence of other osmotically active particles [11].

4. **Ionized calcium** levels should be maintained within the normal range.

J. **Management of blood glucose**

1. **Hyperglycemia.** Glucose tolerance is often impaired during CPB due to the stress response associated with CPB, as well as from insulin resistance induced by hypothermia. Hyperglycemia may exacerbate neuronal injury and increase the risk of wound infection.

Blood glucose should be measured frequently, especially in patients with diabetes mellitus. Glucose containing fluids should be avoided. Blood glucose should optimally be maintained below 180 mg/dL, which may require the infusion of insulin.

2. **Hypoglycemia.** Hypoglycemia should be avoided at all costs during CPB because severe hypoglycemia is associated with neurologic injury within a short period, and the signs of hypoglycemia are masked by both the anesthesia and the hemodynamic changes during CPB. Blood glucose should be measured more frequently if patients are receiving insulin or have received hypoglycemic agents preoperatively on the day of surgery.

V. Rewarming, aortic cross-clamp release, and preparation for weaning

  A. Rewarming. On commencement of rewarming, **additional anesthetics** may be required because the brain rewarms faster than the body core.

CLINICAL PEARL Commencement of rewarming is an appropriate time to reassess anesthetic depth, anticoagulation, arterial blood gases, and likely requirements for weaning.

Additional heparin may be required because the rate of metabolism of heparin returns to normal at normothermia. The extent of **hemodilution** should be re-assessed because oxygen requirements increase during rewarming (see also Section IV.E above).

  B. Release of aortic cross-clamp
   1. **Deairing.** Air may collect in the pulmonary veins, left atrium, or LV, particularly during open chamber procedures. This is aspirated through the aortic root vent prior to cross-clamp release or other vents. Temporarily raising the CVP and inflating the lungs will fill the LV and permit easier surgical aspiration of intracavity air. Residual air can be detected using TEE. Flushing the surgical field with CO_2 prior to cardiac chamber closure may reduce residual air, as CO_2 is reabsorbed much faster than air.
   2. **Blood pressure.** Hypertension should be avoided at the time of aortic cross-clamp release. Transient hypotension may occur after the release of the cross-clamp, due to residual cardioplegia or metabolites returning to the circulation as the myocardium is reperfused.

  C. Preparation for weaning from CPB. In preparation for weaning from CPB, cardiac **pacing equipment** is attached and checked, **electrolytes and acid–base** disturbances are corrected if necessary, an adequate **Hb** is ensured, and additional **inotropic drug infusions** (e.g., epinephrine, dobutamine) required for the weaning process are prepared and attached to the patient. If **loading doses** of inodilators (e.g., milrinone) or calcium sensitizers (e.g., levosimendan) are required, these should be given before completion of CPB. If the negative inotropic effects of volatile agents are a concern, they should be ceased before weaning commences, and other agents used to maintain adequate anesthesia. Anesthetic management of weaning from CPB is covered in Chapter 8.

VI. Organ protection during CPB (see also Chapter 20)

  A. Renal protection. The most important renal protective strategy is to ensure adequate renal perfusion during CPB by **optimal fluid loading, appropriate pump flow rates**, close attention to the **renal perfusion pressure**, and avoidance of intravascular **hemolysis and hemoglobinuria**. Numerous strategies have been proposed to reduce the incidence or severity of acute kidney injury during CPB, although there is no high-level evidence to support their routine use [13]). **Mannitol**, low-dose dopamine, furosemide, prostaglandin E, and fenoldopam (a selective dopamine-1 receptor agonist) have been advocated for use in high-risk patients during CPB, particularly if oliguria is present. Fenoldopam 0.05 to 0.10 μg/kg/min showed early promise in some but not all clinical trials [14]. N-acetylcysteine (a free-radical scavenger), steroids, calcium antagonists, and urinary alkalinization have also been tried. **Hemolysis and hemoglobinuria** are managed by correcting the cause where possible and by promoting diuresis.

B. **Brain protection** during CPB involves ensuring adequate **cerebral perfusion pressure** (MAP – CVP) and oxygen delivery, with measures to prevent hypotension and increases in either CVP or intracranial pressure (which will reduce cerebral perfusion pressure). Causes of raised CVP should be identified and corrected. Mild or moderate **hypothermia** is often used to provide additional protection. **Deep hypothermia** with anterograde or retrograde cerebral perfusion is used if circulatory arrest is required (see also Section IV.E above). Care is taken to **avoid emboli,** both particulate (e.g., atheroma) and gaseous, by meticulous surgical and perfusion technique. **Jugular venous oxygen saturation** and **cerebral oximetry** using NIRS can be used to guide the efficacy of interventions. Brain protection is covered in detail in Chapter 26.

C. **Myocardial protection.** See IV.G above.

D. **Inflammatory response to CPB.** CPB is one of the main factors contributing to the inflammatory response associated with cardiac surgery [15]. Reactions are usually mild or subclinical but may be severe in some cases and contribute to brain, lung, renal, or myocardial injury. For a detailed discussion of this inflammatory response to CPB and cardiac surgery, see Chapter 20.

   1. **Etiology**

      a. **Exposure of blood to circuit components.** The extensive contact between circulating blood and the extracorporeal circuit results in variable amounts of thrombin generation, activation of complement, release of cytokines, and expression of immune mediators, all of which may contribute to a systemic inflammatory response syndrome.

      b. **Return of shed blood to the CPB circuit** via cardiotomy suction. Shed blood is in contact with mediastinal tissues (e.g., pericardium) and air and is exposed to shear stress when suction is used. It is a potent source of activated coagulation factors and proinflammatory mediators. It may also cause hypotension when returned to the bypass circuit. Unless bleeding is brisk or stasis is minimal, shed blood should not be returned directly to the CPB circuit. A cell saver can be used to wash shed blood in order to conserve RBCs.

      c. **Ischemia** due to inadequate tissue perfusion or organ protection, including **ischemia–reperfusion injury**.

   2. **Prevention**

   Severe reactions are difficult to predict or prevent. Adequate anticoagulation, organ perfusion, and myocardial protection are fundamental. Strategies to reduce the inflammatory response include the use of **biocompatible heparin-coated circuits**, minimization of cardiotomy suction (unless the shed blood is washed), the use of miniature bypass circuits, centrifugal pumps, steroids, and leukodepletion filters. Fibrinolysis can be reduced by the use of **aminocaproic or tranexamic acid**. Novel anti-inflammatory agents (e.g., pexelizumab) remain investigational. Although many of these strategies have been effective in attenuating the inflammatory response to CPB, few have been shown to reduce major complications in the postoperative period.

   3. **Management**

   Low SVR and evidence of capillary leak may be observed during CPB, but most inflammatory reactions manifest post-CPB. No specific therapy is available and management is supportive.

E. **Lung protection** (see also Chapter 20). Numerous strategies have been proposed to ameliorate lung injury by minimizing the inflammatory response (see Section VI.D) [13]. These include modification of the circuit (e.g., minimized and surface-coated circuits, leukofiltration, ultrafiltration, minimizing use of cardiotomy suction) and administration of anti-inflammatory agents (e.g., steroids) and intermittent pulmonary perfusion. While many of these appear to decrease markers of inflammation and may improve oxygenation (PaO_2/FiO_2 ratio), none have been shown to significantly improve clinical outcome. As for other surgery, the use of lung protective ventilation (e.g., low tidal volume, PEEP, lower FiO_2, and frequent recruitment maneuvers) pre- and post-CPB are recommended [16,17].

F. **Splanchnic and gastrointestinal protection.** Although CPB is known to reduce splanchnic blood flow, there are currently no specific interventions that have been shown to consistently protect the gastrointestinal system [13,18]. Strategies include optimizing perfusion and oxygen delivery (see Section II.E) and minimizing the inflammatory response to CPB (see Section VI.D and also Chapter 20).

VII. **Prevention and management of adverse events, complications, and catastrophes associated with CPB** (see also Chapter 20)

The safe conduct of perfusion requires vigilance on the parts of the perfusionist, anesthesiologist, and cardiac surgeon to ensure that perfusion-related problems are prevented where possible and diagnosed early and managed quickly if they occur [19]. Appropriate training, expertise, and accreditation of all personnel are required, and adherence to protocols and checklists is encouraged. The following complications must be actively sought during initiation of CPB. They may, however, occur at any time during CPB. While they may be rare, the outcomes are potentially disastrous and **prevention is paramount**.

A. **Malposition of arterial cannula**

1. **Aortic dissection.** If the cannula orifice is situated within the arterial wall, not in the true lumen, there is a risk of aortic dissection upon commencement of CPB.

CLINICAL PEARL   Adequate expertise and vigilance of all personnel are required to prevent CPB catastrophes, along with mandatory safety precautions and checks.

Therefore, either arterial cannula pressure or pressure in the arterial tubing proximal to it should always be monitored, and **pressure and pulsatility** checked **before starting CPB**. If the pressure in the aortic cannula does not match the systemic pressure, CPB must not commence until the cannula position has been corrected. If the pressure gradient across the aortic cannula exceeds the recommended range for the flow/cannula combination, either cannula malposition or aortic dissection should be strongly considered. For femoral arterial cannulation, TEE can be used to confirm the presence of the guidewire in the distal aortic lumen prior to advancement of the cannula. If CPB has commenced and a dissection has occurred or is suspected, CPB must cease, the aortic cannula be repositioned, and the dissection repaired if necessary.

---

2. **Carotid or innominate artery hyperperfusion** (Fig. 7.2) can occur if the aortic cannula outflow is too close to the innominate artery or left carotid artery. Deleterious effects include cerebral edema or possibly even arterial rupture from the high flows and pressures. Prevention is surgical; use of a short aortic cannula with a flange may help prevent this complication. If a longer cannula is used, the tip position may be visible in the aortic arch using TEE. The diagnosis is suggested by facial flushing, pupillary dilation, and conjunctival chemosis (edema). There is likely to be accompanying low blood pressure in a left radial or femoral arterial catheter and **hypertension** in a right radial arterial catheter due to innominate artery hyperperfusion. The surgeon must reposition the arterial cannula, and measures to reduce cerebral edema (e.g., mannitol, head-up position) may be required.

B. **Reversed cannulation.** Venous drainage connected to the arterial cannula with arterial inflow into the right atrium or vena cava is very unlikely in adults, due to **different size tubing** for arterial and venous drainage. This complication is avoided also by ensuring that arterial pressures are observed in the arterial outflow line before commencing CPB. Reversed cannulation will result in very **low systemic pressures** and **high venous pressures**. More importantly, negative pressure in the aortic cannula risks the **entrainment of air**, which **must be avoided at all costs**. Reverse rotation of roller pumps must also be avoided. Management requires cessation of CPB, placing the patient in a steep head-down position, deairing the cannulas, and executing a massive gas embolism protocol if necessary (Table 7.3).

C. **Obstruction to venous return.** Sudden reduced venous drainage from the patient during CPB will **lower the reservoir level**, increasing the risk of **air embolism**. At the same time, the venous pressures in the patient will rise, reducing perfusion pressure to organs. To avoid

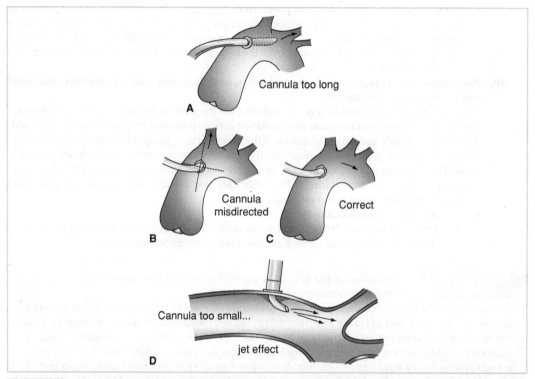

FIGURE 7.2 Potential aortic cannulation problems. **A:** Cannula extends into carotid owing to excessive length, causing excessive carotid flow. **B:** Angle of cannula insertion is improper, which also causes carotid hypoperfusion. **C:** Correct placement. **D:** Cannula diameter is too small; high-velocity jet of blood may damage intima and occlude a vessel. (Redrawn from Moores WY. Cardiopulmonary bypass strategies in patients with severe aortic disease. In: Utley JR, ed. *Pathophysiology and Techniques of Cardiopulmonary Bypass. Vol. 2.* Baltimore, MD: Williams & Wilkins; 1983:190, with permission.)

emptying the venous reservoir further, the perfusionist must reduce the perfusion flow rate, further **reducing organ perfusion**. Alternatively, large fluid volumes must be added to the reservoir. For this reason, the cause must be determined immediately and the **venous drainage restored as quickly as possible**. Most centers use electronic monitors for low reservoir volume, which may include automatic feedback to stop roller pump operation as a safety mechanism (see Section VII.E.1.a).

1. **Air lock.** A sudden reduction in venous blood draining into the venous reservoir may be caused by the presence of large air bubbles within the venous drainage cannula. This creates an "air lock" due to the lower pressure gradient and the surface tension in the air–blood interface. The air lock is overcome by sequentially elevating the venous tubing allowing the air bubble to rise (float to the surface), followed by lowering the tubing to allow the weight of the column of blood to force the bubble distally toward the reservoir.

2. **Mechanical.** Lifting of the heart within the chest by the surgeon often impedes venous drainage. The venous cannula may be malpositioned or kinked inadvertently during surgical manipulations. If reduced venous drainage is observed, the surgeon must be notified immediately and appropriate venous drainage restored urgently.

D. High pressure in the arterial pump line. Normally, arterial inflow line pressure proximal to the aortic cannula is up to three times the patient's arterial pressure (or higher for femoral cannulae), due to high resistance in the tubing and arterial cannula. However, kinking of the inflow line during pump operation will further increase the pressure, risking disruption of the tubing

TABLE 7.3 Massive gas embolism emergency protocol[a]

I. **Stop CPB** immediately (perfusionist), clamp arterial and venous lines, notify entire operating room team of emergency situation

II. Place patient in steep **head-down** position (anesthesiologist)

III. **Locate and isolate source of air**—if from pressurized CPB component, confirm isolation from patient before purging air (surgeon and perfusionist)

IV. Remove aortic cannula; **vent air** from aortic cannulation site (surgeon)

V. **Deair** arterial cannula and pump line and refill with fluid (perfusionist)

If massive cerebral air embolism seems unlikely:

VI. Confirm sufficient volume in CPB reservoir and consider resuming CPB with aortic root venting, administer vasopressors to raise perfusion pressure (hydrostatic pressure shrinks bubbles; also, bubbles occluding arterial bifurcations are pushed into one vessel, opening the other branch), set blender to 100% O_2

VII. Express coronary air by massage and needle venting

VIII. Consider cooling to 20°C for 45 min (increases gas solubility, decreases metabolic demands)

IX. Complete surgical procedure as appropriate to overall clinical situation, rewarm patient, separate slowly from CPB

X. **Continue ventilating the patient with 100% O_2** for at least 6 h (to maximize the blood–alveolar gradient for elimination of N_2)

If massive air embolism seems likely, initiate retrograde perfusion protocol:

I. Institute hypothermic **retrograde SVC perfusion** by connecting arterial pump line to the SVC cannula with caval tape tightened. Blood at 20–24°C is injected into the SVC at 1–2 L/min or more, and air plus blood is drained from the aortic root cannulation site to the pump (Fig. 7.3). Ensure that retrograde perfusion pressure does not exceed 30 mm Hg

II. **Carotid compression** is performed intermittently during retrograde SVC perfusion to allow retrograde purging of air from the **vertebral** arteries (Fig. 7.4)

III. Maintain retrograde SVC perfusion for at least 1–2 min. Continue for an additional 1–2 min if air continues to exit from aorta

IV. In **extensive** systemic air injection accidents in which emboli to splanchnic, renal, or femoral circulation are suspected, **retrograde IVC perfusion** may be performed **after** head deairing procedures are completed. This is performed while the **carotid arteries are clamped** and the patient is in **head-up position** to facilitate removal of air through the aortic root vent but prevent re-embolization of the brain

V. When no additional air can be expelled, **resume anterograde CPB** as in steps VI–X above

Medication considerations

I. **Corticosteroids** may be administered, although this is controversial. The usual dose of methylprednisolone is 30 mg/kg

II. **Barbiturate coma** should be considered if the embolism occurred during warm CPB and if the myocardium will be able to tolerate the significant negative inotropy. Thiopental or pentobarbital, 10 mg/kg loading dose plus infusion at 1–3 mg/kg/hr, may be used empirically. If EEG monitoring is available, titration of barbiturate to an EEG burst suppression (1 burst/min) pattern is preferable

III. Consider additional mannitol 12.5–25 g

Postoperative considerations

I. Consider hyperbaric oxygen treatment (6 atm recommended by US Navy Diving tables) and make any necessary transportation arrangements

II. Consult a neurologist

III. Consider early awakening for neurologic examination vs. sustained barbiturate coma and/or sustained ventilation with 100% O_2

IV. Perform brain CT scan or MRI as advised by neurologist if patient is sufficiently stable

V. Continue resuscitative efforts unless patient is diagnosed as brain dead or unless sustained support becomes futile for other reasons (e.g., multiorgan failure)

[a]This protocol should be reviewed together by all members of the cardiac team periodically.
CPB, cardiopulmonary bypass; CT, computerized tomography; EEG, electroencephalogram; IVC, inferior vena cava; MRI, magnetic resonance imaging; SVC, superior vena cava.
Modified from Mills NL, Ochsner JL. Massive air embolism during cardiopulmonary bypass: causes, prevention, and management. *J Thorac Cardiovasc Surg.* 1980;80(5):708–717; Kurusz M, Mills NL. Management of unusual problems encountered in initiating and maintaining cardiopulmonary bypass. In: Gravlee GP, Davis RF, Kurusz M, et al., eds. *Cardiopulmonary Bypass: Principles and Practice.* 2nd ed. Philadelphia, PA: Lippincott Williams & Wilkins; 2000:596.

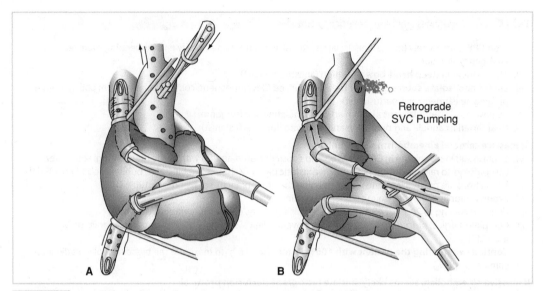

FIGURE 7.3 Retrograde perfusion in the treatment of massive air embolism. **A:** Massive arterial gas embolism has occurred. **B:** Bubbles in the arterial tree are flushed out by performing retrograde body perfusion into the SVC by connecting the deaired arterial pump line to the SVC cannula (and tightening caval tapes). Blood and bubbles exit the aorta from the cannulation wound. SVC, superior vena cava. (Redrawn from Mills NL, Ochsner JL. Massive air embolism during cardiopulmonary bypass: causes, prevention, and management. *J Thorac Cardiovasc Surg*. 1980;80:713, with permission.)

or connections, especially if the line is inadvertently clamped. For this reason, a high-pressure alarm is used, often with automatic feedback to stop roller pump operation.

E. **Massive gas embolism.** Most massive (macroscopic) gas emboli [19,20] consist of air, although oxygen emboli can be generated by a defective or clotted oxygenator (for further discussion of this and CPB safety devices, see Chapter 20). Use of a vented arterial line filter is an important safety device that can help prevent gas emboli reaching the patient; its routine use is strongly recommended. Centrifugal pumps provide an additional level of safety because massive air entry proximal to the pump will empty the pump chamber and render the centrifugal force ineffective. Nevertheless, the risk is not removed. Because of the high risk of stroke, myocardial infarction, or death after massive gas embolism, **prevention is of utmost importance**.

1. **Etiology**

   a. **Empty or low oxygenator reservoir level.** Air may be pumped from an empty reservoir. Avoiding this scenario is one of the key tasks of the perfusionist. There are also alarms to alert staff when the oxygenator reservoir level is reaching an unsafe level. Many such alarms are linked to an automatic cessation of the arterial roller pump. Vortexing can permit air entrainment and embolism when the reservoir blood level is very low but not empty. This is **the most important cause of bypass catastrophes** when utilizing a closed reservoir system. A high-risk period for air embolism or entrainment is at the time of separation from CPB, when the oxygenator reservoir level is often low.

   b. **Leaks in the negative pressure part of the CPB circuit** (between the oxygenator reservoir and the arterial pump) may result in air entrainment—for example, clotted or defective oxygenator, disruption of tubing connections.

   c. **Entrainment of air around the aortic cannula.** This may occur during cannula insertion. Entrainment can also occur via this route if negative pressure in the arterial cannula is allowed to develop during periods of no flow (e.g., before or after the onset of CPB). To prevent negative pressure and draining blood from the patient, the aortic cannula must be clamped during all periods when the arterial pump is inactive.

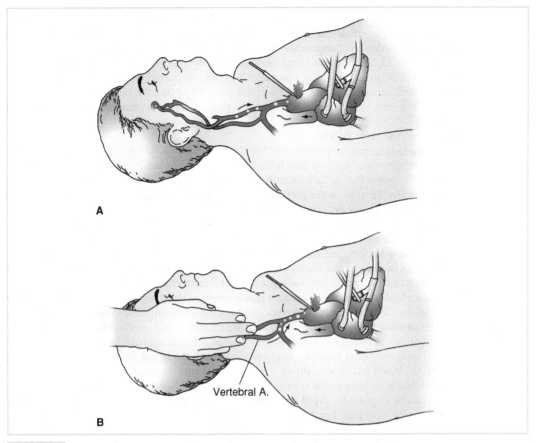

FIGURE 7.4 Carotid (**A**) and vertebral (**B**) artery deairing during retrograde perfusion. In the management of massive arterial gas embolism, steep head-down position helps to flush bubbles out of the *carotid arteries*. Application of intermittent pressure to the carotid arteries increases retrograde *vertebral artery* flow, which helps to evacuate bubbles. (Redrawn from Mills NL, Ochsner JL. Massive air embolism during cardiopulmonary bypass: Causes, prevention, and management. *J Thorac Cardiovasc Surg*. 1980;80:713, with permission.)

    d. **Inadequate deairing** prior to aortic cross-clamp release. This is particularly important for open-chamber procedures.

    e. **Reversed roller pump** flow in vent line or arterial cannula.

    f. **Pressurized cardiotomy reservoir** (causing retrograde flow of air through a nonocclusive vent line roller head into heart or aorta)

    g. **Runaway pump head** (switch inoperative; must unplug pump and crank by hand)

    h. **Other causes** not related specifically to CPB include an improper flushing technique for arterial or left atrial pressure monitoring lines, **paradoxical embolism** of venous air across atrial or ventricular septal defects. Occasionally, a **persistent left SVC** communicates with the left atrium (IV air from a left-sided IV may enter the systemic circulation through this SVC).

  2. **Prevention.** Vigilance is required. Safety devices and alarms must be activated.

  3. **Diagnosis.** Gas embolism is diagnosed mostly by visual inspection. The extent of gas embolism can be gauged by signs of myocardial or other organ ischemia.

  4. **Management.** A massive gas embolus emergency protocol should be available and followed by all staff [20]. See Table 7.3, Figures 7.3 and 7.4.

F. **Failure of oxygen supply.** Inadequate oxygenator gas flow or a hypoxic mixture will result in arterial hypoxemia. The blood in the arterial line will appear dark, and the lower PO_2 will register on in-line PO_2 or Hb oxygen saturation monitors. An oxygen analyzer can be incorporated in the oxygenator gas inflow line as an early alert for hypoxic mixtures, but this will not detect a distal disconnection. A disconnection of the sweep gas will result in a sudden drop in oxygenator exhaust CO_2 level if this is being monitored (see Section IV.A.2). The O_2 supply should be restored immediately, connecting a portable O_2 cylinder to the oxygenator if necessary. If a delay is anticipated, either separate from CPB (if still possible) or cool the patient maximally until O_2 supply is restored. Ventilation with **room air** is preferable to no ventilation at all, if immediate restoration of O_2 supply is not possible.

G. **Pump or oxygenator failure**

1. **Pump failure** may be due to electrical or mechanical failure, tubing rupture or disconnection, or automatic shut off by a bubble or low reservoir detector. A runaway pump head may raise the pump flow to its maximum inappropriately, and the pump control switch will be inoperative. For systems designed to be used with an electromagnetic or ultrasonic transducer, failure of the sensor can prevent one from knowing the actual pump flow rate. Miscalibration of the arterial pump or flowmeter may lead to inadequate (or excessive) blood flow. An open shunt between the arterial line and the venous reservoir will result in decreased effective pump flow. If the occlusion of a roller pump is improperly set, excessive regurgitation occurs (causing hemolysis) and the forward flow is reduced. In the event of electrical failure, CPB pumps usually have battery backup and can be hand cranked if necessary until current is restored. Mechanical failure requires **replacement of the pump**. In case of a runaway pump head, the CPB machine must be unplugged and the tubing switched to a different roller head.

2. **Oxygenator failure** may be due to a manufacturing defect, mechanical obstruction from clot or debris, disruption of the oxygenator shell (trauma, spill of volatile liquid anesthetic), or leakage of water from the heat exchanger into the blood. The diagnosis is based on arterial blood gas abnormalities, acidosis, blood leak, excessive hemolysis, or high pre-membrane pressures. For severe failure, the oxygenator must be replaced. A protocol should be in place for **rapid oxygenator replacement**. If body perfusion will be low or absent for more than 1 or 2 minutes and if the patient cannot be immediately weaned from CPB, then hypothermia to 18° to 20°C should be induced if possible and consideration given to brain, myocardial, and renal protection during the oxygenator replacement. Open cardiac massage may be necessary, depending on the stage of the operation.

H. **Clotted oxygenator or circuit.** This serious event can interfere with gas exchange, prevent CPB flow, or cause massive gas embolus. The main cause is **inadequate anticoagulation**, which may result from **inadequate dose, heparin resistance**, or the inadvertent administration of **protamine during CPB**. This potentially lethal catastrophe should not occur if adequate anticoagulation is confirmed before initiating CPB and at frequent intervals thereafter. It can be diagnosed by visual observation of clot in the oxygenator or high arterial line pressure (evidence of partially clotted arterial line filter). There may also be clues to inadequate heparinization by **the presence of clot in the surgical field**. Management involves cessation of CPB and replacement of the oxygenator and tubing if necessary. If the patient is not cold, open cardiopulmonary resuscitation and topical hypothermia may be required. The patient should then be reheparinized using a different lot of heparin if possible, and satisfactory anticoagulation confirmed before reinstituting CPB.

I. **Dislodgment of cannula or tubing rupture.** With appropriate vigilance and monitoring, this should never occur. Management requires cessation of flow until the cannula is repositioned or the tubing is replaced and re-priming of the lines if necessary.

J. **Heater–cooler malfunction.** If inappropriate water inflow or arterial blood temperatures are observed, the heater–cooler and its tubing should be checked and replaced, if necessary. If heater–cooler malfunction can be excluded, the oxygenator should be checked.

VIII. **Minimally invasive surgical techniques requiring CPB**

CPB for minimally invasive procedures follows the same principles as conventional CPB but requires additional instrumentation and monitoring due to the limited surgical exposure [21]. Irrespective of the technique used, frequent interaction between surgeon, perfusionist, and anesthesiologist is required for a successful outcome (see Chapter 13).

> **CLINICAL PEARL**   Minimally invasive procedures require additional instrumentation and monitoring due to the limited surgical access, typically including TEE guidance for cannula placement.

A. **Port-access surgery.** Typically the cannulae are inserted peripherally (e.g., femoral artery and vein). The venous cannula is advanced into the RA in order to drain both the SVC and IVC. This is performed using a guidewire technique and requires TEE guidance. Insertion of a separate SVC cannula via the internal jugular vein using TEE guidance may also be required. VAVD is often necessary for peripheral venous cannulation. An aortic occlusion catheter may be used instead of an aortic cross-clamp. This is placed in the ascending aorta under fluoroscopic or TEE guidance. An endocoronary sinus catheter is inserted via the jugular approach under TEE guidance for delivery of retrograde cardioplegia, and a PA vent catheter is inserted to decompress the heart through the left atrium. Correct position of the inflated aortic occlusion catheter balloon should be checked regularly using TEE. Loss of the right radial arterial pressure trace may indicate cephalad migration of the balloon.

B. **Minithoracotomy.** If a small incision is used (e.g., hemisternotomy, anterior thoracotomy), it may be possible to use modified arterial and even venous cannulas inserted transthoracically and a modified aortic cross-clamp or a combination of peripheral and central cannulation. An aortic root vent for anterograde cardioplegia can also be inserted, and a coronary sinus catheter for retrograde cardioplegia if no other route is possible.

C. **Minimally invasive mitral valve surgery.** In this procedure, arterial and venous cannulae are inserted peripherally, and CPB is instituted prior to a right minithoracotomy [22]. TEE guidance is used to ensure that the venous cannula enters or crosses the right atrium to drain the SVC as well as the IVC. Due to the increased length and decreased diameter of the venous cannula, VAVD is typically required. If the right atrium is opened (e.g., for tricuspid valve surgery), a separate SVC cannula (often inserted percutaneously) may be required. With the onset of CPB, ventilation of the lungs is no longer required. Collapse of the right lung on opening of the chest provides surgical access to the heart and great vessels. Alternatively, a double lumen endobronchial tube or bronchial blocker can be used to deflate the right lung earlier while ventilating the left lung. An aortic root cannula for the administration of cardioplegia can then be placed, followed by an aortic cross-clamp. Access to the mitral valve is obtained through the left atrium. CPB management is otherwise unchanged, although before final separation from CPB, a trial separation is undertaken to ensure satisfactory mitral valve function (as assessed by TEE). For further details, see Chapter 13.

D. **Minimally invasive aortic valve surgery.** This can be performed through a partial (upper) sternotomy with extension of the sternotomy incision into a right intercostal space (e.g., third intercostal space) [23]. Alternatively, the procedure can be performed through a right anterior thoracotomy (e.g., second intercostal space). For the latter, a double-lumen endobronchial tube or bronchial blocker may be required to collapse the right lung to permit surgical access prior to CPB.

E. **Choice of cardioplegia.** With minimally invasive procedures, repeated administration of cardioplegia may be technically more difficult or distracting. For this reason, the use of a single dose of a longer lasting solution such as Custodiol is often preferred (see Section IV.G.1). However, ECG monitoring for return of electrical activity is still required, giving a second dose if necessary. Care must be taken to ensure that surgical retractors do not impede cardioplegia distribution to all areas of the heart. Due to the larger volumes required, ultrafiltration is often used to remove excess water [11,21]. Additional bicarbonate and calcium are often required prior to separation from CPB.

IX. **Management of unusual or rare conditions affecting bypass**

A. **Sickle cell trait and disease [19,24].** The congenital presence of abnormal HbS as the trait (heterozygote, Hb-AS) but especially as the disease (homozygote, Hb-SS) allows RBCs to undergo sickle transformation and occlude the microvasculature or lyse. RBC sickling may be induced by exposure to hypoxemia, vascular stasis, hyperosmolarity, or acidosis. Although anesthesia for noncardiac surgery is well tolerated in sickle trait patients, the risks are higher for operations requiring CPB. While **sickle cell trait** patients are at low risk for RBC sickling, **sickle cell disease** patients develop RBC sickling at O_2 saturations less than 85% and are at risk for developing potentially fatal thromboses during CPB, unless appropriate measures are taken. Hypoxia, acidosis, and conditions leading to vascular stasis (e.g., hypovolemia, dehydration) should be avoided or minimized in all patients with **sickle cell trait or disease.** CPB should be avoided if alternative treatment options are available (e.g., off-pump surgery). If CPB is required, hypothermia and cold cardioplegia should ideally be avoided. Preoperative transfusion to a Hb >10 g/dL using donor HbA RBCs will improve oxygen carriage and reduce the percentage of HbS. For deep hypothermia, exchange transfusion may be required. Expert preoperative hematologic consultation is advised for sickle cell disease patients before CPB.

B. **Cold agglutinin disease [19,25].** Autoantibodies against RBCs in patients with cold agglutinin disease are activated by cold exposure below a **critical temperature**. Below this temperature, hemagglutination will occur, resulting in **vascular occlusion** with organ ischemia or infarction. Low titers of antibodies with a low critical temperature (e.g., <28°C) are common but of little clinical relevance. In contrast, patients who have **high titers** of antibodies with a **high critical temperature** are at risk of hemagglutination perioperatively, especially during **hypothermic CPB.** The organ at greatest risk of damage is the myocardium because RBCs are exposed to extreme hypothermia (4° to 8°C) during the preparation of **blood cardioplegia** solution. Aggregates thus formed may be infused into the coronary vasculature, causing severe microcirculatory occlusion and preventing distribution of cardioplegia. If cold agglutinins are suspected preoperatively, careful assessment by a hematologist is warranted, including characterizing the type of antibody, its titer, and its critical temperature. CPB should be avoided if alternative strategies (e.g., off-pump surgery) are feasible. If CPB is required, **systemic temperatures** should be maintained *above* the critical temperature. Systemic temperatures of 28°C or higher are generally safe in asymptomatic patients. **DHCA** is feasible, provided the coldest blood temperature is several degrees warmer than the critical temperature. Cardioplegia management includes **avoidance of cold blood cardioplegia**. If a reduction of the patient's core temperature below their critical temperature for hemagglutinin formation is unavoidable, preoperative **plasmapheresis** may be required.

C. **Cold urticaria [26].** Patients with this disorder develop systemic histamine release and generalized urticaria in response to cold exposure. Cold CPB should be avoided if possible because marked histamine release occurs during CPB rewarming and can cause hemodynamic instability. If cold CPB is unavoidable, the cardiovascular responses to histamine can be prevented by pretreatment with H_1- and H_2-receptor blockades; concomitant steroid administration may be useful.

D. **Malignant hyperthermia (MH) [27,28].** An acute MH crisis may occur in susceptible patients exposed to triggering agents and in rare cases, may manifest for the first time during CPB. The mainstay of management is prevention, by avoiding triggering agents. During CPB, the usual early signs of an MH crisis, of hyperthermia, rigidity, and tachycardia, may be absent due to the use of hypothermia and cardioplegia. However, the increased skeletal muscle metabolism associated with the disorder may cause a mixed metabolic and respiratory acidosis, hyperkalemia, and rhabdomyolysis with myoglobinuria (and late renal failure) even during CPB. Recognition of MH crisis can be difficult, particularly during the rewarming phase when temperature is expected to increase. **A high index of suspicion** is required for patients with known MH susceptibility. **Management** involves ceasing triggering agents, cooling to reduce hyperthermia, correction of acid–base and electrolyte changes, and the early administration of dantrolene (1 to 2 mg/kg IV initially, with further doses as required titrated to effect). Active cooling and treatment of other MH complications may be necessary in the post-CPB period.

E. **Hereditary angioedema [29].** A deficiency or abnormality in function of an endogenous inhibitor of the C1 esterase complement protein leads to exaggerated complement pathway activation after even minor stress, resulting in edema of the airway, face, gastrointestinal tract, and extremities. CPB can cause fatal complement activation in patients with hereditary angioedema; peak activation follows protamine administration. In the past, management of acute episodes has been mainly supportive because epinephrine, steroids, and histamine antagonists are of little benefit, and fresh frozen plasma may exacerbate the reaction by providing additional complement substrates. Subacute and chronic therapies include androgens (stanozolol) and antifibrinolytics. A purified human C1 esterase inhibitor replacement protein (C1-INHRP) concentrate (Cinryze, ViroPharma, Exton, PA) is now available for prophylaxis against and treatment of acute episodes, and another purified C1-INH concentrate (Berinert, CSL Behring, King of Prussia, PA) is available for treatment. Other drugs have been introduced recently to block bradykinin B_2 receptors or inhibitor plasma kallikrein and reduce the severity of reactions.

F. **Pregnancy [30].** Cardiac surgery with CPB during pregnancy involves a high risk of fetal demise or morbidity. Longer duration of CPB appears to increase the risk to the fetus. Fetal heart rate monitoring is mandatory in the second and third trimesters. Uterine contractile activity should be monitored using a tocodynamometer applied to the maternal abdomen. Maintaining an increased perfusion pressure (e.g., >70 mm Hg) is advocated because uterine blood flow is not autoregulated. Using increases in pump flow to elevate the blood pressure may be preferable to using pressor drugs, due to the risk of uterine artery vasoconstriction with α-adrenergic stimulation. Toward term, left uterine displacement is necessary. Fetal bradycardia not related to hypothermia may indicate placental hypoperfusion and should be treated promptly by increasing the pump flow and perfusion pressure. **Tocolytic drugs** such as magnesium sulfate, ritodrine, or terbutaline may be necessary. **Inotropic drugs** ideally should not have unbalanced α-vasoconstrictor or uterine-contracting activity.

G. **Jehovah's Witnesses** may accept CPB so long as there is a continuous circuit and any blood that is not in circulation is not retransfused. Therefore, it is important to ensure continuous circulation of blood from commencement of CPB until full separation, with no transfusion of residual blood once CPB has ceased.

REFERENCES

1. **Zheng F, Sheinberg R, Yee MS, et al. Cerebral near-infra-red spectroscopy and neurological outcomes in adult cardiac surgery: a systematic review.** *Anesth Analg.* 2013;116(3):663–676.
2. Murkin JM. Cerebral oximetry: monitoring the brain as the index organ. *Anesthesiology.* 2011;114(1):12–13.
3. Frässdorf J, De Hert S, Schlack W. Anaesthesia and myocardial ischaemia/reperfusion injury. *Br J Anaesth.* 2009;103(1):89–98.
4. Graham J, Gibbs NM, Weightman WM. Relationship between temperature corrected oxygenator exhaust PCO_2 and arterial PCO_2 during hypothermic cardiopulmonary bypass. *Anaesth Intensive Care.* 2005;33(5):457–461.
5. Baulig W, Seifert B, Schmid ER, et al. Comparison of spectral entropy and bispectral index electroencephalography in coronary artery bypass surgery. *J Cardiothor Vasc Anesth.* 2010;24(4):544–549.
6. **Murphy GS, Hessel EA 2nd, Groom RC. Optimal perfusion during cardiopulmonary bypass: an evidence-based approach.** *Anesth Analg.* 2009;108(5):1394–1417.
7. Joshi B, Ono M, Brown C, et al. Predicting the limits of cerebral autoregulation during cardiopulmonary bypass. *Anesth Analg.* 2012;114(3):503–510.
8. Gravlee GP, Angert KC, Tucker WY, et al. Early anticoagulation peak and rapid distribution after intravenous heparin. *Anesthesiology.* 1988;68(1):126–129.
9. **Ho KM, Tan JA. Benefits and risks of maintaining normothermia during cardiopulmonary bypass in adult cardiac surgery: a systematic review.** *Cardiovasc Ther.* 2011;29(4):260–279.
10. Engelman R, Baker RA, Likosky DS, et al. The STS/SCA/AmSECT: clinical practice guidelines for cardiopulmonary bypass—temperature management during cardiopulmonary bypass. *Ann Thorac Surg.* 2015;100(2):748–757.
11. Edelman JJ, Seco M, Dunne B, et al. Custodiol for myocardial protection and preservation: a systematic review. *Ann Cardiothoracic Surg.* 2013;2(6):717–728.
12. Nadolny EM, Svennson LG. Carbon dioxide field flooding techniques for open heart surgery: monitoring and minimizing potential adverse effects. *Perfusion.* 2000;15(2):151–153.
13. Grocott HP, Stafford-Smith M, Mora-Mangano CT. Cardiopulmonary bypass management and organ protection. In: Kaplan JA, Augoustides JGT, Manecke Jr GR, et al., eds. *Kaplan's Cardiac Anesthesia for Cardiac and Noncardiac Surgery.* 7th ed. Philadelphia, PA: Elsevier; 2016:1111–1161.
14. Ranucci M, De Benedetti D, Biachini C, et al. Effects of fenoldopam infusion in complex cardiac operations: a prospective, double-blind, placebo-controlled study. *Minerva Anesthesiol.* 2010;76(4):249–259.
15. Levy JH, Tanaka KA. Inflammatory response to cardiopulmonary bypass. *Ann Thorac Surg.* 2003;75(2):S715–S720.
16. Bignami E, Guarnieri M, Saglietti F, et al. Mechanical ventilation during cardiopulmonary bypass. *J Cardiothorac Vasc Anesth.* 2016;30(6):1668–1675.
17. Apostolakis EE, Koletsis EN, Baikoussis NG, et al. Strategies to prevent intraoperative lung injury during cardiopulmonary bypass. *J Cardiothorac Surg.* 2010;5:1.
18. Allen SJ. Gastrointestinal complications and cardiac surgery. *J Extra Corpor Technol.* 2014;46(2):142–149.

19. **Kurusz M, Mills NL, Davis RF. Unusual problems in cardiopulmonary bypass. In: Gravlee GR, Davis RF, Hammon JW, et al., eds. *Cardiopulmonary Bypass and Mechanical Support*. 4th ed. Philadelphia, PA: Wolters Kluwer; 2016:569–601.**

20. Mills NL, Ochsner JL. Massive air embolism during cardiopulmonary bypass: causes, prevention, and management. *J Thorac Cardiovasc Surg.* 1980;80(5):708–717.

21. **Kypson AP, Sanderson Jr DA, Nifong LW, et al. Cardiopulmonary bypass and myocardial protection for minimally invasive cardiac surgery. In: Gravlee GR, Davis RF, Hammon JW, et al., eds. *Cardiopulmonary Bypass and Mechanical Support*. 4th ed. Philadelphia, PA: Wolters Kluwer; 2016:569–601.**

22. Walther T, Falk V, Mohr FW. Minimally invasive mitral valve surgery. *J Cardiovasc Surg (Torino).* 2004;45(5):487–495.

23. **Glauber M, Ferrarini M, Miceli A. Minimally invasive aortic surgery: state of the art and future directions. *Ann Cardiothoracic Surg.* 2013;4(1):26–32.**

24. Firth PG, Head CA. Sickle cell disease and anesthesia. *Anesthesiology.* 2004;101(3):766–785.

25. Atkinson VP, Soeding P, Horne G, et al. Cold agglutinins in cardiac surgery: management of myocardial protection and cardiopulmonary bypass. *Ann Thorac Surg.* 2008;85(1):310–311.

26. Lancey RA, Schaefer OP, McCormick MJ. Coronary artery bypass grafting and aortic valve replacement with cold cardioplegia in a patient with cold-induced urticaria. *Ann Allergy Asthma Immunol.* 2004;92(2):273–275.

27. Larach DR, High KM, Larach MG, et al. Cardiopulmonary bypass interference with dantrolene prophylaxis of malignant hyperthermia. *J Cardiothorac Anesth.* 1987;1(5):448–453.

28. Metterlein T, Zink W, Kranke E, et al. Cardiopulmonary bypass in malignant hyperthermia susceptible patients: a systematic review of published cases. *J Thorac Cardiovasc Surg.* 2011;141(6):1488–1495.

29. Levy JH, Freiberger DJ, Roback J. Hereditary angioedema: current and emerging option. *Anesth Analg.* 2010;110(5):1271–1280.

30. Chandrasekhar S, Cook CR, Collard CD. Cardiac surgery in the parturient. *Anesth Analg.* 2009;108(3):777–785.

8

The Postcardiopulmonary Bypass Period: Weaning to ICU Transport

Benjamin N. Morris, Chandrika R. Garner, and Roger L. Royster

KEY POINTS

1. Core temperature (nasopharyngeal or bladder) should be greater than 36°C before terminating cardiopulmonary bypass (CPB). Discontinuation of CPB at temperatures less than 36°C increases the risk of rebound hypothermia in the intensive care unit (ICU). However, the nasopharyngeal temperature should not exceed 37°C, as this will increase the risk of postoperative central nervous system dysfunction. Using nasopharyngeal temperature to avoid hyperthermia and the rectal/bladder temperature to assure adequate rewarming may be the safest technique.

(continued)

2. Visualization of the heart, directly to assess right ventricular (RV) function and volume status, as well as with transesophageal echocardiography (TEE) to rule out air and to assess valve and ventricular function is important before terminating CPB.

3. The first attempt to terminate CPB is usually the best one. Optimize all central venous pressure (CVP) mnemonic parameters before CPB termination. Consider prophylactic inotropes in patients with markedly reduced ventricular function.

4. Protamine should not be given until the heart has been successfully weaned from CPB. A struggling heart after CPB discontinuation could require reinstitution of CPB.

5. Vasoplegic syndrome is a severe form of post-CPB vasodilation characterized by low arterial pressure, normal to high cardiac output (CO), normal right-side filling pressures, and low systemic vascular resistance (SVR) that is refractory to pressor therapy.

6. When evaluating hypoxemia after CPB, the possibility of a right-to-left shunt through a patent foramen ovale must be considered and evaluated with TEE.

7. New-onset renal dysfunction requiring dialysis after CPB increases mortality almost eightfold. Maintenance of a higher mean arterial pressure (MAP) on pump in patients with pre-existing renal insufficiency may be protective in some patients.

I. Introduction

Terminating cardiopulmonary bypass (CPB) requires the anesthesiologist to apply the basic tenets of cardiovascular physiology and pharmacology. The goal is a smooth transition from the mechanical pump to the heart as the source of blood flow and pressure. Weaning from the pump involves optimizing cardiovascular variables including preload, afterload, heart rate (HR) and rhythm, and contractility as in the pre-CPB period. However, the time period for optimization is compressed to minutes or seconds, and decisions must be made quickly to avoid myocardial injury or damage to the other major organ systems.

II. Preparation for termination of bypass: central venous pressure (CVP) mnemonic

The major objectives in preparing for termination of CPB can be remembered with the aid of the mnemonic **CVP shown in** Table 8.1. One can also call this "C6V4P6" as a reminder of the number of items for each letter.

A. Cold

Core temperature (nasopharyngeal or rectal/bladder) should be greater than 36°C before terminating CPB. Rectal or bladder temperature should be at least 35° to 36°C [1]. Ending CPB when cold causes prolonged hypothermia from equilibration of the cooler, vessel-poor group (imperfectly represented by rectal or bladder temperature) with the warmer and better perfused vessel-rich group (represented by nasopharyngeal or esophageal temperature). Nasopharyngeal temperature correlates with brain temperature but may be artificially elevated during rapid rewarming and should not be used for determining the temperature at which CPB is discontinued unless it has been stable for 15 to 20 minutes. Venous return temperature can be used in a similar manner to help confirm core temperature. The nasopharyngeal temperature should not exceed 37°C, as this will increase the risk of postoperative central nervous system

TABLE 8.1	The major objectives in preparing for termination of CPB can be remembered with the aid of the mnemonic CVP	
C	**V**	**P**
Cold	Ventilation	Predictors
Conduction	Vaporizer	Protamine
Calcium	Volume expanders	Pressure
Cardiac output (CO)	Visualization	Pressors
Cells		Pacer
Coagulation		Potassium

CPB, cardiopulmonary bypass; CVP, central venous pressure.

dysfunction. Using nasopharyngeal temperature to avoid hyperthermia and the rectal/bladder temperature to avoid underwarming may be the safest technique.

B. **Conduction**

Cardiac rate and rhythm must be controlled as follows:

1. **Rate**

   a. HR of 80 to 100 beats per minute (bpm) may be needed for adequate cardiac output (CO) post-CPB because of reduced ventricular compliance and inability to increase stroke volume. In coronary artery bypass graft (CABG) procedures, complete revascularization allows a higher rate (80 to 100 bpm) after CPB, with less risk of ischemia than before CPB. Patients with severely limited stroke volume (aneurysmectomy or after ventricular remodeling) may require even higher rates.

   b. Sinus bradycardia may be treated with atropine or an inotropic drug, but epicardial pacing is more reliable and is most commonly employed.

   c. Sinus tachycardia of more than 120 bpm should be avoided. Often increasing preload before termination of CPB will reflexively decrease the HR to an acceptable level. Other etiologies of sinus tachycardia must be addressed. Common etiologies include:

      (1) Hypoxia

      (2) Hypercapnia

      (3) Medications (inotropes, anticholinergics)

      (4) Light anesthesia, awareness

         (a) "Fast track" anesthesia with its lower medication dosing schedule requires special attention to this complication. An additional dose of narcotic and benzodiazepine, or hypnotic (propofol infusion) should be considered during the rewarming period if tachycardia is present. Bispectral index (BIS) or depth of anesthesia monitors may be helpful in guiding therapy. A dexmedetomidine infusion can also be considered.

      (5) Anemia

      (6) Ischemia: ST and T-wave changes indicative of ischemia should be treated and the surgeon should be notified. A nitroglycerin (NTG) infusion and/or an increase in the perfusion pressure often improves the situation. Refractory causes include residual air or graft occlusions. If coronary air is suspected, briefly increasing the perfusion pressure to a mean of 90 mm Hg may improve the situation.

2. **Rhythm**

   a. Normal sinus rhythm is preferable. In patients with poorly compliant, thick-walled ventricles (associated with aortic stenosis, hypertension, or ischemia), the atrial "kick" may contribute up to 40% of stroke volume (and thus CO), so attaining synchronized atrial contraction (sinus rhythm, atrial, or atrioventricular [AV] sequential pacing) is very important before attempting CPB termination. Atrial pacing is acceptable if there is no AV block, but often atrial and ventricular leads are needed. Atrial pacing may not be possible initially because the atria often require longer to recover from cardioplegia than the ventricles and have a higher pacing threshold.

   b. Supraventricular tachycardias (SVTs, >120 bpm) such as regular narrow-QRS atrial flutter and atrial fibrillation, should be cardioverted with synchronized internal cardioversion before terminating CPB. Atrial flutter and other SVTs from the atrial or AV node may be converted with overdrive pacing.

   c. Esmolol, verapamil, amiodarone, or adenosine may be used to chemically cardiovert or to control the ventricular response rate. An undesired decrease in contractility may occur with all of these agents except adenosine.

   d. Third-degree AV block requires AV sequential pacing, although atropine occasionally may be effective.

   e. Ventricular dysrhythmias are treated as indicated (see Chapters 2 and 18).

C. **Calcium**

Calcium should be immediately available to treat hypocalcemia and hyperkalemia, which commonly occur after CPB. However, the routine administration of calcium post-CPB is not recommended.

1. **Mechanism of action.** Most studies suggest that calcium produces an elevation in systemic vascular resistance (SVR) when the ionized Ca^{++} level is in the low–normal range or higher [2]. Despite this increase in afterload, contractility is maintained. At very low ionized calcium levels (<0.8 mM), contractility is increased by calcium administration. Elevating calcium levels will also help counteract the negative physiologic actions of hyperkalemia. The usual and safest initial dose is 5 mg/kg of calcium chloride ($CaCl_2$).

2. **Measurement.** Ionized Ca^{++} levels should be evaluated after rewarming to help direct therapy. Citrated blood cardioplegia reperfusion solutions can lower blood Ca^{++} levels substantially (normal range 1 to 1.3 mmol/dL). Calcium levels are affected by pH: Low pH will increase Ca^{++} levels, whereas elevated pH will decrease Ca^{++} levels. Correction of pH should be attempted before treating abnormal values.

3. **Risks of calcium administration**
   a. Arrhythmias: Especially patients taking digoxin (now uncommon) may experience life-threatening arrhythmias.
   b. Inhibition of the hemodynamic action of inotropes (e.g., epinephrine, dobutamine) has been reported.
   c. Coronary artery spasm might occur in rare susceptible patients.
   d. Augmentation of reperfusion injury is possible in the already calcium overloaded myocardium. Calcium administration should be avoided unless there is hyperkalemia or ionized calcium is less than 0.8 mM.

D. **Cardiac output (CO)**
Evaluating cardiac function is vital after CPB. CO may be obtained from a pulmonary artery (PA) catheter or estimated by using transesophageal echocardiography (TEE). **If a continuous CO PA catheter is used, it may take more than 3 minutes to obtain the first CO after CPB.** If the patient is stable, this is acceptable; if not, the equipment for a manual determination should be used initially.

E. **Cells**
1. The hemoglobin concentration should be measured after rewarming. If it is 6.5 g/dL or less before terminating CPB, blood administration should be considered to maintain O_2-carrying capacity after CPB. If the venous reservoir contains a large amount of blood, this blood may be concentrated by a cell saver and given back to the patient after CPB, which could preclude the need for blood transfusion. Patients with residual coronary stenoses, anticipated low CO, or end-organ damage may benefit from a higher hemoglobin concentration such as 8 g/dL.
2. Two units of packed red blood cells (PRBCs) should be immediately available for use once the CPB pump volume is exhausted. If excessive bleeding is anticipated (see Section F below), then additional units should be on hand.

F. **Coagulation**
Anticipate possible coagulation abnormalities prior to discontinuation of CPB. Blood coagulation components (e.g., platelets and fresh frozen plasma [FFP]) should await complete heparin neutralization and be guided by the clinical situation and laboratory findings (e.g., thromboelastogram, prothrombin time, partial thromboplastin time, platelet count).
1. Patients at risk include:
   a. Patients taking platelet inhibitors (clopidogrel, prasugrel, ticlopidine, aspirin) [3]
   b. Patients having emergency surgery and who have been exposed to:
      (1) Thrombolytic agents (alteplase, tenecteplase)
      (2) Antiplatelet glycoprotein IIb/IIIa agents (abciximab, eptifibatide, tirofiban)
      (3) Direct thrombin inhibitors (bivalirudin, dabigatran, argatroban)
      (4) Warfarin
      (5) Factor Xa inhibitors (apixaban, rivaroxaban)
   c. Patients with chronic renal failure
   d. Long "pump run," for example, redo or complex operation
   e. Low body mass index (BMI)
   f. Extreme hypothermia on CPB
   g. Excessive bleeding with previous cardiac surgery [4]

2. Platelets and FFP should be available if indicated (as above).
3. Desmopressin acetate (DDAVP) can be used to increase platelet aggregation in patients with chronic renal failure and in acquired von Willebrand disease which occurs with aortic stenosis or left ventricular–assist devices (LVADs). In patients without pre-existing platelet abnormalities, DDAVP has little effect on blood loss or replacement in CABG patients but may be effective in open-chamber surgery.

> **CLINICAL PEARL** DDAVP can improve clot formation and platelet function in patients having aortic valve surgery and in patients with LV-assist devices having heart transplants.

4. Plasma, fibrinogen concentrates or cryoprecipitate should be available if indicated for the treatment of appropriate factor deficiencies.
5. Factor concentrates (specifically rVIIA and prothrombin complex concentrates [PCCs]) have been used in cases of severe refractory bleeding. Possible complications are related to increased risk of thrombosis (coronary occlusion, graft occlusion, stroke).

G. **Ventilation**
1. Adequate oxygenation and ventilation while the patient is on CPB must be ensured by checking arterial and venous blood gas measurements at routine intervals. Arterial pH should be between 7.3 and 7.5 at normothermia before CPB separation.
2. The lungs should be reexpanded with two to three sustained breaths to a peak pressure of 30 cm H_2O with visual confirmation of bilateral lung expansion and resolution of atelectasis. In patients with internal mammary artery grafts, care must be taken to prevent lung overdistention, which may cause graft avulsion. Coordinate this maneuver with the surgical team. An estimate of lung compliance should be made (see Section VII). The surgeon may need to evacuate any hemothorax or pneumothorax.
3. Inspired oxygen fraction (FiO_2) should be 100%. If air was used during CPB to prevent atelectasis, it should be discontinued. Nitrous oxide should never be used during or after cannulation, because it can increase the size of air emboli [5].
4. Confirm that the pulse oximeter is working once pulsatile flow returns. Pulse oximeter probes (especially on fingers) may not work, however, despite pulsatile flow in a patient who is still cold and peripherally vasoconstricted.
5. All respiratory monitors should be on-line (apnea, peak inspiratory pressure [PIP], FiO_2, end-tidal CO_2 [$ETCO_2$]).
6. Mechanical ventilation must be started before an attempt to terminate CPB. The timing for commencement of mechanical ventilation while the patient is still on CPB remains controversial. Some practitioners believe that ventilation should begin when arterial or pulmonary pulsatile blood flow resumes in order to avoid hypoxemia. However, this may not be necessary in normothermic, nearly full-flow bypass and may cause severe respiratory alkalosis of pulmonary venous blood. The pulse oximeter or the CPB circuit venous oxygen tension also can be used to assess the need for ventilation during partial CPB.
7. Auscultation of breath sounds will confirm air movement and may reveal wheezing, rales, or rhonchi. Visual confirmation of bilateral lung expansion is important. Appropriate treatment (suctioning, bronchodilators) should be instituted before terminating CPB. Bronchoscopy may occasionally be needed for mucus plugging in patients with lung disease.

H. **Vaporizer**
Inhalation agents used during CPB for blood pressure (BP) control ordinarily should be turned down or off at least 10 minutes before terminating CPB. These agents will decrease contractility and confuse the etiology of myocardial dysfunction postbypass.

I. **Volume expanders**
Albumin or crystalloid solutions should be available to increase preload if blood products are not indicated.

J. Visualization of the heart

Primarily the right atrium and ventricle are visible from the surgical field. TEE importantly provides a more detailed examination. It is possible to evaluate the following parameters:

1. **Contractility.** An experienced observer can often estimate right ventricle (RV) contractility by just looking at the heart in the chest, but left ventricle (LV) visualization is more limited. Both RV and LV wall-motion abnormalities from ischemia or infarct should be compared to pre-CPB observations.

2. **Distention** of the chambers can be seen with both methods.

3. **Residual air** in left-sided structures (e.g., left atrium [LA], LV, pulmonary veins). TEE imaging during and after ventilation will confirm the location of residual air. Air evacuation maneuvers should be performed prior to termination of bypass to prevent a coronary air event.

4. **Conduction.** Direct observation of the atria and ventricles can often help differentiate arrhythmias, AV dyssynchrony, or pacemaker malfunction more easily than using the electrocardiogram (ECG). TEE visualization of the LA appendage may prove especially helpful in this regard. A four-chamber view is most helpful.

5. **Valvular function** or perivalvular leaks should be identified by TEE before attempting CPB termination so that repair can be accomplished if needed.

K. Predictors and factors contributing to adverse cardiovascular outcome

1. Assess the patient's risk for difficult weaning from CPB. Risk factors that can be identified before terminating CPB include [6]:

    a. Preoperative left ventricular ejection fraction (LVEF) less than 45% or diastolic dysfunction

    b. Renal disease: Increased morbidity and mortality correlates with preoperative creatinine concentration.

    c. Female patient undergoing CABG (tendency for incomplete revascularization due to smaller more diseased coronary arteries)

    d. Elderly patient

    e. Congestive heart failure (usually related to valvular or myocardial dysfunction)

    f. Emergent surgery

        (1) Ongoing ischemia or evolving infarct

        (2) Failed closed intervention (angioplasty/stent/valvuloplasty)

    g. Prolonged CPB duration (≥2 hours)

    h. Inadequate surgical repair

        (1) Incomplete coronary revascularization

            (a) Small vessels (not graftable or poor "runoff")

            (b) Distal disease (especially in diabetic patients)

        (2) Valvular disease

            (a) Valve replacement with very small valve (high transvalvular pressure gradient post-CPB)

            (b) Suboptimal valve repair (residual regurgitation or stenosis)

    i. **Incomplete myocardial preservation during cross-clamping**

        (1) ECG not asystolic (incomplete diastolic arrest)

        (2) Prolonged ventricular fibrillation before cross-clamping

        (3) Warm myocardium

            (a) LV hypertrophy (incomplete cardioplegia)

            (b) High-grade coronary stenoses (no cardioplegia to that area of heart)

            (c) Choice of grafting order (grafts should ideally be performed first in an area of the heart served by a high-grade lesion in the absence of retrograde cardioplegia, so cardioplegia may be infused early)

            (d) Noncoronary collateral flow washing out cardioplegia

            (e) Poor LV venting causing cardiac distention (aortic insufficiency if using anterograde cardioplegia)

            (f) Inadequate topical cooling

            (g) Left-sided superior vena cava with retrograde cardioplegia

    j. Prolonged ventricular failure

    k. Impaired myocardial perfusion before and after cross-clamping

        (1) Sustained low perfusion pressure on CPB (less than 50 mm Hg)

        (2) Ventricular distention

        (3) Emboli (air, clot, particulate)

            (a) From ventriculotomy or improper deairing of coronary grafts

  2. **Additional preparations for high-risk patients**

    a. One common practice is to have a syringe of ephedrine (5 mg/mL) or dilute epinephrine prepared (4 to 10 μg/mL). Boluses can be used until a decision is made regarding the need for further inotropes.

    b. Discuss the need for additional invasive monitoring with the surgeon (i.e., LA or central aortic catheter).

    c. Check for immediate availability of other inotropic or vasoactive medications: epinephrine, dobutamine, milrinone, norepinephrine, vasopressin, nitric oxide (NO), or inhaled epoprostenol (Flolan).

    d. As appropriate to the anticipated level of difficulty separating from CPB, check for immediate availability of an intra-aortic balloon pump (IABP). Consider placement of a femoral arterial catheter prebypass to facilitate its rapid insertion and possibly for improved BP monitoring.

    e. Consider starting an inotropic infusion or an IABP before terminating CPB in patients with poor contractility. Note that the Frank–Starling law implies that an empty heart will not beat very forcefully. Often a sluggishly contracting heart will start to "snap" once it is filled.

    f. **"The first attempt at terminating CPB is the best one."** Optimizing all CVP mnemonic parameters before CPB termination is strongly advised. If in doubt, start an inotrope. Preemptive use of milrinone has been shown to improve cardiac function during and after cardiac surgery. A milrinone bolus without an infusion can be sufficient in marginal candidates [7].

    g. **Ischemic preconditioning/postconditioning.** The heart will react to a low level ischemic stress and subsequent exposure to free radicals by becoming more "resistant" to further ischemic injury. This can be attempted intraoperatively [8,9].

        (1) Inhalational agents (isoflurane and sevoflurane have been most studied) can mimic this effect.

            (a) This can be accomplished by using the agent at 1 to 2.5 MAC for 5 to 10 minutes after initiating CPB but before aortic cross-clamping and cardioplegia administration.

            (b) Others suggest using sevoflurane pre-CPB, during CPB, and post-CPB instead of using a propofol infusion [10].

        (2) Ketamine, nicorandil, and the "statins" have also been studied with beneficial results [11].

        (3) Postischemic conditioning by brief sequential ischemia and reperfusion episodes has also been suggested in this setting [12].

L. **Protamine**

The protamine dose should be calculated and drawn up in a syringe or should be ready as an infusion. Premature use of protamine is catastrophic. Protamine should be prominently labeled and should not be placed where routine medications are stored to avoid accidental use. The surgeon, anesthesiologist, and perfusionist must all coordinate the use of this medication.

CLINICAL PEARL Given the potential catastrophic consequences of premature administration of protamine, there should be a team approach such that the surgeon, anesthesiologist, and perfusionist are all made aware via a "time-out" or similar approach so that appropriate steps can be taken by all parties.

M. **Pressure**

Check the zeroing and level of all transducers before terminating CPB.

1. **Arterial pressure.** Recognize that radial artery catheters may underestimate central aortic pressure following rewarming [13]. In the absence of aortoiliac occlusive disease, femoral artery catheters do not share this limitation. An aortic root vent, if present, may be connected to a transducer also. If the radial arterial catheter is not functioning, a needle placed in the aorta or aortic cannula can be transduced during and after termination of CPB until the cannula is removed.

2. **PA pressure.** Ensure that the catheter has not migrated distally to a wedge position. Often the PA catheter must be withdrawn 3 to 5 cm even if this was done at CPB initiation.

N. **Pressors and inotropes**

1. Medications that are likely to be used should be readily available, including a vasodilator (e.g., NTG) and a potent inotropic agent (e.g., dobutamine, epinephrine, milrinone).

2. NTG and phenylephrine should always be available to infuse after CPB as they are commonly used. Some practitioners use prophylactic NTG infusion (approximately 25 to 50 µg/min) for all coronary revascularization procedures to prevent coronary spasm and to enhance noncoronary collateral flow in cases of incomplete revascularization. It also can be used as a venodilator to allow additional CPB pump volume to be infused after CPB.

3. Volumetric infusion pumps deliver vasoactive substances with the highest accuracy and reproducibility.

O. **Pacer**

An external pacemaker should be in the room, checked, and set to the initial settings by the anesthesiologist. A pacemaker often is needed for treatment of relative bradycardia or asystole. In patients with heart block, AV sequential pacing is strongly advised to retain a synchronized atrial contraction. Use of a DDD pacer, when available, is recommended. Temporary biventricular pacing in patients with reduced EF is used in some centers.

P. **Potassium**

Blood chemistries should be checked before terminating CPB.

1. **Hyperkalemia** may induce conduction abnormalities and decreases in contractility. This is more common after long cross-clamp times when large amounts of potassium cardioplegia solution are more likely to be used, and the risk is higher in patients with renal dysfunction.

2. **Hypokalemia** can cause arrhythmias and should be treated if less than 3.5 mEq/L and there is adequate urine output after CPB.

3. **Glucose** levels should be checked and treatment undertaken for hyperglycemia in all patients, not just diabetic patients. Hyperglycemia may contribute to central nervous system dysfunction, poor wound healing, and cardiac morbidity. The optimal glucose level is controversial. Some advocate "aggressive treatment" and suggest a glucose level at or below 110 mg/dL. Most authors try to maintain a level less than 150 mg/mL due to concerns that more aggressive control may lead to complications related to hypoglycemia and possibly higher mortality [14].

4. Ionized Ca^{++} levels are discussed in Section II.C above.

5. Other electrolytes should be evaluated as needed. In particular, low levels of magnesium are common after CPB and have been associated with arrhythmias, coronary vasospasm, and postoperative hypertension. Magnesium (2 to 4 g) can be administered into the pump prior to emergence from CPB [15].

CLINICAL PEARL Magnesium administered into the CPB circuit can increase serum magnesium levels and reduce the need for postoperative magnesium administration, which may cause weakness in a recently extubated patient.

III. **Sequence of events immediately before terminating cardiopulmonary bypass (CPB)**

Weaning from bypass describes the transition from total CPB to a final condition in which the heart provides 100% of the work. The transition should be gradual, recognizing that cardiac function post-CPB is not usually normal. At times, though, cardiac function may improve after bypass if ischemia is relieved or valvular dysfunction repaired.

A. **Final checklist before terminating CPB**
   1. **Confirm**
      a. Ventilation
         (1) Lungs are ventilated with 100% O_2 with visual confirmation, and $ETCO_2$ is present.
         (2) Ventilatory alarms are enabled.
         (3) Pulse oximetry is working. Change in monitoring location (e.g., earlobe or nasal septum) may be necessary.
      b. The patient is sufficiently rewarmed.
      c. The heart, great vessels, and grafts have been properly deaired.
      d. The patient is in optimal metabolic condition.
      e. All equipment and medications are ready.
   2. Do not proceed until these criteria have been met.
   3. Weaning from CPB requires utmost concentration and vigilance by the anesthesiologist, and all distractions should be eliminated. **Turn the music down and limit extraneous conversations.**

B. **What to look at during weaning**
   Key information can be obtained from four sources: the invasive pressure display, the heart itself, the TEE, and the ECG.
   1. **Invasive pressure display**
      a. Pressure waveforms (arterial, central venous pressure [CVP], and PA or LA, if used) are best displayed using overlapping traces. Advantages of this display format include the following:
         (1) Coronary perfusion pressure is graphically depicted as the vertical height between the arterial diastolic pressure and the filling pressure (PA diastolic or LA mean) during diastole.
         (2) The vertical separation between the PA mean and CVP waveforms estimates RV work.
         (3) The slope of the rise in central aortic pressure during systole may give some indication of LV contractility and is most easily appreciated if the waveform is not compressed.
         (4) Valvular regurgitation can be diagnosed by examining CVP, pulmonary capillary wedge pressure (PCWP), or LA waveforms (e.g., mitral regurgitation may produce V waves in LA and PCWP tracings) as well as by TEE.
      b. **Arterial pressure.** The systolic and mean systemic arterial pressures should be checked continuously.
         (1) The systolic pressure describes the pressure generated by the heart's own contraction.
         (2) Before CPB separation, the mean pressure describes the work performed by the bypass pump and the vascular tone. After separation, it reflects the cardiac work and vascular tone. SVR can be easily calculated on pump, mean arterial pressure (MAP)/flow, prior to separation.
         (3) The diastolic pressure reflects vascular tone and gives an indication of coronary perfusion pressure.
         (4) The pulse pressure reflects the mechanical work done by the heart. As the heart assumes more of the circulatory work, this pressure difference increases. LV failure is suggested by a decreased pulse pressure.
         (5) Difficulty in weaning (poor LV function) may be reflected by a low pulse pressure or systolic minus mean pressure difference in the presence of high atrial filling pressures when the venous return line is partially occluded.
         (6) It is important to remember that a radial artery catheter may not be accurate following CPB. During the first 30 minutes after CPB, the radial artery tends to underestimate both the systolic and mean central aortic pressures. The surgeon

can often confirm that there is a pressure difference by palpating the aorta. Clinically significant radial artery hypotension should be confirmed by a noninvasive BP reading or with a central aortic or femoral artery pressure measurement before treatment or resumption of CPB.

   c. **CVP.** This provides an index of right heart filling before and during weaning. High CVP suggests right heart dysfunction secondary to poor myocardial protection or pulmonary hypertension.

   d. **PA pressures.** When pulmonary vascular resistance (PVR) is normal, PA diastolic pressure (PADP) can give a good indication of left heart filling pressure with volume confirmed by TEE. Pulmonary hypertension usually indicates elevated PVR and RV afterload. This needs to be treated when the RV looks sluggish or is failing. NTG and inhaled NO or epoprostenol may be necessary to treat pulmonary hypertension without decreasing systemic MAP, which best reflects RV perfusion pressure.

     (1) **Inspection of the heart visually or by TEE** provides valuable information about contractility, wall-motion abnormalities, conduction, preload, valvular function, and quality of surgical repair.

     (2) **ECG** changes (e.g., heart block, dysrhythmias, or ischemia occur frequently, mandating frequent examination).

     (3) **TEE.** The midpapillary transverse view is best for obtaining or estimating LVEF, preload, and regional wall-motion abnormalities. The four-chamber view can reveal valvular function and conduction abnormalities.

     (4) **Ventilation and oxygenation.** Routine airway management issues as well as problems in the other major organ systems must not be overlooked. The partial pressure of carbon dioxide ($PaCO_2$) should be kept at or below 40 mm Hg in the post-CPB period. Minor elevations in $PaCO_2$ can increase PVR significantly. This is most important when RV failure is noted.

IV. Sequence of events during weaning from CPB

CLINICAL PEARL   TEE is a valuable tool for real-time assessment of LV filling and function during weaning from CPB.

  A. Step 1: Impeding venous return to the pump

    1. **Consequences of partial venous occlusion.** Slowly the venous line is partially occluded (by the surgeon or perfusionist). This increase in venous line resistance causes right atrial pressure to rise and diverts blood flow through the tricuspid valve into the RV instead of draining into the pump circuit. According to the Frank–Starling law, CO increases as preload rises; as a result, the heart begins to eject blood more forcefully as the heart fills and enlarges.

    2. **Preload.** The amount of venous line occlusion is adjusted carefully to attain and maintain optimal LV end-diastolic volume (LVEDV, or LV preload).

     a. **Estimating preload.** With the use of TEE, LV volume can be assessed in real time. In the absence of TEE, LVEDV can only be estimated from pressures measured by a central venous or PA catheter. With a PA catheter in place, both PADP and PCWP estimate LA pressure (LAP). The relationship of LVEDV to LAP, PCWP, and PADP can be quite variable after bypass secondary to changes in LV diastolic compliance. PVR also affects PADP. Decreased LV compliance is caused by myocardial edema and ischemia. Therefore, PADP, PCWP, and LAP are relatively poor indicators of LVEDV in the post-CPB period.

     b. **Optimal preload** is the lowest value that provides an adequate CO. Preload greater than the optimal value may cause:

      (1) Ventricular distention and increased wall tension (increased myocardial oxygen consumption [MvO_2])

      (2) Decreased coronary perfusion pressure (Coronary perfusion pressure = diastolic BP – LVEDP)

      (3) Excessive or decreased CO, depending on the position on the Starling curve

      (4) Pulmonary edema

  c. Typical weaning filling pressures. For patients with good LV function preoperatively, PCWP of 8 to 12 mm Hg or CVP of 6 to 12 mm Hg often suffices. Abnormal contractility or diastolic stiffness may necessitate much higher filling pressures to achieve adequate filling volumes (20 mm Hg or higher), but in such cases it is imperative to monitor left heart filling by a PA or LA line, or by TEE. Preoperative PADP and CVP can be useful in determining appropriate pressures for weaning.

  d. CVP/LAP ratio. Normally, the CVP is equal or lower than the LAP, which is usually estimated by the PADP (CVP/LAP ratio less than or equal to 1). If the ratio is elevated (greater than 1), this strongly suggests RV dysfunction, and the intraventricular septum may be forced toward the left in diastole, limiting LV filling and CO. This "septal shift" often can be diagnosed by TEE as well. In this situation, termination of CPB may be impossible until the ratio is normalized by improving RV function [16].

B. Step 2: Lowering pump flow into the aorta

  1. Attaining partial bypass. The rise in preload causes the heart to begin to contribute to the CO. This condition is termed partial bypass because the venous blood draining into the right atrium divides into two paths: Some goes into the pump circuit, and some passes through the RV and lungs and is ejected into the aorta by the LV.

    a. Some institutions advocate keeping the patient on partial CPB for several minutes to wash vasoactive substances from the lungs before terminating CPB and to provide a gradual transition to normal RV and LV workloads.

  2. Reduced pump outflow requirement. Because two sources of blood are now supplying the aorta, the amount of arterial blood returned from the pump to the patient can be reduced as native CO increases to maintain total aortic blood flow. Therefore, the perfusionist is able to lower the pump flow rate in increments of 0.5 to 1 L/min, resulting in gradual reductions in pump flow rate while cardiac function and hemodynamics are carefully monitored.

  3. Readjusting venous line resistance. Some adjustment in the venous line resistance may be needed to maintain a constant filling pressure as the heart is given more work to perform. Also, as arterial pump outflow is reduced, less venous inflow is needed to keep the venous reservoir from being pumped dry. Therefore, the venous line clamp can be progressively tightened to achieve the desired increase in preload.

C. Step 3: Terminating bypass

If the heart is generating an adequate systolic pressure (typically 90 to 100 mm Hg for an adult) at an acceptable preload with pump flows of 1 L/min or less, the patient is ready for a trial without CPB, and bypass is terminated. The pump is stopped and the venous cannula is clamped. If hemodynamics are not satisfactory, CPB is reinstituted, and management of cardiovascular decompensation is begun.

V. Sequence of events immediately after terminating CPB

A. Preload: Infusing blood from the pump

If cardiac performance is inadequate, small increases in preload may be beneficial. For adult patients, volume is transferred in 50- to 100-mL increments from the venous pump reservoir to the patient through the aortic cannula. Before volume infusion, the aortic cannula should be inspected for air bubbles within its lumen. Increments of 10 to 50 mL are used in pediatric patients. During volume infusions from the pump, the BP, filling pressure, and heart should be watched closely. Continuous infusion is contraindicated because overdistention of the heart may occur and the oxygenator reservoir may be emptied, thus potentially infusing air into the patient.

  1. The almost instantaneous infusion of volume by the pump allows for evaluation of LV function. One can assume that during the infusion there is no change in SVR. According to the formula

$$BP = CO \times SVR$$

If you make SVR a constant, then:

$$BP = CO$$

    a. An increase in BP with a small volume infusion must indicate an increase in CO.

2. **If BP and CO do not change** with increased preload, the patient probably is at the top (flat part) of the Frank–Starling curve, and further volume infusion is unlikely to provide benefit.

3. **If BP does rise**, the rise is probably due to a rise in CO, and further volume administration may be beneficial. In this manner, the optimal preload can be titrated after CPB. TEE can help assess RV size and function with volume administration.

4. Three factors often contribute to a need to give volume after CPB:

    a. Continued rewarming of peripheral vascular beds results in vasodilation.

    b. Changes in LV diastolic compliance alter optimal filling pressure.

    c. Ongoing bleeding.

B. Measuring cardiac function

1. Before removing the aortic cannula or administering protamine, cardiac function should be assessed, because an adequate BP can occur in the setting of low CO and a high SVR. Cardiac function may be assessed by measuring CO or by TEE. The derived cardiac index (CI) (CO/body surface area) should be calculated. In general, a CI of more than 2 L/min/m^2 should be present to consider permanent termination of CPB, although an index of greater than 2.2 usually is considered "normal." If HR is high, a normal CO can exist despite a low stroke volume. Therefore, a calculation of the stroke volume index (CI/HR) can be useful (normal is greater than 40 mL/beat/m^2).

2. **Measuring patient perfusion.** Signs of adequate tissue perfusion after CPB should be sought. Within the first 5 to 10 minutes after terminating CPB, arterial blood gases and pH should be measured, looking for lactic acidosis or gas exchange abnormalities. Mixed venous oxygen saturation (SvO$_2$) indicates global body O$_2$ supply–demand balance. Urine output indicates adequacy of renal perfusion and normally rises after CPB; lack of such a rise should be evaluated and treated immediately. The ideal perfusion pressure for adequate tissue perfusion should be individualized. Patients with renal insufficiency, cerebrovascular disease, or hypertension may require higher perfusion pressures, although the increased BP may worsen bleeding.

3. **Afterload and aortic impedance.** In the presence of good LV function (and the absence of myocardial ischemia), the anesthesiologist should avoid elevated afterload (as reflected by systolic BP) to prevent excessive stress on the aortic suture lines and to reduce surgical bleeding. In adults, the usual desired range for systolic BP is 100 to 130 mm Hg. With impaired LV function or valvular regurgitation, SVR should be reduced to the lowest level possible while maintaining adequate BP for organ perfusion. Reducing the aortic impedance improves LV ejection and lowers systolic LV wall stress and myocardial O$_2$ demand. Impedance is related to BP and SVR, and lowering SVR can result in increased CO with no change in BP.

C. Removing the cannulas

1. **Venous cannula(s).** The presence of a large cannula(s) in the right atrium or in the vena cava will impair venous return to the heart, and if cardiac function is reasonable, the venous cannula should be removed as soon as possible. Removing the cannula will allow the perfusionist to "reprime" the pump and allow for further volume infusion through the aortic cannula. Typically, the venous cannula(s) are removed prior to the initiation of protamine to prevent contamination of the pump with protamine.

2. **Aortic cannula.** Removal of the aortic cannula should usually wait until at least half of the protamine dose has been infused and cardiovascular stability confirmed.

D. Cardiovascular decompensation

CLINICAL PEARL   RV failure can be diagnosed by TEE or by visual assessment of RV contraction and distention.

1. Refer to Chapter 2 for specific drug pharmacology and doses.
2. Failure of the LV or RV, both of which are recovering from the insult of CPB, together with low SVR are the most common causes of cardiovascular insufficiency during the weaning process.

   a. LV failure

     (1) The differential diagnosis of LV failure after CPB is listed in Table 8.2.

     (2) Treatment of LV failure during weaning from CPB includes:

       (a) Inotropic drug administration. Most commonly epinephrine or milrinone is chosen as a first-line agent, although some institutions advocate the use of dopamine or dobutamine initially. Regardless of choice, a bolus of epinephrine 4 to 10 µg (or alternatively ephedrine 5 to 20 mg) can be given to increase contractility and BP while commencing infusion of an inotrope.

         (i) Epinephrine (>3 mcg/min) or dopamine (>3 mcg/kg/min) may be appropriate if HR is normal and SVR is low or normal.

         (ii) Dobutamine or milrinone may be more appropriate if SVR is increased.

         (iii) Low-dose epinephrine or milrinone may be appropriate if HR is elevated.

         (iv) Dobutamine or dopamine may be more appropriate if HR is low and pacing is not being used.

         (v) Norepinephrine or phenylephrine may be appropriate if SVR is low and CO is normal or elevated.

         (vi) Milrinone will significantly reduce SVR, so the use of an arterial vasoconstrictor (phenylephrine, norepinephrine, or vasopressin) often is necessary.

         (vii) In the setting of post-CPB hypocalcemia, calcium can be an excellent inotrope (and vasoconstrictor).

       (b) Start NTG if ischemia is present (also consider use of short-acting β-blockers).

   b. RV failure

     (1) Diagnosis

       (a) Active pumping by the RV is mandatory for optimal cardiovascular function, particularly in the presence of elevated PA pressures.

       (b) TEE can be particularly useful in the detection of RV failure. The RV will appear distended and hypocontractile.

       (c) The RV can be directly visualized over the drape when a sternotomy has been performed. Function and volume of the RV can be assessed by the surgical and anesthesiology teams in this way.

       (d) **Patients most at risk include those with**

         (i) Pulmonary hypertension

           (a) Chronic mitral valve disease

           (b) Left-to-right shunts (atrial septal defect, ventricular septal defect)

           (c) Massive pulmonary embolism

           (d) Air embolism

           (e) Primary pulmonary hypertension

           (f) Acute or chronic mitral regurgitation
- Valvular dysfunction
- Papillary muscle rupture

           (g) Diastolic LV dysfunction

         (ii) RV ischemia or infarct or poor myocardial protection

         (iii) RV outflow obstruction

         (iv) Tricuspid regurgitation

       (e) Physiologic findings

         (i) Depressed CI.

         (ii) Inappropriate elevation in CVP compared to PCWP (unless biventricular failure exists).

TABLE 8.2 Differential diagnosis of LV failure after CPB

I. Ischemia
   A. Graft failure
       1. Clot, particulate in graft
       2. Distal suture causing constriction
       3. Kinking of graft
       4. Air in graft
       5. Graft sewn in backward (no flow through valves)
       6. Inadequate flow through internal mammary artery
   B. Inadequate coronary blood flow
       1. Incomplete revascularization (secondary to distal disease or inoperable vessels)
       2. Inadequate coronary perfusion pressure
       3. Emboli in native coronary arteries—air or particulate matter (clot, atherosclerotic plaque)
       4. Coronary artery spasm
       5. Tachycardia (decreased diastolic filling time)
       6. Increased myocardial O_2 demand
       7. Surgical injury to native coronary artery
   C. Myocardial ischemia leading to myocardial damage
       1. Incomplete myocardial preservation during CPB
       2. Evolving myocardial infarction
II. Valve failure
   A. Prosthetic valve
       1. Sewn in backward
       2. Perivalvular leak
       3. Mechanical obstruction (immobile disk)
   B. Native valve—acute mitral regurgitation (papillary muscle ischemia or rupture)
III. Inadequate gas exchange
   A. Hypoxemia
       1. Inadequate Fio_2
       2. Residual atelectasis
       3. Mechanical ventilator failure
       4. Airway disconnection
       5. Severe bronchospasm
       6. Pulmonary edema ("pump lung" or ARDS)
   B. Hypoventilation
IV. Preload
   A. Inadequate preload
       1. Hypovolemia
       2. Loss of atrial contraction (loss of sinus rhythm)
   B. Excessive preload (can lead to distention of cardiac structures)
V. Reperfusion injury
VI. Ventricular septal defect
VII. Miscellaneous causes of decreased contractility
   A. Medications
       1. β-Blockade
       2. Calcium channel blockers
       3. Inhalational agents
   B. Acidemia
   C. Electrolyte abnormalities
       1. Hyperkalemia
       2. Hypocalcemia
   D. Pre-existing LV failure

CPB, cardiopulmonary bypass; LV, left ventricular; ARDS, adult respiratory distress syndrome.

(iii) Increased PVR (more than 2.5 Wood units or greater than 200 dynes sec/cm^5; contributes to RV failure, but does not result from it).

(iv) **Pulmonary hypertension; leads to RV failure, but true RV failure results in high CVP with low PA pressures.**

> **CLINICAL PEARL** Pulmonary hypertension can cause RV failure. However, good RV function and increases in CO can also increase PA pressures.

(v) Increase in CVP relative to PA pressure is a sign of RV failure.

c. **Treatment** [17]

(1) Treat signs of ischemia (e.g., inferior ST changes, regional RV wall-motion disturbance).

(a) Start NTG infusion if systemic BP permits.

(b) Increase coronary perfusion pressure by increasing systemic diastolic pressure with a vasopressor.

(2) Increased preload usually is required but must be judicious in the setting of RV failure.

(3) Increase inotropic support. Milrinone, dobutamine, and isoproterenol are often effective because any of these will increase RV contractility and decrease PVR.

(4) Use adjuncts to decrease PVR [18].

(a) Hyperventilation will induce hypocapnia and decrease PVR. This should be accomplished by means of a high respiratory rate rather than an increase in inflation pressure, which may increase PVR.

(b) Avoid hypoxemia, which will induce pulmonary vasoconstriction.

(c) Avoid acidemia.

(d) Maintain normal core temperature.

(e) Use pulmonary vasodilators (NTG, nitroprusside, epoprostenol [Flolan]) [19].

(5) Administer NO by inhalation (10 to 40 ppm). Prostaglandin E_1 prostacyclin (PGE$_1$—epoprostenol) by inhalation. The benefit of inhaled (rather than intravenous [IV]) pulmonary vasodilators is that well-ventilated areas will have the most vasodilation, which improves V/Q matching.

(6) Use an RV-assist device.

E. **Inappropriate vasodilation**

Inappropriate vasodilation may prevent achievement of an adequate BP despite an acceptable or elevated CI.

1. Causes include:

a. Pre-existing medications (calcium channel blockers, angiotensin-converting enzyme [ACE] inhibitors)

b. Electrolyte abnormalities

c. Acid–base disturbances

d. Sepsis

e. Pre-existing diseases (chronic hepatic or renal disease)

f. Hyperthermia

g. Idiopathic condition (poorly characterized factors related to CPB)

2. Excessive hemodilution (e.g., Hgb concentration 7 g/dL or lower) decreases viscosity and lowers the apparent SVR.

3. Management includes vasoconstrictors (e.g., phenylephrine, vasopressin, or norepinephrine) and red blood cell (RBC) transfusion when appropriate.

4. **Vasoplegic syndrome** is a severe form of post-CPB dilation characterized by low MAP, normal to high CO, normal right-sided filling pressures, and low SVR which is refractory to pressor therapy. Pre-CPB risk factors include higher patient EuroSCORE, preoperative use of β-blockers and ACE inhibitors, pre-CPB hypotension, and pressor use. Unexpected hypotension after starting CPB may predict this syndrome [20]. The syndrome is associated

with an increased overall mortality. Frequently increasing concentrations of norepinephrine or norepinephrine combined with vasopressin are used to treat this syndrome. However, high doses of norepinephrine may compromise organ perfusion [21]. NO inhibition with methylene blue has been used as salvage therapy in these cases. A dose of 2 mg/kg can be given over 20 minutes. Methylene blue is an inhibitor of monoamine oxidase (MAO), and therefore should not be given to patients who are on MAO inhibitors or selective serotonin reuptake inhibitors due to the risk of inducing serotonin syndrome [22].

F. Resumption of CPB

  1. The decision to resume CPB after a trial of native circulation should not be taken lightly, because there are potential dangers to resuming CPB (inadequate heparinization, hemolysis, worsening coagulopathy, and vasoplegia after a second bypass run). Nevertheless, CPB must be restarted before permanent ischemic organ damage occurs (heart, brain, kidneys). TEE can rapidly facilitate diagnosis and treatment of common problems such as inadequate preload, thereby potentially preventing resumption of CPB. If severe cardiovascular derangements continue for a prolonged period, reinstitution of CPB is indicated. While the patient is on CPB, diagnosis and treatment should continue but may proceed without markedly increasing the risk of organ failure.

  a. A variation on this theme is rapid return to full CPB after an unpromising weaning effort or a very brief but unreassuring trial of native circulation. This can enable institution of appropriate pharmacologic or mechanical support with less immediacy and drama.

  2. Heparin should be given as needed based on the last activated clotting time measurement made while the patient was on CPB. If any protamine was given, a full dose of heparin, 300 to 400 units/kg, is needed before resuming CPB.

  3. During the period that it takes to reestablish CPB, it is important to maintain coronary and cerebral perfusion with inotropes and vasopressors. In extreme circumstances, it may be necessary for the surgical assistant to initiate open-chest massage if the cannulas were already removed.

  4. When CPB is reinitiated, consideration should be given to discontinuation of inotropes and vasopressors, because patients in this situation may become hypertensive. If BP elevation is marked, the perfusionist can lower pump flow briefly while appropriate vasodilator therapy is given or until such time as the effect of these pressors remits (typically less than 5 minutes). Resumption of extracorporeal circulation importantly lowers myocardial oxygen requirements. Maintenance of a reasonable perfusion pressure is critical to allow adequate O_2 delivery to potentially ischemic cells. If MAP is inadequate (e.g., <60 mm Hg), this should be achieved with a pure α-agent such as phenylephrine. Despite lower O_2 requirements and adequate supply, the ischemic cell may not be able to utilize O_2 efficiently. If this is thought to be the case, the use of secondary cardioplegia should be considered.

  5. Additional recovery and reversal of damage can occur if the heart is rearrested with warm-blood–enriched cardioplegia for a brief period.

  6. Any mechanical factors that could compromise cardiac performance must be sought and surgically corrected.

  a. Ongoing ischemia based on ECG changes or TEE wall-motion abnormalities may indicate graft occlusion and may require surgical reevaluation for graft patency. A Doppler probe can be used to assess flow.

  b. Valvular abnormalities can be assessed by TEE. Perivalvular leaks, prosthetic valve malfunction, or residual stenosis/regurgitation should be assessed.

  7. Unsuccessful weaning may necessitate the addition of more aggressive inotropic support. Additional myocardial reperfusion time on CPB may also circumvent or reduce this need.

  8. Additional monitoring. LAP is a better estimate of left ventricular end diastolic pressure (LVEDP) than PA pressures. Aortic or femoral arterial pressures may be more accurate than radial arterial pressures. TEE or epicardial echocardiography can provide valuable data on function and filling.

9. Consideration of separation from bypass should be made only after the surgeon is assured that technical difficulties did not account for impaired myocardial performance and that the heart is "adequately rested." If the second attempt to wean is unsuccessful, continue to optimize preload and afterload with vasodilators or volume infusion as needed.

   a. **IABP** will augment diastolic BP, increase coronary perfusion, and decrease afterload, and should be considered. It is relatively contraindicated in thoracic aortic surgery or in the presence of mobile atheroma in the aorta seen on TEE.

   b. Chest closure may adversely affect hemodynamics (see Section V.E).

   c. If available, ventricular-assist devices or extracorporeal membrane oxygenation (ECMO) can be life-saving after failed attempts to separate the patient from CPB. These are generally used either to rest the "stunned myocardium" or as a bridge to heart transplantation (see Chapter 22).

VI. Cardiovascular considerations after successful weaning from CPB

The post-CPB period represents a time in which the myocardium is recovering from the insult of surgery, CPB, and its attendant inflammatory effects. During this period, major physiologic and surgical changes occur that need to be understood in order to develop proper therapeutic approaches.

A. Reperfusion injury

Reperfusion injury describes a series of functional, structural, and metabolic alterations that result from reperfusion of myocardium after a period of temporary ischemia. The potential for this type of injury exists for all cardiac procedures where the aorta is clamped. The damage is characterized by:

1. Cytosolic accumulation of calcium

2. Marked cell swelling (myocardial edema), which decreases postischemic blood flow and ventricular compliance

3. Generation of free radicals resulting from reintroduction of O_2 during reperfusion. These oxygen free radicals can cause membrane damage by lipid peroxidation. Various strategies are used to minimize injury, including reoxygenation with warm blood to start aerobic metabolism as well as other evolving strategies [23].

B. Decannulation

When the patient is hemodynamically stable after separation from CPB, the venous cannula(s) is (are) removed. Blood loss and atrial dysrhythmias are the most common complications during repair of the atrial cannula site. After infusion of the appropriate volume of blood from the pump, the aortic cannula is clamped and removed. To minimize blood loss and prevent possible aortic disruption, the BP is frequently lowered (systolic pressure usually less than 100 mm Hg) to reduce tension on the aortic wall. If, during aortic cannula removal, there is significant blood loss resulting in hemodynamic deterioration, a cannula may quickly be reinserted into the right atrium and the appropriate volume infused to achieve stability. Protamine administration is usually started prior to aortic cannula removal in case it adversely affects hemodynamics, but most surgeons remove it before its completion owing to the risk for intra-aortic clot and embolism.

C. Manipulation of the heart

The heart often is lifted after bypass to allow examination or repair of the distal anastomotic sites. The sequelae of this action include impaired venous return, atrial and ventricular dysrhythmias, and decreased ventricular ejection; all may result in systemic hypotension. Manipulation such as this should be limited to brief periods in order to avoid hemodynamic deterioration. If the BP drops substantially, a good technique is to simply call out the systolic pressure or MAP, which subtly conveys the need for the surgeon to put the heart back down. If the heart is slow to recover after such maneuvers, there may be a need to limit cardiac manipulation. Overtreatment of these hypotensive episodes with the administration of catecholamine or calcium boluses should be avoided, as it often results in hypertension once manipulation is stopped. Very high BP at this stage can lead to graft disruption and increased bleeding.

D. **Myocardial ischemia**

1. Coronary artery spasm. Ischemia in the postbypass period may derive from spasm of the native coronary arteries or an internal mammary artery graft. This typically manifests as regional wall-motion abnormalities on TEE or as ST-segment elevation, although dysrhythmias, severe hypotension, and cardiac arrest may also occur as sequelae. Mechanisms that have been proposed include intense coronary vasoconstriction from hypothermia, local trauma, respiratory alkalosis, excess sympathetic stimulation of the α-adrenergic receptors on the coronary vessels, release of vasoconstricting agents from platelets (thromboxane), and injury to native vascular endothelium with the loss of endogenous vascular relaxing factors (i.e., endothelium-derived relaxing factor and prostacyclin). Therapeutic modalities that have been used successfully to treat coronary spasm include intracoronary administration of drugs including NTG and papaverine; or systemic administration of NTG, calcium channel blockers (e.g., nicardipine), and other phosphodiesterase inhibitors (milrinone).

2. Mechanical obstruction. Compression of vein or internal mammary artery grafts can produce myocardial ischemia and should be considered. Ventilation with large tidal volumes can intermittently impair internal mammary artery graft flow, and overdistended lung can disrupt the graft at the anastomotic site.

3. Air in grafts. Due to improper deairing of grafts or the LV, air bubbles can impede blood flow through the grafts. Manifestations are typically the same as with other causes of ischemia, including ST-segment changes, regional wall-motion abnormalities on TEE, hypotension, or dysrhythmias. Surgeons can often see air in the coronary arteries to confirm the suspected diagnosis. Primary treatment is to increase coronary perfusion pressure with increased aortic diastolic pressure (e.g., administer a vasopressor), but consideration should also be given to decreasing LVEDP with a vasodilator such as NTG. Myocardial rest with a return to CPB may be needed.

4. Inadequate revascularization. This may result from poor target coronary arteries available to the surgeon to graft or planned combination surgical and percutaneous revascularization (more common with off-pump procedures). Treatment of inadequate or incomplete revascularization is similar to medical therapy for coronary artery disease, including maximizing coronary perfusion pressure and decreasing LVEDP, using vasopressors, vasodilators, and inotropes as needed.

E. **Chest closure**

During chest closure, hemodynamic deterioration may ensue. In general, patients with normal RV and LV function and adequate intravascular volume tolerate closure without problems. Some patients experience mild hypotension and will respond promptly to volume administration. In individuals with poor ventricular function or patients currently receiving inotropic agents, additional volume or inotropic support may be required to maintain similar hemodynamics. If these interventions fail, the surgeon may be required to reopen the chest. TEE can be especially useful to determine the causes of hemodynamic instability, including myocardial ischemia with new wall-motion abnormalities or hypovolemia. Chest closure may cause cardiovascular deterioration for the following reasons:

1. In patients who have significant myocardial edema, closure will impair RV function and venous return.

2. Edematous, overdistended lungs can lead to a tamponade-like effect after closure in patients with severe chronic obstructive lung disease (COPD). Ongoing bronchospasm, low pulmonary compliance, and positive end-expiratory pressure (PEEP) may contribute to this, as may noncompliant chest walls from obesity or advanced age.

3. A source of bleeding not identified before adaptation of the sternal borders can lead to cardiac tamponade.

4. Chest closure may kink a vein or internal mammary artery graft to cause ischemia in the jeopardized area of the myocardium. If these mechanical problems are eliminated and hemodynamics remain compromised, the chest may need to be reopened temporarily. If repeated closure efforts fail, a sterile dressing can be placed to cover the open chest and

the patient brought to the intensive care unit (ICU) in this condition. The chest can then be closed in the future, typically within 24 to 48 hours.

F. **Management of hemodynamics in the postbypass period**

Proper management of patients in the postbypass period involves continuous assessment of five hemodynamic variables as summarized in Figure 8.1. These are preload, rate, rhythm, contractility, and afterload. Although cardiovascular collapse after bypass is uncommon, should it occur, it is most likely that a technical problem (ischemia, valvular dysfunction) or severe metabolic derangement exists. TEE can help make the correct diagnosis. If cardiovascular deterioration is unresponsive to maximal inotropic therapy [24] and no immediately reversible cause can be identified, then reinstitution of CPB will be necessary.

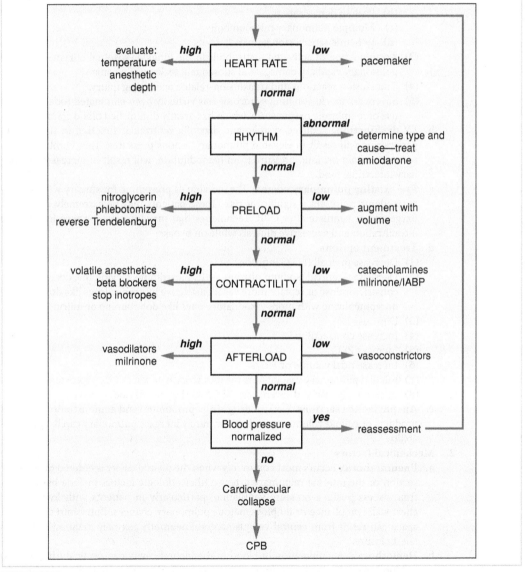

FIGURE 8.1 Management scheme for cardiovascular dysfunction in the postbypass period. CPB, cardiopulmonary bypass; IABP, intra-aortic balloon pump.

VII. Noncardiovascular considerations

A. Respiratory system

1. **Pulmonary edema**

    a. **Post-CPB pulmonary dysfunction.** Originally described in its most severe form as postperfusion lung syndrome ("pump lung"), pulmonary dysfunction after CPB is a common event. The alveolar–arterial (A–a) O_2 gradient increases after bypass and becomes greatest at approximately 18 to 48 hours postoperatively. The etiology of this ventilation–perfusion mismatch is presumed to be multifactorial, ultimately leading to an increase in noncardiogenic pulmonary interstitial fluid and resultant hypoxemia and possibly hypercapnia as well. Etiologic factors include:

        (1) Prolonged atelectasis and subsequent loss of surfactant

        (2) Hypoxic damage to lung tissue, and pulmonary vasculitis caused by:

            (a) Hemolyzed blood

            (b) Protein denaturation

            (c) Multiple pulmonary microemboli

            (d) Ischemic reperfusion injury

        (3) Accumulation of activated neutrophils in the lungs. Lysosomal enzymes produce pulmonary capillary damage and subsequent leakage of plasma.

        (4) Transfusion reactions and transfusion-related acute lung injury.

        (5) Severe postperfusion lung syndrome has virtually been eliminated today with the use of membrane oxygenators, which has greatly diminished blood trauma.

    b. **LV dysfunction.** Reduced systolic and diastolic ventricular function in the postbypass period will result in elevated pulmonary venous pressures. This, combined with reduced colloid osmotic pressure from hemodilution, will result in increased pulmonary interstitial fluid.

    c. **Pre-existing pulmonary edema.** The individuals presenting for surgery with pulmonary edema represent a significant risk. These patients may be extremely difficult to oxygenate or ventilate after CPB. Techniques that may improve oxygenation include ultrafiltration and aggressive diuresis while on bypass.

    d. **Treatment options**

        (1) Decrease preload (NTG infusion)

        (2) Decrease afterload (sodium nitroprusside, nicardipine, clevidipine, decrease vasoconstrictor dose or replace more vasoconstrictive inotropic drugs like dopamine or norepinephrine with more vasodilatory ones like dobutamine or milrinone).

        (3) Diuresis

        (4) Increase contractility

        (5) Increase PEEP

        (6) Increase tidal volume or Fio_2

        (7) Inhaled pulmonary vasodilators for refractory hypoxia (NO, epoprostenol)

        (8) In extremely rare and severe cases, ECMO therapy may be necessary.

    e. **Anaphylactic reactions.** Certain drugs (e.g., protamine) and administration of blood products or colloid volume expanders may rarely increase pulmonary capillary permeability.

2. **Mechanical factors**

    a. **Pneumothorax** occurs most commonly when the pleural cavity is entered during dissection of the internal mammary artery. Other etiologic factors include barotrauma from excess positive-pressure ventilation, particularly in patients with low lung or chest wall compliance or emphysematous pulmonary changes. Entry into the pleural space can result from central venous access. Pneumothorax may manifest only after chest closure.

    b. **Hemothorax.** Accumulation of blood in the pleural cavity can occur during bypass, as blood from the mediastinum frequently overfills the pericardial "sling." It also may occur with dissection of the internal mammary artery before administration of heparin, which results in the collection of clot in the pleural space. The pleural space can be inspected with TEE and visually in the surgical field, and adequate removal of blood and clot is imperative before termination of CPB and before chest closure.

c. **Movement of the endotracheal tube.** Draping the patient for cardiac procedures often obscures part of the head and the endotracheal tube from our direct vision. Even when the endotracheal tube is visible from the head of the operating table, the surgeon may unintentionally push on it in an attempt to gain better exposure, which may displace it. Therefore, it is important to intermittently reconfirm proper positioning by checking all connections, observing bilateral chest movement, and visualizing or auscultating one or both lung fields if the pleural cavities are exposed. Since partial obstruction or disconnection can be subtle, $ETCO_2$ and pulse oximeter monitoring may fail to detect them.

d. **Obstruction of the tracheobronchial tree**

(1) **Mucus plug.** Dry inspissated secretions may accumulate in the tracheobronchial tree or endotracheal tube, and partially or completely obstruct the airway. In most cases, this can be diagnosed and managed by suctioning the airway with a small catheter. It may be necessary to use bronchoscopy to perform guided therapy.

(2) **Blood.** Injury to the upper airway or trachea due to laryngoscopy, placement of an endotracheal tube, or an unrecognized pre-existent airway lesion followed by heparinization may result in aspiration of blood. If significant, this can result in varying degrees of airway obstruction. More likely, however, the blood will be aspirated into the distal airways and alveoli, causing marked ventilation–perfusion mismatch. Blood also may appear in the airway due to perforation of the PA from a PA catheter. Risk factors for catheter-induced PA rupture include surgical manipulation of the heart, advanced patient age, anticoagulation, hypothermia, and pulmonary hypertension.

3. **Increase in dead space**

a. The most common cause is air trapping from bronchospasm but may be related to other factors. The $ETCO_2$ tracing can confirm an obstructive pattern, and the $ETCO_2$–$PaCO_2$ difference increases. In severe cases the gradient may be 15 to 25 mm Hg.

b. **Etiology**

(1) Bronchospasm

(a) Pre-existing asthma or COPD

(b) New onset

(i) Mechanical

(a) Endotracheal tube (carinal irritation)

(b) Secretions or blood

(ii) Chemical

(a) Medications

(b) Histamine release

(c) Inflammation

(d) Allergic/anaphylactoid

(2) Adult respiratory distress syndrome (ARDS)

(3) Transfusion related

(4) Decreased CO

(5) Pulmonary embolus

(a) Thrombus unlikely, but possible after protamine administration

(b) Air entrainment

c. **Treatment for bronchospasm**

(1) **Remove the offending agent**

(2) Inhaled β_2 agonists (albuterol, salmeterol)

(3) Inhaled anticholinergic agents—ipratropium bromide

(4) Epinephrine

(5) Corticosteroids (IV or inhaled)

(6) Consider theophylline in chronic patients

(7) Magnesium

(8) Ventilatory changes (longer expiratory time, lower respiratory rate)

(9) Potent inhalational anesthetic agents if CI is adequate

4. **Intrapulmonary shunt**

a. **Atelectasis.** Perhaps the most common cause of decreased arterial oxygenation post-bypass is atelectasis. Although diffuse, chest radiographs postoperatively frequently reveal a pattern of left lower lobe infiltration and atelectasis. The likely explanation is that application of ice causes temporary phrenic nerve injury with subsequent paralysis of the left diaphragm. During CPB, applying PEEP or even ventilating with low tidal volumes (<200 mL) is associated with higher PaO_2 post-CPB. However, you may be asked to limit ventilation if it impairs surgical exposure. After CPB, recruitment maneuvers with addition of PEEP can be utilized to minimize atelectasis while resuming normal ventilation (6 mL/kg).

b. **Inhibition of hypoxic pulmonary vasoconstriction.** Hypoxic pulmonary vasoconstriction is the mechanism believed to be responsible for the increase in PVR in regions of atelectasis. This protective mechanism can be attenuated or inhibited by the use of vasodilators (nitroprusside, NTG) and inotropes used to improve hemodynamic status.

5. **Intracardiac shunt.** When evaluating hypoxemia after CPB, the possibility of a right-to-left shunt must always be considered. Decreased RV contractility and compliance after CPB, in the presence of increased PVR associated with PEEP, will frequently elevate right atrial pressures above those on the left side. This equalization or reversal of pressure is the mechanism by which a patent foramen is opened. TEE should easily facilitate identification of a new interatrial shunt.

B. **Hematologic system**

Management of the coagulation system and blood conservation is just below cardiovascular stability in terms of priority and decision making during this time period. Blood product management should be a joint decision by the surgical, intensive care, and anesthesia teams based on individual patient needs and guided by available coagulation testing to tailor therapy. Institutional algorithms have been shown to be useful for preventing excessive blood product use in cardiac surgery. Please see Chapters 9 and 21 for detailed discussion of these topics.

C. **Renal system**

1. **Effects of CPB on the kidneys.** Many of the variables introduced with initiation of CPB affect the renal system. Hemodilution and/or hemolysis reduce renal vascular resistance, resulting in increased flow to the outer renal cortex and subsequent enhanced urine flow. Hemolysis also releases free hemoglobin, which can cause renal injury. If systemic hypothermia is used as a form of myocardial protection, renal vascular resistance increases and renal blood flow, glomerular filtration rate, and free water clearance all decrease. During CPB, nonpulsatile flow, decreased perfusion pressure, and embolic phenomena from aortic plaque can also decrease renal blood flow. The decrease is most likely in patients with renal artery stenosis. CPB-induced inflammation can also worsen renal outcome. It is important to prevent this complication, because new-onset renal dysfunction requiring dialysis will increase mortality almost eightfold [25].

2. **Postbypass renal dysfunction.** Certain factors have been identified that place patients at risk for renal dysfunction in the postbypass period. These include elevated preoperative serum creatinine, combined valve and CABG, advanced age, and diabetes. Prolonged bypass times and decreased CI post-CPB place patients at risk.

3. **Management.** Pharmacologic therapy may have some benefit in patients with severe preexisting renal dysfunction or failure. While these therapies may not prevent acute kidney injury (AKI), they can temporize hypervolemia and hyperkalemia. A frequent observation is that urine flow is diminished during bypass compared with the individuals who have normal renal function. Renal insufficiency may result in significant hyperkalemia and accumulation of extracellular fluid.

4. Treatment options include:
    a. Furosemide (initial dose 10 to 20 mg) or mannitol (0.5 to 1 g/kg).
    b. Fenoldopam (0.05 to 0.1 μg/kg/min) will increase renal blood flow and may provide an important therapeutic option. It may cause unacceptable hypotension.
    c. Ultrafiltration can be performed on CPB to remove excess volume.
    d. Despite these interventions, some patients may require dialysis in the early postoperative period.

D. **Central nervous system**
    1. **Anesthetic depth.** The modern assessment of anesthetic depth with the BIS or other monitors may add important information for optimal anesthetic management. In the postbypass period, there are varying levels of surgical stimulation, with the highest being the placement of sternal wires and chest closure. If an increase in depth of anesthesia is needed, the choice of agent(s) will depend primarily on the patient's hemodynamic status.
    2. **Small doses of opioids or benzodiazepines** can be titrated incrementally in patients with stable hemodynamics. Additionally, the judicious use of a volatile agent may be considered, particularly in patients who are hypertensive with a reasonable CI.
    3. Many anesthesiologists are using a propofol infusion with good results after CPB. The infusion can be started upon rewarming and continue until and through the initial ICU stay. An infusion of 25 to 50 μg/kg/min is usually acceptable but can be titrated as indicated. Another alternative is dexmedetomidine, starting at doses of 0.2 to 0.5 μg/kg/hr, again titrating as indicated.
    4. It must be remembered that all patients have some degree of postbypass ventricular dysfunction. Even small doses of narcotics and propofol have the potential to cause adverse hemodynamic consequences.
    5. **Neuromuscular blockade.** Patients frequently require additional neuromuscular relaxation in the postbypass period. The main objective is to prevent shivering, which can increase O_2 consumption by as much as 500%. Frequent monitoring of the train of four is necessary. Renal and hepatic functions can deteriorate in the face of cardiovascular compromise, which can be a consideration in the choice or dosing of neuromuscular blocking agent (e.g., rocuronium vs. cisatracurium). Temperature changes, blood loss, cardiac function, and adjuvant medications can also affect the pharmacokinetics and plasma levels of neuromuscular relaxants.
    6. Fast-track protocols in some hospitals allow for muscle relaxant reversal in the operating room (OR) or after admission to the ICU. The cardiovascular side effects of reversal, such as HR changes, should be anticipated.

E. **Metabolic considerations**
    1. **Electrolyte disturbances**
        a. **Hypokalemia** is a relatively common electrolyte abnormality in the postbypass period. Although the etiologic factors are numerous, only those unique to bypass will be mentioned. The kidney represents a major source of potassium loss. Both the preoperative and intraoperative use of diuretics, including mannitol administration, promotes significant potassium wasting. Glucose may be administered as a myocardial substrate during bypass. If significant hyperglycemia occurs, an osmotic diuresis with potassium loss will ensue. Hypokalemia may also result from the shift of potassium to the intracellular space. Such a shift may occur with alkalemia from either hyperventilation or excess bicarbonate administration, and with concomitant administration of insulin in a diabetic patient.

        In addition, the use of inotropes capable of stimulating β_2-adrenergic receptors will promote an intracellular shift of potassium. Treatment will vary depending on the severity of hypokalemia. Commonly, potassium levels tend to rise modestly without treatment due to redistribution and blood product administration. In most instances, IV administration at rates up to 10 mEq/hr (in adults) will be effective. In life-threatening situations, potassium may be administered at a rate up to 20 mEq/hr with continuous cardiac monitoring. **Adequate renal function**, initially assessed by urine output, should be confirmed prior to initiating potassium replacement.

TABLE 8.3   Treatment of hyperkalemia

1. Diuresis-loop diuretic (furosemide 10–40 mg), higher doses if patient on chronic therapy
2. Sodium bicarbonate, 1–2 mEq/kg in children and one ampule (50 mEq) in adults
3. Infusion of dextrose and insulin, 1–2 g glucose per kilogram with 0.3 units regular insulin per gram of glucose in children; 25 g (1 ampule of D50) of glucose and 10 units of regular insulin in adults
4. Calcium, 20 mg/kg of calcium gluconate over a 5-min period for children and 5–10 mg/kg of calcium chloride for adults

    b. Hyperkalemia occurs uncommonly after bypass. In most cases, hyperkalemia occurs when large doses of cardioplegic agents are administered, particularly in patients with impaired renal function. Hyperkalemia may persist in the postbypass period but generally resolves spontaneously without intervention. Depending on the cardiac rhythm, moderate hyperkalemia (potassium levels between 6 and 7 mEq/L) may require therapy with one of the treatment modalities listed in Table 8.3. With severe hyperkalemia (potassium levels greater than 7 mEq/L), therapeutic interventions will be needed.

    c. Hypocalcemia can occur after bypass. Common etiologic factors include hemodilution from the pump prime, particularly in children; acute alkalemia; and calcium sequestration from blood product administration. Alkalemia that occurs with hyperventilation or rapid administration of parenteral bicarbonate enhances calcium binding to protein. Sequestration of calcium occurs with administration of a large volume of blood that contains the chelating agent citrate. Severe hypocalcemia results in myocardial depression and vasodilation.

        (1) Calcium administration after CPB is indicated in the presence of severe hyperkalemia or in cases of hypotension associated with low serum ionized calcium. Calcium may be administered as 10% $CaCl_2$ (272 mg of elemental calcium) in a dose of 5 to 10 mg/kg. The typical adult dose is 500 to 1,000 mg. Calcium gluconate in incremental doses of 10 mg/kg may also be used.

    d. Hypomagnesemia commonly occurs in patients undergoing cardiac surgery. England et al. suggested that large quantities of magnesium-free fluids with subsequent hemodilution most likely contribute to this observation [15]. Other etiologic factors include loss of the cation in the extracorporeal circuit and redistribution of magnesium to other body stores. In a randomized, controlled trial (patients in the treatment group receiving 2 g of magnesium chloride after termination of CPB), magnesium-treated patients had a lower incidence of postoperative ventricular dysrhythmias and an increased CI in the early postoperative period [15]. Therefore, many centers will give magnesium prior to terminating CPB.

  2. Hyperglycemia. The stress response places all patients at risk for developing hyperglycemia during cardiac surgery [26]. Diabetics, particularly those who are insulin dependent, usually require an intraoperative insulin infusion to maintain glucose hemostasis. Inotropes, particularly epinephrine, may contribute to hyperglycemia after bypass by stimulating hepatic glycogenolysis and gluconeogenesis. The deleterious effects associated with hyperglycemia include: an osmotic diuresis and its attendant electrolyte abnormalities; exacerbation of both focal and global ischemic, neurologic and cardiac injury; and coma (if severe).

F. Postbypass temperature regulation

  1. Hypothermia. All patients who undergo hypothermic CPB experience variable degrees of hypothermia in the postbypass period, with profound effects on the cardiovascular system, particularly in individuals with borderline cardiac reserve. As the temperature decreases, arteriolar tone will increase, resulting in elevated SVR. The hemodynamic consequences include hypertension, decreased CO, and increased MvO_2. If shivering occurs, total body O_2 consumption increases. Coagulopathy is also associated with hypothermia.

  2. Etiology of postbypass hypothermia. Hypothermic CPB causes a vasoconstricted state. During rewarming, many of the peripheral vascular beds (i.e., muscle and subcutaneous fat) may not adequately dilate and therefore can act as a hypothermic reservoir, which will eventually equilibrate with the central circulation. Opening and warming these vascular beds with pharmacologic vasodilation during rewarming may diminish the "after-drop" in core temperature. The decrease in temperature usually reaches its nadir 80 to 90 minutes after bypass.

   3. Prevention and treatment of hypothermia. The most effective way to attenuate postbypass hypothermia is to be assured that effective rewarming occurs during CPB. If circulatory arrest was used, rewarming will be significantly delayed.

   The most effective way to maintain temperature postbypass is the forced-air heater. Underbody techniques are perhaps most useful, because in many cardiac surgical procedures anterior access is limited to the head and neck due to the surgical drapes. Covering the head improves warming. A lower body cover can be used after the vein sites are dressed if necessary. Other techniques that have been suggested to attenuate hypothermia include heating inspired gases, use of an IV fluid warmer, increasing ambient temperature, and using warm irrigation fluids in the chest cavity and warming blankets. The contribution of these techniques to either postbypass hypothermia prevention or to active rewarming is likely to be minor, but they may aid in maintaining the patient's temperature until he or she leaves the OR.

   4. Hyperthermia should be avoided, since it will exacerbate cerebral ischemic injury, during either aggressive warming on CPB, after CPB, or in the ICU. The core or nasopharyngeal temperature should not exceed 37°C.

VIII. **Preparing for transport**

   A. **Moving the patient to the transport or intensive care unit (ICU) bed in the operating room (OR)**

   After the chest is closed and all dressings are applied, the patient must be moved to the transport bed. This requires a coordinated effort to minimize the risk of complications. Monitor lines can be lost, inotropic support disconnected, and ventilation can be interrupted with devastating consequences during this seemingly easy process. There is a lapse in cardiovascular monitoring during transfer to a mobile or transport monitor. Disconnect monitoring devices sequentially, so there is an "active" monitor to assess the patient at all times.

   1. Complications of transfer

   a. Tracheal extubation

   b. Coronary air embolism from bubble dislodgement (after open cardiac procedures) leading to ischemia or ventricular fibrillation

   c. Arterial line or PA catheter removal

   d. IABP line disruption

   e. Pacemaker wire dislocation or disconnection

   f. Loss of IV lines

   g. Monitors (pulse oximeter probe, ECG lead) pulled off

   h. Patient fall

   i. Corneal injury (e.g., from wires, tubing)

   j. Loss of vasoactive or inotrope infusions

   k. Chest tube or urinary catheter dislodgement

   l. Venodilation with resultant hypotension

   m. Loss of O_2 supply (empty O_2 tank)

   n. Inadequate manual ventilation (observe for adequate chest wall expansion)

   B. **Transport to the ICU**

   Emergency equipment and medications must be collected prior to transport. The type of equipment necessary is related to the distance traveled. A move 5 floors away from the OR is much different than one 50 ft away. See Table 8.4 for a suggested list of equipment/medications. Murphy's law is in play here. There are case reports of cardiac arrest and extubation in compromising situations. We have experienced an IABP failure in an elevator with adverse consequences. The patient must be monitored and adequate ventilation ensured during transport no matter the distance transported. Minimum monitoring requirements include: ECG, arterial line, and pulse oximetry.

   Fast-tracking (early extubation) approaches are discussed in Chapter 25. In highly selected patients, such as patients with atrial septal defect repairs and off-pump single-vessel bypass

TABLE 8.4 Suggested emergency equipment for transport
■ **Airway equipment**
Endotracheal tube
Laryngoscope blades
Tube changer/stylet (optional)
Bag/valve/mask device
Oxygen tank
PEEP valve (not optional if PEEP 10 cm H$_2$O or higher)
■ **Medications**
Phenylephrine for bolus
Ephedrine or epinephrine (4 μg/mL)
Epinephrine (1 mg) vial if unstable
Atropine
Muscle relaxant of choice
Succinylcholine
Narcotic of choice
■ **Personnel**
Trained personnel to monitor/troubleshoot IABP or LVAD/RVAD
Adequate personnel to attend to IV poles and bed movement

PEEP, positive end-expiratory pressure; IABP, intra-aortic balloon pump; LVAD, left ventricular–assist device; RVAD, right ventricular–assist device; IV, intravenous.

grafting which have either short CPB runs or brief ischemic times, some cardiac surgical teams may choose to extubate the trachea in the cardiac OR. Patients with long CPB runs and ischemic times are not good candidates for OR extubation because of potential cardiac and cerebral complications which may not manifest at this time. Our view is that extubation in the OR most often unnecessarily complicates the early postoperative period without patient benefit.

CLINICAL PEARL During transport, bring various syringes with a pressor, an inotrope, and antihypertensive agents, as this can be a time of extreme hemodynamic lability.

C. **Admission to the ICU**

Most institutions will call a standardized report to the ICU prior to transport. This report will document ventilatory settings, inotrope and vasoactive infusions, and vital signs. This information allows time for preparation. Most ICUs will continue to use the infusion bags from the OR. If your infusion volumes are getting low, we recommend replacing them prior to transport, otherwise alert ICU personnel to have replacement medication infusions available prior to leaving the OR. **The loss of a critical inotrope at this juncture can be devastating.**

After the patient is safely transferred to the ICU, permanent monitoring is reinstituted sequentially. Document the pertinent vital signs in the anesthesia record and to whom you gave the report. At this point in time, the anesthesia team knows the most about the patient's physiology. If hemodynamic instability is noted, you are in the best position to provide the treatment of choice. *Take control of the situation.*

When giving the report, give those accepting care of the patient any additional information you feel would help them. For example, you may have seen the CI fall when the PADP was less than 15 mm Hg because of diastolic dysfunction. Let the ICU team know, so they won't have to "reinvent the wheel" and find out for themselves, putting the patient in harm's way.

Continued bleeding during transport can induce hypovolemia and increase fluid requirements. LV dysfunction may improve over time and inotropic support, which is necessary in the OR, may need to be weaned to avoid hypertensive complications. Continue care until you are satisfied that the patient's condition is stable.

REFERENCES

1. Nussmeier NA. Management of temperature during and after cardiac surgery. *Tex Heart Inst J.* 2005;32(4):472–476.
2. Royster RL, Butterworth JF 4th, Prielipp RC, et al. A randomized, blinded, placebo-controlled evaluation of calcium chloride and epinephrine for inotropic support after emergence from cardiopulmonary bypass. *Anesth Analg.* 1992;74(1):3–13.
3. Carroll RC, Chavez JJ, Snider CC, et al. Correlation of perioperative platelet function and coagulation tests with bleeding after cardiopulmonary bypass surgery. *J Lab Clin Med.* 2006;147(4):197–204.
4. Nuttall GA, Henderson N, Quinn M, et al. Excessive bleeding and transfusion in a prior cardiac surgery is associated with excessive bleeding and transfusion in the next surgery. *Anesth Analg.* 2006;102(4):1012–1017.
5. Steinlechner B, Zeidler P, Base E, et al. Patients with severe aortic valve stenosis and impaired platelet function benefit from preoperative desmopressin infusion. *Ann Thorac Surg.* 2011;91(5):1420–1426.
6. **Bernard F, Denault A, Babin D, et al. Diastolic dysfunction is predictive of difficult weaning from cardiopulmonary bypass. *Anesth Analg.* 2001;92(2):291–298.**
7. Kikura M, Sato S. The efficacy of preemptive milrinone or amrinone therapy in patients undergoing coronary artery bypass grafting. *Anesth Analg.* 2002;94(1):22–30.
8. **Riess ML, Stowe DF, Warltier DC. Cardiac pharmacological preconditioning with volatile anesthetics: from bench to bedside? *Am J Physiol Heart Circ Physiol.* 2004;286(5):H1603–H1607.**
9. Cromheecke S, Pepermans V, Hendrickx E, et al. Cardioprotective properties of sevoflurane in patients undergoing aortic valve replacement with cardiopulmonary bypass. *Anesth Analg.* 2006;103(2):289–296.
10. Tsang A, Hausenloy DJ, Yellon DM. Myocardial postconditioning: reperfusion injury revisited. *Am J Physiol Heart Circ Physiol.* 2005;289(1):H2–H7.
11. Zaugg M, Schaub MC, Foëx P. Myocardial injury and its prevention in the perioperative setting. *Br J Anaesthesia.* 2004;93(1):21–33.
12. **Jivraj N, Liew F, Marber M. Ischaemic postconditioning: cardiac protection after the event. *Anaesthesia.* 2015;70(5): 598–612.**
13. Mohr R, Lavee J, Goor DA. Inaccuracy of radial artery pressure measurement after cardiac operations. *J Thorac Cardiovasc Surg.* 1987;94(2):286–290.
14. **NICE-SUGAR Study Investigators; Finfer S, Chittock DR, Su SY, et al. Intensive versus conventional glucose control in critically ill patients. *N Engl J Med.* 2009;360(13):1283–1297.**
15. England MR, Gordon G, Salem M, et al. Magnesium administration and dysrhythmias after cardiac surgery. A placebo-controlled, double blind, randomized trial. *JAMA.* 1992;268(17):2395–2402.
16. Kopman EA, Ferguson TB. Interaction of right and left ventricular filling pressures at the termination of cardiopulmonary bypass. Central venous pressure/pulmonary capillary wedge pressure ratio. *J Thorac Cardiovasc Surg.* 1985;89(5):706–708.
17. Rimeika D, Sanchez-Crespo A, Nyren S, et al. Iloprost inhalation redistributes pulmonary perfusion and decreases arterial oxygenation in healthy volunteers. *Acta Anaesthesiol Scand.* 2009;53(9):1158–1166.
18. **Haj RM, Cinco JE, Mazer CD. Treatment of pulmonary hypertension with selective pulmonary vasodilators. *Curr Opinion Anaesthesiol.* 2006;19(1):88–95.**
19. De Wet CJ, Affleck DG, Jacobsohn E, et al. Inhaled prostacyclin is safe, effective, and affordable in patients with pulmonary hypertension, right heart dysfunction, and refractory hypoxemia after cardiothoracic surgery. *J Thorac Cardiovasc Surg.* 2004;127(4):1058–1067.
20. Levin MA, Lin HM, Castillo JG, et al. Early-on cardiopulmonary bypass hypotension and other factors associated with vasoplegic syndrome. *Circulation.* 2009;120(17):1664–1671.
21. **Hajjar LA, Vincent JL, Barbosa Gomes Galas FR, et al. Vasopressin versus norepinephrine in patients with vasoplegic shock after cardiac surgery. *Anesthesiology.* 2017;126(1):85–93.**
22. Mehaffey JH, Johnston LE, Hawkins RB, et al. Methylene blue for vasoplegic syndrome after cardiac operation: Early administration improves survival. *Ann Thorac Surg.* 2017;104(1):36–41.
23. Chello M, Patti G, Candura D, et al. Effects of atorvastatin on systemic inflammatory response after coronary bypass surgery. *Crit Care Med.* 2006;34(3):660–667.
24. Bailey JM, Levy JH, Hug CC. Cardiac surgical pharmacology. In: Edmunds H, ed. *Adult Cardiac Surgery.* New York: McGraw-Hill; 1997:225–254.
25. Cooper WA, O'Brien SM, Thourani VH, et al. Impact of renal dysfunction on outcomes of coronary artery bypass surgery: results from the Society of Thoracic Surgeons National Adult Cardiac Database. *Circulation.* 2006;113(8):1063–1070.
26. **Reddy P, Duggar B, Butterworth J. Blood glucose management in the patient undergoing cardiac surgery: A review. *World J Cardiol.* 2014;6(11):1209–1217.**

9 Blood Management

Nadia B. Hensley, Megan P. Kostibas, Steven M. Frank, and Colleen G. Koch

KEY POINTS

1. Blood transfusion is the most common procedure performed in US hospitals and has been named one of the top five overused procedures by The Joint Commission.
2. Both anemia and transfusion carry significant risks. Balancing these risks is the key to appropriate blood transfusion decisions.
3. Despite published guidelines, clinical transfusion practice still varies substantially among clinicians and centers and often falls outside recommended guidelines.
4. Transfusion-related acute lung injury (TRALI) is the most frequent cause of mortality from blood transfusion. The second most frequent cause of mortality is transfusion-associated circulatory overload (TACO).
5. Two large hemoglobin trigger trials in cardiac surgery support the use of a restrictive transfusion strategy with hemoglobin triggers of 7.5 to 8 g/dL; no improvement in primary outcomes was attained with higher triggers (9 to 10 g/dL).
6. Red blood cell (RBC) storage duration has been associated with adverse outcomes in retrospective studies; however, recent prospective clinical trials have not shown better outcomes with fresh blood than with standard-issue blood. The oldest blood (35 to 42 days) is still untested.
7. Of all blood components, platelets are associated with the highest risk and cost. Bacterial sepsis is the most common adverse event, given that platelets are stored at room temperature.

"**BLOOD TRANSFUSION IS LIKE MARRIAGE:** *it should not be entered upon lightly, unadvisedly or wantonly or more often than is absolutely necessary.*"

—*R. Beale* [1]

I. Background

Blood transfusion is the most common procedure performed in US hospitals and has been named one of the top five overused procedures by The Joint Commission. Competing risks form the core of perioperative transfusion. Patients face tangible complication risks if hemoglobin values fall too low, and different but equally real risks when exposed to allogeneic blood transfusion. The risks of both anemia and transfusion vary depending on the patient's comorbidities, degree of and ability to tolerate anemia, and surgical procedure. In the dynamic milieu of the operating rooms, clinicians caring for cardiovascular surgical patients encounter challenging transfusion decisions daily. No measures can definitively direct transfusion decisions; rather clinical judgment based on the balance of perceived risks and benefits must guide individual transfusion decisions. Given this background, the substantial variability of transfusion even within a single institution becomes understandable [2,3].

A. **Practice patterns vary widely for transfusion of all three major blood components in cardiac surgery.**

   1. **The wide variation in transfusion practice patterns was highlighted in a nationwide study in 2010. More than 100,000 patients undergoing isolated coronary artery bypass graft surgery were included from almost 800 hospitals** [3]. Such variability often serves as the impetus for evidence-based guidelines that are intended to reconcile disparate evidence.

   2. The most widely cited guideline for transfusion practice in cardiac surgery is the guideline for blood transfusion and blood conservation published jointly by the Society of Thoracic Surgeons (STS) and Society of Cardiovascular Anesthesiologists, which was last updated in 2011 [4].

B. **Patient blood management (PBM) programs**

   1. **PBM programs are somewhat new but are being implemented in many hospitals with the goal of reducing risks, improving outcomes, and lowering costs** [5].

   2. The Society for Advancement of Blood Management defines PBM as "the timely application of evidence-based medical and surgical concepts designed to maintain hemoglobin concentration, optimize hemostasis, and minimize blood loss in an effort to improve patient outcome."

   3. The primary goal of PBM is to reduce unnecessary transfusions. Several methods of blood conservation discussed in this chapter are being effectively utilized in PBM programs.

   4. The Joint Commission, along with AABB (formerly the American Association of Blood Banks), introduced a certification for PBM in 2016. Certification enables hospitals to be recognized for successfully implementing these valuable methods of care that are considered advancements in patient safety and quality.

CLINICAL PEARL   Anemia, bleeding, and transfusion are all associated with adverse outcomes. It is therefore important to treat and prevent anemia, to minimize bleeding, and transfuse blood and blood components according to evidence-based indications.

C. **Complications of transfusion**

   1. Complications of transfusion have always been a major concern, highlighted by the threat of transfusion-transmitted viral infections, such as human immunodeficiency virus (HIV), which peaked in 1983 [6]. Now, with nucleic acid testing for HIV and hepatitis C, the risk for transmission of these viruses is similar to that of dying from an airline crash or lightning strike [7].

   2. The decrease in infection risk has led some to assume that blood is incredibly safe; however, transfusion poses much more common and potentially life-threatening events that should be recognized.

   3. **The Food and Drug Administration's (FDA) summary of fatalities related to transfusion for fiscal year 2015 listed transfusion-related acute lung injury (TRALI) and transfusion-associated circulatory overload (TACO) as the first and second most frequent causes of mortality from transfusion** (Fig. 9.1) [8]. Between 2011 and 2015, 38% of deaths were from TRALI, and 24% were from TACO. Hemolytic transfusion reactions (HTR) caused by non-ABO (14%) and ABO (7.5%) incompatibilities were also causes for mortality, followed by microbial contamination and allergic/anaphylactic reactions.

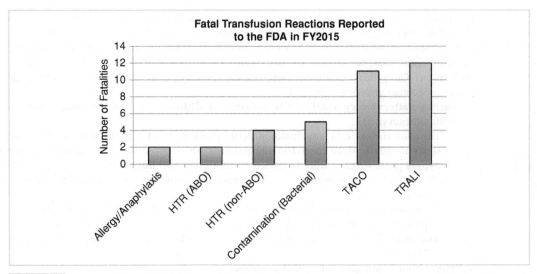

FIGURE 9.1 In a report from the FDA [8], transfusion-related acute lung injury (TRALI) represented the most frequently reported cause of transfusion-related mortality, and transfusion-associated circulatory overload (TACO) was the second most common cause [19]. FDA, Food and Drug Administration; HTR (non-ABO), hemolytic transfusion reactions unrelated to ABO incompatibility; HTR (ABO), hemolytic transfusion reactions related to ABO incompatibility; FY2015, Fiscal Year 2015.

    a. TRALI, which is primarily a clinical diagnosis, can vary from mild to severe. It is defined by the presence of hypoxemia and pulmonary edema on x-ray within 6 hours after transfusion. The purported mechanism for TRALI likely involves human leukocyte antigen (HLA) incompatibility, which triggers a cytokine-mediated inflammatory response in the lungs that looks clinically like a number of pulmonary edema–causing conditions; thus some believe that TRALI is underreported [9,10]. The incidence has been reported as about 1 in 5,000 transfusions; however, recent data from the Mayo Clinic suggest that TRALI or possible TRALI may occur in as many as 1 in 100 transfusions [11].

    b. TACO, like TRALI, also presents as pulmonary edema; therefore the two syndromes are often hard to differentiate. TACO is thought to occur in approximately 1 in 100 transfusions, but it may also be underreported. The Mayo group has reported a frequency as high as 5 in 100 transfusions [12]. TACO can be difficult to differentiate from heart failure or generalized intravascular volume overload, all of which can present with the same clinical picture.

  4. **A recent investigation noted that TRALI, a diagnosis of exclusion, can be difficult to diagnose in patients undergoing cardiac surgery.** The authors reported greater pulmonary morbidity in the postoperative period for patients transfused with RBCs and fresh-frozen plasma (FFP); this pulmonary morbidity may have been related to TRALI, TACO, both, or neither. Nevertheless, transfusion of either RBCs or FFP was independently associated with pulmonary morbidity in the postoperative period [13].

  5. Stokes and colleagues [14] recently examined the effect of bleeding-related complications, blood product use, and costs on a population of inpatient surgical patients. They documented that inadequate surgical hemostasis leads to bleeding complications as well as transfusion. The authors were able to rank incremental cost per hospitalization associated with bleeding-related complications and adjust for covariates. Their findings support the need for further implementation of blood conservation strategies.

  6. **Bleeding complications and the associated need for reoperation correlate with increased morbidity in cardiac surgical patients.** Recent work attempted to delineate whether increased morbidity risk was related to the reoperation, blood transfusion, or both.

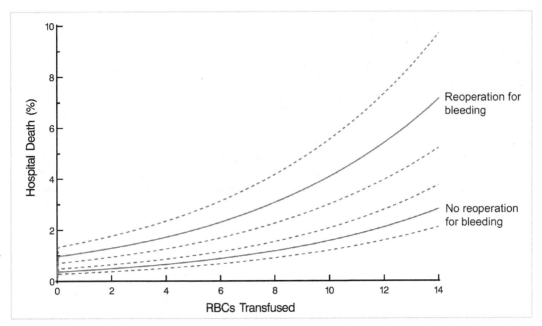

FIGURE 9.2 Predicted probability of operative mortality stratified by reoperation for bleeding and RBC transfusion. RBC transfusion and reoperation for bleeding were independently associated with increased mortality. RBCs, red blood cells. (Reprinted with permission from Vivacqua A, Koch CG, Yousuf AM, et al. Morbidity of bleeding after cardiac surgery: is it blood transfusion, reoperation for bleeding, or both? *Ann Thorac Surg.* 2011;91:1780–1790.)

The patients who underwent reoperation had greater subsequent morbidity, increased resource utilization, and higher in-hospital mortality even after risk adjustment (Fig. 9.2) [15].

7. A recent investigation in patients undergoing noncardiac thoracic surgery showed that postoperative outcomes were worse in patients transfused with 1 to 2 units of RBCs than in those who received no transfusion. The negative effect of transfusion was dose dependent and was associated with increased morbidity and resource utilization. The authors urged clinicians to be cautious in transfusing patients for mild degrees of anemia [16].

CLINICAL PEARL   TRALI and TACO are the leading two causes of transfusion-related death. HTR and bacterial sepsis are the next most common causes.

II. **Red blood cell (RBC) transfusion and clinical outcomes**

RBC units contain red cells that have been separated from whole blood by centrifugation or apheresis (Table 9.1) [17]. Isbister and colleagues reported on the abundance of data supporting morbidity risk associated with transfusion, yet noted that transfusion remains "ingrained" in current medical practice almost as a "default" position [18]. Furthermore, establishing causation between RBC transfusion and morbidity is difficult because of the potential for confounding in cohort study designs. Some argue that the etiology of poor outcomes relates to the fact that "sicker" patients receive a transfusion rather than to the RBC product itself. Recently, several large studies have examined clinical outcomes related to transfusion to determine the ideal hemoglobin thresholds for transfusion in postoperative cardiac surgery patients and whether prolonged RBC storage is associated with adverse outcomes. In addition, the AABB has recently updated its red cell transfusion guidelines, which are relevant to cardiac surgery [19].

A. **Hemoglobin transfusion trigger trials**

1. **In the past decade, practice has moved toward transfusing less blood to patients, including those undergoing cardiac surgery.** This change in practice is supported by

TABLE 9.1   Fast facts: RBCs from American Red Cross compendium [17]

Fast facts: RBC units	
Concentrated from whole blood	By centrifugation or collected by apheresis
Hematocrit	55–65% or 65–80%
Plasma content	20–100 mL
Typical volume	300–400 mL
Volume of Hb	50–80 g
Iron content	**Approximately 250 mg**
1 unit RBC transfusion	Increases hematocrit by 3%
Perioperative/periprocedural/critically ill indications for RBC transfusion	**When Hb is <6 g/dL in a young healthy patient; when Hb is <7 g/dL in critically ill patients; 7–8 g/dL in patients with cardiovascular disease**
Indication intermediate Hb 6–10 g/dL	Based on patient symptoms, comorbidities, ongoing bleeding, or end organ ischemia

Hb, hemoglobin; RBC, red blood cell.

large randomized trials showing noninferiority when a restrictive transfusion strategy is compared to a liberal strategy. The two large studies carried out in cardiac surgical patients were the Transfusion Requirements after Cardiac Surgery (TRACS) Trial in 2010 [20], and the Transfusion Indication Threshold Reduction (TITRe2) in 2015 [21]. Both studies focused on postoperative transfusion triggers, and neither demonstrated a difference in the primary outcomes between a liberal and a restrictive transfusion strategy.

a. TRACS trial
   (1) Compared hematocrit of 24% (restrictive) to hematocrit of 30% (liberal).
   (2) Primary outcome was a composite of morbidity and mortality.
   (3) The primary outcome occurred with similar frequency in the liberal (10%) and restrictive (11%) groups ($P = 0.85$). The various event rates in the two groups are shown in Figure 9.3.

b. TITRe2 trial
   (1) Compared hemoglobin triggers of 7.5 g/dL (restrictive) and 9.0 g/dL (liberal).
   (2) Primary outcome was a serious infection or ischemic event.

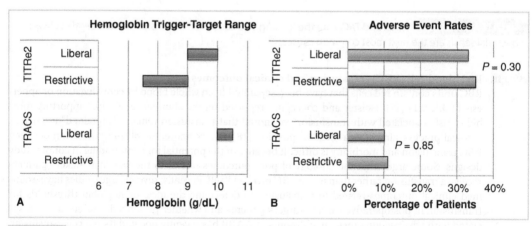

FIGURE 9.3 Hemoglobin and primary outcome data are shown for the liberal and restrictive transfusion groups in the TRACS and the TITRe2 trials [20,21]. In postoperative cardiac surgery patients, adverse event rates for the primary outcome (as defined by these trials) were similar in the groups assigned to a lower (restrictive) or a higher (liberal) hemoglobin transfusion threshold (**panel B**). In **panel A**, the left edge of the *red bars* represents the hemoglobin trigger (prior to transfusion), and the right edge of the *red bars* represents the hemoglobin target (after transfusion).

(3) The primary outcome occurred with similar frequency in the liberal (33.0%) and restrictive (35.1%) groups ($P = 0.30$). The primary event rates after 90 days are shown in Figure 9.3.

(4) The fact that outcome event rates were similar in the restrictive and liberal transfusion groups strongly supports use of a restrictive approach, as we only add risk and cost by administering more blood than is necessary. Although the restrictive group had a higher mortality at 90 days postoperatively in the TITRe2 trial (4.2 vs. 2.6%, $P = 0.045$), this was a secondary outcome with no statistical adjustment for multiple comparisons, making the significance questionable. This finding suggests we may not fully understand tolerable lower levels of hemoglobin in high-risk patients.

  c. A recent meta-analysis [22] of randomized controlled trials (RCTs) involving transfusion triggers reported that restrictive thresholds may place patients at risk for adverse postoperative outcomes. The methods differed from those of other studies in that the authors used a context-specific approach (i.e., they separated groups for analysis according to patient characteristics and clinical settings). Risk ratios (RRs) were calculated for the following 30-day complications: inadequate oxygen supply, mortality, a composite of both, and infections. Thirty-one trials were regrouped into five context-specific risk strata. In patients undergoing cardiac/vascular procedures, restrictive strategies possibly increased the risk of events reflecting inadequate oxygen supply (RR, 1.09 [95% Confidence Intervals (CI) 0.97 and 1.22]); mortality (RR, 1.39 [CI 0.95, 2.04]); whereas the composite risk of events did reach statistical significance (RR 1.12, [CI 1.01, 1.24]). Restrictive transfusion strategies also led to higher RRs among elderly orthopedic patients. Given the limitations of meta-analyses, this finding does not clearly support a liberal transfusion strategy in cardiac surgery patients.

2. One caveat is that when patients are actively bleeding, they will need to be transfused more liberally because whatever hemoglobin threshold is chosen, transfusion must at least keep pace with the bleeding.

CLINICAL PEARL Two large randomized trials, comparing restrictive transfusion triggers (hemoglobin 7.5 to 8 g/dL) to liberal transfusion triggers (hemoglobin 9 to 10 g/dL) in postoperative cardiac surgery patients, showed no difference in the primary outcome that was measured. This supports giving less blood, since we only add risk and cost when giving more blood than is necessary.

B. **Intraoperative transfusion triggers**
  1. In contrast to the postoperative setting, the ideal intraoperative hemoglobin transfusion trigger for cardiac surgical patients has not been rigorously studied.
  2. The STS and Society of Cardiovascular Anesthesiologists Blood Conservation Clinical Practice Guidelines [4] suggest a lower limit of 6 g/dL for patients on cardiopulmonary bypass (CPB) with moderate hypothermia, although they recognize that high-risk patients may need higher hemoglobin levels. This recommendation is supported by relatively weak evidence in the guideline.
  3. Some centers have begun monitoring cerebral tissue oxygen content with near-infrared spectroscopy technology; however, no conclusive evidence shows that this type of monitoring can reliably guide transfusion therapy.
  4. By lowering metabolic rate, hypothermic bypass reduces oxygen demands for all vital organs, meaning that lower hemoglobin levels will be tolerated. However, some groups now use either very mild or no systemic hypothermia. Instead they use selective regional cooling of the chest cavity, leaving the brain and kidneys at normal temperature.
  5. Additional studies are needed to determine the ideal hemoglobin levels during CPB.
C. **RBC storage duration**
  1. **As storage duration increases, RBCs undergo alterations in both structural shape and biochemical properties.** Implications of these time-dependent changes may contribute to

adverse clinical outcomes associated with RBC transfusion. However, findings from clinical and experimental animal studies have been inconsistent [23–25].

2. Although 6 weeks is the approved shelf life for ADSOL (additive solution)-preserved RBCs in the United States, according to a recent survey, the mean storage duration of RBC units has increased from 19.4 days in 2011, to 22.7 days in 2013 [26]. This increase may be due to an overall decrease in blood utilization nationwide by about 20% over the past decade, resulting in blood units sitting on the shelf longer before being used. Blood banks still operate on the "first-in, first-out" inventory management strategy, meaning that the oldest units get issued preferentially.

3. Survival of red cells after transfusion is an important variable, as it relates to their functionality. The current FDA-approved 42-day storage duration limit is based on a requirement that 75% of RBCs remain in circulation for 24 hours after transfusion, with less than 1% hemolysis. The requirement does not consider the cells' functional state. With fresh blood, RBC survival is approximately 90% at 24 hours posttransfusion. As storage duration increases, 24-hour survival (i.e., circulatory retention) decreases [27,28].

4. Laboratory investigation

   a. As storage time increases, RBCs exhibit degradation in structural shape, membrane deformability, aggregability, and metabolic function. The entire host of changes is referred to as the "storage lesion," which contributes to limited posttransfusion RBC survival and potentially to impaired oxygen delivery via the microcirculation.

   b. A number of biochemical changes occur over time in stored RBCs. Levels of S-nitrosothiols decrease 2 to 3 hours after collection. After several days of storage, lactate, potassium, and free hemoglobin progressively increase, whereas pH decreases [29]. 2,3-Diphosphoglycerate (2,3-DPG) levels decrease by approximately 95% from baseline by halfway through the approved shelf life (at 21 days) [30]. This depletion causes a left shift in the hemoglobin–oxygen saturation curve, which impedes the off-loading of oxygen from the hemoglobin molecule at the tissue level. It is unclear how rapidly 2,3-DPG is replenished after transfusion, but studies suggest that a complete return to baseline requires 24 to 72 hours.

   c. Storage-induced reduction in RBC membrane structural integrity (reduced deformability and increased fragility) is thought to be related to intra-RBC energy source depletion. RBC membrane deformability is significantly decreased by about halfway through the shelf life [31]. This loss of deformability may impede blood flow through small capillaries, which are as small as 5 microns in diameter, because the RBC itself is 7 microns in diameter.

   d. Release of cell-free hemoglobin and microparticles can lead to increased consumption of nitric oxide (NO) [32] and unwanted vasoconstriction in ischemic vascular beds. Some investigators have proposed insufficient NO bioavailability as an explanation for the increased morbidity and mortality observed after transfusion [33].

   e. Relevy and colleagues [34] showed that not only was RBC membrane deformability impaired, but RBC endothelial adherence was also increased. These findings suggest that transfusion of rheologically impaired RBCs might be detrimental for oxygen delivery, particularly in patients with cardiovascular disease.

   f. In a study of canines with induced sepsis, Solomon et al. [35] showed that mortality was greater in animals that received RBCs near the end of the 42-day shelf life than in those that received fresh blood. The mechanism they proposed was an increase in hemolysis and NO depletion from free hemoglobin in the circulation.

   g. In a recent mouse study, blood stored for ≥35 days was associated with increased non-transferrin-bound iron (free iron), whereas blood stored <35 days showed no significant increase in free iron [36]. The authors suggested that this free iron could promote infections, and that consideration should be given to limiting storage duration to 35 days.

5. Clinical investigation

   a. Many clinical studies, including retrospective observational studies and prospective RCTs, have examined the effect of RBC storage duration on patient outcomes.

6

Multiple retrospective studies have shown better outcomes with fresher blood, whereas five recent RCTs have shown no benefit to fresher blood.

b. **In a 2008 retrospective investigation that included over 6,000 cardiac surgical patients at a single center, patients who received exclusively older blood exhibited 39% greater in-hospital mortality and 33% greater 1-year mortality than did patients who received exclusively fresher blood (20 vs. 10 days median storage)** [25]. Prolonged intubation, sepsis, and composite morbidity were also increased. **This pivotal study was the impetus for the large RCTs carried out in a variety of settings, including adult cardiac surgical patients (the RECESS trial)** [37], **critically ill adult ICU patients (the ABLE study)** [38], **and the largest study to date, which enrolled all types of hospitalized patients (the INFORM study with over 20,000 patients)** [39]. **Each of these trials found no difference in any major clinical outcomes, although few patients were administered blood near the end of the allowed storage duration limit (35 to 42 days).**

c. A recent study with over 23,000 transfused patients, although retrospective, showed that administering the oldest blood in the bank (35 to 42 days storage) to the sickest patients in the hospital (those requiring ICU stays) resulted in higher mortality, but administering "middle age" blood even to high-risk patients, or the oldest blood to healthier patients did not increase mortality [40].

d. Most European countries allow a 35-day storage duration limit, whereas the United States continues to allow 42 days of RBC storage.

CLINICAL PEARL The recent randomized trials showing no difference in outcomes between blood stored for shorter and longer duration included few patients receiving blood near the end of the shelf life (35 to 42 days storage). The primary findings show that very fresh blood and blood stored for a medium duration are associated with similar outcomes.

III. Component therapy

A. **Restrictive RBC transfusion practices** have become a standard of care; yet, evidence-based indications for the use of blood component therapy such as FFP and platelet concentrate transfusion have been more limited [41]. After donation, whole blood is separated into components, which are stored at different temperatures. Though RBCs can be stored for up to 42 days at 1° to 6°C, platelets are stored at room temperature for a much shorter storage duration of 5 days. Plasma and cryoprecipitate can be stored frozen for 1 year.

1. Use of predetermined ratios of component therapy to RBCs has gained increased attention as a result of recent research into military and civilian trauma resuscitation. These investigations focus on earlier and increased use of component therapy. For example, using a strategy of 1:1:1 RBCs to FFP to platelets is thought to prevent dilutional coagulopathy.

2. Liumbruno and colleagues [42] provided detailed recommendations for transfusion of FFP and platelets in a number of clinical settings.

3. Mitra et al. [43] reported increased initial survival in association with higher FFP:RBC ratios. However, those authors also noted that this association is difficult to interpret because of an inherent survival bias.

4. Sperry and colleagues [44] associated FFP:RBC ratios ≥1:1.5 with lower mortality after massive transfusion. In a population of patients who had serious blunt injury and required ≥8 units of RBCs, survival was better. However, the risk of acute respiratory distress syndrome was also higher.

5. Though retrospective evidence supports the premise that survival increases with more aggressive use of plasma and platelets in massive transfusion, only recently (in 2015) was a large prospective randomized trial [45] published comparing lower to higher ratios of FFP and platelets to RBCs. The results of this study are described below in Section III.E.3, under massive transfusion.

TABLE 9.2 Fast facts: platelets from American Red Cross compendium [17]

Fast facts: Platelets	
Derived from whole blood	5.5×10^{10} platelets per bag
Plasma content (whole blood derived)	40–70 mL
Apheresis platelets	3.0×10^{11} platelets per bag
Plasma content (apheresis derived)	100–500 mL
Average platelet count increase in (70 kg) adult per each random donor platelet transfusion	5,000–10,000/μL
In general, appropriate indication for transfusion	Platelet count <50,000/μL with active bleeding or invasive procedures/surgery
In cardiac surgery, appropriate indication for transfusion	Platelet count <100,000/μL and microvascular bleeding, or impaired platelet function

B. **Platelet therapy** (Table 9.2)

1. General recommendations for platelet therapy stress that platelet transfusion cannot be based simply on platelet count. In general, for major surgical procedures or during massive transfusion (e.g., replacement of one or more blood volumes), a platelet count of at least 50,000/μL is recommended [46]. A standard dose of platelets for adults is approximately one unit per 10 kg body weight. Transfusing six units of platelets harvested from whole blood increases the platelet count by approximately 30,000/μL (Table 9.2) [17]. This "dose" corresponds roughly with the number of platelets collected by apheresis from a single donor. Platelets do not require crossmatching or ABO/Rh compatibility, but some blood banks preferentially transfuse ABO- and Rh-compatible platelets when feasible. When patients do not show the expected increase in platelet counts, they may need HLA-matched units, as HLA antibodies in the recipient are associated with platelet refractoriness. Since transfusion of WBCs causes HLA incompatibility, some centers elect to leukoreduce platelets.

2. **Of all the major blood components, platelets are associated with the highest risk and cost. The foremost major adverse outcome with platelet transfusion is bacterial sepsis. One in 3,000 platelet concentrates may have bacterial contamination, with an estimated mortality from sepsis occurring in between 1 in 17,000 and 1 in 61,000 transfusions** [47].

    a. Room temperature storage is the primary reason that platelets are more likely to have bacterial growth than other blood components. Therefore, platelets are routinely cultured before transfusion is allowed.

    b. Newer methods of reducing bacterial contamination include pathogen reduction technology with either a psoralen compound or riboflavin, followed by treatment with UV light, which reduces risk for virtually all viral, bacterial, and other pathogens (e.g., babesiosis, Zika virus). Pathogen reduction, however, is not yet widespread, given that it was only FDA approved in late 2014.

    c. TRALI has been associated with platelet transfusion more than with other blood components because TRALI reduction strategies have excluded women from donating plasma, but not platelets, and women have a higher rate of HLA antibodies owing to fetal blood exposure during childbirth.

3. As with RBCs, storage leads to changes in platelet structural and biochemical properties over time. A recent study found no increase in short-term adverse outcomes with increasing platelet storage time [48]. These authors and others reviewed current challenges of maintaining adequate platelet inventory with the limit of 5 days' storage and also described platelet storage lesion and the interesting controversy surrounding the proposed extension of platelet storage to 7 days (e.g., the increased risk for bacterial contamination over time is well described). Recently the FDA approved 7-day storage for platelets, but only if a secondary test is used for rapid bacterial detection on the day of transfusion [46,49].

TABLE 9.3   Fast facts: fresh plasma from American Red Cross compendium [17]

Fast facts: FFP	
Noncellular portion of blood	From whole blood or apheresis
Volume of 1 unit (approximate)	250 mL
Frozen at −18°C	Within 6–8 hrs of collection
Contains all coagulation factors	At usual plasma concentration (1 unit of activity/mL of plasma)
Thawed and used or stored at 1°–6°C for 24 hrs	
Transfusion should be guided by coagulation testing	Prothrombin time >1.5 × normal, activated partial thromboplastin time >1.5 × normal, or factor assay <25%
Dose	10–20 mL/kg
Selected indications	Massive transfusion with coagulopathic bleeding, active bleeding due to coagulation multiple factor deficiency, severe bleeding due to warfarin therapy

FFP, fresh-frozen plasma.

CLINICAL PEARL   Platelets impose the highest risk and cost of all the blood components. The primary risk is bacterial sepsis, which is increased relative to the other blood components since platelets are stored at room temperature.

C. **Fresh-frozen plasma** (Table 9.3) [17]
1. FFP refers to human donor plasma that is separated and frozen at −18°C within 8 hours of collection; frozen plasma-24 (FP-24) refers to plasma separated and frozen at −18°C within 24 hours of collection. FFP from a collection of whole blood has a volume of approximately 300 mL and can be stored for up to 1 year. Both products contain necessary plasma coagulation factors that are maintained after thawing and storage at 1° to 6°C for up to 5 days. In general, the dose of FFP is 10 to 20 mL/kg [50]. FFP should be ABO compatible but does not require crossmatching.
2. **Excessive blood loss, coagulation factor consumption, and specific deficiencies in coagulation factors are among a number of factors that can lead to inadequate hemostasis and the need for an FFP transfusion, particularly when specific factor concentrates are unavailable.** In patients who require massive transfusion, it is well recognized that the use of crystalloids, colloids, and RBCs can lead to a dilutional coagulopathy, and that this condition can potentially lead to disseminated intravascular coagulation. A number of publications address limited adherence to published guidelines and rational use of FFP transfusion [51]. **When surgical bleeding is excessive, it has been suggested that clinicians guide their FFP use and dosing by point-of-care testing coagulation studies rather than by preset formulas** (see also Chapter 21).
3. Interestingly, Holland and Brooks [52] reported that FFP transfusion failed to change the international normalized ratio (INR) in patients with a minimally prolonged INR (<1.6); INR decreased only with treatment of the disease causing the elevated INR.
4. Prophylactic use of FFP is not supported by evidence from good-quality RCTs. **Evidence indicates that prophylactic plasma for transfusion is not effective across a range of clinical settings** [51].
5. Although the INR test is routinely used to determine when FFP is given, the INR was designed to follow anticoagulant dosing with vitamin K antagonist drugs, and is likely too sensitive and inadequately specific to guide FFP dosing accurately. For example, in our experience, until the INR is 2.0 or higher, the thromboelastogram (TEG) will usually be normal, suggesting that coagulation is unimpaired.
D. **Cryoprecipitate** (Table 9.4) [17]
1. When FFP is thawed for 24 hours at 1° to 6°C, high–molecular-weight proteins separate out from the plasma; this precipitate can be frozen at −18°C for up to 1 year.

TABLE 9.4   Fast facts: cryoprecipitate, from American Red Cross compendium [17]

Fast facts: Cryoprecipitate	
Unit is prepared from 1 unit of FFP at 1°–6°C	Recovering cold insoluble precipitate
Refrozen within 1 hr	
Contains concentrated levels of	Fibrinogen, Factor VIII:C, Factor VIII:vWF, Factor XIII, and fibronectin
Factor VIII:C in 1 unit	At least 80 IU
Fibrinogen in 1 unit	Minimum of 150 mg
Plasma volume of 1 unit	5–20 mL
Dose and response from 1 pool or "bag" (5 units)	Fibrinogen increases by approximately 50 mg/dL for average adult
Selected indications	Bleeding associated with fibrinogen deficiencies; massive transfusion when fibrinogen <150–200 mg/dL

2. One bag of cryoprecipitate contains 10 to 15 mL of insoluble protein.

3. Cryoprecipitate contains Factors I (fibrinogen), VIII, and XIII, von Willebrand Factor, fibronectin, and platelet microparticles.

4. **Cryoprecipitate is most commonly used as a concentrated source of fibrinogen**, except in some European countries where fibrinogen concentrate is approved (and preferred) to treat acquired fibrinogen deficiency [53]. In the United States, fibrinogen concentrate is approved by the FDA only for congenital, not acquired, deficiency.

5. Hypofibrinogenemia occurs in patients undergoing cardiac surgery, most often in those with hemorrhage. In such patients, even a balanced ratio of RBCs, FFP, and platelets will eventually result in fibrinogen deficiency, as FFP has some fibrinogen, but not enough to maintain normal levels during massive transfusions. Depending upon the weight of the recipient, 10 pooled units of cryoprecipitate will increase plasma fibrinogen by 70 to 100 mg/dL [50,53].

6. Recent guidelines for treating hemorrhage suggest that fibrinogen levels be maintained above 150 to 200 mg/dL. Ideally, viscoelastic point-of-care testing is used to guide such therapies, focusing on clot strength (α-angle and maximum amplitude).

E. **Massive transfusion and component ratios**

1. The formal definition of massive transfusion is one entire blood volume replacement in a 24-hour time period. When a patient undergoes massive transfusion or experiences any other large, rapid blood loss, it is important to administer an optimal ratio of blood components to avoid dilutional coagulopathy.

2. Given the complexity of cardiac surgery and extracorporeal support, the incidence of massive transfusion is substantial, especially in tertiary referral centers that perform revision cardiac surgeries, transplants, and extracorporeal life support (ECMO).

3. Most studies in this area have been retrospective and focused on trauma patients with active hemorrhage. These studies support using a high ratio of plasma and platelets to RBCs in order to reconstitute a mixture similar to that of whole blood. **The recently completed PROPPR study showed that in actively bleeding trauma patients, the primary outcomes of 24-hour and 30-day mortality were similar in the 1:1:1 and the 1:1:2 groups (platelet:plasma:RBC ratios)** [45]. However, early exsanguination, which was the predominant cause of death, occurred less frequently in the 1:1:1 group. This secondary outcome suggests that a balanced ratio of components, similar to whole blood, was efficacious in improving outcomes. Whether this finding applies to massive hemorrhage in cardiac surgical patients is unclear, as trauma patients may have unique characteristics. Nonetheless, many providers will use a 1:1:1 ratio when transfusing one or more blood volumes over a short period. Ideally, the ratio can be tailored based on laboratory testing, including viscoelastic (TEG or rotational thromboelastometry [ROTEM]) testing, to avoid coagulopathy.

IV. **Blood conservation measures**

A. **Preoperative anemia management**

1. **Best practices for PBM include the diagnosis and treatment of preoperative anemia with the goal of reducing the need for allogeneic transfusion** [54]. This type of care

applies primarily to elective surgical patients because there is insufficient time for medical treatment in urgent or emergent cases, which are not infrequent in cardiac surgery.

2. For patients undergoing elective surgery, effective and specific treatments, such as iron replacement for iron deficiency (either oral or intravenous), can make a difference.

3. Erythropoietic stimulating agents (e.g., erythropoietin or darbepoetin) can also be used to increase hemoglobin levels preoperatively [55], although the FDA warnings for thrombotic events and promotion of tumor growth should be considered when weighing the risks and benefits of such therapies.

4. One must rule out GI malignancy as the underlying cause of iron deficiency in the anemia workup.

B. **Antifibrinolytics**

The use of lysine analogs, ε-aminocaproic acid (EACA) and tranexamic acid (TXA), suppresses pathologic hyperfibrinolysis associated with CPB [56]. **In a 2011 Cochrane review, Henry et al. [57] conducted a meta-analysis on antifibrinolytic use that included 34 studies of TXA, 11 studies of EACA, and 6 trials comparing the two. The findings showed that TXA use was associated with a 32% reduction in the need for allogeneic blood transfusion. Those who received EACA had a 30% reduction.** On average, patients who received either TXA or EACA saw reductions in both intraoperative and postoperative blood loss. Although both drugs are relatively inexpensive, TXA costs approximately 10 times more for an equivalent dose. Neither drug has been shown to increase thrombotic events, however TXA in high doses is associated with increased risk for seizures [58]. These drugs have now replaced aprotinin as the drugs of choice because aprotinin was removed from the US marketplace in 2008 for safety concerns (increased mortality) after the BART trial [59]. Although controversial, in 2011 aprotinin was reintroduced and marketed across Canada and Europe, after debate over the methods used to reclassify the primary outcomes in the BART study.

CLINICAL PEARL   Antifibrinolytic drugs are commonly used intraoperatively to reduce bleeding and transfusion requirements in cardiac surgery patients. There is no evidence that they are associated with increased venous thromboembolic events.

C. **Acute normovolemic hemodilution (ANH)**

1. For ANH, a certain amount of blood is withdrawn from a patient before heparinization and CPB, and the intravascular volume is replaced to maintain isovolemia. The autologous whole blood is then readministered, usually after CPB. The use of ANH reduces requirements for allogeneic transfusion by preserving RBCs, coagulation factors, and platelets and improving perfusion during CPB by decreasing blood viscosity [60].

2. **Barile et al. [61] conducted a meta-analysis of 29 RCTs that included 2,439 patients to compare the use of ANH with standard intraoperative care. They assessed the number of allogeneic RBC units transfused, rate of perioperative transfusion, and estimated total blood loss.** They found that ANH reduced the number of allogeneic RBC units used, the incidence of transfusion, and the amount of bleeding.

3. **ANH is associated with reduced allogeneic transfusion, most notably when associated with >800 mL of ANH phlebotomy.** In a multicenter, observational study of over 13,000 patients [62], researchers found that at all volumes of ANH, the number of allogeneic transfusions was reduced. Perhaps unsurprisingly, this reduction became more pronounced with increased ANH volume removal. They also noted a lower rate of plasma and platelet transfusion in those who had ANH, as well as less acute kidney injury and lower rates of prolonged length of stay.

4. In a retrospective study that included 2,058 patients, Zhou et al. [63] found that even those who underwent low-volume ANH (5 to 8 mL/kg) required significantly fewer RBC units intraoperatively. This reduction did not carry over to a reduction in FFP or platelet transfusions, postoperative or total perioperative allogeneic transfusions, or significant difference in postoperative outcomes.

5. Other studies have not demonstrated a reduction in transfusion requirements with ANH [64,65]. It is also important to note potential confounding variables. For example, patients who undergo ANH tend to be younger and male, have a larger body surface area, have less preoperative anemia, and have lower STS mortality scores.

6. In the 2011 STS guidelines on perioperative blood transfusion and conservation in cardiac surgery, the evidence supporting ANH was considered class IIb. Accordingly, the guidelines indicated that ANH could be considered as part of a multipronged approach to blood conservation [4].

D. **Methods used by perfusionists**
   1. Cell salvage
      a. Cell salvage is a technique in which whole blood from a patient is centrifuged to collect platelets and other clotting factors into the cell-washing supernatant.
      b. Dr. Denton Cooley [66] first described salvage of autologous blood during cardiac surgery in the 1960s.
      c. Modern day cell salvage has been used since the early 1980s in cardiac surgery as a method to reduce transfusion of allogeneic blood products.
      d. Numerous RCTs have examined whether cell salvage decreases the risk of allogeneic blood product transfusion. In one meta-analysis, Wang et al. [67] investigated 31 RCTs and found that the use of cell salvage significantly reduced the odds of any allogeneic blood product transfusion (OR, 0.63; 95% CI, 0.43 to 0.94; $P = 0.02$) compared with no cell salvage. There has been concern that removal of platelets and clotting factors during cell salvage could increase the risk of a cardiac surgical patient requiring transfusion of these products. However, Wang et al. [67] discovered that the mean units of FFP ($P = 0.18$) and platelets ($P = 0.26$) transfused did not differ significantly between those who did and did not receive cell salvage. Similarly, **a Cochrane review in 2010 found that the risk of allogeneic blood transfusion was reduced by an average of 34% in cardiac surgical patients who received cell salvage** [68]. **In addition, the use of cell salvage saved an average of one RBC unit per patient.**
      e. Cell salvage has become a standard of care in cardiac surgery owing to the recent emphasis on blood conservation. In addition, salvaged RBCs may be higher in quality than stored (banked) RBCs. Compared with banked RBCs, salvaged blood has normal levels of 2,3-DPG, no left shift in the hemoglobin–oxygen saturation curve, and better cell membrane deformability [31,69].
   2. Modified ultrafiltration
      a. Membrane oxygenators activate the coagulation cascade, dilute platelets and clotting factors, and induce fibrinolysis and systemic inflammatory response syndrome. Various studies have attempted to mitigate these risks with a technique known as modified ultrafiltration (MUF), which has been shown to reduce postoperative blood loss and blood product utilization.
      b. MUF involves use of a hydrostatic pressure gradient to remove water and some low–molecular-weight substances from plasma, producing protein-rich whole blood to be returned to the patient after the cessation of CPB. When this technique is used during CPB, it is considered conventional ultrafiltration, or zero-balance ultrafiltration (Z-BUF). The ultrafiltration occurs on the arterial side of the pump after blood has been pressurized by the roller pump and gone through the oxygenator membrane. The outlet is connected to the patient's venous line as blood reenters the patient's right atrium after passing through the hemofilter.
      c. MUF was created by pediatric cardiac surgeons who were attempting to reduce the hemodilutional effects of CPB, which are particularly pronounced in children but also occur in adults. **In a meta-analysis that compared MUF to no ultrafiltration, Boodhwani et al. [70] demonstrated that MUF significantly reduced transfusion requirements.** In a prospective randomized trial of 573 patients, Luciani et al. [71] found not only that the mean volume of RBCs transfused for each patient was lower

but also that the proportion of patients who did not receive any blood products was higher with MUF (51.8% vs. 38.1%, $P = 0.001$).

    d. MUF is a blood conservation strategy that is likely underutilized in adults and has become the standard of care for pediatric cardiac surgical patients.

3. Zero-balance ultrafiltration

    a. For Z-BUF, or conventional ultrafiltration, ultrafiltration occurs during CPB, and the ultrafiltrate is replaced with an equal volume of balanced electrolyte solution. The Z-BUF filter unit is connected to the CPB pump, takes blood from a premembrane port, and runs in parallel to the main cardiopulmonary circuit. To prevent patient blood flow from dropping, the arterial pump rate is increased to compensate for the blood flow through the hemofilter.

    b. The main theoretical advantage is that Z-BUF can be used to reduce the inflammatory mediators that are activated when blood contacts a foreign surface. Thus, this technique might decrease lung injury, neurologic inflammation, bleeding, and acute kidney injury, as well as other indicators of morbidity. A recent meta-analysis of RCTs showed no significant difference in ICU length of stay, duration of ventilation, chest tube output, and other parameters between patients who received Z-BUF and those who received no hemofiltration [72].

4. Low-volume CPB circuits

    a. Smaller-diameter and shorter-length tubing as well as low-volume oxygenators can reduce the hemodilution that occurs when patients are placed on CPB.

    b. Such low-volume circuits result in blood conservation and can reduce transfusion requirements.

5. Retrograde autologous prime

    a. By using the patient's own venous blood to prime the CPB circuit by retrograde flow, a reduction in hemodilution can be achieved, resulting in less anemia and transfusion requirements.

CLINICAL PEARL   Perfusionists play a prominent role in achieving blood conservation in cardiac surgery patients. There are several methods they can employ to reduce the incidence of anemia and transfusion.

E. Viscoelastic testing

    a. TEG and ROTEM are viscoelastic hemostatic assays that are used to assess whole blood clot formation: initiation, propagation, strength, and dissolution. The diagnosis of a specific cause of coagulopathic bleeding allows for targeted hemostatic correction, and potentially prevents the use of unwarranted blood products. Early utilization of TEG and ROTEM (while the patient is still on CPB), allows for prompt decision making about FFP, platelets, and cryoprecipitate transfusions.

    b. **Transfusion algorithms that use TEG and ROTEM parameters have been shown to reduce transfusion requirements in cardiac surgery** [73,74]. One of the first prospective, randomized trials to compare the algorithmic use of TEG ($n = 53$) and standard routine laboratory testing ($n = 52$) showed that, although intraoperative transfusion rates did not differ significantly, the TEG group had fewer postoperative and total transfusions [73]. Early and specific identification of hemostasis abnormalities by TEG might have enabled physicians to proactively improve hemostasis.

    c. More recent studies have continued to show that TEG/ROTEM reduces the need for transfusion, but also potentially correlates with a reduced mortality [75]. Conventional viscoelastic testing methods are unable to detect the effect of antiplatelet medications (P2Y12 inhibitors or aspirin) on platelet function. Though controversial and arguably lacking sufficient evidence, the use of point-of-care platelet function tests or platelet mapping has been suggested as an additional modality to assess platelet dysfunction caused by antiplatelet agents and CPB [76,77]. Corredor et al. [78] examined whether the various point-of-care platelet function tests predicted blood loss and/or blood product utilization after cardiac surgery, and whether this testing along with blood management algorithms (TEG/ROTEM) leads to improved patient outcomes. The authors found that platelet mapping use within a blood transfusion algorithm resulted in a significant reduction in bleeding at longest follow-up, and reduced transfusion of RBCs and FFP. Additional large, randomized trials are needed to confirm these results.

V. Conclusion

Although transfusion is a necessary treatment strategy for selected patients, it is associated with a number of morbidity risks, as is anemia. Recent work suggests moving from the current blood banking, "supply-centric" perspective to a "patient-centric" blood management approach. Implementation of institutional PBM protocols enhances practitioners' knowledge base and the consistency of transfusion practices while encouraging a more restrictive approach to blood utilization.

REFERENCES

1. Beal RW. The rational use of blood. *Aust N Z J Surg*. 1976;46(4):309–313.
2. Frank SM, Savage WJ, Rothschild JA, et al. Variability in blood and blood component utilization as assessed by an anesthesia information management system. *Anesthesiology*. 2012;117(1):99–106.
3. **Bennett-Guerrero E, Zhao Y, O'Brien SM, et al. Variation in use of blood transfusion in coronary artery bypass graft surgery.** *JAMA*. **2010;304(14):1568–1575.**
4. Ferraris VA, Brown JR, Despotis GJ, et al. 2011 update to the Society of Thoracic Surgeons and the Society of Cardiovascular Anesthesiologists blood conservation clinical practice guidelines. *Ann Thorac Surg*. 2011;91(3):944–982.
5. Waters JH, Ness PM. Patient blood management: a growing challenge and opportunity. *Transfusion*. 2011;51(5):902–903.
6. Vamvakas EC, Blajchman MA. Transfusion-related mortality: the ongoing risks of allogeneic blood transfusion and the available strategies for their prevention. *Blood*. 2009;113(15):3406–3417.
7. Carson JL, Grossman BJ, Kleinman S, et al. Red blood cell transfusion: a clinical practice guideline from the AABB. *Ann Intern Med*. 2012;157(1):48–58.
8. **Fatalities reported to the FDA following blood collection and transfusion. Annual summary for fiscal year 2015. Available from https://www.fda.gov/BiologicsBloodVaccines/SafetyAvailability/ReportaProblem/TransfusionDonationFatalities/default.htm. Accessed March 4, 2018.**
9. Toy P, Lowell C. TRALI—definition, mechanisms, incidence and clinical relevance. *Best Pract Res Clin Anaesthesiol*. 2007; 21(2):183–193.
10. Popovsky MA. Pulmonary consequences of transfusion: TRALI and TACO. *Transfus Apher Sci*. 2006;34(3):243–244.
11. Clifford L, Jia Q, Subramanian A, et al. Characterizing the epidemiology of postoperative transfusion-related acute lung injury. *Anesthesiology*. 2015;122(1):12–20.
12. Clifford L, Jia Q, Yadav H, et al. Characterizing the epidemiology of perioperative transfusion-associated circulatory overload. *Anesthesiology*. 2015;122(1):21–28.
13. Koch C, Li L, Figueroa P, et al. Transfusion and pulmonary morbidity after cardiac surgery. *Ann Thorac Surg*. 2009;88(5): 1410–1418.
14. Stokes ME, Ye X, Shah M, et al. Impact of bleeding-related complications and/or blood product transfusions on hospital costs in inpatient surgical patients. *BMC Health Serv Res*. 2011;11:135.
15. Vivacqua A, Koch CG, Yousuf AM, et al. Morbidity of bleeding after cardiac surgery: is it blood transfusion, reoperation for bleeding, or both? *Ann Thorac Surg*. 2011;91(6):1780–1790.
16. Ferraris VA, Davenport DL, Saha SP, et al. Intraoperative transfusion of small amounts of blood heralds worse postoperative outcome in patients having noncardiac thoracic operations. *Ann Thorac Surg*. 2011;91(6):1674–1680.
17. American Red Cross. A compendium of transfusion practice guidelines. Third edition 2017. Available from https://p.widencdn.net/maopz6/TransfusionPractices-Compendium_3rdEdition. Accessed April 16, 2017.
18. Isbister JP, Shander A, Spahn DR, et al. Adverse blood transfusion outcomes: establishing causation. *Transfus Med Rev*. 2011; 25(2):89–101.
19. **Carson JL, Guyatt G, Heddle NM, et al. Clinical practice guidelines from the AABB: red blood cell transfusion thresholds and storage.** *JAMA*. **2016;316(19):2025–2035.**
20. **Hajjar LA, Vincent JL, Galas FR, et al. Transfusion requirements after cardiac surgery: the TRACS randomized controlled trial.** *JAMA*. **2010;304(14):1559–1567.**
21. **Murphy GJ, Pike K, Rogers CA, et al. Liberal or restrictive transfusion after cardiac surgery.** *N Engl J Med*. **2015; 372(11):997–1008.**
22. Hovaguimian F, Myles PS. Restrictive versus liberal transfusion strategy in the perioperative and acute care settings: a context-specific systematic review and meta-analysis of randomized controlled trials. *Anesthesiology*. 2016;125(1):46–61.
23. Raat NJ, Verhoeven AJ, Mik EG, et al. The effect of storage time of human red cells on intestinal microcirculatory oxygenation in a rat isovolemic exchange model. *Crit Care Med*. 2005;33(1):39–45.
24. Yap CH, Lau L, Krishnaswamy M, et al. Age of transfused red cells and early outcomes after cardiac surgery. *Ann Thorac Surg*. 2008;86(2):554–559.
25. Koch CG, Li L, Sessler DI, et al. Duration of red-cell storage and complications after cardiac surgery. *N Engl J Med*. 2008;358(12): 1229–1239.

26. Whitaker B, Rajbhandary S, Kleinman S, et al. Trends in United States blood collection and transfusion: results from the 2013 AABB blood collection, utilization, and patient blood management survey. *Transfusion*. 2016;56(9):2173–2183.

27. Simon ER. Adenine in blood banking. *Transfusion*. 1977;17(4):317–325.

28. Hamasaki N, Yamamoto M. Red blood cell function and blood storage. *Vox Sang*. 2000;79(4):191–197.

29. Bennett-Guerrero E, Veldman TH, Doctor A, et al. Evolution of adverse changes in stored RBCs. *PNAS*. 2007;104(43):17063–17068.

30. Scott AV, Nagababu E, Johnson DJ, et al. 2,3-Diphosphoglycerate concentrations in autologous salvaged versus stored red blood cells and in surgical patients after transfusion. *Anesth Analg*. 2016;122(3):616–623.

31. Frank SM, Abazyan B, Ono M, et al. Decreased erythrocyte deformability after transfusion and the effects of erythrocyte storage duration. *Anesth Analg*. 2013;116(5):975–981.

32. Kim-Shapiro DB, Lee J, Gladwin MT. Storage lesion: role of red blood cell breakdown. *Transfusion*. 2011;51(4):844–851.

33. Roback JD, Neuman RB, Quyyumi A, et al. Insufficient nitric oxide bioavailability: a hypothesis to explain adverse effects of red blood cell transfusion. *Transfusion*. 2011;51(4):859–866.

34. Relevy H, Koshkaryev A, Manny N, et al. Blood banking-induced alteration of red blood cell flow properties. *Transfusion*. 2008;48(1):136–146.

35. Solomon SB, Wang D, Sun J, et al. Mortality increases after massive exchange transfusion with older stored blood in canines with experimental pneumonia. *Blood*. 2013;121(9):1663–1672.

36. Rapido F, Brittenham GM, Bandyopadhyay S, et al. Prolonged red cell storage before transfusion increases extravascular hemolysis. *J Clin Invest*. 2017;127(1):375–382.

37. **Steiner ME, Ness PM, Assmann SF, et al. Effects of red-cell storage duration on patients undergoing cardiac surgery. *N Engl J Med*. 2015;372(15):1419–1429.**

38. Lacroix J, Hebert PC, Fergusson DA, et al. Age of transfused blood in critically ill adults. *N Engl J Med*. 2015;372(15):1410–1418.

39. Heddle NM, Cook RJ, Arnold DM, et al. Effect of short-term vs. long-term blood storage on mortality after transfusion. *N Engl J Med*. 2016;375(20):1937–1945.

40. Goel R, Johnson DJ, Scott AV, et al. Red blood cells stored 35 days or more are associated with adverse outcomes in high-risk patients. *Transfusion*. 2016;56(7):1690–1698.

41. Gajic O, Dzik WH, Toy P. Fresh frozen plasma and platelet transfusion for nonbleeding patients in the intensive care unit: benefit or harm? *Crit Care Med*. 2006;34(5 Suppl):S170–S173.

42. Liumbruno G, Bennardello F, Lattanzio A, et al. Recommendations for the transfusion of plasma and platelets. *Blood Transfus*. 2009;7(2):132–150.

43. Mitra B, Mori A, Cameron PA, et al. Fresh frozen plasma (FFP) use during massive blood transfusion in trauma resuscitation. *Injury*. 2010;41(1):35–39.

44. Sperry JL, Ochoa JB, Gunn SR, et al. An FFP:PRBC transfusion ratio >/= 1:1.5 is associated with a lower risk of mortality after massive transfusion. *J Trauma*. 2008;65(5):986–993.

45. **Holcomb JB, Tilley BC, Baraniuk S, et al. Transfusion of plasma, platelets, and red blood cells in a 1:1:1 vs a 1:1:2 ratio and mortality in patients with severe trauma: the PROPPR randomized clinical trial. *JAMA*. 2015;313(5):471–482.**

46. **Kaufman RM, Djulbegovic B, Gernsheimer T, et al. Platelet transfusion: a clinical practice guideline from the AABB. *Ann Intern Med*. 2015;162(3):205–213.**

47. Stroncek DF, Rebulla P. Platelet transfusions. *Lancet*. 2007;370(9585):427–438.

48. Welsby IJ, Lockhart E, Phillips-Bute B, et al. Storage age of transfused platelets and outcomes after cardiac surgery. *Transfusion*. 2010;50(11):2311–2317.

49. Kleinman S, Dumont LJ, Tomasulo P, et al. The impact of discontinuation of 7-day storage of apheresis platelets (PASSPORT) on recipient safety: an illustration of the need for proper risk assessments. *Transfusion*. 2009;49(5):903–912.

50. Stanworth SJ. The evidence-based use of FFP and cryoprecipitate for abnormalities of coagulation tests and clinical coagulopathy. *Hematology Am Soc Hematol Educ Program*. 2007:179–186.

51. Roback JD, Caldwell S, Carson J, et al. Evidence-based practice guidelines for plasma transfusion. *Transfusion*. 2010;50(6):1227–1239.

52. Holland LL, Brooks JP. Toward rational fresh frozen plasma transfusion: the effect of plasma transfusion on coagulation test results. *Am J Clin Pathol*. 2006;126(1):133–139.

53. Callum JL, Karkouti K, Lin Y. Cryoprecipitate: the current state of knowledge. *Transfus Med Rev*. 2009;23(3):177–188.

54. Guinn NR, Guercio JR, Hopkins TJ, et al. How do we develop and implement a preoperative anemia clinic designed to improve perioperative outcomes and reduce cost? *Transfusion*. 2016;56(2):297–303.

55. Yoo YC, Shim JK, Kim JC, et al. Effect of single recombinant human erythropoietin injection on transfusion requirements in preoperatively anemic patients undergoing valvular heart surgery. *Anesthesiology*. 2011;115(5):929–937.

56. Pustavoitau A, Faraday N. Pro: antifibrinolytics should be used in routine cardiac cases using cardiopulmonary bypass (unless contraindicated). *J Cardiothorac Vasc Anesth*. 2016;30(1):245–247.

57. Henry DA, Carless PA, Moxey AJ, et al. Anti-fibrinolytic use for minimising perioperative allogeneic blood transfusion. *Cochrane Database Syst Rev*. 2011:CD001886.

58. Myles PS, Smith JA, Forbes A, et al. Tranexamic acid in patients undergoing coronary-artery surgery. *N Engl J Med*. 2017;376(2):136–148.

59. Mangano DT, Tudor IC, Dietzel C; Multicenter Study of Perioperative Ischemia Research Group; Ischemia Research and Education Foundation. The risk associated with aprotinin in cardiac surgery. *N Engl J Med*. 2006;354(4):353–365.

60. Grant MC, Resar LM, Frank SM. The efficacy and utility of acute normovolemic hemodilution. *Anesth Analg*. 2015;121(6):1412–1414.

61. Barile L, Fominskiy E, Di Tomasso N, et al. Acute normovolemic hemodilution reduces allogeneic red blood cell transfusion in cardiac surgery: a systematic review and meta-analysis of randomized trials. *Anesth Analg.* 2017;124(3):743–752.

62. Goldberg J, Paugh TA, Dickinson TA, et al. Greater volume of acute normovolemic hemodilution may aid in reducing blood transfusions after cardiac surgery. *Ann Thorac Surg.* 2015;100(5):1581–1587.

63. Zhou ZF, Jia XP, Sun K, et al. Mild volume acute normovolemic hemodilution is associated with lower intraoperative transfusion and postoperative pulmonary infection in patients undergoing cardiac surgery—a retrospective, propensity matching study. *BMC Anesthesiol.* 2017;17(1):13.

64. Hohn L, Schweizer A, Licker M, et al. Absence of beneficial effect of acute normovolemic hemodilution combined with aprotinin on allogeneic blood transfusion requirements in cardiac surgery. *Anesthesiology.* 2002;96(2):276–282.

65. Curley GF, Shehata N, Mazer CD, et al. Transfusion triggers for guiding RBC transfusion for cardiovascular surgery: a systematic review and meta-analysis. *Crit Care Med.* 2014;42(12):2611–2624.

66. Cooley DA, Crawford ES, Howell JF, et al. Open heart surgery in Jehovah's Witnesses. *Am J Cardiol.* 1964;13:779–781.

67. Wang G, Bainbridge D, Martin J, et al. The efficacy of an intraoperative cell saver during cardiac surgery: a meta-analysis of randomized trials. *Anesth Analg.* 2009;109(2):320–330.

68. **Carless PA, Henry DA, Moxey AJ, et al. Cell salvage for minimising perioperative allogeneic blood transfusion. *Cochrane Database Syst Rev.* 2010(4):CD001888.**

69. Salaria ON, Barodka VM, Hogue CW, et al. Impaired red blood cell deformability after transfusion of stored allogeneic blood but not autologous salvaged blood in cardiac surgery patients. *Anesth Analg.* 2014;118(6):1179–1187.

70. Boodhwani M, Williams K, Babaev A, et al. Ultrafiltration reduces blood transfusions following cardiac surgery: a meta-analysis. *Eur J Cardiothorac Surg.* 2006;30(6):892–897.

71. Luciani GB, Menon T, Vecchi B, et al. Modified ultrafiltration reduces morbidity after adult cardiac operations: a prospective, randomized clinical trial. *Circulation.* 2001;104(12 Suppl 1):I253–I259.

72. Zhu X, Ji B, Wang G, et al. The effects of zero-balance ultrafiltration on postoperative recovery after cardiopulmonary bypass: a meta-analysis of randomized controlled trials. *Perfusion.* 2012;27(5):386–392.

73. **Shore-Lesserson L, Manspeizer HE, DePerio M, et al. Thromboelastography-guided transfusion algorithm reduces transfusions in complex cardiac surgery. *Anesth Analg.* 1999;88(2):312–319.**

74. Wasowicz M, McCluskey SA, Wijeysundera DN, et al. The incremental value of thromboelastography for prediction of excessive blood loss after cardiac surgery: an observational study. *Anesth Analg.* 2010;111(2):331–338.

75. Wikkelso A, Wetterslev J, Moller AM, et al. Thromboelastography (TEG) or rotational thromboelastometry (ROTEM) to monitor haemostatic treatment in bleeding patients: a systematic review with meta-analysis and trial sequential analysis. *Anaesthesia.* 2017;72(4):519–531.

76. Kwak YL, Kim JC, Choi YS, et al. Clopidogrel responsiveness regardless of the discontinuation date predicts increased blood loss and transfusion requirement after off-pump coronary artery bypass graft surgery. *J Am Coll Cardiol.* 2010;56(24):1994–2002.

77. Preisman S, Kogan A, Itzkovsky K, et al. Modified thromboelastography evaluation of platelet dysfunction in patients undergoing coronary artery surgery. *Eur J Cardiothorac Surg.* 2010;37(6):1367–1374.

78. Corredor C, Wasowicz M, Karkouti K, et al. The role of point-of-care platelet function testing in predicting postoperative bleeding following cardiac surgery: a systematic review and meta-analysis. *Anaesthesia.* 2015;70(6):715–731.

Anesthetic Management for Specific Disorders and Procedures

10

Anesthetic Management of Myocardial Revascularization

Michael S. Green, Gary Okum, and Jay C. Horrow

KEY POINTS

1. Supply of oxygen to the myocardium is determined by arterial oxygen content of blood and coronary blood flow (CBF).
2. The three main determinants of myocardial oxygen demand are heart rate, contractility, and wall stress.
3. A doubling of heart rate more than doubles the myocardial oxygen demand owing to an associated small increase in contractility.
4. Wall stress varies directly with pressure and radius and inversely with wall thickness.

5. Regional wall-motion abnormalities (RWMAs) occur <1 minute after onset of ischemia, before electrocardiogram (ECG) changes.
6. Although off-pump, compared to on-pump **coronary artery bypass grafting** (CABG), makes no difference in mortality and quality of life, it associates with shorter durations of mechanical ventilation and of hospital stay, and with less morbidity.
7. Myocardial ischemia can occur at any time during CABG: before, during, and after bypass.
8. A brief, intentional period of myocardial ischemia ("preconditioning") may protect against the damage caused by subsequent prolonged ischemia and tissue reperfusion.
9. Hybrid operating rooms (OR) incorporate catheterization facilities; they allow a surgical approach to the left anterior descending (LAD) artery combined with a noninvasive approach to other vessels.

I. Introduction

A. Prevalence and economic impact of coronary artery disease

Despite declining rates in the last several decades, coronary heart disease remains the leading cause of death in the United States, with the prevalence of 16.5 million for an angina pectoris or myocardial infarction diagnosis in 2017 [1].

Cardiovascular disease consumes almost 17% of health care spending on major illness in the United States, with recently estimated expenditures at $317 billion [2], and nearly a fifth of disability disbursements from the Social Security Administration [1].

B. Symptoms and progression of coronary artery disease

Unlike valvular heart disease, coronary artery disease presents with symptoms that are more variable and progress with more sudden, discrete events such as angina or myocardial infarction. Angina pectoris precedes only 18% of myocardial infarctions [1]. Many patients who have silent ischemia require diligence for detection and prompt treatment perioperatively.

C. Historical perspective of coronary artery bypass grafting (CABG)

Early unsuccessful or suboptimal attempts at myocardial revascularization took place before the 1960s. The first successful attempt at myocardial revascularization occurred in 1967, when Favalaro and Effler at the Cleveland Clinic performed reversed saphenous vein bypass grafting procedures. In 1968, Green anastomosed the internal mammary artery (IMA) directly to a coronary artery. IMA grafting enjoyed a resurgence of interest in the late 1970s and early 1980s following demonstration of higher graft patency rates and better long-term survival compared to vein grafts. During these decades, high-dose fentanyl anesthesia largely supplanted morphine-based and inhalation-based techniques, allowing operation on more fragile patients at the expense of many hours of mechanical ventilation after operation.

The 1990s ushered in an interest in enhanced recovery ("fast-track") cardiac surgery, accompanied by bypass-sparing myocardial stabilization devices, "keyhole" surgery, limited sternotomy incisions, and improvements in clinical outcome [3]. By 2000, transesophageal echocardiography (TEE) had established a role for monitoring ischemia during coronary revascularization as an adjunct to the electrocardiogram (ECG) and pulmonary arterial (PA) catheter; by 2015, it had replaced the PA catheter for many applications.

From 2005 to 2015, refinement of drug-eluting intracoronary stents and invention of potent antiplatelet drugs reduced the risk of stent thrombosis, resulting in sharp declines in the number of coronary artery operative procedures. Only in recent years have operation numbers recovered, now applied to patients with anatomy too complex for single or multivessel stents.

D. Evaluating risk of morbidity and mortality for CABG surgery

1. **Risk factor models.** Risk stratification tools differ in the weights assigned to individual factors, and in the factors considered for inclusion in a model of increased perioperative morbidity or mortality. Among the reported models, poor left ventricular (LV) function, including a history of congestive heart failure or LV ejection fraction less than 30%, advanced age, obesity, emergency surgery, concomitant valve surgery, prior cardiac surgery, history of diabetes, and history of renal failure feature prominently [4,5]. Some

TABLE 10.1 Risk factor inclusion in various risk stratification models for coronary artery bypass grafting (CABG)

	Montreal	Cleveland	Newark	New York	Northern New England	Society of Thoracic Surgeons
Emergency	+	+	+	+	+	+
Poor left ventricular (LV) function/ congestive heart failure	+	+	+	+	+	+
Redo operation	+	+	+	+	+	+
Gender/small size	–	+	+	+	+	+
Valve disease	–	+	+	+	–	–
Advanced age	+	+	+	+	+	+
Renal disease	–	+	+	+	+	–
Obesity	+	–	+	–	–	–

reports also link these factors to increased length of stay and increased hospital costs. Table 10.1 presents several risk stratification tools.

2. **Model evaluation.** No model can completely capture the risk of caring for sicker patients. The American College of Cardiology/American Heart Association (ACC/AHA) assigns a level IIA recommendation (level of evidence C) to the use of models for prediction of morbidity and mortality [6]. Some models do not allow for adequate flexibility concerning the dynamic nature of patient physiology during the preoperative period. For example, a patient's LV ejection fraction at the time of cardiac catheterization will be used in the evaluation process instead of that derived from TEE at the time of surgery.

II. Myocardial oxygen supply

A. **Introduction**

The viability and function of the heart depend upon the relatively delicate balance of oxygen supply and demand. The cardiac anesthesiologist can manipulate these determinants perioperatively to benefit the patient. The myocardium maximally extracts O_2 from arterial blood at rest, with a coronary sinus blood PO_2 of 27 mm Hg, and saturation less than 50%. Upon exertion or hemodynamic stress, the only way to increase O_2 supply acutely to meet the greater myocardial energy demand is by increasing the coronary blood flow (CBF). When CBF does not increase sufficiently, anaerobic metabolism and ischemia ensue. The following approach achieves the clinical goal of ensuring that O_2 supply at least matches demand:

1. Optimize the determinants of myocardial O_2 supply and demand.
2. Select anesthetics and adjuvant agents and techniques according to their effects on O_2 supply and demand.
3. Monitor for ischemia to detect its occurrence early and intervene rapidly.

B. **Coronary artery anatomy**

1. **Left main coronary artery.** A thorough understanding of the coronary artery anatomy and the distribution of myocardial blood flow allows an understanding of the extent and degree of myocardium at risk for ischemia and infarction during surgery. The blood supply to the myocardium derives from the aorta through two main coronary arteries (see Fig. 10.1), the left and right coronary arteries. The left main coronary artery extends for a short distance (0 to 40 mm) before dividing, between the aorta and PA, into the left anterior descending (LAD) artery and the circumflex coronary artery.

2. **Left anterior descending coronary artery.** The LAD coronary artery begins as a continuation of the left main coronary artery and courses down the interventricular groove, giving rise to the diagonal and septal branches. The septal branches vary in number and size, and provide the predominant blood supply to the interventricular septum. The septal branches also supply the bundle branches and the Purkinje system. One to three diagonal branches of variable size distribute blood to the anterolateral aspect of the heart. The LAD artery usually terminates at the apex of the LV.

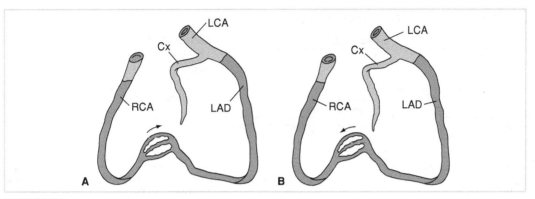

FIGURE 10.1 Two examples of possible left main "equivalency." Two-vessel coronary disease with an occluded left anterior descending coronary artery (LAD) and myocardium jeopardized by a right coronary artery (RCA) stenosis (**A**) or an occluded RCA and myocardium jeopardized by a stenotic LAD (**B**). Cx, circumflex coronary artery; LCA, left coronary artery. Darker shading indicates occlusion or severe stenosis. (From Hutter AM Jr. Is there a left main equivalent? *Circulation.* 1980;62(2):207–211, with permission.)

3. **Circumflex coronary artery.** The circumflex artery courses through the left atrioventricular groove giving rise to one to three obtuse marginal branches, which supply the lateral wall of the LV. In 15% of patients, the circumflex artery gives rise to the posterior descending coronary artery ("left dominant"). In 45% of patients, the sinus node artery arises from the circumflex distribution.

4. **Right coronary artery (RCA).** The RCA traverses the right atrioventricular groove. It gives rise to acute marginal branches that supply the right anterior wall of the right ventricle (RV). In approximately **85% of individuals**, the RCA gives rise to the **posterior descending artery** to supply the posterior inferior aspect of the LV (right dominant system). Thus, in the majority of the population, the RCA supplies a significant portion of blood flow to the LV, while in the other 15% of the population, the posterior-inferior aspect of the LV is supplied by the circumflex coronary artery (left dominant system) or both right coronary and circumflex arteries (codominant system). The sinus node artery arises from the RCA in 55% of patients. The atrioventricular node artery derives from the dominant coronary artery and is responsible for blood supply to the node, the bundle of His, and the proximal part of the bundle branches.

C. **Determinants of myocardial oxygen supply**

In broad terms, the supply of oxygen to the myocardium is determined by the arterial oxygen content of the blood and the blood flow in the coronary arteries.

1. **O_2 content = (hemoglobin) (1.34) (% saturation) + (0.003) (PO_2)**

Maximal O_2 content therefore involves having a high hemoglobin level, highly saturated blood, and a high PO_2, although a high PO_2 is quantitatively less important than a high O_2 saturation. Normothermia, normal pH, and high levels of 2,3-diphosphoglyceric acid all favor tissue release of O_2.

2. **Determinants of blood flow in normal coronary arteries.** CBF varies directly with the **pressure differential** across the coronary bed (coronary perfusion pressure [CPP]) and inversely with coronary vascular resistance (CVR): CBF = CPP/CVR. However, CBF is autoregulated (i.e., resistance varying directly with perfusion pressure) so that flow is relatively independent of CPP between 50 and 150 mm Hg but is pressure dependent outside of this range. Metabolic, autonomic, hormonal, and anatomic parameters alter CVR, and hydraulic factors influence CPP. Coronary stenoses also increase CVR.

a. **Control of CVR.** Factors affecting CVR are outlined in Table 10.2.

(1) **Metabolic factors.** When increased coronary flow is required secondary to increased myocardial workload, metabolic control factors are primarily responsible. Hydrogen ion, CO_2, lactate, and adenosine all may play a role in metabolic regulation of CBF by inducing changes in CVR [7].

TABLE 10.2 Control of coronary vascular resistance

	Increase CVR	Decrease CVR
Metabolic	$\uparrow O_2, \downarrow CO_2, \downarrow H^+$	$\downarrow O_2, \uparrow CO_2, \uparrow H^+$ Lactate Adenosine
Autonomic nervous system	$\uparrow$ α-Adrenergic tone $\uparrow$ Cholinergic tone	$\uparrow$ β-Adrenergic tone
Hormonal	$\uparrow$ Vasopressin (antidiuretic hormone) $\uparrow$ Angiotensin $\uparrow$ Thromboxane	$\uparrow$ Prostacyclin
Endothelial modulation		$\uparrow$ Nitric oxide $\uparrow$ Endothelium-derived hyperpolarizing factor $\uparrow$ Prostaglandin I_2

$\uparrow$, increased; $\downarrow$, decreased; CVR, coronary vascular resistance.

(2) **Autonomic nervous system.** The coronary arteries and arterioles possess α- and β-**adrenergic** receptors. In general, α_1-receptors are responsible for coronary vasoconstriction, whereas β-receptors mediate a vasodilatory effect. α_2-Receptors on endothelial cells and muscarinic signaling appear to be involved in a nitric oxide–mediated decrease in coronary vascular tone [8]. An increased population of α-receptors may cause episodes of coronary spasm in individuals with nonobstructed coronaries. α_1-Mediated constriction of the coronary circulation may counter some of the metabolic vasodilation, especially in the resting basal state. However, under most circumstances such as increasing demand or ischemia, metabolic control factors will override α-mediated vasoconstriction.

(3) **Hormonal factors.** Two stress hormones, vasopressin (antidiuretic hormone) and angiotensin, are potent coronary vasoconstrictors. However, blood levels of these hormones during major stress may be insufficient to produce significant coronary vasoconstriction. Thromboxane participates in thrombosis and coronary vasospasm during myocardial infarction. Prostaglandin I_2 (PGI$_2$) decreases coronary vascular tone.

(4) **Endothelial modulation.** Nitric oxide triggers a cyclic guanosine monophosphate (c-GMP)–mediated vasodilatory effect on vascular smooth muscle, and may also contribute to vessel patency and blood flow by inhibiting platelet adhesion. PGI$_2$ and endothelium-derived hyperpolarizing factor also cause relaxation of vascular smooth muscle.

(5) **Anatomic factors**

    (a) **Capillary/myocyte ratio.** Only three- to four-fifths of available myocardial capillaries function during normal conditions. During exercise, episodes of hypoxia, or extreme myocardial O_2 demand, the additional unopened capillaries are recruited and increase blood flow, causing a decrease in CVR and in diffusion distance of O_2 to a given myocyte. This adaptation, along with coronary vasodilation, contributes to coronary vascular reserve.

    (b) **Coronary collaterals.** Coronary collateral channels exist in the human myocardium. Under most circumstances, they are nonfunctional. However, in the presence of impeded CBF, these coronary channels may enlarge over time and become functional.

(6) **Other factors affecting CVR.** CVR may be partly regulated by myogenic control of vessel diameter, which dynamically responds to the distending pressure inside the vessel. CVR increases with the increased blood viscosity caused by high hematocrit or hypothermia. Thus, hemodilution should accompany induced hypothermia. There is a transmural gradient of vascular tone, with vascular resistance being lower in the subendocardium than in the subepicardium [7].

b. **Hydraulic factors and subendocardial blood flow**
   (1) **LV subendocardial blood flow.** Unlike CBF in the low-pressure RV system, LV subendocardial blood flow is intermittent and occurs only during diastole. Because of the increased intracavitary pressure and excessive subendocardial myocyte shortening, subendocardial arterioles are essentially closed during systole. **Of the total LV coronary flow, 85% occurs during diastole and 15% occurs in systole (primarily in the epicardial region).** Thus, the majority of blood flow to the epicardial and middle layers of the LV and **all** the blood flow to the endocardium occur during diastole.
   (2) **Coronary perfusion pressure (CPP).** CPP equals the arterial driving pressure less the back-pressure to flow across the coronary bed. For the LV, the driving pressure is the aortic blood pressure during diastole. The back-pressure to flow depends on the area of myocardium under consideration. Because the endocardium is the area most prone to ischemia, attention focuses on its flow, and thus the usual formula for CPP uses left ventricular end-diastolic pressure (LVEDP) as back-pressure instead of right atrial pressure (RAP), despite the fact that most coronary venous blood returns to the heart via the coronary sinus:

$$CPP = \text{Aortic diastolic pressure} - LVEDP$$

Because diastole shortens relative to systole as heart rate increases, subendocardial blood flow is decreased at extremely rapid heart rates. Figure 10.2 demonstrates the total time per minute spent in diastole as a function of heart rate. Elevations in LVEDP (e.g., heart failure, ischemia) also will impede subendocardial blood flow. **Thus, to optimize CPP, one should aim for normal-to-high diastolic blood pressure, low LVEDP, and low heart rate.**

3. **Determinants of myocardial blood flow in stenotic coronaries.** In addition to the physiologic determinants of myocardial blood flow in normal coronary arteries, stenotic vessels add pathologic determinants of myocardial blood flow. Stenoses locally increase CVR and decrease CBF, although ischemia-induced arteriolar vasodilation decreases CVR downstream of stenosis in a compensatory effort to maintain blood flow. Reduction in CBF in stenotic vessels is a function of the length and degree of stenosis, presence or absence of collaterals, pattern of stenosis, and presence of certain coexisting disease states, such as diabetes mellitus and hypertension, which predispose to microcirculatory pathology and ventricular hypertrophy, respectively.

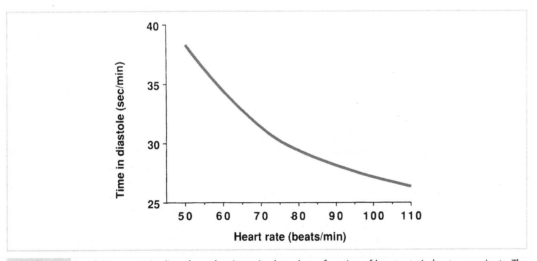

FIGURE 10.2 Total time spent in diastole each minute is plotted as a function of heart rate in beats per minute. The reduction in diastolic interval leads to diminished left ventricular (LV) blood flow as heart rate increases.

In particular, some patients present with a vasospastic component, which may aggravate a fixed lesion or even create anginal symptoms in patients with angiographically clear vessels.

a. Poiseuille's law determines the hemodynamic significance of a coronary obstruction in long (segmental) lesions. Given the same decrease in cross-sectional area, a longer segmental stenosis of a coronary artery reduces flow more than a short one.

b. Because CBF is reduced in proportion to the fourth power of the vessel diameter, a 50% diameter decrease in lumen size decreases flow to 1/16th its initial value, which is hemodynamically consistent with symptoms of angina on exertion. A 75% reduction in diameter at angiography corresponds to a greater than 98% reduction in flow, and corresponds clinically to symptoms of angina at rest.

c. Sequential lesions in the same coronary artery impact coronary flow in an additive fashion.

d. With longstanding coronary obstruction, collateral circulation often develops. For low-grade obstructive lesions, these channels supply enough blood flow to prevent ischemia. However, as the degree of coronary stenosis increases, the collateral channels may not be adequate.

e. Certain patterns of stenoses have important clinical implications related to the amount of myocardium supplied and placed in jeopardy by the stenotic lesion(s). A left main coronary stenosis limits blood flow to a large amount of the LV muscle mass. High-grade, very proximal stenotic lesions of both the circumflex and LAD systems have the same physiologic implications as does a left main stenosis. Prognostically, however, a left main stenosis is grimmer because rupture of a single atheroma will compromise a larger amount of myocardium. In addition, similar "left main equivalent" situations may exist when a severely stenosed coronary provides collateral blood flow to a region with a totally occluded vessel (Fig. 10.1). In addition to discrete focal and segmental coronary lesions in graftable vessels, diffuse distal disease may lessen the effectiveness of bypassing proximal coronary obstructions.

III. **Myocardial oxygen demand**

Direct measurement of myocardial oxygen demand is not feasible in the clinical setting. The three major determinants of myocardial O_2 demand are heart rate, contractility, and wall stress.

A. **Heart rate**

If a relatively fixed amount of O_2 were consumed per heartbeat, one would expect the O_2 demand per minute to increase linearly with heart rate. Thus, a doubling of heart rate would yield a doubling of O_2 demand. In fact, demand more than doubles with a twofold increase in heart rate. The source of this additional O_2 demand is the staircase phenomenon, in which increased heart rate causes a small increase in contractility and increases in contractility mean more O_2 consumed (see Section III.B below). As the functional impact of myocardial ischemia is virtually immediate, the impact of heart rate is best considered in the context of the balance between oxygen supply and demand per beat rather than per minute, which underscores the importance of the simultaneous small increase in O_2 demand and substantial decrease in O_2 supply associated with even a modest increase in heart rate.

B. **Contractility**

More O_2 is used by a highly contractile heart compared with a more relaxed heart.

1. **Quantitative assessment.** Strictly defined, the contractile state of the heart is a dynamic intrinsic characteristic that is not influenced by preload or afterload. Previous attempts to measure contractility using physiologic variables include the rate of rise of LV pressure, (dP/dt), and its value normalized to chamber pressure ([dP/dt]/P). Neither succeeds. Clinically it is possible to quantify dP/dt echocardiographically by measuring the rate of rise in the velocity of the mitral regurgitant jet using Doppler technology. Unfortunately, loading conditions and chamber compliance significantly affect the acceleration of the mitral regurgitant jet. In addition, although mitral regurgitation frequently is observed echocardiographically, it is not universally present. Contractility can be approximated in a load-independent fashion using the slope of the end-systolic pressure–volume

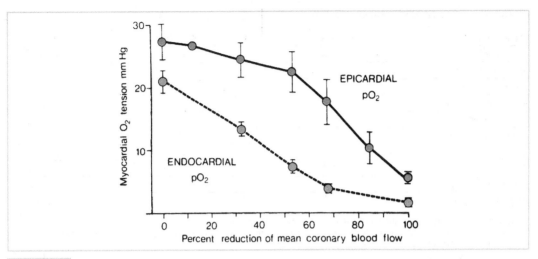

FIGURE 10.3 Relationship of subendocardial O_2 supply (represented by myocardial O_2 tension) to reductions in coronary blood flow (CBF). Demonstrated is the increased vulnerability of the subendocardial zone compared to the epicardial zone. (Modified from Winbury MM, Howe BB. Stenosis: regional myocardial ischemia and reserve. In: Winbury MM, Abiko Y, eds. *Ischemic myocardium and antianginal drugs.* New York: Raven; 1979:59.)

relationships of a family of LV pressure–volume loops. This method usually is not available in clinical settings.

2. **Qualitative measures.** One can easily observe the contractile state of the heart when the pericardium is open. Remember, though, that the RV is more easily and most often viewed this way, whereas the LV is more obscured. TEE provides a means for qualitative estimation of LV contractility. Clinically, we infer good contractility when the arterial pressure tracing rises briskly. However, the shape of the radial arterial tracing is heavily influenced by the system's resonant frequency, damping by air bubbles in the tubing, compliance of the arterial tree, reflections of pressure waves from arterioles, and other confounders.

3. **Increased subendocardial myocyte shortening.** Myocytes in the subendocardial region undergo more shortening than those in other areas because of geometric factors. Because they operate at a higher contractile state, they have greater oxidative metabolism. Subendocardial vessels, already maximally dilated, cannot respond to increased demand and intermittent limitations of blood flow in the subendocardial region. Thus, myocardial O_2 tension falls first here (Fig. 10.3), and this region is more susceptible to ischemia.

C. **Wall stress**

The stress in the ventricular wall depends on the pressure in the ventricle during contraction (afterload), the chamber size (preload), and the wall thickness. The calculation for a sphere (which we shall assume for the shape of the ventricle, for the sake of simplicity) comes from Laplace's law:

Wall stress = Pressure × radius/(2 × wall thickness)

1. **Chamber pressure.** Oxygen demand increases with chamber pressure. Doubling the pressure doubles the O_2 demand. Systemic blood pressure usually reflects the chamber pressure; thus, we equate systemic blood pressure with LV afterload. The heart's true afterload is more complex, because elastic and inertial components also affect ejection. In aortic stenosis, however, the LV experiences very high chamber pressures despite more modest systemic pressures. The clinical goal is to keep afterload (and thus wall stress) low.

2. **Chamber size.** Doubling the ventricular volume increases the radius by only 26% (volume varies with the radius cubed). Thus, increased chamber size is associated with more modest increases in O_2 demand. Nevertheless, because preload determines ventricular size, we desire a low preload to keep wall stress (and thus O_2 demand) low. Much of the benefit of nitroglycerin stems from venodilation and its attendant decrease in preload.

TABLE 10.3 Regulation of O_2 supply and demand

Parameter	Demand	Supply	O_2 balance
Low heart rate	↓	↑	Positive
Low RAP or PCWP	↓	↑[a]	Positive
High heart rate	↑	↓	Negative
High RAP or PCWP	↑	↓	Negative
High temperature	↑	0	Negative
Low temperature	↑↓	↓	Variable
Low MAP	↓	↓	Variable
High MAP	↑	↑	Variable
Low hemoglobin	↓	↓↑	Variable
High hemoglobin	↑	↑↓	Variable

[a]However, a drastic decrease in filling pressure will decrease cardiac output.
↑, increased; ↓, decreased; ↑↓, may increase or decrease; 0, unchanged; MAP, mean arterial pressure; PCWP, pulmonary capillary wedge pressure; RAP, right atrial pressure.

3. **Wall thickness.** A thicker wall means less stress over any part of the wall. Ventricular hypertrophy serves to decrease wall stress, although the additional tissue requires more O_2 overall. Hypertrophy occurs in response to the elevated afterload that occurs in chronic systemic hypertension or aortic stenosis. Although wall thickness is essentially uncontrollable clinically, its effects should be considered. LV aneurysms, seen after transmural infarction, increase wall stress because of their effect on LV volume (radius) and reduced wall thickness.

D. **Summary**

The factors that increase O_2 demand are increases in heart rate, chamber size, chamber pressure, and contractility. Table 10.3 and Figure 10.4 summarize the myocardial supply and demand relationship. Note that tachycardia and increases in LVEDP both lead to increased demand and decreased supply of oxygen.

IV. **Monitoring for myocardial ischemia**

A. **Introduction**

Typical monitoring for CABG surgery includes the standard American Society of Anesthesiologists (ASA) monitors and invasive arterial blood pressure monitoring. The most recent (2010) ASA/SCA practice guidelines recommend that TEE be *considered* for all CABG patients unless probe placement is contraindicated [9]. The use of PA catheters for routine CABG has become variable. Detection and treatment of intraoperative ischemia is critically important because intraoperative ischemia is an independent predictor of postoperative myocardial infarction [10]. Only half of intraoperative ischemic events can be related to a hemodynamic alteration and none can be detected by the presence of angina in anesthetized patients. Reduced or negative lactate extraction in a regional myocardial circulatory bed, while diagnostic of ischemia, cannot be routinely measured. Thus, we seek clues that ischemia leaves in its wake: changes on the ECG, PA pressure changes, and myocardial wall-motion abnormalities.

CLINICAL PEARL Trends in physiologic variables often predict a patient's status better than absolute numbers.

B. **Electrocardiogram (ECG) monitoring**

1. **Introduction.** TEE detection of wall-motion abnormalities has not replaced continuous multi-lead ECG monitoring as a standard monitor of intraoperative ischemia. ECG monitoring is inexpensive, easy to use and read, can be automated, and is available before and during the induction of anesthesia, when the TEE probe is not in place, and may be

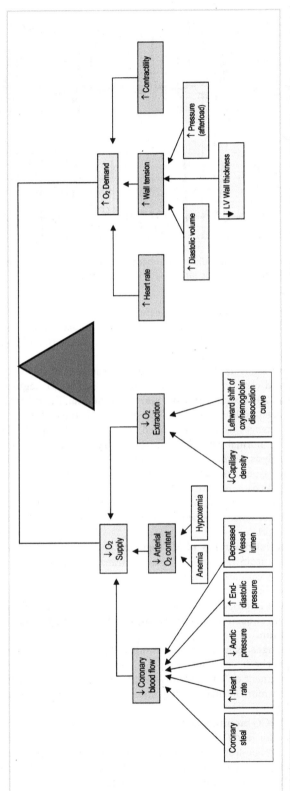

FIGURE 10.4 Summary of factors that affect myocardial oxygen supply and demand. (Adapted from Crystal GJ. Cardiovascular physiology. In: Miller RD, ed. *Atlas of anesthesia: vol. VIII. Cardiothoracic anesthesia.* Philadelphia, PA: Churchill Livingstone; 1999: 1:1, with permission.)

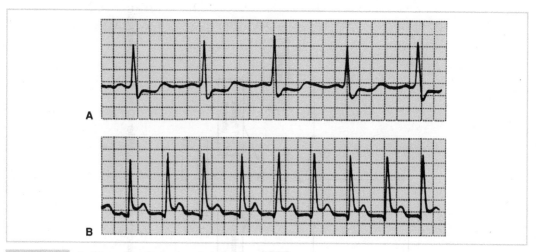

FIGURE 10.5 **A:** ST-segment depression, an indicator of subendocardial ischemia. **B:** Transmural ischemia, one cause of ST-segment elevation, produces the pattern appearing in the lower tracing.

carried through to the intensive care unit (ICU) setting, where TEE monitoring is impractical. ECG changes are less sensitive to ischemia: They occur later in the temporal cascade of events that follow myocardial ischemia, especially with lesser degrees of coronary supply/demand mismatch.

2. **ST-segment analysis.** Depression of the ST segment of the ECG denotes endocardial ischemia, and elevation denotes transmural ischemia. **ST-segment changes occur at least 60 to 120 seconds after the start of ischemia.** The reference for the ST segment usually is taken as 80 ms after the J-point, which is the end of the QRS wave (Fig. 10.5). Significant changes usually are defined as 0.1 mV or 1 mm of ST-segment elevation or depression at normal gain. ECG monitoring systems include automated real-time ST-segment analysis. Although this feature constitutes a definite advance in the "human engineering" aspects of ischemia monitoring, the machine is only as smart as the person interpreting its data. Beware of intraventricular conduction delays, bundle branch blocks, and ventricular pacing, all of which can render ST-segment analysis invalid. Check the machine's determination of where the ST segment occurs: 80 ms after the J-point is not always appropriate.

    a. **Differential diagnosis of ST-segment changes.** ST-segment elevation (Fig. 10.5) may arise from the several causes of transmural ischemia (atherosclerotic disease, coronary vasospasm, intracoronary air), or from pericarditis or ventricular aneurysm. One also must consider improper lead placement, particularly reversal of limb and leg leads, and improper selection of electronic filtering. **The diagnostic mode should always be chosen on machines equipped with a diagnostic–monitor mode selection option.**

3. **T-wave changes.** New T-wave alterations (flipped or flattened) may indicate ischemia. These may not be detected by viewing the ST segment alone. Likewise, pseudonormalization of the ST segment or T wave (an ischemic-looking tracing in a patient without ischemia changing to a more normal-looking one) may indicate a new onset of ischemia and should be treated appropriately.

4. **Multi-lead ECG monitoring.** Simultaneous observation of an inferior lead (II, III, or aVF) and an anterior lead (V_5: 5th intercostal space, anterior axillary line) provides detection superior to single-lead monitoring, together detecting approximately 90% of ischemic events. Ischemia limited to the posterior segments of the LV is difficult to detect with standard ECG monitoring. Modified chest leads may be necessary when the surgical incision precludes usual placement.

C. **Pulmonary artery (PA) pressure monitoring**

1. **General indications for a PA catheter for revascularization procedures.** PA catheters provide central delivery of infusions (typically via a side port introducer or a proximal lumen in the catheter), measurement of blood temperature and chamber pressures, and calculations of cardiac output, vascular resistance, and RV ejection fraction (with special catheters equipped with particularly fast thermistors). Some catheters also continuously measure mixed venous oxygen saturation. Observational studies conclude that PA catheterization does not affect outcome [11,12]. When clinicians were denied intraoperative access to PA catheter data unless the situation met strict criteria, access occurred in only 23% of patients, and management changed in fewer than 9% of all cases [13]. Even if shown unnecessary for the intraoperative management of routine coronary bypass surgery, PA catheters achieve utility postoperatively, when TEE cannot be utilized.

2. **Detection of ischemia: PA pressures.** The absolute PA pressure is not diagnostic of ischemia. Pulmonary hypertension, whether primary or secondary to chronic ischemia, hypertension, or to valvular heart disease, is not uncommon. PA pressures or pulmonary capillary occlusion pressures (PCWP) commonly exceed upper levels of normal due to chronic obstructive pulmonary disease (COPD), dependent catheter locations in the lung, or mitral stenosis, making elevated PA and PCWP pressures less reliable in the diagnosis of ischemia [14]. The shape of the transduced pressure waveform, however, is more predictive. Appearance of a new V wave on the PCWP waveform indicates functional mitral regurgitation, which is due to "new" ischemic papillary muscle dysfunction. It may occur before or even in the absence of ECG changes. However, detection of changes on the pulmonary capillary occlusion waveform requires frequent balloon inflation (wedging), introducing additional risk of vessel rupture. Often ischemia may be detected by a change in the shape of the PA tracing, obviating the need for frequent wedging.

CLINICAL PEARL   Look at the waveforms on the monitor first; if believable, then look at the digital readouts.

D. **Transesophageal echocardiography (TEE)**

1. **General indications for TEE during revascularization procedures.** TEE can assess ventricular preload and contractility, detect myocardial ischemia-induced regional wall-motion abnormalities (RWMAs), evaluate the aortic cannulation site, detect concomitant valve pathology, detect the presence and pathophysiologic effect of pericardial effusion, aid the placement of intra-aortic balloon catheters and coronary sinus catheters, and detect the presence of ventricular aneurysms and ventricular septal defects. TEE has become an invaluable clinical tool and has achieved routine intraoperative use during CABG at most institutions. New RWMAs after bypass correlate with adverse outcomes. See Chapter 5 for a detailed discussion of intraoperative TEE.

2. **Detection of myocardial ischemia with TEE RWMAs**

   a. **Introduction.** The heart **develops abnormal motion less than 1 minute following perfusion defects** [15]. RWMAs resulting from myocardial ischemia temporally precede both ECG and PAP changes. TEE simultaneously interrogates regions of the heart representative of all three major coronary arteries, including the posterior wall, which is not easily monitored with ECG. This is most easily accomplished in the short-axis, midpapillary muscle view. Some ischemia, confined to regions not visualized with this view, will escape detection unless one performs a comprehensive examination in multiple planes.

   b. **Limitations of monitoring RWMAs**

      (1) **Tethering.** Nonischemic tissue adjacent to ischemic tissue may move abnormally because it is attached to poorly moving tissue, thus exaggerating an RWMA.

      (2) **Pacing/bundle branch blocks.** Abnormal ventricular depolarization sequences not only affect ST-segment analysis (see Section IV.B.2), but also alter wall motion, and can mimic RWMA.

(3) **Interventricular septum.** Normal septal motion depends on appropriate ventricular loading conditions, the presence of pericardium, and normal electrical conduction.

(4) **Stunned myocardium.** Adequately perfused myocardium may exhibit RWMA if recovering from recent ischemia, thus prompting inappropriate therapeutic intervention.

(5) **Induction/ICU.** TEE use is not practical during induction of anesthesia or for continuous ICU monitoring.

> **CLINICAL PEARL**   Make observation of the surgical field and basic hemodynamics a priority, especially when performing TEE intraoperatively.

(6) **Diastolic LV filling patterns.** Unfortunately, ventricular filling patterns depend on ventricular loading conditions and the site of Doppler interrogation within the ventricular inflow tract, limiting its utility as a monitor for ischemia.

c. **Intraoperative stress TEE.** Low-dose dobutamine (2.5 μg/kg/min), when administered for 3 to 5 minutes, improves coronary flow without significantly affecting demand. The resultant myocardial energetics improve existing wall-motion abnormalities. Demonstration of contractile reserve using intraoperative stress echo then directs revascularization efforts to regions of myocardium able to benefit from the additional blood supply.

d. **Contrast echocardiography.** Intracoronary injection of sonicated albumin allows imaging of perfused myocardium, providing a tool to identify stunned myocardium, thus avoiding needless therapeutic intervention. At present, contrast agents are not approved by the U.S. Food and Drug Administration for this indication. Routine clinical use awaits resolution of some technical imaging issues. A microbubble contrast injection technique has also been described [16].

3. **Detection of infarction complications.** TEE can detect complications of ischemia/infarction such as acute mitral insufficiency, ventricular septal defect, and pericardial effusion.

V. **Anesthetic effects on myocardial oxygen supply and demand**
Outcome studies in cardiac surgery fail to reveal an effect of particular anesthetic agents [17,18]. Cardiac anesthesiologists, keenly aware of the impact of anesthetic agents on myocardial oxygen supply/demand dynamics, effectively monitor for and treat myocardial ischemia, thus accommodating for any such effects.

A. **Intravenous nonopioid agents**
1. **Propofol.** Propofol decreases systemic vascular resistance (SVR) and cardiac contractility and increases heart rate.

2. **Ketamine.** Ketamine increases sympathetic tone, leading to **increases in SVR, filling pressures, contractility, and heart rate.** Myocardial O_2 demand strongly increases, whereas O_2 supply only slightly augments, thus producing ischemia. However, a patient already maximally sympathetically stimulated responds with decreased contractility and vasodilation. Ketamine is not recommended for routine use in patients with ischemic heart disease. However, it is sometimes used in patients with cardiac tamponade, because of its ability to preserve heart rate, contractility, and SVR.

3. **Etomidate.** Induction doses of etomidate (0.2 to 0.3 mg/kg) **do not alter heart rate or cardiac output,** although mild peripheral vasodilation may lower blood pressure slightly. As such, it is an ideal drug for rapid induction of anesthesia in patients with ischemic heart disease. Etomidate offers little protection from the increases in heart rate and blood pressure that accompany intubation. It is usually necessary to supplement etomidate with other agents (e.g., opioids, benzodiazepines, volatile agents, β-blockers, and nitroglycerin) in order to control the hemodynamic profile and prevent myocardial oxygen supply/demand imbalance. An induction dose blocks adrenal steroidogenesis for at least 6 hours.

4. **Benzodiazepines.** Midazolam (0.2 mg/kg) or diazepam (0.5 mg/kg) may be used to induce anesthesia. Although both agents are compatible with the goal of maintaining hemodynamic stability, blood pressure may decrease more with midazolam due to more potent peripheral vasodilation. Negative inotropic effects are inconsequential. Blood pressure and filling pressures decrease with induction, whereas the heart rate remains essentially unchanged. Addition of induction doses of a benzodiazepine to a moderate-dose opioid technique, however, may result in profound peripheral vasodilation and hypotension.

5. **α_2-Adrenergic agonists.** Centrally acting α_2-adrenergic agonists result in a reduction in stress-mediated neurohumoral responses, and therefore are associated with decreases in heart rate and blood pressure [19]. These agents typically are used during maintenance of anesthesia or postoperatively. Preoperative oral clonidine reduces perioperative myocardial ischemia in patients undergoing CABG surgery, but occasionally results in significant intraoperative hypotension. Dexmedetomidine possesses greater α_2-selectivity than clonidine. Both agents have sedative and antinociceptive properties. Use of α_2-adrenergic agonists is associated with a reduced opioid requirement. In addition, α_2-adrenergic agonists do not cause respiratory depression.

B. **Volatile agents**

In general, volatile anesthetics decrease both O_2 supply and demand. The net effect on the myocardial supply/demand balance depends upon the hemodynamic profile that prevails at the time of administration.

1. **Heart rate.** Sevoflurane has negligible effect on heart rate. Desflurane and isoflurane often increase heart rate, although isoflurane decreases heart rate if its associated decrease in SVR is not profound, if the carotid baroreceptor function is impaired, or if the patient is fully β-blocked. In the steady state, the cardiovascular actions of desflurane are similar to those of isoflurane. However, during rapid desflurane induction without opioids, heart rate and systemic and PA blood pressures may increase and require therapeutic intervention.

   Desflurane use for inhalation induction is unwise due to a significant increase in heart rate, particularly with rapid escalation of the inspired concentration. Junctional rhythms may occur with any volatile agent; they deprive the heart of an atrial "kick," leading to decreased stroke volume, cardiac output, and CBF, offsetting the salubrious effects of low heart rate.

2. **Contractility.** All volatile anesthetics decrease contractility, lowering O_2 demand. However, isoflurane, desflurane, and sevoflurane cause less depression than halothane or enflurane. In decompensated hearts, all volatile anesthetics impair ventricular function.

3. **Afterload.** Decreases in cardiac output and SVR with volatile anesthesia result in decreased systemic blood pressure. Venodilation and blunted contractility account for the decrease in cardiac output. All volatile anesthetics vasodilate, but SVR decreases least with halothane. Both O_2 supply and O_2 demand decrease.

4. **Preload.** Volatile agents maintain filling pressures. Therefore, CPP (diastolic aortic pressure minus LVEDP) may decrease during volatile anesthesia.

5. **Coronary steal.** A coronary "steal" phenomenon has been described in which dilation of normal vascular beds diverts blood away from other beds that are ischemic and thus maximally dilated. Steal-prone anatomy may exist in 23% of the patients undergoing CABG [20]. Coronary steal has been observed in canine models of steal-prone coronary anatomy with isoflurane administration under circumstances in which collateral flow is pressure dependent. It is doubtful that isoflurane-induced coronary steal is clinically significant in patients undergoing coronary revascularization surgery as long as hypotension and consequent pressure-dependent coronary artery perfusion are avoided. Coronary steal has not been reported with halothane, enflurane, or desflurane.

6. **Preconditioning.** Volatile anesthetics may confer a degree of preconditioning-like protective effect against ischemia–reperfusion injury in human myocardial tissue [21] and reduce late cardiac events following cardiac surgery [22] (see Section VII.D.6).

C. **Nitrous oxide**

The mild negative inotropic effects of nitrous oxide decrease contractility, producing a reduction in both O_2 supply and demand. Nitrous oxide inhibition of norepinephrine uptake in the lung may explain the increased plasma norepinephrine levels and associated increase in pulmonary vascular pressures and resistance seen with nitrous oxide administration [23]. Adding nitrous oxide to an opioid-oxygen anesthetic decreases SVR due, in part, to the removal of the vasoconstrictive effects of 100% O_2. The sympathomimetic effects of nitrous oxide counterbalance any direct depression of contractility except in patients with poor LV function in whom the myocardium already is highly stimulated intrinsically.

If nitrous oxide is used in a technique that provides a "light" anesthetic that is inadequate to cover attendant stimulation, increases in SVR and afterload ensue.

D. Opioids

1. **Heart rate.** All opioids except meperidine decrease heart rate by centrally mediated vagotonia; meperidine has an atropine-like effect. The dose of drug and speed of injection affect the degree of bradycardia. The result is decreased O_2 demand. By releasing histamine, morphine or meperidine may elicit a reflex tachycardia that decreases O_2 supply and increases O_2 demand.

2. **Contractility.** Aside from meperidine, which decreases contractility, the opioids have little effect on contractility in clinical doses.

3. **Afterload.** In compromised patients, who often depend on elevated sympathetic tone to maintain cardiac output and systemic resistance, the loss of sympathetic tone associated with opioid induction of anesthesia may result in a sudden drop in blood pressure and consequent decreases in both O_2 supply and demand. Concomitant midazolam use augments the decreased SVR with opioid induction.

4. **Preload.** Despite a lack of histamine-releasing properties, fentanyl and sufentanil reduce preload when administered in either moderate (25 µg/kg for fentanyl) or larger doses by decreasing intrinsic sympathetic tone. Oxygen demand is decreased.

5. **Hyperdynamic state.** Following surgical incision and especially with sternotomy, elevations of heart rate, blood pressure, and cardiac output with or without decreased filling pressures are common during pure opioid-oxygen anesthetic techniques in patients with good ventricular function. This high-supply/high-demand state may be less preferable than the low-supply/low-demand state achieved with volatile anesthetic agents. Additional opioid, which often fails to treat the hypertension associated with a hyperdynamic cardiac state, may decrease systemic blood pressure excessively when hypertension originates from increased SVR alone.

E. Muscle relaxants

1. **Succinylcholine.** This drug may cause a variety of **dysrhythmias** (bradycardia, tachycardia, extrasystoles), which negatively affect myocardial O_2 balance, although most often it is hemodynamically benign.

2. **Pancuronium.** Heart rate increases 20% when pancuronium accompanies a volatile anesthetic, but effectively neutralizes the bradycardia that accompanies a high-dose opioid technique. With declining use of high-dose opioid techniques, many institutions have removed pancuronium from their formularies, in favor of vecuronium, rocuronium, and cisatracurium.

3. **Vecuronium.** Vecuronium has a **flat cardiovascular profile** that is ideal with a low- or moderate-dose opioid anesthetic supplemented by a volatile agent. Bradycardia occurs when it accompanies the **rapid** injection of high doses of the highly lipid-soluble opioids.

4. **Rocuronium.** Rocuronium's mild vagolytic action is typically clinically insignificant, and rocuronium administration does not cause significant hemodynamic perturbations.

5. **Cisatracurium.** Cisatracurium lacks significant cardiovascular effects. The majority of metabolism is via Hofmann elimination, with ester hydrolysis making a minor contribution. Evidence supports faster neuromuscular recovery with cisatracurium versus rocuronium or vecuronium in both adults and children [24,25], although this difference is likely insignificant in view of the duration of coronary artery procedures.

F. Summary

Pure volatile anesthesia provides a **low-supply/low-demand** environment. The opioid-oxygen technique provides a **high-supply/high-demand** environment. Success with either technique depends on maintaining proper balance, with O_2 supply exceeding demand. Techniques utilizing modest doses of opioid with propofol or low doses of volatile anesthetics are commonly used. These techniques permit rapid recovery from anesthesia while requiring careful attention to hemodynamic control to avoid intraoperative ischemia, and diligent monitoring to detect and treat it.

VI. Anesthetic approach for myocardial revascularization procedures

A. Fast-track cardiac anesthesia is defined as techniques leading to early endotracheal extubation, typically within 6 hours of completion of surgery.

1. **Inclusion guidelines.** Early fast-track initiatives excluded patients with obesity, moderate-to-severe pulmonary disease, emergency operations, poor ventricular function, combined procedures, re-operations, or advanced age—about 40% to 60% of surgical revascularization patients. Application to sicker and riskier patients has progressed, so that most patients now have an opportunity for early extubation, the exceptions usually being those with hemodynamic compromise, intraoperative complications, or difficult airways [26].

2. **Anesthetic management** (Table 10.4)

   a. **Premedication.** Long-acting agents are preferentially avoided. Same-day admission patients have inadequate time for sedation with slow-onset agents. Midazolam (0.03 to 0.07 mg/kg IV) usually suffices to allay anxiety.

   b. **Intraoperative anesthetic agent management**

   (1) **Induction of anesthesia.** Etomidate or propofol accomplishes induction. Supplementation with a volatile agent or fentanyl (up to 7 µg/kg) provides more stable hemodynamics for tracheal intubation. Esmolol or nitroglycerin can prevent or treat a breakthrough hyperdynamic state.

   Intrathecal or epidural analgesia, placed preoperatively, facilitates recovery by decreasing the perioperative opioid requirements [27]. Regarding the potential for neuraxial hematoma formation, current American Society of Regional Anesthesia and Pain Medicine (ASRA) guidelines recommend 1 hour between needle insertion and administration of IV heparin, an interval easily achieved in coronary artery surgery [28]. Intrathecal lumbar injection of preservative-free morphine 5 µg/kg via a 25 g or smaller needle is also quick, effective, and appropriate for these patients already committed to postoperative intensive care.

   (2) **Maintenance of anesthesia.** Volatile agent supplementation limits the total opioid dose to 10 to 15 µg/kg fentanyl (or its approximate equivalent using sufentanil). The ultra–short-acting opioid remifentanil provides good hemodynamic stability, adequate attenuation of the neurohumoral stress response, and early awakening. However, a short half-life and rapid tolerance necessitate substantial opioid administration postoperatively. Reliance on a volatile agent can lead to a hyperdynamic state during transport or upon ICU arrival, potentially prompting the use of long-duration sedatives by the ICU staff.

TABLE 10.4   Typical fast-track cardiac anesthetic

Induction	Etomidate—or—	0.3 mg/kg
	Propofol	2–3 mg/kg
	Fentanyl	0–10 µg/kg
	Midazolam	0–0.05 mg/kg
	Succinylcholine—or—	1 mg/kg
	Rocuronium	0.6–1.2 mg/kg
Maintenance	Fentanyl	5–10 µg/kg
	Midazolam	0.05 mg/kg
	Rocuronium	To maintain train-of-four count of 1 or 2
	Propofol	0–30 µg/kg/min
	Volatile agent	0.5–1 minimum alveolar concentration
Intensive care unit (ICU)	Propofol—or—	0–30 µg/kg/min
	Dexmedetomidine	0.5–1 µg/kg/hr

α_2-Agonists (e.g., dexmedetomidine and clonidine) are used adjunctively to reduce the neurohumoral stress response and for their sedative and antinociceptive properties. These agents reduce the anesthetic requirement and thus facilitate more rapid emergence. Further, a dexmedetomidine infusion can be continued postoperatively without compromising early extubation, thus facilitating both ICU transition and fast tracking.

c. **Intraoperative awareness.** Significant intraoperative awareness occurs in 0.3% of fast-track patients, similar to that observed in general surgery [29]. When using moderate doses of opioids, matching the depth of anesthesia to the operative stimulus at different times will avoid harmful hemodynamic responses; volatile agents provide this flexibility. A vaporizer attached to the cardiopulmonary bypass (CPB) circuit facilitates appropriate anesthetic depth during bypass with moderate hypothermia. The role of continuous processed EEG monitoring such as bispectral index (BIS, Aspect Medical Systems, Natick, MA, USA) remains unclear, although many centers have embraced its use.

d. **Temperature homeostasis.** Early extubation is unwise in the hypothermic patient: Arrhythmia, coagulopathy, shivering, and increased oxygen consumption complicate postoperative care and delay discharge [30]. Fluid-filled warming blankets and heated-humidified breathing circuits fail to preserve heat in the face of the huge caloric deficits of cardiac surgical patients who undergo moderate hypothermia (28° to 32°C) during CPB. Intravenous (IV) fluid warmers can significantly attenuate core temperature reduction during cardiac surgery if infused volumes are substantial [31]. The CPB circuit heat exchanger provides the best means of restoring body temperature. Prior to separation from CPB, targeting a PA blood temperature greater than 37°C and a bladder temperature greater than 35°C reduces hypothermic "rebound." Forced hot-air convective warming helps during off-bypass revascularization, despite the minimal body surface available. Maintaining OR temperature as warm as can be reasonably tolerated by operative personnel prevents heat loss.

e. **Hemostasis.** To prevent bleeding after operation, supplement scrupulous surgical attention to hemostasis with pharmacologic hemostatic agents such as aminocaproic acid or tranexamic acid (see Chapter 19). Many centers restrict use of these agents to revascularization that involves CPB.

f. **Intraoperative extubation.** In the absence of ventricular impairment, hemodynamic instability, hypothermia, or significant coagulopathy, one can consider extubation in the OR prior to transport. One nonrandomized, underpowered study claimed intraoperative extubation did not reduce ICU length of stay [32]. With careful patient selection, immediate extubation offers the potential for shorter ICU and hospital stays [33], although the benefit to using this approach remains debatable. Strategic use of opioids at induction and judicious use after sternal wiring enables adequate ventilation while providing satisfactory analgesia. One technique combines intrathecal morphine (300 to 500 µg) prior to an induction using sufentanil (150 to 250 µg IV) with morphine (0 to 10 mg IV) at sternal reapposition. Rapid awakening can be facilitated by substituting nitrous oxide or desflurane for isoflurane or sevoflurane upon placement of sternal wires. With this technique, ICU personnel must be willing to tolerate the mild to moderate respiratory acidosis ($PaCO_2$ up to 50 mm Hg) seen in patients with adequate opioid analgesia immediately after extubation. Patients remaining intubated need adequate sedation or anesthesia to last through the transport and for at least 30 minutes beyond in order to avoid hypertension, tachycardia, and coughing in the semi-controlled environment of tangled access lines and rolling beds.

CLINICAL PEARL Plan ahead for tracheal extubation. When extubating in the OR titrate analgesics in advance and prepare ICU staff to accept the mild respiratory acidosis accompanies adequate analgesia.

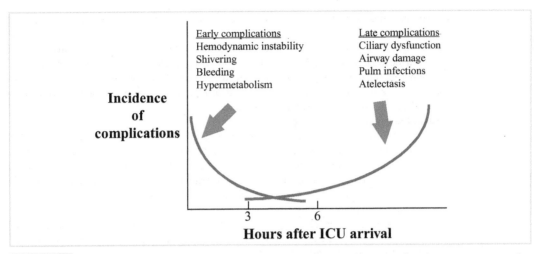

FIGURE 10.6 Early and late immediate postoperative complications seen in patients undergoing coronary revascularization. Pulm, pulmonary; ICU, intensive care unit. (Adapted from Higgins T. Pro: early endotracheal extubation is preferable to late extubation in patients following coronary artery surgery. *J Cardiothorac Vasc Anesth.* 1992;6(4):488–493.)

3. **ICU management.** A traditional fast-track approach requires sedation with a relatively short-acting agent until the patient is ready for tracheal extubation, ideally with an agent devoid of significant hemodynamic effect. For an uncomplicated patient, tailor the level of sedation for extubation 4 to 6 hours after arrival, during which time the patient recovers from myocardial stunning, achieves normothermia, and demonstrates perioperative hemostasis (Fig. 10.6).

Propofol provides a smooth transition from intraoperative anesthesia to postoperative sedation. It is easy to titrate, with quick onset and offset of action, and minor hemodynamic effects at sedative doses. Supplemental nitroglycerin, nitroprusside, or clevidipine infusions can titrate blood pressure rapidly. Compared to low-dose morphine, sufentanil analgesia in the early ICU period resulted in fewer and less severe ischemic events [34]. When administered as a continuous infusion, dexmedetomidine, mimics natural sleep and significantly reduces use of analgesics, β-blockers, antiemetics, epinephrine, and diuretics [35]. Studies comparing the safety and efficacy of dexmedetomidine and propofol for ICU sedation (including endpoints such as analgesic requirement reduction and hemodynamic changes) fail to substantiate the superiority of either approach [36,37], and show no difference in ventilator weaning time [36].

CLINICAL PEARL   Monitor hemodynamics continuously during transfer from the OR. Actively treat important hemodynamic changes and pain during transfer.

4. **Clinical and economic benefits**
   a. **Clinical benefits of enhanced recovery.** Early extubation may be associated with reduced postoperative lung atelectasis and improved pulmonary shunt fraction, and yields greater patient satisfaction as long as appropriate analgesia is maintained. Positive-pressure ventilation has deleterious effects on cardiac output and organ perfusion that may be minimized by early extubation. Early chest tube removal facilitates patient mobilization.
   b. **Economic benefits.** Early extubation protocols reduce ICU and hospital lengths of stay, and thus can reduce the cost of hospitalization by as much as 25% [37,38].
B. **Off-bypass revascularization**
   Off-pump coronary artery bypass (OPCAB) utilizes venous or arterial conduits to the coronary arteries via sternotomy but without CPB. See Section VI.D.2 for a discussion of port

access surgery and Section VI.D.3 for minimally invasive direct coronary artery bypasses (MIDCAB).

1. **Technique.** Following sternotomy and anticoagulation, the surgeon places distal anastomoses using myocardial stabilizers. With the heart continuing to fill, beat, and contract, a section is immobilized sufficiently to permit vascular sutures for distal anastomoses. If needed, an aortic side clamp permits placement of proximal anastomoses. Reapproximation of the sternum and layered closure complete the surgical procedure.

2. **Advantages and Disadvantages**
   a. **Graft patency.** Randomized studies comparing OPCAB to conventional CABG with CPB yield differing results [39,40] with respect to short- and long-term graft patency. Grafts to the right coronary circulation appear more likely to lose patency with OPCAB. Outcomes over 6 to 8 years did not differ between on pump versus OPCAB in an experienced center [41]. Most available data from randomized controlled studies derive from patients with expected mortality of 1% to 2%.
   b. Level IA evidence-based criteria suggest that mortality and quality-of-life markers do not differ, whereas the duration of ventilation, hospital length of stay, and overall morbidity are decreased with OPCAB.
   c. Somewhat weaker evidence supports decreased blood loss and transfusion requirements, decreased myocardial enzyme release up to 24 hours, less renal dysfunction, fewer coagulation abnormalities, and lower incidences of atrial fibrillation and cognitive impairment with OPCAB [42].
   d. **Hemodynamic instability.** During performance of circumflex or inferior anastomoses (i.e., on the posterior surface of the heart), maintaining hemodynamic stability may prove challenging despite frequent manipulation of patient position, volume status, and vasopressors. This difficulty derives from torsion of the heart or geometry incompatible with effective ejection. Ventricular fibrillation may occur suddenly during this time.

3. Patient selection for OPCAB varies widely among institutions. Examples of local criteria include:
   a. Patients with anterior lesions only, thus limiting the risks of hemodynamic compromise and potential subsequent graft occlusion associated with inferior anastomoses.
   b. Avoidance of CPB to minimize the risk for stroke and renal failure (i.e., for those patients with large amounts of aortic plaque, severe vascular disease in general, or with renal insufficiency).
   c. **None or all.** Some surgeons choose to perform all CABGs as OPCABs, while others consistently utilize CPB.

4. **Preoperative assessment.** More so than with conventional CABG, with OPCAB knowledge of the intended placement of grafts and functional myocardial reserve prepares the anesthesia team for the extent of physiologic trespass and its expected impact on homeostasis.
   a. Interruption of flow when grafting proximal coronary artery stenoses can impact a large amount of myocardium.
   b. Interruption of flow to vessels with high-grade lesions may have little impact owing to formation of collateral circulation.

5. Monitoring for a given OPCAB patient should be at least as extensive as for conventional CABG due to the added stress of cumulative myocardial ischemia during vessel occlusion and grafting. Twisting or "flipping" the heart changes its electrical axis, making it difficult to diagnose ischemia via ECG criteria, and also thwarting acquisition of standard TEE images. Thermodilution will still accurately measure cardiac output.

6. **Fast-track criteria apply.** See Section VI.A regarding choice of anesthetic agents and techniques to facilitate early extubation, awakening, and safe transfer from intensive care environments. Occasionally, an OPCAB case converts to one using CPB; for this reason, some caregivers avoid techniques they would not employ in the presence of full heparinization, such as epidural anesthesia.

7. **Temperature.** Without the heat exchanger of the CPB machine to transfer calories to the patient, temperature management focuses on prevention of heat loss and use of forced air on available surfaces, even if only head and shoulders. The so-called "second skin" underbody warming approaches can be used as well. See Section VI.A.2.d for additional guidance.

8. Heparin management varies among institutions. Some target an ACT twice that of baseline, as for noncoronary vascular surgery. Others aim for a minimum of 300 seconds, whereas some administer doses as they would for the conduct of CPB. Protamine doses should aim to neutralize the heparin administered, because bleeding with OPCAB remains nearly as much a threat to successful surgery as it does with conventional CABG. However, CPB affects platelet function adversely and activates the fibrinolytic system more than does OPCAB.

9. Specific maneuvers to provide adequate hemodynamics.

    a. Intravascular volume loading and head down tilt (modified Trendelenburg position) augment preload to counter obstructed venous return from torqued or flipped cardiac positioning during performance of distal anastomoses.

    b. Vasoconstrictors or vasoconstricting inotropes (e.g., phenylephrine, norepinephrine, epinephrine) likewise can maintain CPP and collateral flow during vessel occlusion.

    c. **Controlled hypotension.** When the surgeon sutures proximal anastomoses using an aortic side clamp, systolic pressures less than 100 mm Hg will help prevent aortic dissection. Vasodilators and volatile anesthetics plus normovolemia and head-up tilt can facilitate this.

C. **Regional anesthesia adjuncts**

1. **Intrathecal opioid.** Placement of 300 to 500 μg of preservative-free morphine via lumbar puncture immediately prior to induction of general anesthesia provides lasting, preemptive analgesia. Larger doses increase the risks of postoperative pruritus, nausea, and ventilatory depression peaking around 6 to 10 hours after administration. Minimize the possibility of neuraxial bleeding and compression as follows:

    a. Time the administration of heparin to occur at least 1 hour following puncture, especially if blood returns in the spinal needle [28]. Some centers delay operation by 24 hours if a large bore needle (e.g., 22 g or larger) has been used.

    b. Use a small gauge spinal needle—25 g or smaller.

    c. Do not persist if identification of the intrathecal space proves difficult.

2. **Epidural opioid and/or local anesthesia.** After identifying the epidural space, up to 5 mg of preservative-free morphine can provide preemptive analgesia. Because the larger epidural needle increases the risk of bleeding and of significant hematoma formation following heparin administration, most practitioners avoid this approach.

3. **Precautions.** Potent antiplatelet therapy (e.g., clopidogrel, prasugrel, ticagrelor) not halted at least 7 days before the day of surgery raises concern in performing neuraxial procedures, as does a therapeutic INR (greater than 1.5) from vitamin K antagonist therapy.

4. Neuraxial preemptive analgesia may facilitate early extubation by facilitating adequate ventilation. Nevertheless, expect a patient breathing spontaneously immediately after a very-early-extubation technique to have a $PaCO_2$ as high as 50 mm Hg, which is similar to that of noncardiac surgical patients with adequate opioid-based analgesia in the PACU.

D. **Special circumstances**

1. **Radial artery conduits.** Confirm before placing monitoring catheters whether or not the surgeon intends to utilize this conduit, and if so, mark the operative upper extremity clearly to avoid placing either intravenous or radial arterial catheters there. Some protocols call for diltiazem infusions as prophylaxis against arterial spasm in the radial graft; be aware of the accompanying systemic vasodilation.

2. **Port access surgery.** This approach utilizes a small thoracotomy incision, endoscopic instruments inserted through small ports, and TEE placement of endovascular devices to facilitate CPB. This technique is more frequently employed when valvular surgery is performed than coronary revascularization.

3. **MIDCAB.** An anterior thoracotomy incision permits access for harvesting of the left IMA and its anastomosis to the LAD coronary artery without CPB. Although this is technically a variation on OPCAB, typically it is called MIDCAB.

4. **Urgent coronary artery bypass surgery**
   a. **Patient profile.** Patients who present for urgent coronary artery bypass surgery usually have ongoing ischemia, including actively infarcting tissue, frequently with hemodynamic instability.
   b. **Induction and monitoring.** If the patient's condition requires rapid establishment of CPB, utilize existing femoral catheters (from cardiac catheterization laboratory) for monitoring and intravenous access rather than delay surgery.

> **CLINICAL PEARL** With active ischemia, time equals myocardium: Be flexible with sequencing placement of arterial and other catheters with the induction of anesthesia and surgical incision.

   c. **Anesthetic management.** In the hypotensive patient, consider etomidate for induction and potent longer-acting amnestics (e.g., lorazepam) as adjuncts. Make every effort to institute CPB without delay.

5. Patients with **poor ventricular function** (ejection fraction less than 35%) receive reduced or no premedication. Severe ventricular compromise may require inotrope administration before induction. Popular induction techniques employ etomidate or slow titration of opioids (150 to 250 μg fentanyl every 30 seconds).

6. **Left main disease or its equivalent.** These patients generally fare better with a high-supply/high-demand anesthetic technique rather than a low-supply/low-demand technique (see Section V.F). Maintain diastolic blood pressure during induction and until revascularization is completed with the aid of phenylephrine or other vasopressors to ensure adequate oxygen balance.

7. **CABG for patients previously treated with antiplatelet medications.** Patients treated with potent antiplatelet agents (platelet glycoprotein receptor antagonists, clopidogrel, prasugrel, ticagrelor, vorapaxar) are at risk for significant coagulopathy and consequent bleeding. Empirical platelet infusions can avoid catastrophic blood loss and high transfusion requirements.

8. **CABG for patients with heparin-induced thrombocytopenia.** See Chapter 21.

9. **Redo CABG procedures.** More bleeding, perioperative ischemia, infarction, and pump failure accompany repeat operations. Adherence of the RV to the sternum may result in sudden, extensive hemorrhage during surgical dissection. Table 10.5 summarizes these special concerns, their causes, and appropriate perioperative anesthetic management.

10. Concomitant acute ischemic mitral regurgitation arises from ischemic papillary muscle dysfunction or ruptured chordae tendineae, with attendant hemodynamic instability. Operation is nearly always urgent (see Section VI.D.4). The accompanying tachycardia, high LVEDP, and increased contractility all worsen myocardial oxygen supply/demand balance. Intra-aortic balloon counterpulsation frequently stabilizes these patients sufficiently to permit survival until the institution of CPB.

VII. **Causes and treatment of perioperative myocardial ischemia** (Table 10.6).
   A. **Causes of ischemia in the prebypass period**
      1. **Specific high-risk anesthetic-surgical events.** Events precipitating ischemia in the prebypass period include endotracheal intubation, surgical stress (skin incision, sternal split), cannulation, and initiation of bypass [10]. Episodes of ischemia may occur during these high-risk events even in the absence of hemodynamic changes [10].
      2. **Hemodynamic abnormalities.** Some episodes of ischemia during high-risk periods arise from hemodynamic abnormalities, especially tachycardia (greater than 100 beats/min). Minimize hemodynamic alterations to prevent myocardial ischemia. Intraoperative ischemia triples the likelihood of perioperative infarction.

TABLE 10.5 Perioperative management of the myocardial revascularization reoperation patient

Perioperative problem	Cause	Management
Bleeding	Pericardial adhesions Preoperative antiplatelet or anticoagulant medication	Large-bore IV access Blood readily available and checked in the OR Careful dissection on reopening chest Femoral area exposed and ready for emergency cannulation Anticipated need for clotting factors and platelets in the postbypass period Availability of blood salvage equipment (cell saver) Prophylactic antifibrinolytic therapy
Ischemia or infarction	Increased incidence of unstable angina Long period before bypass instituted Thrombus in vein grafts embolize to native vessels Interruption of vein graft flow (associated with 50–60% mortality) Longer bypass and cross-clamp times Increased amount of noncoronary collateral flow	Close monitoring of ischemia (ECG, PA catheter, two-dimensional TEE) Expeditious treatment of ischemia once detected Careful manipulation of vein grafts; retrograde cardioplegia Careful dissection around vein grafts Minimal cross-clamp time Mean perfusion pressure <60 mm Hg when cross-clamp is applied to limit noncoronary flow
Pump failure after bypass	Perioperative ischemia and infarction	Same as above Treat ischemia aggressively after bypass to improve myocardial function Anticipate need for intravenous inotropic and mechanical support

ECG, electrocardiogram; IV, intravenous; OR, operating room; PA, pulmonary artery; TEE, transesophageal echocardiography.

3. **Coronary spasm.** Coronary artery spasm in a normal vessel or around an atherosclerotic lesion causes ischemia. Intense sympathetic stimulation, light levels of anesthesia, and surgical manipulation may theoretically trigger coronary vasospasm.

4. **Spontaneous thrombus formation.** Atherosclerotic plaque rupture with thrombus formation occludes coronary vessels. Although uncommon, this may occur at any time, including in the operating room prior to revascularization.

B. **Causes of ischemia during bypass**

1. **Periods without aortic cross-clamp.** Hemodynamic alterations rarely lead to ischemia during CPB. However, mechanical factors and ventricular fibrillation can sharply decrease oxygen supply or increase its demand, respectively. Air or microparticles (thrombus,

TABLE 10.6 Causes of perioperative ischemia in the myocardial revascularization patient

Prebypass	Bypass	Postbypass
Hemodynamic alterations[a]	Hemodynamic alterations[a]	Hemodynamic alterations[a]
Coronary spasm	Coronary spasm Cardioplegic arrest	Coronary spasm
Thrombus formation	Emboli (air, thrombus particulate matter)	Thrombus (native vessel, graft)
High-risk anesthetic-surgical events[b]	Ventricular fibrillation Ventricular distention Surgical complications[b]	Surgical complications[b] Incomplete revascularization Excessive use of inotropes Distention of the lungs leading to occlusion of internal mammary artery (IMA) graft flow

[a]Includes tachycardia, hypotension, hypertension, ventricular distention.
[b]See text for details.

plastic, and other foreign material) present in the CPB circuit may embolize to the coronary circulation. Whenever the heart or aorta is opened, air embolism to the native coronary circulation can occur.

2. **During aortic cross-clamp.** Ischemia occurs regardless of the myocardial preservation technique. The potential for ischemic injury and subsequent infarction increases with cross-clamp time, and varies with the techniques and protective solutions used for myocardial preservation. Washout of cold cardioplegic solution owing to excessive noncoronary collateral flow may lead to ischemia. Electrical and mechanical quiescence during this period precludes monitoring for ischemia.

3. **After cross-clamp removal**
   a. **Surgical and technical complications**
      (1) Inadvertent incision of the coronary artery back wall, leading to coronary dissection
      (2) Improper handling of the vein graft with endothelial cell loss, leading to graft thrombus formation
      (3) Twisting of vein grafts
      (4) Faulty anastomosis of the vein graft to the coronary artery, including
         (a) Suturing the artery closed while grafting or poor-quality anastomoses
         (b) Inadequate vein graft length, leading to stretching of the vein when the heart is filled
         (c) Excess length of vein graft, leading to vein kinking
   b. **Etiology** of ST-segment elevation after cross-clamp removal. This arises from residual electrophysiologic effects of cardioplegia, coronary artery air or atheromatous debris embolus, or coronary artery spasm. Appearance in the inferior leads (i.e., right coronary distribution) implicates air embolism, because air seeks the high (anterior) location of the right coronary ostium. Ventricular aneurysm and pericarditis also cause persistent ST-segment elevations.

C. **Causes of ischemia in the postbypass period**
   1. **Incomplete revascularization**
      a. **Ungraftable vessels.** The region of myocardium supplied by the unrevascularized stenotic vessel may develop ischemia after CPB because of the added insult of ischemic arrest.
      b. **Diffuse distal disease.** Revascularization rarely restores effective flow in this scenario, which often occurs in chronic diabetes. Early vein graft closure owing to poor runoff in the small distal vessels further complicates care.
      c. **Stress.** Ischemia occurrence depends on attention to oxygen supply and demand balance, rather than the degree of analgesia or sedation provided [26,34]. This includes inappropriate inotrope use, including calcium, during separation from CPB or thereafter.
   2. **Coronary spasm.** Coronary artery spasm can occur in the postbypass period, most commonly in right coronary arteries that are not diseased. Surgical manipulation and exogenous and endogenous catecholamines can contribute to this problem.
   3. **Mechanical factors.** These include vein graft kinking or stretching, or occlusion of IMA flow from overinflation of the lungs.
   4. **Thrombus formation.** See Section VII.A.4. Postsurgical hypercoagulability may contribute to clot formation.

D. **Treatment of myocardial ischemia** (Table 10.7)
   1. **Treatment of ischemia secondary to hemodynamic abnormalities**
      a. Increase or decrease anesthetic depth.
      b. Administer vasodilators or vasopressors when SVR is either high or low, respectively, assuming euvolemia.
      c. Administer a β-blocker, specifically esmolol (for short half-life), to treat tachycardia.
      d. Use atrioventricular sequential pacing. Specifically in the postbypass period, this can be extremely beneficial to improve rate, rhythm, and hemodynamic stability.

TABLE 10.7   Treatment of ischemia
Adequate oxygenation
Hemodynamic stability (e.g., adequate anesthetic depth)
Surgical correction

Specific pharmacologic treatment
   Nitroglycerin
   Calcium channel blockers
   β-Blockers (esmolol)
   Heparin

Inotropic support (ischemia secondary to a failing ventricle)

Mechanical support
   Intra-aortic balloon pump
   LV assist device
   RV assist device

    e. Use inotropes for ventricular failure, diagnosed by decreased cardiac output and increased ventricular filling pressures. Pump failure leads to severe decreases in CPP because diastolic blood pressure is decreased and LVEDP is increased. Indiscriminate use of inotropes may aggravate ischemia. Therefore, preload and heart rate and rhythm should be optimized before using inotropes.

    f. Especially if heparin has not yet been neutralized, consider resuming CPB for a short period to facilitate myocardial recovery and/or to facilitate initiation of circulatory support with an inotrope or intra-aortic balloon pump.

2. Correction of surgical complications and mechanical problems

    a. Avoid overinflation of the lungs when an IMA graft is present.

    b. Increasing systemic blood pressure with a vasoconstrictor such as phenylephrine can push intracoronary air through the vasculature and restore blood flow to regions not perfused because of the intravascular air lock.

3. Treatment of coronary spasm. IV nitroglycerin, diltiazem, and nicardipine can treat coronary spasm. For specific doses of each drug for this indication, refer to Chapter 2.

4. Specific pharmacologic treatment of ischemia. This treatment includes (a) nitroglycerin, (b) β-blockers, and (c) calcium channel blockers. Prophylactic IV nitroglycerin finds use after CPB in incompletely revascularized patients, patients with severe distal coronary disease, and diabetic patients. Because ischemia frequently occurs from thrombus formation on an atheroma, many nonsurgical patients receive heparin as acute therapy and antiplatelet agents (most commonly aspirin) for long-term prophylaxis. These agents should be withheld after bypass until the threat of surgical hemorrhage ceases.

5. Mechanical support. Refer to Chapter 22 for a complete discussion of circulatory assist devices.

    a. Intra-aortic balloon pumps. Intra-aortic balloon counterpulsation increases CPP and decreases LV afterload. Patients with impaired ventricular function benefit from improved pump performance in addition to relief of ischemia.

    b. RV and LV assist devices. These devices may be useful for treating severe ischemia caused by myocardial failure or ischemia that led to myocardial failure. Their use as treatment of ischemia is still in question.

6. Ischemic preconditioning is a technique that may be useful in protecting against myocardial injury or stunning.

    a. Myocardial injury. Tissue injury results from ischemia and subsequent tissue reperfusion may involve a reduction in adenosine triphosphate (ATP) levels, free oxygen radicals, calcium-mediated injury, nitric oxide, heat shock proteins, a form of protein kinase C, mitogen-activated protein kinases, and mitochondrial ATP-dependent potassium channels.

b. Preconditioning. A brief period of tissue ischemia may protect against the damage caused by subsequent prolonged ischemia and tissue reperfusion. The benefit of this ischemic preconditioning occurs in both experimental animals and humans. Endogenously produced adenosine may mediate ischemic preconditioning via enhanced preservation of ATP, inhibition of platelet and neutrophil-mediated inflammatory tissue injury, vasodilation, and decreased basal cellular energy requirements related to intracellular hyperpolarization [20].

c. Early versus late preconditioning. In experimental models, the early, classic form of preconditioning lasts 2 to 3 hours after the ischemic event. Typically the period of ischemia and subsequent period of reperfusion each last about five minutes. Four such cycles (total 40 minutes) reduce infarct size from a subsequent 40-minute ischemic period by 75%. The time required to precondition for each anastomosis to mitigate sequelae from an anticipated 5 to 15 minutes of vessel occlusion creates logistic challenges in clinical practice.

d. Role of inhalational anesthetics. Halothane, isoflurane, desflurane, and sevoflurane decrease the deleterious effects of ischemia, in a manner similar to ischemic preconditioning.

VIII. Anesthesia for hybrid cardiac procedures

A. Impetus for hybrid facilities

The majority of patients requiring coronary revascularization can now be treated with nonsurgical interventions, thanks to advances in stent design, stent drug elution, oral antiplatelet drug therapy, and interventional access techniques. However, anatomic and other technical factors still render complex lesions better managed surgically. Many cardiac centers have hybrid operating rooms combining space, lighting, monitoring, and supplies of a cardiac surgical suite with that of an imaging-equipped interventional laboratory. These facilities allow combined surgical anastomosis and catheter-based interventions without moving the patient. Most typically, the LAD artery is revascularized surgically, based on data indicating better patency, while other grafts may be individualized either to surgical or catheter approaches based on patient-specific factors. These hybrid facilities afford excellent anesthetizing conditions for transcatheter valve, vascular endograft, electrophysiology, neurovascular, and other procedures, thus justifying their cost to moderately sized institutions.

B. Hybrid room design considerations

1. **Stakeholders.** Planning a hybrid space requires involvement of all stakeholders: anesthesiologists, cardiologists, nurses and nurse specialists, radiologists, surgeons, perfusionists, and administrators.

2. **Location.** Placement depends on hospital geography. Anesthesiologists usually prefer the facility in proximity to the main surgical suite, thus providing easy access to backup equipment and resources, and often near cardiac intensive care. However, local considerations may supervene.

3. **Size.** A hybrid room should be at least 1,600 sq ft to accommodate imaging equipment, scrub area, and control room, as well as the number of people (up to 20) who may participate in the procedure.

4. **Special features.** Floor reinforcements and additional lead shielding may be required. The numerous personnel require many well-positioned auxiliary monitors to view vital data. Positioning surgical lights amid imaging equipment and monitors demands considerable **design expertise** (Fig. 10.7).

C. Rationale for hybrid procedures

1. **The problem: Immediate graft failure.** Hybrid procedures allow for immediate correction of graft occlusion. Graft failure prior to discharge from the hospital occurs in 5% to 20% of patients. These failures arise from vein valves impeding flow, IMA dissections, vein graft kinking, or incorrect graft placement. About 6% of grafts imaged immediately after surgery have issues addressed by interventional techniques, minor adjustments, or surgical revision.

2. **Long-term results.** A case-control study compared 141 consecutive hybrid patients with disease not amenable to CABG alone or percutaneous coronary intervention (PCI)

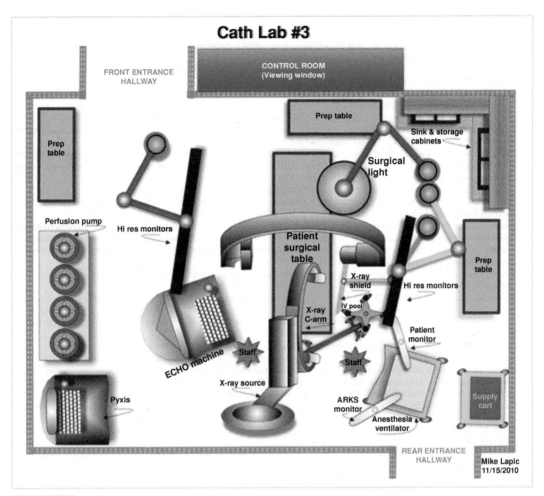

FIGURE 10.7 An example of a setup for a hybrid operating room. ARKS, anesthesia information system.

alone to matched CABG and PCI cohorts. The hybrid patients underwent LAD surgical grafting using the LIMA followed by PCI of other lesions. At 3 years' follow-up, repeat revascularization occurred in 6 hybrid, 3 CABG, and 18 PCI patients; and death in 1, 4, and 5 patients, respectively [43]. The markedly different anatomic and physiologic states of the cases relative to the selected controls limit clinical inference from this study.

3. **Other potential advantages** include avoidance of aortic manipulation, fewer transfusions, and especially compared to OPCAB, less hemodynamic compromise.

D. **Indications for hybrid CABG**

The most recent ACC/AHA guidelines [44] give a Class IIA recommendation (level of evidence B) for hybrid CABG in the following situations:

1. Limitations to traditional CABG, such as a heavily calcified proximal aorta or poor surgical target vessels (but amenable to PCI).
2. Lack of suitable graft conduits.
3. Unfavorable LAD for PCI (excessive tortuosity or chronic occlusion).

E. **Anesthetic implications**

The working environment may pose a challenge to those accustomed to a traditional cardiac operating room. This is especially true if the hybrid OR is not located in proximity to the main cardiac ORs. Routine avoidance of a full median sternotomy and the brief duration of bypass support early extubation, so the anesthetic should be designed to allow for that.

REFERENCES

1. **Benjamin EJ, Blaha MJ, Chiuve SE, et al. Heart disease and stroke statistics-2017 update. A report from the American Heart Association. *Circulation*. 2017;135(10):e204–228.**
2. Benjamin EJ, Blaha MJ, Chiuve SE, et al. Heart disease and stroke statistics-2017 update. A report from the American Heart Association. *Circulation*. 2017;135(10):e444.
3. Cheng DC, Wall C, Djaiani G, et al. Randomized assessment of resource use in fast-track cardiac surgery 1-year after hospital discharge. *Anesthesiology*. 2003;98(3):651–657.
4. Higgins TL. Quantifying risk and assessing outcome in cardiac surgery. *J Cardiothorac Vasc Anesth*. 1998;12(3):330–340.
5. Dupuis JY, Wang F, Nathan H, et al. The cardiac anesthesia risk evaluation score: a clinically useful predictor of mortality and morbidity after cardiac surgery. *Anesthesiology*. 2001;94(2):194–204.
6. **Eagle KA, Guyton RA, Davidoff R, et al. ACC/AHA 2004 guideline update for coronary artery bypass graft surgery: Summary Article: A report of the American College of Cardiology/American Heart Association Task Force on Practice Guidelines. *Circulation*. 2004;110:1168–1176.**
7. Dole WP. Autoregulation of the coronary circulation. *Prog Cardiovasc Dis*. 1987;29(4):293–323.
8. Berkowitz DE. Vascular function: From human physiology to molecular biology. In: Schwinn DA, ed. *New Advances in Vascular Biology and Molecular Cardiovascular Medicine*. Baltimore, MD: Williams & Wilkins; 1998:25–47.
9. **American Society of Anesthesiologists and Society of Cardiovascular Anesthesiologists Task Force on Transesophageal Echocardiography. Practice guidelines for perioperative transesophageal echocardiography. A report by the American Society of Anesthesiologists and the Society of Cardiovascular Anesthesiologists Task Force on Transesophageal Echocardiography. *Anesthesiology*. 2010;112(5):1084–1096.**
10. Slogoff S, Keats AS. Does perioperative myocardial ischemia lead to postoperative myocardial infarction? *Anesthesiology*. 1985;62(2):107–114.
11. Tuman KJ, McCarthy RJ, Spiess BD, et al. Effect of pulmonary artery catheterization on outcome in patients undergoing coronary artery surgery. *Anesthesiology*. 1989;70(2):199–206.
12. Connors AF Jr, Speroff T, Dawson NV, et al. The effectiveness of right heart catheterization in the initial care of critically ill patients. SUPPORT Investigators. *JAMA*. 1996;276(11):889–897.
13. Djaianai G, Karski J, Yudin M, et al. Clinical outcomes in patients undergoing elective coronary artery bypass graft surgery with and without utilization of pulmonary artery catheter-generated data. *J Cardiothorac Vasc Anesth*. 2006;20(3):307–310.
14. **American Society of Anesthesiologists Task Force on Pulmonary Artery Catheterization. Practice guidelines for pulmonary artery catheterization: An updated report by the American Society of Anesthesiologists Task Force on Pulmonary Artery Catheterization. *Anesthesiology*. 2003;99(4):988–1014.**
15. Shanewise JS. How to reliably detect ischemia in the intensive care unit and operating room. *Semin Cardiothorac Vasc Anesth*. 2006;10(1):101–109.
16. Ward RP, Lang RM. Myocardial contrast echocardiography in acute coronary syndromes. *Curr Opinion Cardiol*. 2002; 17(5):455–463.
17. Slogoff S, Keats AS. Randomized trial of primary anesthetic agents on outcome of coronary artery bypass operations. *Anesthesiology*. 1989;70(2):179–188.
18. Tuman KJ, McCarthy RJ, Spiess BD, et al. Does choice of anesthetic agent significantly affect outcome after coronary artery surgery? *Anesthesiology*. 1989;70(2):189–198.
19. Mukhtar AM, Obayah EM, Hassona AM. The use of dexmedetomidine in pediatric cardiac surgery. *Anesth Analg*. 2006; 103(1):52–56.
20. **Buffington CW, Davis KB, Gillispie S, et al. The prevalence of steal-prone anatomy in patients with coronary artery disease: an analysis of the Coronary Artery Surgery Study Registry. *Anesthesiology*. 1988;69(5):721–727.**
21. Lee HT. Mechanisms of ischemic preconditioning and clinical implications for multiorgan-reperfusion injury. *J Cardiothorac Vasc Anesth*. 1999;13(1):78–91.
22. Garcia C, Julier K, Bestmann L, et al. Preconditioning with sevoflurane decreases PECAM-1 expression and improves one-year cardiovascular outcome in coronary artery bypass graft surgery. *Br J Anaesth*. 2005;94(2):159–165.
23. Rorie DK, Tyce GM, Sill JC. Increased norepinephrine release from dog pulmonary artery caused by nitrous oxide. *Anesth Analg*. 1986;65(6):560–564.
24. Reich DL, Hollinger I, Harrington DJ, et al. Comparison of cisatracurium and vecuronium by infusion in neonates and small infants after congenital heart surgery. *Anesthesiology*. 2004;101(5):1122–1127.
25. Jellish WS, Brody M, Sawicki K, et al. Recovery from neuromuscular blockade after either bolus and prolonged infusions of cisatracurium or rocuronium using either isoflurane or propofol-based anesthetics. *Anesth Analg*. 2000;91(5):1250–1255.
26. Prakash O, Johson B, Meij S, et al. Criteria for early extubation after intracardiac surgery in adults. *Anesth Analg*. 1977;56(5): 703–708.
27. Scott NB, Turfrey DJ, Ray DA, et al. A prospective randomized study of the potential benefits of thoracic epidural anesthesia and analgesia in patients undergoing coronary artery bypass grafting. *Anesth Analg*. 2001;93(3):528–535.
28. **Horlocker TT, Wedel DJ, Rowlingson JC, et al. Regional anesthesia in the patient receiving antithrombotic or thrombolytic therapy. *Reg Anesth Pain Med*. 2010;35(1):64–101.**
29. Dowd NP, Cheng DC, Karski JM, et al. Intraoperative awareness in fast track cardiac anesthesia. *Anesthesiology*. 1998; 89(5):1068–1073.
30. Leslie K, Sessler DI. The implications of hypothermia for early tracheal extubation following cardiac surgery. *J Cardiothorac Vasc Anesth*. 1998;12(6 Suppl 2):30–34.
31. Ginsberg S, Solina A, Papp D, et al. A prospective comparison of three heat preservation methods for patients undergoing hypothermic cardiopulmonary bypass. *J Cardiothorac Vasc Anesth*. 2000;14(5):501–505.

32. Montes FR, Sanchez SI, Giraldo JC, et al. The lack of benefit of tracheal extubation in the operating room after coronary artery bypass surgery. *Anesth Analg.* 2000;91(4):776–780.
33. Chamchad D, Horrow JC, Nachamchik L, et al. The impact of immediate extubation in the operating room after cardiac surgery on intensive care and hospital lengths of stay. *J Cardiothorac Vasc Anesth.* 2010;24(5):780–784.
34. **Mangano DT, Siliciano D, Hollenberg M, et al. Postoperative myocardial ischemia: therapeutic trials using intensive analgesia following surgery. The Study of Perioperative Ischemia (SPI) Research Group. *Anesthesiology.* 1992; 76(3):342–353.**
35. Her DL, Sum-Ping ST, England M. ICU sedation after coronary artery bypass graft surgery: Dexmedetomidine-based versus propofol-based sedation regimens. *J Cardiothorac Vasc Anesth.* 2003;17(5):576–584.
36. Anger KE, Szumita PM, Baroletti SA, et al. Evaluation of dexmedetomidine versus propofol-based sedation therapy in mechanically ventilated cardiac surgery patients at a tertiary academic medical center. *Crit Pathw Cardiol.* 2010;9(4):221–226.
37. Hawkes CA, Dhileepan S, Foxcroft D. Early extubation for adult cardiac surgical patients. *Cochrane Database Syst Rev.* 2003;(4): CD003587.
38. **Cheng DC, Karski J, Peniston C, et al. Early tracheal extubation after coronary artery bypass graft surgery reduces costs and improves resource use. A prospective, randomized, controlled trial. *Anesthesiology.* 1996;85(6):1300–1310.**
39. Khan NE, DeSouza A, Mister R, et al. A randomized comparison of off-pump and on-pump multivessel coronary-artery bypass surgery. *N Engl J Med.* 2004;350(1):21–28.
40. Puskas JD, Williams WH, Mahoney EM, et al. Off-pump vs conventional coronary artery bypass grafting. Early and 1-year graft patency, cost, and quality-of-life outcomes. A randomized trial. *JAMA.* 2004;291(15):1841–1849.
41. Puskas J, Williams W, O'Donnell R, et al. Off-pump and on-pump coronary artery bypass grafting are associated with similar graft patency, myocardial ischemia, and freedom from reintervention: long-term follow-up of a randomized trial. *Ann Thor Surg.* 2011;91(6):1836–1842.
42. **Sellkez FW, DiMaio JM, Caplan LR, et al; American Heart Association. Comparing on-pump and off-pump coronary artery bypass grafting: numerous studies but few conclusions: a scientific statement from the American Heart Association council on cardiovascular surgery and anesthesia in collaboration with the interdisciplinary working group on quality of care and outcomes research. *Circulation.* 2005;111(21):2858–2864.**
43. Shen L, Hu S, Wang H, et al. One-stop hybrid coronary revascularization versus coronary artery bypass grafting and percutaneous coronary intervention for the treatment of multivessel coronary artery disease: 3-year follow-up results from a single institution. *J Am Coll Cardiol.* 2013;61(25):2525–2533.
44. Hillis LD, Smith P, Anderson J, et al. 2011 ACC/AHA Guideline for Coronary Artery Bypass Graft Surgery. *Circulation.* 2010; 124:(23), e676.

11 Anesthetic Management for the Surgical and Interventional Treatment of Aortic Valvular Heart Disease

Benjamin C. Tuck and Matthew M. Townsley

KEY POINTS

1. All valvular lesions can potentially lead to changes in cardiac loading conditions (i.e., volume and/or pressure overload) and a well-planned anesthetic must compensate for this through the manipulation of several hemodynamic variables. Most importantly, these include heart rate and rhythm, preload, afterload, and cardiac contractility.

2. During transcatheter aortic valve replacement (TAVR), there may be periods of acute hemodynamic instability as a result of the device occluding the already narrow valve, the creation of acute aortic regurgitation (AR) during balloon valvuloplasty, massive bleeding from dissection of major vasculature, damage to the left ventricle or mitral valve, or acute occlusion of a coronary ostium.

3. Because atrial contraction contributes up to 40% of left ventricular filling in patients with aortic stenosis (AS) and hypertrophic cardiomyopathy (HCM), it is essential to maintain sinus rhythm and treat arrhythmias aggressively in both of these conditions.

4. In patients with AS, the early use of α-adrenergic agonists, such as phenylephrine, is indicated to prevent drops in blood pressure that can quickly lead to severe hemodynamic compromise and cardiac arrest.

5. The dynamic left ventricular outflow tract (LVOT) obstruction caused by systolic anterior motion (SAM) of the mitral valve occurs proximal to the aortic valve (i.e., subaortic) in mid-to-late systole. The degree of obstruction is directly proportional to LV contractility and inversely proportional to LV preload (end-diastolic volume) and afterload. Specifically, decreases in systemic vascular resistance (SVR) and preload, as well as increases in contractility and heart rate will precipitate or worsen SAM/LVOT obstruction.

6. Patients with severe, acute AR are not capable of maintaining sufficient forward stroke volume and often develop sudden and severe dyspnea, hemodynamic instability, and deteriorate rapidly. Patients with chronic AR may be asymptomatic for many years.

7. The hemodynamic requirements for combined AS and mitral regurgitation (MR) are contradictory. Because AS will most frequently lead to potential cardiovascular collapse, it should be given priority when managing hemodynamic parameters.

I. Introduction

At most major cardiac centers, the surgical volume for valve procedures has remained stable, and the management of patients with valvular heart disease continues to evolve with advances in both catheter-based and surgical interventions. This is especially true for aortic valve disease, as transcatheter aortic valve replacement (TAVR) has revolutionized the surgical approach to aortic stenosis (AS), which is the most common valve lesion in the United States. The role of the anesthesiologist continues to evolve and expand with these advancements as well. In particular, the less invasive nature of TAVR, as compared to surgical aortic valve replacement (AVR), has changed the landscape of patients presenting for AVR. The growing elderly population and/or those with significant comorbidities, who would not previously have been operative candidates, are now presenting for valve replacement at a growing rate. Thus, the cardiac anesthesiologist is now increasingly called upon to provide care for a more complicated and challenging patient population with aortic valve disease. In addition, as experience with TAVR continues to grow, there may eventually be further expansion of indications for this procedure into a younger and healthier patient population. In fact, the PARTNER 3 trial is currently underway evaluating the safety and effectiveness of the SAPIEN 3 (Edwards Lifesciences, Irvine, California) transcatheter heart valve in low-risk patients with AS. Importantly, advancements in the technology and experience with these catheter-based techniques require modifications of the anesthetic technique as well, as many centers are performing TAVR procedures with moderate anesthesia care or no sedation at all. Clearly, this introduces a completely new set of considerations for the safe and effective perioperative management of valve replacement in these patients. As TAVR continues to evolve, however, open surgical AVR still remains one of the most common cardiac surgical procedures performed at the present time.

Regardless of the procedural approach, the goal of aortic valve intervention is to improve symptoms and/or survival, in addition to minimizing the risk of complications such as irreversible ventricular dysfunction, stroke, pulmonary hypertension, and dysrhythmias [1]. The anesthetic management of aortic valve disease is often quite challenging, as both AS and aortic regurgitation (AR) frequently lead to pathophysiologic changes in the heart with profound hemodynamic consequences. All valvular lesions can potentially lead to changes in cardiac loading conditions (i.e., volume and/or pressure overload) and a well-planned anesthetic must compensate for this through the manipulation of several hemodynamic variables [2]. Most importantly, these include heart rate and rhythm, preload, afterload, and cardiac contractility. In addition, it is essential to consider the time course of the disease, as the clinical presentation and management considerations will vary dramatically in the setting of acute versus chronic valvular disorders.

This chapter will review the physiologic implications of both AS and AR and the practical approach to the management of these patients. Additionally, hypertrophic cardiomyopathy (HCM) will be discussed, as the hallmark of the obstructive form of this condition is dynamic subaortic stenosis. A section addressing prosthetic valves will conclude the chapter with a review of the most common types of prostheses utilized for AVR.

II. Stenotic versus regurgitant lesions

A. Valvular stenosis. Stenotic lesions lead to pathology associated with pressure overload. Narrowing of the orifice of a cardiac valve will ultimately lead to obstruction of blood flow through the valve. This obstruction translates into an increase in blood flow velocity as it approaches the stenotic valve orifice. The pattern of blood flow is distinctly different in the regions proximal and distal to a stenotic valve. The high-velocity flow proximal to the stenosis is laminar and organized; while distal to the stenosis it becomes turbulent and disorganized. In addition, the increased blood flow velocities observed in valvular stenosis translate into an increase in the pressure gradient across the valve. The simplified Bernoulli equation helps to explain this relationship. In this equation, the pressure gradient through the stenotic valve can be estimated by multiplying the peak velocity squared times four:

$$\text{Pressure gradient } (\Delta) = 4 * \text{Peak blood flow velocity (v) squared}$$

squared times four:

$$(\Delta P = 4v^2)$$

The simplified Bernoulli equation allows blood flow velocities measured by Doppler echocardiography to be converted into pressure gradients that can be used to quantify the severity of valvular stenosis. It is also important to understand that valvular obstruction can be of two primary types: fixed versus dynamic. In fixed obstruction (i.e., true valvular AS, subaortic membrane), the degree of obstruction to blood flow remains constant throughout the cardiac cycle and is not affected by the loading conditions of the heart. With dynamic obstruction (i.e., hypertrophic obstructive cardiomyopathy [HOCM] with dynamic subaortic stenosis), obstruction is only present for part of the cardiac cycle, primarily occurring in mid-to-late systole. The degree of obstruction is highly dependent on loading conditions, changing in severity as loading conditions change.

B. Valvular regurgitation. Regurgitant lesions lead to pathology associated with volume overload, resulting in chamber dilatation and eccentric hypertrophy (wall thickness increases in proportion to the increase in LV chamber size). Clinically, although this chamber remodeling will initially allow the left ventricle (LV) to compensate for the increased volume load, it will lead to an eventual decline in LV systolic function that can ultimately lead to irreversible LV failure. Effective perioperative management of valvular regurgitation is facilitated by understanding how preload, afterload, and heart rate each affect the contributions of the forward stroke volume (flow reaching the peripheral circulation) and regurgitant stroke volume (retrograde flow back across the valve) to the overall total stroke volume of the ventricle [3]. Hemodynamic management of these patients should aim to optimize the forward stroke volume, while minimizing the amount of regurgitant stroke volume.

III. Structural and functional response to valvular heart disease

The anesthetic management of patients undergoing aortic valve surgery requires a thorough understanding of the hemodynamic changes associated with valvular heart disease, as well as the cardiac remodeling imposed by an abnormal aortic valve.

A. Cardiac remodeling includes changes in the size, shape, and function of the heart in response to an acute or chronic cardiac injury. In valvular heart disease, cardiac injury is usually caused by alterations in ventricular loading conditions. Depending on the nature of the valvular pathology, the ventricle will be subject to either pressure or volume overload, or both. This leads to cardiac remodeling in the form of chamber dilation and ventricular hypertrophy. In addition to mechanical stress, cardiac remodeling results from the activation of neurohumoral factors, enzymes such as angiotensin II, ion channels, and oxidative stress [4]. Intended initially as an adaptive response to maintain cardiac performance, remodeling eventually leads to decompensation and deterioration in ventricular function. Ventricular hypertrophy is defined as increased LV mass. Ventricular hypertrophy can be either concentric or eccentric. Pressure overload usually results in concentric ventricular hypertrophy, which means that ventricular mass is increased by myocardial thickening while ventricular volume is not increased. Concentric versus eccentric hypertrophy can be determined using echocardiography. LV mass index >95 g/m^2 for women and >115 g/m^2 for men defines hypertrophy.

If relative wall thickness is >0.42, the hypertrophy is concentric. If <0.42, the hypertrophy is eccentric. Concentric hypertrophy reduces wall stress that results from the chronic pressure overload. Recall the law of Laplace to understand how this compensatory hypertrophy results in reduced wall stress, where:

$$\text{LV wall stress} = \frac{\text{LV pressure} \times \text{LV radius}}{2 \times \text{LV wall thickness}}$$

AS is a fixed obstruction at the level of the aortic valve and causes increased afterload for the LV, which increases the LV intracavitary pressure. The resultant increase in LV wall stress is mitigated by the increased LV wall thickness as demonstrated in the equation above. Concentric hypertrophy has the beneficial effect of reducing LV wall stress and avoiding a significant decline in LV systolic function. The cost of LV hypertrophy, however, is a reduction in LV compliance, which leads to diastolic dysfunction with an increase in LV end-diastolic pressure (LVEDP) and greater risk for subendocardial ischemia.

Volume overload, on the other hand, leads to eccentric hypertrophy, where the increase in ventricular mass is associated with ventricular cavity dilatation. In this scenario, myocardial thickness increases in proportion to the increase in ventricular chamber radius.

B. **Ventricular function.** To anticipate the effect of valvular lesions on ventricular function, it is helpful to separate ventricular function into its two distinct components [2]:
  1. **Systolic function** represents the ventricle's ability to eject blood into the systemic circulation.
     a. **Contractility** can be defined as the intrinsic ability of the myocardium to contract and generate force. Contractility itself is independent of preload and afterload. Normal contractility means that a ventricle of normal size and normal preload can generate sufficient stroke volume at rest and during exercise.
     b. **Preload** can be defined as the load placed on the myocardium before contraction. This load results from a combination of diastolic volume and filling pressure and can be expressed as end-diastolic wall stress.
     c. **Afterload** is the load placed on the myocardium during contraction. This load results from the combination of systolic volume and generated pressure and can be expressed as end-systolic wall stress.
  2. **Diastolic function** represents the ventricle's ability to accept inflowing blood. Diastolic function consists of a combination of relaxation and compliance. In general, normal diastolic function means that the ventricle accepts normal diastolic volume at normal filling pressure. When diastolic dysfunction occurs, maintaining normal ventricular diastolic volume requires elevated ventricular filling pressure. Both systolic and diastolic function require energy and can be compromised by ventricular ischemia.

IV. **Pressure–volume loops** may be utilized to illustrate LV function and performance. These loops are constructed by plotting ventricular pressure (y axis) versus ventricular volume (x axis) over the course of a complete cardiac cycle (Fig. 11.1). The presence of valvular heart disease alters the normal pressure–volume loop tracing, representing changes in ventricular physiology and loading conditions imposed by valvular pathology. The ventricle adapts differently to each valvular lesion, and characteristic patterns of the pressure–volume loop help to illustrate these changes.

V. **Aortic stenosis (AS)**
  A. **Natural history**
    1. **Etiology.** The normal adult aortic valve has three cusps, with an aortic valve area of 2.6 to 3.5 cm^2, representing a normal aortic valve index of 2 cm^2/m^2. AS may result from congenital or acquired valvular heart disease. Congenital AS is classified as valvular, subvalvular, or supravalvular based on the anatomic location of the stenotic lesion. Subvalvular and supravalvular aortic stenoses are usually caused by a membrane or muscular band. Congenital valvular AS may occur with a unicuspid, bicuspid, or a tricuspid aortic valve with partial commissural fusion. Aortic valves with supernumerary cusps (greater than 3 cusps) have also been reported.

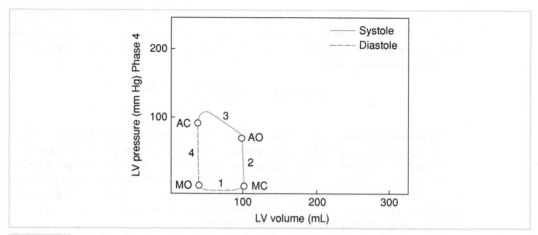

FIGURE 11.1 Normal pressure–volume loop. The first segment of the ventricular pressure–volume loop (Phase 1) represents diastolic filling of the left ventricle. The next two segments represent the two stages of ventricular systole: isovolumic contraction (Phase 2) and ventricular ejection (Phase 3). The final segment of the loop corresponds to isovolumic relaxation of the left ventricle, which precedes ventricular filling and the start of the next cardiac cycle. The isovolumic relaxation and ventricular filling phases constitute the two phases of diastole. Both end-systolic volume at the time of aortic valve closure (AC) and end-diastolic volume at the time of mitral valve closure (MC) are represented as distinct points on the loop. MO, mitral valve opening; AO, aortic valve opening; LV, left ventricle. (Modified from Jackson JM, Thomas SJ, Lowenstein E. Anesthetic management of patients with valvular heart disease. *Semin Anesth.* 1982;1:240.)

A congenitally bicuspid aortic valve occurs in approximately 1% to 2% of the general population, making it the most common congenital valvular malformation. Calcification of a congenitally bicuspid valve results in the early onset of AS and represents the most common cause of AS among patients younger than 70 years of age [5]. Estimates suggest that bicuspid aortic valve disease accounts for approximately 50% of all valve replacements for AS in the United States and Europe [6]. Commonly associated findings in patients with bicuspid aortic valves include abnormalities of the aorta, including aortic coarctation, aortic root dilatation, and an increased risk of aortic dissection.

Of the acquired aortic stenoses, senile degeneration is the most common cause in the developed world. The fibrotic and calcific change that occurs in the aortic valve prior to flow obstruction is known as aortic sclerosis, and the incidence of this may be as high as 25% of individuals over the age of 65 years and 50% of individuals over the age of 85. Epidemiologic data suggest that the incidence of severe AS may be as high as 3.4% in individuals over the age of 75 in developed countries [7]. The calcification seen with senile degeneration of the aortic valve also appears to have an inflammatory component as well, similar to that observed with coronary artery disease (CAD) [2]. While rheumatic AS is now rarely seen in the developed world, it remains an important cause of AS in developing countries. However, senile calcific disease is the most prevalent etiology of AS worldwide. Additionally, rheumatic AS is usually associated with some degree of AR and frequently affects the mitral valve as well. Less frequent causes of AS include atherosclerosis, end-stage renal disease, and rheumatoid arthritis.

A characteristic finding of senile valvular degeneration is progression of the calcification from the base of the valve toward the edge, as opposed to rheumatic degeneration in which calcification spreads from the edge toward the base.

2. **Symptoms.** Unicuspid AS often presents in infancy. Patients with rheumatic AS may be asymptomatic for 40 years or more. Congenital bicuspid aortic valves in the majority of cases must undergo calcific degeneration to become stenotic. The time of onset and speed of progression of calcific degeneration vary from patient to patient. This is why patients with congenitally bicuspid aortic valves may develop symptomatic AS anytime between the ages of 15 and 65, and even later in life. Degenerative stenosis of a tricuspid aortic valve

usually develops in the seventh or eighth decade of life. Asymptomatic patients with AS have an excellent prognosis. Patients with even severe AS may stay asymptomatic for many years and carry a small risk of sudden death, which does not exceed the risk of operation. However, the onset of any one of the following triad of symptoms is an ominous sign and indicates a life expectancy of less than 5 years:

a. **Angina pectoris.** Angina is the initial symptom in approximately two-thirds of patients with severe AS. Angina and dyspnea secondary to AS alone initially occur with exertion [8]. Life expectancy when angina develops is about 5 years.

b. **Syncope.** Syncope is the first symptom in 15% to 30% of patients. Once syncope appears, the average life expectancy is 3 to 4 years.

c. **Congestive heart failure.** Once signs of LV failure occur, the average life expectancy is only 1 to 2 years.

B. **Pathophysiology**

1. **Heart remodeling.** As stenosis progresses, the maintenance of normal stroke volume is associated with an increasing systolic pressure gradient between the LV and the aorta. The LV systolic pressure (LVSP) increases to as much as 300 mm Hg, whereas the aortic systolic pressure and stroke volume remain relatively normal. This pressure gradient results in a compensatory concentric LV hypertrophy. Occasionally, as stenosis progresses, eccentric LV hypertrophy may develop and result in impaired LV systolic function.

2. **Hemodynamic changes**

a. **Arterial pressure.** In severe AS, the arterial pulse pressure usually is reduced to less than 50 mm Hg. The systolic pressure rise is delayed with a late peak and a prominent anacrotic notch. As stenosis increases in severity, the anacrotic notch occurs lower in the ascending arterial pressure trace. The dicrotic notch is relatively small or absent.

b. **Pulmonary arterial wedge pressure.** Because of the elevated LVEDP, which stretches the mitral valve annulus, a prominent V wave can be observed, but with progression of the disease and the development of left atrial hypertrophy, a prominent A wave becomes the dominant feature.

3. **Pressure–volume loop in aortic stenosis** (Fig. 11.2)

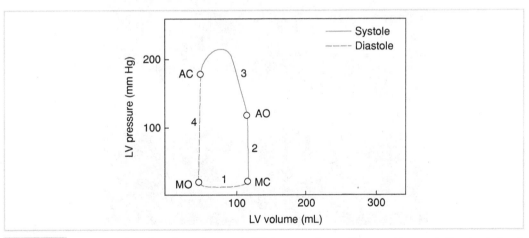

FIGURE 11.2 Pressure–volume loop in aortic stenosis (AS). In comparison to the normal loop, note the elevated peak systolic pressure necessary to generate a normal stroke volume in the face of the elevated pressure gradient through the aortic valve. Also, end-diastolic pressure is elevated with a steeper diastolic slope, reflecting diastolic dysfunction with altered left ventricular compliance. Phase 1, diastolic filling; phase 2, isovolumic contraction; phase 3, ventricular ejection; phase 4, isovolumic relaxation. MO, mitral valve opening; MC, mitral valve closure; AO, aortic valve opening; AC, aortic valve closure; LV, left ventricle. (Modified from Jackson JM, Thomas SJ, Lowenstein E. Anesthetic management of patients with valvular heart disease. *Semin Anesth.* 1982;1:241.)

TABLE 11.1   Assessment of AS severity with echocardiography

Measurement	Aortic sclerosis	Mild AS	Moderate AS	Severe AS
Aortic valve area (cm²)	2.6–3.5	>1.5	1.0–1.5	<1.0
Mean gradient (mm Hg)	<10	<20	20–40	>40
Indexed aortic valve area (cm²/m²)	2.0	>0.85	0.60–0.85	<0.6
Peak velocity of blood flow through aortic valve (m/sec)	<2.6	2.6–3.0	3–4	>4

AS, aortic stenosis.
Adapted from Baumgartner H, Hung J, Bermejo J, et al. Echocardiographic assessment of valve stenosis: EAE/ASE recommendations for clinical practice. *J Am Soc Echocardiogr.* 2009;22(1):1–23.

C. **Preoperative evaluation and assessment of severity**
   1. **Echocardiographic evaluation (Echocardiographic criteria—see Table 11.1)**
      Echocardiography is now the standard modality for quantifying the severity of AS. With the exception of rare cases where echocardiography is nondiagnostic or discrepant with clinical data, cardiac catheterization is no longer recommended for this purpose. The most commonly utilized methods for quantifying AS severity with echocardiography include measurement of the peak blood flow velocity of the AS jet, mean gradient across the aortic valve, and determination of aortic valve area. In AS, the valve area can be measured by the direct planimetry and continuity equation methods. The pressure gradient can be measured using a simplified Bernoulli equation (Fig. 11.3).

      Transesophageal echocardiography (TEE) is particularly useful in patients with poor transthoracic windows or in patients with complex cardiac pathology (e.g., a combination of subaortic and valvular stenoses). It is also useful when precise planimetry of the aortic valve area is necessary or when infective endocarditis is suspected. Supplemental Videos 11.1 and 11.2 demonstrate TEE images of a severely stenotic aortic valve, with both 2D imaging and color flow Doppler.

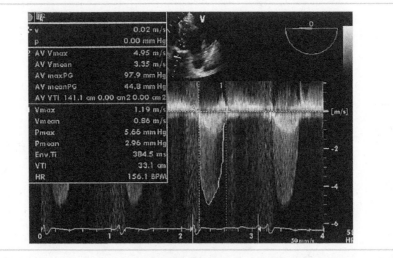

FIGURE 11.3 Severe aortic stenosis (AS), showing determination of the aortic valve (AV) gradient using the Bernoulli equation. This image displays a deep transgastric long-axis TEE view with a continuous wave Doppler beam aligned through the left ventricular outflow tract (LVOT) and AV. Tracing 2 on the spectral display (outer traced envelope) represents blood flow through the severely stenotic AV, with a mean velocity (AV Vmean) of 3.35 m/sec and mean AV pressure gradient (AV mean PG) of 44.8 mm Hg. A mean PG ≥40 mm Hg is consistent with severe AS. (Reprinted with permission from Perrino AC, Reeves ST, eds. *A Practical Approach to Transesophageal Echocardiography.* 2nd ed. Philadelphia, PA: Lippincott Williams & Wilkins; 2008:246.)

2. Most patients with severe AS will have a mean transvalvular gradient >40 mm Hg and peak velocity >4 m/sec. However, up to 30% of patients with an aortic valve area (AVA) <1 cm^2 may have transvalvular gradients and velocities less than the cutoffs for severe stenosis [7].

   a. *Classical* low-flow, low-gradient severe AS describes a scenario in which a patient has a low left ventricular ejection fraction (LVEF) resulting in a low-flow state (defined as stroke volume index <35 mL/m^2) and mean gradient <40 mm Hg, peak velocity <4 m/sec, and AVA <1 cm^2. In this scenario, dobutamine stress echocardiography (DSE) should be performed. If the addition of inotropic support results in a mean gradient >40 mm Hg and the calculated AVA remains less than 1 cm^2, the diagnosis of true severe AS is confirmed. If the mean gradient remains less than 40 mm Hg, but the calculated AVA increases to greater than 1 cm^2, then a diagnosis of pseudosevere AS is made. Pseudosevere AS is primarily an issue of LV dysfunction and AVR is not indicated.

   b. *Paradoxical* low-flow, low-gradient severe AS describes a scenario in which a patient with normal LVEF has an AVA <1 cm^2, mean gradient <40 mm Hg, and peak velocity <4 m/sec. In this case, the patient has a low-flow state (stroke volume index <35 mL/m^2) because of small stroke volumes secondary to concentric remodeling and impaired diastolic filling. Low-dose DSE may be useful in confirming this diagnosis as well.

   c. However, if DSE fails to increase the flow across the aortic valve and the discordant values remain, it is possible to calculate a projected AVA based on normal flow. For patients that fail to increase the stroke volume by 20% with dobutamine, the mortality for surgical AVR is high. Additionally, multidetector computed tomography (CT) can be used to quantitate the calcification of the aortic valve, and a calcium score can be used to predict the risk of stenosis progression.

> **CLINICAL PEARL**   In the patient with AS and low LV ejection fraction, it is critical to understand that although the pressure gradients generated with echocardiography may not suggest criteria for severe AS, these patients with low-flow, low-gradient AS represent a high-risk patient population.

3. If cardiac catheterization data are utilized, the mean pressure gradient may be measured from a direct transaortic measurement, and the aortic valve area may be calculated using the Gorlin formula.

D. Timing and type of intervention

1. The timing of intervention is based upon the stage of the disease, and the stage of disease takes into account not only the severity determined by echocardiography but also the presence or absence of symptoms. Table 11.2 summarizes indications for valve replacement.

2. Due to the high risk of sudden death and limited life expectancy, symptomatic patients should undergo surgery. Asymptomatic patients with severe AS may be monitored closely until symptoms develop. However, the risk of waiting should be carefully weighed against the risk of surgery. For example, prior to elective noncardiac surgery under general or neuraxial anesthesia, asymptomatic patients with severe AS should be considered for aortic valve surgery.

3. Patients with moderate AS should have aortic valve surgery if they happen to require another cardiac operation, such as coronary artery bypass grafting (CABG), because the rate of progression of AS is approximately 0.1 cm^2 per year and the risk of having to redo cardiac surgery is substantially higher than the risk of the primary operation. Similarly, if a patient undergoing aortic valve surgery has significant CAD, CABG should be performed simultaneously. In patients over age 80 years, the risk of AVR alone is approximately the same as the risk of combined AVR and CABG [9].

4. A commissural incision or balloon aortic valvuloplasty is often the first procedure performed in young patients with severe noncalcific aortic valve stenosis, even if they are asymptomatic [8]. This operation frequently results in some residual AS and AR. Eventually, most patients require a subsequent prosthetic valve replacement. In older adult patients with

TABLE 11.2   Recommendations for timing of AVR in aortic stenosis (AS)

Class I indications

Symptomatic patients with severe high-gradient AS who have symptoms by history or on exercise testing

Asymptomatic patients with severe AS and LVEF <50%

Severe AS when undergoing other cardiac surgery

Class IIa indications

Asymptomatic patients with very severe AS (aortic velocity ≥5 m/sec) and low surgical risk

Asymptomatic patients with severe AS and decreased exercise tolerance or a fall in blood pressure with exercise

Asymptomatic patients with low-flow/low-gradient severe AS with reduced LVEF with low-dose dobutamine stress study showing an aortic velocity ≥4 m/sec (mean pressure gradient ≥40 mm Hg) with a valve area ≤1 cm^2 at any dobutamine dose

Symptomatic patients who have low-flow/low-gradient severe AS who are normotensive and have an LVEF ≥50% if clinical, hemodynamic, and anatomic data support valve obstruction as the most likely cause of symptoms

Patients with moderate AS (aortic velocity 3–3.9 m/sec) who are undergoing other cardiac surgery

Class IIb indication

Asymptomatic patients with severe AS and rapid disease progression and low surgical risk

AVR, aortic valve replacement; LVEF, left ventricular ejection fraction.
Adapted from Nishimura RA, Otto CM, Bonow RO, et al. 2014 AHA/ACC guideline for the management of patients with valvular heart disease: executive summary. *JACC.* 2014;63(22):2444.

calcific AS, valve replacement is the primary operation. In young adults, a viable alternative to AVR is the Ross (switch) procedure. In the Ross procedure, the diseased aortic valve is replaced with the patient's normal pulmonary valve, and the pulmonary valve is replaced with a pulmonary homograft. This more complex procedure avoids the need for systemic anticoagulation and extends the time until reoperation is required by several decades.

5. Surgical intervention should not be denied to patients almost no matter how severe the symptoms because irreversible LV failure occurs only very late in the disease process.

6. **Balloon aortic valvuloplasty** in adults with advanced disease often results in significant AR and early restenosis and is reserved for patients with severe comorbidity.

7. **Transcatheter aortic valve replacement (TAVR).** Although surgical replacement of the aortic valve is the treatment of choice for patients with severe AS, some patients are at very high risk for mortality or major morbidity with surgery. TAVR is a less invasive alternative performed without cardiopulmonary bypass (CPB), in which a bioprosthetic valve is implanted within the native aortic valve via a catheter introduced through a major artery or the apex of the LV [10]. Both techniques require brief cessation of the patient's cardiac output via rapid pacing during positioning of the device. Hemodynamic instability is not uncommon and necessitates prompt recognition and treatment. The 30-day mortality is 7%, while at 1-year post-TAVR, the stroke rate is 4.1% and the overall mortality is 23.7% [11].

   a. There are two valves currently available:

      (1) Edwards SAPIEN valve (Edwards Lifesciences, Irvine, CA): Transfemoral or transapical deployment. This valve requires rapid ventricular pacing during deployment and is expanded with a balloon. Thus, the cardiac output is zero during deployment.

      (2) CoreValve ReValving System (Medtronic, Minneapolis, MN): Transfemoral deployment. This valve is self-expanding and does not require rapid ventricular pacing to deploy. The LV continues to eject during deployment.

   b. **Contraindications.** Contraindications used in clinical trials to date include acute myocardial infarction within 1 month, congenital unicuspid or bicuspid valve, mixed aortic valve disease (stenosis and regurgitation), HCM, LV ejection fraction below 20%, native aortic annulus size outside of the manufacturer's recommended range, severe vascular disease precluding safe placement of the introducer sheath (for the transfemoral approach), cerebrovascular event within 6 months, and need for emergency surgery.

c. **Hybrid operating room** [12,13]. Cardiovascular hybrid surgery, which includes TAVR, is a rapidly evolving field where less invasive surgical approaches are combined with interventional cardiology techniques in the same setting. Such procedures require a combination of high-quality imaging modalities found in a cardiac catheterization suite (fluoroscopy, navigation systems, post-processing capabilities, high-resolution invasive monitoring, intracardiac and intravascular ultrasound, echocardiography, etc.) in addition to the ability to perform open surgery under general anesthesia, including the use of CPB. These procedures require close collaboration and communication among multidisciplinary teams including interventional cardiologists, surgeons, anesthesiologists, perfusionists, technicians, and nursing staff, some of whom may be distant from the operating field. Thus, the presence of multiple monitor panels in areas visible to all and advanced communication systems are critical. Large amounts of space and careful planning of room layout are crucial for all of the equipment to be readily accessible and to allow unobstructed access to the patient (see Chapter 10). In addition, both the radiation safety requirements of the cardiac catheterization suite and the hygienic standards of the operating room must be met. These many demands have led to the creation of specialized hybrid operating rooms (Fig. 10.7).

d. **Surgical approaches** (Fig. 11.4) [14–16]

(1) **Retrograde or transfemoral approach**

(a) The right femoral artery is accessed for device deployment. The left femoral artery and vein are accessed to provide for hemodynamic monitoring, transvenous pacing, contrast administration, and preparation for emergent CPB.

(b) Heparin (100 to 150 units/kg) is given intravenously, titrating therapy to an activated clotting time (ACT) of about 300 seconds.

(c) A guidewire is advanced across the aortic valve, and the balloon angioplasty catheter is advanced over the wire.

(d) Ventricular pacing at about 200 beats/min (bpm) creates a low cardiac output state (Fig. 11.5). In combination with apnea, a motionless field is obtained during inflation of the balloon, after which ventilation is resumed and pacing is terminated.

(e) The valve catheter is positioned using fluoroscopy and TEE. Rapid ventricular pacing and apnea are used during valve deployment.

(f) Fluoroscopy and TEE are used to assess valve position and function and to check for leak.

(2) **Antegrade transapical approach**

(a) This more invasive approach is reserved for patients with peripheral arterial disease which would not accommodate the introducer and valve deployment systems.

(b) The left femoral artery and vein are accessed as mentioned earlier.

(c) The LV apex is exposed via left anterolateral thoracotomy. TEE may facilitate identification of the apex.

(d) Heparin is given with the same ACT targets described earlier.

(e) A needle is inserted through the LV apex, through which a guidewire is passed through the aortic valve under fluoroscopic and TEE guidance.

(f) A balloon valvuloplasty catheter is introduced over the guidewire and positioned in the aortic valve. Similar to the retrograde approach, rapid ventricular pacing and apnea are initiated to create a motionless field during inflation.

(g) The valvuloplasty sheath is then replaced by the device introducer sheath through which the prosthetic valve is deployed in a similar fashion.

■ Percutaneous aortic valve replacement

Percutaneous aortic valve replacement is done via a retrograde, antegrade, or transapical approach. Each has its challenges. In all three approaches, the positioning of the prosthetic valve is determined by the patient's native valvular structure and anatomy and is guided by fluoroscopic imaging, supra-aortic angiography, and transesophageal echocardiography. Current prosthetic valves are made from equine or bovine pericardial tissue.

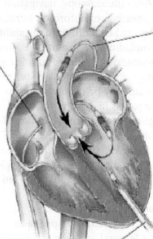

Retrograde or transfemoral technique
The catheter is advanced to the stenotic aortic valve via the femoral artery.

Advantages
Faster, technically easier than antegrade approach

Disadvantages
Potential for injury to the aortofemoral vessels
Crossing the stenotic aortic valve can be challenging

Antegrade technique
The catheter is advanced via the femoral vein, traversing the interatrial septum and the mitral valve, and is positioned within the diseased aortic valve.

Advantages
Femoral vein accommodates the large catheter sheath
Easy management of peripheral access site

Disadvantages
Risk of mitral valve injury and severe mitral valve regurgitation
Correctly positioning the prosthetic valve can be challenging

This technique is no longer in use.

Transapical technique
A valve delivery system is inserted via a small intercostal incision. The apex of the left ventricle is punctured, and the prosthetic valve is positioned within the stenotic aortic valve.

Advantages
Access to the stenotic valve is more direct
Avoids potential complications of a large peripheral access site

Disadvantages
Potential for complications related to puncture of the left ventricle
Requires general anesthesia and chest tubes

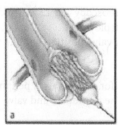
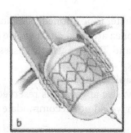
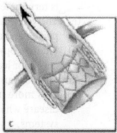

The aortic valve prosthesis is placed at mid-position in the patient's aortic valve so as not to impinge on the coronary ostia or to impede the motion of the anterior mitral leaflet (a). The prosthesis is deployed by inflating (b), rapidly deflating, and quickly withdrawing the delivery balloon (c).

CCF
Medical Illustrator: Joseph Pangrace ©2008

FIGURE 11.4 Approaches to transcatheter aortic valve replacement (TAVR).

(3) Other approaches

(a) A transaxillary approach has been described as an alternative for patients with severe iliofemoral arterial disease [17]. Preoperative CT imaging is obtained to ensure that the vasculature is suitable for this approach. Access is obtained via surgical cutdown, and the valve is deployed similar to the retrograde (transfemoral approach).

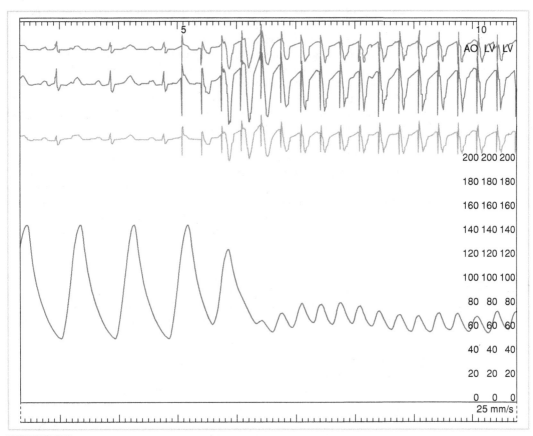

FIGURE 11.5 Hemodynamics during rapid ventricular pacing. The bottom waveform is taken from the arterial catheter. AO, aorta; LV, left ventricle.

(b) Transaortic approach via ministernotomy has also been reported. In the authors' institution, this is the most commonly used alternative approach when peripheral vascular disease prevents a transfemoral technique.

(c) Recently, a transcarotid approach has been used in patients who are not candidates for the other approaches.

e. Anesthetic considerations

(1) In addition to standard monitors, large-bore venous access and invasive blood pressure monitoring are essential. For the ongoing clinical trials, a pulmonary artery catheter (PAC) is usually placed; however, the catheter is withdrawn during the procedure itself as it interferes with the fluoroscopic image. TEE is helpful as a monitor and guide for valve placement, but transthoracic imaging or fluoroscopy alone may be used in patients having the procedure done via the retrograde transfemoral approach, using local anesthesia and sedation.

(2) Blood should be readily available, as massive hemorrhage from arterial injury can occur acutely.

(3) Radiolucent defibrillation pads should be placed prior to draping the patient, in case the need arises for cardioversion or defibrillation.

(4) With the transapical and transaortic approaches, general anesthesia is necessary. Lung isolation may be helpful for surgical exposure but is not absolutely needed. For the retrograde approach, local or regional anesthesia with MAC may be adequate, but each patient should be assessed on an individual basis. The advantages of using local/regional anesthesia with sedation include the ability to assess neurologic status,

avoidance of airway manipulation, and a more rapid early recovery. However, general anesthesia may be more comfortable for the patient, provide immobility during valve deployment, and provide a secure airway in the event of complications and the need for emergent CPB [18–20]. General anesthesia is especially helpful when TEE is used, and some clinicians see this as the "tipping point" for its selection. With either method of anesthesia, the goal is for the patient to recover rapidly. Shorter-acting anesthetic agents along with other adjuncts, such as intercostal nerve blocks performed under direct vision by the surgical team (transapical approach), will help accomplish this goal.

2

(5) During the procedure, there may be periods of acute hemodynamic instability as a result of the device occluding the already narrow valve, the creation of acute AR during valvuloplasty, massive bleeding from dissection of major vasculature, damage to the LV or mitral valve, or acute occlusion of a coronary ostium. Arrhythmias are common during insertion of guidewires and catheters into the LV. Clear communication with the surgical team is of the utmost importance in order to treat appropriately and to avoid "overshooting" with vasopressors. Sometimes the solution is as simple as repositioning the catheter.

> **CLINICAL PEARL** Acute, dramatic hemodynamic changes are common during TAVR, for both patient-related and procedure-related causes, making it essential to communicate with the surgical team so that they can contribute to diagnosis and treatment of these changes.

(6) Normothermia should be actively maintained with the use of forced air warming blankets and fluid warmers as needed.

(7) TEE is used to assess global cardiac function, measure the aortic root for sizing of the prosthesis, screen for aortic disease, facilitate proper valve positioning, and identify complications of the procedure such as paravalvular leak (Supplemental Video 11.3), tamponade, or coronary occlusion [11,21].

   f. **Complications** [22,23]. Major complications of TAVR include stroke, vascular damage including dissection, rupture of the aortic root, occlusion of coronary ostia, cardiac conduction abnormalities, damage to other cardiac structures such as the mitral valve, embolization of the prosthesis requiring emergent surgical retrieval, and massive blood loss from vascular damage or rupture of the LV. Paravalvular leak is more common after TAVR than open surgery, probably because diseased, calcified tissue that may hinder optimal valve deployment is not removed. Paravalvular leaks may be treated with balloon reinflation to better appose the stented prosthesis to the aortic annulus.

   g. **Outcomes** [9,24]. For nonsurgical candidates, TAVR has been associated with an improvement of symptoms and mortality at 1 year as compared to medical management. For patients at too high risk for surgical AVR, TAVR has transformed the management and led to significant reductions in mortality. The success of TAVR in this population has led to considerable interest in its use for lower-risk patients. However, paravalvular regurgitation remains a limitation with TAVR, and even mild residual postoperative paravalvular leak may increase mortality. Also, there appears to be a higher incidence of heart block, stroke, and major vascular complications with TAVR. As the transcatheter prostheses evolve, it is likely that this technique will eventually be available for low-risk populations. Currently, only high-risk patients or intermediate-risk patients who are enrolled in clinical trials are considered for TAVR. We look forward to more long-term outcome data as the procedure becomes more common.

8. **Surgical (open) aortic valve replacement**

   a. Patients who require AVR and who do not qualify for (or sometimes who do not choose) TAVR require a traditional open aortic valve replacement, which is most often

TABLE 11.3 Hemodynamic goals for management of AS

	LV preload	Heart rate	Contractility	SVR	Pulmonary vascular resistance
AS	↑	↓ (sinus)	Maintain constant	↑	Maintain constant

AS, aortic stenosis; SVR, systemic vascular resistance.

performed using a median sternotomy and cardiopulmonary bypass. Minimally invasive surgical approaches to aortic valve replacement are presented in Chapter 13.

   b. Anesthetic considerations are as discussed above for TAVR (see Section V.D.7.e). Goals of perioperative management are generally the same as for TAVR (see Section V.E).

   c. Types of valves are discussed in Section IX.

E. Goals of intraoperative management

   1. Hemodynamic profile (Table 11.3)

     a. LV preload. Due to the decreased LV compliance as well as the increased LVEDP and LV end-diastolic volume (LVEDV), preload augmentation is necessary to maintain a normal stroke volume.

     b. Heart rate. Extremes of heart rate are not tolerated well. A high heart rate can lead to decreased coronary perfusion. A low heart rate can limit cardiac output in these patients with a fixed stroke volume. If a choice must be made, however, low heart rates (50 to 70 beats/min) are preferred to rapid heart rates (greater than 90 beats/min) to allow time for systolic ejection across a stenotic aortic valve. Because atrial contraction contributes up to 40% of LV filling, due to decreased LV compliance and impaired early filling during diastole, it is essential to maintain a sinus rhythm. Supraventricular dysrhythmias should be treated aggressively, if necessary, with synchronized DC shock because both tachycardia and the loss of effective atrial contraction can lead to rapid reduction of cardiac output.

     c. Contractility. Stroke volume is maintained through preservation of a heightened contractile state. β-Blockade is not well tolerated and can lead to an increase in LVEDV and a decrease in cardiac output significant enough to induce clinical deterioration.

     d. Systemic vascular resistance (SVR). Most of the afterload to LV ejection is caused by the stenotic aortic valve itself and thus is fixed. Systemic blood pressure reduction does little to decrease LV afterload. In addition, patients with hemodynamically significant AS cannot increase cardiac output in response to a drop in SVR. Thus, arterial hypotension may rapidly develop in response to the majority of anesthetics. Finally, when hypotension develops, the hypertrophied myocardium of the patient with AS is at great risk for subendocardial ischemia because coronary perfusion depends on maintenance of an adequate systemic diastolic perfusion pressure. Therefore, the early use of α-adrenergic agonists such as phenylephrine is indicated to prevent drops in blood pressure that can lead quickly to sudden death.

     e. Pulmonary vascular resistance. Except for end-stage AS, pulmonary artery pressures remain relatively normal. Special intervention for stabilizing pulmonary vascular resistance is not necessary.

   2. Anesthetic techniques

   3. An experienced cardiac surgeon should be present, and perfusionists should be prepared before induction of anesthesia, should rapid cardiovascular deterioration necessitate emergency use of CPB.

   4. Placement of external defibrillator pads should be considered to allow for rapid defibrillation if cardiovascular collapse occurs on induction or prior to sternotomy.

   5. Preinduction arterial line placement is standard practice at most institutions and is generally well tolerated with light premedication and local anesthetic infiltration.

Invasive blood pressure monitoring facilitates early recognition and intervention if any hemodynamic instability occurs during induction.

6. During induction of anesthesia, in order to maintain hemodynamic stability, medications should be carefully titrated to a fine line between a reasonable depth of anesthesia and hemodynamic stability.

> **CLINICAL PEARL** During induction of general anesthesia for the patient with AS (or any other valvular lesion), it is less important to focus on the use of specific anesthetic agents or vasopressor drugs, as it is to proceed with a regimen/plan that aims to achieve and optimize specific hemodynamic goals (i.e., related to choosing a drug regimen based on overall optimization of heart rate/rhythm, SVR, inotropy).

7. During the maintenance stage of anesthesia, anesthetic agents causing myocardial depression, blood pressure reduction, tachycardia, or dysrhythmias can lead to rapid deterioration. A narcotic-based anesthetic usually is chosen for this reason. Low concentrations of volatile anesthetics are usually safe.

8. If the patient develops signs or symptoms of ischemia, nitroglycerin should be used with caution because its effect on preload or arterial pressure may actually make things worse.

9. **Thermodilution cardiac output.** PACs are helpful in evaluating the cardiac output of patients prior to repair/replacement of the aortic valve. The pulmonary capillary wedge pressure (PCWP), however, may overestimate preload of a noncompliant LV. Mixed venous oxygen saturation monitoring via an oximetric PAC may be used to provide a continuous index of cardiac output. However, because the post-bypass management is not likely to be marked by myocardial failure or low output states, this technique may be best reserved for other patients who may be at higher risk of post-bypass hemodynamic complications.

10. There is also a small risk of life-threatening arrhythmias leading to drug-resistant hypotension during passage of a PAC through the right atrium and ventricle. In the absence of pre-existing left bundle branch block or tachyarrhythmias, a PAC may be placed under continuous rhythm monitoring, perhaps, after placement of transcutaneous pacing electrodes. In the presence of pre-existing abnormal rhythms or conduction disturbances, however, the most conservative approach dictates leaving the catheter tip in a central venous position until the chest is open, when internal defibrillator pads can be easily applied and CPB can be initiated within a few minutes, if necessary.

11. **TEE** is useful for intraoperative monitoring of LV function, preload, and afterload. TEE can predict prosthetic aortic valve size based on the LV outflow tract width. It is also very helpful in the detection of air and facilitating deairing prior to weaning from CPB. TEE is the method of choice for the post-bypass assessment of a prosthetic valve for paravalvular regurgitation and prosthetic valve stenosis. It is important to remember that Doppler-derived blood flow velocities and pressure gradients must be interpreted in light of the altered loading conditions seen in the dynamic operating room setting.

12. In the presence of myocardial hypertrophy, adequate myocardial preservation with cardioplegic solution during bypass is a challenging task. A combination of antegrade cardioplegia administered via coronary ostia and retrograde cardioplegia via the coronary sinus has an important role in preserving myocardial integrity.

13. In the absence of preoperative ventricular dysfunction and associated coronary disease, inotropic support often is not required after CPB because valve replacement decreases ventricular afterload.

F. **Postoperative care.** After a sharp drop in the aortic valve gradient, PCWP and LVEDP immediately decrease and stroke volume rises. Myocardial function improves rapidly, although the hypertrophied ventricle may still require an elevated preload to function normally. Over a period of several months, LV hypertrophy regresses. It must be remembered that a properly sized and functionally prosthetic aortic valve may cause an elevated mean pressure gradient (i.e., ~7 to 19 mm Hg).

1. TAVR patients who receive general anesthesia often are extubated in the operating room or shortly after arrival in the intensive care unit.

2. Patients undergoing open aortic valve replacements are less often extubated in the operating room, but may be fast-tracked (see Chapter 10) if conditions permit.

VI. Hypertrophic cardiomyopathy (HCM)

  A. Natural history

    1. **Etiology and classification.** HCM is a relatively common genetic cardiac disorder, affecting approximately 0.2% of the general population worldwide. This equates to roughly 1 case in every 500 births, with some estimates now suggesting an even greater prevalence of HCM, with increased awareness and screening. Outside of the medical community, its link to the sudden deaths of young, otherwise healthy athletes has generated mainstream notoriety and attention for the condition. Nomenclature and classification schemes related to HCM have historically been somewhat confusing, with several different names being used to describe this disease state (i.e., idiopathic hypertrophic subaortic stenosis [IHSS], asymmetric septal hypertrophy, muscular subaortic stenosis). Since ventricular hypertrophy may occur in a number of different patterns and not just confined to the ventricular septum, HCM is now recognized as the preferred term for describing this disorder. Additionally, despite the classic association of HCM with dynamic obstruction to systolic outflow through the left ventricular outflow tract (LVOT), only ~25% of patients with HCM exhibit this subvalvular obstruction. The term HOCM is used to refer to this subset of HCM patients.

      HCM is a familial disease, inherited in an autosomal dominant fashion with variable penetrance. Mutations in a number of different genes encoding various components of cardiac sarcomere proteins have been identified as a cause for HCM. Most common are mutations involving the β-myosin heavy chain, myosin-binding protein C, troponin T, troponin I, and tropomyosin α-1 chain.

    2. **Symptoms.** Patients with HCM may present with a wide range of symptoms, with many having no symptoms at all. The most common presenting symptom is dyspnea on exertion, with poor exercise tolerance. Patients may also experience syncope, presyncope, chest pain, fatigue, and palpitations. While LVOT obstruction may cause symptoms, there is no clear relationship between the degree of LVOT obstruction and the occurrence or severity of symptoms. Other equally important causes of symptoms include diastolic dysfunction, dysrhythmias, mitral regurgitation (MR), and an imbalance of myocardial oxygen supply and demand. Unfortunately, the initial presenting symptom in many patients is sudden cardiac death, usually due to ventricular fibrillation. While all patients with HCM are at risk for sudden death, the highest-risk groups include those with a family history of HCM and young patients undergoing significant physical exertion. This has led to increased and improved measures to screen for HCM in young athletes and patients with a family history of the disorder.

  B. Pathophysiology. By definition, HCM involves an abnormal thickening of the myocardium without a clearly identifiable cause for the hypertrophy (i.e., chronic hypertension, AS). There is an absence of chamber dilation and in most cases, normal-to-hyperdynamic LV systolic function is present. In addition, there are important histologic derangements, including abnormal cellular architecture and disarray of the cardiac myocytes, interstitial fibrosis, increased connective tissue, and patchy myocardial scarring, although this information is rarely available preoperatively. These cellular abnormalities contribute significantly to problems with diastolic filling, including decreased chamber compliance and impaired relaxation. Even more importantly, these histopathologic abnormalities lead to a derangement in the electrophysiology of the heart capable of inducing the potentially catastrophic dysrhythmias seen in these patients. HCM patients are prone to both atrial and ventricular dysrhythmias, with ventricular fibrillation representing the most common cause of sudden death.

In the subset of patients with outflow tract obstruction, systolic anterior motion (SAM) of the anterior mitral valve leaflet (AML) is the underlying cause for dynamic outflow tract obstruction. Severe hypertrophy of the ventricular septum results in narrowing of the LVOT, whose borders are formed by the septum and the anterior leaflet of the mitral valve (Fig. 11.6). During systole, further narrowing of the LVOT occurs due to septal thickening with ventricular contraction. This leads to an increase in the blood flow velocity and pressure gradient through the narrowed outflow tract. An important distinction between this condition and AS is that the pre-existing ventricular hypertrophy leads to the elevated pressure gradient in HCM, as opposed to the stenotic orifice leading to ventricular hypertrophy in AS.

Basal septal hypertrophy also leads to a decreased distance between the AML and the septum. Additionally, patients with HCM tend to have hypertrophied, anteriorly displaced papillary muscles along with elongated mitral valve leaflets. This shifts the mitral apparatus toward the septum, causing the posterior mitral valve leaflet (PML) to coapt closer to the base of the AML, when the two valve leaflets oppose one another during systole. The result of this altered coaptation is excess, slack AML tissue extending beyond the coaptation point. Rapid blood flow creates hydraulic forces (Venturi effect)

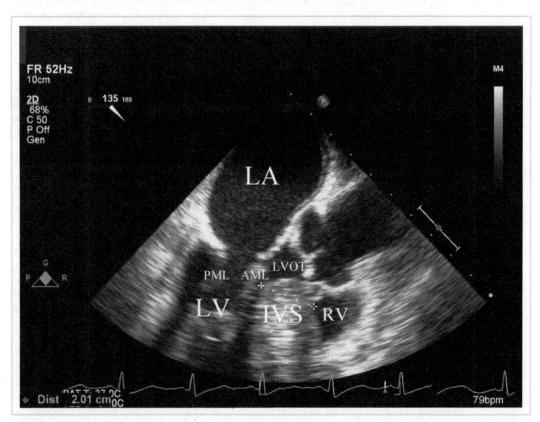

FIGURE 11.6 Basal septal hypertrophy in a patient with hypertrophic cardiomyopathy (HCM). Caliper measurement of the basal septum (*dotted white line*) demonstrates severe hypertrophy (2.01 cm) visualized in a midesophageal long-axis (ME LAX) TEE view. LA, left atrium; PML, posterior mitral valve leaflet; AML, anterior mitral valve leaflet; LVOT, left ventricular outflow tract; LV, left ventricle; IVS, interventricular septum; RV, right ventricle. (Reprinted with permission from Hymel BJ, Townsley MM. Echocardiographic assessment of systolic anterior motion of the mitral valve. *Anesth Analg.* 2014;118(6):1197–1201, Figure 11.1, p. 1198.)

capable of pulling this slack anterior mitral leaflet tissue into the LVOT. Although the Venturi effect has long been hypothesized as the primary mechanism of SAM, it is likely that a drag force generated by LV contraction pulls the anteriorly displaced, slack leaflet tissue into the LVOT in early systole. In fact, this drag force (i.e., pushing/sweeping of the mitral valve leaflet) into the outflow tract is now believed to be the predominant cause of SAM. SAM leads to dynamic obstruction, in which the degree of obstruction varies based upon cardiac loading conditions and contractility. Specifically, the extent of LVOT obstruction is a function of the mitral valve leaflet physically contacting the septum in order to obstruct flow. Therefore, the degree of obstruction correlates directly with the onset, extent, and duration of mitral–septal contact. The obstruction occurs proximal to the aortic valve (subaortic) in mid-to-late systole, with the degree of obstruction directly proportional to LV contractility and inversely proportional to LV preload (end-diastolic volume) and afterload. Specifically, decreases in SVR and preload, as well as increases in contractility and heart rate will precipitate or worsen SAM/LVOT obstruction.

A further consequence of SAM is a **posteriorly** directed jet of MR that results from the abnormal mitral valve leaflet motion. During SAM, the distal portion of the AML remains in the LVOT during systole, as opposed to coapting with the PML in systole. This essentially creates a funnel, formed by the distal portions of both mitral valve leaflets, that directs regurgitant flow posteriorly through this channel. MR in this scenario occurs after the onset of SAM, with its severity primarily related to the degree of LVOT obstruction. Therefore, maneuvers to alleviate LVOT obstruction will also lead to improvement or resolution of the MR. In addition to LVOT obstruction, dynamic mid-cavitary obstruction can also occur in patients with HCM. This typically occurs in patients with concentric hypertrophy most pronounced at the mid-LV level. Intracavitary pressures/obstruction are affected by the same hemodynamic conditions as SAM/dynamic LVOT obstruction.

While dynamic LVOT obstruction is seen in only a subset of HCM patients, most will exhibit diastolic dysfunction secondary to ventricular hypertrophy, as well as hypertrophy and disarray of the myocytes. Early diastolic filling is impaired secondary to this poor diastolic compliance, making atrial contraction, and thus maintenance of sinus rhythm, critical for adequate diastolic filling. Mismatch of oxygen supply and demand is a frequent occurrence in HCM that predisposes to ischemia. The hypertrophied myocardium represents a large muscle mass, and there is increased oxygen demand associated with elevated ventricular pressures and wall tension.

C. **Preoperative evaluation and assessment of severity.** Echocardiography allows for assessment of the location and severity of hypertrophy and helps determine the necessity and feasibility of potential surgical intervention. When patients with HOCM present for surgical myomectomy, the baseline intraoperative TEE exam is a critical component of the procedure. The extent of basal septal hypertrophy is assessed in a midesophageal long-axis (ME LAX) view at end-diastole (Fig. 11.6). Additionally, a nonstandard ME five-chamber view may also be used. While normal LV thickness is ≤1 cm, many patients will often present with severe basal septal hypertrophy in excess of 2 cm. The diameter of the LVOT, as well as the distance from mitral coaptation point to the septum (C-sept distance) is also measured. Both a narrow LVOT (≤2.0 cm) and small C-sept distance (≤2.5 cm) have been identified as risk factors for the development of hemodynamically significant SAM. Both of the above-mentioned views can be used to evaluate for the presence of SAM (Supplemental Video 11.4). In the presence of SAM, color flow Doppler will demonstrate high-velocity, turbulent flow (aliasing) in the LVOT. Additionally, a posteriorly directed jet of MR is also frequently observed as a consequence of the SAM, resulting in a characteristic "Y-shaped" color flow Doppler (CFD) pattern (Supplemental Video 11.5).

CWD measurements of the peak LVOT velocity and pressure gradient, in either a deep transgastric LAX or transgastric LAX view, quantifies the severity of subaortic obstruction. With dynamic LVOT obstruction, the Doppler profile demonstrates a late peaking, "dagger-shaped" envelope of high-velocity flow due to the onset of obstruction in

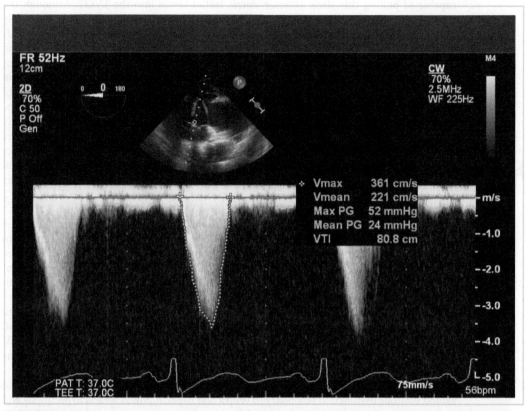

FIGURE 11.7 Dynamic left ventricular outflow tract (LVOT) obstruction. Continuous wave Doppler tracing of blood flow through the LVOT in a patient with hypertrophic cardiomyopathy (HCM), demonstrating a high-velocity Doppler flow profile with a delayed peak ("dagger shaped") consistent with dynamic LVOT obstruction peaking in mid-to-late systole. The peak gradient (max PG) is significantly elevated at 52 mm Hg. (Reprinted with permission from Hymel BJ, Townsley MM. Echocardiographic assessment of systolic anterior motion of the mitral valve. *Anesth Analg.* 2014;118(6):1197–1201, Figure 11.2, p. 1199.)

mid-to-late systole (Fig. 11.7). A mean gradient of ≥30 mm Hg is considered significant. In addition to the mitral coaptation defect associated with SAM, the mitral apparatus itself may be abnormal in HCM patients and should be thoroughly examined. LV systolic function is typically normal or hyperdynamic and diastolic function is almost always abnormal.

D. **Timing and type of intervention.** The mainstay of medical therapy for HCM involves treatment with β-blockers, which help reduce LVOT obstruction due to their negative inotropic effects and reduction in heart rate. Calcium channel blockers are also frequently utilized for their favorable effect on diastolic compliance. The most critical intervention in patients identified as high risk for malignant dysrhythmias is placement of an automated implantable cardioverter–defibrillator. Other nonsurgical approaches to decrease outflow obstruction include dual-chamber pacing and ethanol ablation of the ventricular septum. Surgical treatment involves removal of septal muscle tissue to widen the LVOT via septal myomectomy and may occasionally involve modification of the mitral valve apparatus or mitral valve repair/replacement. Following myomectomy, the intraoperative TEE exam allows for immediate assessment of the adequacy of surgical intervention. Expected findings are a significant reduction in the LVOT gradient by continuous wave Doppler (CWD), as well as thinning of the septum/widening of the LVOT and resolution of SAM.

E. **Goals of perioperative management**
1. **Hemodynamic profile** (Table 11.3)
   a. **LV preload.** Any condition that leads to a decrease in LV cavity size can potentially exacerbate dynamic LVOT obstruction, as this places the septum and anterior mitral leaflet in closer proximity, narrowing the outflow tract and increasing the potential for SAM and obstruction. In this regard, preload augmentation is essential to help maintain ventricular volume. Additionally, similar to AS, diastolic dysfunction will lead to decreased LV compliance with increased LVEDP, which will necessitate adequate preload to maintain a normal stroke volume. Treatment with nitroglycerin, or other vasodilators, should be avoided, as it may dangerously reduce cardiac output.
   b. **Heart rate.** It is essential to avoid tachycardia in patients with HCM because it leads to a reduction in ventricular volume, exacerbation of dynamic LVOT obstruction, and increased oxygen demand. Decreased heart rates are beneficial, as this prolongs diastole and allows more time for ventricular filling. Maintenance of sinus rhythm and the atrial contraction component of ventricular filling is critical due to reduced early diastolic filling because of reduced LV compliance.
   c. **Contractility.** Decreases in myocardial contractility help reduce outflow obstruction. β-Blockade, volatile anesthetics, and avoidance of sympathetic stimulation are all potentially beneficial. The use of intraoperative inotropic agents can increase contractility, worsen LVOT obstruction, and lead to severe hemodynamic instability. Thus, they should be avoided.

CLINICAL PEARL   HOCM is one of the few clinical scenarios in which agents with positive inotropic effects can lead to clinical deterioration.

   d. **Systemic vascular resistance.** Decreases in afterload must be promptly and aggressively treated with vasopressors, such as phenylephrine or vasopressin. Hypotension can be especially detrimental in this population because diastolic dysfunction leads to increased LVEDP, requiring an increased blood pressure to provide adequate coronary perfusion pressure (CPP):

$$CPP = \text{Diastolic blood pressure (aorta)} - LVEDP$$

   e. **Pulmonary vascular resistance.** Pulmonary artery pressures remain relatively normal in most patients. Specific intervention for stabilizing pulmonary vascular resistance is typically not necessary.
2. **Anesthetic technique**
   a. **Premedication.** Many of these patients are on maintenance therapy with β-blockers or calcium channel blockers, which should be given on the day of surgery and continued throughout the perioperative period.
   b. **Induction and maintenance of anesthesia.** During induction and laryngoscopy, careful attention is required to avoid decreases in afterload, as well as sympathetic stimulation leading to increases in heart rate and contractility. Adequate preload must be maintained and all blood or fluid losses should be aggressively replaced. The direct myocardial depressant effect of volatile anesthetics is potentially advantageous.
   c. Patients with HCM are at risk for atrial and ventricular tachyarrhythmias during surgery. Preparation must be in place for immediate cardioversion or defibrillation.
   d. Intraoperative TEE, like preoperative echocardiography, allows visualization of the location and extent of hypertrophy in the septum, the degree of SAM and LVOT obstruction, and quantification of the degree of MR. It is customary to measure the

thickness of the septum at the point of contact with the anterior leaflet, as this information is helpful to the surgeon. Since central venous pressure (CVP) and PCWP measurements will overestimate true volume status, TEE is the most reliable means of accurately assessing volume. The ability to monitor LV systolic function and wall motion is useful, as the oxygen supply–demand relationship is tenuous in these patients making them prone to ischemia. The adequacy of surgical repair and any postrepair complications can also be immediately assessed.

e. **Postoperative care.** Potential complications in the immediate postoperative period following septal myomectomy include residual LVOT obstruction, residual SAM, residual MR, complete heart block, and the creation of a ventricular septal defect (VSD). Unroofing of septal perforator vessels is an expected TEE finding after septal myomectomy and should not be confused with an iatrogenic VSD.

VII. Aortic regurgitation (AR)

A. **Natural history**

1. **Etiology.** AR may be caused by abnormalities of either the aortic valve leaflets or the aorta itself. Problems with the valve leaflets may occur from degenerative, inflammatory, infectious, traumatic, iatrogenic, or congenital etiologies. Specific examples include calcific valve disease, rheumatic disease, endocarditis, a congenitally bicuspid aortic valve, myxomatous valve disease, and systemic inflammatory disorders. Aortic root dilatation, leading to separation and incomplete apposition of the aortic valve leaflets in diastole, can be caused by degenerative aortic dilation, syphilitic aortitis, Marfan syndrome, and aortic dissection. Acute AR is usually caused by aortic dissection, trauma, or aortic valve endocarditis.

A helpful approach to understanding the underlying cause of AR has been described and is based upon a modification of the well-established classification scheme used to classify mechanisms for MR (Carpentier classification). With this approach, three types of AR morphology are described, based upon the motion of the aortic valve leaflets. Type I is associated with normal aortic valve leaflet motion, type II is associated with excessive valve leaflet motion (i.e., leaflet prolapse), and type III is associated with restricted valve leaflet motion (i.e., thickening and/or calcification of leaflets). Type I AR may be further divided into four additional subtypes based upon pathology of the aortic root and aortic valve. Type Ia involves sinotubular junction enlargement and dilatation of the ascending aorta, type Ib involves dilatation of the sinuses of Valsalva and sinotubular junction, type Ic involves dilation of the aortic valve annulus, and type Id involves perforation of the aortic valve leaflet [25].

2. **Symptoms.** Patients with chronic AR may be asymptomatic for many years. However, although they remain asymptomatic, many patients will be undergoing progressive ventricular dilatation with the development of impaired myocardial contractility. Symptoms such as shortness of breath, palpitations, fatigue, and angina usually develop only after significant dilatation and dysfunction of the LV myocardium have occurred. The 10-year mortality for asymptomatic AR varies between 5% and 15%. Once symptoms develop, however, patients progressively deteriorate and have an expected survival around 10 years. Patients with severe acute AR, due to the lack of longstanding compensation, are not capable of maintaining sufficient forward stroke volume. These patients are likely to develop sudden and severe dyspnea, significant pulmonary edema, refractory heart failure, and may deteriorate rapidly due to cardiovascular collapse.

B. **Pathophysiology**

1. **Pathophysiology and natural progression**

a. **Acute AR.** The sudden occurrence of acute AR places a major volume load on the LV. The immediate compensatory mechanism for the maintenance of adequate forward flow is increased sympathetic tone, producing tachycardia and an increased contractile state. Fluid retention increases preload. However, the combination of increased LVEDV, along with increased stroke volume and heart rate may not be sufficient to maintain a normal cardiac output. Rapid deterioration of LV function can occur, necessitating emergency surgical intervention.

CLINICAL PEARL   The patient with acute-onset, severe AR represents an especially high-risk patient population, and the perioperative plan must include preparations to manage sudden cardiac collapse.

        b. Chronic AR. Chronically, AR leads to LV systolic and diastolic volume overload. LV wall tension also increases, precipitating the replication and lengthening of cardiac sarcomeres. This causes the wall thickness to increase in proportion to the increase in LV chamber size in a pattern of eccentric ventricular hypertrophy. Because the LVEDV increases slowly, the LVEDP remains relatively normal. Forward flow is aided by the presence of chronic peripheral vasodilation, which occurs along with a large stroke volume. As the LV dilatation progresses, coronary perfusion finally decreases leading to irreversible LV myocardial tissue damage and dysfunction. The onset of LV dysfunction is followed by an increase in PA pressure with symptoms of dyspnea and congestive heart failure. As a compensatory mechanism for the poor cardiac output and poor coronary perfusion, sympathetic constriction of the periphery occurs to maintain blood pressure, which in turn leads to further decreases in cardiac output.

    2. Pressure wave disturbances

        a. Arterial pressure. Incompetence of the aortic valve leads to regurgitant blood flow from the aorta back into the LV during diastole. This causes a pronounced decline in aortic diastolic blood pressure, translating into a wide pulse pressure. Patients with AR, therefore, show a wide pulse pressure with a rapid rate of rise, a high systolic peak, and a low diastolic pressure. The pulse pressure may be as great as 80 to 100 mm Hg. The rapid upstroke is due to the large stroke volume, and the rapid downstroke is due to the rapid flow of blood from the aorta back into the ventricle and then into the dilated peripheral vessels. The occurrence of a double peaked, or bisferiens pulse trace, is not unusual due to the occurrence of a "tidal" or back wave. It is this wide pulse pressure that leads to the presence of the many eponymous clinical signs associated with AR.

        b. Pulmonary capillary wedge trace. Stretching of the mitral valve annulus may lead to functional MR, a prominent V wave, and a rapid Y descent. In patients with acute AR associated with poor ventricular compliance, LV pressure may increase fast enough to close the mitral valve before end diastole. In this situation, AR raises the LVEDP above left atrial pressure, and the PCWP can significantly underestimate the true LVEDP.

    3. Pressure–volume loop in aortic regurgitation (Fig. 11.8)

  C. Preoperative evaluation and assessment of severity

    1. Historically, the amount of AR was estimated based on angiographic clearance of dye injected into the aortic root. Currently, echocardiography is the method of choice for qualitative, semiquantitative, and quantitative assessment of AR.

        a. Echocardiographic assessment of AR (Table 11.4)

        Supplemental Videos 11.6 and 11.7 demonstrate the appearance of AR as seen on TEE. The severity of AR can be assessed with echocardiography by several techniques (Table 11.5). Qualitative assessment includes the two-dimensional analysis of the aortic valve anatomy, with particular attention to any structural abnormalities of the leaflets. The aortic root and LV cavity should be closely examined for evidence of dilation. CFD allows for visualization of the regurgitant jet, originating at the aortic valve and extending back into the LVOT in diastole. An experienced echocardiographer can often accurately estimate the degree of regurgitation with this initial observation; however, quantitative measurements are made to more accurately assess severity. The vena contracta is, perhaps, the most widely utilized measurement. It represents the narrowest

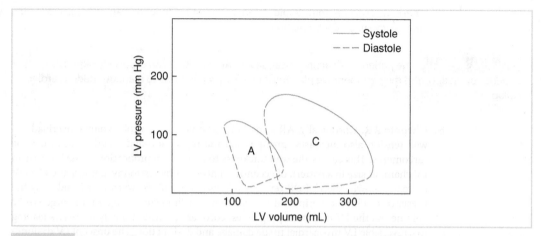

FIGURE 11.8 Pressure–volume loop in acute and chronic AR. Note the rightward shift of the loop in chronic AR (C), reflecting elevated LV volume without a dramatic elevation in filling pressure. In acute AR (A), LV volumes are also increased; however, the ventricle has not adapted to accommodate the increased volumes without elevation of filling pressures. AR, aortic regurgitation. (Modified from Jackson JM, Thomas SJ, Lowenstein E. Anesthetic management of patients with valvular heart disease. *Semin Anesth.* 1982;1:247.)

TABLE 11.4   Hemodynamic goals for management of dynamic subaortic stenosis

	LV preload	Heart rate	Contractility	SVR	Pulmonary vascular resistance
Dynamic subaortic stenosis	↑	↓	↓	↑	Maintain constant

SVR, systemic vascular resistance.

TABLE 11.5   Assessment of AR severity with echocardiography

	Mild	Moderate	Severe
Left ventricular size	Normal[a]	Normal or dilated	Usually dilated[b]
Jet deceleration rate/pressure half-time (msec)[c]	Slow (>500)	Medium (500–200)	Steep (<200)
Diastolic flow reversal in descending thoracic aorta	Brief, early diastolic reversal	Intermediate	Prominent holodiastolic reversal
Vena contracta width (cm)	<0.3	0.3–0.6	>0.6

Grade	Mild (1+)[d]	Mild–moderate (2+)	Moderate–severe (3+)	Severe (4+)
Jet width/LVOT width (%)	<25	25–45	46–64	≥65
Jet CSA/LVOT CSA (%)	<5	5–20	21–59	≥60
Regurgitant volume (mL/beat)	<30	30–44	45–59	≥60
RF (%)	<30	30–39	40–49	≥50
EROA (cm²)	<0.10	0.10–0.19	0.20–0.29	≥3.0

[a]Unless there are other reasons for LV dilation.
[b]The LV is usually dilated in chronic AR. In acute AR, the LV size is often normal since the ventricle has not had time to dilate.
[c]Pressure half-time is shortened with increasing LV diastolic pressure and vasodilator therapy. It may be prolonged with chronic adaptation to severe AR.
[d]Note that there are several echocardiographic parameters that can subclassify regurgitation severity into mild, mild–moderate, moderate–severe, and severe. These subclassifications correspond to the angiographic grades of 1+, 2+, 3+, and 4+, respectively.
AR, aortic regurgitation; LVOT, left ventricular outflow tract; CSA, cross-sectional area; RF, regurgitant fraction; EROA, effective regurgitant orifice area.
Adapted from Zoghbi WA, Adams D, Bonow RO, et al. Recommendations for noninvasive evaluation of native valvular regurgitation: a report from the American Society of Echocardiography developed in collaboration with the Society for Cardiovascular Magnetic Resonance. *J Am Soc Echocardiogr.* 2017;30(4):303–371.

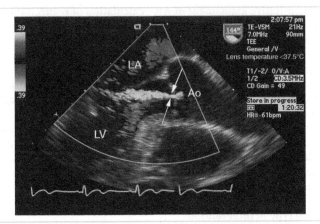

FIGURE 11.9 Vena contracta. Caliper measurement of the narrowest portion of the aortic regurgitant jet, which corresponds to an approximation of the regurgitant orifice area. Ao, aorta; LA, left atrium; LV, left ventricle. (Reprinted with permission from Perrino AC, Reeves ST, eds. *A Practical Approach to Transesophageal Echocardiography*. 2nd ed. Philadelphia, PA: Lippincott Williams & Wilkins, 2008:232, Figure 11.4.)

point of the regurgitant jet and corresponds to the size of the regurgitant orifice. It is a relatively easy measurement to obtain and is also unaffected by changes in preload or afterload (Fig. 11.9). Severity of regurgitation can also be estimated by measuring the extent in which the regurgitant jet occupies the LVOT. The ratio of jet width to LVOT width, or jet area to LVOT area, has been found to correlate well with angiographic assessment (Fig. 11.10). CWD can be used to measure the deceleration rate of the regurgitant jet and the pressure half-time. These measurements are based on the rate of equilibration between aortic and LV pressures. As the severity of AR increases (i.e., regurgitant orifice becomes larger), the more quickly these pressures will equilibrate. Thus, significant AR corresponds to a steep slope of the jet deceleration rate and a short pressure half-time. Severe AR may also be associated with holodiastolic flow reversal in the descending thoracic aorta seen on a pulsed-wave Doppler (PWD) exam.

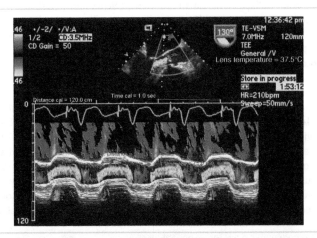

FIGURE 11.10 Color M-mode assessment of AR. Utilizing a ME aortic long-axis view, the width of the regurgitant jet and the LVOT are measured. The ratio of jet width to LVOT width can be used to estimate the severity of the AR. AR, aortic regurgitation; ME, midesophageal; LVOT, left ventricular outflow tract. (Reprinted with permission from Perrino AC, Reeves ST, eds. *A Practical Approach to Transesophageal Echocardiography*. 2nd ed. Philadelphia, PA: Lippincott Williams & Wilkins, 2008; 229, Figure 11.2.)

b. **Quantitative assessment of AR—calculation of regurgitant volume and regurgitant fraction.** A quantitative estimate of the severity of AR may be obtained by calculating the regurgitant volume and regurgitant fraction (RF). The total stroke volume in a patient with AR is the regurgitant volume plus the forward stroke volume actually ejected into the circulation. The regurgitant volume is the amount of blood that flows back through the incompetent aortic valve during each cardiac cycle. It is quantified as the difference between the total stroke volume flowing through the aortic valve and the total *forward* stroke volume through a different valve. This reference valve is most commonly the mitral valve, with Doppler echocardiography being used to calculate the transmitral stroke volume. Total LV stroke volume can be determined with either Doppler echocardiography measurement of flow through the LV outflow tract or it may be derived from the left ventriculogram on cardiac catheterization. The RF, or fraction of each stroke volume flowing back into the LV, equals the ratio of the right ventricle (RV) to the total stroke volume through the regurgitant aortic valve.

D. **Timing and type of intervention**

1. **Acute aortic regurgitation.** Urgent surgical intervention is often indicated in acute AR due to a high incidence of hemodynamic instability. Inotropic support is frequently needed to maintain cardiac output.

2. **Chronic aortic regurgitation.** AVR is recommended for the symptomatic patient with chronic, severe AR, regardless of LV systolic function. Asymptomatic patients with chronic AR and LV systolic function (EF <50%) should also undergo AVR. The asymptomatic patient with normal LV function should be closely followed for the onset of clinical symptoms and with serial echocardiographic examination. These patients should have surgical intervention at the earliest sign of LV dysfunction, as overall outcomes are significantly improved when surgery is performed prior to deterioration of ventricular function. Additionally, evidence of ventricular dilatation (left ventricular end-diastolic diameter >65 mm, left ventricular end-systolic diameter >50 mm) should prompt consideration for surgery, even in the presence of normal LV function [1].

3. **Surgical intervention.** The most frequent approach to surgical treatment of AR is AVR. Experience with aortic valve repair has been limited to only a few highly specialized centers, and the durability of aortic valve repair remains unproven. Although enthusiasm for valve repair in certain patient populations (i.e., young patients with bicuspid aortic valves) has resulted in advances in the technique, the AHA/ACC guidelines only recommend aortic valve repair in specialized centers with proven experience and expertise [1]. In cases in which AR is secondary to aortic root and/or ascending aortic dilatation, valve-sparing replacement of the aorta may effectively resolve AR if there is no significant underlying aortic valve pathology.

E. **Goals of perioperative management**

1. **Hemodynamic management** (Table 11.6)

a. **LV preload.** Due to the increased LV volumes, maintenance of forward flow depends on preload augmentation. Pharmacologic intervention producing venous dilation has the potential to impair cardiac output in these patients by reducing preload.

b. **Heart rate.** Patients with AR show a significant increase in forward cardiac output with an increase in heart rate. Decreased time spent in diastole, as occurs with a faster heart rate, results in a decrease in RF. Actual improvement in subendocardial blood flow is observed with an increased heart rate, owing to a higher systemic diastolic pressure and a lower LVEDP. This explains why a patient who is symptomatic at rest may show an improvement in symptoms with exercise. A heart rate of around 90 beats/min seems to be optimal, improving cardiac output while not inducing ischemia.

TABLE 11.6 Hemodynamic goals for management of AR

	LV preload	Heart rate	Contractile state	SVR	Pulmonary vascular resistance
AR	↑	↑	Maintain	↓	Maintain

SVR, systemic vascular resistance; AR, aortic regurgitation.

    c. **Contractility.** LV contractility must be maintained. In patients with impaired LV function, use of pure β agonists or phosphodiesterase inhibitors can increase stroke volume through a combination of peripheral dilation and increased contractility ("inodilation").

    d. **Systemic vascular resistance.** The forward flow can be improved with afterload reduction. Increases in LV afterload result in increased stroke work and can significantly increase the LVEDP.

    e. **Pulmonary vascular resistance.** Pulmonary vascular pressure remains relatively normal except in patients with end-stage AR associated with severe LV dysfunction.

2. **Anesthetic technique**

    a. **Premedication.** Light premedication is recommended.

    b. **Induction and maintenance.** Serious hemodynamic instability during induction of general anesthesia is less likely with severe AR than with severe AS because arterial vasodilation, which is a major effect of most of the induction drugs, is beneficial in AR and transient hypotension is usually well tolerated. However, the importance of careful titration of induction agents in combination with adequate hydration should not be underestimated. Particular caution is warranted with acute AR, where ventricular decompensation is more likely to occur. The hemodynamic goals for induction and maintenance of anesthesia should be directed at preserving the patient's preload and contractility, maintaining the peripheral arterial dilation, and avoiding bradycardia. Careful attention should be paid to avoiding profound bradycardia/asystole in the period after aortic cannulation and onset of CPB, since the LV is especially prone to distend due to the presence of the AR. Until it is vented surgically, the LV must, therefore, vent itself via systolic ejection.

    c. A PAC is helpful in evaluating the cardiac output of patients prior to repair of the aortic valve and, especially, in the post-bypass period for monitoring and optimizing preload and myocardial function.

    d. **Intraoperative TEE** is beneficial for monitoring LV function and assessment of the severity of regurgitation prior to valve surgery. Specific pathology of the aortic valve leaflets and aortic root can be easily assessed. It is also useful in predicting the appropriate size of a prosthetic valve based on the diameters of the aortic annulus and LV outflow tract. If aortic valve repair is performed, TEE is valuable for providing immediate feedback concerning the integrity of valvular function. In AVR, TEE allows for immediate assessment of any perivalvular regurgitation, as well as the pressure gradient across the newly placed prosthetic valve.

    e. **Use of an intra-aortic balloon pump is contraindicated** in the presence of significant AR because augmentation of the diastolic pressure will increase the amount of regurgitant flow.

    f. **Weaning from cardiopulmonary bypass** may be complicated by LV dysfunction secondary to suboptimal myocardial protection and coronary air embolism. AVR leads to a mild transvalvular gradient because most prosthetic valves have a degree of inherent stenosis. An elevated transvalvular gradient, in combination with a significantly dilated LV, may result in increased afterload, low cardiac output, and may contribute to LV dysfunction. Inotropic support may be indicated in order to maintain cardiac output and avoid further LV dilation and dysfunction. Preload augmentation must be continued to maintain filling of the dilated LV.

3. **Postoperative care.** Immediately following AVR, the LVEDP and LVEDV decrease. However, the LV dilation and eccentric hypertrophy persist. In the early postoperative period, a decline in LV function may necessitate inotropic or intra-aortic balloon pump support. If surgical intervention is delayed until significant LV dysfunction has occurred, the prognosis for long-term survival is poor. The 5-year survival rate for patients whose hearts do not return to a relatively normal size within 6 months following surgical repair is only 43%. If surgery is performed early enough, the heart will return to relatively normal dimensions, and a long-term survival rate of 85% to 90% after 6 years can be expected [2].

VIII. **Mixed valvular lesions.** For all mixed valvular lesions, management decisions emphasize the most severe or the most hemodynamically significant lesion.

A. **AS and mitral stenosis.** Pathophysiologically, the progression of the disease follows a course similar to that seen in patients with pure mitral stenosis with development of pulmonary hypertension and, eventually, RV failure. Symptoms are primarily referable to the pulmonary circulation, including dyspnea, hemoptysis, and atrial fibrillation. This combination of valvular heart disease may lead to underestimation of the severity of the AS because the aortic valve gradient may be relatively low owing to low aortic valvular flow. Such a combination of lesions can be extremely serious because of the limitation of blood flow at two points. Intraoperative management should focus on maintaining adequate preload, preserving sinus rhythm, and avoiding tachydysrhythmias in order to optimize ventricular filling. SVR and systemic blood pressure must be preserved in order to avoid ventricular ischemia.

B. **AS and mitral regurgitation (MR).** MR is not an uncommon finding in the setting of severe AS. With progression of the stenotic lesion, the LVSP increases to overcome the flow obstruction. MR flows from the LV during systole into the left atrium (LA). Elevated LVSP results in a larger gradient between the LV and LA and a subsequent increase in MR. Compensatory ventricular remodeling can further worsen MR, as the mitral valve annulus is distorted. MR may improve after the aortic valve is replaced as the LVSP decreases, and this has led to controversy in the surgical management of moderate, functional MR in the setting of severe AS. In managing these patients, the hemodynamic requirements for AS and MR are contradictory. Because AS is more likely to cause cardiovascular collapse, it should be given priority when managing the hemodynamic variables.

C. **AS and AR.** The combination of AR and AS is not well tolerated because it provides the LV with both severe pressure and volume overloading. These stresses lead to major increases in myocardial oxygen consumption (MVO_2) and, as might be expected, angina pectoris is an early symptom with this combination. Once symptoms develop, the prognosis is similar to that of pure AS.

D. **AR and MR.** The combination of AR and MR occurs frequently, and this combination can cause rapid clinical deterioration. The hemodynamic requirements of AR and MR are similar. The primary problem is providing adequate forward flow into the peripheral circulation. The development of acidosis leading to peripheral vasoconstriction and increased impedance to LV outflow can lead to rapid clinical deterioration. Therefore, keeping the SVR relatively low while maintaining an adequate perfusion pressure is the goal until CPB can be initiated.

E. **Multivalve surgical procedures.** While the surgical management of multivalve disease has continued to improve, these patients still represent a significantly higher-risk group than patients presenting for surgery on a single valve.

IX. **Prosthetic valves**

The decision regarding which prosthetic valve should be used for a particular patient is based upon a variety of factors, including the expected longevity of the patient (mechanical prostheses last longer), the ability of the patient to comply with anticoagulation therapy (mechanical prostheses require ongoing anticoagulation), the anatomy and pathology of the existing valvular disease, and the experience of the operating surgeon [26].

A. **Essential characteristics** of prosthetic heart valves. An ideal prosthetic heart valve mimics the characteristics of the native valve and has excellent hemodynamics, is nonthrombogenic, durable, chemically inert, preserves blood elements, and allows physiologic blood flow. The large number of different prosthetic valves that have been developed means that no ideal valve has yet been found and each valve has its own inherent limitations [27].

B. **Types of prosthetic valves**

1. **Mechanical.** Current mechanical prosthetic valves are durable but thrombogenic. At present, all patients with mechanical prosthetic valves require anticoagulation therapy for the remainder of their lives. Normally, anticoagulation is provided with warfarin sodium, administered at a dose that will elevate the prothrombin time to 1.5 to 2 times control. There are four basic types of mechanical prosthetic valves, the caged ball, caged disc, monocuspid tilting disc, and bicuspid tilting disc valves. Of these, the bicuspid tilting–disc

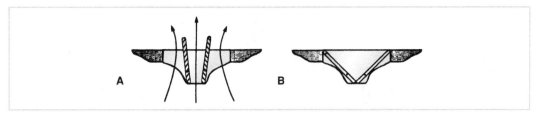

FIGURE 11.11 Bileaflet valve prosthesis showing discs in open (**A**) and closed (**B**) positions. (Reprinted with permission from Hensley FA, Martin DE, Gravlee GR. *A Practical Approach to Cardiac Anesthesia*. 4th ed. Philadelphia, PA: Lippincott Williams and Wilkins; 2008:344.)

valves are in common use today. This valve design is less bulky than its predecessors and provides improved central laminar blood flow.

   a. **Bileaflet tilting–disc valve prosthesis** (Fig. 11.11). In 1977, a bileaflet St. Jude cardiac valve was introduced as a low-profile device to allow central blood flow around two semicircular discs that pivot on supporting struts. When the leaflets open, the opening angle relative to the leaflets ranges from 75 to 90 degrees. Three orifices are present within the valve when open: a smaller central orifice between two larger semicircular orifices on the lateral edges [27]. Due to these size differences, higher flow velocities occur within the smaller central orifice as compared to the two larger outer orifices of the valve. The valve is designed to have an inherent (but small) degree of regurgitant flow originating from backflow from the motion of the occluders and leakage through the components of the prosthesis. This purposeful regurgitant flow is included in the valve to provide "washing jets" to minimize blood stasis and thrombus formation on the valve components [27]. The St. Jude bileaflet tilting–disc valve can be placed in the aortic, mitral, or tricuspid positions. These valves produce low resistance to blood flow and have a lower incidence of thromboembolic complications, though anticoagulation is still necessary. The most popular bileaflet tilting disc is still the St. Jude Medical (Saint Paul, MN). Other bileaflet tilting–disc valve prostheses include the CarboMedics (Sorin Group, Milan, Italy), On-X (MRCI, Austin, TX), and Advancing the Standard (ATS) Medtronic valves.

2. **Bioprosthetic valves.** The Hancock porcine aortic bioprosthesis (now the Medtronic Hancock II stented porcine bioprosthesis) was introduced in 1970, followed by the Ionescu–Shiley bovine pericardial prosthesis in 1974, and the Carpentier–Edwards porcine aortic valve bioprosthesis in 1975. In contrast to modern mechanical prostheses, current bioprostheses are less durable but also less thrombogenic. Long-term anticoagulation for a bioprosthetic valve is usually unnecessary. Bioprosthetic valves in the aortic position last longer than in the mitral position. Because durability is an issue and because their lifespan is longer in older patients, bioprosthetic valves are usually used for patients older than 60 years of age and when anticoagulation is not a desirable option (e.g., when pregnancy is anticipated).

   a. Bioprosthetic valves fall into two types: stented and nonstented. **Stented bioprosthetic** valves constructed from porcine aortic valves or bovine pericardium are placed on a polypropylene stent which is attached to a silicone sewing ring covered with Dacron. These valves allow for improved central annular flow and less turbulence, but the stent does cause some obstruction to forward flow, thereby leading to a residual pressure gradient across the valve. The effective orifice areas of bioprosthetic valves (for a given annulus size) are typically smaller than for bileaflet mechanical valves. A small amount of central regurgitant flow is common in most bioprosthetic valves. Most valves in current production are treated with glutaraldehyde to reduce antigenicity and anticalcification agents or processes [27]. Examples of stented bioprosthetic valves that can be found in clinical use today include the Carpentier–Edwards Perimount (Fig. 11.12), Magna, and S.A.V. valves (Edwards Lifesciences, Irvine, CA); Epic (St. Jude Medical);

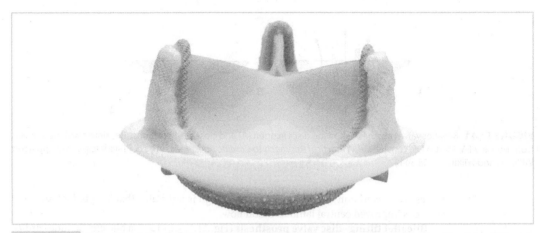

FIGURE 11.12 Carpentier–Edwards Perimount RSR stented pericardial bioprosthetic aortic valve. (Courtesy of Edwards Lifesciences, Irvine, California.) (Reprinted with permission from Hensley FA, Martin DE, Gravlee GR. *A Practical Approach to Cardiac Anesthesia*. 4th ed. Philadelphia, PA: Lippincott Williams and Wilkins; 2008:345.)

Biocor (St. Jude Medical); Hancock II (Medtronic); Mitroflow (Sorin Group); Mosaic (Medtronic); and Trifecta (St. Jude Medical).

   b. Stentless bioprostheses. Stentless valves were developed in order to provide improved hemodynamic characteristics and durability as compared to stented bioprostheses. These valves are constructed from intact porcine aortic valves or bovine pericardium. Stentless bioprosthetic valves are technically more difficult to place and are used almost exclusively in the aortic position. Modern stentless bioprosthetic valves are often used when aortic root replacement is also necessary. The first generation of stentless bioprostheses includes Medtronic Freestyle, Toronto SPV (St. Jude Medical), and Prima–Edwards (Edwards Lifesciences) (Fig. 11.13). Newer generations include the Shelhigh Super Stentless aortic valve (Shelhigh Inc., Union, NJ) and Sorin Pericarbon Freedom valve (Sorin Group), which are easier to implant since they only require one layer of suture for implantation [27].

3. **Sutureless bioprosthetic valves.** Stent-mounted sutureless valves have recently been designed for AVR involving sutureless positioning and anchoring at the site of implantation. These sutureless valves can be used for replacement of either a diseased native valve or dysfunctional prosthetic valve. A primary advantage of these valves lies in the fact that they can be implanted more quickly than other valves, with a significant reduction in aortic cross-clamp and bypass time. Examples include the Perceval (Sorin Group), 3F Enable valve (Medtronic), and Intuity (Edwards Lifesciences) [27].

4. **Human valves.** The first use of a bioprosthesis taken from a cadaver occurred in 1962. However, techniques such as irradiation or chemical treatment used to sterilize and preserve the early homografts for implantation led to a shortened life span. More recently, antibiotic solutions have been used to sterilize human valves, which then are frozen in liquid nitrogen until implantation. Using these techniques, weakness of the prosthesis leading to cusp rupture occurs infrequently, with more than 75% of prostheses lasting for longer than 10 years regardless of patient age. The incidence of prosthetic valve endocarditis and hemolysis resulting from blood flow through the homograft is very low. Anticoagulation is usually not required. Homografts are predominately used in the aortic position, especially when aortic root replacement is necessary and for pulmonary valve replacement in the Ross procedure. Homografts may be most useful in patients younger than 35 and in patients with native valve endocarditis.

5. **Transcatheter valves.** Valves utilized in the TAVR procedure have been introduced and discussed earlier in this chapter. The classification of TAVR valves falls into two main

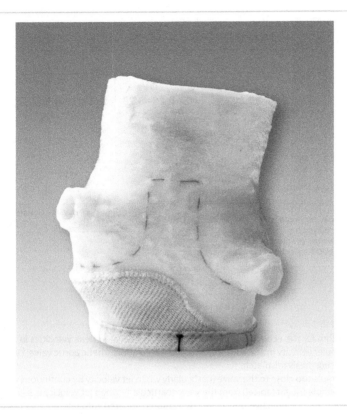

FIGURE 11.13 Edwards Prima Plus stentless bioprosthetic aortic valve. (Courtesy of Edwards Lifesciences, Irvine, California.) (Reprinted with permission from Hensley FA, Martin DE, Gravlee GR. *A Practical Approach to Cardiac Anesthesia.* 4th ed. Philadelphia, PA: Lippincott Williams and Wilkins; 2008:345.)

categories/types: balloon-expandable valves and self-expanding valves. The Edwards valves initially used for the procedure were balloon-expandable valves mounted in a steel frame, available in either 23-mm or 26-mm size. The newer generation of valve is the Edwards SAPIEN XT (Edwards Lifesciences), which is made of bovine pericardium mounted in a cobalt chromium frame. This valve is available in 20-, 23-, 26-, and 29-mm sizes and is implanted using either 18-, 19-, or 22-Fr delivery catheter. Of note, it appears that balloon-expandable valves typically have larger effective orifice areas and lower gradients compared to surgical bioprosthetic valves. As previously discussed, however, paravalvular regurgitation is a more frequent issue with TAVR valves [27].

CoreValve systems (Medtronic) first introduced for this procedure were self-expanding valves made from bovine pericardium in a nitinol, self-expanding frame. Subsequent modifications of this valve have occurred, most notably to allow for true supra-annular placement of the valve. The current, third-generation CoreValve is available in 26-, 29-, and 31-mm sizes and is implanted using an 18-Fr delivery catheter. It appears as though the CoreValve results in larger effective orifice areas and lower gradients than the SAPIEN valves but is more likely to demonstrate paravalvular regurgitation following deployment [27].

C. **Echocardiographic evaluation of prosthetic valves in the aortic position**
  a. **Evaluation for aortic prosthetic valve stenosis**
    (1) The 2D exam should focus on the sewing ring and valve leaflets. Doppler interrogation should determine the mean transvalvular gradient, peak velocity, contour of the jet velocity, acceleration time (AT), Doppler velocity index (DVI), and the effective orifice area of the prosthesis.

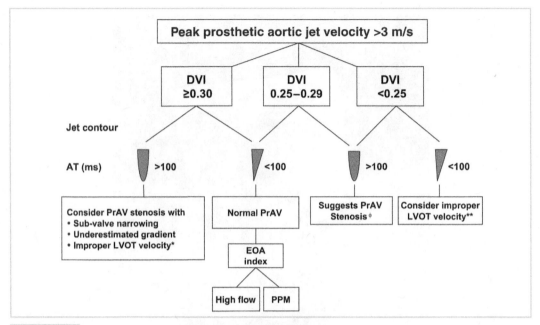

FIGURE 11.14 Algorithm for the echocardiographic evaluation of elevated peak velocities in prosthetic valves in the aortic position. DVI, Doppler velocity index; AT, acceleration time; PrAV, prosthetic aortic valve; LVOT, left ventricular outflow tract; PPM, patient prosthesis mismatch.
*Pulse wave Doppler sample too close to the valve (particularly when jet velocity by continuous wave Doppler is ≥4 m/s.
**Pulse wave Doppler sample too far (apical) from the valve (particularly when jet velocity is 3–3.9 m/s.
◊Stenosis further substantiated by effective orifice area derivation compared with reference values if valve type and size are known.
(Reprinted with permission from Zoghbi WA, Chambers JB, Dumesnil JG, et al. Recommendations for evaluation of prosthetic valves with echocardiography and Doppler ultrasound. *JASE.* 2009;22(9):975–1014, Figure 11.10, p. 990.)

    (2) The following findings are suggestive of significant stenosis: mean gradient >35 mm Hg, peak velocity >4 m/sec, rounded symmetrical contour of the Doppler velocity profile index (as opposed to early peaking triangular shape), AT >100 msec, and DVI <25.

    (3) Occasionally, there are normal prosthetic valves with elevated peak velocities. Figure 11.14 presents a useful algorithm for determining if the conflicting data are due to a high-flow state, measurement error, or patient–prosthesis mismatch (Fig. 11.14).

  b. **Evaluation for aortic prosthetic valve regurgitation**

    (1) The same criteria in determining the severity of native aortic valve regurgitation can be applied to prosthetic aortic valves.

    (2) The 2D evaluation focuses on the sewing ring and valve leaflet motion. Doppler interrogation allows determination of jet width in the LVOT, pressure half time, the presence of holodiastolic flow reversal in the descending thoracic aorta, and calculation of regurgitant volume and RF.

    (3) Transthoracic echocardiography has limited ability to evaluate for posterior paravalvular regurgitation, and TEE may add incremental value if pathology is suspected in this location.

CLINICAL PEARL   When performing TEE for TAVR procedures, it is especially important to assess for the presence and location of paravalvular regurgitation, as this is a common complication of the procedure that may need to be immediately addressed with surgical intervention following initial valve deployment.

TABLE 11.7 Antibiotic recommendations for prophylaxis of bacterial endocarditis

	Agent	Adult dose (30–60 min before procedure)	Pediatric dose[a]
Standard general prophylaxis	Amoxicillin	2 g PO	50 mg/kg/PO
Patients unable to take oral medications	Ampicillin	2 g IV or IM	50 mg/kg IV or IM
Penicillin- and amoxicillin-allergic patients	Cephalexin[b] or clindamycin or azithromycin or clarithromycin	2 g PO 600 mg PO 500 mg PO	50 mg/kg PO 20 mg/kg PO 15 mg/kg PO
Penicillin- and amoxicillin-allergic patients unable to take oral medications	Clindamycin or cefazolin or ceftriaxone	600 mg IV or IM 1 g IV or IM	20 mg/kg IV or IM 50 mg/kg IV or IM

[a]Total pediatric dose should not exceed the adult dose.
[b]Cephalosporins should not be used in patients with immediate-type hypersensitivity reaction (urticaria, angioedema, or anaphylaxis) to penicillins.
Adapted from: Nishimura RA, Otto CM, Bonow RO, et al. 2017 AHA/ACC focused update of the 2014 AHA/ACC guideline for the management of patients with valvular heart disease. *J Am Coll Cardiol.* 2017;70(2):252–289.

X. Prophylaxis of bacterial endocarditis

When an invasive procedure puts the patient with valvular heart disease at risk of bacteremia, precautions should be taken to prevent seeding of an abnormal or artificial valve with bacteria that, once present, are very hard to eradicate. Practically, this concern translates into (a) a strict aseptic technique for all procedures performed in patients with valvular heart disease; (b) elimination of existing sources of infection before implantation of a prosthetic valve; and (c) in selected cases, antibiotic prophylaxis. Guidelines from the American Heart Association and American College of Cardiology on prevention of infective endocarditis limit antibiotic prophylaxis to cardiac conditions associated with the highest risk of infective endocarditis [28]. These conditions include patients with prosthetic cardiac valves (including transcatheter-implanted prostheses and homografts) or material used in heart valve repair (i.e., annuloplasty rings and chords), previous infective endocarditis, unrepaired cyanotic congenital heart disease or repaired congenital heart disease with residual shunts or defects in the proximity of the site of a prosthetic patch or device, and cardiac transplant recipients with valvular disease. Endocarditis prophylaxis is recommended only for "dental procedures that involve manipulation of gingival tissue or the periapical region of teeth or perforation of the oral mucosa." There is no evidence to support the administration of antibiotic prophylaxis in gastrointestinal or genitourinary procedures if there is no known active infection. Guidelines for antibiotic prophylaxis, to be begun 1 hour prior to a procedure, are shown in Table 11.7.

REFERENCES

1. **Nishimura RA, Otto CM, Bonow RO, et al. 2014 AHA/ACC guideline for the management of patients with valvular heart disease: executive summary: a report of the American College of Cardiology/American Heart Association Task Force on Practice Guidelines. *J Am Coll Cardiol.* 2014;63(22):2438–2488.**
2. Cook DJ, Housmans PR, Rehfeldt KH. Valvular heart disease: replacement and repair. In: Kaplan JA, Reich DL, Savino JS, eds. *Kaplan's Cardiac Anesthesia: The Echo Era*, 6th ed. St Louis, MO: Elsevier Saunders; 2011:570–614.
3. Otto CM. Textbook of Clinical Echocardiography. 4th ed. Philadelphia, PA: Elsevier Saunders; 2009:259–325.
4. Galderisi M, de Divitiis O. Risk factor induced cardiovascular remodeling and the effects of angiotensin-converting enzyme inhibitors. *J Cardiovasc Pharmacol.* 2008;51(6):523–531.
5. Roberts WC, Ko JM. Frequency by decades of unicuspid, bicuspid, and tricuspid aortic valves in adults having isolated aortic valve replacement for aortic stenosis, with or without associated aortic regurgitation. *Circulation.* 2005;111(7):920–925.
6. **Baumgartner H, Hung J, Bermejo J, et al. Echocardiographic assessment of valve stenosis: EAE/ASE recommendations for clinical practice. *J Am Soc Echocardiogr.* 2009;22(1):1–23.**
7. **Lindman BR, Clavel MA, Mathieu P, et al. Calcific aortic stenosis. *Nat Rev Dis Primers.* 2016;2:16006.**
8. Otto CM, Bonow RO. Valvular heart disease. In: Bonow RO, Mann DL, Zipes DP, et al., eds. *Braunwald's Heart Disease: A Textbook of Cardiovascular Medicine.* 9th ed. St. Louis, MO: Elsevier, 2011:1468–1530.

9. Maslow A, Casey P, Poppas A, et al. Aortic valve replacement with or without coronary bypass graft surgery: the risk of surgery in patients ≥80 years old. *J Cardiothorac Vasc Anesth.* 2010;24(1):18–24.

10. **Leon MB, Smith CR, Mack M, et al. Transcatheter aortic-valve implantation for aortic stenosis in patients who cannot undergo surgery.** *N Engl J Med.* **2010;363(17):1597–1607.**

11. **Holmes DR Jr, Brennan JM, Rumsfield JS, et al. Clinical outcomes at 1 year following transcatheter aortic valve replacement.** *JAMA.* **2015;313(10):1019–1028.**

12. Kpodonu J. Hybrid cardiovascular suite: the operating room of the future. *J Card Surg.* 2010;25(6):704–709.

13. Kpodonu J, Raney A. The cardiovascular hybrid room: a key component for hybrid interventions and image guided surgery in the emerging specialty of cardiovascular hybrid surgery. *Interact Cardiovasc Thorac Surg.* 2009;9(4):688–692.

14. Singh IM, Shishehbor MH, Christofferson RD, et al. Percutaneous treatment of aortic valve stenosis. *Cleve Clin J Med.* 2008;75(suppl 11);805–812.

15. **Billings FT 4th, Kodali SK, Shanewise JS. Transcatheter aortic valve implantation: anesthetic consideration.** *Anesth Analg.* **2009;108(5):1453–1462.**

16. Heinze H, Sier H, Schafer U, et al. Percutaneous aortic valve replacement: overview and suggestions for anesthetic management. *J Clin Anesth.* 2010;22:373–378.

17. Fraccaro C, Napodano M, Taratini G, et al. Expanding the eligibility for transcatheter aortic valve implantation the trans-subclavian retrograde approach using: the III generation CoreValve revaling system. *JACC Cardiovasc Interv.* 2009;2(9):828–833.

18. Covello RD, Maj G, Landoni G, et al. Anesthetic management of percutaneous aortic valve implantation: focus on challenges encountered and proposed solutions. *J Cardiothor Vasc Anesth.* 2009;23(3):280–285.

19. **Dehedin B, Guinot PG, Ibrahim H, et al. Anesthesia and perioperative management of patients who undergo transfemoral transcatheter aortic valve implantation: an observational study of general versus local/regional anesthesia in 125 consecutive patients.** *J Cardiothorac Vasc Anesth.* **2011;25(6):1036–1043.**

20. Covello RD, Ruggeri L, Landoni G, et al. Transcatheter implantation of an aortic valve: anesthesiological management. *Minerva Anesthesiol.* 2010;76(2):100–108.

21. Chin D. Echocardiography for transcatheter aortic valve replacement. *Eur J Echocardiogr.* 2009;10:21–29.

22. Krishnaswamy A, Tuczu EM, Kapadia SR. Update on transcatheter aortic valve replacement. *Curr Cardiol Rep.* 2010;12(5): 393–403.

23. Abdel-Wahab M, Zahn R, Horack M, et al. Aortic regurgitation after transcatheter aortic valve implantation: incidence and early outcome. Results from the German transcatheter aortic valve interventions registry. *Heart.* 2011;97(11):899–906.

24. **Smith CR, Leon MB, Mack MJ, et al. Transcatheter versus surgical aortic-valve replacement in high-risk patients.** *N Engl J Med.* **2011;364(23):2187–2198.**

25. **Zoghbi WA, Adams D, Bonow RO, et al. Recommendations for noninvasive evaluation of native valvular regurgitation: a report from the American Society of Echocardiography developed in collaboration with the Society for Cardiovascular Magnetic Resonance.** *J Am Soc Echocardiogr.* **2017;30(4):303–371.**

26. Rahimtoola SH. Choice of prosthetic heart valve in adults: an update. *J Am Coll Cardiol.* 2010;55(22):2413–2426.

27. Mahjoub H, Dumesnil JG, Pibarot P. Classification of prosthetic valve types and fluid dynamics. In: Lang RM, Goldstein SA, Kronzon I, et al., eds. *ASE's Comprehensive Echocardiography.* 2nd ed. Philadelphia, PA: Elsevier Saunders; 2016:542–549.

28. **Nishimura RA, Otto CM, Bonow RO, et al. 2017 AHA/ACC focused update of the 2014 AHA/ACC guideline for the management of patients with valvular heart disease.** *J Am Coll Cardiol.* **2017;70(2):252–289.**

12

Anesthetic Management for the Treatment of Mitral and Tricuspid Valvular Heart Disease

Rabia Amir, Yanick Baribeau, and Feroze U. Mahmood

KEY POINTS

1. The increasing utilization of intraoperative transesophageal echocardiography (TEE) has greatly expanded the role of the cardiac anesthesiologist in operations for valve repair and replacement.
2. In patients with mitral stenosis (MS), particular attention should be paid to avoiding any increases in pulmonary artery pressure (PAP) due to inadequate anesthesia or inadvertent acidosis, hypercapnia, or hypoxemia.
3. Bradycardia is harmful in patients with mitral regurgitation (MR), leading to an increase in left ventricular (LV) volume, reduction in forward cardiac output, and an increase in regurgitant fraction (RF). The heart rate should be kept in the normal to elevated range.
4. The severity of MR can be underestimated under the altered loading conditions of general anesthesia. Therefore, it is more appropriate to grade the severity of MR by using the preoperative echocardiographic examination.
5. In patients with tricuspid regurgitation (TR), high airway pressures during pulmonary ventilation and agents that can increase PAP should be avoided. If inotropic support is necessary, dobutamine, isoproterenol, or milrinone, which dilate the pulmonary vasculature, should be used.

I. Introduction

A. Despite the decline in open cardiac surgery volume due to advances in interventional cardiology, valvular heart disease represents 10% to 20% of all cardiac surgical procedures in the United States.

B. Approximately, 2.5% of the population in industrialized countries is affected by valvular heart disease with the likelihood of developing valvular heart disease increasing with age.

C. Valvular heart disease has intraoperative implications in that changes in hemodynamic variables (heart rate and rhythm, preload, afterload, and contractility) should be adequately compensated for physiologic optimization.

D. Intraoperative transesophageal echocardiography (TEE) has expanded the role of the cardiac anesthesiologist during valve repair and replacement surgeries and provides an enhanced physiologic perspective through the dynamic display of anatomy.

E. Additionally, intraoperative TEE provides real-time diagnostic interpretation to guide surgical decision making.

F. Please refer to Chapter 16 for the management of pulmonary valve disease.

II. Stenotic versus regurgitant lesions

A. Valvular stenosis

1. Stenotic lesions are associated with pathology related to pressure overload in the upstream cardiac chamber.

2. The narrowed valvular orifice obstructs blood flow across the valve (during systole in aortic and pulmonary valves; during diastole in mitral and tricuspid valves) resulting in increased proximal pressure buildup. Flow converges as blood reaches the stenotic valve with increased velocity and blood is ejected through the orifice with simultaneous pressure drop and consequent increase in the pressure gradient across the valve.

3. There are two types of valvular obstruction:

   a. Fixed: The degree of obstruction to blood flow is constant throughout the cardiac cycle.

   b. Dynamic: The obstruction is present for only part of the cardiac cycle.

B. Valvular regurgitation

1. Regurgitant lesions cause pathology associated with volume overload that results in chamber dilatation and eccentric hypertrophy.

2. The ventricles initially compensate for the increased volume load with increased stroke volume but eventually function declines and irreversible failure occurs.

3. The hemodynamic management of these patients focuses on maximizing forward stroke volume (FSV) and minimizing regurgitant stroke volume.

III. Structural and functional response to valvular heart disease

A. Cardiac remodeling

1. Cardiac remodeling includes changes in the size, shape, and function of the heart in response to an acute or chronic cardiac injury.

2. Cardiac injury in valvular heart disease is caused by alteration in ventricular loading conditions. The ventricle is subjected to pressure and/or volume overload, leading to cardiac remodeling in the form of ventricular hypertrophy and chamber dilation.

3. Neurohumoral factors and enzymes, such as angiotensin II, ion channels, and oxidative stress, also contribute to cardiac remodeling.

4. Remodeling is initially adaptive but eventually leads to decompensation and deterioration in ventricular function.

5. Ventricular hypertrophy, defined as increased ventricular mass, can be concentric or eccentric.

6. Pressure overload results in concentric ventricular hypertrophy where ventricular mass is increased by myocardial thickening, and ventricular volume stays constant.

7. Conversely, volume overload causes eccentric ventricular hypertrophy where increased ventricular volume raises ventricular mass without changing myocardial wall thickness.

B. Ventricular function

1. Ventricular function is divided into systolic and diastolic functions.

   a. Systolic function

   (1) Represents the ability of the ventricle to contract and eject blood.

   (2) Contractility is the intrinsic ability of the myocardium to contract and generate force, independent of preload and afterload.

   (3) Preload is the stretch placed on myocardium prior to contraction that results from a combination of diastolic volume and filling pressure. It is physiologically expressed as end-diastolic stress.

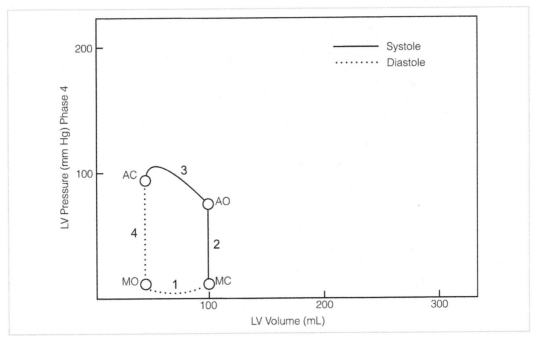

FIGURE 12.1 Normal pressure–volume loop (PV loop). First segment/phase 1 of the PV loop represents diastolic filling of the left ventricle (LV). Phase 2 represents isovolumetric contraction and phase 3 represents ventricular ejection, and both these phases constitute ventricular systole. Phase 4 represents the isovolumetric relaxation of the LV and along with phase 1 constitutes ventricular diastole. AC, aortic valve closure at end systole; MC, mitral valve closure at end diastole; MO, mitral valve opening; AO, aortic valve opening. (Modified from Jackson JM, Thomas SJ, Lowenstein E. Anesthetic management of patients with valvular heart disease. *Semin Anesth.* 1982;1:240.)

      (4) Afterload is the load placed on the myocardium during contraction that occurs from a combination of systolic volume and generated pressure. It is physiologically expressed as end-systolic stress.

  b. Diastolic function

      (1) Represents the ability of the ventricle to accept inflowing blood.

      (2) It consists of a combination of relaxation and compliance.

      (3) Diastolic dysfunction is present when the heart requires higher ventricular filling pressures to maintain normal diastolic ventricular volume.

      (4) Both systolic and diastolic functions require energy and can be compromised by ventricular ischemia.

 C. **Pressure–volume loops (PV loops)**

    PV loops are used to illustrate ventricular function and performance with ventricular pressure plotted on the y axis and the ventricular volume plotted on the x axis for one cardiac cycle (Fig. 12.1). Both stenotic and regurgitant valvular lesions display a characteristic PV loop pattern. Recognizing these patterns can aid in the identification of lesions and helps to understand the altered ventricular physiology and function.

IV. **Valvular heart disease**

 A. **Mitral valve**

  1. Anatomy

    a. The mitral valve apparatus consists of mitral annulus and the suspension network that comprises the leaflets, chordae tendineae and papillary muscles (Fig. 12.2).

    b. The anatomical junction between the left atrium (LA) and left ventricle (LV) is represented by the mitral annulus, which is a three-dimensional (3D), nonplanar,

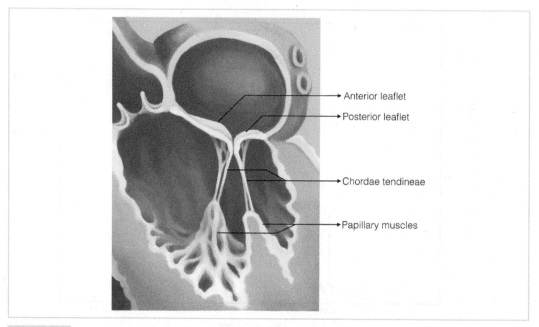

Anterior leaflet

Posterior leaflet

Chordae tendineae

Papillary muscles

FIGURE 12.2 An illustration of the mitral valve apparatus demonstrating the anterior and posterior leaflets along with the suspension network which is comprised of chordae tendineae and papillary muscles.

saddle-shaped, dynamic structure that changes size and shape during the cardiac cycle.

c. The anterior leaflet is attached to one-third of the annulus at its base and the posterior leaflet is attached to the remaining two-thirds. The posterior leaflet is divided by two indentations into three scallops that are named from lateral to medial as P1, P2, and P3, respectively. The anterior leaflet is similarly divided into three segments, A1, A2, and A3, which correspond to the posterior scallops.

d. The leaflets meet at the posteromedial and anterolateral commissures with two groups of papillary muscles situated beneath each commissure. At their free edges, the leaflets are attached to the papillary muscles by the chordae tendineae.

e. The chordae are divided into primary, secondary, and tertiary depending on the location of attachment to the leaflets.

B. Mitral valve stenosis

1. Etiology

a. Mitral stenosis (MS) is the most common valvular sequela of rheumatic heart disease and accounts for approximately 10% of all cases of MS in Europe.

b. Other causes of MS include degenerative (calcific) and congenital MS. However, 99% of surgically excised stenotic mitral valves worldwide are from fibrosis and scarring caused by rheumatic changes [1]. Women are twice as likely to be affected as compared to men.

c. MS has a high mortality rate. Without surgery, 20% of all diagnosed patients are likely to die within 1 year of diagnosis, and 50% die within a decade of being diagnosed with MS.

2. Symptoms

a. Patients with MS from rheumatic heart disease may be asymptomatic for more than two decades after the initial onset of rheumatic fever. Symptoms appear with the development of stenosis over years and initially present during exercise or high cardiac output states.

b. The progression of MS is slow with increasing episodes of fatigue, chest pain, palpitations, shortness of breath, paroxysmal nocturnal dyspnea, pulmonary edema, and hemoptysis, as well as hoarseness due to compression of the left recurrent laryngeal nerve by a distended left atrium (LA) and enlarged pulmonary artery. LA dilatation may also cause dysphagia through esophageal compression.

   c. Stenotic symptoms become more evident with the onset of atrial fibrillation that also increases the risk of LA thrombi and subsequent cerebral or systemic emboli. Chest pain may occur in 10% to 20% of patients with MS but is not a good predictor of coexisting coronary artery disease (CAD), since it may be attributed to other causes such as coronary thromboembolism or pulmonary hypertension.

3. Pathophysiology

   a. Natural progression

      (1) The normal adult mitral valve area (MVA) is 4.0 to 6.0 cm^2 (mitral valve index: 4 to 4.5 cm^2/m^2). The symptoms of MS manifest with progressive decreases in valve area, about 0.1 cm^2 annually. Initially dyspnea may occur with moderate exertion (valve area <2.5 cm^2), along with the LA enlargement and elevated LA volume and pressure that may predispose to atrial fibrillation and increased blood in the pulmonary vasculature. The degree of pulmonary hypertension is a marker of the global hemodynamic consequences of MS, and severe pulmonary hypertension is associated with a reduction in mean survival of <3 years.

      (2) As the valve area further decreases between 1 and 1.5 cm^2, symptoms of MS may be present with mild to moderate exertion. Atrial fibrillation can herald severe congestive heart failure (CHF) via impaired LA contraction that normally contributes up to 30% of LV filling in MS. CHF may also occur secondary to cardiac high-output states with increased cardiac demand that cause rapid elevations of LA and pulmonary artery pressures (PAPs).

      (3) Severe MS with symptoms at rest manifests when valve areas go below 1 cm^2. High LA pressures contribute to increased pulmonary vein resistance and ensuing chronic pulmonary hypertension, right ventricular (RV) dilation, and failure. The dilated, high-pressure RV may also cause left-sided bowing of the interventricular septum, thereby further reducing LV size, limiting stroke volume, impairing cardiac output, and resulting in tricuspid regurgitation (TR) with further dilation.

      (4) The smallest MVA compatible with life is 0.3 to 0.4 cm^2.

   b. Intracardiac hemodynamics and cardiac remodeling

      (1) Significant MS is characterized by a reduced left ventricular end-diastolic volume (LVEDV) and left ventricular end-diastolic pressure (LVEDP) as the blood flow from the LA to the LV is restricted. Reduced filling of the LV decreases stroke volume and LV contractility may also decrease due to chronic LV deconditioning.

   c. Pressure wave disturbances

      (1) In patients with normal sinus rhythm, a large A wave hallmarks MS. If associated MR is present, a pronounced V wave is also seen. The A wave becomes small as LA contractility is impaired as a consequence of severe MS and disappears completely with atrial fibrillation.

      (2) PV loop in MS (Fig. 12.3). Stroke volume is reduced due to decreased LV filling pressures and low end-diastolic and end-systolic volumes.

4. Imaging approach

   a. TTE is most commonly used to demonstrate mitral valve morphology and grade the severity of MS. However, several acquired and congenital abnormalities of the mitral valve are treated with surgery, and TEE is uniquely suited to view the mitral valve intraoperatively due to its location. It is routinely used for preoperative assessment that involves the identification of the mechanism, extent, and severity of lesions affecting the mitral valve, as well as for the determination of postoperative success.

   b. In recent years, 3D echocardiography has opened another dimension of imaging by allowing fast acquisition of images, enhanced visualization of the valvular anatomy, and improved diagnosis of the mechanism of various pathologies. In particular, leaflet pathology is better appreciated with real-time 3D TEE.

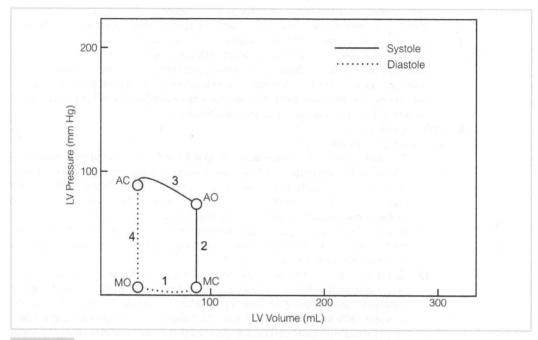

FIGURE 12.3 Pressure–volume loop (PV loop) in mitral stenosis (MS). Due to the reduction in end-diastolic and end-systolic volumes and LV filling pressure, the stroke volume is decreased in MS. AO, aortic valve opening; MC, mitral valve closure; MO, mitral valve opening; AC, aortic valve closure. Phase 1, ventricular filling; phase 2, isovolumetric contraction; phase 3, ventricular ejection; phase 4, isovolumetric relaxation. (Modified from Jackson JM, Thomas SJ, Lowenstein E. Anesthetic management of patients with valvular heart disease. *Semin Anesth.* 1982;1:244.)

    c. A stress test may be used when there is a discrepancy between symptoms and resting Doppler echocardiographic findings.

        (1) TEE findings: Traditionally, the mitral valve is examined with the midesophageal (ME) four-chamber, ME mitral commissural, ME long-axis (LAX), and transgastric (TG) basal short-axis (SAX) views, with and without color flow Doppler (CFD) (Fig. 12.4). Patients with MS secondary to rheumatic fever have distinct

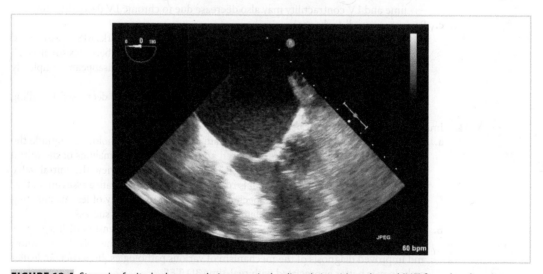

FIGURE 12.4 Stenosis of mitral valve seen during ventricular diastole in midesophageal (ME) four-chamber view.

TABLE 12.1 Echocardiographic grouping follows the echocardiographic and fluoroscopic (calcification) evaluation of the following characteristics: valve mobility, fusion of the subvalvular apparatus, and the amount of leaflet calcification

	Group 1	Group 2	Group 3
Mitral valve anatomy	Pliable, noncalcified anterior mitral anatomy leaflet and mild subvalvular disease (thin chordae ≥10 mm long)	Pliable, noncalcified anterior mitral leaflet and severe subvalvular disease (thickened chordae <10 mm long)	Calcification of mitral valve of any extent, as assessed by fluoroscopy, no matter the state of the subvalvular apparatus

echocardiographic features such as progressive leaflet thickening, calcification, and limited mobility due to chordal and/or commissural fusion. Restricted motion of the anterior mitral valve leaflet in diastole presents as "doming" and is described as a "hockey-stick" appearance. The posterior leaflet may also be identified as immobile with echocardiography (Video 12.1). LA enlargement with spontaneous echo contrast is associated with a low-flow state and should prompt exclusion of thrombi, especially in the LA appendage. MR may also be present and can be qualitatively and quantitatively assessed using TEE.

(2) Assessment of morphologic features with two-dimensional (2D) echocardiography such as leaflet thickness, leaflet mobility and flexibility, leaflet calcification, and commissural and subvalvular fusion can be used for different scoring systems, including the commonly used Wilkins score where each feature is graded on a scale of 1 to 4, yielding a maximal score of 16 [2].

(3) Echocardiographic grouping (Table 12.1) [3] follows the echocardiographic and fluoroscopic (calcification) evaluation of the following characteristics: valve mobility, fusion of the subvalvular apparatus, and the amount of leaflet calcification.

(4) These scores are used to grade mitral valve pathology, determine suitability for treatment options such as percutaneous mitral balloon valvuloplasty, and predict successful repair [4].

5. Assessment of severity
   a. The severity of MS should not be described by a single value but should be evaluated using a multimodality approach that establishes pulmonary pressures, valve areas, and mean Doppler gradients (Table 12.2). These can be calculated using echocardiography and, sometimes, cardiac catheterization to measure the MVA or a diastolic pressure gradient across the mitral valve. The different methods for grading MS severity are summarized in Table 12.2.
   b. Routine assessment of the severity of MS involves the combination of mean gradient using the pressure half-time (PHT) method and planimetry, respectively. However, the mean gradient and systolic PAP cannot be considered as surrogate markers of the severity of MS as they are largely supportive signs.
   c. The most commonly used method is the PHT method, utilizing continuous wave Doppler where prolongation of the PHT corresponds to a decrease in mitral valve orifice area. A normal PHT is relatively short and correlates to the rapid early diastolic filling of the LV and the associated rapid fall in the LA-to-LV pressure gradient during this early filling phase. Since the LA-to-LV pressure gradient is increased for a longer period in MS, the PHT will become more prolonged as the degree of stenosis worsens.
   d. Planimetry involves the direct tracing of the elliptical mitral valve orifice area during mid-diastole utilizing the lowest gain setting to visualize the entire orifice area. The smallest orifice area is determined by scanning the LV from the apex to the base. Two-dimensional parasternal SAX view is routinely used and can be augmented with 3D echo to orient the positioning of the measurement plane.
   e. The continuity equation uses the principle of the conservation of mass but requires a series of measurements that increase the impact of errors of measurements. It is difficult

TABLE 12.2 Quantification of severity of MS

Method	Mild MS	Moderate MS	Severe MS	Limitations
Pressure Half-Time	>1.5 cm²	1–1.5 cm²	<1 cm²	Aortic regurgitation, atrial septal defect, previous surgical/percutaneous mitral valvuloplasty, net LA/LV compliance
Planimetry (in cm²): Tracing the inner edge of the mitral valve orifice in mid-diastole				Underestimation due to high gain
Continuity equation (in cm²) $\pi(D^2/4)$ (VTI aorta [cm]/ VTI mitral [cm])				Limited accuracy and reproducibility, atrial fibrillation, aortic/mitral regurgitation
PISA (in cm²) $MVA = \pi(r^2)(V_{aliasing})/$ peak $V_{mitral} \cdot \alpha/180°$				Technically difficult
Mean pressure gradient across the mitral valve (in mm Hg): Tracing of the Doppler diastolic mitral flow profile	<5	5–10	>10	Dependent on transmitral flow and heart rate
Systolic PAP = TR gradient + RAP, (in mm Hg)	<30	30–50	>50	Underestimation due to misalignment, inaccurate assessment of RAP

Adapted from Bonow RO, Carabello BA, Chatterjee K, et al. 2008 Focused update incorporated into the ACC/AHA 2006 guidelines for the management of patients with valvular heart disease: a report of the American College of Cardiology/American Heart Association Task Force on Practice Guidelines (Writing Committee to Revise the 1998 Guidelines for the Management of Patients With Valvular Heart Disease): endorsed by the Society of Cardiovascular Anesthesiologists, Society for Cardiovascular Angiography and Interventions, and Society of Thoracic Surgeons. *Circulation.* 2008;118(15):e523–e661. LA, left atrium; LV, left ventricle; MR, mitral regurgitation; MS, mitral stenosis; TR, tricuspid regurgitation; PHT, pressure half-time; PAP, pulmonary artery pressure; RAP, right atrial pressure; V, velocity; VTI, velocity time integral; MVA, mitral valve area; PISA, proximal isovelocity surface area.

to use for MS severity since it cannot be used in the presence of atrial fibrillation or significant mitral or aortic regurgitation.

   f. The proximal isovelocity surface area (PISA) method allows the estimation of mitral volume flow by dividing mitral volume flow by the maximum velocity of diastolic mitral flow as assessed by Continuous Wave Doppler interrogation (CWD). While it is technically demanding, it is independent of flow conditions and can be used in the presence of significant regurgitation.

   g. The pressure gradient is dependent on transmitral flow and heart rate and, therefore, may be a less accurate method to evaluate MS severity.

6. Timing and type of intervention

   a. Since irreversible ventricular dysfunction may occur, early surgical intervention is recommended; however, surgery is only recommended for those patients demonstrating symptoms of MS.

   b. For those with mild to moderate MS (MVA 1–1.5 cm²), conservative management with regular clinical and echocardiographic examinations every 2 years is recommended. Patients with severe MS (MVA <1.0 cm²) who are asymptomatic can be assessed annually.

   c. The decision to proceed with surgery depends on the individual and their unique situation, taking into account preoperative risk factors, the mitral valve orifice size, indicators of systemic embolization, the presence and severity of pulmonary hypertension, as well as the lifestyle desired.

   d. Once the systolic PAP surpasses 30 mm Hg, surgical intervention will likely be needed [4]. The four treatment options for rheumatic MS are:

      (1) Mitral valve replacement

      (2) Open mitral commissurotomy

      (3) Closed commissurotomy

      (4) Balloon mitral valvuloplasty

  e. Closed mitral commissurotomy can only be performed for patients without atrial thrombosis, significant valvular calcification, or chordal fusion. It can be performed without cardiopulmonary bypass (CPB); however, this procedure is rarely done in the United States and has been replaced by mitral balloon valvuloplasty as the treatment of choice for rheumatic MS.

  f. Balloon mitral valvuloplasty is a percutaneous interventional procedure routinely performed in the cardiac catheterization laboratory under general anesthesia or conscious sedation. It involves the gradual progression of a balloon catheter through the inter-atrial septum that is inflated at the mitral orifice to split and open fused commissures, increasing MVA. TEE is used in addition to fluoroscopy to guide the catheter and assess possible thrombi formation.

  g. Contraindications to balloon mitral valvuloplasty in addition to CAD that requires coronary artery bypass grafting (CABG) and concomitant severe valvular diseases include MVA >1.5 cm^2, moderate or severe MR, severe calcification, evidence of LA thrombi, and lack of commissural fusion. It is relatively contraindicated in MS not due to commissural fusion [5,6].

  h. Immediate good results are noted in the majority of patients with the MVA enlarging to an average of 1.9 to 2.0 cm^2, after balloon mitral valvuloplasty.

  i. Severe MR, lasting atrial septal defect, and systemic embolism may occur as possible complications of the procedure.

  j. Both commissurotomy and balloon mitral valvuloplasty lower the severity of stenosis, delaying surgical intervention that is eventually required to relieve the stenosis. While anticoagulation is rarely required in this time period and morbidity is lower when compared to an indwelling prosthetic valve, these procedures still carry a significant risk of restenosis.

  k. Mitral valve replacement is required if commissurotomy or balloon mitral valvulo-plasty cannot be performed. In the presence of chronic atrial fibrillation, the maze procedure or the creation of fibrous scar tissue to disrupt atrial reentry pathways in the LA can also be performed during surgical intervention.

7. Goals of perioperative management

  a. Hemodynamic management

    (1) LV preload

      (a) Given the elevated LA pressures and pulmonary vascular congestion of MS, TEE is the ideal modality used to monitor volume status intraoperatively and is preferred over more invasive techniques such as pulmonary artery cath-eters. Adequate preload is necessary to facilitate forward flow across the ste-notic valve. Aggressive fluid loading can exacerbate pre-existing CHF into florid pulmonary edema.

    (2) Heart rate

      (a) While in theory bradycardia assists hemodynamic stability in MS, stroke volume generally cannot match excessively low heart rates. Atrioventricular pacing may be challenging, and a long PR interval of 0.15 to 0.2 msec will pre-vent declines in diastolic flow that could decrease cardiac output. Induction of tachycardia should be avoided.

    (3) Contractility

      (a) End-stage MS may be marked by severe CHF due to LV deconditioning. Atrial filling may also be limited by RV contractility. Both these factors can lower cardiac output, which may be hazardous during surgery. Inotropic support is encouraged prior to initiation and completion of CPB.

    (4) Systemic vascular resistance

      (a) Decreased cardiac outputs in patients with MS result in elevated systemic vas-cular resistance. Afterload reduction in these patients does not improve the forward flow, and it is critical to maintain afterload in the normal range.

(5) Pulmonary vascular resistance (PVR)
  (a) Pulmonary vasoconstriction develops rapidly in these patients in the setting of hypoxia, inadequate anesthesia, hypercapnia, or acidosis due to pre-existing elevated PVR.
b. Anesthetic technique
  (1) Premedicate with caution in these patients to avoid sudden decreases in preload or exacerbation of pre-existing pulmonary hypertension via a slow respiratory drive and concomitant hypoxia and hypercapnia. In the onset of new atrial fibrillation, cardioversion is suggested.
  (2) Proceed cautiously while inserting pulmonary artery catheters for perioperative management in these patients due to the risk of pulmonary artery rupture. Note that wedge pressures are often inaccurate and do not reflect LVEDP. Also monitor PAPs carefully as they may rise suddenly due to causes stated above.

> **CLINICAL PEARL** With severe MS, pulmonary capillary wedge pressure is usually elevated, yet LVEDP is reduced.

  (3) Mitral valve repair can be assessed using TEE. Complications following mitral valve repair such as paravalvular leaks and systolic anterior motion of mitral valve can be recognized early while simultaneously evaluating ventricular function.
  (4) CPB can depress myocardial contractility, including those with normal preoperative LV function. Therefore, fluids should be initiated with care to prevent ventricular failure. Cardiac output can be maintained by using inotropes, vasopressors, and by amiodarone prophylaxis in patients with chronic atrial fibrillation.
c. Postoperative course
  (1) A successful postoperative surgical course is evident as early as postoperative day 1 by a robust cardiac output accompanied by reduced pulmonary arterial and LA pressures as well as reduced PVR. While a mean pressure gradient of 4 to 7 mm Hg usually persists after prosthetic valve replacement, PVR in most patients continues to decrease. Failure of the PAP to decrease is usually a sign of irreversible pulmonary hypertension and/or irreversible LV dysfunction, which are indicators of poor prognosis.

C. **Mitral valve regurgitation**
  1. Natural history
     The spectrum of MR varies from acute forms, in which rapid deterioration of myocardial function can occur, to chronic forms that have slow indolent courses. MR may result from mitral valve leaflet abnormalities, mitral annulus dilation, chordae rupture, papillary muscle disorder, global LV dysfunction, or disproportionate LV enlargement.
  a. Acute MR
     (1) Acute MR may result from papillary muscle dysfunction due to myocardial ischemia or papillary muscle rupture due to myocardial infarction or blunt chest trauma. Chordae tendineae rupture can be caused by myxomatous disease of the mitral valve or acute rheumatic fever. A mitral valve leaflet can acutely deteriorate as a result of infective endocarditis, balloon valvuloplasty, or a penetrating chest injury.
  b. Chronic MR
     (1) *Mitral annulus dilatation* may result from LV dilatation due to dilated or ischemic cardiomyopathy or aortic insufficiency. It can also develop from LA enlargement in patients with diastolic dysfunction, for example, AS or systemic hypertension. Finally, mitral annulus dilatation will eventually exacerbate MR of any other cause secondary to LA and LV enlargement and stretching of the annulus.
     (2) *Disorders of the mitral leaflets* include mitral valve prolapse that may be idiopathic or caused by rheumatic fever or myxomatous degeneration, mitral leaflet damage

TABLE 12.3   Classification scheme used to describe differing mechanisms of mitral regurgitation (MR) based upon the leaflet motion of the valve

Carpentier's classification	Mitral valve motion	Common causes
I	Normal	• Mitral annulus dilatation • Leaflet destruction (endocarditis) • Leaflet perforation or cleft
II	Excessive	• Leaflet prolapse • Flail leaflet
IIIa	Restricted during diastole and systole	• Rheumatic valve disease
IIIb	Restricted during systole only	• Functional MR • Ischemic MR

by infective endocarditis, and restrictive changes due to thickening or calcification from any inflammatory or degenerative process. Restriction can also be caused by disproportionate enlargement of the LV in relation to papillary muscles and chordae tendineae causing incomplete mitral valve closure. This occurs in a majority of cases of ischemic MR.

(3) *Disorders of the subvalvular apparatus.* Rupture or elongation of chordae tendineae may occur in myxomatous degeneration. Rheumatic heart disease may lead to chordae tendineae rupture, thickening, and calcium deposition in the subvalvular apparatus. Depending on the type and number of chordae ruptured, subsequent MR may range from acute to chronic and from mild to severe.

(4) *Functional MR.* MR that occurs in the setting of normal leaflets and chordal structures is frequently due to functional MR. This phenomenon is not fully understood but is most likely the result of global LV dysfunction, which results in disruption of the normal geometric relationship between the mitral valve leaflets, papillary muscles, and LV. The LV dysfunction results in ventricular and annular dilatation and a more spherical appearance of the LV, which ultimately disrupts the normal structure and function of the entire mitral apparatus. Ischemic MR is a type of functional MR that is caused by ischemic heart disease.

c. Carpentier's classification

(1) This widely recognized classification scheme is used to describe differing mechanisms of MR based upon the leaflet motion of the valve (Table 12.3) [7].

2. Pathophysiology

a. Natural progression

(1) Acute

(a) Acute MR often presents as biventricular failure. With the loss of normal LA compliance, rapid rises in LA and PAP lead to pulmonary congestion, pulmonary edema, and right heart failure. Heart rate is also increased in an effort to maintain cardiac output but prevents complete emptying of the LV, raising LV volume and end-diastolic pressure that cause ischemia and further exacerbate LV dysfunction.

(2) Chronic

(a) LA dilatation and eccentric hypertrophy mark the gradual development of chronic MR. Primarily, LV dilation maintains an adequate LVEDP despite increased volume and preserves forward cardiac output by an overall increase in the FSV. However, once LV dilatation and hypertrophy can no longer meet the necessary FSV to maintain cardiac output, LV dysfunction ensues and symptoms of heart failure manifest. LA dilatation also causes widening of the mitral annulus, thereby worsening regurgitation and contributing to elevated PAPs, pulmonary congestion, and ultimately, RV dysfunction and failure. It also results in the development of atrial fibrillation and increases the risk of thrombosis.

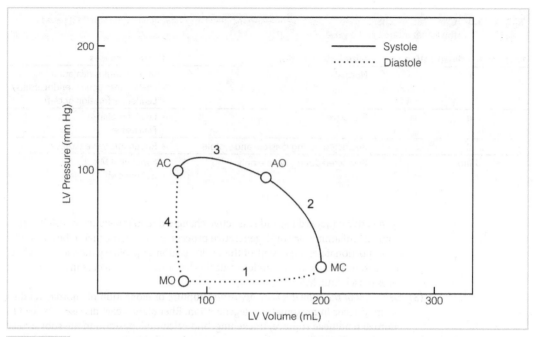

FIGURE 12.5 Pressure–volume loop (PV loop) in acute and chronic mitral regurgitation (MR). In chronic MR, there is an increase in end-diastolic volume without significant increase in LV filling pressures. Whereas in acute MR, the increase in end-diastolic volume is associated with an increase in LV filling pressure. AO, aortic valve opening; MC, mitral valve closure; MO, mitral valve opening; AC, aortic valve closure. Phase 1, ventricular filling; phase 2, isovolumetric contraction; phase 3, ventricular ejection; phase 4, isovolumetric relaxation. (Modified from Jackson JM, Thomas SJ, Lowenstein E. Anesthetic management of patients with valvular heart disease. *Semin Anesth.* 1982;1:248.)

   b. Intracardiac hemodynamics and cardiac remodeling
       (1) In acute MR, maintaining the stroke volume requires dilation of the LA. This is accomplished by an increase in the LVEDP. In contrast, in chronic MR, the LVEDP remains normal until the MR has progressed to a severe stage.
   c. Pressure wave disturbances
       (1) The compliance of the LA, the compliance of the pulmonary vasculature, the amount of pulmonary venous return, and the regurgitant volume, all collectively determine the size of the regurgitant wave ("giant V wave") on pulmonary capillary wedge tracing. V waves develop in patients with acute MR that are absent in patients with chronic disease due to increased atrial compliance. A PV loop characteristic for MR is illustrated in Figure 12.5.
   d. TEE
       (1) The baseline TEE examination should focus on the underlying pathology, while a more thorough examination should focus on the structure and function of the valvular apparatus involved as well as the LV function (Figs. 12.6 and 12.7). The first assessment is necessary for initial surgical decision making. Once it is decided that mitral repair will occur, the TEE examination should focus on identifying any predictors of postrepair systolic anterior motion (SAM), a noted complication of this procedure that can cause critical postoperative hemodynamic instability. Several factors can predispose patients to SAM, such as the presence of a myxomatous mitral valve with redundant leaflets, especially excessive anterior leaflet tissue in a nondilated, hyperdynamic LV. After repair, decreased distance between the mitral valve coaptation point and the ventricular septum (C-sept distance) can also result in SAM [8].

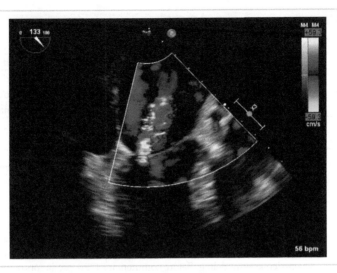

FIGURE 12.6 TEE with color flow Doppler (CFD) interrogation demonstrates regurgitation of mitral valve during ventricular systole.

CLINICAL PEARL The severity of MR is often underestimated under the altered loading conditions of general anesthesia, and so it is more appropriate to grade the severity of MR using the preoperative echo examination.

3. Assessment of severity
   a. Echocardiography has completely replaced the angiocardiographic dye clearance as the preferred method to assess MR severity.
   b. Echocardiographic assessment of MR (Table 12.4)
   c. Quantitative assessment of MR
      (1) The intraoperative approach to MR begins with quantification of the regurgitation with PISA or jet area followed by identification of the mechanism of the lesion based on Carpentier's classification [9].

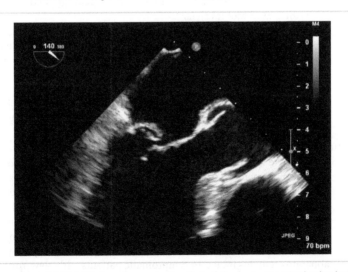

FIGURE 12.7 Midesophageal (ME) LAX view demonstrating flail of the posterior mitral valve leaflet in severe mitral regurgitation (MR). Also see Video 12.2.

TABLE 12.4 Echocardiographic assessment of MR

	Mild	Moderate	Severe
LA size	Normal	Normal or dilated	Usually dilated
LV size	Normal	Normal or dilated	Usually dilated
Morphology of valve	Normal/abnormal	Normal/abnormal	Flail valve, papillary muscle rupture
Jet area	Small	Intermediate	Large or eccentric wall impinging
Vena contracta	<3 mm	—	≥7 mm
PISA	None or small	Intermediate	Large
EROA	>20 mm^2	20–29 mm^2, 30–39 mm^2	40 mm^2
Regurgitant volume	>30 mL	30–39 mL, 40–59 mL	>60 mL

LV, left ventricular; LA, left atrial; MR, mitral regurgitation; PISA, proximal isovelocity surface area; EROA, effective regurgitant orifice area.

(2) The next step involves geometric quantification with determination of annular dimensions, length of the leaflets, ventricular dimensions, and indices of annular leaflet and ventricular remodeling. Before commencing CPB, predictors of repair failure should be analyzed such as mitral annular calcification, severity of annular dilatation, and susceptibility to systolic anterior motion. Once the patient has been separated from CPB, a postrepair evaluation of surgical success is conducted by excluding stenosis with planimetry and PHT and excluding moderate or greater regurgitation [9].

(3) The most conventional methods of MR severity assessment utilize 2D TEE with CFD (Video 12.3). While it is mostly used for diagnosis of MR and not MR quantification, the general assumption remains that the larger the jet area, the more severe the MR. However, this is influenced by technical factors, loading conditions, and jet eccentricity.

(4) The vena contracta is the narrowest point of the area of the jet as it leaves the regurgitant orifice. It is measured with an adapted Nyquist limit for optimal visualization and can be used to grade MR. Vena contracta width of 3 mm indicates mild MR and ≥7 mm is quantified as severe [8]. Its utility is limited, however, since it cannot accurately discriminate mild from moderate or moderate from severe MR. A second method is required if intermediate values are found. Other limitations of this method include the assumption that the regurgitant orifice is circular; its value is unclear in multiple jets.

(5) Flow convergence is the recommended method of quantifying MR, when possible. The Nyquist limit is reduced for PISA visualization and the radius is measured at mid-systole. From this, regurgitant volume and effective regurgitant orifice area (EROA) can be obtained. With these values, MR can be graded into mild, moderate, or severe. It is also possible to make subclassifications of mild to moderate or moderate to severe. This method is especially useful for eccentric jets but also relies on geometrical assumptions of the orifice form. It is influenced by hemodynamics and not valid for multiple jets.

4. Surgical intervention

a. Mitral valve repair is the recommended surgical intervention for MR before mitral valve replacement is attempted. Mitral valve repair is advantageous in that both chronic anticoagulation (with mechanical valves) and future reoperation for prosthetic valve failure (with bioprosthetic valves) are avoided. Most importantly, LV function is better preserved after mitral valve repair. Disruption of the mitral valve apparatus interferes with LV function, leading to LV dysfunction. This situation may arise from a mitral valve replacement and can be avoided by a mitral repair since the apparatus remains intact. In symptomatic patients with New York Heart Association (NYHA) class II heart failure and/or chronic or recurrent atrial fibrillation resulting from MR, surgical intervention is strongly endorsed. In asymptomatic patients, the decision to wait or go ahead for surgery depends on the presence of LV enlargement, dysfunction, and pulmonary hypertension, with the onset of LV dysfunction being the most important indicator for surgery in these patients. A stress echo can be done to search for latent LV dysfunction. If chances of repair are good, early surgery is recommended because good long-term results are likely and anticoagulation is not needed. If CABG is indicated and at least moderate ischemic MR is present, mitral valve repair/replacement at the same time as CABG is beneficial. In this scenario, successful mitral valve repair is often straightforward, requiring only placement of an annuloplasty ring.

b. The MitraClip transcatheter mitral valve repair procedure reduces MR severity and symptoms in patients not suitable for surgery.

c. Suitability for repair

(1) Generally, easily reparable mitral valve lesions include leaflet perforation, mitral valve annulus dilatation, and excessive motion of mitral valve leaflets. Conditions more difficult to repair include restricted leaflet motion, severe calcification, and active infection. The greatest success for mitral valve repairs involves isolated lesions of the posterior mitral valve leaflet.

(2) Three-dimensional echocardiography allows the generation of dynamic LA en face surgical views to help in the diagnosis of MR. A similar LV en face view can be obtained simultaneously among other views. These views aid in establishing Carpentier's classification of MR prior to the initiation of CPB intraoperatively. Accurate diagnosis of valve pathology is provided with display of mitral valve apparatus in CFD. The determination of the etiology of degenerative MR can be accomplished via parameters of mitral valve geometry from real-time 3D echocardiographic images, particularly using the billowing height and volume [9].

(3) *Degenerative MR.* About 70% of the cases of MR result from degenerative valve disease; these valves are considered the most apt for repair. However, the decision to repair a regurgitant mitral valve surgically depends on a number of clinical and echocardiographic factors. Degenerative MR with multiple (≥3) scallop involvement in both leaflets, severe mitral annular calcification especially anteriorly, presence of a large central regurgitant jet, and severe dilatation of the mitral valve (>5 cm) suggest unsuitability for repair. On the other hand, relatively longer posterior and chordal lengths and younger age are encouraging predictors for mitral valve repair surgery [9]. In patients with large valve perforation who have previously suffered from infective endocarditis and in patients with rheumatic valve disease, lack of valve tissue is also a significant predictor of unsuccessful repair.

(4) *Ischemic functional MR.* Significant MR can occur in the presence of normal-appearing mitral valve apparatus due to commissural involvement and posterior leaflet clefts and grooves that appear as >50% and <50% indentations, respectively. Three-dimensional TEE can differentiate these findings from ischemic tethering, further clarifying the etiology of MR. Tethering eventually causes widening of the size of the regurgitant orifice, shifting the coaptation point below the plane of the mitral annulus, resulting in a tented appearance of the valve. Malcoaptation of the leaflets and interscallop regions causes MR, and the degree of tethering can be used as a surrogate marker for the chronicity and significance of MR. During a standard 2D TEE, the distance between the plane of the mitral annulus and the coaptation point during systole is measured in the ME 4-Ch or ME LAX view and is called the tenting height. The tenting height is directly related to MR and a tenting height >0.6 cm is considered abnormal [9]. Three-dimensional echocardiography provides other tenting indices like mitral valve tenting area that is a strong marker for MR severity in ischemic cardiomyopathy patients and tenting volume that correlates well with functional MR caused by dilated cardiomyopathy.

(5) Around half of the patients with ischemic functional MR undergoing repair face the probability of repair failure if they have the following features on intraoperative

TEE: systolic tenting area ≥1.6 cm², severe functional ischemic MR, and mitral diastolic annulus diameter of 37 mm [8]. Preoperative TTE can also point to certain indicators of unsuccessful repair. These include systolic tenting area >2.5 cm², a higher posterior leaflet restriction with a posterior leaflet angle >45 degrees, and coaptation distance >1 cm. A large central jet, multiple central and posteromedial complex jets, and severe LV dilatation also decrease the likelihood of successful MR repair.

5. Goals of perioperative management
   a. Hemodynamic management
      (1) LV preload

CLINICAL PEARL In patients with MR, preload augmentation and maintenance is patient specific and can be accurately determined by evaluating the patient's clinical and hemodynamic response to a fluid load.

(a) Preload augmentation and maintenance is largely patient specific and can be effectively gauged by assessing the patient's clinical and hemodynamic response to a fluid load. However, it is routinely useful in determining appropriate FSV.

(2) Heart rate
   (a) Atrial fibrillation is increasingly common in patients receiving surgical intervention for MR, particularly in those with chronic disease. Low heart rates can be extremely deleterious in this population due to consequent LV volume increase and cardiac output reduction.

(3) Contractility
   (a) The eccentric hypertrophy of MR principally affects the FSV. Clinical deterioration follows LV dysfunction secondary to loss of myocardial contractility. Inotropic agents therefore play a key role in management by augmenting forward flow and diminishing regurgitation via mitral annular contraction.

(4) Systemic vascular resistance
   (a) Afterload reduction is desired since increased afterload leads to an increase in regurgitant fraction (RF) and consequently a reduction in systemic cardiac output.

CLINICAL PEARL PVR is increased in patients with severe MR elevating pulmonary pressure and raising LA pressure.

---

(5) Pulmonary vascular resistance (PVR)
   (a) The importance of each component in elevating PAP can be determined by calculating PVR using the following formula:

$$PVR = 80 \times (\text{mean PAP} - \text{PCWP})/CO$$

PVR = pulmonary vascular resistance
80 = the conversion factor to dynes · sec/cm⁵
PAP = pulmonary artery pressure
PCWP = pulmonary capillary wedge pressure
CO = cardiac output

Avoid situations that may lead to pulmonary constriction such hypercapnia, hypoxia, nitrous oxide, and inadequate anesthesia in patients with high PVR.

b. Anesthetic technique
   (1) Premedication
      (a) Light medication is usually adequate.

(2) Induction and maintenance of general anesthesia.

    (a) The hemodynamic goals for induction and maintenance of anesthesia center around maintaining a heart rate of 90 beats/min by preserving ventricular contractility and controlling systemic vascular resistance. Cautious use of volatile anesthetics, narcotics, and anxiolytics usually involves titration. Pulmonary edema as a consequence of rapid rises in PAP can sometimes occur in intubated patients who have not been appropriately anesthetized.

(3) Pulmonary artery catheters

    (a) Rapid increases in PAPs can occur subsequent to LV dysfunction or pulmonary vasoconstriction. This ventricular dysfunction may be precipitated by ischemia or vasoconstriction secondary to inadequate anesthesia. Pulmonary artery catheters in addition to regulating fluid therapy can also be invaluable in the timely detection and management of these sudden elevations.

    (b) This reversible pulmonary hypertension adequately responds to both nitric oxide as well as hyperventilation with minimal increase in intrathoracic pressures while preserving systemic pressures. Alternatives include inhaled milrinone and prostaglandin E1.

(4) TEE

    (a) Post bypass, TEE is invaluable for the assessment of the adequacy of valvular repair and allows communication with the surgical team to address any significant complications such as paravalvular leaks or significant residual regurgitation.

    (b) Assessment of the mitral valve after repair involves critical decision making and is time sensitive. It is performed immediately post procedure to exclude left ventricular outflow tract obstruction (LVOT) caused by SAM of redundant leaflets or significant regurgitation or stenosis. The echocardiographic principles for postrepair evaluation are the same for both prosthetic and native valves and include multiple ME and TG views of the repaired mitral valve to ensure normal function.

    (c) Successfully repaired mitral valves when judged by the criteria used for native valves should have no more than mild MR immediately after separation from CPB. The most frequent method used for visual quantification of MR in the immediate post-CPB period is jet with CFD. Immediate success of repair is shown by lack of significant stenosis or regurgitation on CFD that also shows instantaneous adequacy of the valve. Other methods of quantification such as EROA or vena contracta are challenging and time consuming due to change in the mitral valve anatomy after repair. Three-dimensional echocardiography further strengthens the accuracy of quantitative evaluations and gives evidence for long-term durability of the valve by providing information on structural integrity.

    (d) Normal leaflet motion and structural stability of the prosthetic device are shown through LA and LV en face views of the mitral valve. The ME LAX view also helps exclude and document the extent of SAM if present. The echocardiographic investigation of SAM consists of 2D confirmation of anterior leaflet motion and LVOT velocity of >2 m/sec, CFD evidence of turbulence with an anteriorly directed eccentric MR jet in LVOT, and early closure of the aortic valve in M-mode. Three-dimensional imaging can further provide conclusive proof of complete or partial LVOT obstruction by SAM over the LVOT in more complex cases.

    (e) Reduction in the MVA occurs after mitral valve repair with annuloplasty. LA/LV compliance and hemodynamic stability fluctuate in the immediate post-CPB period. Thus, the role of the PHT method to calculate MVA after repair is controversial. After a complete physical and CFD examination of the repaired mitral valve is done, MVA should be calculated by Doppler assessment of transvalvular flow. Three-dimensional planimetry accounts for the nonplanar shape of the mitral annulus and has shown promise in tracing out the mitral valve orifice. However, all of these methods have certain limitations and must be interpreted contextually with the given clinical circumstances such as PHT with LVEDV and gradients with cardiac output (transvalvular flow).

   (5) Weaning from CPB

      (a) Postoperatively, LV function is compromised more severely in patients who have received mitral valve replacements due to extensive resection of the subvalvular apparatus. These patients therefore require robust inotropic support compared to their counterparts who have received mitral valve repairs. Post-bypass inotrope use is also determined by several factors including LV ejection fraction, degree of regurgitation, aortic cross-clamp time, and presence of pulmonary hypertension. Rarely intra-aortic balloon pumps may be required to maintain LV structure and function. Prophylactic treatment with amiodarone may ensure maintenance of sinus rhythm and is also commonly used if a maze procedure was performed concurrently.

  c. Postoperative course

    (1) Cardiac output remains dependent on high LA pressures in patients with established MR, despite lowering of PAPs and LA pressure following surgical intervention.

D. Mitral stenosis (MS) and mitral regurgitation (MR)

  1. Rheumatic MS most commonly coexists with MR.

  2. The predominant lesion determines which hemodynamic considerations must be used for decision making in patients with combined MS and MR.

  3. Optimal stabilization requires normalization of afterload, heart rate and contractility, maintenance of adequate preload, and avoidance of agents or conditions that lead to pulmonary constriction.

  4. Patients with multivalve disease are always a higher-risk group than those patients with single-valve lesions.

E. Tricuspid valve stenosis

  1. Natural history

    a. Etiology

      (1) Tricuspid stenosis can be congenital, carcinoid, or most commonly caused by rheumatic valvulitis. Rheumatic tricuspid stenosis is rare and regularly associated with concomitant TR as it almost never exists in isolation. The mitral valve is involved in most cases. Endocardial fibroelastosis, right atrial tumor, systemic lupus erythematosus, and carcinoid syndrome are other causes for tricuspid stenosis.

    b. Symptoms

      (1) Tricuspid stenosis is apparent in the signs and symptoms of right-sided heart failure, which includes peripheral edema, hepatic dysfunction, ascites, hepatomegaly, and jugular venous distention.

  2. Pathophysiology

    a. Natural progression

      (1) Composed of three leaflets (anterior, posterior, and septal), the tricuspid valve is the largest cardiac valve with a normal area of 7 to 9 cm^2 in the typical adult. The normal gradient across the tricuspid valve is only 1 mm Hg. By the time the valve opening decreases to less than 1.5 cm^2, the tricuspid valve has endured significant degradation and severely impaired forward blood flow. As a result, as the stenosis develops, there is a long asymptomatic period. A mean gradient of 3 mm Hg across the tricuspid valve typically correlates to a valve area of 1.5 cm^2. The right atrial pressure (RAP) increases, right atrium dilates, and forward blood flow decreases during progression of the stenosis.

    b. Calculation of severity

      (1) Cardiac catheterization and echocardiography can be used to grade the severity of tricuspid stenosis by calculating orifice area and pressure gradient. A severe

stenosis is indicated in a gradient of 5 mm Hg across the tricuspid valve and tricuspid valve area of 1 cm^2.

    c. TEE

        (1) Patients with rheumatic tricuspid stenosis will demonstrate thickened leaflets with restricted motion and diastolic doming, often accompanied by fusion of the commissures. For functional tricuspid stenosis, a right atrial mass is apparent and responsible for the obstruction of RV inflow. CWD can be used to assess the pressure gradients for the valve and subsequently grade the severity of the stenosis.

3. Surgical intervention

    a. Salt restriction, diuretics, and digitalization reduce surgical risks in patients with severe tricuspid stenosis by improving hepatic function, reducing hepatic congestion, and delaying the surgery. Most patients with tricuspid stenosis have additional valvular lesions that require operation. If pressure gradients exceed 5 mm Hg or valvular area is less than 2 cm^2, tricuspid valve intervention is indicated. A low-profile prosthetic valve may be necessary for extensive calcification. Otherwise, commissurotomy of the tricuspid valve is usually sufficient.

4. Goals of perioperative management

    a. Hemodynamic management

        (1) RV preload

            (a) Adequate preload is key to maintaining forward flow across the stenotic tricuspid valve.

        (2) Heart rate

            (a) Normal sinus rhythms must be maintained in patients with tricuspid stenosis. Both supraventricular tachyarrhythmia and bradycardia can be harmful. The former can cause rapid cardiac deterioration and should be controlled with immediate cardioversion or pharmacologic intervention, while the latter can reduce total forward flow and should be treated pharmacologically or via pacing.

        (3) Contractility

            (a) Adequate cardiac output is maintained by an increase in RV contractility, and tricuspid stenosis impedes initial RV filling. A sudden drop in ventricular contractility can critically restrict cardiac output and increase RAP.

        (4) Systemic vascular resistance

            (a) In patients with limited blood flow over the tricuspid valve, systemic vasodilation can exacerbate hypotension.

        (5) PVR

            (a) Reducing PVR has little benefit in improving forward flow because forward flow limitation is found at the tricuspid valve. Maintaining PVR in the normal range is desired.

    b. Anesthetic technique

        (1) Minimal premedication is indicated.

        (2) In patients with isolated tricuspid stenosis, the anesthetic goals include maintenance of high preload, high afterload, and adequate contractility. In patients with coexisting mitral valve disease, the anesthetic technique usually depends on the type of mitral valve lesion.

        (3) Insertion of a pulmonary artery catheter through the stenotic tricuspid valve can be troublesome and not always warranted. Often, the catheter can be kept in the superior vena cava (SVC) until after bypass and then moved ahead by the surgeon upon completion of tricuspid valve repair/replacement. The catheter can also be floated after weaning from CPB. Clear communication with the surgeon prior to the beginning of the operation is recommended.

(4) During CPB, SVC drainage must be carefully tended to in order to avoid elevated SVC pressure, reduced cerebral perfusion pressure, and subsequent cerebral injury. Central venous pressure monitoring above the SVC tie, as well as intermittent assessment of the patient's head for any signs of edema and venous stasis, is indicated. The pulmonary artery is isolated from the blood flow during CPB, so no drug infusions may be given through associated accessory ports.

> **CLINICAL PEARL** During CPB, the pulmonary artery is isolated from the blood flow preventing drug infusions from being given through associated accessory ports.

(5) Preload augmentation must be continued during the post-CPB period, and inotropic support may be warranted if RV dysfunction becomes apparent [9].

F. **Tricuspid valve regurgitation**

1. Natural history
   a. Isolated TR is uncommon and often seen with drug abuse–related endocarditis, carcinoid syndrome, Ebstein anomaly, connective tissue disorders leading to valve prolapse, or chest trauma. Usually functional TR (FTR) develops secondary to RV failure, pulmonary hypertension, or left-sided cardiac abnormalities, such as end-stage aortic or MS. Severe aortic or mitral valve disease that strains the RV can lead to RV failure with TR. This FTR results either from dilatation of the tricuspid valve annulus or from RV dilatation that restricts the tricuspid valve leaflets.

2. Pathophysiology
   a. Natural progression
      (1) Since RV can compensate for volume overload, isolated TRs are bearable. Many TR symptoms are from an increased RV afterload. When TR is associated with pulmonary hypertension, there is decreased cardiac output due to RV impedance. Atrial fibrillation is also a common concurrent issue in patients with TR.
   b. TEE evaluation and grading of severity of TR
      (1) TEE examination of FTR shows dilatation of RV and the tricuspid valve annulus, along with leaflet restriction due to tethering. Different accompanying conditions have characteristic appearances. For endocarditis, vegetations and valvular perforation are common; rheumatic disease often shows commissural fusion and probable mitral and/or aortic valve involvement; and carcinoid heart disease results in diffuse leaflet thickening, leading to both stenosis and regurgitation with tricuspid and pulmonic valve involvement. In Ebstein anomaly, the tricuspid leaflets are displaced into the RV cavity, reducing its size and forcing the leaflets toward the RV apex. CFD is used to assess the severity of the TR. Similar to MR, however, the severity of the TR is most likely underestimated because of the changes to the loading conditions. Pulse wave Doppler can aid in calculating the severity of the regurgitation via changes in the hepatic vein flow.
   c. Pressure wave abnormalities
      (1) Although central venous pressure tracings may show the presence of giant V, other factors, including the compliance of the right atrium, filling of the right atrium, and regurgitant volume, determine the size of the regurgitant wave.

3. Goals of perioperative management
   a. Hemodynamic management
      (1) RV preload
         (a) Since a drop in central venous pressure can severely limit RV stroke volume, preload augmentation is useful for adequate forward flow.
      (2) Heart rate
         (a) Normal-to-high heart rates are beneficial in these patients to sustain forward flow and prevent peripheral congestion.

    (3) Contractility

        (a) As mentioned previously, TR is usually secondary to RV failure, and since the RV is equipped to accommodate volume but not pressure loads, positive-pressure ventilation, elevated PVR, or suppression of myocardial contractility may all lead to RV failure.

    (4) Systemic vascular resistance

        (a) In the absence of aortic or mitral valve lesions, variations in systemic afterload have little effect on TR.

    (5) PVR

        (a) Decreases in PVR improve RV function and forward blood flow. However, high airway pressures and agents that increase PAP should be avoided, though hyperventilation can be helpful in reducing PVR by producing hypocapnia. Thus, agents that dilate the pulmonary vasculature should be used if inotropic support is necessary. Dobutamine, isoproterenol, or milrinone would be beneficial for this. In addition, inhalation of nitric oxide or epoprostenol may also be helpful for these patients.

  b. Anesthetic technique

    (1) Minimal premedication is indicated.

    (2) In patients with coexisting mitral valve disease, the method of anesthetic is usually dependent upon the mitral valve lesion, as it is with tricuspid stenosis.

    (3) The regurgitant wave has a tendency to push a pulmonary artery catheter in the opposite direction of its insertion, making its entry into the regurgitant tricuspid valve difficult. Cold injectate is ejected retrograde into the atrium rather than the pulmonary artery, which leads to inaccuracy in the determination of cardiac output in the presence of TR.

    (4) Similar to tricuspid stenosis, during CPB, close attention must be paid to the SVC drainage.

    (5) Residual tricuspid stenosis may occur if a prosthetic valve is placed because the valve prosthesis is smaller than the native valve and postbypass preload augmentation may be warranted. In addition, in the immediate postbypass period, the entire stroke volume will have to be ejected against the higher PVR with no pop-off pressure lowering back into the right atrium placing the RV under increased strain. Accordingly, RV failure requiring inotropic support may occur and should be anticipated.

V. Prosthetic valves

The decision to use a prosthetic valve is patient specific and depends on various factors including the expected longevity of the patient (mechanical prostheses last longer), the ability of the patient to comply with anticoagulation therapy (mechanical prostheses require ongoing anticoagulation), the anatomy and pathology of the existing valvular disease, and the experience of the operating surgeon.

A. Essential characteristics

  1. An ideal prosthetic valve is nonthrombogenic, chemically inert, preserves blood elements, and allows physiologic blood flow.

  2. There are many different kinds of prosthetic valves available that can replace tricuspid or mitral valves, but none are without possible complications.

B. Types of prosthetic valves

  1. Mechanical

    a. Although durable, current mechanical valves are thrombogenic. Patients receiving mechanical valves require anticoagulation therapy indefinitely.

    b. Anticoagulation is normally provided with warfarin sodium, administered at a dose that will elevate the prothrombin time to 1.5 to 2 times control.

    c. There are four basic types of mechanical prosthetic valves: the caged ball, caged disc, monocuspid tilting disc, and bicuspid tilting disc valves. Out of these, the bicuspid tilting disc valves are the most common because of their streamlined design as well as improved laminar blood flow.

  (1) Bileaflet tilting disc valve prosthesis

   (a) In 1977, a bileaflet St. Jude cardiac valve was introduced as a low-profile device to allow central blood flow through two semicircular discs that pivot on supporting struts. This valve can be placed in the aortic, mitral, or tricuspid positions.

   (b) These valves produce low resistance to blood flow and have a lower incidence of thromboembolic complications, though anticoagulation is still necessary.

   (c) A few examples of bileaflet tilting disc valve prostheses include the Carbo-Medics, Edwards Tekna, Sorin Bicarbon, and Advancing the Standard (ATS); the St. Jude Medical remains the most popular.

 2. Bioprosthetic valves

  a. The Hancock porcine aortic bioprosthesis (now the Medtronic Hancock II stented porcine bioprosthesis) was introduced in 1970, followed by the Ionescu–Shiley bovine pericardial prosthesis in 1974 and the Carpentier–Edwards porcine aortic valve bioprosthesis in 1975.

  b. Bioprosthetic valves are beneficial because they usually do not require long-term anticoagulation therapy and are less thrombogenic; however, they are less durable as well.

  c. Because of lower durability and because these valves last longer in older patients, they are usually recommended for patients older than 60 years and when anticoagulation is better avoided.

  d. These valves last longer in the aortic position than in the mitral position.

  e. These valves fall into two categories: stented and nonstented.

  (1) Stented bioprosthetic valves

   (a) These valves are constructed from porcine aortic valves or bovine pericardium and are placed on a polypropylene stent attached to a silicone sewing ring covered with polyethylene terephthalate (Dacron).

   (b) These valves allow for improved central annular flow and less turbulence, but the stent does cause some obstruction to forward flow, thereby leading to a residual pressure gradient across the valve.

   (c) Stented valves that can be found in clinical use today include the Carpentier–Edwards perimount, Medtronic Mosaic, Carpentier–Edwards porcine, Hancock porcine, and Medtronic intact porcine.

  (2) Stentless bioprostheses

   (a) Porcine valves fixed in a pressure-free glutaraldehyde solution and without the use of a stent make up the category of stentless bioprostheses.

   (b) The primary types of valves clinically encountered in this category include the St. Jude Medical Toronto SPV stentless porcine, Edwards Prima Plus stentless bioprosthesis, and Medtronic Freestyle stentless porcine.

   (c) Stentless bioprosthetic valves are used almost exclusively in the aortic position and often when aortic root replacement is also necessary. They have excellent hemodynamic characteristics but technically are more difficult to place.

 3. Human valves

  a. The first bioprosthesis was from a cadaver in 1962. Early techniques such as irradiation or chemical treatment used to sterilize and preserve homografts decreased life span.

  b. Antibiotic solutions are used to sterilize human valves that are then frozen in liquid nitrogen until implantation. This method allows more than 75% of prostheses to last longer than 10 years, regardless of patient age, as cusp ruptures from weakness of the prostheses are minimized.

  c. Anticoagulation is often unnecessary and the incidence of prosthetic valve endocarditis and hemolysis from blood flow through the homograft is low.

  d. Homografts are primarily used for aortic or pulmonary valve replacement.

  e. These are most useful in patients younger than 35 and those with native valve endocarditis.

ACKNOWLEDGMENTS

The current version of this chapter is based on the one in the previous edition, and the authors acknowledge with thanks the important contributions of the coauthors in previous editions as well as Jelliffe Jeganathan, MBBS and Yannis Amador, MD in this edition.

REFERENCES

1. Manjunath CN, Srinivas P, Ravindranath KS, et al. Incidence and patterns of valvular heart disease in a tertiary care high-volume cardiac center: a single center experience. *Indian Heart J.* 2014;66(3):320–326.
2. Wilkins GT, Weyman AE, Abascal VM, et al. Percutaneous balloon dilatation of the mitral valve: an analysis of echocardiographic variables related to outcome and the mechanism of dilatation. *Br Heart J.* 1988;60(4):299–308.
3. Lung B, Cormier B, Ducimetière P, et al. Immediate results of percutaneous mitral commissurotomy. A predictive model on a series of 1514 patients. *Circulation.* 1996;94(9):2124–2130.
4. Nishimura RA, Otto CM, Bonow RO, et al. American College of Cardiology/American Heart Association Task Force on Practice Guidelines. 2014 AHA/ACC guideline for the management of patients with valvular heart disease: a report of the American College of Cardiology/American Heart Association Task Force on Practice Guidelines. *J Am Coll Cardiol.* 2014 Jun 10; 63(22):e57–e185.
5. **American College of Cardiology/American Heart Association Task Force on Practice Guidelines, Society of Cardiovascular Anesthesiologists, Society for Cardiovascular Angiography and Interventions, et al. ACC/AHA 2006 guidelines for the management of patients with valvular heart disease: a report of the American College of Cardiology/ American Heart Association Task Force on Practice Guidelines (writing committee to revise the 1998 Guidelines for the Management of Patients with Valvular Heart Disease): developed in collaboration with the Society of Cardiovascular Anesthesiologists: endorsed by the Society for Cardiovascular Angiography and Interventions and the Society of Thoracic Surgeons. *Circulation.* 2006;114(5):e84–e231.**
6. **Wunderlich NC, Beigel R, Siegel RJ. Management of mitral stenosis using 2D and 3D echo-Doppler imaging. *JACC Cardiovasc Imaging.* 2013;6(11):1191–1205.**
7. Stewart WJ, Currie PJ, Salcedo EE, et al. Evaluation of mitral leaflet motion by echocardiography and jet direction by Doppler color flow mapping to determine the mechanisms of mitral regurgitation. *J Am Coll Cardiol.* 1992;20(6):1353–1361.
8. **Lancellotti P, Moura L, Pierard LA, et al; European Association of Echocardiography. European Association of Echocardiography recommendations for the assessment of valvular regurgitation. Part 2: mitral and tricuspid regurgitation (native valve disease). *Eur J Echocardiogr.* 2010;11(4):307–332.**
9. Mahmood F, Matyal R. A quantitative approach to the intraoperative echocardiographic assessment of the mitral valve for repair. *Anesth Analg.* 2015;121(1):34–58.

13

Alternative Approaches to Cardiothoracic Surgery with and without Cardiopulmonary Bypass

Anand R. Mehta, Peter Slinger, James G. Ramsay, Javier H. Campos, and Michael G. Licina

KEY POINTS

1. Off-pump coronary artery bypass grafting (OPCAB) has become a mainstream technique that accounts for as much as 33% of surgical coronary revascularization.
2. OPCAB has not produced the expected reductions in neurologic and renal complications, although it has consistently reduced perioperative blood loss and transfusion.
3. Adjuncts such as intracoronary shunts, ischemic and/or anesthetic preconditioning, and intra-aortic balloon pumps (IABPs) may help to minimize ischemia during OPCAB. Circulatory support with vasoconstrictors and/or inotropic drugs is often required.
4. Transesophageal echocardiography (TEE) monitoring during OPCAB can promptly identify acute ischemia, although transgastric views are often compromised by the cardiac positioning required for distal coronary anastomoses.

5. Anesthetic techniques compatible with fast-tracking are most often used for OPCAB, which typically involves a "balanced" technique utilizing a combination of inhalational anesthetic, modest amounts of opioid, and intermediate-duration muscle relaxation. Excessive use of benzodiazepines and long-acting medications is avoided.

6. Adept positioning of the heart during OPCAB minimizes hemodynamic disturbances from reduced venous return, especially while performing coronary anastomoses within the right coronary and left circumflex arterial distributions. Maintaining adequate intravascular volume is essential.

7. Minimally invasive cardiac valve surgery most often requires CPB, but the incisions are smaller and sometimes off the midline, and cannulation for CPB often utilizes port-access technology. Robotic-assisted techniques can be used for minimally invasive mitral valve replacement or repair.

8. TEE is critical during minimally invasive valve surgery (MIVS) for CPB cannulation and assessment of valve structure and function.

9. Percutaneous approaches to mitral regurgitation (MitraClip), mitral stenosis (balloon mitral valvuloplasty), and aortic stenosis (transcatheter aortic valve implantation [TAVI]) are rapidly growing in popularity. Each approach presents unique challenges to the anesthesiologist; these procedures can be performed either with sedation or general anesthesia, each with its own benefits and risks.

10. Robotic-assisted minimally invasive techniques can be used for coronary artery bypass grafting (CABG) performed either on- or off-cardiopulmonary bypass (CPB).

I. Introduction

The past two decades have witnessed a major evolution in cardiac surgery in parallel with "minimally invasive" and laparoscopic developments in other surgical disciplines [1]. Two major objectives have been a reduction in the use of cardiopulmonary bypass (CPB) for revascularization and a reduction in the invasiveness of the surgical approach. The overall goals are to preserve and enhance the quality of the procedure(s) while providing faster recovery, reduced procedural costs, and reduced morbidity and mortality. The contribution of the anesthesia care team is to facilitate cost-effective early recovery while providing safe, excellent operating conditions both for the patient and the surgeon. Anesthetic techniques and monitoring modalities have needed to evolve with changes in surgical practice. Anesthesiologists have learned more about how to support the circulation during cardiac manipulation and periods of coronary occlusion. We have been charged with monitoring and support while the surgeon operates with minimal exposure while at the same time facilitating early recovery and discharge. The surgical techniques and their anesthetic considerations discussed in this chapter include the following: coronary artery bypass grafting (CABG) without the use of CPB (off-pump CABG [OPCAB] and minimally invasive direct coronary artery bypass [MIDCAB]); minimally invasive valve surgery (MIVS, except see Chapter 11 for transcatheter aortic valve implantation); computer-enhanced, endoscopic robotic-controlled CABG; and robotic noncardiac thoracic surgical procedures. Although not mentioned subsequently, we recommend the routine use of intra-arterial blood pressure monitoring for all of these procedures because of the rapidity and frequency of significant hemodynamic disturbances and the need for frequent assessment of labs (e.g., arterial blood gases, activated clotting times [ACTs], coagulation studies, etc.).

II. Off-pump coronary artery bypass (OPCAB) and minimally invasive direct coronary artery bypass (MIDCAB)

A. Historical perspective

1. **Early revascularization surgery**
    a. Early attempts at coronary artery surgery without the use of CPB included the Vineberg procedure in Canada (tunneling the internal mammary artery [IMA] into the ischemic myocardium) in the 1950s, and internal mammary to coronary anastomosis in the 1960s by Kolessov in Russia.

    b. Sabiston from the United States and Favolaro from South America reported the use of the saphenous vein for aorta-to-coronary artery bypass grafts, performed without CPB, in the same period.

    c. The introduction of CABG in the late 1960s expanded the indications for CPB, which had enabled congenital heart repairs and heart valve surgery since the 1950s. CPB with the use of cardioplegia became the standard of care in the 1970s, providing a motionless field and myocardial "protection" with asystole and hypothermia.

  2. Reports in the early 1990s

    a. South American surgeons with limited resources continued to develop techniques for surgery without CPB, publishing in North American journals in the 1980s and early 1990s. In 1991, Benetti et al. [2] reported on 700 CABG procedures without CPB performed over a 12-year period with very low morbidity and mortality.

    b. North American and European interest grew in the 1990s, fueled by a desire to make surgery more appealing (vs. angioplasty) as well as the need to reduce cost and length of stay. Alterative incisions were explored, and techniques and devices to facilitate surgery on the beating heart were developed. The terms "OPCAB" and "MIDCAB" were coined.

  3. Port-access (or "Heartport")

    a. Simultaneous with attempts to perform CABG without CPB, a group from Stanford University introduced a technique permitting surgery to be done with endoscopic instrumentation through small (1 to 2 cm) ports and a small thoracotomy incision. This was termed port-access surgery or by the trade name of Heartport (Johnson and Johnson, Inc., New Brunswick, NJ, USA). A motionless surgical field was required, necessitating CPB. Extensive use of TEE is required to assist in the placement of and to monitor the position of the various cannulae and the endoaortic balloon (see below).

    b. Port-access cardiac surgery contributed new knowledge in two major areas: Percutaneous, endovascular instrumentation for CPB and instrumentation for performing surgery through a small thoracotomy incision. The latter techniques continue to be developed and modified to permit MIVS through partial sternotomy or thoracotomy incisions.

  4. Minimally invasive direct coronary artery bypass (MIDCAB). A number of alternative incisions to midline sternotomy have facilitated access to specific coronary artery distributions to allow CABG without CPB. **The most popular alternative approach is the left anterior thoracotomy, which allows IMA harvest and grafting to the left anterior descending (LAD) artery territory. This is the procedure usually referred to as MIDCAB.**

  5. North American/European experience after 1998

    a. Initially viewed by most as experimental, off-pump techniques are now established as an acceptable alternative to CABG with CPB. The reported use of OPCAB has been reported to be as high as 33% [3], but the range in practice is wide. Some surgeons perform virtually all revascularizations as OPCAB, which typically refers to a multivessel CABG performed through a median sternotomy without CPB. Most large cardiac surgery practices have at least one surgeon who performs a significant number of OPCAB procedures. The physiology and anesthetic management for OPCAB have been recently reviewed by Chassot et al. [4].

    b. MIDCAB procedures are more technically demanding than OPCAB because they require specialized instrumentation and operating through a small incision. These procedures are done in a smaller number of institutions than OPCAB. Some surgeons harvest the IMA endoscopically before making the small incision to do the coronary anastomosis.

B. Rationale for avoiding sternotomy and cardiopulmonary bypass (CPB) for coronary artery surgery

  1. Reduction in complications

    a. Sewing coronary vessels on the beating heart is technically challenging and not necessarily appropriate for all surgeons [5]. Whether or not there is a benefit of performing on-pump versus OPCAB is a topic of heated debate. Several published randomized trials [6–10] confirm reductions in enzyme release, bleeding, time to extubation, and length of stay. While there are long-term follow-up studies suggesting similar rates of survival and graft patency between the two groups [11,12], other studies suggest that graft patency is lower in off-pump procedures [9,13], with one large randomized controlled trial finding a higher 1-year mortality rate in the off-pump group [13]. Of note, the latter studies came from surgeons less experienced in the off-pump technique. Intraoperative conversion from off-pump to on-pump has been associated with an increase in mortality [14,15]. Although reduction in stroke has been one of the proposed benefits of the technique (due to avoidance of aortic cannulation and cross-clamping), studies do not demonstrate this benefit. Similarly, reduction in renal dysfunction has been proposed but not proved in these studies and in one additional recent publication [16]. In August 2004, an updated guideline for CABG surgery was published by the American College of Cardiology and American Heart Association; this guideline recognizes the potential benefits for avoiding CPB but the need for further data with the lack of proved benefit in randomized controlled trials [17].

b. Avoidance of aortic manipulation and cannulation might reduce embolic complications such as stroke, yet a partial or side-biting aortic clamp may be necessary to perform proximal venous anastomoses in multivessel OPCAB. This can be avoided by using the IMA as the only proximal vessel with its origin intact or with the use of devices designed to avoid the use of a cross-clamp (e.g., the "Heartstring").

c. The whole body "inflammatory response" induced by extracorporeal circulation is avoided with MIDCAB and OPCAB. This approach should result in lower fluid requirements and less coagulopathy and is consistent with lesser volumes of blood loss and transfusion demonstrated in several comparisons of OPCAB to CABG with CPB.

2. **Competition with angioplasty.** Refinements in interventional cardiology and reductions in postprocedure restenosis have allowed an ever-increasing population of patients to have coronary lesions treated in the catheterization laboratory, although long-term outcomes in multivessel coronary disease are slightly better with CABG than with stents. However, patients will often choose the less invasive interventional cardiology approach over surgery if those results are nearly equivalent. Evolution of surgical techniques to provide excellent results with less physiologic trespass may be necessary for coronary artery surgery to survive.

3. **Progress toward truly "minimally invasive" surgery**

a. **Avoidance of CPB is more physiologically important than avoidance of sternotomy**, but postoperative recovery from sternotomy is foremost in patients' minds. The smaller the surgical scar, the better. The MIDCAB addresses this issue, but this approach can only access the LAD and its diagonal branches.

b. Cardiac surgeons have been slow to embrace endoscopic approaches partly because, until recently, existing technology did not provide the range of motion and control required for coronary artery anastomoses.

c. The port-access approach introduced endoscopic techniques to cardiac surgery; surgeons are now working with computer-assisted instruments to perform surgery on the beating heart (see later). Techniques developed for off-pump surgery are likely to contribute to the ability to perform such procedures endoscopically.

C. **Refinement of surgical approach**

1. **Development of modern epicardial stabilizers**

a. In early reports, compressive devices (e.g., metal extensions rigidly attached to the sternal retractor) were used to reduce the motion of the coronary vessel during the cardiac and respiratory cycles. These devices often interfered with cardiac function and were impossible to use for left circumflex coronary artery lesions.

b. Modern devices typically apply gentle pressure or epicardial suction, reducing the effect on myocardial function while providing better fixation of the area immediately surrounding the coronary artery anastomotic site. These devices also allow greater access to arteries on the inferior and posterior surfaces of the heart (Fig. 13.1).

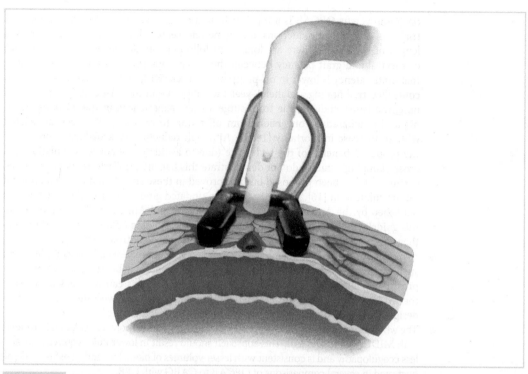

FIGURE 13.1 The Octopus 2 tissue stabilizer (Medtronic Inc., Minneapolis, MN, USA). Through gentle suction the device elevates and pulls the tissue taut, thereby immobilizing the target area. (Courtesy of Medtronic Inc.)

2. **Techniques to position the heart (through midline sternotomy)**

a. Surgery on the anterior wall of the heart (LAD and diagonal branches) usually requires only mild repositioning, such as a laparotomy pad under the cardiac apex. This is associated with minimal effects on cardiac function.

b. Surgery on the right coronary artery (RCA) or the circumflex artery (CX) and its marginal branches requires turning or twisting of the heart. To do this manually (i.e., by an assistant) is cumbersome and is associated with hemodynamic compromise.

c. Use of posterior pericardial traction stitches and a gentle retracting "sock" (web roll wrapped around the apex in a "sling" to pull the heart to either side) greatly improves the hemodynamic tolerance of these abnormal positions.

d. For circumflex vessel distribution surgery, dissection of the right pericardium to prevent the right ventricle (RV) from being compressed as it is being turned allows preservation of hemodynamic function.

3. **Surgical adjuncts to reduce ischemia**

a. Performing CABG surgery on the beating heart requires a mandatory period of coronary occlusion for each distal coronary artery anastomosis.

b. Intracoronary shunts can maintain coronary flow at the possible cost of trauma to the endothelium.

c. "Ischemic preconditioning" involves a brief (e.g., one to four 5-minute periods) occlusion and then the same period of reperfusion before performing the anastomosis. In animal models of myocardial infarction, this technique reduces the area of necrosis. A nearly equivalent physiologic effect can be provided by 1 MAC end-tidal isoflurane [18] or other inhaled agents, which is termed anesthetic or pharmacologic preconditioning. Ischemic preconditioning for 7- to 10-minute occlusions, such as those required for OPCAB and MIDCAB, probably does not provide the same benefit as one might see with longer periods of occlusion, but this technique is employed by some surgeons.

    d. The proximal anastomosis of a vein graft can be performed first in order to allow immediate perfusion once the distal anastomosis is completed.

    e. Regional hypothermia techniques have been described for use during coronary occlusion.

    f. Preoperative insertion of an intra-aortic balloon pump (IABP) has been used for patients with reduced ventricular function requiring multivessel OPCAB.

D. Patient selection: High risk versus low risk

    1. Early reports of OPCAB often described single-vessel or double-vessel bypass performed on low-risk patients. This was promoted as permitting early recovery and discharge.

    2. OPCAB is now promoted for multivessel bypass in patients with risk factors for adverse outcomes. Elderly patients at risk for stroke, patients with severe lung disease, or patients with severe vascular disease and/or renal dysfunction are often selected. As mentioned earlier, scientific studies have not yet demonstrated reduced adverse outcomes with OPCAB in these populations.

    3. Zenati et al. [19] have described combining MIDCAB (i.e., IMA to LAD) with angioplasty/stent to other vessels in high-risk patients.

    4. As mentioned earlier, a small number of surgeons attempt to perform virtually all CABG procedures as OPCAB regardless of preoperative risk status.

E. Anesthetic management

    1. Preoperative assessment

        a. The cardiac catheterization report should be reviewed and the procedure discussed with the surgeon, including the planned sequence of bypass grafts and the potential use of specific adjuncts (e.g., shunts or perfusion-assisted direct coronary artery bypass grafting [PADCAB]). This allows the anesthesiologist to predict the effect of each coronary occlusion, which requires knowledge of the coronary anatomy and its usual nomenclature (Fig. 13.2).

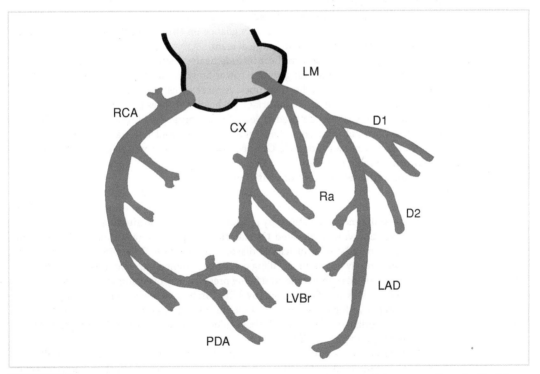

FIGURE 13.2 Coronary anatomy. The main branches from the circumflex artery (*CX*) are named "marginal" or "obtuse marginal" vessels. *D1*, first diagonal; *D2*, second diagonal; *LAD*, left anterior descending artery; *LM*, left main; *PDA*, posterior descending artery; *RCA*, right coronary artery; *LVBr*, LV branch; *Ra*, Ramus intermedius (<40% of individuals).

b. The vessel, location, and degree of stenosis determine the functional response to intraoperative coronary occlusion. Even with a proximal stenosis, an important vessel (e.g., LAD) may supply adequate resting flow to a large area of myocardium. Acute loss of flow to this large area (with surgical occlusion) may cause ventricular failure. A stenosis further down the vessel may be less important for overall ventricular performance.

c. High-grade stenosis (e.g., 90%) is likely to be associated with some collateral blood flow from adjacent regions, as flow through the stenosis may be inadequate even at rest. A 10-minute occlusion of such a vessel may have surprisingly little effect on regional function and hemodynamics because of the collateral flow. A lesser degree of stenosis (e.g., 75% to 80%) may not affect resting flow, hence there may be little or no collateral blood flow. Occlusion of such a vessel may cause severe myocardial dysfunction in the distribution of the vessel.

d. If incisions other than sternotomy are to be employed to access specific coronary regions, positioning of the arms and the body, the potential need for one lung anesthesia, and sites for vascular access need to be discuss. Some surgeons prefer one-lung anesthesia even for a median sternotomy approach to OPCAB.

2. Measures to avoid hypothermia

a. Unlike on-pump CABG, it is difficult to restore heat to a hypothermic OPCAB patient. In order to maintain hemostasis and facilitate early recovery, **prevention of heat loss needs to be planned before the patient enters the room**.

b. While in the preoperative area, the patient should be kept warm with blankets.

c. The operating room should be warmed to the greatest degree tolerated by the operating team (e.g., 75°F or higher). The temperature can be reduced once warming devices have been placed and the patient is fully draped.

d. The period and degree to which the patient remains uncovered for preoperative procedures (e.g., urinary catheter placement) and surgical skin preparation and draping should be minimized. This requires vigilance on the part of the anesthesiology team and frequent reminders to the surgical team.

e. Various adjuncts to preserve heat include heated mattress cover or insert; forced-air warming blankets, including sterile "lower body" blankets placed after vein harvesting; and circumferential heating tubes. A more expensive and possibly more effective option is the use of disposable surface-gel heating devices [20].

f. Fluid warmers should be used at least for the principal intravenous volume infusion "line," if not for all intravenous lines other than those used for intravenous drug infusions.

g. Low fresh-gas flows and circle/CO_2 reabsorption circuits will help prevent heat loss.

3. Monitoring (Table 13.1)

a. Preoperative assessment of ventricular function

(1) Preoperative LV function is a major determinant of the need for extensive monitoring. **Patients with normal or near-normal LV function are less likely to need diagnosis and therapy guided by invasive monitoring.**

(2) A patient with an elevated LV end-diastolic pressure (at cardiac catheterization) may have a "stiff" ventricle, or diastolic dysfunction. This commonly results from hypertrophy or ischemia. Filling pressures obtained intraoperatively must be interpreted in this context (i.e., the filling pressure may overestimate LV preload). Volumetric assessment of preload (by TEE) can be valuable in this situation.

(3) Patients with poor ventricular function may tolerate coronary occlusions poorly. Appropriate responses may be best guided by monitors of cardiac output (CO) and filling pressures, or TEE [21,22].

(4) Repeated occlusions in multiple regions of the myocardium (i.e., for multivessel OPCAB) are likely to result in a cumulative detrimental effect on hemodynamics. There may be a period of myocardial dysfunction requiring inotropic support even in patients with good underlying LV function. The combination of reduced ventricular function and the need for multiple bypass grafts is likely to result in a need

TABLE 13.1 Monitoring approaches for OPCAB and MIDCAB

Monitor	Advantages	Disadvantages	Comment
ECG	• Universal • Simple • Inexpensive • Recognized criteria	• Insensitive • Position dependent (lead and heart) • Incision dependent • Loss of V4–5 (MIDCAB)	• Best if multilead • Should be calibrated • ST-segment trending helpful
Central venous pressure	• Simple • Inexpensive	• Pressure–volume relationship uncertain • Insensitive for LV dysfunction • No CO	• Important for drug infusions • Affected by position of heart and patient • Use of "introducer" allows rapid insertion of PAC
PAC	• LV filling pressure • CO • Options may be helpful (mixed venous O_2 saturation, continuous CO, pacing)	• Pressure–volume relationship uncertain • Expensive • Insensitive for acute regional dysfunction	• Controversial monitor • May prolong ICU stay due to "abnormal numbers"
TEE	• Gold standard for acute ischemia • Verify restoration of function • Guide surgical cannula placement	• Expensive • User dependent • Distracting • May not have good view of heart	• Requires real-time interpretation
CO bioimpedance (BE); ED; AW	• Less invasive than PAC • AW gives stroke volume variation	• No measure of LV filling • ED positional • AW may vary with vascular tone	• BE and stroke volume variation (from AW) questionable with open chest • ED may interfere with TEE (or vice versa)

OPCAB, off-pump coronary artery bypass; ECG, electrocardiogram; MIDCAB, minimally invasive direct coronary artery bypass; LV, left ventricular; ED, esophageal Doppler; CO, cardiac output; PAC, pulmonary artery catheter; ICU, intensive care unit; TEE, transesophageal echocardiography; AW, arterial waveform analysis.

for inotropic and/or vasopressor infusions guided by monitoring with a pulmonary artery catheter (PAC) and/or TEE.

(5) Preoperative placement of a PAC introducer, but with an obturator of some kind or a single- or double-lumen central venous catheter placed through it rather than a PAC may be a reasonable first approach in most patients. This avoids the use of the PAC in uncomplicated patients while allowing for rapid PAC placement should this be desired any time in the perioperative period.

b. **Specific monitors**

(1) Lead V5 of the electrocardiogram (ECG) detects 75% of the ischemia found on all 12 leads. This lead should be monitored in all patients undergoing OPCAB or MIDCAB, as permitted by the surgical incision. Lead II gives clear P waves, but adds little to the sensitivity of ischemia detection.

(2) The PAC is variably useful during OPCAB. For single- or double-vessel bypass in patients with preserved LV function, there can be little justification for this monitor [23]. **The worse the ventricular function and the greater the number of planned bypass grafts, the more likely it is that information from the PAC will be useful.**

(3) Continuous CO from the PAC or other devices and continuous mixed venous oximetry may provide incremental benefit in assessing the adequacy of cardiac function. Use of these devices is often institution-specific or even surgeon/anesthesiologist-specific.

(4) Monitoring with TEE can provide detailed information about the effects of coronary occlusion and recovery, and it provides the earliest, most specific information during acute deterioration and interventions. Acute ventricular dilatation and mitral regurgitation may occur when a large region of the myocardium becomes ischemic, and this is detected immediately with TEE. In addition, distortion of the mitral annulus due to abnormal positioning may cause mitral regurgitation [24]. Obtaining adequate images may be distracting to clinical care. With the heart in an unusual position, images may be difficult or impossible to obtain. A reversible wall-motion abnormality that resolves with restoration of flow is reassuring; however, this does not guarantee a good quality graft or anastomosis.

(5) Normal carbon dioxide (CO_2) elimination requires adequate CO. If ventilation is constant, an acute decline in CO will cause an acute decrease in end-tidal CO_2 concentration.

c. Monitoring for specific procedures

(1) For MIDCAB or other reduced-access procedures, provision must be made for transcutaneous defibrillation and pacing. An important consideration is the requirement to reinflate the lungs for defibrillation during closed-chest surgery to provide tissue (rather than air) for the current to traverse [25].

(2) For port-access surgery (Heartport or related procedures), TEE is required to guide and monitor cannula placement and function.

4. Anesthetic technique

a. Early recovery is usually desired. Extubation immediately or shortly after surgery should be the goal.

b. A vapor-based anesthetic technique facilitates early recovery. Keys to prevention of delayed awakening are as follows: Minimizing the dose of benzodiazepine; use of modest doses of opioids; and avoiding residual paralysis at the end of surgery. Some clinicians use very short-acting opioids such as remifentanil to facilitate early extubation, but this approach requires awareness of the need for effective longer-lasting analgesia at the time of extubation and thereafter. Use of bispectral index (BIS) monitoring can help guide administration of hypnotic agents.

c. Transfer of the intubated yet awakening patient to the intensive care unit (ICU), and early ICU care are facilitated by use of short-acting sedative drugs such as propofol or dexmedetomidine.

d. Thoracic epidural or lumbar spinal anesthetic and analgesic techniques have been promoted by some as suitable adjuncts to off-pump approaches. There are reports of OPCAB procedures done without general anesthesia. Most centers are reluctant to risk major neuraxial techniques immediately before full heparinization for CPB. Use of such techniques is unlikely to shorten postoperative length of stay and has not been shown to provide a measurable benefit.

e. For MIDCAB (thoracotomy), postoperative epidural analgesia [26], paravertebral block, or intercostal blockade may be useful for pain control.

5. Anticipation and management of ischemia

a. Knowledge of the coronary anatomy and surgical plan is essential. This allows appropriate timing of pharmacologic and other interventions before ischemia is induced. **Use of isoflurane (or other volatile inhalational agent) anesthesia can provide pharmacologic "preconditioning,"** as mentioned earlier. The hemodynamic alterations commonly associated with ischemia such as tachycardia (especially in the presence of hypotension) must be avoided. Intravenous β-adrenergic blockade may be beneficial; however, this must be balanced with the possibility of impaired myocardial performance during coronary occlusion.

b. Maintenance of adequate coronary artery perfusion pressure is of great importance in allowing collateral blood flow to ischemic regions. Volume loading and appropriate positioning (see following), alteration of the depth of anesthesia, and/or use of α-adrenergic agonists may all be indicated.

    c. Prophylactic nitrate infusions may interfere with preload (see later).

    d. Early experience without modern stabilizers suggested that bradycardia (to reduce motion) would aid the surgeon. This is no longer an issue. Grafting to the RCA territory (supplying the sinus and AV nodes) can be associated with bradycardia. Thus, although β-adrenergic blockade may be useful to prevent or treat tachycardia, epicardial pacing may be required for ischemia-induced bradycardia.

    e. Anecdotally, patients with compromised ventricular function undergoing multivessel procedures may benefit from "prophylactic" administration of an inotropic medication.

  6. **Intravascular volume loading**

    a. **Positioning of the heart may kink or partially obstruct venous return and/or compress the RV. Intravascular volume loading and head-down (Trendelenburg) position can help reduce this effect** (Fig. 13.3) [27]. Close observation of the heart, filling pressures, and blood pressure to provide feedback to the surgeon is essential.

    b. Intravenous vasodilators (e.g., nitrates) can exacerbate reductions in cardiac filling. More commonly, intravenous vasoconstrictors (phenylephrine, norepinephrine) will be required during abnormal cardiac positions.

  7. **Surgery-anesthesiology interaction.** With all the above considerations, it should be clear that there must be excellent communication between the surgeon and the anesthesiologist for OPCAB or MIDCAB. Anticipation and planning for problems allow the anesthesiologist to intervene in a timely manner. The surgeon must say in advance what he is planning to do. Similarly, changes in cardiac performance and the need for intervention must be continuously communicated to the surgeon. The anesthesiologist must observe the surgical field, watching the procedure as well as the position, size, and function of the heart. An observant, communicative team with basic monitoring (ECG, blood pressure, and central venous pressure) is likely to produce better results than a team that communicates poorly, but uses extensive monitoring.

F. **Anticoagulation**

  1. **Heparin management**

    a. Heparin anticoagulation protocols are institution-specific. Similar to on-pump surgery, there are few data to recommend targeting specific ACT values.

    b. Some surgeons request full heparinization similar to on-pump procedures (i.e., ACT target >400 seconds); others request lower doses of heparin such as would be used for noncardiac vascular procedures (ACT target typically >200 seconds), or something in between. Outcomes appear to be equivalent using either approach, which suggests that ACT targets as high as those used for CPB are unnecessary.

  2. **Protamine reversal**

    a. Extracorporeal circulation induces a postoperative multifactorial defect in coagulation that may reduce early graft thrombosis. When coagulation is reversed after OPCAB or MIDCAB, no such hypocoagulable state exists; indeed, there is evidence that the coagulation system is activated by the stress of surgery, similar to what has been showed for other major procedures [28].

    b. In order to gradually return the coagulation to normal leaving perhaps a little residual heparin effect, reversal may be achieved with incremental doses of protamine. If "full" heparinization has been employed, administration of 50 mg of protamine may bring the ACT down to near 200 seconds, after which small increments (10 to 25 mg) can be given to achieve an ACT that is about 25% to 50% above control (i.e., 150 to 180 seconds).

    c. If the patient is clinically bleeding with an elevated ACT, then heparin should be reversed completely. Even in the absence of clinical bleeding, some cardiac surgeons prefer complete reversal immediately after completion of the grafts.

    d. Prolonged OPCAB procedures may be associated with extensive blood loss and therefore facilitated by the use of cell-saver devices (i.e., washing of salvaged blood so it is free of coagulation proteins and platelets). Over time, this may induce a dilutional coagulopathy similar to what is often seen after CPB.

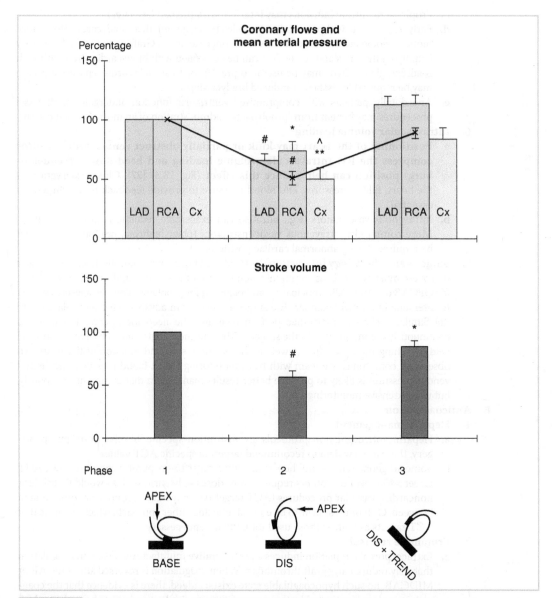

FIGURE 13.3 Relative changes in hemodynamic parameters during vertical displacement of the beating porcine heart by the Medtronic Octopus tissue stabilizer and the effect of head-down tilt. *BASE,* pericardial control position; *Cx,* circumflex coronary artery; *DIS,* displacement of the heart by the Octopus; *DIS + TREND,* Trendelenburg maneuver (20-degree head-down tilt while the heart remains retracted 90 degrees); *LAD,* left anterior descending artery; *RCA,* right coronary artery; x = mean arterial pressure. Statistical comparison with control values: *$p <0.05$; **$p <0.01$; #$p <0.001$; ^$p = 0.046$ versus combined relative value of LAD and RCA flows. (From Grundeman PF, Borst C, van Herwaarden JA, et al. Vertical displacement of the beating heart by the Octopus tissue stabilizer: Influence on coronary flow. *Ann Thorac Surg.* 1998;65: 1348–1352, with permission.)

3. **Antiplatelet therapy**
   a. Thrombosis at the site of vascular anastomoses is initiated by platelet aggregation and adhesion. Similar to strategies that are used in angioplasty/stent procedures, antiplatelet therapy may help reduce early graft thrombosis in CABG, whether done with or without CPB.
   b. A common practice is to administer a dose of aspirin preoperatively. This can be achieved with a suppository if the patient is already anesthetized.

    c. In on-pump CABG, administration of aspirin within 4 hours after the procedure reduces graft thrombosis. This strategy should also be applied to OPCAB and MIDCAB.

    d. There are no published data about the use of newer antiplatelet drugs in this setting. As with all such therapies (including aspirin), the concern for bleeding must be balanced with the desire to prevent graft thrombosis.

  4. Antifibrinolytic therapy. Use of lysine analogs to inhibit fibrinolysis has become common practice with on-pump CABG, as they have been shown to reduce perioperative blood loss. Recent investigations now support the use of these agents during OPCAB as well [29].

G. Recovery

  1. Extubation in the operating room

    a. For uncomplicated procedures, recovery from OPCAB or MIDCAB can be rapid without the requirement for postoperative ventilation or sedation.

    b. Normothermia, hemostasis, and hemodynamic stability must be assured.

    c. Residual anesthesia and paralysis from long-acting agents (e.g., pancuronium, large doses of morphine) must be avoided.

    d. The extra time spent in the operating room to achieve extubation may be more costly than a few hours of postoperative ventilation and sedation.

  2. ICU management

    a. For most patients, early postoperative management can employ the "fast-track" technique where mechanical ventilation is withdrawn within a few hours of surgery, and patients are extubated and possibly mobilized at the bedside late in the day or during the evening of surgery.

    b. ICU stay is driven by institutional practice, but for patients having straightforward, uncomplicated procedures, there may be no need for more than a few hours in a high-intensity nursing area (i.e., postanesthetic care unit or ICU).

    c. If length of stay is reduced, cost will almost certainly be reduced. If there is no significant reduction in stay, the cost of specialized retractor systems may exceed the cost of the disposables required for CPB.

    d. Some surgeons passionately believe that OPCAB is better for their patients; perhaps with time and additional randomized trials, the hoped-for reductions in neurologic events, renal dysfunction, and other adverse outcomes will become apparent.

III. Minimally invasive valve surgery (MIVS)

A. Introduction

The Society of Thoracic Surgeons National Database defines minimally invasive surgery as "any procedure that has not been performed with a full sternotomy and CPB support. All other procedures, on- or off-pump with a small incision or off-pump with a full sternotomy are also considered minimally invasive" [30]. Similar to MIDCAB, the premise of MIVS is that "smaller is better" for valve surgery as well. A partial sternotomy or small thoracotomy with port incisions may achieve some benefits when compared to standard median sternotomy. Similar to OPCAB, alternative approaches were explored in the late 1990s, with the first publication in 1998. Proposed [31,32] but unproved advantages to these approaches include the following:

  1. Reduced hospital length of stay and costs

  2. Quicker return to full activity

  3. Less atrial fibrillation (26% vs. 38% in one report [33])

  4. Less blood transfusion

  5. Same results (mortality, valve function)

  6. Less pain

  7. Earlier ambulation

In addition, the surgical opinion is that reoperation should be easier after MIVS, as the pericardium is not opened over the RV outflow tract. These proposed benefits may be observed with specific surgeons in specific centers; however, there have been no rigorous or randomized studies. The limited data that exist suggest that acute postoperative pulmonary function impairment is not improved by the use of the limited incision. Minimally invasive reoperative

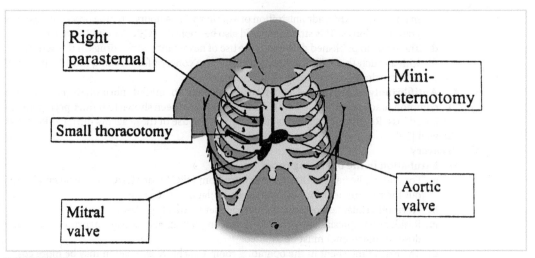

FIGURE 13.4 Incisions for MIVS. The most common approach is the "mini" sternotomy, which extends from the sternal notch part way to the xiphisternum but is diverted to the right at the level of the third or fourth interspace (for the aortic valve), leaving the lower sternum intact. The mitral valve can be accessed through the small right thoracotomy. (From Clements F, Glower DD. Minimally invasive valve surgery. In: Clements F, Shanewise J, eds. *Minimally Invasive Cardiac and Vascular Surgical Techniques. Society of Cardiovascular Anesthesiologists monograph*. Philadelphia, PA: Lippincott Williams & Wilkins; 2001:30.)

aortic valve surgery is a new and successful technique, especially in patients who have had previous cardiac operations using a full sternotomy (e.g., prior CABG). This surgical approach does not disturb the vein grafts or the patent IMAs [34].

B. Surgical approaches (Fig. 13.4)

1. Port-access (Heartport): This approach involves direct surgical visualization and operation through small openings (ports) and a small right horizontal thoracotomy incision for access to the mitral valve or atrial septum. In order to avoid sternotomy, the port-access system uses alternative access sites and cannulae. The aorta is cannulated through a long femoral arterial catheter or a shorter transthoracic aortic catheter. These devices are advanced to the ascending aorta and include an "endo-aortic clamp" or inflatable balloon to achieve aortic occlusion ("cross-clamp") from within. They include a cardioplegia administration port. Venous cannulation is achieved with a long femoral venous catheter, supplemented as needed with a pulmonary artery vent. A coronary sinus catheter is used to administer cardioplegia. Placement of these catheters can be time-consuming and requires imaging with fluoroscopy and/or TEE. A limited number of institutions still use this approach to MIVS. Some reports have raised concerns about device-related aortic dissections as well as endoaortic balloon rupture and dislocation [35].

2. Video-assisted port-assisted (using the port-access cannulae and small incisions with video equipment to visualize and perform valve surgery). This is currently performed in a small number of institutions worldwide.

3. Robotic (see below). This is an evolving technique, particularly for mitral valve repair, with excellent results being reported.

4. Direct-access (small incision—many types: Anterolateral mini-thoracotomy, partial upper or lower sternotomy, right parasternal incision, and others). The right parasternal approach is preferred by some surgeons (especially for aortic valve access) because there is no sternal disruption and it is cosmetically pleasing. The avoidance of sternotomy bleeding into the pericardial sac with associated fibrinogen depletion may result in less perioperative bleeding and less pain that is easier to control, although the need to divide two or more costochondral cartilages with the parasternal approach does induce considerable postoperative pain. As mentioned earlier, avoidance of opening the pericardium over the

RV outflow tract may make future cardiac reoperation easier and safer. One problem with this approach is the sacrifice of the right IMA.

5. The current standard approach for aortic valve surgery using a minimally invasive approach is an "inverse L"-shaped partial sternotomy extending to the third or fourth right intercostal space. In order to bring the entire heart more anteriorly, three to four retention stitches are passed through the pericardial rim and fixed to the skin incision. This may be associated with compression of the right atrium (RA) and a decrease in the venous return to the heart. The arterial cannula for CPB is placed in the ascending aorta. Venous return is established by direct cannulation of the right atrial appendage or by percutaneous femoral vein cannulation of the RA. With the latter cannulation technique, often a two-stage cannula is used with the distal tip placed at the junction of the superior vena cava (SVC) and RA as confirmed by TEE (bicaval view) [36].

6. Minimally invasive mitral valve surgery can use a right anterolateral minithoracotomy for which the patient is positioned supine with slight elevation of the right chest (often using a folded blanket) and extension of the right arm. Optimal visualization the heart requires deflation of the right lung, which is achieved most often by using a double-lumen endobronchial tube. CPB is established via the femoral vessels. The SVC may also be cannulated percutaneously via the right internal jugular vein (IJV). A percutaneous transthoracic aortic cross-clamp is placed through a separate stab incision in the right posterior axillary line [35], and the mitral valve is accessed through the left atrium. Another approach is a right parasternal incision with mitral valve exposure via the RA and interatrial septum.

7. Reduced-size skin/soft tissue incision compared with full median sternotomy can give a more cosmetically pleasing result.

C. **Preoperative assessment**

In addition to understanding the valvular and associated cardiac disease, the anesthesiologist must have a good appreciation for the surgical plan. Nonsternotomy and port-access approaches require specific positioning, including having the arms extended or cephalad either suspended in a sling or resting on an "airplane" type of armrest, and will have implications for peripheral venous, central venous, and arterial catheter placement. Port-access procedures will require planning for fluoroscopic and TEE assistance to guide and monitor placement of catheters.

D. **Monitoring**

1. Central venous catheter versus PAC. Because of pericardial traction and/or compression of the RA, pulmonary artery, or RV outflow tract, the relationship between pressures recorded from central venous or PACs and chamber volumes may be changed. In addition, due to limited ability to palpate around the heart, there may be an increased risk of inadvertently including the PAC in surgical sutures. These considerations must be balanced with the potential need to guide fluid and inotropic therapy perioperatively.

2. TEE. There can be little doubt that TEE monitoring is an integral part of MIVS [36]. With such limited access, the surgeon cannot rely on visual cues about cardiac distension or volume status. Thus, TEE is used in the following ways:

   a. Pre-CPB to determine:
      (1) Valve dysfunction
      (2) Cardiac volume and function
      (3) Arterial cannulation site
      (4) Specialized cannula placement, especially for port access
   b. During CPB for port-access and robotic surgery, TEE is used to monitor appropriate placement of the endoaortic "clamp" and to detect intracardiac air, which can be extensive in MIVS cases.
   c. After CPB, TEE used in the usual manner to assist with identification and management of new-onset ventricular dysfunction, which may occur in as much as 20% of MIVS patients. This is more frequent in patients with significant intracardiac air. TEE is also used to assess valve function and to look for aortic dissection.

E. Specific anesthesiology concerns

Regardless of the type of surgical access to MIVS, there are several common problems that require enhanced awareness:

1. Long surgical learning curve: Be prepared for anything during this period.
2. Limited surgical access (small incision)
   a. Urgent cardiac pacing and direct current cardioversion may need to be done trans-thoracically. Appropriate skin electrodes or patches must be placed before surgery is started.
   b. Big fingers, sponges, or instruments can compress vascular structures, causing large swings in hemodynamics.
   c. "Blind" suture placement can lead to bleeding from posterior sites which can be very difficult to control. Full median sternotomy is occasionally required to control the bleeding.
   d. Inadequate valve repair or replacement: Paravalvular leaks or valve dysfunction secondary to suture-induced valve leaflet sticking can occur.
   e. Errant suture placement may cause coronary artery compromise leading to myocardial ischemia, or may affect the conduction system leading to heart block or dysrhythmias.
   f. De-airing is very difficult, even when guided by TEE. Residual air may embolize to the coronary arteries resulting in acute cardiac decompensation. CO_2 gas is very commonly administered into the operating field to minimize this complication, with varying success.
   g. Tamponade: After chest closure, even a small amount of bleeding can lead to tamponade physiology in the mini-incision area.

F. Postoperative management

The goal is early recovery and extubation. As in MIDCAB and OPCAB, this is governed by a number of factors, including patient stability and temperature, duration of the procedure, and the use of short-acting agents. Extubation in the operating room is possible but uncommon. Certain incisions (i.e., thoracotomy) may lend themselves to the use of paravertebral or intercostal nerve blocks for postoperative pain relief.

G. Percutaneous valve repair/replacement

Percutaneous approaches to mitral regurgitation, mitral stenosis, and aortic stenosis are rapidly growing in popularity. Each approach presents unique challenges to the anesthesiologist.

1. **MitraClip** [37,38]. A clip has been developed for mitral regurgitation which captures the free edges of both mitral valve leaflets, creating a double orifice valve similar to the Alfieri surgical repair. Under general anesthesia, the femoral vein is accessed, and with fluoroscopic and TEE guidance the device is advanced over a guidewire through the interatrial septum and through the regurgitant portion of the mitral valve, where it is deployed. Multiple clips may be used if necessary. Early studies suggest that though the procedure is safe, it may be most beneficial to high-risk surgical candidates with functional MR, as conventional surgical methods are more effective in reducing the severity of MR. Potential complications include hemopericardium leading to tamponade, damage to the mitral valve, device failure requiring surgical repair, device embolization, creation of mitral stenosis, and persistent interatrial shunt from the septal puncture. This procedure continues to be investigated.

2. **Percutaneous balloon mitral valvuloplasty** [39]. Certain patients with symptomatic or severe mitral stenosis may be candidates for percutaneous balloon mitral valvuloplasty as an effective alternative to open surgical mitral commissurotomy. Prior to the procedure, TEE is performed to interrogate the left atrium and left atrial appendage for thrombus which may dislodge during the dilation and lead to systemic embolization. The procedure can be performed using local anesthesia with sedation or general anesthesia. Under fluoroscopic guidance, a guidewire is advanced through the femoral vein into the RA then through the interatrial septum. The balloon catheter is advanced along the guidewire and positioned in the mitral valve. Once properly positioned, the balloon is inflated, thereby dilating the valve. Repeated dilations are performed until there is an improvement of the pressure gradient between the left atrium and LV, significant mitral regurgitation occurs, or echocardiographic assessment reveals adequate fracture of the commissures. Complications include damage

to cardiac structures, hemopericardium leading to tamponade, emboli release, worsening or creation of mitral regurgitation, damage to the subvalvular apparatus, and persistent interatrial shunt. Acute success rates and long-term restenosis rates are comparable to those for open surgical mitral commissurotomy.

3. **Transcatheter Aortic Valve Implantation (TAVI)** [40]. This technique is discussed in Chapter 11. That discussion also includes hybrid operating rooms, which are presented in Chapter 10 as well.

IV. Robotically enhanced cardiac surgery

A. Historical perspective

1. Use of robotics in surgery was initially considered for facilitation of surgical expertise at a site remote from the surgeon (e.g., battlefield, developing country).

2. Robotic cardiac surgery has evolved through advances in telemanipulation technology, endoscopic instruments and visualization tools, and peripheral cannulation techniques [41].

3. Computer-assisted, robotic cardiac surgery in patients was first reported by Loulmet et al. [42] and Reichenspurner et al. [43] in 1999. Carpentier and colleagues performed the first robotically assisted mitral valve surgery in 1997 using a prototype of the da Vinci® system which was followed by the first robotic mitral valve surgery by Chitwood et al. in the United States [44]. Since 2002, the Food and Drug Administration (FDA) has approved the use of the da Vinci system for cardiac surgery [45].

4. Since then, a variety of procedures ranging from multivessel totally endoscopic coronary artery bypass grafting (TECAB), both on-pump and off-pump, to hybrid procedures involving robotic revascularization and PCI have evolved with promising results [46]. Other cardiac surgeries that can be performed using a robotic system include mitral valve surgeries, tricuspid valve surgeries, ASD/PFO closure, atrial mass removal (myxoma). Congenital and catheter-based technologies and surgeries for atrial fibrillation and LV lead placement have also been performed. Suri et al. have provided proof of concept for a robotic-assisted aortic valve replacement using a sutureless bovine pericardial prosthesis (Perceval self-expanding valve) in cadavers [47].

B. Overview

1. Taylor et al. [48] described the complementary capabilities of surgeon and machine.
   a. Surgeons are dextrous, adaptive, fast, and can execute motions over a large geometric scale; they develop judgment and experience. Limiting factors include geometric inaccuracy and inexact exertion of directional force. Performance is compromised by confined spaces or bad exposure. Surgeons get tired, and with age can lose skills and vision.
   b. Machines are precise and untiring. Computer-controlled instruments can be moved through an exactly defined trajectory with controlled forces, facilitating work in confined spaces.

2. Endoscopic surgeries, being minimally invasive, are advantageous by minimizing stress and pain associated with open procedures. Other advantages include early recovery, reduced median length of stay, complications, mortality, cosmetic benefits, decreased bleeding and improved early quality of life [49,50].

3. Robotic approaches to cardiac surgery avoid sternotomy preserving thoracic integrity and function and provide a virgin chest for redo operations via a sternotomy.

C. Technologic advances permitting endoscopic surgery

1. Development of the charge-coupling device (CCD) allows high-resolution video images to be transmitted through optical scopes to the surgeon. Present systems utilize 3D (as compared to 2D for endoscopic procedures) 1080i with 10× magnification imaging displays providing better depth perception.

2. High-intensity xenon and halogen light sources improve visualization of the surgical field.

3. Improved hand instrumentation permits procedures that previously could only be performed through an open incision to be executed by less invasive methods [51].

4. The major limitations of endoscopic instruments are the control of fine motor activity, surgery in a confined space, and a somewhat reduced sensory feedback of tissue resistance

TABLE 13.2 Endoscopic versus computer-enhanced instrumentation systems

Parameter	Conventional endoscopic instruments	Computer-enhanced systems
Degrees of freedom[a]	4	7
Tremor filter[b]	No	Yes
Motion transmission[c]	1:1	1:1 to 5:1
Hand–eye alignment[d]	Poor	Natural
Fulcrum effect[e]	Reversed motion	Not effective
Force ratio (hand/tip)[f]	Large/abnormal/not linear	Programmable/linear
Indexing[g]	Not possible	Possible
Ergonomics	Unfavorable	Favorable

[a]Number of different directions of movement. For instance, if something is capable of moving the x, y, and z directions, then it has three degrees of freedom. The da Vinci can probably move in the x, y, and z directions, plus it can rotate and act like forceps.
[b]Image filter that filters out camera vibrations or filters out surgeon tremors at the control station.
[c]Displacement amplifier to make finer movements possible. At the 5:1 setting, the robot moves 1 cm for every 5-cm movement of the surgeon at the control station.
[d]Assesses hand–eye coordination.
[e]Fulcrum is the point or support on which a lever turns. The conventional instrument is said to be reversed motion, meaning that if the surgeon moves in one direction, the actual motion of the instrument is in the opposite direction.
[f]Feedback physical force the surgeon feels at the control station when operating.
[g]Indexing denotes capability for manual dexterity enhancement.

    or firmness. This becomes very relevant during tissue dissection and knot tying and the surgeon depends on visual cues to ascertain tissue strain [45].

5. Placement of a microprocessor between the surgeon's hand and the tip of the surgical instrument dramatically enhances control and fine movement. Table 13.2 lists the ways in which computerized dexterity enhancement addresses limitations of conventional endoscopy.

6. The addition of a dynamic atrial retractor provides continuous and rapid retraction providing sustained exposure in a tight space along with true dexterity provided by the instruments.

7. Other disadvantages include a steep learning curve, increased operative and CPB times and cost [52]. The technology limits itself to a highly selective group and is contraindicated in patients with significant aortic, iliofemoral arterial disease [53], significant mitral annular calcification (MAC) [54], severe lung disease, chest wall abnormalities with abnormal heart orientation within the chest cavity, previous thoracic procedures (increased adhesion leading to poor exposure), severe pulmonary hypertension and severely reduced ventricular function [55].

D. **Endoscopic robotic-assisted systems**

1. Robotic systems consist of three principal components:
   a. A surgeon console. The surgeon sits at the console and grasps specially designed instrument handles. The surgeon's motions are relayed to a computer processor, which digitizes hand motions.
   b. A computer control system. The digitized information from the computer control system is related in real time to robotic manipulators, which are attached to the operating room table.
   c. Robotic manipulators. These manipulators hold the endoscopic instrument tips, which are inserted into the patient through small ports.

2. Currently, only one robotic system is commercially available: the da Vinci system (Intuitive Surgical, Mountain View, CA, USA).

3. A number of enhancements are required to move robotic systems toward more widespread acceptance.
   a. Development of endoscopic Doppler ultrasonography may aid in internal thoracic (mammary) artery harvesting, especially when the vessel is covered by fat or muscle.
   b. Although providing articulation, the endoscopic stabilizers need refinement to permit easier placement.

    c. Multimodal three-dimensional image visualization and manipulation systems may allow modeling of the range of motion of the robotic arms to individual patient data sets (computerized tomographic (CT) scan, ECG-gated magnetic resonance imaging). This may help optimize port placement and minimize the risk of collisions in the future.

    d. "Virtual" cardiac surgical planning platforms will allow the surgeon to examine the topology of a patient thorax for planning the port placement and the endoscopic procedure.

E. **Anesthetic considerations related to robotic surgery**

Robotic surgery requires the anesthesiologist to interact prospectively with the surgeon and machine to maintain ideal operating conditions, as well as stable hemodynamics and cardiac rhythm in an environment that may change rapidly from regional ischemia and cardiac manipulation. When the patient is fully instrumented and the robotic surgery is under way, direct access to the operative field is very limited and likely to be delayed. Anticipation and excellent communication are especially important where rapid surgical interventions are all but impossible. In general, the less invasive the surgery, the more involved is the team to compensate for the lack of direct visualization.

> **CLINICAL PEARL** Robotic-assisted cardiac surgery in selected patients offers a minimally invasive option with equivalent surgical outcomes and faster recovery times.

    1. Preoperative preparation

        a. Similar to OPCAB or MIDCAB, the anesthesiologist must discuss the procedure with the surgeon to understand the coronary anatomy, what is planned, and what special considerations might be involved (see above).

        b. Specific to robotic surgery are considerations that may be applicable to the robot (e.g., site of ports, location of manipulators, electrical interference).

        c. Peripheral cannulation and remote access perfusion requires additional imaging studies such as Doppler US and CT angiography to determine size and calcification of the peripheral vessels and aorta (atherosclerotic plaques which may embolize with retrograde perfusion) [53].

    2. Monitoring must take into account the patient's pathology (i.e., underlying ventricular function), the surgeon's familiarity with the robotic technique, anticipated problems, and duration of the procedure.

    3. Induction and maintenance of anesthesia

        a. Specific anesthetic techniques are similar to other cardiac surgery settings where rapid emergence from anesthesia is desired ("fast track").

        b. Position is critical for appropriate location of ports and access for robotic manipulators. For TECAB procedures the left hemithorax is elevated. Positioning for mitral valve surgery consists of the patient being supine with the right trunk elevated avoiding excessive stress on neck and shoulders.

        c. One-lung ventilation (OLV) may be employed for better visualization and depends on the surgical procedure. For TECAB the left lung is deflated whereas for mitral valve surgery the right lung is deflated [55]. This may be achieved with a double-lumen tube or a bronchial blocker.

        d. Lung deflation is critical during exposure, assessment and control of bleeding and chest closure. Alternatives to lung isolation are intermittent apnea and establishing CPB prior to exposure [56] (Fig. 13.5).

        e. During robotic CABG surgery, CO_2 is insufflated into the left hemithorax during one-lung anesthesia. The insufflation pressure should be 6 to 8 mm Hg. This sustained positive intrathoracic pressure may mechanically decrease myocardial contractility and/or impair cardiac filling, which is rapidly reversible after the release of CO_2 from the chest cavity [57]. There may be sufficient absorption of CO_2 to induce respiratory acidosis and its attendant potential for tachycardia, dysrhythmias, and pulmonary hypertension. These effects are negated to a certain extent by gradual insufflation, additional

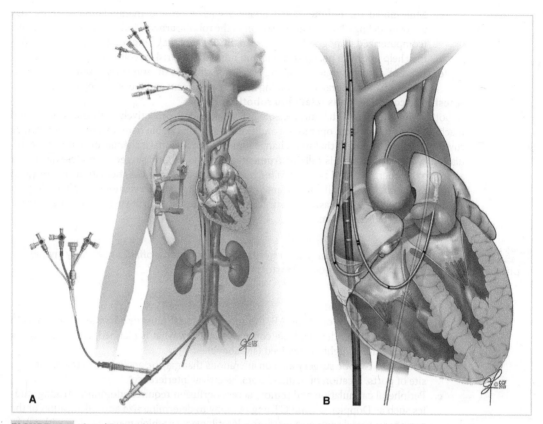

FIGURE 13.5 **A** and **B:** Peripheral cannulation techniques with use of endoballoon and pulmonary artery vent.

fluid boluses, and use of vasopressors and/or inotropes. Reducing the insufflation pressure aids in reversing severe hemodynamic compromise almost immediately [69].

> **CLINICAL PEARL** Lung isolation is essential for better visualization of cardiac structures and instrumentation inside a closed chest.

  f. External defibrillator/pacing pads should be attached to the patient as surgical access to the heart for either of these functions is very limited and delayed [55,56].
  g. Similar to OPCAB and MIDCAB, a multimodal approach should be taken to prevent heat loss. Although robotic procedures often reduce the extent of exposed intrathoracic surfaces as compared to OPCAB or CABG using CPB, the procedures can be lengthy, so the risk for hypothermia remains significant.
  h. Other considerations during robotic cardiac surgery include long operative times and limited access to the patient. If required, CPR must only be provided after all robotic instruments are removed to prevent patient injury [55].

> **CLINICAL PEARL** Access to the patient during the surgical procedure may be limited making resuscitation difficult.

  4. Anticoagulation and reversal. See discussion under "OPCAB and MIDCAB" in Section II.F.
  5. TEE is an essential tool in all robotic cardiac procedures. Limited surgical exposure makes TEE very important during the procedure [55–57]. It is helpful in:

   a. Confirming the preoperative findings

   b. Examination of the visible aorta for severe atheromatous disease which increases the risk of stroke with retrograde perfusion via femoral artery.

   c. Dilatation of the aortic root and or ascending aorta which limits the use of a percutaneous endoballoon.

   d. Presence and quantification of aortic regurgitation necessitating use of a percutaneous retrograde coronary sinus catheter and a percutaneous PA vent. Severe aortic regurgitation may potentially limit the approach because of a lack of adequate ventricular emptying limiting myocardial protection during CPB.

   e. Imaging is critical during remote access perfusion and peripheral cannulation and its associated complications including aortic dissection and cardiac tamponade. Positions of guidewires and cannulae need to be confirmed. Although a peripheral arterial cannula will not be visualized in the descending aorta visualized by TEE, at our institutions we identify the guidewire in the aortic lumen prior to cannulation.

CLINICAL PEARL   TEE is valuable in confirming the surgical diagnosis, monitoring hemodynamics, confirming placement of peripheral cannulation, percutaneous cardioplegia devices, and complications.

---

   f. Ventricular function during capnothorax and volume status.

   g. De-airing and weaning from CPB

   h. Adequacy of the surgical procedure

6. Cannulation, cross-clamping, cardioplegia delivery, and venting techniques [41,45,55].

   a. Venous drainage

   (1) Vacuum-assisted (increases flow by 20% to 40%) venous drainage is achieved by a percutaneously placed femoral venous catheter (22 to 28F) with the tip positioned in the SVC.

   (2) Additional venous drainage may be supplemented via a percutaneous SVC cannula (17F) placed via the right IJV.

   (3) Alternatively, direct venous cannulation may be achieved through a larger incision.

   b. Arterial cannulation

   (1) Arterial cannulation is achieved via the femoral or subclavian artery.

   c. Cross-clamping

   (1) A percutaneously placed aortic endoballoon via the femoral or subclavian artery. Aortic root enlargement, inadequate femoral arterial diameter, and calcium in the ascending aorta may limit its use.

   (2) Positioning of the endoballoon in the aortic root is aided by TEE and an injection of adenosine directly via the device prior to insufflation.

   (3) A fine balance between proximal flow from residual cardiac contraction or infusion of antegrade cardioplegia against the retrograde flow from the arterial inflow determines the motion of the endoballoon in the aortic root and ascending aorta. Migration of the device distally may limit perfusion to the head vessels and inadequate myocardial perfusion. It can be monitored with the use of TEE (limited utility on CPB with air in the chest cavity and an empty heart) and monitoring bilateral arterial pressure tracings. A significant fall in the right arterial pressure tracing (from innominate artery occlusion) indicates distal migration.

   (4) Other complications of endoballoon placement include injury to the aortic valve while positioning and/or with proximal migration.

   (5) Alternatively, a percutaneous transthoracic aortic clamp can be introduced via the right axilla along with the placement of an aortic root vent via the incision.

   (6) Certain procedures may be performed on a beating heart or with induced ventricular fibrillation.

> **CLINICAL PEARL** Robotic cardiac surgery has been made possible due to advances in telemanipulation, peripheral cannulation, and cardioplegia techniques.

   d. Cardioplegia delivery
   (1) Antegrade
      (a) Directly with the use of aortic root cannulation.
      (b) Via the endoballoon.
   (2) Retrograde [58,59]
      (a) Indications for retrograde percutaneous cardioplegia include redo operations, complex procedures with long operative times, a patent LIMA, significant aortic regurgitation, and LV hypertrophy.
      (b) It is commonly introduced via the right IJV percutaneously under TEE (modified bicaval view, deep 4-chamber view, midesophageal 2-chamber or midesophageal bicommissural view), fluoroscopy guidance and by transducing the catheter. Ventricularization of the tracing after balloon inflation suggests it is in the coronary sinus.
      (c) It may be difficult to place in patients with a hypoplastic or thrombosed coronary sinus and a prominent thebesian valve. Cardioplegia delivery may be ineffective in patients with a dilated coronary sinus or incorrectly placed (too deep) catheter.
      (d) It may be displaced by the venous cannula and or by a dynamic atrial catheter.
      (e) Trauma to the coronary sinus can occur during placement, overinflation of the catheter balloon, elevated cardioplegia infusion pressure or aggressive retraction of the heart with the catheter in place.
   e. Venting
   (1) Is achieved via the endoballoon, directly via the ascending aorta with a transthoracic aortic clamp, a percutaneously placed PA vent, or directly via a vent in the LV across the mitral valve in mitral valve surgeries.
   (2) The PA vent is a flimsy non–heparin-coated catheter whose distal tip is positioned in the main PA with the help of TEE and that drains a rate of 50 mL/min (Figs. 13.6 and 13.7).
   f. Postoperative management
   (1) Extubation in the operating room may be possible (see above for OPCAB and MIDCAB).
   (2) If postoperative ventilation is anticipated, plan to change the double-lumen endobronchial tube to a single-lumen endotracheal tube.
   (3) Postoperative pain management will depend on the size and number of port incisions. If a thoracotomy incision was made, intercostal, paravertebral, epidural analgesia, pectoral nerve (PECS) blocks, and serratus anterior blocks can be considered.

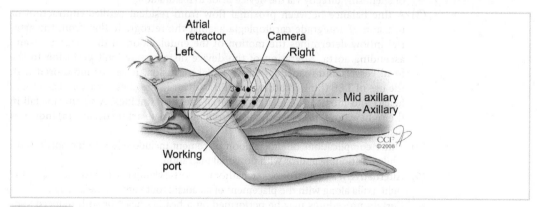

FIGURE 13.6 Surgical access for robotic mitral valve repair.

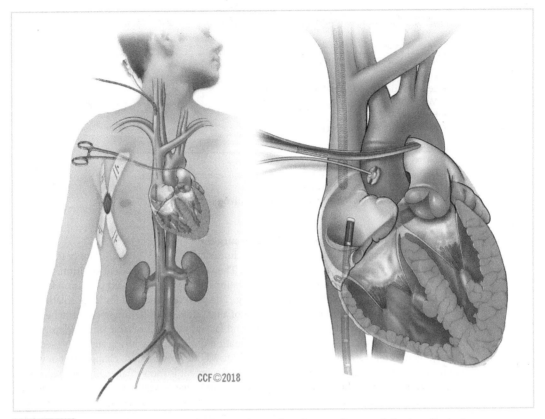

CCF©2018

FIGURE 13.7 Peripheral cannulation techniques with use of aortic cross-clamp and direct cardioplegia.

F. Conversion to sternotomy

Reasons to abandon the robotic approach for a conventional sternotomy include inadequate CPB flows, complications with peripheral access and or remote access perfusion, inadequate exposure, inadequate repair, IMA injury, anastomosis problems, graft kinking, intraoperative ischemia, ventricular failure, and inadequate target exposure due to intramyocardial course of the coronary vessels.

G. Summary

The field of robotically enhanced cardiac surgery will present a wide range of anesthetic challenges as it continues to develop. Anesthesiologists and surgeons alike must adapt to rapidly changing techniques in our continuing efforts to improve clinical outcomes.

V. Anesthesia for robotic noncardiac thoracic surgery

A. Introduction

Robotic surgical procedures are usually performed by two surgeons, the surgeon at the console and the table-side surgeon, who introduces the trocars and connects them with the robotic arms and changes the robotic instruments through the other ports if needed. The size of the robotic trocar is 10 mm for the binocular robotic camera and 8 mm for the instruments. Some of the potential advantages of using a robotic surgical system in thoracic surgery include: shorter hospital length of stay, less pain, less blood loss and transfusion, minimal scarring, faster recovery, and potentially a faster return to normal activities [60]. Table 13.3 displays the advantages and disadvantages of robotic thoracic surgery. Table 13.4 displays the surgical procedures performed in thoracic surgery with the da Vinci robotic surgical system.

TABLE 13.3 Advantages and disadvantages of robotic thoracic surgery
■ **Advantages**
• Shorter hospital length of stay
• Less pain
• Less blood loss and need for transfusion
• Minimal scarring
• Faster recovery
• Faster return to normal activities
■ **Disadvantages**
• Increasing surgical times
• Increased number of operating room personnel needed
• Potential for conversion to open procedure
• Cost and outcomes (need to be compared with other techniques)

B. **Anesthetic implications in robotic thoracic surgery**
The basic principles applied to video-assisted thoracic surgery (VATS) also apply to robotic-assisted thoracic surgery (see also Chapter 26). The combination of patient position, management of OLV techniques, and surgical manipulations alter ventilation and perfusion from the dependent and nondependent or collapsed lung. The preferred method for lung isolation during robotic-assisted thoracic surgery is the use of a left-sided double-lumen endotracheal tube (DLT) because of the greater margin of safety and faster and more reliable lung collapse. Also, it provides ready access for bronchoscopic evaluation of the airway during surgical resection.

In general, careful attention must be given to airway devices because changes in body position may cause tube migration. OLV anesthetic management is more challenging during robotic thoracic surgery due to the presence of the robot chassis that is stationed over the patient. The patient's airway is also usually located far from the anesthesia field. In some instances access to the airway, if needed, is not optimal because of the presence of the robotic arms nearby. In addition, visualization during robotic thoracic surgery may be enhanced by continuous intrathoracic CO_2 insufflation, which may increase airway pressures. When CO_2 is used it should not exceed intrathoracic pressures of 10 to 15 mm Hg. Increasing the intrathoracic pressure (i.e., >25 mm Hg) can compromise venous return and cardiac compliance; also the dependent lung develops higher airway pressures and ventilation can become difficult. During the surgical procedure, the FiO_2 should be maintained at 100% and the peak inspiratory pressure should be kept <30 cm H_2O. The ventilatory parameters should be adjusted to maintain a $PaCO_2$ at approximately 40 mm Hg.

C. **Robotic-assisted surgery and anesthesia for mediastinal masses**
One of the commonest thoracic surgical procedures performed to date with the use of the da Vinci robotic surgical system is thymectomy [61]. Of the patients scheduled for robotic-assisted thymectomy, some have the diagnosis of myasthenia gravis because of the presence of a thymoma. Preparation of the patient for surgery includes neurologic evaluation to assess the patient's neurologic status and optimization of neurologic conditions; continuation of anticholinesterase therapy and plasmapheresis may be indicated in some cases [62]. Precautions regarding anesthetic management include the proper dosing of muscle relaxants and the potential consequences of a large mediastinal mass on oxygenation and ventilation.

TABLE 13.4 Surgical procedures performed in thoracic surgery with the da Vinci robotic surgical system
• Thymectomy
• Mediastinal mass resection
• Nissen fundoplications
• Esophageal dissections
• Esophagectomy
• Pulmonary lobectomy

Positioning the patient for a thymectomy with the use of the robotic system requires specific care and attention. In these cases, the patients are placed in an "incomplete side-up" position at a 30-degree angle right or a left lateral decubitus position with the use of a beanbag. The arm of the elevated side is positioned at the patient's side as far back as possible so the surgeon can gain enough space for the robotic arms. While the robot is in use it is imperative to consider strategies to protect all pressure points and to avoid unnecessary stretching of the elevated arm because this can cause damage to the brachial plexus. Also, because the arm of the robot is in the chest cavity, a complete lung collapse must be maintained throughout the procedure. Robotic surgery with the da Vinci robotic surgical system does not allow for changes in patient position on the operating room table once the robot has been docked. Robotic thymectomy requires that the operating room table be rotated 90 degrees away from the anesthesiologist's field. For this reason access to the airway to make adjustments to the DLT during the surgery can be challenging. In some cases, a bilateral approach may be required. In these cases, the operation is performed in two stages and requires rotating the table 180 degrees to provide the surgeon access to the contralateral chest for the second stage of the operation. The anesthesiologist must be cautious during these changes to avoid problems with the airway and to ensure that the lines and monitor wires have enough slack to accommodate changes in position. The anesthesiologist must be aware during these cases of possible injury to the contralateral pleura, especially if CO_2 capnothorax is being used, as the elevated intrathoracic pressure in the contralateral hemithorax can make ventilation difficult and cause cardiovascular collapse or tension pneumothorax because of malfunction of the chest tube. Special attention must be given to the patient's elevated arm and head to prevent crushing injuries with the robotic arms. One case report [63] showed a brachial plexus injury in an 18-year-old male after robotic-assisted thoracoscopic thymectomy. In this report, the left upper limb was in slight hyperabduction. It is important to keep in mind that hyperabduction of the elevated arm to give optimal space to the operating arm of the robot can lead to a neurologic injury. Close communication between surgeon and anesthesiologist in relation to the positioning and function of the robot is mandatory, and all proper measures must be taken, including the use of soft padding and measures to avoid hyperabduction of the arm. The elevated arm should be protected by using a sling resting device. Operating room staff should always be vigilant of telescope light sources because direct contact of these devices with surgical drapes and the patient's skin can quickly cause serious burns while telescopes and cameras are being changed.

An early report by Bodner et al. [64] involving 13 patients with mediastinal masses resected with the da Vinci robotic surgical system showed no intraoperative complications or surgical mortality. In this series of patients, a complete thymectomy with en bloc removal of all mediastinal fat around the tumor was performed. In this report, cases were restricted to patients with a tumor size less than 10 cm in diameter.

In a report by Savitt et al. [65] involving 14 patients undergoing robotic-assisted thymectomy, all patients received a DLT for selective lung ventilation; in addition, patients were managed with arterial and central venous pressure catheters. Complete thymectomy was performed on all 14 patients. Right-lung deflation was accomplished with selective lung ventilation and CO_2 insufflation to a pressure of 10 to 15 mm Hg to maintain the lung away from the operative area. It is important that the anesthesiologist recognize the effects of CO_2 insufflation in the thoracic cavity. The outcome of this report included no conversion to open thoracotomy, nor any intraoperative complications or deaths; the median hospital stay was 2 days with a range of 1 to 4 days.

In another report, Rückert et al. [66] had zero mortality and an overall postoperative morbidity rate of 2% in 106 consecutive robotic-assisted thymectomies. Therefore, robotic thymectomy appears to be a promising technique for minimally invasive surgery. Length of stay was shorter with robotic thymectomy when compared to the conventional approach via sternotomy.

A recent systematic review and meta-analysis comparing robotic-assisted minimally invasive surgery versus open thymectomy [67] clearly showed that the patients undergoing robotic thymectomy have a reduced hospital length of stay, less intraoperative blood loss, fewer chest-in-tube days, and less postoperative complications when compared to open thymectomy.

In contrast another meta-analysis [68] comparing robotic-assisted thymectomy versus video-assisted thymectomy showed no statistically significant differences in surgery outcomes among the two groups (no significant difference on conversion rates, surgical times or average days or length of stay).

In addition the indications for the use of the robot have been extended for cases with posterior mediastinal tumor where the access can be challenging and these have also reported good outcomes [69].

D. Robotic-assisted pulmonary lobectomy

Since the introduction of the da Vinci robotic surgical system, there has been widespread interest in its use in minimally invasive surgery involving the chest. Lobectomy with lymph node dissection remains the cornerstone of surgical treatment of early-stage cancer. However, due to the use of low-dose CT scans, the number of patients who are diagnosed with early-stage disease each year is increasing; these patients can be treated via lobectomy or segmentectomy. In order to offer more minimally invasive resection options to patients with lung disease, video-assisted lobectomy/segmentectomy and subsequently robotic-assisted lobectomy/segmentectomy approaches have been developed [70].

The robotic-assisted lobectomy/segmentectomy has attracted the interest of thoracic surgeons since its introduction in 2002. Proposed advantages of robotic lobectomy/segmentectomy include: smaller incisions, decreased postoperative pain, faster recovery time, and superior survival when compared to conventional open thoracotomy.

A report by Park et al. [71] showed robotic-assisted thoracic surgical lobectomy to be feasible and safe. In the report, the operation was accomplished with the robotic system in 30 out of 34 scheduled patients. The remaining four patients required conversion to open thoracotomy. Anderson et al. [72] reported a series of 21 patients that underwent robotic lung resection for lung cancer. In this report, the 30-day mortality and conversion rate was 0%. The median operating room time and blood loss were 3.6 hours and 100 mL. The complication rate was 27% and included atrial fibrillation and pneumonia. Gharagozloo et al. [73] reported a series of 100 consecutive robotic-assisted lobectomies for lung cancer and concluded that robotic surgery is feasible for mediastinal, hilar, and pulmonary vascular dissection during video-assisted thoracoscopy lobectomy.

Positioning the patient for a robotic lobectomy includes placing the patient over a bean bag in a maximally flexed lateral decubitus position with the elevated arm slightly extended so that the thoracic cavity can be accessed and no damage to the arm occurs during manipulation of the robotic arms. Patients undergoing robotic lobectomy must have a lung isolation device to achieve OLV. In the vast majority of these cases, a left-sided DLT is used and optimal position is achieved with the flexible fiberoptic bronchoscope. In a few cases in which the airway is deemed to be difficult, an independent bronchial blocker could be used and optimal position achieved with the use of a fiberoptic bronchoscope. Initial thoracic exploration is performed with conventional thoracoscopy to verify tumor location. During robotic-assisted lobectomy, it is mandatory that lung collapse is achieved effectively to allow the surgeon the best field of vision and to avoid unnecessary damage to vessels or lung parenchyma.

All patients undergoing robotic-assisted thoracic lobectomy should have an arterial line. The anesthesiologist must be ready for potential conversion to an open thoracotomy. In the Park report [71], three out of four cases that needed to be converted had minor bleeding; in addition, in one case lung isolation was lost, requiring an open thoracotomy. It is mandatory that the anesthesiologist involved in these cases have experience in placing a DLT and can guarantee optimal position with the aid of flexible fiberoptic bronchoscope. Using intraoperative fiberoptic bronchoscopy to make adjustments to the DLT during surgery is challenging because the table is rotated 180 degrees away from the anesthesiologist's field. The chassis of the robot is often positioned over the patients head leaving a very small area for the anesthesiologist to access the airway.

The report by Gharagozloo et al. [73] reported one nonemergent conversion to open thoracotomy. In this report, postoperative analgesia was managed with the infusion of a local anesthetic (0.5% bupivacaine, 4 mL/hr) through catheters placed in a subpleural tunnel encompassing intercostal spaces 2 through 8. All patients were extubated in the operating room. Mean operating room time was 216 minutes (range 173 to 369). Overall mortality within 30 days was 4.9%, and median length of stay was 4 days. Postoperative complications included atrial fibrillation in four cases, prolonged air leak in two cases, and pleural effusion requiring drainage in two cases—complications that are not different from those occurring with video thoracoscopic surgery.

A meta-analysis [74] in 2015 has evaluated the perioperative outcomes of robotic-assisted thoracoscopic surgery for early-stage lung cancer. This meta-analysis report showed that the morbidity and perioperative 30-day mortality was similar in both groups. A more recent meta-analysis [70] comparing robotic- versus video-assisted lobectomy/segmentectomy for lung cancer showed that robotic lobectomy is a feasible and safe alternative to a video thoracoscopic surgery with a low 30-day mortality and similar morbidity; also this study reported lower open thoracotomy conversion rate, but longer operative time which increases the cost of surgery. Robotic cases surgical times must be shorter with a reduced cost and improve morbidity to become an alternative to other surgical techniques.

Acute and chronic pain after open thoracotomy continues to be a problem. Minimally invasive thoracic surgery approaches result in less tissue trauma, shorter recovery, and improved cosmesis [75]. A recent study [76] evaluating the outcomes of the acute and chronic pain after robotic-, video-assisted thoracoscopic surgery, or open anatomic pulmonary resection showed that robotic and video thoracoscopic surgery (VATS) approach resulted in less acute pain and chronic numbness when compared to open thoracotomy. However, there was no significant difference between robotic or VATS. This report indicates that in terms of pain control, there is no difference regardless which minimally invasive surgery the surgical team chooses and no advantage of one versus the other technique (robotic vs. VATS).

E. **Carbon dioxide (CO_2) insufflation during robotic surgery**

Continuous low-flow insufflation of CO_2 has been demonstrated as an aid for surgical exposure during minimally invasive thoracic procedures. It has been used as the only means of providing surgical exposure to the thoracic cavity (during two-lung ventilation for VATS), or more frequently in conjunction with a DLT or an independent bronchial blocker and OLV. The compression of the lung parenchyma by CO_2 acts as a retractor.

A study by Ohtsuka et al. [77] involving 38 patients undergoing minimally invasive internal mammary harvest during cardiac surgery found significant increases in mean central venous pressure, pulmonary artery pressure, and the pulmonary artery wedge pressure. They also found that with insufflation of the right hemithorax, but not the left side, slight decreases were noted in the mean arterial blood pressure and cardiac index. They concluded that the hemodynamic effect from continuous insufflation of CO_2 at 8 to 10 mm Hg for 30 to 40 minutes is mild in both hemithoraces, although the impact is greater on the right. This information was supported by another study [78]. This study involving 20 patients undergoing thoracoscopic sympathectomy and concluded that compared to the left-sided hemithorax the impact of CO_2 insufflation on the vena cava and the RA during right-sided procedures was associated with reduction of venous return and low cardiac index and stroke volume. The impact of CO_2 insufflation on the respiratory system has also been studied. El-Dawlatly et al. also reported a significant pressure-dependent increase in peak airway pressure and a decrease in dynamic lung compliance but no difference in tidal volume or minute ventilation during volume-controlled ventilation.

Insufflation of CO_2 should only be started after initial thoracoscopic evaluation has ruled out that the port of insufflation has not compromised a vascular structure or the lung parenchyma. Communication between the surgeon, anesthesiologist, and operating room personnel is crucial at this point. Insufflation is ideally started at low pressures of 4 to 5 mm Hg and is gradually increased while monitoring the patient's vital signs. The anesthesiologist should always be aware of the possibility of gas embolization during these cases. In the case of sudden cardiac collapse, the CO_2 flow should be discontinued immediately. Ventilation during CO_2 insufflation should be titrated to keep adequate oxygenation and a normal $PaCO_2$ and pH. Also, damage to the contralateral pleura may occur resulting in CO_2 flow to the contralateral chest, making ventilation difficult and also causing hemodynamic compromise, along with the potential development of subcutaneous emphysema. In addition, venous return compromise or progressive arterial desaturation can occur [79].

F. **Robotic-assisted esophageal surgery and anesthetic implications**

Transthoracic esophagectomy with extended lymph node dissection is associated with higher morbidity rates than transhiatal esophagectomy. Esophagectomy is both a palliative and a potentially curative treatment for esophageal cancer. Minimally invasive esophagectomy has been performed to lessen the biologic impact of surgery and potentially reduce pain. The initial esophagectomy experience with the da Vinci robotic surgical system involved a patient who had a thoracic esophagectomy with wide celiac axis lymphadenectomy. The case was reported by Kernstine et al. [80] and had promising results. Thereafter another report using the da Vinci robotic surgical system has been published of six patients undergoing esophagectomy without intraoperative complications [81]. The surgical approach in this report was performed from the right side of the chest. A left-sided DLT was used to selectively collapse the right lung while, at the same time, ventilation was maintained in the left lung.

In a report by van Hillegersberg et al. [82] involving 21 consecutive patients with esophageal cancer who underwent robotic-assisted thoracoscopic esophagolymphadenectomy, 18 were completed thoracoscopically and 3 required open procedures (because of adhesions or intra-operative hemorrhage). In this case series report, all patients received a left-sided DLT and a thoracic epidural catheter as part of their anesthetic management. Positioning of these patients was in a left lateral decubitus position, and the patient was tilted 45 degrees toward the prone position. Once the robotic thoracoscopic phase was completed, the patient was then put in supine position and a midline laparotomy was performed. A cervical esophagogastrostomy was performed in the neck for the completion of surgery. Of interest in this series is the fact that pulmonary complications occurred in the first 10 cases (60%), caused primarily by left-sided pneumonia and associated acute respiratory distress syndrome in 3 patients (33%). These complications were probably related to barotrauma to the left lung (ventilated lung) attributed to high tidal volumes and high peak inspiratory pressures. In the 11 patients that followed, the same authors modified their OLV ventilator settings to administer continuous positive airway pressure ventilation (5 cm H_2O) to the non-ventilated lung and pressure-controlled OLV; with this approach the respiratory complication rate was reduced to 32%.

A report by Kim et al. [83] described 21 patients who underwent robotic-assisted thoracoscopic esophagectomy performed in a prone position with the use of a Univent® bronchial blocker tube (Fuji Systems Corp, Tokyo Japan). All thoracoscopic procedures were completed with robotic-assisted techniques followed by a cervical esophagogastrostomy. In Kim's report, major complications included anastomotic leakage in four patients, vocal cord paralysis in six patients, and intra-abdominal bleeding in one patient. The prone position led to an increase in central venous pressure and mean pulmonary arterial pressure and a decrease in static lung compliance. The overall conclusion from this report is that robotic assistance esophagectomy in the prone position is technically feasible and safe. Others have reported a robotic-assisted transhiatal esophagectomy technique feasible and safe as well [84].

Another study [85] involved 14 patients who underwent esophagectomy using the da Vinci robotic surgical system in different surgical stages. It showed that for a complete robotic esophagectomy including laparoscopic gastric conduit, the operating room time was an average of 11 hours with a console time by the surgeon of 5 hours, and an estimated mean blood loss of 400 ± 300 mL. In this report after the robotic thoracoscopic part of the surgery was accomplished with the patient in the lateral decubitus position, patients were then placed in supine position and reintubated, and the DLT was replaced with a single-lumen endotracheal tube. The head of each patient was turned upward and to the right, exposing the left neck for the cervical part of the operation. Among the pulmonary complications in the postoperative period, arterial fibrillation occurred in 5 out of 14 patients. In this report, among the recommendations to improve efficiency in these cases is the "use of an experienced anesthesiologist who can efficiently intubate and manage single-lung ventilation and hemodynamically support the patient during the procedure." This follows what Nifong and Chitwood [86] have reported in their editorial views regarding anesthesia and robotics: that a team approach with expertise in these procedures involving nurses, anesthesiologists, and surgeons with an interest in robotic procedures is required.

The data on robotic-assisted esophagectomy suggest that the procedure is safe, feasible, and associated with preoperative outcomes similar to open and minimally invasive esophagectomy. No data, however, demonstrate improved outcomes in terms of operative morbidity,

TABLE 13.5 Complications of robotic-assisted thoracic surgery

References	n = Cases	Operation	Intraoperative complications	Postoperative complications
Rea et al. [87]	33	Thymectomy	0	Chylothorax, $n = 1$ Hemothorax, $n = 1$
Savitt et al. [65]	15	Mediastinal mass resection	0	Atrial fibrillation, $n = 1$
Kernstine et al. [85]	98, 103	Esophagectomy	Conversion to open procedure, $n = 1$	Thoracic duct leak, $n = 3$ Vocal cord paralysis, $n = 3$ Atrial fibrillation, $n = 5$
Rückert et al. [66]	106	Thymectomy	Bleeding, $n = 1$	Phrenic nerve injury, $n = 1$
Pandey et al. [63]	1	Thymectomy	–	Brachial plexus injury
Bodner et al. [81]	14	Mediastinal mass resection	0	Postoperative hoarseness due to lesion to left laryngeal recurrent nerve
Cerfolio et al. [69]	153	Anterior mediastinal Inferior/posterior pathology	0	Conversion to thoracotomy, $n = 1$ Esophageal leak, $n = 1$ Atrial fibrillation, $n = 4$ Pneumothorax, $n = 2$ Prolonged air leak, $n = 1$
Park et al. [71]	34	Lobectomy	Conversion to open thoracotomy, $n = 3$ Lack lung isolation, $n = 1$	Supraventricular arrhythmia, $n = 6$ Bleeding, $n = 1$ Air leak, $n = 1$
Gharagozloo et al. [73]	100	Lobectomy	0	Atrial fibrillation, $n = 4$ Air leak, $n = 2$ Bleeding, $n = 1$ Pleural effusion, $n = 2$
Van Hillegersberg et al. [82]	21	Esophagectomy	Conversion to open procedure, $n = 3$	Pulmonary complication 60%, first 10 cases Pulmonary complication 32%, 11 patients
Kim et al. [83]	21	Esophagectomy	Bleeding, $n = 1$	Anastomotic leakage, $n = 4$ Vocal cord paralysis, $n = 6$
Suda et al. [89]	16	Esophagectomy		Vocal cord paralysis, $n = 6$ Anastomotic leakage, $n = 6$ Pneumonia, $n = 1$
Dunn et al. [88]	40	Esophagectomy		Anastomotic leakage, $n = 10$ Recent laryngeal nerve injury, $n = 14$
Cerfolio et al. [90]	22	Esophagectomy	Conversion from laparoscopy to laparotomy, $n = 1$	Anastomotic leakage, $n = 1$ Atrial fibrillation, $n = 1$

pain, operative time, or total costs. Table 13.5 displays the complications of robotic-assisted thoracic surgery involving the mediastinum lung and esophagus.

Although the outcome of robotic-assisted minimally invasive esophagectomy compared to thoracic minimally invasive esophagectomy is comparable, one of the advantages of using robotic technique is the reduced incidence of vocal cord paralysis. Three-dimensional images enhance identification of the recurrent laryngeal nerve; therefore it could reduce the chance of damaging the nerve. One study [89] reported a reduced incidence of vocal cord paralysis by approximately 50% when a robotic-assisted technique was used (6/38 vs. 15/20). Other reported complications include anastomotic leakage, bleeding, dysrhythmia, and acute lung injury [90].

G. Summary

The use of the da Vinci robotic surgical system in thoracic and esophageal surgery continues to gain acceptance. Although its use has reduced surgical scarring and decreased length of stay, specific indications for use in these areas need to be determined. All reports to date describe the use of lung isolation devices, most often a left-sided DLT, as part of the intraoperative management of thoracic surgery patients to facilitate surgical exposure. In addition, because the surgical approach varies depending on the thoracic procedure, optimal positioning is not standard, and varies among the specific surgical procedures. Vigilance is required with patients' elevated arms to avoid nerve injuries or crush injuries from the robotic arms. Continuous low-flow insufflation of CO_2 has been used as an aid for surgical exposure during minimally invasive thoracic procedures. The potential to convert to an open thoracotomy requires preparation by the surgical team and anesthesiologist. The use of the da Vinci robotic surgical system is expected to grow in the years to come. Prospective studies are needed to define the specific advantages of this robotic system.

REFERENCES

OPCAB and MIDCAB

1. Clements F, Shanewise J, eds. *Minimally Invasive Cardiac and Vascular Surgical Techniques.* Society of Cardiovascular Anesthesiologists Monograph. Philadelphia, PA: Lippincott Williams & Wilkins; 2001.
2. Benetti FJ, Naselli G, Wood M, et al. Direct myocardial revascularization without extracorporeal circulation. *Chest.* 1991; 100(2):312–316.
3. **Mack M, Bachand D, Acuff T, et al. Improved outcomes in coronary artery bypass grafting with beating-heart techniques. *J Thorac Cardiovasc Surg.* 2002;124(3):598–607.**
4. Chassot PG, van der Linden P, Zaugg M, et al. Off-pump coronary artery bypass surgery: physiology and anesthetic management. *Br J Anesth.* 2004;92(3):400–413.
5. Bonchek LI. Off pump coronary bypass: is it for everyone? *J Thorac Cardiovasc Surg.* 2002;124(3):431–434.
6. Angelini GD, Taylor FC, Reeves BC, et al. Early and midterm outcome after off-pump and on-pump surgery in Beating Heart Against Cardioplegic Arrest Studies (BHACAS 1 and 2): a pooled analysis of two randomized controlled trials. *Lancet.* 2002;359(9313):1194–1199.
7. van Dijk D, Nierich AP, Jansen EW, et al. Early outcome after off-pump versus on-pump coronary artery bypass. *Circulation.* 2001;104(15):1761–1766.
8. **Puskas JD, Williams WH, Mahoney EM, et al. Off-pump vs conventional coronary artery bypass grafting: early and 1-year graft patency, cost, and quality-of-life outcomes: a randomized trial. *JAMA.* 2004;291(15):1841–1849.**
9. Khan NE, De Souza A, Mister R, et al. A randomized comparison of off-pump and on-pump multivessel coronary artery bypass surgery. *N Engl J Med.* 2004;350(1):21–28.
10. Puskas JD, Williams WH, Duke PG, et al. Off-pump coronary artery bypass grafting provides complete revascularization with reduced myocardial injury, transfusion requirements, and length of stay: a prospective randomized comparison of two hundred unselected patients undergoing off-pump versus conventional coronary artery bypass grafting. *J Thorac Cardiovasc Surg.* 2003;125(4):797–808.
11. Hueb W, Lopes NH, Pereira AC, et al. Five-year follow-up of a randomized comparison between off-pump and on-pump stable multivessel coronary artery bypass grafting. *Circulation.* 2010;122(suppl 1):S48–S52.
12. Puskas JD, Williams WH, O'Donnell R, et al. Off-pump and on-pump coronary artery bypass grafting are associated with similar graft patency, myocardial ischemia, and freedom from reintervention: long-term follow-up of a randomized trial. *Ann Thorac Surg.* 2011;91(6):1836–1843.
13. Shroyer AL, Grover FL, Hattler B, et al; Veterans Affairs Randomized On/Off Bypass (ROOBY) Study Group. On-pump versus off-pump coronary-artery bypass surgery. *N Engl J Med.* 2009;361(19):1827–1837.
14. Légaré JF, Buth KJ, Hirsch GM. Conversion to on pump from OPCAB is associated with increased mortality: results from a randomized controlled trial. *Eur J Cardiothorac Surg.* 2005;27(2):296–301.
15. Novitzky D, Baltz JH, Hattler B, et al. Outcomes after conversion in the veterans affairs randomized on versus off bypass trial. *Ann Thorac Surg.* 2011;92(6):2147–2154.
16. Schwann NM, Horrow JC, Strong MD 3rd, et al. Does off-pump coronary artery bypass reduce the incidence of clinically evident renal dysfunction after multivessel myocardial revascularization? *Anesth Analg.* 2004;99(4):959–964.
17. Eagle KA, Guyton RA, Davidoff R, et al. ACC/AHA 2004 guideline update for coronary artery bypass graft surgery: summary article: a report of the ACC/AHA Task Force on Practice Guidelines (Committee to Update the 1999 Guidelines on CABG surgery). *Circulation.* 2004;100(9):1168–1176.
18. Cason BA, Gamperl AK, Slocum RE, et al. Anesthetic-induced preconditioning. *Anesthesiology.* 1997;87(5):1182–1190.
19. Zenati M, Cohen HA, Griffith BP. Alternative approach to multivessel coronary disease with integrated coronary revascularization. *J Thorac Cardiovasc Surg.* 1999;117:439–446.
20. Grocott HP, Mathew JP, Carver EH, et al. A randomized controlled trial of the Arctic Sun temperature management system versus conventional methods for preventing hypothermia during off-pump cardiac surgery. *Anesth Analg.* 2004;98(2):298–302.
21. **Resano FG, Stamou SC, Lowery RC, et al. Complete myocardial revascularization on the beating heart with epicardial stabilization: anesthetic considerations. *J Cardiothorac Vasc Anesth.* 2000;14(5):534–539.**
22. Moisés VA, Mesquita CB, Campos O, et al. Importance of intraoperative transesophageal echocardiography during coronary surgery without cardiopulmonary bypass. *J Am Soc Echocardiogr.* 1998;11(12):1139–1144.
23. Djaiani G, Karski J, Yudin M, et al. Clinical outcomes in patients undergoing elective coronary artery bypass graft surgery with and without utilization of pulmonary artery catheter-generated data. *J Cardiothorac Vasc Anesth.* 2006;20(3):307–310.

24. George SJ, Al-Ruzzeh S, Amrani M. Mitral annulus distortion during beating heart surgery: a potential cause for hemodynamic disturbance–a three-dimensional echocardiography reconstruction study. *Ann Thorac Surg.* 2002;73(5):1424–1430.
25. Hatton KW, Kilinski L, Ramiah C, et al. Multiple failed external defibrillation attempts during robot-assisted internal mammary harvest for myocardial revascularization. *Anesth Analg.* 2006;103:1113–1114.
26. Dhole S, Mehta Y, Saxena H, et al. Comparison of continuous thoracic epidural and paravertebral blocks for postoperative analgesia after minimally invasive direct coronary artery bypass surgery. *J Cardiothorac Vasc Anesth.* 2001;15(3):288–292.
27. Gründeman PF, Borst C, van Herwaarden JA, et al. Vertical displacement of the beating heart by the Octopus Tissue Stabilizer: influence on coronary flow. *Ann Thorac Surg.* 1998;65(5):1348–1352.
28. Mariani MA, Gu YJ, Boonstra PW, et al. Procoagulant activity after off-pump coronary operation: is the current anticoagulation adequate? *Ann Thorac Surg.* 1999;67(5):1370–1375.
29. Murphy GJ, Mango E, Lucchetti V, et al. A randomized trial of tranexamic acid in combination with cell salvage plus a meta-analysis of randomized trials evaluating tranexamic acid in off-pump coronary artery bypass grafting. *J Thorac Cardiovasc Surg.* 2006;132(3):475–480.

Minimally Invasive Valve Surgery
30. Caffarelli AD, Robbins RC. Will minimally invasive valve replacement ever really be important? *Curr Op Cardiol.* 2004;19(2): 123–127.
31. Cosgrove DM, Sabik JF, Navia JL. Minimally invasive valve operations. *Ann Thorac Surg.* 1998;65(6):1535–1539.
32. Swerc MF, Benckart DH, Wiechmann RJ, et al. Partial versus full sternotomy for aortic valve replacement. *Ann Thorac Surg.* 1999;68(6):2209–2213.
33. Asher CR, DiMengo JM, Arheart KL, et al. Atrial fibrillation early postoperatively following minimally invasive cardiac valvular surgery. *Am J Cardiol.* 1999;84(6):744–747.
34. Byrne JG, Karavas AN, Filsoufi F, et al. Aortic valve surgery after previous coronary artery bypass grafting with functioning internal mammary artery grafts. *Ann Thorac Surg.* 2002;73(3):779–784.
35. **Walther W, Falk V, Mohr FW. Minimally invasive surgery for valve disease. *Curr Prob Cardiol.* 2006;31(6):399–437.**
36. Secknus MA, Asher CR, Scalia GM, et al. Intraoperative transesophageal echocardiography in minimally invasive cardiac valve surgery. *J Am Soc Echocardiogr.* 1999;12(4):231–236.
37. Feldman T, Foster E, Glower DD, et al. Percutaneous repair or surgery for mitral regurgitation. *N Engl J Med.* 2011;364(15):1395–1406.
38. Treede H, Schirmer J, Rudolph V, et al. A heart team's perspective on interventional mitral valve repair: percutaneous clip implantation as an important adjunct to a surgical mitral valve program for treatment of high-risk patients. *J Thorac Cardiovasc Surg.* 2012;143(1):78–84.
39. **Nobuyoshi M, Arita T, Shirai S, et al. Percutaneous balloon mitral valvuloplasty: a review. *Circulation.* 2009;119(8): e211–e219.**
40. Smith CR, Leon MB, Mack MJ, et al. Transcatheter versus surgical aortic-valve replacement in high-risk patients. *N Engl J Med.* 2011;364(23):2187–2198.

Robotic Cardiac Surgery
41. **Vernick W, Alturi P. Robotic and Minimally Invasive Cardiac Surgery. *Anesthesiol Clin.* 2013;31(2):299–320.**
42. **Loulmet D, Carpentier A, d'Attellis N, et al. Endoscopic coronary artery bypass grafting with the aid of robotic assisted instruments. *J Thorac Cardiovasc Surg.* 1999;118(1):4–10.**
43. Reichenspurner H, Damiano RJ, Mack MJ, et al. Use of the voice-controlled and computer-assisted surgical system ZEUS for endoscopic coronary artery bypass grafting. *J Throac Cardiovasc Surg.* 1999;118:11–16.
44. Chitwood WR Jr, Nifong LW, Elbeery JE, et al. Robotic mitral valve repair: trapezoidal resection and prosthetic annuloplasty with the Da Vinci Surgical System. *J Thorac Cardiovasc Surg.* 2000;120(6):1171–1172.
45. **Rehfeldt KH, Mauermann WJ, Burkhart HM, et al. Robot-assisted mitral valve repair. *J Cardiothorac Vasc Anesth.* 2011;25(4):721–730.**
46. **Bonatti JO, Zimrin D, Lehr EJ, et al. Hybrid Coronary Revascularization Using Robotic Totally Endoscopic Surgery: Perioperative Outcomes and 5-Year Results. *Ann Thorac Surg.* 2012;94(6):1920–1926.**
47. Suri RM, Burkhart HM, Schaff HV. Robot-Assisted Valve replacement using a novel sutureless bovine pericardial prosthesis. Proof of concept as an alternative to percutaneous implantation. *Innovations (Phila).* 2010;5(6):419–423.
48. Taylor, RH, Lavallee S, Burdea GC, et al. *Computer-Integrated Surgery: Technology and Clinical Applications.* Cambridge, MA: The MIT Press; 1996.
49. Yanagawa F, Perez M, Bell T, et al. Critical outcomes in non robotic vs robotic assisted cardiac surgery. *JAMA Surgery.* 2015; 150(8):771–777.
50. Mack MJ. Minimally invasive and robotic surgery. *JAMA.* 2001;285(5):568–572.
51. **Mohr FW, Falk V, Digeler A, et al. Computer-enhanced "robotic" cardiac surgery: experience in 148 patients. *J Thorac Cardiovasc Surg.* 2001;121(5):842–853.**
52. Kaneko T, Chitwood WR Jr, et al. Current readings: Status of robotic cardiac surgery. *Semin Thoracic Surg.* 25(2):165–170.
53. **Moodley S, Schoenhagen P, Gillinov AM, et al. Preoperative multidetector computed tomography angiography for planning minimally invasive robotic mitral valve surgery: impact on decision making. *J Thorac Cardiovasc Surg.* 2013;146(2):262–268.**
54. **Gillinov AM, Suri RM, Mick S, et al. Robotic mitral valve surgery: current limitations and future directions. *Ann Cardiothorac Surg.* 2016;5(6):573–576.**
55. **Deshpande SP, Lehr E, Odonkor P, et al. Anesthetic management of robotically assisted totally endoscopic coronary artery bypass surgery (TECAB). *J Cardiothorac Vasc Anesth.* 2013;27(3):586–599.**
56. Ohtsuka T, Imanaka K, Endsh M, et al. Hemodynamic effects of carbon dioxide insufflation under single-lung ventilation during thoracoscopy. *Ann Thorac Surg.* 1999;68:29–33.

57. Coddens J, Deloof T, Hendrickx J, et al. **Transesophageal echocardiography for port-access surgery.** *J Cardiothorac Vasc Anesth.* **1999;13(5):614–622.**

58. Labriola C, Greco F, et al. Percutaneous coronary sinus catheterization with ProPlege catheter under transesophageal echocardiography and pressure guidance. *J Cardiothorac Vasc Anesth.* 2015;29(3):598–604.

59. Herman CR, Sunadaram B, Goldhammer JE. Misadventures of a retrograde cardioplegia catheter. *J Cardiothorac Vasc Anesth.* 2016;30(6):1614–1617.

Anesthesia for Robotic Non-Cardiac Thoracic Surgery

60. **Campos J. Anesthesia for robotic thoracic surgery. In: Slinger P, ed.** *Principles and Practice of Anesthesia for Thoracic Surgery.* **2nd ed. New York: Springer; 2018:445–452.**

61. Campos JH, Anaesthesia for Robotic Surgery: Mediastinal Mass Resection and Pulmonary Resections. *Anaesth Int Clin.* 2011;19–22.

62. Abel M, Eisenkraft JB. Anesthetic implications of myasthenia gravis. *Mt Sinai J Med.* 2002;69(1–2):31–37.

63. Pandey R, Elakkumanan LB, Garg R, et al. Brachial plexus injury after robotic-assisted thoracoscopic thymectomy. *J Cardiothorac Vasc Anesth.* 2009;23(4):584–586.

64. Bodner J, Wykypiel H, Greiner A, et al. Early experience with robot-assisted surgery for mediastinal masses. *Ann Thorac Surg.* 2004;78(1):259–265.

65. Savitt MA, Gao G, Furnary AP, et al. Application of robotic-assisted techniques to the surgical evaluation and treatment of the anterior mediastinum. *Ann Thorac Surg.* 2005;79(2):450–455.

66. Rückert JC, Ismail M, Swierzy M, et al. Thoracoscopic thymectomy with the da Vinci robotic system for myasthenia gravis. *Ann NY Acad Sci.* 2008;1132:329–335.

67. Buentzel J, Straube C, Heinz, et al. Thymectomy via open surgery or robotic video assisted thoracic surgery: Can a recommendation already be made? *Medicine (Baltimore).* 2017;96(24):e7161.

68. **Buentzel J, Heinz J, Hinterthaner M, et al. Robotic versus thoracoscopic thymectomy: The current evidence.** *Int J Med Robot.* **2017;13(4). doi: 10.1002/rcs.1847**

69. Cerfolio RJ, Bryant AS, Minnich DJ. Operative techniques in robotic thoracic surgery for inferior or posterior mediastinal pathology. *J Thorac Cardiovasc Surg.* 2012;143(5):1138–1143.

70. Liang H, Liang W, Zhao L, et al. Robotic versus video-assisted lobectomy/segmentectomy for lung cancer: A meta-analysis. *Ann Surg.* 16 June 2017.

71. Park BJ, Flores RM, Rusch VW. Robotic assistance for video-assisted thoracic surgical lobectomy: technique and initial results. *J Thorac Cardiovasc Surg.* 2006;131(1):54–59.

72. Anderson CA, Filsoufi F, Aklog L, et al. Robotic-assisted lung resection for malignant disease. *Innovations.* 2007;2:254–258.

73. Gharagozloo F, Margolis M, Tempesta B, et al. Robot-assisted lobectomy for early-stage lung cancer: report of 100 consecutive cases. *Ann Thorac Surg.* 2009;88(2):380–384.

74. **Ye X, Xie L, Chen G, et al. Robotic thoracic surgery versus video-assisted thoracic surgery for lung cancer: a meta-analysis.** *Interact Cardiovasc Thorac Surg.* **2015;21:409–414.**

75. Grogan EL, Jones DR. VATS lobectomy is better than open thoracotomy: what is the evidence for short-term outcomes. *Thorac Surg Clin.* 2008;18(3):249–258.

76. Kwon ST, Zhao L, Reddy RM, et al. Evaluation of acute and chronic pain outcomes after robotic, video-assisted thoracoscopic surgery, or open anatomic pulmonary resection. *J Thorac Cardiovasc Surg.* 2017;154(2):652–659.

77. Ohtsuka T, Nakajima J, Kotsuka Y, et al. Hemodynamic response to intrapleural insufflation with hemipulmonary collapse. *Surg Endosc.* 2001;15:1327–1330.

78. El-Dawlatly AA, Al-Dohayan A, Abdel-Meguid ME, et al. Variations in dynamic lung compliance during endoscopic thoracic sympathectomy with carbon dioxide insufflation. *Clin Auton Res.* 2003;13(1):I94–I97.

79. Campos J, Ueda K. Update on Anesthetic Complications of Robotic Thoracic Surgery. *Minerva Anestesiol.* 2014;80:83–88.

80. Kernstine KH, DeArmond DT, Karimi M, et al. The robotic, 2-stage, 3-field esophagolymphadenectomy. *J Thorac Cardiovasc Surg.* 2004;127:1847–1849.

81. Bodner JC, Zitt M, Ott H, et al. Robotic-assisted thoracoscopic surgery (RATS) for benign and malignant esophageal tumors. *Ann Thorac Surg.* 2005;80:1202–1206.

82. van Hillegersberg R, Boone J, Draaisma WA, et al. First experience with robot-assisted thoracoscopic esophagolymphadenectomy for esophageal cancer. *Surg Endosc.* 2006;20:1435–1439.

83. Kim DJ, Hyung WJ, Lee CY, et al. Thoracoscopic esophagectomy for esophageal cancer: feasibility and safety of robotic assistance in the prone position. *J Thorac Cardiovasc Surg.* 2010;139(1):53–59.

84. Gutt CN, Bintintan VV, Köninger J, et al. Robotic-assisted transhiatal esophagectomy. *Langenbecks Arch Surg.* 2006;391(14):428–434.

85. Kernstine KH, DeArmond DT, Shamoun DM, et al. The first series of completely robotic esophagectomies with three-field lymphadenectomy: initial experience. *Surg Endosc.* 2007;21:2285–2292.

86. Nifong LW, Chitwood WR Jr. Challenges for the anesthesiologist: robotics? *Anesth Analg.* 2003;96(1):1–2.

87. **Rea F, Marulli G, Bortolotti L, et al. Experience with the "da Vinci" robotic system for thymectomy in patients with myasthenia gravis: report of 33 cases.** *Ann Thorac Surg.* **2006;81(2):455–459.**

88. Dunn DH, Johnson EM, Morphew JA, et al. Robot-assisted transhiatal esophagectomy: a 3-year single-center experience. *Dis Esophagus.* 2013;26(2):159–166.

89. Suda K, Ishida Y, Kawamura Y, et al. Robot-assisted thoracoscopic lymphadenectomy along the left recurrent laryngeal nerve for esophageal squamous cell carcinoma in the prone position: technical report and short-term outcomes. *World J Surg.* 2012;36(7):1608–1616.

90. Cerfolio RJ, Bryant AS, Hawn MT. Technical aspects and early results of robotic esophagectomy with chest anastomosis. *J Thorac Cardiovasc Surg.* 2013;145(1):90–96.

14 Anesthetic Management for Thoracic Aortic Aneurysm and Dissection

Amanda A. Fox and John R. Cooper, Jr.

KEY POINTS

1. An aortic dissection usually occurs when blood penetrates the aortic intima, forming either an expanding hematoma within the aortic wall or simply a false channel for blood flow between the medial layer.
2. An aortic aneurysm involves dilation of all three layers of the aortic wall.
3. The term dissecting aneurysm, although commonly used, is often a misnomer because the aorta may not be dilated.
4. Administering a potent arterial vasodilator such as nitroprusside or nicardipine and a β-blocker to decrease left ventricular (LV) ejection velocity is critical to preventing further propagation of aortic dissection, rupture of a torn aorta, or a leaking thoracic aortic aneurysm.
5. Concomitant aortic valve repair or replacement is often needed with repair of aortic dissection or aneurysm. Which procedure is used depends on involvement of the sinus of Valsalva and the aortic annulus.
6. Managing left heart bypass (LHB) can be challenging for the cardiac anesthesiologist while descending thoracic aneurysms or aortic tears are being repaired (see Table 14.11). Transesophageal echocardiography (TEE) is very useful for guiding volume management, because native cardiac output must be preserved to provide adequate blood flow to the brain.
7. Cerebral spinal fluid drainage has been shown in randomized studies to significantly decrease the incidence of postoperative paraplegia and paraparesis in appropriately selected patients who undergo descending thoracic aortic surgery.

ANESTHESIOLOGISTS CARING FOR THORACIC AORTIC surgical patients encounter considerable variation among patients with regard to the cause and location of aortic disease. It is vital that anesthesiologists understand the implications of and the challenges related to these variations in providing optimal perioperative care. Members of both the American Society of Anesthesiologists and the Society of Cardiovascular Anesthesiologists were involved in the multidisciplinary development of the 2010 ACCF/AHA/AATS/ACR/ASA/SCA/SCAI/SIR/STS/SVM Guidelines for the Diagnosis and Management of Patients with Thoracic Aortic Disease [1]. This chapter gives a concise overview of the pathophysiology of thoracic aortic surgery, a review of its surgical approaches and results, and a rational approach to managing patients undergoing thoracic aortic surgery. Surgery on the thoracic aorta, particularly the descending and thoracoabdominal aorta, can require complex anesthetic management. Therefore, each team member must have a clear understanding of what is being planned. Often, all that is required is a brief preoperative conversation among the surgeon, anesthesiologist, nursing team, and perfusionist as to the exact requirements for a particular procedure.

CLINICAL PEARL Anesthetic management of thoracic aneurysms requires knowledge of aortic anatomy, the planned surgical approach, the adjuncts needed, and excellent communication with the surgeon.

I. **Classification and natural history**
  A. **Dissection**

1

An *aortic dissection* usually occurs when blood penetrates the aortic intima, forming either an expanding hematoma (also called a dissecting hematoma) within the aortic wall or simply a false channel for flow between the medial layers. The true lumen of the dissecting aorta is generally not dilated; rather, it is often compressed by the dissection. Because the dissection does not necessarily involve the entire circumference of the aorta, branching vessels may be

2

unaffected, they may be occluded, or they may arise from the false lumen. An *aortic aneurysm* involves dilation of all three layers of the aortic wall and has different pathophysiology and

3

management concerns from those of a dissection. The term *dissecting aneurysm*, although commonly used, is often a misnomer because the aorta frequently is not dilated.

  1. **Incidence and pathophysiology**
    a. **Incidence.** The incidence of dissection in the United States is unclear, mainly because of underreporting; however, European studies have reported an incidence of 3.2 dissections per 100,000 autopsies, and that the incidence increased over time. Also, dissection results in more deaths than does aneurysm rupture [2].
    b. **Predisposing conditions.** The medical conditions predisposing to aortic dissection are listed in Table 14.1 in general order of importance. Interestingly, *atherosclerosis* by itself may not contribute to the risk of subsequent aortic dissection.
    c. **Inciting event.** The onset of aortic dissection has been associated with increased physical activity or emotional stress. Dissection also has been associated with blunt trauma to the chest; however, the temporal relationship between blunt trauma and subsequent dissection has not been well established. Dissection can occur without any physical

TABLE 14.1 Conditions predisposing to aortic dissection

History of hypertension	Present in ≈90% of patients
Advanced age	>60 yrs
Sex	Male preponderance age <60 yrs
Arachnodactyly	Connective tissue disorders (e.g., Marfan syndrome)
Congenital heart disease	Coarctation of aorta, bicuspid aortic valve
Pregnancy	Uncommon
Other causes	Toxins and diet

TABLE 14.2 Sites of primary intimal tears in acute dissection of the aorta (398 autopsy cases)

Site	Percent incidence
Ascending	61
Descending	24
Isthmus	16
Other	8
Arch	9
Abdominal	3
Other	1

Modified from Hirst AE Jr, Johns VJ Jr, Kime W Jr. Dissecting aneurysm of the aorta: a review of 505 cases. *Medicine (Baltimore)*. 1958;37(3):243.

activity. It also can occur during cannulation for cardiopulmonary bypass (CPB), either antegrade from the ascending aorta or retrograde from the femoral artery (FA).

d. **Mechanism of aortic tear.** An intimal tear is the initial event in aortic dissection. The tear usually occurs in a weakened portion of the aortic wall and typically involves the middle and outer layers of the media. In this area of weakening, the aortic wall is more susceptible to shear forces produced by pulsatile blood flow through the aorta. Thus, intimal tears most frequently arise in the areas subject to the greatest mechanical shear forces (Table 14.2): the ascending and isthmic (just distal to the left subclavian artery (LSA)) segments of the aorta, which are particularly vulnerable because they are relatively fixed.

In large autopsy series, however, up to 4% of dissections involved no identifiable intimal disruption. In these cases, rupture of the *vasa vasorum*, the vessels that supply blood to the aortic wall, has been implicated as an alternative cause of dissection. The thin-walled vasa vasorum are located in the outer third of the aortic wall, and their rupture would cause the formation of a medial hematoma and propagation of a dissection in an already diseased vessel, without formation of an intimal tear.

e. **Propagation.** An aortic dissection can propagate within seconds. The factors that contribute to propagation are the hemodynamic forces inherent in pulsatile flow: pulse pressure and ejection velocity of blood.

f. **Exit points.** Exit points are found in a relatively small percentage of dissection cases. Exit-point tears usually occur distal to the intimal tear and represent points at which blood from the false lumen reenters the true lumen. The presence or absence of an exit point does not appear to affect the clinical course.

g. **Involvement of arterial branches.** Aortic dissection can involve the origins of the major branches of the aorta, including the coronary arteries. Their involvement ranges from branch-vessel occlusion due to mechanical compression by the false lumen to propagation of the dissecting hematoma into the arterial branch. The incidence of involvement of the various arterial branches in a large autopsy series is listed in Table 14.3 [3].

2. **DeBakey classification of dissections** (Fig. 14.1). This classification consists of three different types based on the location of the intimal tear and the section of the aorta involved.

a. **Type I.** The intimal tear is located in the ascending portion, but the dissection involves all portions of the thoracic aorta (ascending, arch, and descending) and may extend into the abdominal aorta.

b. **Type II.** The intimal tear is in the ascending aorta, and the dissection involves the ascending aorta only, stopping before the takeoff of the innominate artery.

c. **Type III.** The intimal tear is located in the descending segment. If the dissection involves the descending portion of the thoracic aorta only, starting distal to the origin of the LSA and ending above the diaphragm, it is considered type III A.

TABLE 14.3 Involvement of major arterial branches in aortic dissections

Artery	Percent incidence
Iliac	25.2
Common carotid	14.5
Innominate	12.9
Renal (either)	12.0
Left subclavian	10.9
Mesenteric	8.2
Coronary (either)	7.5
Intercostal	4.0
Celiac	3.2
Lumbar	1.6

Modified from Hirst AE Jr, Johns VJ Jr, Kime W Jr. Dissecting aneurysm of the aorta: a review of 505 cases. *Medicine (Baltimore)*. 1958;37(3):243.

    If the dissection propagates below the diaphragm, it is considered type III B. By definition, type III dissection can extend proximally into the arch, but this is rare.

3. **Stanford (Daily) classification of dissections** (Fig. 14.2). This classification is simpler than DeBakey's and perhaps has more clinical relevance.

    a. **Type A.** Type A dissections are those that have any involvement of the ascending aorta, regardless of where the intimal tear is located or how far the dissection propagates. Clinically, type A dissections run a more virulent course and are generally considered urgent or emergent cases. They are most often managed with open-chest surgical repair.

    b. **Type B.** Type B dissections involve the aorta distal to the origin of the LSA. Many cases can be managed medically or with endovascular (EV) therapy.

4. **Natural history**

    a. **Mortality—untreated.** The survival rate of untreated patients with ascending aortic dissection is dismal, with a 2-day mortality of up to 50% in some series and 3-month

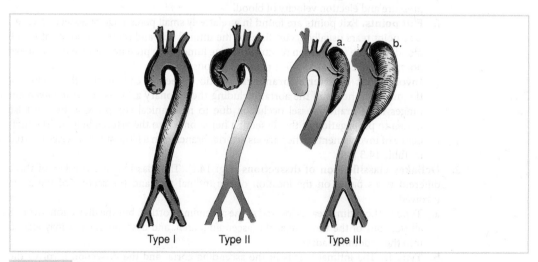

Type I   Type II   Type III

FIGURE 14.1 DeBakey classification of aortic dissections by location: type I, with intimal tear in the ascending portion and dissection extending to descending aorta; type II, ascending intimal tear and dissection limited to ascending aorta; type III, intimal tear distal to left subclavian, but dissection extending for a variable distance, either to the diaphragm (*a*) or to the iliac artery (*b*). (From DeBakey ME, Henly WS, Cooley DA, et al. Surgical management of dissecting aneurysms of the aorta. *J Thorac Cardiovasc Surg.* 1965;49:131, with permission.)

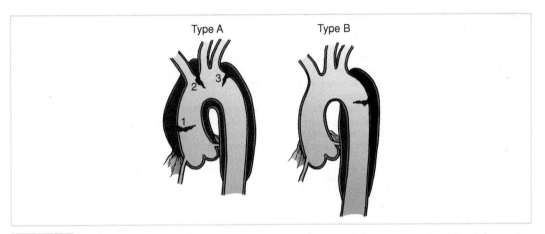

FIGURE 14.2 Stanford (Daily) classification of aortic dissections. Type A describes a dissection involving the ascending aorta regardless of site of intimal tear (*1*, ascending; *2*, arch; *3*, descending). In type B, both the intimal tear and the extension are distal to the left subclavian. (From Miller DC, Stinson EB, Oyer PE, et al. Operative treatment of aortic dissections. Experience with 125 patients over a sixteen-year period. *J Thorac Cardiovasc Surg*. 1979;78:367, with permission.)

mortality approaching 90% [3]. The usual cause of death is rupture of the false lumen into the pleural space or pericardium. Mortality is lower with DeBakey type III or Stanford type B dissection. Other causes of death include progressive cardiac failure (aortic valve involvement), myocardial infarction (coronary artery involvement), stroke (occlusion of cerebral vessels), and bowel gangrene (mesenteric artery occlusion).

    b. **Surgical mortality.** Overall mortality ranges from 3% to 24% and varies with the section of aorta that is affected. Dissection involving the aortic arch carries the highest mortality [2].

B. Aneurysm
  1. **Incidence.** In the European studies cited above, the prevalence of thoracic aneurysm among autopsied patients was approximately 460 in 100,000. In one study, 45% of thoracic aneurysms involved the ascending aorta, 10% the arch, 35% the descending aorta, and 10% the thoracoabdominal aorta [4].
  2. **Classification by location and cause.** In general, the causes and pathophysiology of aortic aneurysm are site dependent (Table 14.4). Most commonly, ascending aortic aneurysms are due to medial degeneration, whereas descending and thoracoabdominal aortic aneurysms result from degenerative conditions associated with atherosclerosis.
  3. **Classification by shape**
    a. **Fusiform.** Fusiform aneurysmal dilation involves the entire circumference of the aortic wall.
    b. **Saccular.** Saccular aneurysms involve only part of the circumference of the aortic wall. Isolated *aortic arch aneurysms* are commonly saccular.
  4. **Natural history.** The natural history of aortic aneurysm is one of progressive dilation, and more than half of aortic aneurysms eventually rupture. The untreated, 5-year rate of survival for patients with thoracic aortic aneurysms ranges from 13% to 39% [2]. Other complications of thoracic aortic aneurysm include mycotic infection, atheroembolism to peripheral vessels, and dissection. This last complication is rare, probably occurring in fewer than 10% of cases. Some predictors of poor prognosis are large aneurysm size (i.e., maximum transverse diameter >10 cm), symptoms, and associated cardiovascular disease, especially coronary artery disease, myocardial infarction, or stroke.

C. Thoracic aortic rupture (tear)
  1. **Etiology.** Most thoracic aortic ruptures occur after trauma—almost always a *deceleration injury* from a motor vehicle accident. Sudden deceleration places great mechanical shear stress on points of the aortic wall that are relatively immobile. Whereas aortic rupture

TABLE 14.4 Causes of aneurysm based on location in the aorta

■ Ascending	
Medial necrosis	Accumulation of mucoid material between elastic elements in the outer third of aortic wall, eventually involving the entire media
Syphilis	Major cause before 1950, distinguished by invasion of the aortic wall by *Treponema pallidum*
Congenital	Secondary to inborn errors in metabolism (Marfan syndrome, Ehlers–Danlos syndrome) leading to generalized defect of connective tissue
Poststenotic dilation	Secondary to long-standing aortic stenosis
Atherosclerosis	Not a major cause in ascending pathology
■ Arch	
Isolated	Atherosclerosis
Associated with ascending disease	Same causes as for disease in ascending aorta
■ Descending	
Atherosclerosis	Begins as intimal disease; major cause of thoracoabdominal and abdominal aneurysm
Congenital	See under Ascending, above
Trauma	Causal relationship difficult to prove; history of blunt trauma may be distant
Infection	Syphilis, *Salmonella,* tuberculosis

Causes are listed in order of frequency.

leads to immediate exsanguination and death in many patients, approximately 10% to 15% of patients maintain integrity of the adventitial covering of the aortic lumen and therefore survive to emergency care. Surgical treatment of these survivors is often successful.

2. **Location.** Most thoracic aortic ruptures occur just distal to the origin of the LSA (isthmus), because of the relative fixation of the aorta at this point by the ligamentum arteriosum (Fig. 14.3). The second most common site of aortic rupture is in the ascending aorta, just distal to the aortic valve.

II. **Diagnosis**

A. **Clinical signs and symptoms** (Table 14.5)

1. **Dissection.** Aortic dissection usually presents with a dramatic onset and a fulminant course. Clinical presentations of Stanford types A and B are listed in Table 14.5.

2. **Aneurysm.** Aneurysms of the ascending aorta, aortic arch, or descending thoracic aorta often are asymptomatic until late in their course. In many circumstances, the aneurysm

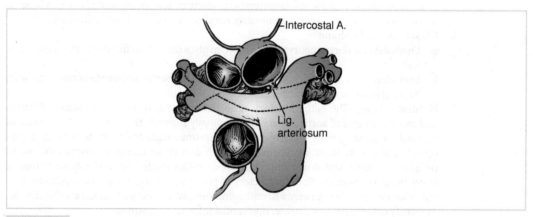

FIGURE 14.3 The heart and great vessels are relatively mobile in the pericardium, whereas the descending aorta is relatively fixed by its anatomic relations. The attachment of the ligamentum (Lig.) arteriosum enhances this immobility and increases the risk of aortic tear due to deceleration injury. A., artery. (From Cooley DA, ed. *Surgical Treatment of Aortic Aneurysms*. Philadelphia, PA: WB Saunders, 1986:186, with permission.)

TABLE 14.5 Presenting clinical signs and symptoms by location and type of aortic pathology

	Aneurysm	Dissection	Aortic tear
General presentation	Chronic symptoms, but leaking or ruptured aneurysm can lead to fulminant course (see Aortic tear for symptoms and signs)	Dramatic onset and fulminant course; symptoms depend on location (type A or type B) Patient presents in shock, anxious, diaphoretic	History of deceleration injury; usually fulminant course (good chance of survival if patient gets to treatment center). Patient can present in hypovolemic shock
Symptoms and signs **Ascending and arch**		**Type A dissection**[a]	
Location of pain	Anterior chest pain secondary to compression of (1) Coronary arteries (2) Sensory mediastinal nerves	Anterior chest pain secondary to (1) Extension of dissection (ripping or tearing sensation) (2) Angina, from dissection of coronaries	Chest pain secondary to compression of structures by enlarging adventitia (the only structure maintaining aortic integrity)
Cardiovascular	CHF symptoms secondary to aortic annular enlargement (1) Widened pulse pressure (2) Diastolic murmur Facial and upper trunk venous congestion secondary to superior vena cava compression BP usually elevated chronically	CHF symptoms: (1) Murmur of aortic valve insufficiency (2) Narrowing of true lumen (increased afterload), systolic ejection murmur BP (1) Hypotension secondary to rupture into the retroperitoneum, intra-abdominal, intrathoracic, or pericardial spaces (2) Hypertension secondary to pain, anxiety Asymmetry of pulses, or pulseless extremity	BP (1) Hypotension from hypovolemia (2) Hypertension from pain
Respiratory	Hoarseness secondary to compression of recurrent laryngeal nerve Dyspnea or stridor due to tracheal compression Hemoptysis due to erosion into trachea Rales secondary to CHF	Hoarseness secondary to compression of recurrent laryngeal nerve Dyspnea and stridor due to tracheal compression Hemoptysis due to erosion into trachea (chronic) Rales secondary to CHF	Lung contusion if chest trauma is significant
Gastrointestinal	Not usually affected	See under Descending	Not usually affected
Renal	Not usually affected	See under Descending	Decreased function secondary to hypotension
Neurologic	Possible because of emboli to carotid artery from aortic valve or aneurysmal segment (see Dissection, at right)	Hemiparesis or hemiplegia secondary to involvement of single carotid artery Reversible or progressive coma	Symptoms related to hypoperfusion

(continued)

TABLE 14.5 Presenting clinical signs and symptoms by location and type of aortic pathology (*continued*)

	Aneurysm	Dissection	Aortic tear
Descending		**Type B dissection**	
Location of pain	Chronic back pain may occur	Located in back, midscapular region	Located in midscapular region
Cardiovascular	BP usually normal or elevated (chronic hypertension)	BP (1) Elevated secondary to pain (common) (2) Hypotension if rupture of dissection has occurred	BP (1) Elevated secondary to pain (especially with other injuries from trauma) (2) Hypotension if hypovolemic
Respiratory	Dyspnea from left main stem bronchial obstruction Hemoptysis due to erosion into left bronchus Hemorrhagic pleural effusion	Dyspnea due to left main stem bronchial obstruction Hemorrhagic pleural effusion	Sequelae of lung contusion or rib fracture
Gastrointestinal	Usually normal	Mimics an acute abdomen (1) Pain, rigid abdomen, nausea, and vomiting (2) Gastrointestinal bleeding Bowel ischemia secondary to compression or dissection of mesenteric or celiac artery	Usually normal
Renal	Renal insufficiency or renovascular hypertension if occlusive aortic disease develops	Ischemia due to involvement of renal arteries in dissection: (1) Infarction and renal failure (2) Renal insufficiency	Renal hypofunction from hypoperfusion or hypovolemia
Neurologic	Usually not affected	Paraparesis or paraplegia possible secondary to occlusion of critical spinal cord blood flow	Paraplegia possible

*Type A dissections may involve the entire aorta; therefore, symptoms of both ascending and descending pathology may be present.
BP, blood pressure; CHF, congestive heart failure.

is not detected until medical evaluation is conducted for an unrelated problem or for a problem related to a complication of the aneurysm.

3. **Traumatic rupture.** Rupture most commonly occurs just distal to the LSA. If the patient survives the initial trauma, signs and symptoms are similar to those of aneurysms of the descending thoracic aorta.

B. **Diagnostic tests**

1. **Electrocardiogram (ECG).** Many patients with aortic disease will have evidence of *left ventricular (LV) hypertrophy on ECG*, secondary to the high incidence of hypertension in these patients. In patients with aortic dissection, the ECG may show ischemic changes caused by coronary artery involvement, or evidence of pericarditis from hemopericardium.

2. **Chest radiograph.** A *widened mediastinum* is a classic radiographic finding with thoracic aortic pathology. Widening of the aortic knob is often seen, with *disparate ascending-to-descending aortic diameter*. A double shadow has been described in patients with aortic dissection, secondary to visualization of the false lumen.

3. **Serum laboratory values.** There are no laboratory findings specifically associated with asymptomatic aortic aneurysms. Aortic dissection or rupture lowers hemoglobin levels. Dissection may raise cardiac enzyme levels by causing coronary artery occlusion, increase blood urea nitrogen and creatine levels through renal artery involvement, and lead to

metabolic acidosis due to low cardiac output or ischemic bowel. Fibrinogen levels may decrease in patients with associated disseminated intravascular coagulation.

4. **Computed tomographic scans and magnetic resonance imaging.** Computed tomography using intravenous (IV) contrast is a useful tool for ascertaining aneurysm size and location and has evolved into the standard modality for diagnosing and planning the surgical repair of aortic dissections and aneurysms. It is also useful for following the progression of aortic disease. Digital images can be manipulated into a three-dimensional form, which can make it easier to assess the lesion and plan repair. Magnetic resonance imaging is extremely sensitive and specific in identifying the entry tear location, presence of false lumen, aortic regurgitation, and pericardial effusion accompanying aortic dissection [5].

5. **Angiography.** This technique has been largely replaced by computed tomography scanning and magnetic resonance imaging but can be useful for delineating the involvement of the coronary arteries, as well as identifying significant coronary artery disease in patients with ascending aortic pathology. Patients with disease of the thoracic aorta often have concurrent coronary artery disease, and bypassing significant lesions may prevent perioperative myocardial infarction and improve ventricular function (VF) when patients are weaned from CPB.

6. **Transesophageal echocardiography (TEE).** TEE has proved highly sensitive and specific for diagnosing aortic dissection. In many cases, pulsed-wave and color flow Doppler imaging can aid in determining the presence, extent, and type of dissection. Identifying a mobile intimal flap constitutes a prompt bedside diagnosis that can be lifesaving. In addition, entry and reentry tears can be located; aortic regurgitation can be identified and quantified, LV function and wall-motion abnormalities can be assessed, pericardial effusion with possible associated cardiac tamponade can be identified, and follow-up studies of the false lumen can be made after therapeutic intervention.

   TEE can also be used to assess many thoracic aortic aneurysms. For ascending or descending thoracic aortic aneurysm in particular, the location, diameter, and extent of the aneurysm, as well as whether the aneurysm contains significant atheroma, can often be well described. TEE can also be used to determine whether the aneurysm is saccular or fusiform in shape. TEE rarely can be used to definitively identify aneurysmal involvement of the aortic arch and distal ascending aorta. This is because the trachea obscures the distal ascending aorta from TEE, and because the entire arch is not usually visible on TEE. Surgeons who desire detailed preoperative imaging of the aortic arch should confer with a radiologist about magnetic resonance or computerized tomographic imaging.

   Because traumatic aortic transection generally occurs just distal to the left subclavian takeoff, it is often easily and rapidly identified by TEE imaging. In addition, aortic transection operations are usually emergencies, so TEE imaging is advantageous because it can be conducted quickly and in most locations in the medical center.

C. **Indications for surgical correction**
   1. **Ascending aorta**
      a. **Dissection.** Acute type A dissection should be surgically corrected, given its virulent course and high associated mortality rate if not surgically treated.
      b. **Aneurysm.** Indications for surgical resection include the following:
         (1) Persistent pain despite a small aneurysm
         (2) Aortic valve involvement producing aortic insufficiency
         (3) Angina from LV strain secondary to aneurysmal involvement of the aortic valve or coronary arteries
         (4) Rapidly expanding aneurysm, or an aneurysm larger than 5 to 5.5 cm in diameter, because the chance of aortic rupture increases with the aneurysm's size
   2. **Aortic arch**
      a. **Dissection.** Acute dissection limited to the aortic arch is rare but is an indication for surgery.
      b. **Aneurysm.** Isolated aneurysm of the aortic arch is rare. However, arch involvement is often seen together with ascending aneurysm (less so with descending aneurysm) and

is thus dealt with at the time of surgical repair of the ascending aortic lesion. Indications to operate on the aortic arch include the following:

(1) Persistent symptoms

(2) Aneurysm larger than 5.5 to 6 cm in transverse diameter

(3) Progressive aneurysmal expansion

3. **Descending aorta**

a. **Dissection.** Some controversy remains concerning the best treatment for an acute type B dissection. Because in-hospital mortality statistics are better for medical versus surgical interventions and similar for medical versus EV management [6], type B dissection often is treated medically in the acute phase, especially if the patient's comorbidities make the risk of surgical mortality prohibitively high. However, patients with type B dissection are treated surgically or with EV repair if they have any of the following complications:

(1) Failure to control hypertension medically

(2) Continued pain (indicating progression of the dissection)

(3) Aneurysm enlargement on chest radiograph, computed tomographic scan, or angiogram

(4) Development of a neurologic deficit

(5) Evidence of renal or gastrointestinal ischemia

(6) Development of aortic insufficiency

b. **Aneurysm.** Indications for surgical or EV repair of descending thoracic aneurysm include the following:

(1) Aneurysm larger than 5.5 to 6 cm in diameter. In patients with known connective tissue disorders, the diameter threshold for repair may be lower [1]

(2) Aneurysm expanding

(3) Aneurysm leaking (causing more fulminant symptoms)

(4) Chronic aneurysm causing persistent pain or other symptoms

III. **Preoperative management of patients requiring surgery of the thoracic aorta**

Emergency preoperative management of *aortic dissection* is discussed below. However, emergency preoperative management is similar for a *leaking thoracic aortic aneurysm* or a *contained thoracic aortic rupture*. Both of these are acute aortic syndromes.

A. **Prioritizing: making the diagnosis versus controlling blood pressure (BP)**

In patients with suspected aortic dissection, aortic tear, or leaking aortic aneurysm, the first priority is always to control the BP and ventricular ejection velocity, because these propagate aortic dissection or rupture. *If dissection is strongly suspected, a definitive diagnosis should be made with radiographic studies after proper monitoring, IV access, hemodynamic stability, and heart rate and BP control have been established (if possible).* During diagnostic procedures, the patient should be monitored closely, with a physician present as clinically indicated. An anesthesiologist, if needed, should become involved as early as possible to lend expertise in monitoring and in airway and hemodynamic management in patients whose clinical condition deteriorates before they reach the operating room. Rapid diagnosis with TEE may save critical minutes in initiating definitive surgical treatment in patients with suspected thoracic aortic dissection or rupture.

B. **Achieving hemodynamic stability and control**

The ideal drug to control BP is administered intravenously, is rapidly acting, has a short half-life, and causes few, if any, side effects. Systolic and diastolic BPs and LV ejection velocity should be reduced, because these factors all can propagate aortic dissection.

1. **Monitoring.** Patients must have an ECG to detect ischemia and dysrhythmias, two large-bore IV catheters for volume resuscitation, an arterial line in the appropriate location (discussed below), and, if time permits, a central venous catheter or pulmonary artery (PA) catheter for monitoring filling pressures and for infusing drugs centrally.

2. **BP-lowering agents**

a. **Vasodilators**

(1) **Nicardipine** is a calcium channel blocker that inhibits calcium influx into vascular smooth muscle and the myocardium. It can be as administered in a single 0.5- to 2-mg IV "push" or as a 5- to 15-mg/hr infusion titrated to the desired effect.

(2) **Nitroglycerin** is a less potent vasodilator than sodium nitroprusside, and it causes more venous than arterial dilation. It can be useful in patients whose ascending aortic pathology is coupled with myocardial ischemia, because nitroglycerin can improve coronary blood flow by inducing coronary artery vasodilation. Infusion dosage usually ranges from 1 to 4 μg/kg/min.

(3) **Nitroprusside** is a useful agent for controlling BP in patients with critical aortic lesions, because its rapid onset and offset make it quickly effective and easily regulated. A vasodilator that relaxes both arterial and venous smooth muscles, it is given as an IV infusion, and although central administration is probably optimal, it can be administered through a peripheral vein with good effect. The usual starting dose is 0.5 to 1 μg/kg/min, titrated to effect. Doses of 8 to 10 μg/kg/min have been associated with cyanide toxicity (see also Chapter 2).

b. **β₁-Antagonists**

   Decreasing LV ejection velocity is important for decreasing risk of propagating aortic dissection. Medications to lower heart rate may be particularly useful for attenuating the reflex tachycardia and increased ventricular contractility that can occur with use of nicardipine or sodium nitroprusside. Vasodilation can increase LV ejection velocity by increasing dP/dt and heart rate. For this reason, β-adrenergic blockade should be used with vasodilators to decrease both tachycardia and contractility.

(1) **Propranolol**, a nonselective β-antagonist, has been used for many years as first-line therapy for reducing LV ejection velocity and can be administered as an IV bolus of 1 mg, but doses of 4 to 8 mg may be required for adequate heart rate control. Propranolol has been somewhat supplanted by selective β₁-antagonists.

(2) **Labetalol** is a combined α- and β-blocker and offers an alternative to the nitroprusside–propranolol combination. It should be given initially as a 5- to 10-mg loading bolus; once the effect has been assessed, the dose is doubled, allowing a few minutes for onset of effect. This process should be repeated until target BP or a total dose of 300 mg is reached. Once target BP and heart rate are achieved with the loading dose, a continuous infusion can be started at 1 mg/min, or a small bolus dose can be given every 10 to 30 minutes to maintain BP control.

(3) **Esmolol** is a β-blocking agent with a short half-life that can be useful in these cases. It is administered as a bolus loading dose of 500 μg/kg over 1 minute and then continued as an infusion starting at 50 μg/kg/min and titrated to effect to a maximum dose of 300 μg/kg/min. Tachyphylaxis is commonly encountered with esmolol.

(4) **Metoprolol**, another β₁-selective agent, is used in doses of 2.5 to 5 mg titrated to effect over a few minutes to a maximum dose of 15 to 20 mg. It provides a longer effect, which may be useful.

3. **Desired endpoints.** To decrease the chance of propagating aortic dissection or rupture, systolic BP should usually be lowered to approximately 100 to 120 mm Hg or to a mean pressure of 70 to 90 mm Hg. Heart rate should be 60 to 80 beats/min. If a PA catheter is in place, the cardiac index can be lowered to a range of 2 to 2.5 L/min/m² to reduce ejection velocity from a hyperdynamic LV.

C. **Bleeding and transfusion**

   Coagulopathy is frequently encountered in the thoracic aortic surgical patient. Many of these patients require left heart bypass (LHB) or full CPB during surgery to help maintain sufficient end-organ perfusion during aortic repair; thus, they also require heparinization. CPB may cause a consumptive coagulopathy and enhanced fibrinolysis, thus increasing blood loss. Patients requiring deep hypothermic circulatory arrest (DHCA) for aortic arch surgery also may have substantial platelet dysfunction secondary to extreme hypothermia. Platelet consumption has also been noted in the abdominal aortic surgical population. In patients undergoing thoracoabdominal aortic aneurysm repairs, "back-bleeding" through intercostal vessels increases blood loss, and very large losses can occur that necessitate transfusion of multiple units of blood products.

1. A total of 8 to 10 units of packed red blood cells should be typed and crossmatched before surgery, and it may be helpful to notify the blood bank that ongoing blood loss could necessitate transfusing additional blood products beyond those units that are initially crossmatched.

2. Using blood-scavenging/reprocessing devices decreases the amount of banked blood transfused, but extensive bleeding and the logistics of effectively scavenging autologous blood during these operations frequently necessitate transfusing packed cells and procoagulant blood products. It is also important to recognize that reprocessed autologous blood is deficient in coagulation factors, so fresh-frozen plasma or other factor replacement treatment may still be needed.

3. Antifibrinolytic therapy during aortic surgery is commonly used but controversial. No adequately powered trials of these drugs have yet been conducted in aortic surgical patients, so it is not totally clear whether antifibrinolytics significantly benefit them, particularly those in whom LHB or no bypass is used and full heparinization is not required [7].

   a. **Tranexamic acid or ε-aminocaproic acid (EACA).** A retrospective study of 72 patients who underwent descending thoracic aortic surgery with LHB and tranexamic acid or EACA infusion versus no antifibrinolytic therapy found no difference in incidence of transfusion or chest tube output; however, these patients also all received intraoperative methylprednisolone and platelet-rich plasmapheresis before aortic repair [7]. The authors did find that intraoperative hypothermia independently predicted chest tube output and that lower preoperative hemoglobin levels, older age, and longer cross-clamp time independently predicted transfusion. Larger prospective randomized studies are needed to determine whether tranexamic acid and EACA effectively reduce bleeding and do not cause thrombotic or other complications in thoracic aortic operations.

   b. On the basis of available data, we can neither recommend nor advise against using antifibrinolytic therapies in thoracic aortic surgery. Potential thrombotic risks, including neurocognitive and renal dysfunction, are of concern, and the clinician should weigh these risks against the benefits of potential decreases in transfusion.

D. **Assessment of other organ systems**

1. **Neurologic.** Preoperatively, the patient should be monitored closely for change in neurologic status, as this is an indication for immediate surgical intervention.

> **CLINICAL PEARL** Involvement of the artery of Adamkiewicz can lead to lower-extremity paralysis, whereas propagation of a dissection into a cerebral vessel can result in a change in mental status or cause stroke symptoms.

2. **Renal.** Urine output should be monitored, because development of anuria or oliguria in a euvolemic patient is an indication for immediate surgical intervention.

3. **Gastrointestinal.** Serial abdominal examinations should be performed, and blood gases should be analyzed routinely to assess changes in acid–base status. Ischemic bowel can cause significant metabolic acidosis.

E. **Use of pain medications**

Patients with aortic dissection may be anxious and in severe pain. Pain relief is not only important for patient comfort but also beneficial in controlling BP and heart rate. Oversedation should be avoided so that ongoing patient assessments can be made. In addition to neurologic or abdominal symptoms, worsening of back pain may indicate aneurysm expansion or further aortic dissection and is regarded by many surgeons as an emergent situation.

IV. **Surgical and anesthetic considerations**

A. **Goal of surgical therapy (for aortic dissection, aneurysm, or rupture)**

> **CLINICAL PEARL** The foremost goal in treating acute aortic disruption is controlling hemorrhage. Once control is achieved, the objectives of managing both acute and chronic lesions are to repair the diseased aorta and to restore its relations with major arterial branches.

Thoracic aortic aneurysm is usually treated by replacing the entire diseased segment of the aorta with a synthetic graft and then reimplanting major arterial branches into the graft, if necessary. When repairing an aortic dissection, the goal is to resect the segment of the aorta that contains the intimal tear. When this segment is removed, it may be possible to obliterate the origin of the false lumen and interpose graft material.

CLINICAL PEARL It usually is not possible or necessary to replace the entire dissecting portion of aorta because, if the origin of dissection is controlled, reexpansion of the true lumen usually compresses and obliterates the false lumen. With contained aortic rupture, the objective is to resect the area of the aorta that ruptured and either reanastomose the natural aorta to itself in an end-to-end fashion or interpose graft material for the repair.

    B. **Overview of intraoperative anesthetic management (for aortic dissection, aneurysm, or rupture)**

      1. **Key principles**

        a. **Managing BP.** BP control should be sought during the transition from the preoperative to the intraoperative period. Such control is important in light of the surgical and anesthetic manipulations that will profoundly affect BP during the procedure.

        b. **Monitoring of organ ischemia.** If possible, the central nervous system, heart, kidneys, and lungs should be monitored for adequacy of perfusion. The liver and gut cannot be monitored continuously, but their metabolic functions can be checked periodically.

        c. **Treating coexisting disease.** Patients with aortic pathology often have associated cardiovascular and systemic diseases (Table 14.6).

        d. **Controlling bleeding.** Patients undergoing aortic surgery often have an inflammatory response to foreign graft material and CPB or LHB. This inflammation can interact with the coagulation cascade and lead to significant perioperative coagulopathy. Furthermore, patients with acute dissection and lower fibrinogen and platelet counts may already have a consumptive process from the clotting that often occurs in the false lumen. Coagulation abnormalities and their treatment are discussed in Chapter 21.

      2. **Induction and anesthetic agents.** Many thoracic aortic operations are emergent procedures that require aspiration precautions while the airway is being secured. However, the rapid-sequence induction and intubation typically done for patients with full stomachs may not be appropriate for patients with thoracic aortic pathology, as wide swings in hemodynamics can occur. A "modified" rapid-sequence induction may be preferable, titration of anesthetic induction drugs to better control BP (i.e., avoid hypertension) while laryngoscopy is being performed. Use of nonparticulate antacids, H_2-blockers, and metoclopramide should be considered before anesthesia is induced. Other anesthetic

TABLE 14.6	Incidence of coexisting diseases in patients with aortic pathology presenting for surgery	
Coronary artery disease		66%
Hypertension		42%
Chronic obstructive pulmonary disease		23%
Peripheral vascular disease		22%
Cerebrovascular disease		14%
Diabetes mellitus		8%
Other aneurysms		4%
Chronic renal disease		3%

Modified from Romagnoli A, Cooper JR Jr. Anesthesia for aortic operations. *Cleve Clinic Q.* 1981;48(1):147–152.

TABLE 14.7 Anesthetic and surgical management for thoracic aortic surgery

	Surgical site		
	Ascending	**Arch**	**Descending**
Surgical approach	Median sternotomy	Median sternotomy	Left thoracotomy
Perfusion	CPB—aortic cannula distal to lesion, or in femoral or right axillary artery	CPB—FA cannula or right axillary artery cannula	Simple cross-clamp Heparinized Gott shunt ECC with LHB or CPB (femoral–femoral)
Involvement of the following:			
Aortic valve	Sometimes	Sometimes	No
Coronary arteries	Sometimes	Sometimes	No
Pericardium	Sometimes	Sometimes	No
Invasive monitoring	Left radial or femoral arterial catheter PA catheter[b]	Arterial catheter—either arm, or femoral[a] PA catheter[b]	Proximal arterial (right radial or brachial) Distal arterial (femoral)[b] PA catheter[b]
Special techniques	Renal preservation EEG	DHCA Cerebral protection (DHCA, DHCA with RCP, or anterograde cerebral perfusion) Renal preservation EEG	MEPs[b] One-lung ventilation Renal preservation CSF drainage[b]
Common complications	Bleeding Cardiac dysfunction	Bleeding Hypotension from cerebral protective doses of thiopental Neurologic deficits	Bleeding Paralysis Renal failure Cardiac dysfunction

[a]Depends on whether the left subclavian or innominate arteries are involved in the pathologic process or if axillary arterial cannulation is used. If there is uncertainty preoperatively, use a FA catheter.
[b]Optional, depending on physician's preferences.
CPB, cardiopulmonary bypass; CSF, cerebrospinal fluid; DHCA, deep hypothermic circulatory arrest; ECC, extracorporeal circulation; FA, femoral artery; EEG, electroencephalogram; LHB, left heart bypass; MEPs, motor-evoked potentials; PA, pulmonary artery; RCP, retrograde cerebral perfusion.

considerations and agents are described more fully in Section IV.D. Despite precautions, marked changes in hemodynamics are common when the patient's airway is being secured, and vasoactive drugs (e.g., nitroglycerin, esmolol) should be available to immediately treat an undesirable hemodynamic response to intubation.

   3. **Importance of site of lesion** (Table 14.7). Although the principles of anesthetic induction and maintenance are similar for all aortic lesions, knowing the location of the thoracic aortic lesion is also important for intraoperative management.

C. Ascending aortic surgery

   1. **Surgical approach.** Ascending aortic surgery is conducted through a midline sternotomy.

   2. **Cardiopulmonary bypass (CPB).** CPB is required because of proximal aortic involvement.

     a. If the aneurysm ends in the proximal or middle portion of the ascending aorta, the arterial cannula for CPB can be placed in the upper ascending aorta or proximal arch.

CLINICAL PEARL   Many ascending aneurysms extend into the proximal aortic arch. This extension may not be detected until the aorta is exposed, so further management for arch surgery may be needed.

     b. If the entire ascending aorta is involved, the FA can be cannulated, because an *aortic cannula cannot be placed distal to the lesion without jeopardizing perfusion to the great vessels. Arterial flow on CPB in this case is retrograde from the FA toward the great vessels. Another, newer approach is to cannulate the right axillary, innominate, or, occasionally, right carotid artery, allowing blood to flow retrograde into the innominate artery and then antegrade into the aorta.*

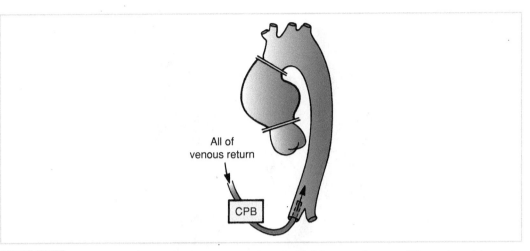

FIGURE 14.4 Circulatory support and clamp placement for surgery of the ascending aorta if femoral arterial cannulation is used; the distal clamp must be distal to the diseased segment. This may be the only clamp required. CPB, cardiopulmonary bypass. (From Benumof JL. Intraoperative considerations for special thoracic surgery cases. In: Benumof JL, ed. *Anesthesia for Thoracic Surgery*. Philadelphia, PA: WB Saunders, 1987:384, with permission.)

    c. Venous cannulation is usually done through the right atrium (RA); however, femoral venous cannulation may be necessary if the aneurysm is very large and obscures the atrium.

  3. **Aortic valve involvement.** Aortic valvuloplasty or valve replacement is often needed with repair of ascending aortic dissection or aneurysm. Which procedure is used depends on the degree of involvement of the sinuses of Valsalva and the aortic annulus.

  4. **Coronary artery involvement.** Ascending aortic dissection or aneurysm may involve the coronary arteries. Aortic dissection can cause coronary occlusion if an expanding false lumen compresses the coronary ostia; such occlusion necessitates surgical coronary artery bypass grafting to restore myocardial blood flow. In cases of proximal aortic aneurysm, displacement of the coronary arteries from their normal position distal to the aortic annulus usually requires coronary artery reimplantation into the reconstructed aortic tube graft, or coronary artery bypass grafting.

  5. **Surgical techniques.** An example of the usual cross-clamp placement used in surgery of the ascending aorta is shown in Figure 14.4. Note that the distal clamp is placed more distally than it is in coronary artery bypass surgery, and the clamped segments might include part of the innominate artery. If aortic insufficiency is present, a large portion of the cardioplegia solution infused into the aortic root will flow through the incompetent aortic valve and into the LV instead of into the coronary arteries. This can cause distention of the LV with increased myocardial oxygen utilization and diminished myocardial protection from reduced distribution of cardioplegia. For these reasons, an aortotomy is often performed immediately after aortic cross-clamping, with direct infusion of cardioplegia into individual coronary arteries. Many centers also use retrograde coronary sinus perfusion for cardioplegia administration as an alternative or in addition to an antegrade technique.

    If the aortic valve and annulus are both normal size and unaffected by concurrent ascending aortic pathology, surgery is limited to replacing the diseased section of the aorta with graft material. If the annulus is normal size but the aortic valve is incompetent, the valve may be resuspended or replaced. If both aortic insufficiency and annular dilation are present, either a composite graft (i.e., a tube graft with an integral artificial valve) or an aortic valve replacement with a graft sewn to the native annulus can be used. If the aortic root is replaced, the coronary arteries must be reimplanted into the wall of a composite graft. In contrast, if the sinuses of Valsalva are spared by doing a separate aortic valve replacement

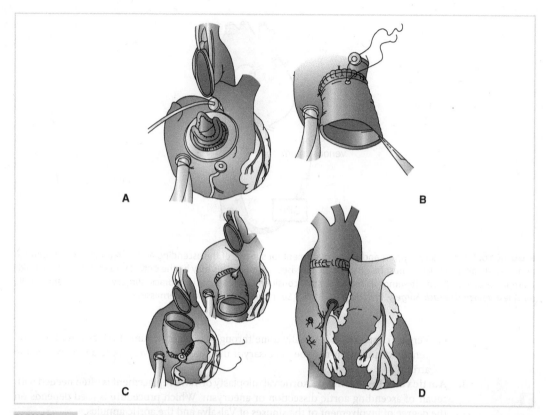

FIGURE 14.5 Surgical repair of ascending aortic aneurysm or dissection. **A:** Aortic valve has been replaced and the aorta is transected at native annulus, leaving "buttons" of aortic wall around coronary ostia. **B:** Graft material anastomosed to the annulus, with left coronary reimplantation. **C:** Completion of left and beginning of right coronary reimplantation. **D:** Completion of distal graft anastomosis. (From Miller DC, Stinson EB, Oyer PE, et al. Concomitant resection of ascending aortic aneurysm and replacement of the aortic valve—operative results and long-term results with "conventional" techniques in ninety patients. *J Thorac Cardiovasc Surg.* 1980;79:394, with permission.)

and then a supracoronary tube graft, the coronary arteries may not need to be reimplanted (Fig. 14.5). The posterior wall of the native aneurysm can be wrapped around the graft material and sewn in place to help with hemostasis.

In patients with ascending dissection, the aortic root is opened and the site of the intimal tear is located. The section of the aorta that includes the intimal tear is excised, and the edges of the true and false lumens are sewn together. Graft is used to replace the excised portion of the aorta.

6. **Complications.** Complications include any that can occur with an operation involving CPB and an open ventricle:
   a. Air emboli
   b. Atheromatous or clot emboli
   c. LV dysfunction secondary to inadequate myocardial protection during aortic cross-clamping. Myocardial dysfunction can, of course, occur despite all protective efforts.
   d. Myocardial infarction or myocardial ischemia secondary to technical problems with reimplantation of the coronaries
   e. Renal or respiratory failure
   f. Coagulopathy
   g. Hemorrhage, especially from suture lines, which can be especially difficult to control in certain locations

D. Anesthetic considerations for ascending aortic surgery
1. **Monitoring**
   a. **Arterial line placement.** The ascending aortic lesion or procedures for its repair may involve the innominate artery, so a left radial or femoral arterial line is inserted for direct BP monitoring. Also, if right axillary cannulation is used, arterial pressure measurement will be falsely elevated because of increased flow (see below) if the right radial artery is cannulated.
   b. **ECG.** Five-lead, calibrated ECG should be used to monitor both leads II and V_5 for ischemic changes.
   c. **PA catheter.** Because of the advanced age of many of these patients and the presence of severe systemic disease that may lead to pulmonary hypertension or low cardiac output, a PA catheter may be useful in selected patients, particularly in the perioperative period.
   d. **TEE.** In addition to its preoperative diagnostic importance, TEE is a useful and often necessary adjunct for the intraoperative management of these patients. Hypovolemia, hypocontractility, myocardial ischemia, intracardiac air, the location of an intimal tear, and the presence and extent of valvular dysfunction can all be detected and assessed with TEE. Caution should be exercised when placing this probe in patients with a large ascending aortic aneurysm, because of the theoretical risk of rupture.
   e. **Neuromonitoring**
      (1) **Electroencephalogram (EEG).** Either raw or processed electroencephalographic data may be helpful for judging the adequacy of cerebral perfusion during CPB. Monitoring the bispectral index might help to assess the depth of anesthesia during these procedures, but the benefits of such monitoring are unproven.
      (2) **Cerebral near-infrared spectroscopy or oximetry** is also employed by many in these cases. See the arch aneurysm section for further discussion.
      (3) **Temperature.** When correctly placed at the back of the oropharynx, a nasopharyngeal or oropharyngeal temperature probe probably gives the anesthesiologist the best overall approximation of brain temperature.
   f. **Renal monitoring.** As with all cases involving CPB, urine output should be monitored.
2. **Induction and anesthetic agents.** See Table 14.8.
3. **Cooling and rewarming.** Hypothermic CPB is used in most cases of ascending aneurysm. If femoral cannulation is to be used and the FA is small, a smaller cannula may be needed. This may delay cooling and rewarming, because blood flows on CPB will have to be lower to avoid excessive arterial line pressures between the roller pump and the arterial cannula.
E. Aortic arch surgery
1. **Surgical approach.** The arch is exposed through a median sternotomy.
2. **Cardiopulmonary bypass (CPB).** In most cases, CPB with femoral or right axillary arterial cannulation and right atrial venous cannulation is required.
3. **Technique.** Typical aortic clamp placement for this procedure is shown in Figure 14.6. Note that blood flow to the innominate, left carotid, and LSA will cease during resection of the aneurysmal or dissected section of the aortic arch, thus necessitating DHCA.

   The attachments of the arch vessels are often excised en bloc so that all three vessels are located on one "button" of tissue (Fig. 14.7). This facilitates rapid reimplantation and reestablishment of blood flow through the arch vessels. Once the distal arch anastomosis is completed, the surgeon sutures the aortic button containing the arch vessels to the graft that is replacing the diseased aortic arch. The aortic cross-clamp can then be placed on the graft proximal to the arch vessels, after which the arch portion of the aortic graft is deaired, and blood flow is reestablished to the cerebral vessels via the arterial CPB cannula. The proximal aortic arch anastomosis is then completed.
4. **Cerebral protection.** As discussed above, resection of the aortic arch requires interrupting or altering cerebral blood flow, which may contribute to postoperative stroke

TABLE 14.8 Anesthetic considerations and choice of anesthetic agent for surgery of the aorta

Patient variables	Opioids[a]	Volatile agent[b]	Other IV agents
Full stomach	Rapid acting (especially sufentanil, alfentanil)	Prolonged induction	Rapid acting if tolerated
Hemodynamic instability	Minimal myocardial depression Potent analgesics useful for treating intraoperative hypertension	Dose-dependent myocardial depression Indicated if hypertensive with adequate cardiac output	T, P: Myocardial depression M, E: Minimal myocardial depression K: Worsens hypertension
Ventricular function (VF)	Indicated with poor VF	Use in patients with good VF	M, E, and K maintain VF Avoid T, P if VF is poor
Neurologic function	Decrease CMRo$_2$	Decrease CMRo$_2$, especially isoflurane; unclear in vivo protective effects	T, P decrease CMRo$_2$, probably protective, used with hypothermic arrest or open ventricle
Myocardial ischemia (coronary involvement)	Oxygen balance: Increases supply/demand ratio and therefore will have adverse effects in presence of hypertension	Decrease supply/demand ratio but will have negative effect in presence of hypotension	T, P: Adversely affect supply secondary to hypotension K: Increases oxygen demand, decreases supply (secondary to tachycardia)

[a]Refers to fentanyl, sufentanil, and alfentanil.
[b]Halothane, sevoflurane, desflurane, and isoflurane.
CMRo$_2$, cerebral metabolic rate of oxygen consumption; E, etomidate; IV, intravenous; K, ketamine; M, midazolam; P, propofol; T, thiopental.

and neurocognitive dysfunction—both significant causes of morbidity and mortality in patients undergoing aortic arch surgery. Although various surgical approaches are used to reduce cerebral ischemia, all include lowering patient temperature with CPB to decrease the cerebral metabolic rate, the corresponding oxygen demand, and the production of toxic metabolites.

a. DHCA is used for arch surgery, because blood flow through the aorta to the brain can be stopped and surgical exposure is maximized. DHCA requires cooling the patient's core temperature to 15° to 22°C, depending on the anticipated complexity and

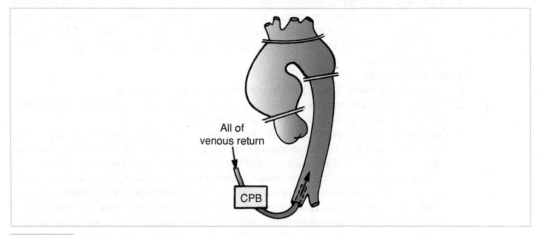

FIGURE 14.6 Representation of cannula and clamp placement for surgery of the aortic arch if femoral bypass is used. Proximal clamp is placed to arrest the heart. Distal clamp isolates the arch so that the distal anastomosis can be performed. Middle clamp on major branches isolates the head vessels so that en bloc attachment to graft is possible. The distal and arch anastomoses may be performed without clamps by using circulatory arrest. CPB, cardiopulmonary bypass. (From Benumof JL. Intraoperative considerations for special thoracic surgery cases. In: Benumof JL, ed. *Anesthesia for Thoracic Surgery*. Philadelphia, PA: WB Saunders, 1987:384, with permission.)

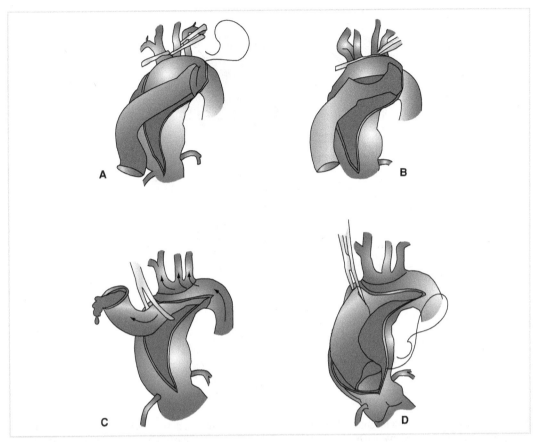

FIGURE 14.7 Aortic arch replacement. **A:** The distal suture line is completed first, followed by (**B**) reattachment of the arch vessels. **C:** Flow is reestablished to these vessels by moving the clamp more proximally. **D:** The proximal suture line is completed. (From Crawford ES, Saleh SA. Transverse aortic arch aneurysm—improved results of treatment employing new modifications of aortic reconstruction and hypokalemic cerebral circulatory arrest. *Ann Surg*. 1981;194:186, with permission.)

duration of the procedure and the adjunctive technique used (antegrade or retrograde cerebral perfusion [RCP]). Turning off CPB and partially draining the patient's blood volume into the venous reservoir provides a bloodless surgical field while protecting the brain and other organs, such as the kidneys, for up to 40 minutes [8], or perhaps longer. DHCA has improved outcomes of aortic arch surgery but is associated with longer CPB times, which are needed to adequately cool and rewarm the patient. Animal studies suggest that it is important to rewarm patients relatively slowly after DHCA, and also not to rewarm the brain above 37°C, because this increases the risk of cerebral injury [9].

CLINICAL PEARL   Because patients can undergo DHCA for only a limited time before suffering cerebral injury, many surgeons use either selective retrograde or antegrade cerebral perfusion (ACP) as an adjunct to DHCA to prolong the "safe time" allowed for complicated reconstruction of the aortic arch and its branch vessels while circulation to the rest of the body is stopped.

   b. **Retrograde cerebral perfusion (RCP) necessitates individual caval cannulation.** At circulatory arrest, the arterial line of the CPB circuit is connected to the superior vena caval cannula, through which low flows are directed to maintain a central venous pressure (CVP) of approximately 20 mm Hg, although this pressure is not necessarily

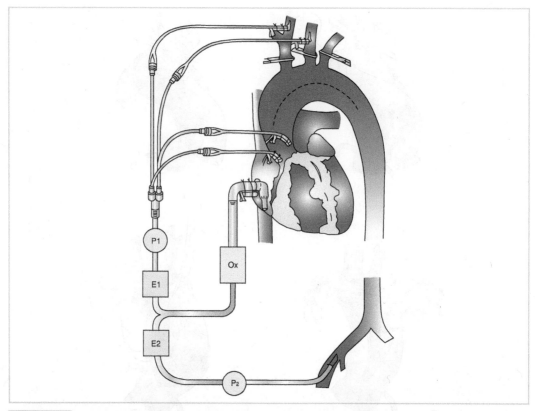

FIGURE 14.8 Perfusion circuit for anterograde cerebral perfusion for aortic arch surgery. Venous blood from the right atrium (RA) drains to the oxygenator (*Ox*), and is cooled to 28°C by heat exchange (*E2*) before passing via the main roller pump (*P2*) to a femoral artery (FA). A second circuit derived from the oxygenator with a separate heat exchanger (*E1*) and roller pump (*P1*) provides blood at 6° to 12°C to the brachiocephalic and coronary arteries. (From Bachet J, Guilmet D, Goudot B, et al. Antegrade cerebral perfusion with cold blood: a 13 year experience. *Ann Thorac Surg.* 1999;67:1875, with permission.)

associated with better outcomes. Advantages of RCP include relative simplicity, uniform cerebral cooling, efficient deairing of the cerebral vessels (thus reducing the risk of embolism), and provision of oxygen and energy substrates. Outcome studies have identified three risk factors for mortality and morbidity in RCP during DHCA: time on CPB, urgency of surgery, and patient age [10]. Controversy exists as to how much flow is actually directed to the brain and how much flow courses through the extracranial vessels.

c. **Antegrade cerebral perfusion (ACP).** With this technique, the brain is selectively perfused via the innominate or carotid arteries. One method of administering ACP is to take blood from the CPB circuit's oxygenator and deliver it via arterial access to the brain by using a roller pump separate from the one used for CPB (Fig. 14.8). Many centers use this same technique to deliver antegrade or retrograde cardioplegia.

Figure 14.8 depicts direct cannulation of both carotid arteries for ACP, but this technique has been simplified in many practices by cannulating the right axillary artery or other arteries, as discussed above, instead of the FA for placement of the arterial line from the CPB circuit. This is usually done by anastomosing (end to side) a tube graft to the axillary artery and attaching the arterial line from the pump to the graft. After CPB is initiated and the patient is cooled, at the time of circulatory arrest the base of the innominate artery is clamped and ACP is delivered

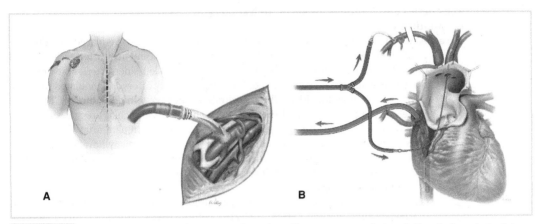

FIGURE 14.9 Antegrade cerebral perfusion (ACP) by right axillary artery cannulation. **A:** Detail of surgical cutdown and graft anastomosis to the right axillary artery, showing relationship to the sternal incision. **B:** Direction of blood flow when the right axillary artery is used for ACP. The brain is perfused via the right carotid artery and (optionally) via the left carotid artery from a balloon-tipped catheter inserted through the surgical field into the base of the artery. Venous return to the pump is via the right atrium (RA). Note occlusion of the base of the innominate artery, allowing opening of the ascending aorta and aortic arch. (Printed with permission from Baylor College of Medicine.)

at lower flow rates (e.g., 10 mL/kg/min) through the axillary artery cannula and thus up the right carotid artery (Fig. 14.9). This allows bilateral cerebral perfusion, assuming that the circle of Willis is intact. If the integrity of collateral blood flow to the left cerebral hemisphere is uncertain, the left common carotid also can be cannulated directly through the surgical field, as shown. Pressure during this method of ACP can be monitored with a right radial arterial line as noted previously, but monitoring pressure and maintaining a certain pressure are not known to improve outcome. Some centers use near-infrared spectroscopy to monitor unilateral cerebral perfusion during ACP via the right carotid. Results of a small study suggest that this may be effective [11].

Cannulating the right axillary artery instead of the FA to provide CPB before and after circulatory arrest reduces the risk of systemic atheroembolism. This is because right axillary artery cannulation provides antegrade aortic flow, whereas FA cannulation produces retrograde flow through an often atherosclerotic descending aorta [12].

Additionally, DHCA is required only for completion of the distal and arch anastomoses. Then the aortic graft can be clamped proximally and full CPB perfusion reinitiated to the rest of the body while the proximal anastomosis and any concomitant aortic valve procedure are performed.

Many groups accept ACP as the safest method of brain protection during arch surgery [13]. ACP may take advantage of autoregulation of cerebral blood flow, which is thought to remain intact even at low temperatures when α-stat blood gas management is used. With intact autoregulation, physiologic protection against complications of hyperperfusion will be active. However, proponents of pH-stat blood gas management argue that the cerebral vasodilation that accompanies elevated pCO_2 produces more uniform cooling and perfusion of the brain (see Chapter 26). There is considerable variation among centers.

5. **Complications.** Complications of aortic arch surgery include those of any procedure in which CPB is used. Irreversible cerebral ischemia is a distinct possibility with this type of surgery. Hemostatic difficulties may be increased secondary to the multiple suture lines, long CPB times, and prolonged periods of intraoperative hypothermia.

F. **Anesthetic considerations for aortic arch surgery**
1. **Monitoring**
    a. **Arterial blood pressure (BP).** An intra-arterial catheter can be placed in either the right or left radial artery, depending on which of the head and neck arteries that extend off of the aortic arch are involved. If both the right- and left-sided arteries are involved, the FA may need to be catheterized. If the right axillary artery is cannulated for CPB, right radial arterial line BPs will not accurately reflect systemic BP during CPB. Conversely, some have advocated monitoring right radial or brachial pressures to assess flow during ACP via the right axillary artery or the innominate artery. There is no consensus on this point. Also, with profound hypothermia, many have found that the radial artery does not provide accurate pressures for a period during rewarming, and they electively and preemptively insert a femoral arterial catheter.
    b. **Neurologic monitors**
        (1) Electroencephalography (EEG) is often used to ensure that the patient has been cooled such that the EEG is isoelectric before DHCA. Propofol is given by some anesthesiologists to achieve or extend this isoelectric state.
        (2) Nasal or oropharyngeal temperature can be used to monitor brain cooling; however, nasopharyngeal temperature generally gives the most accurate estimate of brain temperature [14].
        (3) Near-infrared regional spectroscopy (NIRS). This technology measures frontal cerebral oxygenation through light transmittance. Although the technology is complex, it is easily applied and seems to be most useful as a trend monitor during ascending aortic and arch surgery, particularly when ACP is used. Significant reductions in left-sided sensor values compared with right-sided ones may indicate an incomplete circle of Willis. We have found that these values are usually restored when separate left carotid perfusion begins. Clear outcome data are not yet available, however. Longer periods of lower cerebral oxygenation during DHCA, as indicated by NIRS, have been associated with longer postoperative hospital stays. Large, well-designed prospective studies are needed to validate the efficacy of these approaches [15,16].
    c. **Transesophageal echocardiography (TEE).** As in ascending aortic surgery (see Section IV.D.1), TEE provides useful information during arch procedures.
2. **Choice of anesthetic agents.** See Table 14.8.
3. **Management of hypothermic circulatory arrest.** The technique involves core cooling to a temperature as low as 15° to 20°C. Such low temperatures are used less often now than in the past; currently, some large centers use a target temperature of 24°C, pack the head in ice, use pharmacologic adjuncts to aid in cerebral protection, avoid glucose-containing solutions, and use appropriate monitoring for selective cerebral perfusion. More details are provided in Chapter 26.
4. **Complications.** Complications related directly to anesthesia for aortic arch surgery are uncommon.

G. **Descending thoracic and thoracoabdominal aortic surgery**
1. **Surgical approach.** Aneurysms of the descending thoracic aorta frequently extend into the abdominal cavity and involve the entire aorta. They are often grouped according to Crawford classification (Fig. 14.10). The affected segment of aorta can be exposed through a left thoracotomy incision alone or a thoracoabdominal incision. Extent IV aneurysms involve the supraceliac abdominal aorta but still require low thoracic aortic clamping. For aneurysms of any extent, the patient is placed in a full right lateral decubitus position with the hips rolled slightly to the left so that the femoral vessels can be cannulated for LHB or CPB if necessary. When positioning the patient, it is important to protect pressure points by measures such as using an axillary roll, placing pillows between the knees, and padding the head and elbows. It is also important to maintain the occiput in line with the thoracic spine to prevent traction on the brachial plexus. Various methods can be used to position the left arm.

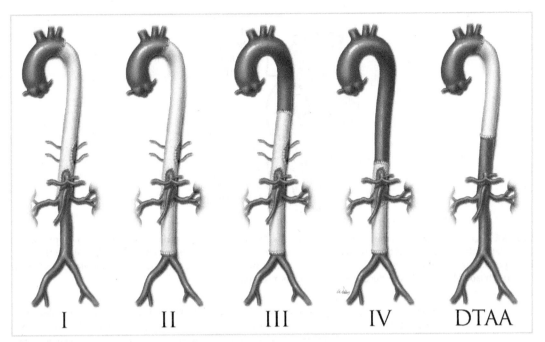

FIGURE 14.10 The Crawford classification of repair for thoracoabdominal aortic aneurysm surgery, with a descending thoracic aortic repair for comparison. The descending aortic repair does not extend beyond the diaphragm, whereas all the others do. Extent I aneurysms involve an area that begins just distal to the left subclavian artery (LSA) and extends to most or all of the abdominal visceral vessels but not the infrarenal aorta. Extent II aneurysms also begin distal to the left subclavian and involve most of the aorta above the abdominal bifurcation. Extent III lesions begin in the midthoracic aorta and involve various lengths of the abdominal aorta. Finally, Extent IV lesions originate above the celiac axis and end below the renal arteries; these aneurysms necessitate a thoracoabdominal approach for proximal aortic cross-clamping. DTAA, descending thoracic aortic aneurysm. (Reproduced with permission from Baylor College of Medicine.)

2. **Surgical techniques.** Regardless of whether a patient has a descending thoracic aortic aneurysm, a thoracoabdominal aneurysm, a dissection, or aortic rupture, surgical repair usually involves placing aortic cross-clamps both above and below the affected region of the aorta and then opening the aorta and replacing the diseased segment with a graft.

   a. **Simple cross-clamping.** Some groups report success with cross-clamping the aorta above and below the lesion without using additional measures to provide perfusion distal to the aortic lesion. This technique has the advantage of simplifying the operation and reducing the amount of heparin needed (Fig. 14.11) because more heparin is required when bypass circuits are used. An obvious disadvantage is potentially compromising flow to the distal aorta and its perfused organs when the simple cross-clamp technique is used. This approach is more often used with less extensively diseased segments, such as aneurysms confined to descending thoracic aorta, and Extent III and IV thoracoabdominal aneurysms.

   Clamping the descending thoracic aorta generally causes marked hemodynamic changes: profound *hypertension* in the proximal aorta and *hypotension* distal to the cross-clamp. The increase in afterload that occurs when the majority of the cardiac output goes only to the arteries perfusing the head and upper extremities can cause acutely elevated LV filling pressures and a corresponding progressive decline in cardiac output. Presumably, LV failure can result if afterload remains elevated for a significant length of time. Furthermore, hypertension in the proximal aorta could precipitate a catastrophic cerebral event, particularly in patients with unidentified cerebral aneurysm. Mean arterial pressure (MAP) distal to the aortic cross-clamp may decrease to less than 10% to 20% of the patient's baseline BP, causing an obvious decline in renal

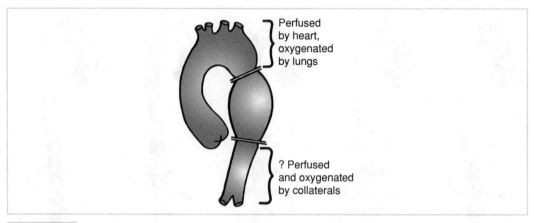

Perfused by heart, oxygenated by lungs

? Perfused and oxygenated by collaterals

FIGURE 14.11 Illustration of simple cross-clamp placement for repair of descending aortic aneurysm or dissection. Distal clamp placement dictates that flow to the spinal cord and major organs proceeds through collateral vessels. (From Benumof JL. Intraoperative considerations for special thoracic surgery cases. In: Benumof JL, ed. *Anesthesia for Thoracic Surgery*. Philadelphia, PA: WB Saunders, 1987:384, with permission.)

perfusion and, perhaps, spinal cord perfusion. The physiology of aortic cross-clamping can change depending on the actual site of the clamp and is influenced by many factors, a discussion of which is beyond the scope of this chapter. Gelman's review of the subject remains an excellent reference [17].

Aortic coarctation repair is another procedure in which simple cross-clamping is often used. Chronic obstruction of distal aortic blood flow, such as that which occurs with aortic coarctation, generally results in well-developed collateral flow and lessens the hemodynamic changes usually encountered when a cross-clamp is placed on the descending thoracic aorta. This is illustrated by BP measurements taken proximal and distal to the aortic cross-clamp in a series of patients with aortic coarctation versus descending thoracic aortic aneurysm (Table 14.9) [18].

Another simple method of aortic cross-clamping is an "open" technique, in which no cross-clamp is placed distal to the aortic pathology. This technique allows direct inspection of the distal aorta for debris such as thrombus and atheroma, and graft material can be anastomosed in an oblique fashion that reincorporates the maximal number of intercostal arteries.

TABLE 14.9   Proximal versus distal blood pressure (BP) in simple aortic clamp

	Proximal systolic/diastolic; mean (mm Hg)	Distal mean (mm Hg)
Coarctation	160/85; 110	23
	145/80; 102	54
	150/85; 107	18
	155/80; 105	36
Average	152/82; 106	33
Thoracic aneurysm	260/160; 194	12
	240/135; 170	8
	245/150; 182	24
	235/140; 172	4
	240/155; 184	10
	255/160; 192	6
Average	245/150; 182	10

Modified from Romagnoli A, Cooper JR Jr. Anesthesia for aortic operations. *Cleve Clinic Q.* 1981;48(1):147–152.

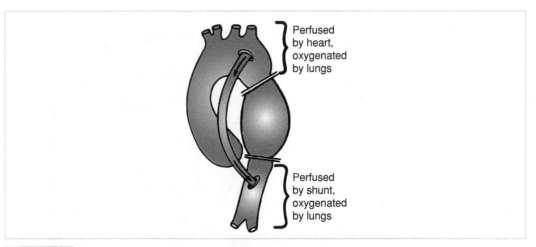

FIGURE 14.12 Placement of a heparin-coated vascular shunt from proximal to distal aorta during repair of descending aneurysm or dissection. (From Benumof JL. Intraoperative considerations for special thoracic surgery cases. In: Benumof JL, ed. *Anesthesia for Thoracic Surgery*. Philadelphia, PA: WB Saunders, 1987:384, with permission.)

    b. Shunts. Placing a heparin-bonded (Gott) extracorporeal shunt from the LV, aortic arch, or LSA to the FA (Fig. 14.12) provides decompression of the proximal aorta and perfusion to the distal aorta. Systemic heparinization usually is not required. However, there may be technical difficulties with placement and kinking of the shunt, which can result in inadequate distal flows. Also, relatively small shunt diameters can limit blood flow and, thereby, limit how much proximal LV decompression and augmentation of distal aortic perfusion can be accomplished.

    c. Extracorporeal circulation (ECC). Historically, the first method used for distal aortic perfusion and proximal decompression in the repair of descending thoracic aortic lesions was ECC. There are several ways to perform ECC, but all involve removal of blood from the patient, passage into an extracorporeal pump, and reinfusion into the FA or another site to provide perfusion distal to the aortic cross-clamp (Fig. 14.13). An alternative technique is perfusing the body of the aneurysm with ECC while

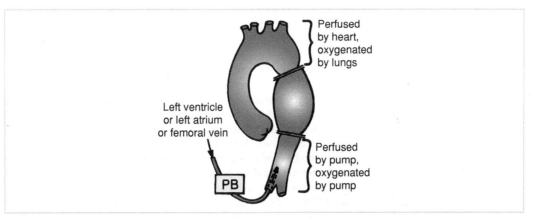

FIGURE 14.13 Partial bypass (*PB*) (or extracorporeal circulation [ECC]) method for maintaining distal perfusion pressure and preventing proximal hypertension. Oxygenated blood can be taken directly from the LV or atrium (or aortic arch) and pumped either by roller head or centrifugal pump into the femoral artery (FA). Alternatively, unoxygenated blood can be taken from the femoral vein (FV), passed through a separate oxygenator, and pumped into the FA. Use of an oxygenator dictates the use of a full heparinizing dose. (From Benumof JL. Intraoperative considerations for special thoracic surgery cases. In: Benumof JL, ed. *Anesthesia for Thoracic Surgery*. Philadelphia, PA: WB Saunders, 1987:384, with permission.)

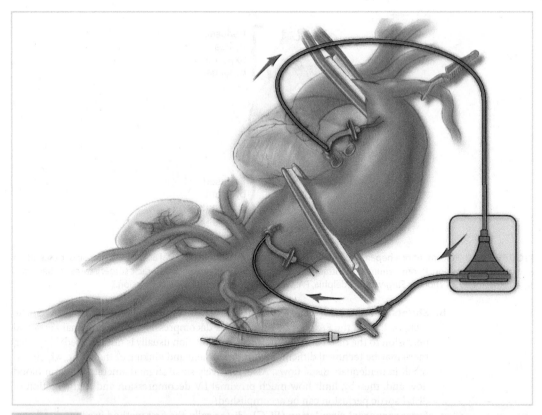

FIGURE 14.14 Left heart bypass (LHB). Perfusing the aneurysm allows completion of the proximal anastomosis while distal perfusion is maintained. After the aneurysm is opened, perfusion of the celiac, superior mesenteric, and renal arteries may be performed by individual cannulation before these arteries are attached to the graft. (From Coselli JS, LeMaire SA. Tips for successful outcomes for descending thoracic and thoracoabdominal aortic aneurysm procedures. *Semin Vasc Surg.* 2008;21:13–20, with permission.)

the proximal anastomosis is being performed and then opening the aneurysm and perfusing the major visceral vessels individually until they can be incorporated into the anastomosis.

Blood can be drained from the patient into the extracorporeal pump via the femoral vein (FV), which is technically the easiest site to access for surgery on the descending thoracic aorta. However, using a systemic venous drainage site necessitates placing an oxygenator in the ECC circuit to provide oxygenated blood for reinfusion. This form of CPB in conjunction with DHCA may be necessary to repair descending thoracic aortic aneurysms that involve the distal aortic arch.

Alternatively, LHB can be used. A pulmonary vein or the left atrium (LA), LV apex, or left axillary artery can be cannulated to carry oxygenated patient blood to the ECC pump; this blood is then returned via the distal aorta, the body of the aneurysm, or the FA. This technique does not require an oxygenator in the LHB circuit (Fig. 14.14).

Both of these ECC techniques have disadvantages. Using an oxygenator requires complete systemic heparinization, which is associated with increased risk of hemorrhage, especially into the left lung. Left atrial or ventricular cannulation for LHB without an oxygenator may allow the use of less heparin, but this approach increases the risk of systemic air embolism. Also, in the venous to arterial circulation CPB technique, a heat exchanger is included in the ECC circuit, which helps to avoid significant perioperative hypothermia and corresponding coagulopathy, although some degree of

TABLE 14.10 Options for increasing distal perfusion in descending aortic surgery

Blood removed from	Blood infused into	Heparinized shunt	Perfusion apparatus		Extracorporeal bypass	
			Roller	Centrifugal	Oxygenator	Heparin (ACT)[a]
LV, AoA, LSA	FA, DAo	Yes	No	No	No	None (nl)
FV	FA, DAo	No	Either		Yes	Full (>480)
LA, AoA, LSA, LV	FA, DAo	No	No	Yes	No	Minimum (nl–250)[b]

[a]Refers to the activated clotting time (in seconds); if used, optimum ACT is controversial.
[b]Some groups will not use heparin when using a centrifugal pump.
AoA, aortic arch; DAo, descending aorta; FA, femoral artery; FV, femoral vein; LA, left atrium; nl, normal; LSA, left subclavian artery; LV, left ventricle.

hypothermia is probably advantageous for spinal cord protection. When LHB is used, a heat exchanger is often not added to the ECC circuit. Table 14.10 summarizes the possible cannulation sites and the major differences between heparinized shunts and ECC for perfusion distal to the aortic cross-clamp.

3. **Complications of descending thoracic aortic repairs**

   a. **Cardiac.** The rate of major cardiac morbidity and mortality was approximately 12% in one large series of thoracoabdominal aneurysm repairs [19].

   b. **Hemorrhage.** Significant perioperative bleeding is a common complication.

   c. **Renal failure.** The incidence of renal failure in large case series ranges from 13% to 18% [19,20]. The mortality rate is substantially higher in patients with postoperative renal failure [19]. The cause is presumed to be a decrease in renal blood flow during aortic cross-clamping. However, renal failure can still occur despite apparently adequate perfusion (heparinized shunt or ECC). Pre-existing renal dysfunction increases a patient's risk of postoperative renal failure.

   d. **Paraplegia.** The reported incidence of paraplegia after open surgical repair descending thoracic or thoracoabdominal aortic aneurysms ranges from 0.5% to 38% [19–21]. The cause is either complete interruption of blood supply or prolonged hypoperfusion (>30 minutes) of the spinal cord via the anterior spinal artery. The anterior spinal artery is formed by fusion of the vertebral arteries and is the major blood supply to the anterior spinal cord. As the anterior spinal artery traverses the spinal cord from cephalad to caudad, it receives collateral blood supply from radicular branches of the intercostal arteries (Fig. 14.15). In most patients, one radicular arterial branch, known as the *great radicular artery (of Adamkiewicz)*, provides a major portion of the blood supply to the midportion of the spinal cord. It can arise anywhere from T_5 to below L_1. Unfortunately, this vessel is difficult to identify by angiography or by inspection during surgery. Interruption of flow can lead to paraplegia, depending on the contribution of other collateral arteries to spinal cord perfusion. With anterior spinal artery hypoperfusion, an *anterior spinal syndrome* can result, in which motor function is usually completely lost (anterior horns) but some sensation may remain intact (posterior columns).

   e. **Miscellaneous.** Other significant complications can arise during surgery of the descending thoracic aorta. Some of these are specific to the type of aortic pathology being addressed. For example, death from multiorgan trauma and failure is a major entity in patients who initially survive traumatic aortic rupture. Furthermore, thoracic aortic surgical patients are more likely to succumb to respiratory failure or multiorgan failure than are patients with isolated abdominal aortic disease. Patients who undergo thoracoabdominal aortic repair may develop postoperative diaphragmatic dysfunction. Cerebrovascular accidents are seen in a small number of these patients. Also, left vocal cord paralysis due to recurrent laryngeal nerve damage commonly occurs during descending thoracic aortic surgery because of the proximity of the nerve to the site of the aneurysm.

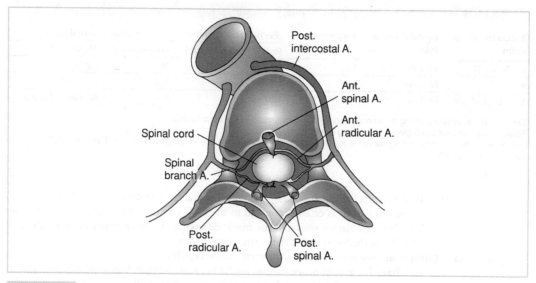

FIGURE 14.15 Anatomic drawing of the contribution of the radicular arteries to spinal cord blood flow. If the posterior intercostal artery is involved in a dissection or is sacrificed to facilitate repair of aortic pathology, critical blood supply may be lost, causing spinal cord ischemia. A., artery. (From Cooley DA, ed. *Surgical Treatment of Aortic Aneurysms.* Philadelphia, PA: WB Saunders, 1986:92, with permission.)

CLINICAL PEARL   All descending thoracic and thoracoabdominal aneurysms can be associated with major complications, but Crawford Extent II lesions involve more potential hazards because more of the aorta is affected.

H. Anesthetic considerations in descending thoracic aortic surgery

   1. **General considerations.** Providing anesthesia for descending thoracic aortic surgery can be extremely demanding because of profound hemodynamic changes and compromised perfusion of organs distal to the aortic cross-clamp. Anesthesia for descending thoracic aortic surgery is summarized in several good reviews [22,23].

   2. **Monitoring**

      a. **Arterial blood pressure (BP).** A right radial or brachial arterial catheter is needed to monitor pressures above the proximal clamp because aortic cross-clamping may occlude the LSA. To assess perfusion distal to the lower aortic cross-clamp, many centers place a FA catheter in addition to the right radial or brachial catheter to monitor pressure below the distal clamp. If the LHB technique of ECC is used, the left FA is typically cannulated for distal perfusion of the aorta, and the right FA can be used for monitoring BP.

      b. **Ventricular function (VF).** Some operative teams monitor LV function during proximal aortic cross-clamping. A TEE can be useful for directly assessing LV function and volume, but occasionally, the TEE probe in the esophagus can interfere with surgical placement of retractors or clamps. In those cases, TEE cannot be used. A PA catheter allows indirect assessment of LV filling and cardiac output, presuming that the right heart and tricuspid valve function well and the patient does not have pulmonary hypertension. However, a PA catheter is not as helpful as TEE for intraoperative real-time patient monitoring.

      c. **Other monitors.** ECG lead V_5 cannot be used because of the surgical approach, which limits the assessment of anterior myocardial ischemia. However, TEE may allow good assessment of anterior LV wall motion.

3. **One-lung anesthesia.** To provide good surgical access, double-lumen endobronchial tubes allow deflation of the left lung during surgery on the descending thoracic and thoracoabdominal aorta. This not only improves surgical exposure but also protects the left lung from trauma associated with surgical manipulation. Furthermore, if trauma to the left lung leads to hemorrhage into the airway, the double-lumen tube can protect the right lung from blood spillage. A left-sided double-lumen endotracheal tube is generally easier for the anesthesiologist to place and is most often used for operations on the descending thoracic aorta. However, in some patients, the aortic aneurysm distorts the trachea or left main stem bronchus to the degree that placing a left-sided double-lumen tube is impossible. Patients with aortic rupture may also have a distorted left main stem bronchus. Right-sided double-lumen endobronchial tubes may be used, but proper alignment with the right upper lobe bronchus should be checked with a fiberoptic bronchoscope. Alternatively, a single-lumen endotracheal tube with an endobronchial blocker can be used when a double-lumen tube cannot be placed, or when exchanging a double-lumen tube for a single-lumen endotracheal tube is anticipated to be challenging (i.e., the patient has a difficult intubation before undergoing an operation that involves major transfusion and fluid resuscitation). For a detailed description of double-lumen and endobronchial blocker tube placement and single-lung ventilation, see Chapter 15.

4. **Anesthetic management before and during aortic cross-clamping.** Before the aorta is cross-clamped, mannitol (0.5 g/kg) is often administered to try to provide some renal protection during aortic cross-clamping, when kidney perfusion may be poor. Even when shunting or ECC is used, changes in the distribution of renal blood flow may make efforts at renal protection prudent.

   After the aortic cross-clamp is applied, it is important to closely monitor acid–base status with serial arterial blood gas measurements, as it is common for metabolic acidosis to develop because of hypoperfusion of critical organ beds. Acidosis should be treated aggressively with sodium bicarbonate and with attempts to increase distal aortic perfusion pressure if LHB or shunting is used (particularly if the patient is normothermic). If simple aortic cross-clamping without shunting or ECC is used, proximal hypertension should be controlled, again with awareness that distal organ flow may be diminished. In treating proximal hypertension, regional blood flow studies have shown that infusing nitroprusside may decrease renal and spinal cord blood flow in a dose-related fashion. Ideally, aortic cross-clamp time (regardless of technique) should be less than 30 minutes, because the incidence of complications, especially paraplegia, starts to increase substantially beyond this time.

   If a heparinized shunt is used and proximal *hypertension* cannot be treated without producing subsequent distal *hypotension* (<60 mm Hg), the surgeon should be made aware that there could be a technical problem with the shunt's placement. If LHB is used, pump speed can be increased to reduce proximal hypertension by moving blood volume from the proximal to the distal aorta. This also increases lower-body perfusion. Usually, little or no pharmacologic intervention is needed during LHB, because changing the pump speed allows rapid control of proximal and distal aortic pressures. Table 14.11 lists the treatment options for several clinical scenarios when using ECC.

   Before the surgeon removes the aortic cross-clamp, the patient should be adequately volume resuscitated, and a vasopressor should be available in case substantial hypotension occurs after the aorta is unclamped.

> **CLINICAL PEARL**   The anesthesiologist must be constantly aware of the stage of the operation so that major events such as clamping and unclamping of the aorta are anticipated.

5. **Declamping shock.** When *simple cross-clamping* of the aorta is used, subsequent unclamping can have serious and even life-threatening consequences, usually from severe hypotension or myocardial depression. Declamping syndrome has several theoretical

TABLE 14.11 Management of extracorporeal circulation for surgery of the descending aorta

Proximal arterial pressure	Distal arterial pressure	Pulmonary wedge pressure	Treatment
↑	↓	↓	Volume; increase pump flow
↑	↓	↑	Increase pump flow
↑	↑	↓	Volume; vasodilator
↑	↑	↑	Vasodilator; diuretic; maintain pump flow, hold volume in pump reservoir (if in use)
↓	↓	↓	Volume; look for partial occlusion of arterial outflow cannula (if reservoir in use)
↓	↓	↑	Increase pump flow; inotrope
↓	↑	↑	Decrease pump flow; inotrope; diuretic
↓	↑	↓	Decrease pump flow; may need volume

causes, including washout of acid metabolites, vasodilator substances, sequestration of blood in the gut or lower extremities, and reactive hyperemia.

CLINICAL PEARL   The usual cause, however, is relative or absolute hypovolemia.

Anesthesiologists may be fooled into underresuscitating patients while the aortic cross-clamp is on because of high proximal arterial pressures. To attenuate the effects of clamp removal, the patient's volume should be optimized, particularly in the 10 to 15 minutes before unclamping. This includes elevating filling pressures by infusing blood products, colloid, or crystalloids. Some advocate prophylactic bicarbonate administration just before clamp removal to minimize myocardial depression from "washout acidosis." It is advisable for the surgeon to release the cross-clamp slowly over a period of 1 to 2 minutes to allow enough time for compensatory hemodynamic changes to occur and for the anesthesiologist to determine whether further volume resuscitation is indicated.

Vasopressors may be needed to compensate for hypotension after the aortic cross-clamp is removed, but the anesthesiologist should take care not to "overshoot" the target BP, as even transient hypertension can result in significant bleeding from the aortic suture lines. With a volume-resuscitated patient and a slow cross-clamp release, any significant postclamp hypotension usually is short lived and well tolerated. If hypotension is severe, the easiest intervention is reapplying the clamp and further volume infusion.

If shunts or ECC are used, declamping hypotension is usually mild, as the vascular bed below the clamp is less "empty," and there will be less proximal to distal aortic volume shifting after the aortic cross-clamp is released. If a volume reservoir is used in the bypass circuit, ECC also provides a means for rapid volume infusion after the aortic cross-clamp is removed. Some type of rapid infusion device is most useful in these cases.

6. **Fluid therapy and transfusion.** Even patients undergoing elective repair of a descending thoracic aneurysm (vs. aortic rupture or dissection) may be relatively hypovolemic.

Despite proximal and distal control of portions of the aorta undergoing surgical repair, blood loss can be considerable in these cases because of backbleeding from the intercostal arteries, which are often ligated when the aorta is opened. Use of intraoperative cell-scavenging devices has become common and has reduced the need for banked blood transfusions. However, large-volume blood loss can occur rapidly in these operations, and banked blood transfusions are often needed. As long as liver perfusion is adequate, even with a large blood loss, citrate toxicity usually is not a problem because of rapid "first-pass" metabolism in the liver.

CLINICAL PEARL   However, thoracic aneurysm repair, particularly with simple clamping, presents a unique situation because hepatic arterial blood flow to the liver is compromised, perhaps for an extended period. In this circumstance, transfusing banked blood may rapidly produce citrate toxicity, resulting in myocardial depression that requires vigilant calcium chloride infusion.

   7.   **Spinal cord protection.** In addition to the use of ECC, shunts, and expeditious surgery, several other methods have been promoted to protect the spinal cord during aortic cross-clamping.

   a.   **Maintaining perfusion pressure.** Some groups prefer to maintain the perfusion pressure of the distal aorta in the range of 40 to 60 mm Hg to increase blood flow to the middle and lower spinal cord. This practice should be regarded as controversial because at present, few data exist regarding outcome. *No method used to maintain blood flow to the distal aorta (i.e., shunt or partial bypass [PB]) guarantees that spinal cord blood flow, and therefore function, will be preserved.* Proximal and distal clamp placement to isolate the diseased aortic segment may include critical intercostal vessels that provide blood flow to the spinal cord, the loss of which is not compensated for by distal aortic perfusion. In addition, distal perfusion may be hindered by atherosclerotic disease in the abdominal aorta, which can also compromise blood flow to the kidneys and spinal cord. Finally, these crucial arterial vessels may be disrupted in gaining surgical exposure.

   b.   **Somatosensory-evoked potentials (SEPs).** SEPs have been promoted as a means of assessing functional status of the spinal cord during periods of possible ischemia. Briefly, SEPs are evoked in the brainstem and cerebral cortex by stimulating a peripheral nerve. Normal SEPs seem to indicate the integrity of the posterior (sensory) columns. However, SEPs have several shortcomings. First, during aortic surgery, the *anterior* (motor) horns are more at risk. Perhaps for this reason, patients who reportedly had normal SEPs during cross-clamping were subsequently found to have paraplegia. Second, it must be remembered that many anesthetics, including all of the halogenated drugs, nitrous oxide, and several IV drugs (e.g., thiopental, propofol), alter the amplitude and latency of the SEP. Ongoing dialogue should therefore occur between the anesthesiologist and the individual(s) performing and evaluating the neuromonitoring during the operation to create an anesthetic plan that will be compatible with effective SEP monitoring (e.g., one-half minimum alveolar concentration of volatile anesthetic). In addition, if simple cross-clamping is used, peripheral nerve ischemia will interfere with SEP interpretation.

      Although it has been used intraoperatively to help identify intercostal arteries that should be reimplanted to preserve spinal cord perfusion, SEP monitoring has not been shown to decrease the incidence of postoperative paraplegia.

   c.   **Motor-evoked potentials (MEPs).** Because of the noted deficiencies in SEPs monitoring, using MEPs has been advocated as a potentially superior method of monitoring for spinal cord ischemia, because MEP monitoring can accurately assess the integrity of the anterior horn of the spinal cord. However, because the central nerve roots cannot be accessed for direct stimulation during thoracic surgery, transcranial stimulation over the motor cortex is used. In addition to being cumbersome, this method has been reported to trigger seizures in susceptible patients. However, some groups have successfully used MEPs, particularly as an adjunct to SEPs, to detect spinal cord injury in patients undergoing thoracic and thoracoabdominal aortic aneurysm repair. Although studies have shown these neuromonitoring techniques to be helpful for predicting spinal cord injury during operations on the thoracic aorta, these monitoring methods cannot definitively rule out intraoperative spinal cord injury that will result in paraplegia. Therefore, these methods should be used in addition to, not instead of, intraoperative spinal cord protection strategies such as cerebrospinal fluid (CSF) drainage and other efforts to maintain arterial perfusion of the spinal cord [24–26]. As with

SEP monitoring, MEP monitoring requires good communication between the anesthesiologist and the neuromonitoring personnel, particularly because neuromuscular blockade cannot be used during intervals when MEP assessment is needed.

d. **Hypothermia.** Allowing the core body temperature to passively drift down to 32° to 34°C during surgery lowers the metabolic rate of the spinal cord tissue, possibly providing some protection from reduced or interrupted blood flow. Usually, temperature can be reduced adequately by exposing the patient to a cool operating room. Other methods such as topical cooling (cooling blankets, bags of crushed ice) and cold saline gastric lavage also may be used. Controlling temperature precisely is difficult, though. At temperatures below 32°C, the myocardium may become more prone to ventricular arrhythmias, and hypothermia increases the risk of coagulopathy. Despite these potential problems, using vigorous methods to rewarm the patient is ill advised because of the risk of rapidly warming neural tissue that may be ischemic.

e. **CSF drainage.** Spinal cord damage may also be mediated by the increases in CSF pressure (CSFP) that often accompany aortic cross-clamping. CSFP can increase to levels as high as the mean distal **aortic** pressure. Spinal cord perfusion pressure (SCPP) is proportional to the patient's MAP minus the CSFP or CVP—whichever is highest. SCPP may be reduced to zero during aortic cross-clamping. One approach to improving perfusion is placing a lumbar spinal drain, which not only allows measurement of the CSFP, but also, by removal of CSF, reduces CSFP and increases SCPP, which apparently reduces the risk of paraplegia [27]. In a randomized controlled trial, CSF drainage significantly decreased postoperative paraplegia and paraparesis rates in 145 patients who underwent surgical repair of Extent I or II thoracoabdominal aneurysm: 13% and 2.6% of patients experienced postoperative paraplegia or paraparesis in the control group versus the spinal drain group, respectively [21]. A meta-analysis of 10 clinical trials of CSF drainage and its effect on spinal cord injury rates after open thoracoabdominal aortic aneurysm repair suggests a reduction in the short-term spinal cord injury rate, although the effects on longer-term spinal cord injury in this meta-analysis (5 studies with long-term data) were not statistically significant [28].

(1) **Potential complications of spinal drain placement.** Draining CSF in patients with elevated intraspinal pressure can provide a gradient for herniation of cerebral structures. Also, CSF drainage, particularly more rapid CSF drainage to lower CSFPs, can cause intracranial bleeding from traction of the brain on the meninges, torn bridging veins, and the formation of subdural hematomas [29,30]. Risk of intracranial bleeding can be decreased by maintaining CSFP above at least 10 cm H_2O (7.4 mm Hg) during CSF drainage [29]. To reduce the incidence of intracranial hemorrhage and subdural hematoma, some centers have changed their indications for perioperative CSF drainage in patients with no indications of spinal cord injury (e.g., changes on intraoperative SEP or MEP monitoring, postoperative paraplegia). For these patients, CSF drainage is now targeted to less aggressive minimum CSFP thresholds, such as 10 to 15 mm Hg, and the rate of drainage is not to exceed 15 mL/hr even if CSFP is above the minimum. If the patients develop paraplegia postoperatively, CSF drainage is then liberalized to try to provoke resolution of the paralysis. If a subdural hematoma develops and CSF is still leaking from the insertion site after drain removal, an epidural blood patch may be warranted at the site [29]. In addition, spinal drain placement followed by systemic heparinization could lead to the formation of an epidural hematoma at the insertion site [30]. This is of more concern in patients who are undergoing concurrent aortic arch and descending thoracic aortic repairs that involve CPB with full heparinization and DHCA and who are, thus, at increased risk of bleeding. Another risk associated with drain placement is catheter fracture in the subarachnoid space.

(2) **Technique for inserting and monitoring spinal drains.** A variety of spinal drain catheters are commercially available, but the insertion technique is similar for all. Spinal drain catheters are generally placed according to anatomic landmarks

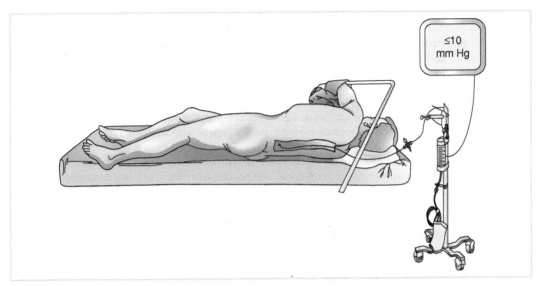

FIGURE 14.16 Intraoperative cerebrospinal fluid (CSF) drainage during thoracoabdominal aortic repair. (From Safi HJ, Miller CC III, Huynh TT, et al. Distal aortic perfusion and CSF drainage for thoracoabdominal and descending thoracic aortic repair: ten years of organ protection. *Ann Surg.* 2003;238:372–380, with permission.)

through a 14G (or smaller) Touhy needle that has been inserted into the subarachnoid space at a lumbar interspace (usually L_3 to L_4 or L_4 to L_5). Once the catheter is threaded into the subarachnoid space and the needle is removed, the drain is attached to a stopcock that allows toggling between CSFP measurement and drainage collection (Fig. 14.16). Some practitioners drain CSF intermittently to reduce CSFP, while others prefer to allow continuous drainage whenever the CSFP exceeds a predetermined set point.

CLINICAL PEARL Although many try maintaining CSFP at 8 to 10 mm Hg to balance the benefit of increasing SCPP against the risk of supratentorial bleeding with a lower CSFP, there is no consensus in the literature regarding what the optimal target CSFP is or how much CSF should be drained over a set time period.

(3) **Postoperative spinal drain management.** There is also no consensus regarding when spinal drains should be removed. This is of concern because 30% or more of all neurologic deficits have delayed onset [31]. Spinal drains are commonly left in for 48 to 72 hours postoperatively [21] and are replaced if neurologic deficits occur after the drain is removed. In addition to maintaining CSFP at 10 to 15 mm Hg in the postoperative setting, efforts must be made to avoid systemic hypotension and associated decreased spinal cord perfusion. If delayed-onset paraparesis or paraplegia evolves, systemic hypotension should be treated and CSF drained. This combination of measures can result in some recovery of neurologic function. As with any patient with a dural puncture, headaches related to residual CSF leaks may be expected, and some will require therapy with epidural blood patches. Reviewing experience at the Texas Heart Institute, we found that the incidences of post–dural puncture headaches and need for an epidural blood patch were elevated in patients with connective tissue diseases such as Marfan syndrome [32].

(4) **Other methods of spinal cord protection.** Additional "protective" measures, such as IV steroids, pharmacologic suppression of spinal cord function through IV

or intrathecal drug administration, local hypothermia, and free radical scavengers, are not widely used or are considered experimental.

8. **Pain relief.** Thoracic and thoracoabdominal aortic surgical patients can be given IV opioid and oral analgesics to relieve postoperative pain. Anesthesiologists may also consider using thoracic epidural anesthesia as an adjunctive perioperative pain control measure, although, depending on the length of the surgical incision, analgesic coverage may not be complete. Whereas thoracic epidural analgesia can potentially enhance perioperative pain control, the risk of additional significant complications associated with thoracic epidural placement should also be considered. In a patient who will undergo partial or even full heparinization and who may have significant intraoperative and early postoperative coagulopathy, instrumenting the epidural space can increase the risk of epidural hematoma (just as placing a spinal drain does). This possibility is particularly worrisome because these patients already have a primary risk of significant neurologic complications. Additionally, using a thoracic epidural may mask neurologic complications related to the removal of a CSF drainage catheter [33]. Thoracic epidural use can delay the diagnosis and treatment of spinal cord ischemia, such as when a patient cannot move his or her legs postoperatively, and the possibility of epidural hematoma or motor blockade related to local anesthesia must also be considered.

9. **Preventing renal failure.** Many patients who require thoracoabdominal aortic repair also present with renal dysfunction. It is therefore important to try to prevent the development of acute or chronic renal failure during the perioperative period. Renal failure is thought to be caused by ischemia from interruption of blood flow during clamping, although embolism remains another possibility. Using CPB or a shunt may be protective, but definitive outcome data are lacking, and renal failure can still occur despite the use of these surgical adjuncts. Adequate volume loading is probably important for renal protection, and some clinicians also use mannitol. In some centers, cold crystalloid or cold blood renal perfusion is administered during thoracoabdominal aneurysm repair. If the renal arteries can be surgically exposed during periods of the operation when renal arterial blood flow is interrupted, perfusate can be administered with a roller-head pump into perfusion catheters that are inserted into the renal arteries [34].

I. **Endovascular (EV) graft repair of the thoracic aorta**

Successful EV graft abdominal aortic aneurysm repair was first reported in 1991 [35]. Since then, EV graft design has improved to allow reliable deployment in the higher-pulse pressure zones of the thoracic aorta, permitting EV repair of thoracic aortic aneurysms and dissections that were previously only reparable with open procedures. This progress has continued to the present with advances in equipment design, including reduced introducer and graft sizes, and increased use of percutaneous vessel-closure devices rather than surgical cutdown for vessel access. There has also been a progressive increase in "hybrid" procedures combining EV intervention with an adjunctive surgical procedure that is less extensive than a purely surgical operation would be (e.g., use of an EV graft to treat a thoracic aneurysm plus a carotid-to-subclavian bypass because the EV graft occludes the origin of the LSA). This has led to EV therapy of more complex aortic arch and descending thoracic aortic lesions.

1. **Surgical approach.** Placing EV grafts in the thoracic aorta generally requires femoral arterial access through which fluoroscopically guided wires and catheters can be passed to allow optimal EV graft positioning. The FA can be accessed percutaneously, or it can be exposed and isolated via a small groin incision. If the FA is too small or stenotic to accommodate the relatively large thoracic EV graft delivery system, retroperitoneal dissection may be required to attain access to the iliac artery. There are reports of EV grafts being placed in the descending thoracic aorta via alternative arterial access sites such as the axillary arteries, but the FA remains the typical access site for EV graft delivery. The delivery system is positioned fluoroscopically at the desired implantation site, and when the delivery device is withdrawn, the endograft expands at this final aortic position. After EV graft deployment, fluoroscopy and TEE are generally used to reassess for blood leakage

around the graft. Patients are positioned supine on the fluoroscopy table throughout the procedure.

2. **Surgical techniques**

   a. Patients must be systemically anticoagulated, usually with heparin, during the procedure.

   b. It is important that patients do not move during angiography, particularly during EV graft deployment. Sometimes, the interventionalist will ask the anesthesiologist to hold respirations during the procedure so that the portion of the aorta in which the EV graft will be deployed can be more closely assessed. This is one reason why EV graft placement in the descending thoracic aorta is usually performed with general anesthesia.

   c. EV grafts are designed to withstand the continuous forward and pulsatile forces of blood flow in the aorta. Advances have led to the development of self-expanding stents that reliably adhere to the aortic wall after deployment and do not require temporarily occlusive balloon inflation in the aorta. This removes the risks of proximal hypertension associated with occluding the thoracic aorta.

   d. EV graft design is evolving rapidly; therefore, the number of patients ineligible for EV grafts is decreasing. However, limitations remain regarding who can receive an EV graft in the descending thoracic aorta. The patient's aortic pathology must ideally have a proximal "landing zone" at least 10 to 15 mm in length and a diameter no greater than that of the largest available EV graft. Many descending thoracic aneurysms and dissections involve the distal aortic arch, including the takeoff of the LSA. EV stent grafts are now placed that cover the ostia of the LSA, but prophylactic preprocedural LSA transposition or left subclavian-to-left common carotid artery bypass is frequently performed as noted above to prevent post–EV graft complications, including left arm ischemia, stroke, and spinal cord ischemia [36,37]. These complications can occur because the LSA not only is the main source of blood flow to the left arm but also branches into the vertebral artery (which contributes to the blood flow to the posterior portion of the circle of Willis), the left internal mammary artery, and costocervical trunk [36]. Myocardial ischemia in patients who have a patent left internal mammary arterial bypass graft is also possible when the LSA takeoff is covered by an EV graft [36]. It is important to note that stroke can also occur as a complication of LSA transposition or left subclavian-to-left common carotid artery bypass, so patients' cerebral blood flow anatomy and institutional comfort with the procedure should be considered before LSA revascularization is performed [36]. The distal site for EV graft attachment needs to be nonaneurysmal and also of sufficient length. Furthermore, fenestrated stents can be used to accommodate aortic side branches [38], but the location of these side branches still must be carefully evaluated and considered when one is selecting and placing EV grafts. Aortic tortuosity, calcification, and atheromatous disease are also considerations in determining whether a patient is an appropriate candidate for EV graft placement.

3. **Advantages of EV graft repair**

   a. Reduced mortality. Randomized controlled trials have shown significantly decreased mortality in patients who undergo EV repair of abdominal aortic aneurysms [39,40]. Nonrandomized studies of descending thoracic aorta repair have associated EV grafting with significantly lower 30-day mortality than open surgical repair; however, this mortality benefit may not persist at 1 year after thoracic aortic repair [41]. The randomized controlled INvestigation of STEnt grafts in Aortic Dissection (INSTEAD) trial reported no significant 2-year mortality advantage for EV stenting versus medical therapy alone in patients with uncomplicated type B dissection [42]. However, in a 5-year follow-up study of the INSTEAD patients, rates of aorta-specific mortality and progression of aortic disease were significantly lower in those who underwent EV repair rather than optimal medical management [43].

b. **Reduced morbidity.** Patients have substantially less blood loss with EV procedures and are spared the prolonged recovery and pulmonary complications that are often associated with large thoracoabdominal incisions. EV procedures also allow greater hemodynamic stability and lower ischemic risk to the heart and other organs than open repairs do. Patients with pulmonary and cardiac comorbidities that would eliminate them as candidates for open repair are often acceptable candidates for thoracic aortic EV graft placement. A meta-analysis of 42 nonrandomized studies that included 5,888 patients with aneurysm, trauma, or dissection of the descending thoracic aorta revealed that patients who underwent EV repair versus open surgical repair had significantly less perioperative paraplegia, cardiac complications, transfusions, reoperation for bleeding, renal dysfunction, and pneumonia, and a shorter hospital length of stay [41]. In addition, many patients who undergo EV repair require substantially shorter intensive care unit stays [44,45].

4. **Complications of EV repair**

   a. **Emergency conversion to open repair** may be necessary if the aorta is ruptured or dissected during manipulations to place the EV graft, or if the EV graft becomes malpositioned such that it poses a substantial risk of visceral ischemia.

   b. **Bleeding.** Although blood loss during EV repair of the thoracic aorta is markedly less (by approximately 500 mL) [45] than during open surgery, bleeding does occur from the FA introducer when it is traversed by wires and catheters during EV repair. Because many patients with thoracic aortic disease have comorbidities that make anemia especially undesirable, significant bleeding warrants periprocedural blood transfusion. Large-volume blood loss can also occur if the internal iliac artery is damaged during removal of a large-diameter graft-deployment device. Massive blood loss should be anticipated in patients with aortic rupture.

   c. **Endoleak.** Endoleak occurs when blood continues to flow into the aneurysmal sac after EV graft placement. It confers continued risk of aortic rupture and thus requires early identification and intervention. If identified, responses range from observation over several months to see whether the leak resolves spontaneously, to another EV procedure to occlude the source of the leak, to, in some cases, open surgical repair. The degree of intervention depends on the type of leak identified. Type I endoleak occurs with an inadequate seal between the EV graft and the wall of the aorta at either the proximal or distal attachment sites, such that there is persistent flow into the native aneurysm. Type II endoleak occurs when the portion of the aorta that was to be excluded by the graft fills in a retrograde fashion from back-bleeding collateral vessels, such as the lumbar or inferior mesenteric arteries. No definitive approach exists for addressing type II endoleak: both observation and side-branch embolization are used. Type III endoleak results from EV graft failure and requires conversion to open repair so that the EV graft does not dislodge.

   d. **Stroke.** The incidence of periprocedural stroke is ~5% [41] and appears to be highest in patients whose EV graft is placed in the region of the distal arch that includes the takeoff of the LSA. Among patients who undergo EV graft placement across the LSA, stroke risk may be lower in those who undergo a staged carotid-to-subclavian artery bypass procedure first, as this may prevent vertebrobasilar arterial insufficiency and potential ensuing posterior cerebral infarction [36]. Stroke risk is elevated in patients who have a history of stroke, whose computed tomography scans reveal severe atheromatous disease of the aortic arch, or in whom EV grafting involves the distal aortic arch [46]. For these reasons, it seems likely that stroke is secondary to embolic events that result from intra-aortic or carotid arterial manipulation during positioning and deployment of the EV graft.

   e. **Paraplegia.** Although some data suggest that risk of lower-extremity paraparesis or paralysis is lower in patients undergoing EV graft versus open thoracic aortic repair, its incidence is still 3% to 4% [41,45,47]. Many surgeons and interventional radiologists, therefore, prefer that a lumbar spinal drain be placed before the procedure and that

CSF drainage be conducted in the same manner described in Section IV.H.7.e for open thoracoabdominal operations.

f. **Contrast nephropathy (CN).** Whereas patients who undergo open aortic surgical repair are susceptible to postoperative acute renal failure from ischemia during aortic cross-clamping, patients who undergo EV graft repair are susceptible to CN. Patients with pre-existing renal insufficiency, especially those with diabetic nephropathy, are particularly susceptible to CN [48]. Older age, hypertension, repeat contrast exposure within a short time, use of high-osmolality contrast, and preprocedural medications such as nonsteroidal anti-inflammatory drugs and angiotensin-converting enzyme (ACE) inhibitors also increase patients' risk of CN [48]. Although the pathogenesis of CN is not completely understood, it appears to be related to decreased renal medullary perfusion and associated ischemia, as well as a direct toxic effect of contrast on the renal epithelial cells. We refer the reader to two excellent reviews of CN for a more detailed discussion [48,49].

J. **Anesthetic considerations for patients undergoing EV stent graft repair of the thoracic aorta**
1. **General considerations**
   a. Although thoracic aortic EV graft placement is minimally invasive, the possibility of aortic rupture, dissection, or malposition of the EV graft should be considered when the location for the procedure is selected and the anesthetic approach is chosen, because any of these complications would necessitate urgent or emergent conversion to an open procedure. If the procedure must be conducted in an imaging suite because no available operating room has appropriate angiographic equipment, the entire care team involved in the procedure must be familiar with plans for resuscitation and for transport to the operating room. If a cardiac or vascular surgeon is not performing the EV graft procedure, one should be immediately available if conversion to open surgery is necessary.
   b. Although there are reports of placing thoracic aortic EV grafts under regional anesthesia, this approach has several disadvantages in comparison to general anesthesia.
      (1) Should emergency conversion to open aortic repair be necessary, this conversion will be slowed by the need to establish airway control before positioning the patient for the operation.
      (2) If the patient is intubated at the start of the procedure and the surgeon believes that the patient is at substantial risk for open conversion, the anesthesiologist can place a bronchial blocker in the left main stem bronchus without inflating it. The bronchial blocker could then be quickly inflated during emergency conversion to provide single-lung ventilation.
      (3) Many thoracic aortic EV graft procedures are too lengthy for regional anesthesia.
      (4) General anesthesia with endotracheal intubation allows the anesthesiologist or cardiologist to conduct TEE evaluation throughout the procedure. This is particularly useful in assessing for endoleaks and for differentiating slow leakage associated with the porosity of the EV stent graft from true high-velocity persistent endoleak [50,51]. In patients undergoing EV stent graft placement for complicated type B dissection, TEE can also be helpful for repositioning the guidewire from the false to the true lumen and for detecting new intimal tears in the thoracic aorta after EV stent placement [50]. Such new distal aortic tears might require additional EV stents to be placed.

2. **Monitoring.** All patients should have standard ASA monitors and a radial arterial line for BP monitoring to help maintain hemodynamic stability. The majority of patients presenting for thoracic aortic EV grafts have significant cardiovascular comorbidities that warrant tight hemodynamic control. Furthermore, surgeons may request transient, mild hypotension during stent deployment to help prevent graft migration. In the event that emergent conversion to open surgery is needed, an arterial line will be extremely useful in guiding volume resuscitation and possible cardiopulmonary resuscitation. The site of

arterial access for stent delivery should be discussed with the surgical team because, if the iliofemoral vasculature is not adequate for the procedure, they may choose to deliver the stent via a brachial artery instead. Typically, a right radial arterial line is ideal for hemodynamic monitoring because it allows monitoring of arterial pressure proximal to the distal aortic arch. Central venous access for monitoring right atrial pressure and effectively administering vasoactive drugs is reasonable for most patients. Some centers monitor SEPs and/or MEPs, as well as CSFP, during placement of thoracic aortic EV grafts. Urine output should be monitored to help assess adequacy of fluid administration during what can often be long procedures. A fluid warmer and warming blanket should be used if possible to help prevent hypothermia, and oropharyngeal temperature should be monitored.

3. **Fluid therapy and transfusion**
   a. Large-bore IV access should be established in case rapid volume resuscitation is needed.
   b. Crossmatched, packed red blood cells should be available.
   c. A system for rapidly infusing blood products and other fluids should be immediately available in cases in which volume resuscitation is needed.

4. **Cerebrospinal fluid (CSF) drainage.** Risk of paraplegia or paraparesis after EV graft placement remains approximately 3% to 4%, as noted above, particularly if long segments of the descending thoracic aorta are involved in EV graft placement or if the patient has previously undergone abdominal aortic aneurysm repair [52,53]. Therefore, many surgeons, interventionalists, and anesthesiologists prefer to place and manage lumbar spinal drains for EV graft procedures in the manner described above. IV fluids and vasopressor drugs should be administered to maintain higher MAP. As with patients who undergo open surgical repair of the descending thoracic aorta, delayed-onset paraparesis or paraplegia can occur in patients who receive EV stent grafts [52,53], so patients should undergo frequent postprocedural neurologic examination; if signs of spinal cord ischemia/injury are detected, aggressive efforts should be made to increase MAP and to drain more CSF.

5. **Contrast nephropathy (CN).** Because EV grafting of the thoracic aorta is often a long procedure that involves a substantial volume of IV contrast, the anesthesiologist should consider strategies to attenuate the risk of CN, particularly in patients with renal insufficiency.
   a. **Hydration.** Studies suggest that preprocedural hydration with 0.9% normal saline mitigates patients' risk of CN [48]. There is no consensus regarding duration of IV 0.9% normal saline infusion before or after the procedure, but avoiding hypovolemia in these patients during the procedure is advisable [49].
   b. **N-acetylcysteine (NAC).** NAC has antioxidant and vasodilatory effects. Some studies have shown a benefit of pretreating patients with NAC for 24 hours before procedures requiring IV contrast, while other studies have shown no such benefit [48,49].
   c. **Diuretics.** Diuretic use does not seem to prevent CN. Some advocate that, if possible, diuretics be withdrawn for the 24 hours before procedures requiring contrast [48] because of concern that they may increase the risk of CN.
   d. **Dopamine and fenoldopam.** Neither of these drugs has been found to prevent CN in human studies [48].

K. **Future trends**

Just as the past several decades of treatment of aortic diseases have been marked by innovation and the refinement of surgical and anesthetic techniques, so also will future years. The most promising developments continue to be made in the area of EV stenting of aneurysmal, dissected, or traumatically transected segments of the aorta. EV stent graft technology will probably continue to advance, with the industry focusing on newer fenestrated grafts that will not obstruct blood flow to important aortic side branches, and other grafts that are able to adhere to curved portions of the aorta, such as the aortic arch. There will also probably be innovations regarding alternate arterial access points for inserting EV stent–deployment devices. Hopefully, greater strides will also be made toward even better protection strategies for organs (i.e., spinal cord, gut, and kidneys), including novel approaches to mitigating end-organ ischemia–reperfusion injury.

Anesthetic developments will focus on refining understanding of the physiology of organ preservation and the pharmacology needed to achieve this. Such advances should continue to improve the survival of patients with thoracic aortic disease.

REFERENCES

1. **Hiratzka LF, Bakris GL, Beckman JA, et al. 2010 ACCF/AHA/AATS/ACR/ASA/SCA/SCAI/SIR/STS/SVM guidelines for the diagnosis and management of patients with thoracic aortic disease: a report of the American College of Cardiology Foundation/American Heart Association Task Force on Practice Guidelines, American Association for Thoracic Surgery, American College of Radiology, American Stroke Association, Society of Cardiovascular Anesthesiologists, Society for Cardiovascular Angiography and Interventions, Society of Interventional Radiology, Society of Thoracic Surgeons, and Society for Vascular Medicine. *Circulation*. 2010;121(13):e266–e369.**
2. Kouchoukos NT, Dougenis D. Surgery of the thoracic aorta. *N Engl J Med*. 1997;336(26):1876–1888.
3. Hirst AE Jr, Johns VJ Jr, Kime SW Jr. Dissecting aneurysm of the aorta: a review of 505 cases. *Medicine (Baltimore)*. 1958;37(3):217–279.
4. Bickerstaff LK, Pairolero PC, Hollier LH, et al. Thoracic aortic aneurysms: a population-based study. *Surgery*. 1982;92(6):1103–1108.
5. Hartnell GG. Imaging of aortic aneurysms and dissection: CT and MRI. *J Thorac Imaging*. 2001;16(1):35–46.
6. Nauta FJ, Trimarchi S, Kamman AV, et al. Update in the management of type B aortic dissection. *Vasc Med*. 2016;21(3):251–263.
7. Shore-Lesserson L, Bodian C, Vela-Cantos F, et al. Antifibrinolytic use and bleeding during surgery on the descending thoracic aorta: a multivariate analysis. *J Cardiothorac Vasc Anesth*. 2005;19(4):453–458.
8. Svensson LG, Crawford ES, Hess KR, et al. Deep hypothermia with circulatory arrest. Determinants of stroke and early mortality in 656 patients. *J Thorac Cardiovasc Surg*. 1993;106(1):19–28; discussion 28–31.
9. Shum-Tim D, Nagashima M, Shinoka T, et al. Postischemic hyperthermia exacerbates neurologic injury after deep hypothermic circulatory arrest. *J Thorac Cardiovasc Surg*. 1998;116(5):780–792.
10. Ueda Y, Okita Y, Aomi S, et al. Retrograde cerebral perfusion for aortic arch surgery: analysis of risk factors. *Ann Thorac Surg*. 1999;67(6):1879–1882; discussion 1891–1894.
11. Urbanski PP, Lenos A, Kolowca M, et al. Near-infrared spectroscopy for neuromonitoring of unilateral cerebral perfusion. *Eur J Cardiothorac Surg*. 2013;43(6):1140–1144.
12. **Strauch JT, Spielvogel D, Lauten A, et al. Axillary artery cannulation: routine use in ascending aorta and aortic arch replacement. *Ann Thorac Surg*. 2004;78(1):103–108; discussion 103–108.**
13. Bachet J, Guilmet D, Goudot B, et al. Antegrade cerebral perfusion with cold blood: a 13-year experience. *Ann Thorac Surg*. 1999;67(6):1874–1878; discussion 1891–1894.
14. Nussmeier NA, Cheng W, Marino M, et al. Temperature during cardiopulmonary bypass: the discrepancies between monitored sites. *Anesth Analg*. 2006;103:1373–1379.
15. Harrer M, Waldenberger FR, Weiss G, et al. Aortic arch surgery using bilateral antegrade selective cerebral perfusion in combination with near-infrared spectroscopy. *Eur J Cardiothorac Surg*. 2010;38(5):561–567.
16. Murkin JM, Arango M. Near-infrared spectroscopy as an index of brain and tissue oxygenation. *Br J Anaesth*. 2009;103(Suppl 1):i3–i13.
17. **Gelman S. The pathophysiology of aortic cross-clamping and unclamping. *Anesthesiology*. 1995;82(4):1026–1060.**
18. Romagnoli A, Cooper JR Jr. Anesthesia for aortic operations. *Cleve Clin Q*. 1981;48(1):147–152.
19. Cambria RP, Clouse WD, Davison JK, et al. Thoracoabdominal aneurysm repair: results with 337 operations performed over a 15-year interval. *Ann Surg*. 2002;236(4):471–479; discussion 479.
20. Svensson LG, Crawford ES, Hess KR, et al. Experience with 1509 patients undergoing thoracoabdominal aortic operations. *J Vasc Surg*. 1993;17(2):357–368; discussion 368–370.
21. **Coselli JS, LeMaire SA, Köksoy C, et al. Cerebrospinal fluid drainage reduces paraplegia after thoracoabdominal aortic aneurysm repair: results of a randomized clinical trial. *J Vasc Surg*. 2002;35(4):631–639.**
22. O'Connor CJ, Rothenberg DM. Anesthetic considerations for descending thoracic aortic surgery: part 1. *J Cardiothorac Vasc Anesth*. 1995;9(5):581–588.
23. O'Connor CJ, Rothenberg DM. Anesthetic considerations for descending thoracic aortic surgery: part II. *J Cardiothorac Vasc Anesth*. 1995;9(6):734–747.
24. Horiuchi T, Kawaguchi M, Inoue S, et al. Assessment of intraoperative motor evoked potentials for predicting postoperative paraplegia in thoracic and thoracoabdominal aortic aneurysm repair. *J Anesth*. 2011;25(1):18–28.
25. Keyhani K, Miller CC 3rd, Estrera AL, et al. Analysis of motor and somatosensory evoked potentials during thoracic and thoracoabdominal aortic aneurysm repair. *J Vasc Surg*. 2009;49(1):36–41.
26. Min HK, Sung K, Yang JH, et al. Can intraoperative motor-evoked potentials predict all the spinal cord ischemia during moderate hypothermic beating heart descending thoracic or thoraco-abdominal aortic surgery? *J Card Surg*. 2010;25(5):542–547.
27. Ling E, Arellano R. Systematic overview of the evidence supporting the use of cerebrospinal fluid drainage in thoracoabdominal aneurysm surgery for prevention of paraplegia. *Anesthesiology*. 2000;93(4):1115–1122.
28. **Khan NR, Smalley Z, Nesvick CL, et al. The use of lumbar drains in preventing spinal cord injury following thoracoabdominal aortic aneurysm repair: an updated systematic review and meta-analysis. *J Neurosurg Spine*. 2016;25(3):383–393.**
29. Dardik A, Perler BA, Roseborough GS, et al. Subdural hematoma after thoracoabdominal aortic aneurysm repair: an underreported complication of spinal fluid drainage? *J Vasc Surg*. 2002;36(1):47–50.

30. Murakami H, Yoshida K, Hino Y, et al. Complications of cerebrospinal fluid drainage in thoracoabdominal aortic aneurysm repair. *J Vasc Surg.* 2004;39(1):243–245.

31. Wong DR, Coselli JS, Amerman K, et al. Delayed spinal cord deficits after thoracoabdominal aortic aneurysm repair. *Ann Thorac Surg.* 2007;83(4):1345–1355; discussion 1355.

32. **Youngblood SC, Tolpin DA, LeMaire SA, et al. Complications of cerebrospinal fluid drainage after thoracic aortic surgery: a review of 504 patients over 5 years. *J Thorac Cardiovasc Surg.* 2013;146(1):166–171.**

33. Heller LB, Chaney MA. Paraplegia immediately following removal of a cerebrospinal fluid drainage catheter in a patient after thoracoabdominal aortic aneurysm surgery. *Anesthesiology.* 2001;95(5):1285–1287.

34. **Coselli JS. Strategies for renal and visceral protection in thoracoabdominal aortic surgery. *J Thorac Cardiovasc Surg.* 2010;140(6 Suppl):S147–S149; discussion S185–S190.**

35. Parodi JC, Palmaz JC, Barone HD. Transfemoral intraluminal graft implantation for abdominal aortic aneurysms. *Ann Vasc Surg.* 1991;5(6):491–499.

36. Rehman SM, Vecht JA, Perera R, et al. How to manage the left subclavian artery during endovascular stenting of the thoracic aorta. *Eur J Cardiothorac Surg.* 2011;39(4):507–518.

37. Weigang E, Parker JA, Czerny M, et al. Should intentional endovascular stent-graft coverage of the left subclavian artery be preceded by prophylactic revascularisation? *Eur J Cardiothorac Surg.* 2011;40(4):858–868.

38. Eagleton MJ, Follansbee M, Wolski K, et al. Fenestrated and branched endovascular aneurysm repair outcomes for type II and III thoracoabdominal aortic aneurysms. *J Vasc Surg.* 2016;63(4):930–942.

39. Greenhalgh RM, Brown LC, Kwong GP, et al. Comparison of endovascular aneurysm repair with open repair in patients with abdominal aortic aneurysm (EVAR trial 1), 30-day operative mortality results: randomised controlled trial. *Lancet.* 2004;364(9437):843–848.

40. Prinssen M, Verhoeven EL, Buth J, et al. A randomized trial comparing conventional and endovascular repair of abdominal aortic aneurysms. *N Engl J Med.* 2004;351(16):1607–1618.

41. **Cheng D, Martin J, Shennib H, et al. Endovascular aortic repair versus open surgical repair for descending thoracic aortic disease: a systematic review and meta-analysis of comparative studies. *J Am Coll Cardiol.* 2010;55(10):986–1001.**

42. Nienaber CA, Rousseau H, Eggebrecht H, et al. Randomized comparison of strategies for type B aortic dissection: the INvestigation of STEnt Grafts in Aortic Dissection (INSTEAD) trial. *Circulation.* 2009;120(25):2519–2528.

43. **Nienaber CA, Kische S, Rousseau H, et al. Endovascular repair of type B aortic dissection: long-term results of the randomized investigation of stent grafts in aortic dissection trial. *Circ Cardiovasc Interv.* 2013;6(4):407–416.**

44. Gopaldas RR, Huh J, Dao TK, et al. Superior nationwide outcomes of endovascular versus open repair for isolated descending thoracic aortic aneurysm in 11,669 patients. *J Thorac Cardiovasc Surg.* 2010;140(5):1001–1010.

45. Makaroun MS, Dillavou ED, Kee ST, et al. Endovascular treatment of thoracic aortic aneurysms: results of the phase II multicenter trial of the GORE TAG thoracic endoprosthesis. *J Vasc Surg.* 2005;41(1):1–9.

46. Gutsche JT, Cheung AT, McGarvey ML, et al. Risk factors for perioperative stroke after thoracic endovascular aortic repair. *Ann Thorac Surg.* 2007;84(4):1195–1200; discussion 1200.

47. Leurs LJ, Bell R, Degrieck Y, et al. Endovascular treatment of thoracic aortic diseases: combined experience from the EUROSTAR and United Kingdom Thoracic Endograft registries. *J Vasc Surg.* 2004;40(4):670–679; discussion 679–680.

48. Maeder M, Klein M, Fehr T, et al. Contrast nephropathy: review focusing on prevention. *J Am Coll Cardiol.* 2004;44(9):1763–1771.

49. Barrett BJ, Parfrey PS. Clinical practice. Preventing nephropathy induced by contrast medium. *N Engl J Med.* 2006;354(4):379–386.

50. Rocchi G, Lofiego C, Biagini E, et al. Transesophageal echocardiography-guided algorithm for stent-graft implantation in aortic dissection. *J Vasc Surg.* 2004;40(5):880–885.

51. **Swaminathan M, Lineberger CK, McCann RL, et al. The importance of intraoperative transesophageal echocardiography in endovascular repair of thoracic aortic aneurysms. *Anesth Analg.* 2003;97(6):1566–1572.**

52. Baril DT, Carroccio A, Ellozy SH, et al. Endovascular thoracic aortic repair and previous or concomitant abdominal aortic repair: is the increased risk of spinal cord ischemia real? *Ann Vasc Surg.* 2006;20(2):188–194.

53. Gravereaux EC, Faries PL, Burks JA, et al. Risk of spinal cord ischemia after endograft repair of thoracic aortic aneurysms. *J Vasc Surg.* 2001;34(6):997–1003.

15

Anesthetic Management for Surgery of the Lungs and Mediastinum

Peter Slinger and Erin A. Sullivan

KEY POINTS

1. Preoperatively, respiratory function should be assessed in three related but independent areas: respiratory mechanics, gas exchange, and cardiopulmonary interaction.
2. The most useful preoperative predictor of difficult endobronchial intubation is the chest film.
3. The most important predictor of PaO_2 during one-lung ventilation (OLV) is the PaO_2 during two-lung ventilation in the lateral position before OLV.
4. Absolute indications for lung isolation include purulent secretions, massive pulmonary hemorrhage, bronchopleural fistula, blebs, and bullae (blood, pus, and air).
5. Iatrogenic injury has been estimated to occur in 0.5 to 2 per 1,000 cases using double-lumen tubes (DLTs).
6. The rapidity of the fall in PaO_2 after the onset of OLV is an indicator of the risk of subsequent desaturation.
7. Because of the risk of increased shunt and pulmonary edema in the dependent lung, no volume should be given for theoretical third-space losses during thoracotomy.
8. Desaturation during bilateral lung procedures is particularly a problem during the second period of OLV.

(continued)

9. The postoperative mortality following pneumonectomy is 17% in patients who develop arrhythmias versus 2% in those without this complication.
10. During induction of general anesthesia in patients with an anterior mediastinal mass, airway obstruction is the most common and feared complication.
11. Hemoptysis in a patient with a PA catheter must be assumed to be caused by perforation of a pulmonary vessel by the catheter until proven otherwise. The mortality rate may exceed 50%.
12. In a patient with pulmonary hypertension, abrupt cessation of treatment with a prostacyclin analog can result in potentially catastrophic rebound pulmonary hypertension.
13. Lung volume reduction surgery (LVRS) is a viable option for a select group of emphysema patients. Goals of treatment include improvements in dyspnea, exercise tolerance, quality of life, and prolonged patient survival.

I. Preoperative assessment

A. Overview

Advances in anesthetic management, surgical techniques, and perioperative care have expanded the envelope of patients now considered to be operable. The principles described apply to all types of pulmonary resections and other chest surgery. In patients with malignancy, the risk/benefit ratio of canceling or delaying surgery pending other investigation/therapy is always complicated by the risk of further spread of cancer during any interval before resection.

1. **Risk assessment.** It is the anesthesiologist's responsibility to use the preoperative assessment to identify patients at elevated risk and then to use that risk assessment to stratify perioperative management and focus resources on the high-risk patients to improve their outcome. This is the primary function of the preanesthetic assessment.

2. **Initial and final assessments.** Commonly, the patient is initially assessed in a clinic and often not by the member of the anesthesia staff who will administer the anesthesia. The actual contact with the responsible anesthesiologist may be only 10 to 15 minutes before induction. It is necessary to organize and standardize the approach to preoperative evaluation for these patients into two temporally disconnected phases: the initial (clinic) assessment and the final (day-of-admission) assessment.

3. **"Lung-sparing" surgery.** Postoperative preservation of respiratory function has been shown to be proportional to the amount of functioning lung parenchyma preserved. To assess patients with limited pulmonary function, the anesthesiologist must understand these surgical options in addition to conventional lobectomy and pneumonectomy.

   Prethoracotomy assessment involves all aspects of a complete anesthetic assessment: past history, allergies, medications, and upper airway. Respiratory complications comprise the major cause of perioperative morbidity and mortality in thoracic surgery. Atelectasis, pneumonia, and respiratory failure occur in 15% to 20% of patients, and cardiac complications (e.g., arrhythmia and ischemia) occur in 10% to 15% of them.

B. Risk stratification

1. **Assessment of respiratory function.** The best assessment of respiratory function comes from a history of the patient's quality of life. An asymptomatic American Society of Anesthesiologists (ASA) class I or II patient with full exercise capacity does not need screening cardiorespiratory testing. Assess respiratory function in three related but independent areas (see Fig. 15.1).

   a. **Lung mechanics.** The most valid single test [1] for postthoracotomy respiratory complications is the predicted postoperative forced expiratory volume in 1 second (ppoFEV$_1$%), which is calculated as follows:

   $$\text{ppoFEV}_1\% = \text{preop. FEV}_1\% \times (1 - \%\text{functional lung tissue removed}/100)$$

   Consider the right upper and middle lobes combined as approximately equivalent to each of the other three lobes and the right lung as 10% larger than the left lung.

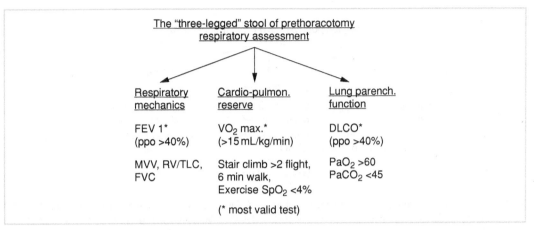

The "three-legged" stool of prethoracotomy respiratory assessment

FIGURE 15.1 "Three-legged" stool of prethoracotomy respiratory assessment. pulmon., pulmonary; parench., parenchymal; ppo, predicted postoperative; FEV 1, forced expiratory volume in 1 second; MVV, maximum voluntary ventilation; RV/TLC, residual volume/total lung capacity; FVC, forced vital capacity; VO_2 max, maximum oxygen consumption; SpO_2, oxygen saturation by pulse oximetry; DLCO, diffusing capacity for carbon monoxide; PaO_2, arterial partial pressure of oxygen; $PaCO_2$, arterial partial pressure of carbon dioxide.

Low risk = $ppoFEV_1$ >40% of preoperative predicted FEV_1
Moderate risk = $ppoFEV_1$ 30% to 40% of preoperative predicted FEV_1
High risk = $ppoFEV_1$ <30% of preoperative predicted FEV_1

b. **Pulmonary parenchymal function.** Traditionally, arterial blood gas (ABG) data such as preoperative PaO_2 less than 60 mm Hg or $PaCO_2$ greater than 45 mm Hg have been used as cutoff values for pulmonary resection. Cancer resections now have been successfully done or even combined with volume reduction in patients who do not meet these criteria, although they remain useful as warning indicators of increased risk. The most useful test of the gas exchange capacity of the lungs is the diffusing capacity for carbon monoxide (DLCO). DLCO correlates with the total functioning surface area of alveolar–capillary interface. A ppoDLCO less than 40% correlates with both increased respiratory and cardiac complications [2].

c. **Cardiopulmonary interaction.** The traditional test in ambulatory patients is stair climbing. The ability to climb three flights or more is associated with decreased mortality. Formal laboratory exercise testing is currently the "gold standard" for assessment of cardiopulmonary function. The maximal oxygen consumption (VO_2 max) is the most valid exercise predictor of postthoracotomy outcome. An estimate of VO_2 max can be made by dividing the distance walked in meters in 6 minutes (6MWT) by 30 (i.e., 450 m/30 = 15 mL/kg/min):

Low risk = VO_2 max >20 mL/kg/min
Moderate risk = VO_2 max = 15 to 20 mL/kg/min
High risk = VO_2 max <15 mL/kg/min

CLINICAL PEARL Patients who can climb at least three flights of stairs without stopping or who can walk at least 600 m in 6 minutes most often have a low risk of perioperative mortality following pulmonary resection.

d. **Ventilation–perfusion scintigraphy** is particularly useful in pneumonectomy patients and should be considered for any patient who has $ppoFEV_1$ less than 40%. Assessments of $ppoFEV_1$, DLCO, and VO_2 max can be upgraded if the lung region to be resected is nonfunctioning.

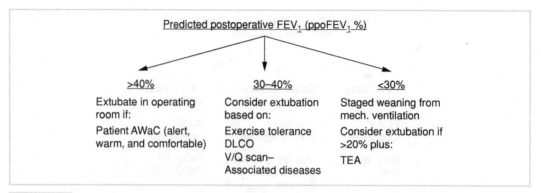

FIGURE 15.2 Postthoracotomy anesthetic management. FEV_1, forced expiratory volume in 1 second; ppo, predicted postoperative; DLCO, diffusing capacity for carbon monoxide; TEA, thoracic epidural analgesia; V/Q, ventilation/perfusion; mech., mechanical.

    e. **Split-lung function studies.** These tests have not shown sufficient predictive validity for universal adoption in potential lung resection patients.

    f. **Combination of tests** (Fig. 15.2). If a patient has $ppoFEV_1$ greater than 40%, it should be possible for the patient to be extubated in the operating room at the conclusion of surgery, assuming the patient is alert, warm, and comfortable ("AWaC"). If $ppoFEV_1$ is greater than 30% and exercise tolerance and lung parenchymal function exceed the increased risk thresholds, then extubation in the operating room should be possible depending on the status of associated diseases. Patients with $ppoFEV_1$ 20% to 30% and favorable predicted cardiorespiratory and parenchymal function can be considered for early extubation if thoracic epidural analgesia (TEA) is used.

2. **Intercurrent medical conditions**

    a. **Age.** For patients older than 80 years, the rate of respiratory complications (40%) is double that expected in a younger population, and the rate of cardiac complications (40%), particularly arrhythmias, nearly triples. The mortality from pneumonectomy (22% in patients older than 70 years), particularly right pneumonectomy, is excessive.

> **CLINICAL PEARL**   As compared to that for middle-aged patients, the risk of pulmonary complications in patients over 80 years of age doubles and the risk of cardiac complications almost triples.

    b. **Cardiac disease**

       (1) **Ischemia.** Pulmonary resection is generally regarded as an intermediate-risk procedure for perioperative ischemia. Beyond the standard history, physical examination, and electrocardiogram, routine screening for cardiac disease does not appear to be cost effective for prethoracotomy patients. Noninvasive testing is indicated in patients with active cardiac conditions (unstable ischemia, recent infarction, decompensated heart failure, severe valvular disease, significant arrhythmia), multiple clinical predictors of cardiac risk (stable angina, remote infarction, previous congestive failure, diabetes, renal insufficiency, or cerebrovascular disease), or in the elderly. Lung resection surgery should ideally be delayed 4 to 6 weeks after placement of a bare-metal coronary artery stent and 6 to 12 months after a drug-eluting stent. After a myocardial infarction, limiting the delay to 4 to 6 weeks in a medically stable and fully investigated and optimized patient seems acceptable.

       (2) **Arrhythmia.** Atrial fibrillation is a common complication (10% to 15%) of pulmonary resection surgery. Factors correlating with an increased incidence of arrhythmia are the amount of lung tissue resected, age, intraoperative blood loss, esophagectomy, and intrapericardial dissection. American Association of Thoracic

Surgery guidelines recommend continuation of β-blockers in patients already receiving them and replacement of magnesium in any patient with low magnesium stores. For patients at increased risk of arrhythmias, perioperative diltiazem and postoperative amiodarone prophylaxis should be considered [3].

c. **Chronic obstructive pulmonary disease (COPD).** Assessment of the severity of COPD is based on $FEV_1\%$ predicted, as follows—stage I: greater than 50%; stage II: 35% to 50%; and stage III: less than 35%. The following factors in COPD need to be considered.

(1) **Respiratory drive.** Many stage II or III COPD patients have an elevated $PaCO_2$ at rest. It is not possible to differentiate "CO_2 retainers" from nonretainers on the basis of history, physical examination, or spirometry. These patients need an ABG preoperatively. Supplemental oxygen causes the $PaCO_2$ to increase in CO_2 retainers by a combination of decreased respiratory drive and increased dead space.

CLINICAL PEARL In patients with advanced COPD, neither history, physical examination, nor FEV_1 predicts chronic CO_2 retention.

---

(2) **Nocturnal hypoxemia.** COPD patients desaturate more frequently and severely than normal patients during sleep. This results from the rapid/shallow breathing pattern that occurs during rapid eye movement sleep.

(3) **Right ventricular (RV) dysfunction.** Cor pulmonale occurs in 40% of adult COPD patients with FEV_1 less than 1 L and in 70% with FEV_1 less than 0.6 L. COPD patients who have resting PaO_2 less than 55 mm Hg and those who desaturate to less than 44 mm Hg with exercise (SpO_2 approximately 75%) should receive supplemental home oxygen. The goal of supplemental oxygen is to maintain PaO_2 at 60 to 65 mm Hg. Pneumonectomy candidates with $ppoFEV_1$ less than 40% should have transthoracic echocardiography to assess right heart function. Elevation of right heart pressures places these patients in a very high-risk group.

3. **Preoperative therapy of chronic obstructive pulmonary disease (COPD).** The four complications of COPD that must be actively sought and treated at the initial prethoracotomy assessment are atelectasis, bronchospasm, chest infection, and pulmonary edema. Patients with COPD have fewer postoperative pulmonary complications when a perioperative program of chest physiotherapy is initiated preoperatively. Pulmonary complications decrease in thoracic surgical patients who are not smoking versus those who continue to smoke up until the time of surgery.

4. **Lung cancer considerations.** At the time of initial assessment, cancer patients should be assessed for the "4 M's" associated with malignancy: **M**ass effects, **M**etabolic abnormalities, **M**etastases, and **M**edications. Prior use of medications that can exacerbate oxygen-induced pulmonary toxicity, such as bleomycin, should be considered (Table 15.1).

5. **Postoperative analgesia.** The risks and benefits of the various forms of postthoracotomy analgesia should be explained to the patient at the time of initial preanesthetic assessment. Potential contraindications to specific methods of analgesia should be determined, such as coagulation problems, sepsis, and neurologic disorders. If the patient will receive prophylactic anticoagulants and epidural analgesia is elected, appropriate timing of anticoagulant

---

TABLE 15.1 Anesthetic considerations in lung cancer patients (the "4 M's")

I. **Mass effects:** Obstructive pneumonia, superior vena cava syndrome, tracheobronchial distortion, Pancoast syndrome, recurrent laryngeal nerve or phrenic nerve paresis

II. **Metabolic effects:** Lambert–Eaton syndrome, hypercalcemia, hyponatremia, Cushing syndrome

III. **Metastases:** Particularly to brain, bone, liver, and adrenal gland

IV. **Medications:** Chemotherapy agents, pulmonary toxicity (bleomycin, mitomycin), cardiac toxicity (doxorubicin), renal toxicity (cis-platinum)

TABLE 15.2 Summary of preanesthetic assessment

Initial preanesthetic assessment for pulmonary resection
I. All patients: Exercise tolerance, ppoFEV$_1$%, discuss postoperative analgesia, D/C smoking
II. Patients with ppoFEV$_1$ <40%: DLCO, V/Q scan, VO$_2$ max
III. Cancer patients: The "4 M's": Mass effects, metabolic effects, metastases, medications
IV. COPD patients: ABG, physiotherapy, bronchodilators

Final preanesthetic assessment for pulmonary resection
I. Review initial assessment and test results
II. Assess difficulty of lung isolation: Chest x-ray film, CT scan
III. Assess risk of hypoxemia during OLV

CT, computed tomographic; D/C, discontinue; DLCO, diffusing capacity for carbon monoxide; ppoFEV$_1$, predicted postoperative forced expiratory volume in 1 second; V/Q, ventilation/perfusion; VO$_2$ max, maximum oxygen consumption; COPD, chronic obstructive pulmonary disease; ABG, arterial blood gas; OLV, one-lung ventilation.

administration and neuraxial catheter placement must be arranged. American Society of Regional Anesthesia guidelines suggest excluding prophylactic heparin administration during a "window" of 2 to 4 hours before to 1 hour after epidural catheter placement. Low-molecular-weight heparin precautions are less clear, but an interval of 24 hours before catheter placement is recommended.

6. **Premedication.** Avoid inadvertent withdrawal of drugs that are being taken for concurrent medical conditions (bronchodilators, antihypertensives, β-blockers). For esophageal reflux surgery, oral antacid and H$_2$-blockers are routinely ordered preoperatively. Mild sedation, such as an intravenous (IV) short-acting benzodiazepine, is often given immediately before placement of invasive monitoring lines and catheters. In patients with copious secretions, an antisialagogue (e.g., glycopyrrolate 0.2 mg IV) is useful to facilitate fiberoptic bronchoscopy (FOB) for positioning of a double-lumen tube (DLT) or bronchial blocker (BB).

CLINICAL PEARL In patients with copious secretions, prophylactic glycopyrrolate often facilitates visualization for FOB-assisted DLT positioning.

7. **Final preoperative assessment.** The final preoperative anesthetic assessment is made immediately before the patient is brought to the operating room. Review the data from the initial prethoracotomy assessment (Table 15.2) and the results of tests ordered at that time. Two other concerns for thoracic anesthesia need to be assessed: (i) The potential for difficult lung isolation and (ii) the risk of desaturation during one-lung ventilation (OLV).
   a. **Assessment of difficult endobronchial intubation.** The most useful predictor of difficult endobronchial intubation is the chest imaging. Clinically important tracheal or bronchial distortions or compression from tumors or previous surgery can usually be detected on plain chest radiographs (CXRs). Distal airway (including distal trachea and proximal bronchi) problems not detectable on the plain x-ray film may be visualized on chest computed tomographic (CT) scans. These abnormalities often will not be mentioned in a written or verbal report from the radiologist or surgeon. The anesthesiologist must examine the chest image before placing a DLT or BB.
   b. **Prediction of desaturation during one-lung ventilation (OLV).** It is possible to determine patients at high risk for desaturation during OLV for thoracic surgery. Factors that correlate with desaturation during OLV are listed in Table 15.3. The most

TABLE 15.3 Factors that correlate with an increased risk of desaturation during OLV

I. High percentage of ventilation (V) or perfusion (Q) to the operative lung on preoperative V/Q scan
II. Poor PaO$_2$ during two-lung ventilation, particularly in the lateral position intraoperatively
III. Right-sided surgery
IV. Good preoperative spirometry (FEV$_1$ or FVC)

V/Q, ventilation/perfusion; FEV$_1$, forced expiratory volume in 1 second; FVC, forced vital capacity; OLV, one-lung ventilation.

important predictor of PaO_2 during OLV is the PaO_2 during two-lung ventilation in the lateral position before OLV. The proportion of perfusion or ventilation to the nonoperated lung on preoperative ventilation/perfusion (V/Q) scans also correlates with the PaO_2 during OLV. The side of the thoracotomy has an effect on PaO_2 during OLV. With the left lung being 10% smaller than the right lung, there is less shunt when the left lung is collapsed. The degree of obstructive lung disease correlates inversely with PaO_2 during OLV. Patients with more severe airflow limitation on preoperative spirometry tend to have a better PaO_2 during OLV. This is related to the development of auto positive end-expiratory pressure (PEEP) during OLV in the obstructed patients.

Stratifying the perioperative risks allows the anesthesiologist to develop a systematic approach to these patients that can be used to guide anesthetic management (Fig. 15.2).

II. Intraoperative management

A. Lung separation

There are three basic options for lung separation: single-lumen endobronchial tubes (EBTs), DLTs (left- or right-sided) (see Figs. 15.3 and 15.4), and BBs. The second half of the 20th century has seen refinements of the DLT from that of Carlens to a tube specifically designed for intraoperative use (Robertshaw) with larger, D-shaped lumens and without a carinal hook. Current disposable polyvinyl chloride DLTs have incorporated high-volume/low-pressure tracheal and bronchial cuffs. Recently, there has been a revival of interest in BBs due to several factors: new blocker designs (see Figs. 15.5 and 15.6) [4] and greater familiarity of anesthesiologists with fiberoptic placement of BBs (see Fig. 15.7).

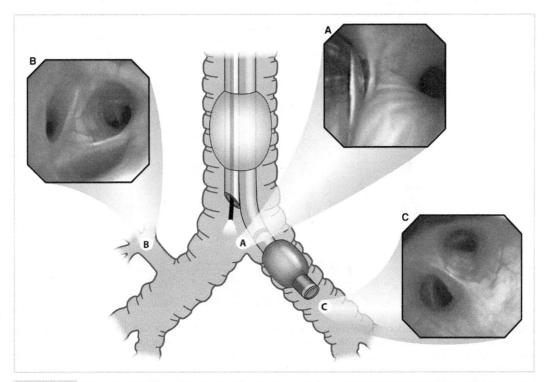

FIGURE 15.3 The optimal position of a left-sided double-lumen endotracheal tube (ETT). **A:** Unobstructed view of the entrance of the right mainstem bronchus as seen from the tracheal lumen. **B:** Take-off of the right upper lobe bronchus with the three segments. **C:** Unobstructed view of the left upper and left lower bronchus as seen from the bronchial lumen. (Reproduced from Campos J. Lung isolation. In: Slinger P, ed. *Principles and Practice of Thoracic Anesthesia*. New York: Springer; 2011, with kind permission of Springer Science + Business Media.)

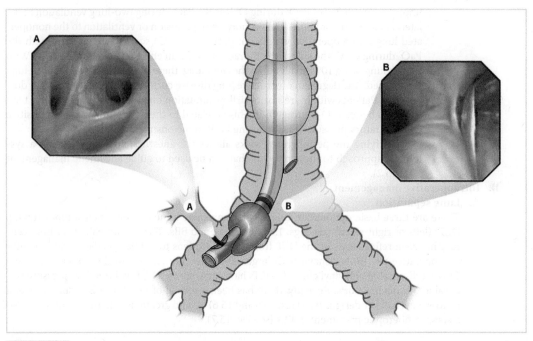

FIGURE 15.4 Optimal position of a right-sided double-lumen endotracheal tube (ETT) as seen with a fiberoptic bronchoscope. **A:** View of the right upper lobe bronchus seen through the ventilating side slot of the bronchial lumen. **B:** View of the carina showing the left mainstem bronchus and the bronchial lumen in the right mainstem bronchus seen from the tracheal lumen. (Reproduced from Campos J. Lung isolation. In: Slinger P, ed. *Principles and Practice of Thoracic Anesthesia.* New York: Springer; 2011, with permission of Springer Science + Business Media.)

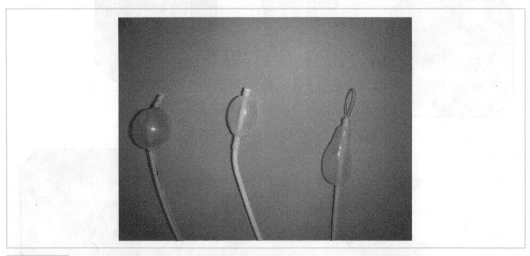

FIGURE 15.5 Three of the endobronchial blockers currently available in North America. **Left:** The Cohen® tip-deflecting endobronchial blocker (Cook Critical Care, Bloomington, IN, USA), which allows anesthesiologists to establish one-lung ventilation (OLV) by directing its flexible tip left or right into the desired bronchus using a control wheel device on the proximal end of the blocker in combination with fiberoptic bronchoscopic (FOB) guidance. **Middle:** The Fuji Uniblocker® (Fuji Corp., Tokyo, Japan). It has a fixed distal curve that allows it to be rotated for manipulation into position with FOB guidance. Unlike its predecessor, the Univent blocker, the Uniblocker is used with a standard endotracheal tube (ETT). **Right:** The wire-guided endobronchial blocker (Arndt® bronchial blocker; Cook Critical Care) introduced in 1999. It contains a wire loop in the inner lumen; when used as a snare with a fiberoptic bronchoscope, it allows directed placement. The snare is then removed, and the 1.4-mm lumen may be used as a suction channel or for oxygen insufflation. (Reproduced from Campos J. Lung isolation. In: Slinger P, ed. *Principles and Practice of Thoracic Anesthesia.* New York: Springer; 2011, with kind permission of Springer Science + Business Media.)

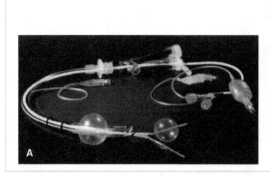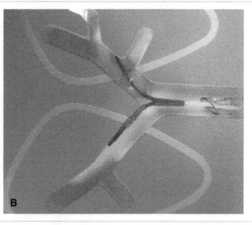

FIGURE 15.6 A, B: The recently introduced EZ Blocker (Teleflex, Wayne, PA, USA). This bronchial blocker (BB) has two blockers and is placed at the carina with fiberoptic guidance and the corresponding cuff to the operative lung is inflated when required.

1. **Indications for lung separation.** Absolute indications for lung isolation include purulent secretions, massive pulmonary hemorrhage, and bronchopleural fistula, blebs, and bullae (blood, pus, and air). More commonly, lung separation is provided intraoperatively to facilitate surgical exposure.

2. **Techniques of lung separation.** The optimal methods for lung isolation are listed in Table 15.4. Because it is impossible to describe one technique as best in all indications for OLV, the various indications are considered separately.

   a. **Elective pulmonary resection, right-sided.** The first choice is a left DLT. The widest margin of safety in positioning is with left DLTs. With blind positioning, the incidence of malposition can exceed 20% but is correctable in virtually all cases by fiberoptic adjustment. During OLV, this technique maintains continuous access to the nonventilated lung for suctioning, fiberoptic monitoring of position, and continuous positive airway pressure (CPAP). There are two possible alternatives: (i) Single-lumen EBT: a

TABLE 15.4 Selection of airway device for lung isolation

Surgery	Primary choice[a]	Secondary options (in order of preference)
Pulmonary resection, right sided	Left DLT	BB, EBT
Pulmonary resection, left sided, not pneumonectomy	Left DLT	BB, right DLT
Pulmonary resection, left-sided pneumonectomy/left main bronchial surgery	Right DLT	BB, left DLT
Thoracoscopy	Left DLT	Right DLT, BB, EBT
Pulmonary hemorrhage	DLT/BB/EBT	
Bronchopleural fistula/abscess	Left DLT	Right DLT, BB, EBT
Esophageal, thoracic aortic, transthoracic vertebral surgery	Left DLT/BB	Right DLT, EBT
Lung transplantation, bilateral/right single	Left DLT	EBT, BB
Lung transplantation, left single	Right DLT	BB, left DLT
Abnormal upper airway, left thoracotomy	BB	Right DLT/left DLT, EBT
Abnormal upper airway, right thoracotomy	EBT/BB	Left DLT/right DLT

[a]Options separated by a slash (/) are equivalent choices.
BB, bronchial blocker ipsilateral to side of surgery; EBT, single-lumen tube placed endobronchially contralateral to surgery; left DLT, left-sided double-lumen tube; right DLT, right-sided double-lumen tube.

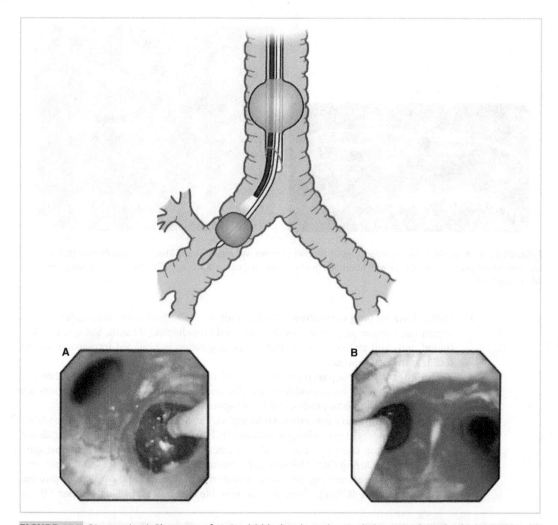

FIGURE 15.7 Diagram (**top**): Placement of an Arndt® blocker through a single-lumen endotracheal tube (ETT) in the right mainstem bronchus with the fiberoptic bronchoscope. Photographs (**bottom**): Optimal position of an endobronchial blocker in the right (**A**) or left (**B**) mainstem bronchus as seen through a fiberoptic bronchoscope. Note that the right-sided placement is deliberately closer to the carina in an effort to avoid overlapping the origin of the right upper lobe bronchus. (Reproduced from Campos J. Lung isolation. In: Slinger P, ed. *Principles and Practice of Thoracic Anesthesia*. New York: Springer; 2011, with kind permission of Springer Science + Business Media.)

standard 7.5-mm diameter, 32-cm long endotracheal tube (ETT) can be advanced over an FOB into the left main stem bronchus. (ii) A BB can be placed external to or intraluminally with an ETT.

   b. **Elective pulmonary resection, left-sided**

   (1) **Not pneumonectomy.** There is no obvious best choice between a BB and a left DLT. Use of a left DLT for a left thoracotomy can be associated with obstruction of the tracheal lumen by the lateral tracheal wall and subsequent problems with gas exchange in the ventilated lung. A right DLT is an alternate choice.

   (2) **Left pneumonectomy.** When a pneumonectomy is foreseen, a right DLT is the best choice. A right DLT will permit the surgeon to palpate the left hilum during OLV without interference from a tube or blocker in the left main stem bronchus. The disposable right DLTs currently available in North America vary greatly

in design, depending on the manufacturer (Mallinckrodt, Rusch, Kendall). The Mallinckrodt design currently is the most reliable. All three designs include a ventilating side slot (fenestration) in the distal bronchial lumen for right upper lobe ventilation. Optimal positioning technique includes bronchoscopically confirming that this fenestration aligns with the right upper lobe orifice as shown in Figure 15.4. If left lung isolation is impossible despite extremely high pressures in the right DLT bronchial cuff, a Fogarty catheter can be passed into the left main bronchus as a BB. As an alternative, there is no clear preference between a left DLT or BB. These all require repositioning before clamping the left main stem bronchus.

   c. **Thoracoscopy.** Lung biopsies, wedge resection, bleb/bullae resections, and some lobectomies can be done using video-assisted thoracoscopic surgery (VATS). During open thoracotomy, the lung can be compressed by the surgeon to facilitate collapse before inflation of a BB. A left DLT is generally preferred for thoracoscopy.

   d. **Pulmonary hemorrhage.** Life-threatening pulmonary hemorrhage can result from a wide variety of causes, such as aspergillosis, tuberculosis, and pulmonary artery (PA) catheter trauma. The primary risk for these patients is asphyxiation, and first-line treatment is lung isolation and suctioning the lower airways. Lung isolation can be with a DLT, BB, or single-lumen EBT, depending on availability and the clinical circumstances. Tracheobronchial hemorrhage from blunt chest trauma usually resolves with suctioning; only rarely is lung isolation necessary.

   e. **Bronchopleural fistula.** The anesthesiologist is faced with the triple problem of avoiding tension pneumothorax, ensuring adequate ventilation, and protecting the healthy lung from any fluid collection in the involved hemithorax. Management depends on the site of the fistula and the urgency of the clinical situation. For a peripheral bronchopleural fistula in a stable patient, a BB may be acceptable. For a large central fistula and in urgent situations, the most rapid and reliable method of securing one-lung isolation and ventilation is a DLT. In life-threatening situations, a DLT can be placed in awake patients with direct FOB guidance.

CLINICAL PEARL   Because positive pressure ventilation risks tension pneumothorax in patients with bronchopleural fistula (and massive air leak in the presence of a chest tube), either preservation of spontaneous ventilation until lung isolation is achieved or rapid attainment of lung isolation is highly recommended.

   f. **Purulent secretions** (lung abscess, hydatid cysts). Lobar or segmental blockade is ideal. Loss of lung isolation in these cases is not merely a surgical inconvenience but may be life threatening. A left DLT is usually preferred.

   g. **Nonpulmonary thoracic surgery.** Thoracic aortic and esophageal surgeries require OLV. Because there is no risk of ventilated-lung contamination, a left DLT and a BB are equivalent choices.

   h. **Bronchial surgery.** An intrabronchial tumor, bronchial trauma, or bronchial sleeve resection during a lobectomy requires that the surgeon have intraluminal access to the ipsilateral main stem bronchus. Either a single-lumen EBT or a DLT in the ventilated lung is preferred.

   i. Unilateral lung lavage, independent lung ventilation, and lung transplantation are all best accomplished with a left DLT.

  3. **Upper airway abnormalities.** It is occasionally necessary to provide OLV in patients who have abnormal upper airways due to previous surgery or trauma or in patients who are known for difficult intubations. There are four basic options for these patients: (i) Fiberoptic-guided intubation with a DLT, (ii) secure the airway with an ETT and then use a "tube exchanger" to place a DLT, (iii) use a BB, and (iv) use an uncut single-lumen tube as an EBT.

    The optimal choice will depend on the patient and the operation. At all times, it is best to maintain spontaneous ventilation and to do nothing blindly in the presence of blood or pus. Awake FOB intubation with a DLT requires thorough topical anesthesia of the airway. It is important when using a tube exchanger to have a second person perform a direct laryngoscopy to expose as much of the glottis as possible during the tube change. Direct laryngoscopy decreases the angles between the oropharynx and trachea and reduces the chance of trauma to the airway from the DLT. Videolaryngoscopes are very useful for this.

BBs are often the best choice for these patients. If the ET tube is too narrow to easily accommodate both a bronchoscope and a BB, the BB can be introduced through the glottis independently external to the ET tube with fiberoptic guidance. Bilateral BBs can be used for bilateral resections or the same blocker can be manipulated from side to side. Bilateral single-lumen EBTs or BBs can be used for lung isolation in patients with tracheal fistulas, trauma, or other abnormalities in the region of the carina. Smaller DLTs (32, 28, and 26 Fr) are available, but they will not permit passage of an FOB of the diameter commonly available to monitor positioning (3.5 to 4.0 mm). An ETT designed for microlaryngoscopy (5- to 6-mm inner diameter [ID] and greater than 30 cm long) can be used as an EBT, with FOB positioning, but beware of right upper lobe obstruction if placed in the right mainstem bronchus. If the patient's trachea can accept a 7-mm ETT, a Fogarty catheter (8-Fr venous thrombectomy catheter with a 10-mL balloon) can be passed through the ETT via an FOB adapter for use as a BB.

4. **Chest trauma.** It is common in both open and closed chest trauma to have some hemoptysis from alveolar hemorrhage. The majority of these cases can be managed without lung isolation after bronchoscopy and suction. The majority of the deaths in these patients are due to their other injuries and not from airway hemorrhage or air embolus. Lung isolation may be helpful in some cases, but if resources and time are limited, the priority must be the resuscitation of the patient.

5. **Avoiding iatrogenic airway injury.** Iatrogenic injury has been estimated to occur in 0.5 to 2 per 1,000 cases with DLTs [5].

   a. **Examine the chest x-ray film or computed tomography (CT) scan,** which can help predict the majority of difficult endobronchial intubations.

   b. **Use an appropriate size tube.** Too small a tube will make lung isolation difficult. Too large a tube is more likely to cause trauma. Useful guidelines for DLT sizes in adults are as follows:

      (1) Females' height <1.6 m (63 in): 35 Fr (possibly 32 Fr if <1.5 m)

      (2) Females >1.6 m: 37 Fr

      (3) Males <1.7 m (67 in): 39 Fr (possibly 37 Fr if <1.6 m)

      (4) Males >1.7 m: 41 Fr

> **CLINICAL PEARL** Avoid the natural tendency to place a DLT that is too small because this often complicates tube positioning, successful lung isolation, and suctioning.

   c. **Depth of insertion of DLT.** Tracheobronchial dimensions correlate with height. The average depth at insertion, from the teeth, for a left DLT is 29 cm in an adult and varies ±1 cm for each 10 cm of patient height above/below 170 cm.

   d. **Avoid nitrous oxide.** Nitrous oxide 70% can increase the bronchial cuff volume by 5 to 16 mL intraoperatively.

   e. **Inflate the bronchial cuff/blocker only to the minimal volume required for lung isolation and for the minimal time.** This volume is usually less than 3 mL for a DLT bronchial cuff and <7 mL for a BB. Inflating the bronchial cuff does not stabilize the DLT position when the patient is turned to the lateral position.

      (1) Endobronchial intubation must be done gently and with fiberoptic guidance if resistance is met. A significant number of case reports of airway injury are from cases of esophageal surgery, where the elastic supporting tissue may be weakened (e.g., by preoperative radiation treatments) and predisposed to rupture from DLT placement.

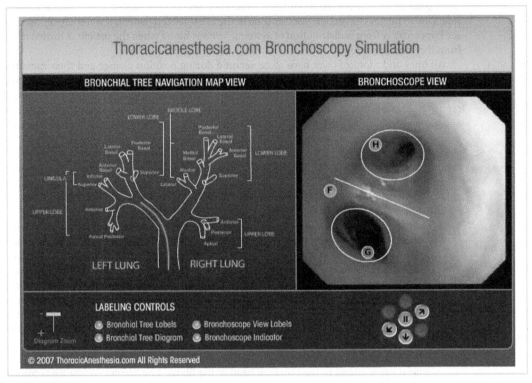

FIGURE 15.8 The free online bronchoscopy simulator at www.pie.med.utoronto.ca. The user can navigate the tracheobronchial tree using real-time video by clicking on the *lighted directional arrows* under the "Bronchoscopic view" (**right**). Clicking on the labels on the "Bronchoscopic view" gives details of the anatomy seen. The process is aided by the "Bronchial Tree Navigational Map" (**left**), which shows the simultaneous location of the bronchoscope as the *orange line* in the airway. (Reproduced from Campos J. Lung isolation. In: Slinger P, ed. *Principles and Practice of Thoracic Anesthesia*. New York: Springer; 2011, with kind permission of Springer Science + Business Media.)

    6. Other complications of lung separation

        a. Malpositioning. Initial malpositioning of DLTs with blind placement can occur in greater than 30% of cases. Verification and adjustment with FOB immediately before initiating OLV is mandatory because these tubes will migrate during patient positioning. Malpositioning after the start of OLV due to dislodgment is more of a problem with BBs than DLTs.

        b. Airway resistance. The resistance from a 37-Fr DLT during two-lung ventilation is less than that of an 8-mm ID ETT but exceeds that of a 9-mm ETT. For short periods of postoperative ventilation and weaning, airflow resistance is not a problem with a DLT.

    7. The **ABCs** of lung separation will always apply:

        a. Know the tracheobronchial **a**natomy [6].

        b. Use the fiberoptic **b**ronchoscope (see Fig. 15.8) [7].

        c. Look at the **c**hest x-ray film and **C**T scan in advance.

B. Positioning

The majority of thoracic procedures are performed with the patient in the lateral position, but, depending on the surgical technique, a semisupine or semiprone lateral position may be used. It is awkward to induce anesthesia in the lateral position; thus, monitors will be placed and anesthesia will be usually induced in the supine position and the anesthetized patient will then be repositioned for surgery. It is possible to induce anesthesia in the lateral position, but semilateral positioning is preferable if tolerated. This may rarely be indicated with unilateral lung diseases, such as bronchiectasis or hemoptysis, until lung isolation can be achieved. However, even these patients will have to be repositioned and the diseased lung turned to the nondependent side. Due to the loss of venous vascular tone in the anesthetized patient, it is not uncommon to see hypotension from redistribution of systemic venous blood when the patient is turned to or from the lateral position.

All lines and monitors will have to be secured during position change and their function reassessed after repositioning. The anesthesiologist should take responsibility for the head, neck, and airway during position change and must be in charge of the operating team to direct repositioning. It is useful to make an initial "head-to-toe" survey of the patient after induction and intubation, checking oxygenation, ventilation, hemodynamics, lines, monitors, and potential nerve injuries. This survey must be repeated after repositioning. It is nearly impossible to avoid some movement of a DLT or BB during repositioning. The patient's head, neck, and EBT should be turned en bloc with the patient's thoracolumbar spine. The margin of error in positioning EBTs or blockers is often so narrow that even small movements can have significant clinical implications. EBT/blocker position and adequacy of ventilation must be rechecked by auscultation and FOB after patient repositioning.

1. **Neurovascular complications.** The brachial plexus is the site of the majority of intraoperative nerve injuries related to the lateral position. The brachial plexus is fixed at two points: proximally by the transverse process of the cervical vertebrae and distally by the axillary fascia. This two-point fixation plus the extreme mobility of neighboring skeletal and muscular structures make the brachial plexus extremely liable to injury. The patient should be positioned with padding under the dependent thorax to keep the weight of the upper body off the dependent arm brachial plexus. This padding will exacerbate the pressure on the brachial plexus if it migrates superiorly into the axilla. It is useful to survey the patient from the side of the table immediately after the patient is turned to ensure that the entire vertebral column is aligned properly.

   The dependent leg should be slightly flexed with padding under the knee to protect the peroneal nerve lateral to the proximal head of the fibula. The nondependent leg is placed in a neutral straight position and padding placed between it and the dependent leg. The dependent leg must be observed for vascular compression. Excessively tight strapping at the hip level can compress the sciatic nerve of the nondependent leg. A "head-to-toe" protocol to monitor for possible neurovascular injuries related to the lateral decubitus position is given in Table 15.5. In general, the goal for this exercise is to avoid stretching or compressing nerves and compressing arteries or veins.

2. **Physiologic changes in the lateral position**

   a. **Ventilation.** Significant changes in ventilation develop between the lungs when the patient is placed in the lateral position. The compliance curves of the two lungs are different because of their difference in size. The lateral position, anesthesia, paralysis, and opening the thorax all combine to magnify these differences between the lungs.

   In a spontaneously breathing patient, ventilation of the dependent lung will increase approximately 10% when the patient is turned to the lateral position. Once the patient is anesthetized and paralyzed, ventilation of the dependent lung will decrease 15%.

TABLE 15.5   Avoiding neurovascular injuries specific to the lateral position

Routine "head-to-toe" survey
  I. Dependent eye
  II. Dependent ear pinna
  III. Cervical spine alignment
  IV. Dependent arm: (i) Brachial plexus, (ii) circulation
  V. Nondependent arm[a]: (i) Brachial plexus, (ii) circulation
  VI. Nondependent leg sciatic nerve
  VII. Dependent leg: (i) Peroneal nerve, (ii) circulation

[a]Neurovascular injuries of the nondependent arm are more likely to occur if the arm is suspended or held in an independently positioned armrest.

TABLE 15.6   Intraoperative complications that occur with increased frequency during thoracotomy

Complication	Etiology
I. Hypoxemia	Intrapulmonary shunt during one-lung ventilation (OLV)
II. Sudden severe hypotension	Surgical compression of the heart or great vessels
III. Sudden changes in ventilating pressure or volume	Movement of endobronchial tube (EBT)/blocker, air leak
IV. Arrhythmias	Direct mechanical irritation of the heart
V. Bronchospasm	Direct airway stimulation, increased frequency of reactive airways disease
VI. Massive hemorrhage	Surgical blood loss from great vessels or inflamed pleura
VII. Hypothermia	Heat loss from the open hemithorax

The compliance of the entire respiratory system will increase once the nondependent hemithorax is open, yet will decrease from interpleural insufflation in a VATS.

Applying PEEP to both lungs in the lateral position, PEEP preferentially goes to the most compliant lung regions and hyperinflates the nondependent lung without causing any improvement in gas exchange. In the lateral position, atelectasis will develop in a mean of 5% of total lung volume, all in the dependent lung.

    b. Perfusion. Turning the patient to the lateral position decreases the blood flow of the nondependent lung due to gravity by approximately 10% of the total pulmonary blood flow.

The matching of ventilation and perfusion will usually decrease in the lateral position compared to the supine position. Pulmonary arteriovenous shunt usually increases from approximately 5% in the supine position to 10% to 15% in the lateral position.

C. Intraoperative monitoring

    1. General to all pulmonary resections. The majority are major operative procedures of moderate duration (2 to 4 hours) and performed in the lateral position either with induced pneumothorax (VATS) or open. Consideration for monitoring and maintenance of body temperature and fluid volume should be given to all of these cases. All cases should have standard ASA monitoring. Additional monitoring is guided by a knowledge of which complications are likely to occur (Table 15.6).

    2. Specific to certain types of resection. There are complications that are more prone to occur with certain resections, such as hemorrhage from an extrapleural pneumonectomy, contralateral lung soiling with resection of a cyst or bronchiectasis, air leak hypoventilation, or tension pneumothorax with a bronchopleural fistula.

    3. Oxygenation. Significant arterial oxygen desaturation (less than 90%) during OLV occurs in approximately 1% of the surgical population with a high inspired oxygen concentration (FiO_2) of 1. Pulse oximetry (SpO_2) has not negated the need for direct measurement of arterial PaO_2 via intermittent blood gases in the majority of thoracotomy patients. PaO_2 offers a more useful estimate of the margin of safety above desaturation than SpO_2. The rapidity of the fall in PaO_2 after the onset of OLV is an indicator of the risk of subsequent desaturation. Consequently, we recommend measuring PaO_2 by ABG before OLV and 20 minutes after the start of OLV.

    4. Capnometry. End-tidal CO_2 ($P_{et}CO_2$) is a less reliable indicator of the $PaCO_2$ during OLV than during two-lung ventilation, and the $P_{a\text{-}et}CO_2$ gradient increases during OLV. As the patient is turned to the lateral position, the $P_{et}CO_2$ of the nondependent lung falls relative to the dependent lung because of increased perfusion of the dependent lung and increased dead space of the nondependent lung. At the onset of OLV, the $P_{et}CO_2$ of the dependent lung usually falls transiently, as all the minute ventilation is transferred to this lung. The $P_{et}CO_2$ then rises as the fractional perfusion is increased to this dependent lung by collapse and pulmonary vasoconstriction of the nonventilated lung. If there is no correction of minute ventilation, the net result will be increased baseline $PaCO_2$ and $P_{et}CO_2$, with an increased gradient. Severe (greater than 5 mm Hg) or prolonged falls in $P_{et}CO_2$ indicate a maldistribution of perfusion between ventilated and nonventilated lungs and may be an early warning of a patient who will desaturate during OLV.

5. **Invasive hemodynamic monitoring**

   a. **Arterial catheter.** There is a significant incidence of transient severe hypotension from surgical compression of the heart or great vessels during intrathoracic procedures. For this reason, plus the utility of intermittent ABG sampling, it is useful to have beat-to-beat assessment of systemic blood pressure during many thoracic surgery cases. Exceptions are limited procedures such as "wedge" segmental resections and/or thoracoscopic resections in younger/healthier patients. For most thoracotomies, placement of a radial artery catheter can be in either the dependent or nondependent arm.

   b. **Central venous pressures (CVPs).** CVP readings obtained intraoperatively with the chest open are not reliable indicators of right atrial pressure or RV preload. It is our practice to routinely place CVP lines in pneumonectomy patients, but not for lesser resections unless there is significant other concurrent illness or risk of bleeding. Our choice is to use the right internal jugular vein with ultrasound guidance to minimize the risk of pneumothorax (as compared to subclavian vein CVP placement) for CVP access unless there is a contraindication.

   c. **Pulmonary artery (PA) catheters.** The risk/benefit ratio for the routine use of PA catheters for pulmonary resection surgery favors their infrequent use, such as patients with life-threatening coexisting cardiac disease or possibly active septicemia. Several recently developed systems of noninvasive cardiac output monitoring may prove equally useful for this purpose (e.g., FloTrac®, Edwards Lifesciences, Irvine, CA, USA).

6. **Fiberoptic bronchoscopy (FOB).** Significant malpositions of left-sided or right-sided DLTs that can lead to desaturation during OLV are often not detected by auscultation or other traditional methods of confirming placement. Positioning of DLTs or BBs should be confirmed after placing the patient in the surgical position because a substantial percentage of tubes/blockers migrate during repositioning of the patient.

CLINICAL PEARL Head and neck extension or rotation during patient repositioning risks displacement of a previously perfectly positioned DLT.

---

7. **Continuous spirometry.** Side-stream spirometry monitors inspiratory and expiratory pressures, volume, and flow interactions during anesthesia. The adequacy of lung isolation can be monitored by breath-to-breath comparison of inspiratory and expiratory tidal volumes. This also gives a sense of the magnitude of air leaks from the ventilated lung. Changes in the position of a DLT can be detected by changes in the pressure–volume loops.

D. **Anesthetic technique**

Any anesthetic technique that provides safe and stable general anesthesia for major surgery can and has been used for lung resection. Many centers use combined regional (e.g., TEA or paravertebral blocks) and general anesthesia for thoracic surgery. Commonly, neuromuscular blockers are used, but they are not essential to the safe conduct of thoracotomies or to DLT management.

1. **Intravenous (IV) fluids.** Because of hydrostatic effects, excessive administration of IV fluids can cause increased shunt and lead to pulmonary edema of the dependent lung. Because the dependent lung is the lung that must carry on gas exchange during OLV, it is best to be as judicious as possible with fluid administration. IV fluids are administered to replace volume deficits and for maintenance only during lung resection anesthesia. No volume is given for theoretical third-space losses during thoracotomy (Table 15.7).

2. **Nitrous oxide.** Nitrous oxide/oxygen mixtures are more prone to cause atelectasis in poorly ventilated lung regions than oxygen by itself. The optimal method to prevent dependent lung atelectasis is the use of air/oxygen mixtures during both two-lung ventilation and OLV, titrating the FiO_2 to avoid hypoxemia. Nitrous oxide also tends to increase PA pressures in patients who have pulmonary hypertension.

TABLE 15.7   Fluid management for pulmonary resection surgery

   I. Total positive fluid balance in the first 24 hrs perioperatively should not exceed 20 mL/kg.
  II. For an average adult patient, crystalloid administration should be limited to <3 L in the first 24 hrs.
 III. No fluid administration for "third-space" fluid losses during pulmonary resection
  IV. Urine output >0.5 mL/kg/hr is unnecessary.
   V. If increased tissue perfusion is needed postoperatively, it is preferable to use invasive monitoring
      and inotropes rather than to cause fluid overload.

3. **Temperature.** Maintenance of body temperature can be a problem during thoracic surgery because of heat loss from the open hemithorax. This is particularly a problem at the extremes of the age spectrum. Most of the body's physiologic functions, including hypoxic pulmonary vasoconstriction (HPV), are inhibited during hypothermia. Increasing the ambient room temperature and using lower and upper body forced-air patient warmers are the best methods to prevent inadvertent intraoperative hypothermia.

4. **Prevention of bronchospasm.** Due to the high incidence of coexisting reactive airways disease in the thoracic surgical population, it is generally advisable to use an anesthetic technique that decreases bronchial irritability. This is particularly important because the added airway manipulation caused by placement of a DLT or BB potently triggers bronchoconstriction. Avoid manipulation of the airway in a lightly anesthetized patient, use bronchodilating anesthetics, and avoid drugs which release histamine.

   For IV induction of anesthesia, either propofol or ketamine diminishes bronchospasm. For maintenance of anesthesia, propofol and/or any of the volatile anesthetics will diminish bronchial reactivity. Sevoflurane may be the most potent bronchodilator of the volatile anesthetics.

5. **Coronary artery disease.** Since a large proportion of lung resection population is composed of elderly patients and smokers, there is a high coincidence of coronary artery disease. This will be a major factor in the choice of the anesthetic technique for many thoracic surgery patients. The anesthetic technique should optimize the myocardial oxygen supply/demand ratio by maintaining arterial oxygenation and diastolic blood pressure while avoiding unnecessary increases in myocardial contractility and heart rate. TEA/analgesia may help to achieve these goals.

E. **Management of one-lung ventilation (OLV)**

1. **Hypoxemia.** There is an incidence of <4% of hypoxemia (arterial saturation <90%) during OLV for thoracic surgery. Hypoxemia is more likely to occur when OLV is in the supine position.

2. **Hypoxic pulmonary vasoconstriction (HPV).** HPV is thought to decrease the blood flow to the nonventilated lung by 50%. The stimulus for HPV is primarily the alveolar oxygen tension (PAO_2), which stimulates precapillary vasoconstriction to redistribute pulmonary blood flow away from hypoxemic lung regions via a pathway involving nitric oxide (NO) and/or cyclooxygenase synthesis inhibition. All of the volatile anesthetics inhibit HPV. This inhibition is dose dependent. Isoflurane, sevoflurane, and desflurane cause less inhibition than older volatile agents such as halothane [8]. No clinical benefit has been shown for total IV anesthesia beyond that seen with isoflurane 1 MAC (minimum alveolar concentration) or less. HPV is decreased by all vasodilators such as nitroglycerin and nitroprusside. In general, vasodilators can be expected to cause a deterioration in PaO_2 during OLV.

3. **Cardiac output.** The net effects of an increase in cardiac output during OLV tend to favor an increase in PaO_2. However, elevation of cardiac output beyond physiologic needs tends to oppose HPV and may cause PaO_2 to fall.

4. **Ventilation during one-lung anesthesia.** It is possible to improve gas exchange for selected individual patients by altering the ventilatory variables that are under the control of the anesthesiologist: tidal volume, rate, inspiratory/expiratory ratio, $PaCO_2$, peak and plateau airway pressures, and PEEP (Table 15.8).

TABLE 15.8   Recommended ventilation parameters for OLV

Parameter	Suggested	Note
Tidal volume	5–6 mL/kg (ideal body weight)	Maintain Peak airway pressure <35 cm H_2O Plateau airway pressure <25 cm H_2O
PEEP	5 cm H_2O (recruitment maneuver at start of OLV and as needed)	Avoid added PEEP in patients with moderate–severe COPD who have auto-PEEP
Respiratory rate	12/min, adjust based on $PaCO_2$	$P_{a\text{-}et}CO_2$ gradient usually will increase 1–3 mm Hg during OLV. Mild hypercapnia ($PaCO_2$ 50–55 mm Hg) is OK
Mode	Volume or pressure control	Patients at risk for lung injury (pneumonectomy, lung transplantation, bullae): pressure-control ventilation preferred
FiO_2	0.8–1.0 initially	Add air to decrease FiO_2 guided by oxygen saturation after 20 min of stable OLV

PEEP, positive end-expiratory pressure; OLV, one-lung ventilation; COPD, chronic obstructive pulmonary disease; $P_{a\text{-}et}CO_2$, arterial end-tidal CO_2 partial pressure; $PaCO_2$, arterial partial pressure of CO_2; FiO_2, inspired oxygen concentration.

    a. Respiratory acid–base status. The overall efficacy of HPV is optimal with normal pH and $PaCO_2$.

    b. Tidal volume. A 5 to 6 mL/kg ideal body weight for OLV is a reasonable starting point. The tidal volume should be adjusted during OLV to keep the airway peak pressure less than 35 cm H_2O and the plateau airway pressure less than 25 cm H_2O.

CLINICAL PEARL   A common misconception is that tidal volume should be substantially reduced when converting from two-lung ventilation to OLV.

    c. Positive end-expiratory pressure (PEEP). Most patients with either normal or supranormal (restrictive lung disease) lung elastic recoil will benefit from low levels (5 cm H_2O) of PEEP during OLV. A recruitment maneuver (e.g., static inflation to 20 cm H_2O for 20 seconds, observing for hypotension) to the ventilated lung is useful at the start of OLV. Auto-PEEP is prone to occur in patients with decreased lung elastic recoil, such as those with emphysema. Auto-PEEP is difficult to detect using currently available anesthetic ventilators but can be estimated with a manually applied prolonged expiratory phase with zero end-expiratory pressure. Applied PEEP combines with auto-PEEP in an unpredictable fashion.

    d. Volume control versus pressure control. Pressure-control OLV is useful in patients with severe obstructive disease and to limit airway pressure in patients with blebs, bullae, or fresh resections in the lung, and also in patients at risk of acute lung injury (pneumonectomies, lung transplantation). When using pressure-control OLV without setting a guaranteed minimum tidal volume, it is important to set an alarm for minimum tidal volume (e.g., 3 mL/kg ideal body weight).

    e. Inspired oxygen concentration (FiO_2). The FiO_2 should be increased at the start of OLV to 0.8 to 1.0 and then can be decreased as tolerated over the next 20 minutes.

  5. Treatment of hypoxemia during one-lung ventilation (OLV) (see Table 15.9)
In cases of severe and/or acute desaturation, resume two-lung ventilation immediately, deflate the bronchial cuff or blocker, and then check the position of the DLT or BB with FOB. In cases of desaturation that have not become life-threatening:

    a. Increase inspired oxygen concentration (FiO_2). The first-line therapy is to increase the FiO_2, which is an option in essentially all patients except those who received bleomycin or similar therapy that potentiates pulmonary oxygen toxicity.

    b. Positive end-expiratory pressure (PEEP). PEEP to the ventilated dependent lung will improve oxygenation in patients with normal lung mechanics and those with increased elastic recoil due to restrictive lung diseases. Apply a recruitment maneuver to the ventilated lung before application of PEEP.

TABLE 15.9 Treatment options for hypoxemia during OLV

Severe/acute: Resume two-lung ventilation

Gradual desaturation:
- **I.** Assure $FiO_2 = 1$
- **II.** Check position of DLT/BB with FOB
- **III.** Optimize cardiac output
- **IV.** Recruitment maneuver of ventilated lung
- **V.** Apply PEEP 5 cm H_2O to ventilated lung (except COPD)
- **VI.** Apply CPAP 1–2 cm H_2O to nonventilated lung (recruitment maneuver first, avoid during VATS)
- **VII.** Intermittent reinflation of nonventilated lung
- **VIII.** Partial ventilation of nonventilated lung:
  - **A.** Segmental oxygen insufflation via FOB
  - **B.** Lobar reinflation
  - **C.** Lobar collapse
  - **D.** Oxygen insufflation
  - **E.** High-frequency ventilation
- **IX.** Mechanical restriction of nonventilated lung pulmonary blood flow

OLV, one-lung ventilation; FiO_2, inspired oxygen concentration; DLT, double-lumen tube; BB, bronchial blocker; FOB, fiberoptic bronchoscopy; PEEP, positive end-expiratory pressure; COPD, chronic obstructive pulmonary disease; CPAP, continuous positive airway pressure.

c. **Pharmacologic manipulations.** Increasing cardiac output will result in a small but clinically useful increase in both PvO_2 and PaO_2 if cardiac output has decreased. Eliminating potent vasodilators, such as nitroglycerin and halothane, will improve oxygenation during OLV. Selective pulmonary vasodilators such as NO have not yet proven to be reliable.

d. **Continuous positive airway pressure (CPAP)** must be applied to a fully inflated or reinflated lung for optimal effect. When CPAP is applied to a fully inflated lung, as little as 2 to 3 cm H_2O can be used. All that is required is a CPAP valve and an oxygen source. Ideally, the circuit should permit variation of the CPAP level and should include a reservoir bag to allow easy reinflation of the nonventilated lung and a manometer to measure the actual CPAP supplied. Such circuits are commercially available or can be readily constructed. When the bronchus of the operative lung is obstructed or open to atmosphere, CPAP will not improve oxygenation. During thoracoscopic surgery, CPAP can significantly interfere with surgery.

CLINICAL PEARL When CPAP is applied to the nondependent, surgical lung to treat hypoxemia, the lung must first be reinflated.

e. **Alternative ventilation methods.** Several alternative methods of OLV, all of which involve partial ventilation of the nonventilated lung, have been described. All improve oxygenation during OLV. These techniques are useful in patients who are particularly at risk for desaturation, such as those with previous pulmonary resections of the contralateral lung.

(1) Oxygen insufflation (5 L/min) for brief periods via the suction channel of an FOB to partially recruit a segment of the nonventilated lung remote from the site of surgery (e.g., a basilar segment of the lower lobe for upper lobe surgery). This is particularly useful in VATS [9]. Surgeon's direct observation is useful to prevent over-reinflation.

(2) Selective lobar collapse of only the operative lobe in the open hemithorax by placement of a blocker in the appropriate lobar bronchus of the ipsilateral operative lung.

(3) Differential lung ventilation by only partially occluding the lumen of the DLT to the operative lung.

(4) Intermittent reinflation of the nonventilated lung by regular reexpansion of the operative lung via an attached CPAP circuit.

(5) Conventional OLV of the nonoperative lung and high-frequency jet ventilation of the operative lung.

f. **Mechanical restriction of pulmonary blood flow.** It is possible for the surgeon to directly compress or clamp the blood flow to the nonventilated lung. This can be done temporarily in emergency desaturation situations or definitively in cases of pneumonectomy or lung transplantation. Another technique is inflation of a PA catheter balloon in the main PA of the operative lung.

6. **Prevention of hypoxemia.** The treatments outlined as therapy for hypoxemia can be used prophylactically to prevent hypoxemia in patients who are at high risk for desaturation during OLV. Desaturation during bilateral lung procedures is particularly a problem during a second period of OLV (e.g., bilateral thoracotomy). It is advisable to operate first on the lung that has better gas exchange. For the majority of patients, this means operating on the right side first.

III. **Specific procedures**

A. **Thoracotomy**

1. **Operations**

a. **Lobectomy.** Lobectomy is the most common pulmonary resection for lung cancer. Early functional loss exceeds the amount of lung tissue resected, but function recovers over a period of 6 weeks so that the final net loss of respiratory function is equivalent to the amount of functioning lung tissue excised. The recovery of pulmonary function after thoracotomy is unique because it shows a plateau with no early recovery during the first 72 hours postoperatively. This period coincides with the occurrence of the majority of postthoracotomy respiratory complications (atelectasis, pneumonia), which are the major causes of mortality after pulmonary resection. These complications are particularly associated with lobectomy and its variations, probably due to the transient dysfunction that occurs in the remaining lobe(s). The right middle lobe is particularly at risk for these complications after a right upper lobectomy and can develop torsion about its bronchovascular pedicle or lobar bronchial kinking as it expands into the apex of the right hemithorax.

b. **Sleeve lobectomy.** A sleeve lobectomy is the excision of a lobe plus the adjacent segment of mainstem bronchus with bronchoplastic repair of the bronchus by end-to-end anastomosis to preserve the distal functioning pulmonary parenchyma. It is done to preserve functioning lung tissue when the tumor encroaches to less than 2 cm from the lobar bronchial orifices, precluding simple lobectomy. This procedure is usually done for right upper lobe tumors but can be used for other lobes. The anesthetic implications of this procedure are that, most often, no airway catheter (single lumen or DLT) or BB can be placed in the ipsilateral main stem bronchus, although some surgeons prefer to use a carefully positioned left-sided DLT during left upper lobe sleeve lobectomies. Mucus clearance across the bronchial anastomosis may be impaired after sleeve resection, and local tumor recurrence is a problem.

c. **Bilobectomy.** In the right lung, a bilobectomy may be used to conserve either a functioning upper or lower lobe when the tumor extends across the lobar fissure or for malignancies involving the bronchus intermedius (the portion of the right main stem bronchus distal to the right upper lobe orifice). The complication rate is slightly higher than for a simple lobectomy but is less than for a pneumonectomy. The incidence of cardiac dysrhythmias increases postoperatively versus lobectomy, whereas the incidence of respiratory complications remains the same. The residual lobe cannot completely fill the hemithorax, and all patients will have a degree of pneumothorax that can be expected to resolve gradually.

d. **Pneumonectomy.** Complete removal of the lung is required when a lobectomy or its modifications is not adequate to remove the local disease and/or ipsilateral lymph node metastases. Atelectasis and pneumonia occur after pneumonectomy, as they do

TABLE 15.10 Postpneumonectomy pulmonary edema

Incidence 2–4% of pneumonectomies
Case fatality >50%
Incidence right > left pneumonectomy (3–4:1)
Clinical onset 2–3 days postoperatively
Associated with increased pulmonary capillary permeability
Not associated with increased PA pressures
Exacerbation by fluid overload

PA, pulmonary artery.

after lobectomy, but may be less of a problem because of the absence of residual parenchymal dysfunction on the operative side. The mortality rate after pneumonectomy exceeds that for lobectomy because of complications that are more likely with pneumonectomy.

(1) **Postpneumonectomy pulmonary edema.** This syndrome presents clinically with dyspnea and an increased alveolar–arterial oxygen gradient on the second or third postoperative day [10] and has a high fatality rate. Radiologic changes precede clinical symptoms by approximately 24 hours. The factors that are known about this syndrome are listed in Table 15.10. Excessive perioperative administration of IV crystalloids or colloids can exacerbate it. However, there is no evidence that judicious amounts of fluids cause this problem. The residual nonoperated lung has an increased pulmonary capillary permeability after pneumonectomy that is not seen in the nonoperated lung after lobectomy. The cause of this increased permeability may be related to surgical lymphatic damage, capillary stress injury from increased flow, or increased airway pressure and hyperinflation of the ventilated lung during OLV. The majority of lobectomies have the potential to become a pneumonectomy, so caution is needed with fluids in most thoracic cases.

(2) **Atrial fibrillation.** Up to 50% of postpneumonectomy patients will develop supraventricular arrhythmias in the first week postoperatively, the majority of which are atrial fibrillation. The perioperative mortality is 17% in patients who develop arrhythmias versus 2% in those without them. The etiology seems to depend on two factors: RV strain and increased sympathetic nervous activity. Similar arrhythmias occur with a lesser incidence after lesser pulmonary resections. Prophylactic digoxin is not effective in preventing them [11].

(3) **Mechanical effects.** A variety of potentially lethal intrathoracic mechanical derangements of cardiorespiratory function can occur after pneumonectomy. The most important of these is cardiac herniation through an incompletely closed pericardium. This is particularly a risk after right pneumonectomy and presents with acute severe hypotension in the immediate postoperative period. The only useful therapy is immediate reoperation to return the heart into the pericardium. A subacute form of cardiac herniation can occur after a left pneumonectomy and presents with a picture of myocardial ischemia as the apex of the heart herniates through the pericardial defect and compresses the coronary arteries. Less acute presentations of cardiovascular or respiratory symptoms may develop related to shifts of the mediastinum that can compress the great vessels or airways after pneumonectomy.

CLINICAL PEARL If sudden, severe hypotension occurs in the early postoperative period after pneumonectomy, a diagnosis of cardiac herniation should be assumed unless proven otherwise.

e. **Sleeve pneumonectomy.** Tumors involving the most proximal portions of the main stem bronchus and the carina may require a sleeve pneumonectomy. These are performed most commonly for right-sided tumors and usually can be performed without cardiopulmonary bypass (CPB) via a right thoracotomy. A long single-lumen EBT can be advanced into the left main stem bronchus during the period of anastomosis, or the lung can be ventilated via a separate sterile ETT and circuit that is passed into the operating field and used for temporary intubation of the open distal bronchus. High-frequency positive pressure ventilation (HFPPV) also has been used for this procedure.

Because the carina is surgically more accessible from the right side, left sleeve pneu-monectomies are commonly performed as a two-stage operation, first a left thoracot-omy and pneumonectomy, and then a right thoracotomy for the carinal excision. The complication rate and mortality are higher and the 5-year survival significantly lower than for nonsleeve pneumonectomies.

f. **Lesser resections (segmentectomy, wedge).** These procedures are commonly per-formed in the elderly or in patients with limited cardiopulmonary reserves to preserve functioning pulmonary parenchyma. These lesser resections are associated with a lower 5-year survival rate compared to lobectomy due to locoregional recurrence of cancer. The decrease of pulmonary function (FEV_1) for lesser resections is in propor-tion to the amount of lung tissue removed. Lesser resections are acceptable therapy for nonmalignant lung lesions.

g. **Extended resections.** Portions of the chest wall, diaphragm, pericardium, left atrium, vena cava, brachial plexus, or vertebral body may be excised with adjacent lung tumor. Resection of any of these structures has important anesthetic implications for choice and placement of intraoperative monitors and lines and for postoperative manage-ment.

h. **Subsequent pulmonary resections.** Lung resection surgery after previous lung resection is increasingly frequent. These operations can be performed for either benign or malignant disease. Ten percent of lung cancer patients can be expected to develop a second primary tumor. Prediction of postoperative lung function for these patients is accurate based on the assessment of preoperative function (lung mechanics, gas exchange, and cardiopulmonary reserve) and estimation of the amount of functional lung tissue removed at surgery (Fig. 15.1). Lobectomy after pneumonectomy can be performed safely if the patient meets minimal standards for predicted postoperative pulmonary function. Intraoperative collapse of the ipsilateral lung is not possible, but surgery can be facilitated by selective lobar or segment bronchial blockade or the use of HFPPV.

Completion pneumonectomy after a previous ipsilateral resection for cancer has a greater than 40% 5-year survival rate. Intraoperative hemorrhage is the specific anes-thetic concern with this procedure, as more than 50% of patients experience blood loss of greater than 1,000 mL. Hemorrhage is particularly a problem in completion pneumonectomy for nonmalignant lung disease (lung abscess, bronchiectasis, tuber-culosis). Inflammatory lung disease tends to destroy the tissue planes around the hilum and makes the surgical dissection more difficult, with an attendant increase in periop-erative mortality.

i. **Incomplete resections.** In general, a lung cancer patient's prognosis is not improved from an incomplete resection. There are several exceptions. Incompletely resected tumors with direct mediastinal invasion or tumors of the superior sulcus may ben-efit if the resection is combined with adjuvant brachytherapy or external irradiation. Also, if the residual tumor is limited to microscopic involvement of the cut mucosal margin of the bronchus, 5-year survival is increased beyond that seen without surgery. Incomplete resections may be indicated for palliation in cases of airway obstruction or hemoptysis if these are not amenable to endoscopic or radiologic procedures.

j. **Adjuvant and neoadjuvant therapy.** The benefits of pre- and/or postoperative pro-phylactic chemotherapy and/or radiotherapy are unclear for lung cancer patients who have undergone complete resections. Thoracic irradiation is usually given to patients with resected N_2 node involvement disease. Chemotherapy may be of some benefit after resection of advanced adenocarcinoma. Neoadjuvant cisplatin-based regimens

TABLE 15.11 Surgical approaches for pulmonary resections

Incision	Pro	Con
Posterolateral thoracotomy	Excellent exposure to entire operative hemithorax	Postoperative pain; ± respiration dysfunction (short and long term)
Lateral muscle-sparing thoracotomy	Decreased postoperative pain	Increased incidence of wound seromas
Anterolateral thoracotomy	Better access for laparotomy, resuscitation, or contralateral thoracotomy, especially in trauma	Limited access to posterior thorax
Axillary thoracotomy	Decreased pain; adequate access for first rib resection, sympathectomy, apical blebs, or bullae	Limited exposure
Sternotomy	Decreased pain, bilateral access	Decreased exposure of posterior structures
Transsternal bilateral ("clamshell")	Good exposure for bilateral lung transplantation	Postoperative pain and chest wall dysfunction
Video-assisted thoracoscopic (VATS)/robotic surgery	Less postoperative pain and respiratory dysfunction	Technically difficult with lung adhesions

for marginally resectable stage IIIa or IIIb disease are currently under investigation. Preoperative radiotherapy does not appear to offer any survival benefits and makes the surgery technically more difficult.

2. **Surgical approaches.** Any given pulmonary resection can be accomplished by a variety of different surgical approaches. The approach used in an individual case depends on the interaction of several factors, which include the site and pathology of the lesion(s) and the training and experience of the surgical team. Each approach has specific anesthetic implications. Common thoracic surgical approaches and their generally accepted advantages and disadvantages are listed in Table 15.11.

   a. **Posterolateral thoracotomy.** For decades, this was the traditional incision in thoracic surgery. The patient is placed in the lateral decubitus position. Chest access is usually via the fifth or sixth intercostal space. The left seventh or eighth space may be used for access to the esophageal hiatus. The serratus anterior, latissimus dorsi, and trapezius muscles all are partially divided during incision, with subsequent postoperative pain and disability. Chest access may be obtained directly through an intercostal space or by excision of a rib. Exposure to all ipsilateral intrathoracic structures is excellent.

   b. **Muscle-sparing lateral thoracotomy.** The lateral muscle-sparing thoracotomy has been advocated to reduce the pain and disability associated with a standard posterolateral thoracotomy. The skin incision may or may not be smaller, but an extensive subcutaneous dissection is required to mobilize the latissimus and serratus muscles.

   c. **Anterolateral thoracotomy.** This is a particularly useful incision in trauma because it allows complete access to the patient for ongoing resuscitation and does not require repositioning for laparotomy or exploration of the contralateral chest. Exposure to the posterior hemithorax is limited in comparison to a posterolateral incision. Because this approach requires incision of only the pectoralis muscles, pain and shoulder disability may be less than with a standard thoracotomy.

   d. **Axillary thoracotomy.** The transaxillary approach provides access only to the apical areas of the hemithorax. The ipsilateral arm must be draped free or suspended, and access to this arm will be limited intraoperatively. Thus, it is preferable for vascular access and monitoring to use the contralateral arm. Postoperative pain and disability are less than with a standard thoracotomy. This is an adequate incision for first rib resection, resection of apical bullae/blebs, or thoracic sympathectomy.

e. **Median sternotomy.** This incision, which is the standard for cardiac surgery, has potential benefits for certain thoracic procedures. Bilateral excisions for metastases and bullae are best performed via this incision. It has been demonstrated that postoperative spirometry is superior and pain is less after median sternotomy than thoracotomy. Most pulmonary resections can be performed via a median sternotomy, which obviates the need for a separate incision in cases of combined cardiac and thoracic surgery (see Section III.J). Certain procedures are more difficult via a median sternotomy, including procedures performed for superior sulcus tumors, tumors with posterior chest wall extension, and left lower lobe tumors. OLV is more of a necessity for surgical exposure than for lateral thoracotomies because of the limited surgical access, and oxygen desaturation is more common with OLV in the supine than the lateral position.

f. **Transsternal bilateral thoracotomy (the "clamshell" incision).** This is the common incision for bilateral lung transplantation. Because of increased pain and postoperative chest wall dysfunction, it is not commonly used for other intrathoracic procedures. It has been used for resection of bilateral metastases, pericardiectomy, resection of a posterior ventricular aneurysm, and cardiac surgery in a patient with a tracheotomy.

B. **Video-assisted thoracoscopic surgery (VATS)**

Essentially any surgical procedure that is performed via thoracotomy has been attempted by VATS. VATS has been advocated for pulmonary resection of lung cancer in patients with limited respiratory reserves because of decreased postoperative pain and loss of early postoperative spirometric respiratory function that is only approximately half of that seen when the same operation is performed by thoracotomy. VATS is the procedure of choice for resection of nonmalignant pulmonary lesions (blebs, bullae, granulomas). VATS will probably become the commonest procedure for the majority of cancer resections. Also, VATS is used for sympathectomy for palmar hyperhidrosis and for the intrathoracic portion of esophagogastrectomy. Bilateral VATS can be performed in the supine position for apical lesions, but for most operations, bilateral VATS requires change from one lateral position to the other intraoperatively. Robotic thoracic surgery is being used increasingly for minimally invasive procedures due to better visualization (see also Chapter 13 for further discussion of robotic thoracic surgery).

Some procedures are attempted by VATS initially with conversion to thoracotomy if the surgery proves impractical. OLV with complete collapse of the operative lung is more of a priority than for open thoracotomy, and application of CPAP to the nonventilated lung is more detrimental to surgery than in open thoracotomy. To aid collapse of the lung, particularly in patients with COPD and poor lung elastic recoil, it is best to ventilate with oxygen instead of air/oxygen mixtures during the period of two-lung ventilation before lung collapse and to apply suction (-20 cm H_2O) to the nonventilated lung after the start of OLV until collapse is complete. Postoperative management is essentially the same as for thoracotomy, and most patients initially will have chest drains. The amount of postoperative pain after VATS varies greatly depending on the surgical procedure performed. Simple wedge excisions will have only the pain of several small intercostal incisions and the chest drain(s), and this can usually be easily managed with oral medications. Pleural abrasions or instillation of pleural sclerosing agents, which are often done for recurrent pneumothoraces or effusions, are extremely painful and may require full postoperative analgesic management, up to and including TEA, in patients with limited pulmonary function.

> **CLINICAL PEARL** Complete collapse of the operative lung is more critical to VATS than to open thoracotomies, and the application of CPAP to that lung is relatively contraindicated because it severely compromises surgical exposure.

C. **Bronchopleural fistula**

A persistent communication between the airway and the interpleural space can develop after medical conditions, such as rupture of a bleb or bulla, infection, or malignancy. Bronchopleural fistula can develop as a postoperative complication after lung surgery. The large majority of persistent lung air leaks will heal with drainage and conservative management.

Surgical intervention is indicated when conservative therapy is unable to permit adequate gas exchange (this is more likely to occur in the immediate postoperative period, particularly after pneumonectomy) or when conventional chest tube drainage and suction are unable to reexpand the ipsilateral lung, or for a second ipsilateral or first contralateral pneumothorax.

There are three specific **anesthetic goals** in all patients with a bronchopleural fistula:

1. Healthy lung regions must be protected from soiling by extrapleural fluid from the affected hemithorax (e.g., coexisting empyema).
2. The ventilation technique must avoid development of a tension pneumothorax in the affected hemithorax.
3. The anesthetic technique must ensure adequate alveolar gas exchange in the presence of a low-resistance air leak.

To achieve these goals, there are two **management principles** that should be used in essentially all cases:

1. A functioning chest drain should be placed before the induction of anesthesia and connected to an underwater seal without suction.
2. A method of lung separation should be placed so that the fistula can be isolated as necessary intraoperatively.

After placement of a chest drain, there are three **options for induction** of anesthesia [12]:

1. A single-lumen or double-lumen EBT or blocker can be placed in an awake patient with topical anesthesia and its position checked fiberoptically before induction. This is often not the best choice in a patient with severely compromised gas exchange because maintaining adequate oxygenation in an already hypoxemic patient can be a problem during awake intubation.
2. Induction of anesthesia, maintaining spontaneous ventilation until lung isolation is secured. A spontaneous ventilation induction may not be desirable if there is a risk of aspiration and in patients with compromised hemodynamics.
3. IV induction of general anesthesia and muscle relaxation after meticulous preoxygenation and manual ventilation using small tidal volumes and low airway pressures until the lung isolation is confirmed. The efficiency of this technique can be improved by using a bronchoscope to guide DLT placement during intubation.

   The air leak through a bronchopleural fistula is dependent on the pressure gradient between the mean airway pressure at the site of the fistula and the interpleural space. High-frequency ventilation, with and without lung or lobar blockade, has been used in certain cases. High-frequency techniques may permit relatively lower proximal mean airway pressures than conventional mechanical ventilation and may be more useful in large central air leaks.

D. **Bullae and blebs**

   Whenever positive-pressure ventilation is applied to the airway of a patient with a bulla or bleb, there is the risk of lesion rupture and development of a tension pneumothorax that will require drainage and may progress to a bronchopleural fistula. The anesthetic considerations are similar to those for a patient with a bronchopleural fistula, except that it is best not to place a chest drain prophylactically because the chest tube may enter the bulla and create a fistula and there is not the risk of soiling healthy lung regions from extrapleural fluid that exists with fistulas. For induction of anesthesia, it is usually optimal to maintain spontaneous ventilation until the lung or lobe with the bulla or bleb is isolated. When there is a risk of aspiration or it is believed that the patient's gas exchange or hemodynamics may not permit spontaneous ventilation for induction, the anesthesiologist will need to use small tidal volumes and low airway pressures during positive-pressure ventilation until the airway is isolated. Nitrous oxide will diffuse into a bleb or bulla, causing it to enlarge, and must be avoided.

E. **Abscesses, bronchiectasis, cysts, and empyema**

   As with bronchopleural fistulas, there is the risk of soiling healthy lung regions by uncontrolled spillage from these lesions. Lung isolation is a primary requirement for anesthesia, and the anesthetic principles and management are similar to those described for fistulas. When an intrathoracic space-occupying lesion is removed, there is the potential for reexpansion pulmonary edema to develop after reinflation of the ipsilateral lung. A slow and gradual reinflation may decrease the severity of this complication.

F. Mediastinoscopy

Cervical mediastinoscopy is a diagnostic sampling of the mediastinal nodes to assess if a pulmonary resection will improve outcome. Basically, it is an attempt to differentiate between stage I or II and stage III lung cancer because the benefits of surgery vary tremendously between these stages. Mediastinoscopy can avoid some but not all unnecessary exploratory thoracotomies. Mediastinoscopy is often omitted from the cancer staging if the CT scan of the mediastinum is negative (mediastinal nodes less than 1 cm in the short axis). Because there are a significant number of false-positive results on cancer staging with CT scan, all patients with positive mediastinal nodes on CT should have a mediastinoscopy.

Mediastinoscopy can be done during a separate anesthetic before pulmonary resection, often as an outpatient, or after induction of anesthesia preceding pulmonary resection. Apart from the specific anesthetic considerations of mediastinoscopy itself, the anesthetic implication of starting the case with these diagnostic procedures is that the resection may be aborted based on the initial mediastinoscopy findings. The likelihood of not proceeding to thoracotomy must enter into each individual assessment of risk/benefit when considering placing an epidural catheter before induction.

Mediastinoscopy is most commonly done via a cervical approach with an incision in the suprasternal notch. Any structure in the upper chest can be injured during the procedure, including great vessels, pleura (pneumothorax), nerves (recurrent laryngeal), and airways.

Hemorrhage is the most frequent major complication, particularly due to inadvertent PA biopsy, and this must always be considered with respect to vascular access, monitoring, and the availability of means for resuscitation. Fortunately, significant hemorrhage during mediastinoscopy can usually be tamponaded temporarily by the surgeon when resuscitation is required. In only a minority of mediastinoscopy hemorrhages is it necessary to proceed to thoracotomy for surgical control of bleeding.

A frequent complication of cervical mediastinoscopy is transient compression of the brachiocephalic (innominate) artery by the mediastinoscope. The surgeon is usually unaware that this is occurring, so it is essential to incorporate continuous pulse monitoring in the right arm (pulse oximetry, arterial line, or palpation) into the anesthetic plan. The surgeon can then be immediately notified and avoid the risk of cerebral ischemia in patients who may not have good collateral cerebral circulation.

> **CLINICAL PEARL** During mediastinoscopy, continuous pulse monitoring in the right arm is essential to early recognition of innominate artery compression.

Because of the different pattern of lymphatic drainage of the left upper lobe, patients with left upper lobe tumors often will have an anterior left parasternal mediastinoscopy or median sternotomy instead of or in addition to a cervical mediastinoscopy. The serious complications associated with cervical mediastinoscopy are not as frequent with parasternal mediastinoscopy.

Endobronchial ultrasound (EBUS)-guided mediastinal nodal biopsies via an FOB are increasingly used as an alternative to traditional mediastinoscopy as a lung cancer–staging procedure. These can be performed awake with topical anesthesia of the airway or under general anesthesia.

G. Anterior mediastinal mass

Patients with anterior mediastinal masses present unique problems to the anesthesiologist. A large number of such patients require anesthesia for biopsy of these masses by mediastinoscopy or VATS, or they may require definitive resection via sternotomy or thoracotomy. Tumors of the anterior mediastinum include thymoma, teratoma, lymphoma, cystic hygroma, bronchogenic cyst, and thyroid tumors. Anterior mediastinal masses may cause obstruction of major airways, main pulmonary arteries, atria, and the superior vena cava. Any one of these complications can be life threatening. During induction of general anesthesia in patients with an anterior mediastinal mass, airway obstruction is the most common and feared complication.

It is important to note that the point of tracheal compression usually occurs distal to the ETT. A history of supine dyspnea or cough should alert the clinician to the possibility of airway obstruction upon induction of anesthesia. Life-threatening complications may occur in the absence of symptoms. The other major complication is cardiovascular collapse secondary to compression of the heart or major vessels. Symptoms of supine syncope suggest vascular compression. Death upon induction of general anesthesia in patients with an anterior mediastinal mass is always a risk. Anesthetic deaths have mainly been reported in children. These deaths may be the result of the more compressible cartilaginous structure of the airway in children or because of the difficulty in obtaining a history of positional symptoms in children.

The most important diagnostic test in the patient with an anterior mediastinal mass is the CT scan of the trachea and chest. Children with tracheobronchial compression greater than 50% on CT cannot be safely given general anesthesia [13]. Flow–volume loops, specifically exacerbation of a variable intrathoracic obstruction pattern (expiratory plateau) when supine, are unreliable for predicting which patients will have intraoperative airway complications. Echocardiography is indicated for patients with vascular compressive symptoms.

Management. General anesthesia will exacerbate extrinsic intrathoracic airway compression in at least three ways. First, reduced lung volume occurs during general anesthesia; second, bronchial smooth muscle relaxes during general anesthesia allowing greater compressibility of large airways; and third, paralysis eliminates the caudal movement of the diaphragm seen during spontaneous ventilation. This reduces or eliminates the normal transpleural pressure gradient that dilates the airways during inspiration and minimizes the effects of extrinsic intrathoracic airway compression.

Management of these patients is guided by their symptoms (Tables 15.12 to 15.14) and the CT scan. All of these patients need a step-by-step induction of anesthesia with continuous monitoring of gas exchange and hemodynamics. This **"NPIC" (Noli Pontes Ignii Consumere, i.e., don't burn your bridges)** anesthetic induction can be an inhalation induction with a volatile agent such as sevoflurane or IV titration of propofol with or without ketamine, which maintains spontaneous ventilation until either the airway is definitively secured or the procedure is completed [14]. Awake intubation of the trachea before induction is a possibility in some adult patients if the CT scan shows an area of noncompressed distal trachea to which the ETT can be advanced before induction. If muscle relaxants are required, ventilation should first be gradually taken over manually to assure that positive-pressure ventilation is possible and only then can a muscle relaxant be administered. Development of airway or vascular compression requires that the patient be awakened as rapidly as possible and then other options for the surgery to be explored. Intraoperative life-threatening airway compression has usually responded to one of two therapies: either **repositioning** of the patient (which should be determined before induction if there is one side or position that causes less compression) or **rigid bronchoscopy** and ventilation distal to the obstruction. This means that an experienced bronchoscopist and equipment must always be immediately available in the operating room with these cases.

CLINICAL PEARL Loss of airway during induction of a patient with an anterior mediastinal mass requires rapid rescue by repositioning the patient or by rigid bronchoscopy.

TABLE 15.12 Grading scale for symptoms in patients with an anterior mediastinal mass

Asymptomatic
Mild: Can lie supine with some cough/pressure sensation
Moderate: Can lie supine for short periods but not indefinitely
Severe: Cannot tolerate supine position

TABLE 15.13 Anterior mediastinal mass patient safety stratification for "NPIC" general anesthesia

A. Safe	**I.** Asymptomatic adult
	II. CT minimum tracheal/bronchial diameter >50% of normal
B. Unsafe	**I.** Severely symptomatic adult or child
	II. Children with CT tracheal/bronchial diameter <50% of normal
C. Uncertain	**I.** Mild/moderate symptomatic adult
	II. Asymptomatic adult with CT tracheal/bronchial diameter <50% of normal
	III. Mild/moderate symptomatic child with CT tracheal/bronchial diameter >50% of normal
	IV. Adult or child unable to give history

CT, computed tomography; NPIC, Noli Pontes Ignii Consumere (i.e., Don't burn your bridges).

Femorofemoral CPB before induction of anesthesia is a possibility for some patients who are considered "unsafe" for "NPIC" general anesthesia. The concept of CPB "standby" during attempted induction of anesthesia is fraught with danger because there is not enough time after a sudden airway collapse to establish CPB before hypoxic cerebral injury occurs [15]. Other options for "unsafe" patients include local anesthetic biopsy of the mediastinal mass or biopsy of another node (e.g., supraclavicular), preoperative radiotherapy with a nonradiated "window" for subsequent biopsy, preoperative chemotherapy or short-course steroids, and CT-guided biopsy of mass or drainage of a cyst.

H. Tracheal and bronchial stenting

Regional narrowing of the trachea or bronchi can be treated temporarily or definitively by placement of tracheal or bronchial stents [16]. The only previous options for these lesions were dilation, laser excision, or surgical excision. Airway stenting is an option for palliation of patients with mediastinal masses pending other therapy. There are two major varieties of stent: metallic and silastic (Dumon). Both are commonly placed during rigid bronchoscopy, although there is an option to place the self-expanding metallic stents with flexible FOB. The metallic stents are more stable and more resistant to dislocation in the airway but are difficult (often impossible) to remove once placed. Thus, metallic stents are commonly only used for palliation in malignant airway obstructions.

Anesthetic management for tracheal stenting is similar to management of patients with mediastinal masses. General anesthesia with muscle relaxation is optimal, but in patients with severe symptoms of airway obstruction, induction of anesthesia should follow a step-by-step "NPIC" protocol as discussed above.

I. Tracheal resection

Anatomically, the trachea has a necessary structural rigidity and a segmental blood supply that complicate its resection and repair. Many different prosthetic designs and materials have been evaluated as tracheal substitutes. Because of unresolved problems with anatomic disruption, poor healing, and infection, end-to-end anastomosis of the trachea remains the ideal method of repair.

Endotracheal intubation and resulting strictures were once the primary cause of the need for tracheal resection, but using less irritating ETT materials and limiting the duration of

TABLE 15.14 Anterior mediastinal mass management for all "uncertain" patients for "NPIC" general anesthesia

I. Secure airway beyond stenosis awake if feasible
II. Rigid bronchoscope and surgeon available at induction
III. Laryngeal mask airway available
IV. Determine optimal positioning of patient
V. Preserve spontaneous respiration capability until tolerance for positive pressure ventilation is proven
VI. Monitor for airway compromise postoperatively "NPIC"

NPIC, Noli Pontes Ignii Consumere (i.e., Don't burn your bridges).

prolonged endotracheal intubation have decreased this complication. Benign and malignant tumors (e.g., adenocarcinomas and cylindromas) constitute the remaining indications for tracheal resection.

For a controlled and methodical operation on the trachea, full control of the airway must be maintained at all times. Cooperation between the surgeon and anesthesiologist is of utmost importance. Both should visualize the lesion preoperatively (CT and bronchoscopy). With preoperative planning and discussions, they can avoid unnecessary hasty procedures that might compromise the end result or worse. Benign lesions can be dilated preoperatively to allow the passage of a small ETT through the lesion. Operatively, the area below the lesion is addressed first. If the degree of obstruction increases, a sterile ETT can be placed directly from the surgical field. The patient should be spontaneously ventilating at the end of the case to allow for extubation. Some surgeons will temporarily place a Montgomery "T" tube distal to the anastomosis with the side arm of the "T" brought out anteriorly through the neck incision to ensure gas exchange in case of proximal tracheoglottic obstruction or edema. Some surgeons will leave a temporary "chin retention" suture for several days postoperatively. This heavy suture between the chin and the sternum restricts head extension and limits traction on the fresh tracheal anastomosis. CPB greatly complicates the conduct of the operation and has largely been unnecessary.

J. Pulmonary hemorrhage

Massive hemoptysis is defined as expectoration of >200 mL of blood in 24 to 48 hours. The commonest causes are carcinoma, bronchiectasis, and trauma (blunt, penetrating, or secondary to a PA catheter). Death can occur quickly due to asphyxia. Management requires four sequential steps: lung isolation, resuscitation, diagnosis, and definitive treatment. The anesthesiologist is often called to deal with these cases outside of the operating room. There is no consensus on the best method of lung isolation. The initial method for lung isolation will depend on the availability of appropriate equipment and an assessment of the patient's airway. All three basic methods of lung isolation have been used: DLTs, single-lumen EBTs, and BBs. FOB is usually not helpful to position EBTs or blockers in the presence of torrential pulmonary hemorrhage, and lung isolation must be guided by clinical signs (primarily auscultation). DLTs will achieve rapid and secure lung isolation. Even if a left-sided tube enters the right mainstem bronchus, only the right upper lobe will be obstructed. However, suctioning large amounts of blood or clots is difficult through the narrow lumens of a DLT. An option is initial placement of a single-lumen tube for oxygenation and suctioning and then replacement with a DLT either by laryngoscopy or with an appropriate tube exchanger. An uncut single-lumen ETT can be advanced directly into the right mainstem bronchus or rotated 90 degrees counterclockwise for advancement into the left mainstem bronchus (less reliable than right-mainstem intubation). A BB will normally pass easily into the right mainstem bronchus and is useful for right-sided hemorrhage (90% of PA catheter–induced hemorrhages are right sided). After lung isolation and resuscitation have been achieved, both diagnosis and definitive therapy are now most commonly performed by radiologists [17] (except for blunt and penetrating trauma).

1. **Pulmonary artery (PA) catheter–induced hemorrhage.** Hemoptysis in a patient with a PA catheter must be assumed to be caused by perforation of a pulmonary vessel by the catheter until proven otherwise. The mortality rate may exceed 50%. This complication seems to be occurring less than previously, possibly related to stricter indications for the use of PA catheters and more appropriate management of PA catheters with less reliance on wedge pressure measurements. Therapy for PA catheter–induced hemorrhage should follow an organized protocol with some variation depending on the severity of the hemorrhage (see Table 15.15).

2. **During weaning from cardiopulmonary bypass(CPB):** Weaning from CPB is one of the times when PA catheter–induced hemorrhage is most likely to occur. Management of the PA catheter during CPB by routinely withdrawing the catheter 2 to 3 cm to avoid wedging during CPB may decrease the risk of this complication. When hemoptysis does occur in this situation, there are several management options available (see Fig. 15.9). The anesthesiologist should resist the temptation to rapidly reverse the anticoagulation in order to quickly get off CPB since this can lead to disaster. Resumption of full CPB ensures

TABLE 15.15   Management of the patient with a PA catheter–induced pulmonary hemorrhage

I. Initially position the patient with the bleeding lung dependent.
II. Endotracheal intubation, oxygenation, airway toilet
III. Lung isolation. Endobronchial DLT or single-lumen tube or BB
IV. Withdraw the PA catheter several centimeters, leaving it in the main PA. Do not inflate the balloon (except with fluoroscopic guidance).
V. Position the patient with the isolated bleeding lung nondependent. PEEP to the bleeding lung if possible.
VI. Transport to medical imaging for diagnosis and embolization if feasible.

BB, bronchial blocker; PA, pulmonary artery; PEEP, positive end-expiratory pressure.

oxygenation while the tracheobronchial tree is suctioned and then visualized with FOB. The use of a PA vent or full-flow CPB may be required to decrease the pulmonary blood flow sufficiently to define the bleeding site (usually the right lower lobe). The pleural cavity should be opened to assess the lung parenchymal damage. When possible, conservative management with lung isolation constitutes optimal therapy. In patients with persistent hemorrhage who are not candidates for lung resection, temporary lobar PA occlusion with a vascular loop may be an option.

K. Posttracheostomy hemorrhage

Hemorrhage in the immediate postoperative period following a tracheostomy is usually from local vessels such as the anterior jugular or inferior thyroid veins. Massive hemorrhage 1 to 6 weeks postoperatively is most commonly due to tracheo-innominate artery fistula [18]. A small sentinel bleed occurs in most patients before a massive bleed. The management protocol for tracheo-innominate artery fistula is outlined in Table 15.16.

IV. Pulmonary thromboendarterectomy (PTE)

A. Overview

PTE, a complete endarterectomy of the pulmonary vascular tree, is the definitive treatment for chronic thromboembolic pulmonary hypertension (CTEPH). Pulmonary embolism (PE)

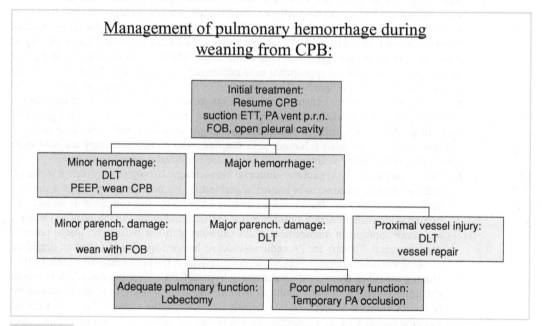

FIGURE 15.9 Management of pulmonary hemorrhage during weaning from cardiopulmonary bypass. BB, bronchial blocker; CPB, cardiopulmonary bypass; DLT, double-lumen tube; ETT, endotracheal tube; PA, pulmonary artery; FOB, fiber-optic bronchoscopy; PEEP, positive end-expiratory pressure; parench., lung parenchyma; p.r.n. (pro re nata), as needed.

TABLE 15.16   Management of tracheo-innominate artery fistula hemorrhage

1. Overinflate the tracheostomy cuff to tamponade the hemorrhage. If this fails:
2. Replace the tracheostomy tube with an oral ETT. Position the cuff with FOB guidance just above the carina.
3. Digital compression of the innominate artery against the posterior sternum using a finger passed through the tracheostomy stoma. If this fails:
4. Slow withdrawal of the ETT and overinflation of the cuff to tamponade.
5. Then proceed with definitive therapy: sternotomy and ligation of the innominate artery.

ETT, endotracheal tube; FOB, fiberoptic bronchoscopy.

is a relatively common cardiovascular event, and in a small percentage of cases it leads to a chronic condition in which repeated microemboli lead to accumulation of connective and elastic tissue on the surface of the pulmonary vessels with resultant end-stage lung disease due to pulmonary hypertension [19]. The only potentially curative options are lung transplantation and PTE, with PTE preferred because of its favorable long-term morbidity and mortality profile. Surgical mortality rates vary in the range of 3% to 6% [20]. The most common symptom of CTEPH is exertional dyspnea. Other symptoms may include chest tightness, hemoptysis, and peripheral edema.

Preoperative evaluation includes CXR, pulmonary function testing, right heart catheterization with pulmonary angiography, high-resolution magnetic resonance imaging, ABG analysis, V/Q scanning, and echocardiography. Diffusing capacity (DLCO) is often reduced and may be the only abnormality on pulmonary function testing. Pulmonary arterial pressures are elevated (mean >25 mm Hg) and sometimes are suprasystemic. Resting cardiac output is often low. Many patients exhibit hypoxia, particularly with exercise. $PaCO_2$ is often slightly reduced, although dead space ventilation is increased. With transthoracic echocardiography, an estimate of PA systolic pressure is provided by Doppler interrogation of the tricuspid regurgitant envelope. Echocardiographic findings include RV enlargement, leftward displacement of the interventricular septum, and encroachment of the enlarged right ventricle (RV) on the left ventricle (LV).

Pulmonary angiography is the gold standard to confirm the diagnosis and to determine the surgical accessibility of thromboembolic disease. Many CTEPH patients receive medical pulmonary vasodilator therapy. This therapy may consist of phosphodiesterase 5 inhibition (e.g., sildenafil), endothelin-1 inhibition (e.g., bosentan), and prostacyclin analogs (e.g., iloprost, epoprostenol, treprostinil). It is prudent to continue these medications preoperatively and to consider their use postoperatively if the surgical result is suboptimal. Abrupt cessation of a prostacyclin analog can result in potentially catastrophic rebound pulmonary hypertension.

B. **Surgical procedure**

PTE is performed through a midline sternotomy and requires CPB with deep hypothermic circulatory arrest (DHCA) in most centers. (Details of anesthetic and CPB management at the Toronto General Hospital are presented in Tables 15.17 and 15.18.) CPB is established with cannulation of the ascending aorta and the inferior and superior vena cava. Circulatory arrest is limited to 20-minute epochs. If additional arrest time is necessary, reperfusion is carried out at 18°C core temperature for a minimum of 10 minutes.

CLINICAL PEARL   In chronic pulmonary thromboembolic disease, the development of prominent bronchial arterial collaterals requires the use of circulatory arrest during pulmonary thromboembolectomy.

C. **Anesthetic management**

The majority of lines and monitors are placed preinduction due to the risk of hemodynamic collapse on induction. Because of the high right-sided pressures, the coronary blood supply to the RV is at risk. Maintenance of adequate mean systemic arterial pressure, systemic vascular resistance (SVR), inotropic state, and normal sinus rhythm is critical. Markedly elevated PA systolic pressures (>2/3 systemic), RVEDP (>14 mm Hg), severe tricuspid regurgitation, and

TABLE 15.17   Pulmonary thromboendarterectomy anesthesia, key points (Toronto General Hospital protocol)

I. Pre-induction
Cooling/warming blanket below patient, supine back head–elevated position
Peripheral large-bore venous access, arterial line (radial + femoral postinduction)
Right internal jugular access, oximetric PA catheter, in vitro calibration
Baseline ABG, ACT, SvO$_2$, CI, and PVR; defibrillation pads

II. Induction of anesthesia[a]
Intubation with single-lumen ETT
Urinary catheter with temperature probe
Forced air warming blanket on legs (not connected)
Triple-lumen CVP postinduction for postoperative access (subclavian preferred site)
Naso- or oropharyngeal probe for temperature
Neuromonitoring as per institutional protocol for other CPB cases
Drugs
   Midazolam + fentanyl (or sufentanil) + ketamine (or etomidate)
   Propofol infusion ± volatile anesthetic
   Methylprednisolone 1 g on induction (30 mg/kg in some centers)
   Cephalosporin 1 g if <80 kg, 2 g if >80 kg (repeat q4h), or vancomycin 1 g (more if >80 kg)
   Tranexamic acid 30 mg/kg loading dose plus infusion of 16 mg/kg/hr on CPB[b]
   Heparin 400 U/kg to raise and maintain ACT >480 sec

III. TEE
Assess RV/LV function, PFO, intracardiac, and PA thrombi
Assess aortic and mitral valve functions
Monitor intracardiac air emboli during weaning
Reassess post-CPB

IV. Post-CPB
Pressure control ventilation, VT 6–7 mL/kg, PEEP 5 cm, decrease FiO$_2$ as tolerated
Minimal doses of furosemide (5–10 mg) if indicated (to avoid excessive diuresis once patient is warmed), aim for
   urine output greater than 1 L while on CPB, total 1.5–2 L at the end of the procedure
Norepinephrine ± vasopressin to wean off CPB, limit cardiac index to 2.0–2.5 L/min/m^2 to decrease pulmonary
   reperfusion injury
Epinephrine if indicated to raise CI, aim at SvO$_2$ greater than 60%
Protamine to reverse heparin, platelets, and clotting factors only for indication (these patients usually have a
   thrombophilia[b]). Bleeding post-CPB is not common despite long CPB times
NG tube after TEE probe removed, FOB at end of case

[a]In patients with very high PA pressures: Risk of hemodynamic collapse on induction, induction after urinary catheter, patient prepped and draped.
[b]Because of thrombophilia, some centers do not use prophylactic antifibrinolytic agents.
PA, pulmonary artery; ABG, arterial blood gas; PVR, pulmonary vascular resistance; ETT, endotracheal tube; CVP, central venous pressure catheter; CPB, cardiopulmonary bypass; PEEP, positive end-expiratory pressure; TEE, transesophageal echocardiography; ACT, activated clotting time; SvO$_2$, mixed venous oxygen saturation; RV/LV, right ventricular/left ventricular; PFO, patent foramen ovale; CI, cardiac index; NG, nasogastric; FOB, fiberoptic bronchoscopy; VT, tidal volume; L, liter.

preoperative pulmonary vascular resistance (PVR) >1,000 dyne sec cm^{-5} are signs of impending decompensation. In order to ensure adequate RV coronary perfusion, a combined vasopressor/inotrope (e.g., norepinephrine) is begun prior to induction with additional inotropic support (e.g., dobutamine or epinephrine) as indicated. Generally, patients with CTEPH have fixed PVR because of mechanical obstruction. However, high PVR can still be exacerbated by factors that increase PVR (e.g., hypoxia, hypercarbia, acidosis, pain, and anxiety). Thus, these stressors should be minimized during induction and the pre-CPB period. Attempts to lower the PVR pharmacologically (e.g., nitroglycerin, nitroprusside) should generally be avoided as they have minimal efficacy in treating CTEPH and can dangerously jeopardize the coronary perfusion pressure to the RV myocardium. Direct pulmonary vasodilators such as NO and prostaglandins, which may be useful in the medical management of patients with other types of pulmonary hypertension, generally show limited benefit for pulmonary endarterectomy patients in the perioperative period.

TABLE 15.18 Pulmonary thromboendarterectomy CPB, Toronto General Hospital protocol

Key points
Initiation
  Standard CPB prime, retrograde autologous prime if hemodynamically stable
  Hemodilution to a hematocrit of 28–30% during cooling
  Perfusion index: 2.4–2.5 L/min/m^2 and about 1.7 L/m^2 during hypothermia
  Aim for mean BP of 70–90 mm Hg during CPB if possible
  Thiopental 10 mg/kg in CPB circuit just before aortic cross-clamp[a]
  Cardioplegia every 30–45 min
  Start cooling to 18–20°C (rectal) once on full bypass
  Head and neck packed in ice or cooling blanket, eyes protected
  Circulatory arrest when PA back-bleeding from bronchial arteries obstructs surgical view
  All anesthesia monitoring/access lines closed to the patient prior to circulatory arrest
  Lung recruitment maneuver as pump turned off
  Two episodes of circulatory arrest of maximum 20 min each

Rewarming
  Start slow warming to 37°C, warming rate <1°C/3min (CPB waterbath–rectal temperature gradient <8°C)
  Unclamp LV and PA vent
  Ventilation with PEEP 5 cm H$_2$O, pressure control ventilation, tidal volume 6 mL/kg, FiO$_2$ 0.21, and respiratory rate
    of 15/min

Weaning
Once 37°C reached
  Slowly wean CPB
  Aim for cardiac index of 2.0–2.5 L/min/m^2 maximum
  Aim for SvO$_2$ of greater than 60%
  Aim for hematocrit of 30% by the end of the rewarming period
  Aim for total urine output of 1.5–2 L at the end of the procedure

[a]Propofol (e.g., 5 mg/kg) can also be used.
CPB, cardiopulmonary bypass; PA, pulmonary artery; PEEP, positive end-expiratory pressure; BP, blood pressure; LV, left
ventricular; SvO$_2$, mixed venous oxygen saturation.

End-tidal carbon dioxide (ETCO$_2$) is a poor measure of ventilation adequacy in these patients both pre- and post-CPB, since dead space ventilation is an integral part of the disease process. Transesophageal echocardiography (TEE) is valuable in monitoring and assessing cardiac function and filling during PTE.

The process of separation from CPB is similar to other surgeries involving CPB. Modest vasopressor/inotropic support (e.g., norepinephrine 0.01 to 0.05 µg/kg/min and/or epinephrine 0.02 to 0.05 µg/kg/min) is often necessary initially because of the long hypothermic period and long aortic cross-clamp time. If the surgery has only been partially successful because of small-vessel disease, pulmonary vasodilators such as inhaled prostacyclin or NO should be considered. Most often, improvement in the cardiac index is seen with a dramatic decrease in PA pressures and a drop in the PVR.

D. **Post-cardiopulmonary bypass (CPB)**

Frothy sputum, if present, likely indicates the onset of reperfusion pulmonary edema. In this case, the ETT is suctioned, FOB is used to evaluate any intrapulmonary source of bleeding, and increasing amounts of PEEP are applied beginning with 5 cm H$_2$O. If bleeding is minor and peripheral, a BB can be placed in the appropriate lobar bronchus. If severe bleeding persists and is predominantly unilateral, lung isolation (double-lumen EBT) and independent lung ventilation are considered, as well as other interventions such as topical vasopressors.

V. **Lung volume reduction surgery (LVRS)**

According to the National Heart, Blood, and Lung Institute, approximately 13.5 million persons in the United States are afflicted with COPD, and 3.1 million of these patients have emphysema (Cure Researchtm.com, http://www.cureresearch.com) as the primary manifestation. Airflow

13

obstruction associated with chronic bronchitis or emphysema occurs due to a loss of the elastic recoil properties of the lung and chest wall. As the disease progresses, patients become increasingly debilitated. They exhibit symptoms of severe dyspnea, require supplemental oxygen, and display poor exercise tolerance. LVRS offers a select group of patients the possibility of improved exercise tolerance, reduction in dyspnea, improved quality of life, and extended life span. It has been suggested that LVRS may provide these patients with a benefit that otherwise cannot be achieved by any means other than lung transplantation.

A. **History of lung volume reduction surgery (LVRS)**

    1. In 1957, Otto Brantigan, MD, described a surgical technique for patients with end-stage emphysema that was designed to alleviate symptoms of severe dyspnea and exercise intolerance. He reasoned that by excising the nonfunctional lung tissue, the compressive effects exerted on normal lung tissue could be relieved to improve V/Q matching. Unfortunately, the operative mortality was significant and no objective measures of benefit could be documented. Thus, early LVRS was abandoned as a viable therapy for patients with end-stage emphysema until 1993.

    2. In 1996, Joel Cooper, MD, authored an editorial advocating the technique of LVRS as a "logical, physiologically sound procedure of demonstrable benefit for a selected group of patients with no alternative therapy" [21,22]. He further stated that the successful application of LVRS was "made possible through an improved understanding of pulmonary physiology, improved anesthetic and surgical techniques, and lessons learned from experience with lung transplantation." Although Dr. Cooper touted the benefits of LVRS for certain patients, he did not minimize the surgical risk and suggested that this was not a procedure to be performed in all healthcare centers across the country. Additionally, he advocated that COPD patients who would otherwise qualify for lung transplantation should be simultaneously evaluated for LVRS so that they would receive the procedure proving to be most appropriate. Dr. Cooper's proposals led to the design and implementation of the National Emphysema Treatment Trial (NETT).

B. **The National Emphysema Treatment Trial (NETT)**

The NETT was conducted from January 1998 to July 2002; 3,777 patients were evaluated and 1,218 patients were ultimately randomized to receive either LVRS or medical therapy.

    1. The **primary objective** of the NETT was to determine if the addition of LVRS to medical therapy improves patient survival and increases exercise capacity.

    2. **Secondary objectives** included defining the profile of patients likely to benefit from LVRS and determining if LVRS improves quality of life, reduces debilitating symptoms, and improves overall pulmonary function.

    3. A successful procedure was defined as a **60% to 70% increase in FEV_1 by 3 months postoperatively that is sustained for at least 1 year; decreased total lung capacity (TLC) and residual volume; improved exercise tolerance; and significant reduction in supplemental oxygen requirement.**

C. **Results.** Of the 608 patients assigned to LVRS, 580 underwent surgery (406 via median sternotomy; 174 VATS). Among the 610 patients assigned to medical therapy alone, 33 underwent LVRS outside the study and 15 received lung transplantation [23]. Overall mortality was 0.11 deaths per person-year in both treatment groups. After 24 months, exercise capacity improved more than 10 W in 15% of patients in the surgery group compared with 3% in the medical therapy–alone group. After exclusion of 140 patients at high risk for death from surgery [21], overall mortality in the surgery group was 0.09 deaths per person-year versus 0.10 in the medical group. Among patients with predominantly upper lobe emphysema and low baseline exercise capacity, mortality was lower in the surgery group than in the medical therapy–alone group.

D. **Conclusions.** The data from the trial suggested that, overall, LVRS increased the chance of improved exercise capacity but did not demonstrate a survival advantage as compared with medical therapy alone. There was a survival advantage demonstrated for those patients with both predominantly upper lobe emphysema and low baseline exercise capacity. Patients with non–upper lobe emphysema and high baseline exercise capacity were found to be poor candidates for LVRS because of the increase in mortality and negligible functional gain [24].

E. **The Cochrane Airways Group** recently published a review of all available randomized clinical trials comparing the effectiveness of LVRS versus nonsurgical standard therapy to improve outcomes in patients with severe diffuse emphysema [25]. This review includes 11 studies and 1,760 participants. This review concluded that LVRS may be effective for selected patients with severe emphysema and may lead to better health status and lung function outcomes, specifically for patients with upper lobe–predominant emphysema with low exercise capacity. The procedure is associated with risks of early mortality and adverse events (persistent air leaks, pulmonary morbidity [e.g., pneumonia] and cardiovascular morbidity). Although LVRS increases quality-associated life years, it is relatively costly.

F. **Anesthetic management for lung volume reduction surgery (LVRS).** Anesthesiology expertise is essential to successful outcomes for patients undergoing LVRS. Our expertise in cardiopulmonary physiology, pharmacology, and pain management allows us to minimize postoperative complications.

1. **Preoperative assessment.** All patients scheduled for LVRS receive the following preoperative physiologic studies: (a) Standard pulmonary function studies; (b) plethysmographic measurement of lung volumes; (c) standardized 6-minute walk test; (d) ABG values; (e) quantitative nuclear lung perfusion scans; and (f) radionuclide cardiac ventriculogram and/or dobutamine stress echocardiogram.

2. **Preoperative pulmonary rehabilitation program.** After the initial preoperative evaluation, all patients are enrolled in a pulmonary rehabilitation program for a minimum of 6 weeks before surgical intervention.

3. **Monitors.** In addition to the standard monitors, large-bore IV access and an arterial catheter are recommended. The use of central venous catheters and PA catheters should be considered on an individual patient basis.

4. The judicious use of **TEA**, both intraoperatively and postoperatively, affords advantages as follows: (a) Preserved ability to cough and clear secretions, thus decreasing atelectasis and possibly reducing pulmonary infection; (b) decreased airway resistance; (c) improved phrenic nerve function; (d) stabilization of coronary endothelial function; (e) improved myocardial perfusion; (f) earlier return of bowel function; (g) preservation of immunocompetence; and (h) decreased cost of perioperative care through reduction of perioperative complications. Best results are obtained with catheters placed in the T4–T5 or T5–T6 spinal interspaces.

   a. **Intraoperative TEA.** TEA can be used as an adjunct to general anesthesia. Local anesthetics, such as 2% lidocaine, 0.5% ropivacaine, or 0.25% bupivacaine, provide optimal surgical conditions. The local anesthetics can be delivered via intermittent bolus or as a continuous infusion.

      (1) Because persistent air leaks may be a problem in the postoperative period and may be exacerbated by positive-pressure ventilation, it is optimal to extubate the patients either at the conclusion of surgery or as soon as possible thereafter.

      (2) Caution must be exercised if opioids are added to the infusate because they have the potential to severely depress the patient's respiratory efforts.

   b. **Postoperative TEA.** TEA provides superior postoperative analgesia for both median sternotomy and bilateral thoracoscopic surgical procedures. A reduced concentration of local anesthetic plus a small dose of opioids delivered by continuous infusion is suggested (e.g., 0.2% ropivacaine plus 0.01 mg/mL hydromorphone).

   c. **Paravertebral nerve blocks** (PVNB) may be used as an alternative to TEA. They may be performed either by multiple injections or by inserting a catheter into the paravertebral space for use with a continuous infusion of local anesthetic. This technique requires the use of a multimodal analgesic regimen including IV opioids and nonsteroidal anti-inflammatory agents. The effect of PVN on morbidity and mortality following thoracic surgery, in particular LVRS, has yet to be determined.

5. **A left-sided double-lumen EBT** should be used to secure the patient's airway.

6. **General anesthesia.** Induction of general anesthesia can be conducted with agents that promote hemodynamic homeostasis. An example is etomidate 0.2 mg/kg plus an easily reversible nondepolarizing neuromuscular blocking agent such as rocuronium.

Maintenance anesthesia may consist of low doses of a volatile agent (e.g., 0.2–0.4% end-tidal isoflurane) and oxygen in addition to TEA. The anesthetic plan for each patient should be individualized appropriately.

7. **Postoperative management.** Problems that should be anticipated in the postoperative period include (a) oversedation, (b) accumulation of airway secretions, (c) pneumothorax, (d) bronchospasm, (e) PE, (f) pneumonia, (g) persistent air leaks, (h) arrhythmias, (i) myocardial infarction, and (j) PE. Reintubation and mechanical ventilation are associated with high morbidity and mortality. Several measures can be taken to minimize these adverse side effects:

   a. Judicious pulmonary toilet
   b. Bronchodilators
   c. Effective analgesia with TEA or PVNB/multimodal analgesia
   d. Avoidance of systemic corticosteroids

G. **Endobronchial valves and blockers for lung volume reduction.** Although LVRS has been shown to benefit patients with a heterogeneous pattern of emphysema, this constitutes only about 20% of patients who are eligible candidates for this treatment. Procedures for bronchoscopic LVRS have been developed to treat patients with heterogeneous and homogeneous patterns of emphysema. Endobronchial treatment has been studied for more than a decade and has been approved in several countries throughout the world; however, it still remains an investigational therapy in the United States. The rationale for this minimally invasive approach is that, by endobronchially obstructing the emphysematous segments of the lung, collapse of these areas should occur. This should reduce hyperinflation and alleviate symptoms without the need for surgery. Currently available bronchoscopic techniques include endobronchial blockers/valves, biologic glues, and airway bypass. Although significant improvements can be achieved with endobronchial valves/blockers, the results have not been as substantial as those obtained with surgical LVRS.

H. **Conclusions.** LVRS is a viable option for a select group of emphysema patients, and endobronchial valves and blockers that are undergoing clinical trials hold much promise as a treatment alternative for all emphysema patients. Regardless of the selection of treatment modality, the goals remain the same: improvements in dyspnea, exercise tolerance, quality of life, and prolonged survival.

The anesthesiologist must be actively engaged in the perioperative management of these patients. Patient history and preoperative status as well as the results obtained from the evaluation of CXRs, high-resolution CT scans, and right heart catheterizations should be carefully weighed when planning these procedures.

REFERENCES

1. **Choi H, Mazzone P. Preoperative evaluation of the patient with lung cancer being considered for lung resection.** *Curr Opin Anesthesiol.* **2015;28(1):18–25.**
2. **Brunelli A, Kim AW, Berger KI, et al. Physiologic evaluation of the patient with lung cancer being considered for resectional surgery. Diagnosis and management of lung cancer, 3rd ed. American College of Chest Physicians evidence-based clinical practice guidelines.** *Chest.* **2013;143(5 Suppl):e166S–e190S.**
3. **Frendl G, Sodickson AC, Chung MK, et al. 2014 AATS guidelines for the prevention and management of perioperative atrial fibrillation and flutter for thoracic surgical procedures.** *J Thorac Cardiovasc Surg.* **2014;148(3):772–791.**
4. Campos JH. An update on bronchial blockers during lung separation techniques in adults. *Anesth Analg.* 2003;97(5): 1266–1274.
5. Knoll H, Ziegeler S, Schreiber JU, et al. Airway injuries after one-lung ventilation: a comparison between double-lumen tube and endobronchial blocker: a randomized, prospective, controlled trial. *Anesthesiology.* 2006;105(3):471–477.
6. **Campos JH, Hallam E, Van Natta T, et al. Devices for lung isolation used by anesthesiologists with limited thoracic experience: comparison of double-lumen endotracheal tube, Univent torque control blocker, and Arndt wire-guided endobronchial blocker.** *Anesthesiology.* **2006;104:261–266.**
7. **Slinger P. Fiberoptic bronchoscopic positioning of double lumen tubes.** *J Cardiothorac Anesth.* **1989;3:486–496. For photographs see "Bronchoscopic positioning of Double-Lumen Tubes" in the Living Library section at the website www.thoracicanesthesia.com.**
8. **Karzai W, Schwarzkopf K. Hypoxemia during one-lung ventilation.** *Anesthesiology.* **2009;110(6):1402–1411.**
9. Ku CM, Slinger P, Waddell TK. A novel method of treating hypoxemia during one-lung ventilation for thoracoscopic surgery. *J Cardiothorac Vasc Anesth.* 2009;23(6):850–852.

10. Slinger P. Postpneumonectomy pulmonary edema: good news, bad news. *Anesthesiology*. 2006;105(1):2–5.

11. Amar D, Roistacher N, Burt ME, et al. Effects of diltiazem versus digoxin on dysrhythmias and cardiac function after pneumonectomy. *Ann Thorac Surg*. 1997;63(5):1374–1381.

12. Riley RH, Wood BM. Induction of anesthesia in a patient with a bronchopleural fistula. *Anaesth Intensive Care*. 1994;22(5): 625–626.

13. Shamberger RC, Hozman RS, Griscom NT, et al. Prospective evaluation by computed tomography and pulmonary function tests of children with mediastinal masses. *Surgery*. 1995;118(3):468–471.

14. Frawley G, Low J, Brown TC. Anaesthesia for an anterior mediastinal mass with ketamine and midazolam infusion. *Anaesth Intensive Care*. 1995;23(5):610–612.

15. Turkoz A, Gulcan O, Tercan F, et al. Hemodynamic collapse caused by a large unruptured aneurysm of the ascending aorta in an 18 year old. *Anesth Analg*. 2006;102(4):1040–1042.

16. Licker M, Schweizer A, Nicolet G, et al. Anesthesia of a patient with an obstructing tracheal mass: a new way to manage the airway. *Acta Anaesthesiol Scand*. 1997;41:84–86.

17. **Fortin M, Turcotte R, Gleeton O, et al. Catheter induced pulmonary artery rupture; using balloon occlusion to avoid lung isolation.** *J Cardiothorac Vasc Anesth*. **2006;20(3):376–378.**

18. **Grant CA, Dempsey G, Harrison J, et al. Tracheoinnominate artery fistula after percutaneous tracheostomy: three case reports and a clinical review.** *Br J Anaesth*. **2006;96(1):127–131.**

19. **Manecke G, Banks D, Madani M, et al. Pulmonary thrombo-endarterectomy. In: Slinger P, ed.** *Principles and Practice of Anesthesia for Thoracic Surgery*. **New York: Springer; 2011.**

20. de Perrot M, McRae K, Shargall Y, et al. Early postoperative pulmonary vascular compliance predicts outcome after pulmonary endarterectomy for chronic thromboembolic pulmonary hypertension. *Chest*. 2011;140(1):34–41.

21. Meyers BF, Yusen RD, Guthrie TJ, et al. Outcome of bilateral lung volume reduction in patients with emphysema potentially eligible for lung transplantation. *J Thorac Cardiovasc Surg*. 2001;122(1):10–17.

22. Cooper JD, Lefrak SS. Is volume reduction surgery appropriate in the treatment of emphysema? Yes. *Am J Respir Crit Care Med*. 1996;153(4 Pt 1):1201–1204.

23. Fishman A, Martinez F, Naunheim K, et al; National Emphysema Treatment Trial Research Group. A randomized trial comparing lung-volume-reduction surgery with medical therapy for severe emphysema. *N Engl J Med*. 2003;348(21):2059–2073.

24. National Emphysema Treatment Trial Research Group, Fishman A, Fessler H. Patients at high risk of death after lung-volume-reduction surgery. *N Engl J Med*. 2001;345(15):1075–1083.

25. **van Agteren JE, Carson KV, Tiong LU, et al. Lung volume reduction surgery for diffuse emphysema.** *Cochrane Database Syst Rev*. **2016;10:CD001001.**

16

Anesthetic Management for Adult Patients with Congenital Heart Disease

Laurie K. Davies, S. Adil Husain, and Nathaen S. Weitzel

I. Introduction

In 1938, Robert Gross performed the first ligation of a patent ductus arteriosus (PDA), thus initiating a major advance in congenital heart surgery and paving the way for development of modern surgical techniques [1]. Major improvements followed, which manifested as continuous reductions in mortality between that time and the 1980s. In 2000, the 32nd Bethesda Conference report generated from the American College of Cardiology indicated that approximately 85% of patients operated on with congenital heart disease (CHD) survived to adulthood [2]. That report estimated that 800,000 patients with adult congenital heart disease (ACHD) were living in the United States in 2000. More recent data suggest that the number of adults living with CHD in the United States now approaches 1.5 million [3] (Fig. 16.1). These reports highlight the importance of an emerging problem in our healthcare system, which is developing a seamless model for transition of CHD patient care from pediatric to adult heart centers. There has been a widespread call for an increased number of physicians capable of providing continuity of care for these patients in an outpatient setting, as well as during the perioperative period. This chapter will focus on anesthesia-specific issues facing ACHD patients in the perioperative period.

II. Epidemiology

A. Defining ACHD

Attempts to establish prevalence and even mortality data for ACHD depend on defining which patients to include. A strict definition of ACHD was proposed by Mitchell et al., "a gross structural abnormality of the heart or intrathoracic great vessels that is actually or possibly of functional significance" [4]. This definition excludes persistent left-sided vena cava, abnormalities of major arteries, bicuspid aortic valve (AV) disease, mitral valve prolapse, and the like [5].

B. Classification

A pathologic categorization scheme divides CHD patients into categories of great, moderate, and simple complexity [6,7] (Table 16.1). These categories are particularly helpful in neonatal disease. In ACHD, a different categorization may be more clinically relevant. These three categories are listed below [8]:

1. **"Complete" Repair**
   a. Examples include repaired atrial septal defect (ASD), ventricular septal defect (VSD), and PDA without hemodynamic sequelae.
   b. It must be kept in mind, however, that it is rare that any cardiac surgical repair is considered curative, as there are long-term sequelae in most of these ACHD patients.

2. **Partial surgical correction or palliation**
   a. Examples include palliative repairs such as Fontan, tetralogy of Fallot (ToF), and transposition of great arteries (TGA) (e.g., Mustard or Senning repair), leaving hemodynamic or physiologic compromise.

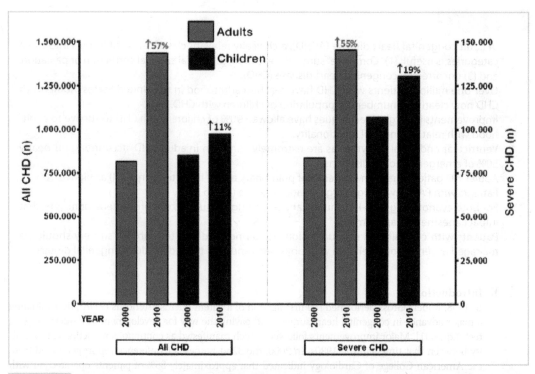

FIGURE 16.1 Estimated numbers of adults and children living with CHD in the United States between 2000 and 2010. There has been a substantial increase in the number of adults living with CHD compared to a smaller increase in children. Numbers were extrapolated from estimated population prevalence from the province of Quebec, Canada, and the USA population in 2000 and 2010. CHD, congenital heart disease. (From Alshawabkeh LI, Opotowsky AR. Burden of heart failure in adults with congenital heart disease. *Curr Heart Fail Rep.* 2016;13:247–254.)

3. **Uncorrected CHD**
   a. Examples include minor ASD, minor VSD, Ebstein anomaly, or undiagnosed ACHD due to limited healthcare access as child.
C. **Prevalence**
   1. Almost 1 in 100 babies is born with CHD. The actual number of adult patients with congenital heart defects is difficult to obtain; however, recent estimates suggest that the ACHD population of patients in Europe is estimated at 2.3 million. A longitudinal study in Canada reported a near 70% increase in the number of adults alive with CHD over the period from 2000 to 2010. Extrapolating their findings suggests that the adult population of CHD patients in the United states is approximately 1.5 million [3,5,9]. Significant improvements in surgical techniques have allowed many patients (up to 90% of children with CHD) to survive to adulthood, and maintain relatively normal function [3,5,9].
   2. **Select populations**
      a. A recent estimate from Canada [3] reported a CHD prevalence of 13.11 cases per 1,000 children and 6.12 cases per 1,000 adults. Selecting out patients with complex CHD (Table 16.1) reduces these estimates to 1.76 per 1,000 children and 0.62 per 1,000 adults. From 2000 to 2010, they noted an increase in prevalence of all CHD and severe CHD in both children and adults; however, a much larger increase was documented in adults than in children. The proportion of subjects with CHD who were adults increased from 54% in 2000 to 66% in 2010.
      b. ACHD becomes a significant issue in certain populations such as obstetrics where patients with CHD now represent the majority (60% to 80%) of obstetric patients with

TABLE 16.1 ACHD classification [7]

Simple	Moderate complexity	Great complexity

• Minor ASD
• Minor VSD
• Mild PS
• Congenital valve disease
• Aortic or mitral
	• Anomalous pulmonary venous drainage
	• AV canal defects
	• ToF
	• Ebstein anomaly
	• Coarctation of aorta
	• Right ventricular outflow obstruction
	• ASD
	  • Ostium primum
	  • Sinus venosus
	• Persistent PDA
	• PV disease
	  • Stenotic or regurgitant lesions
	• Fistula:
	  • Aorto–LV
	  • Sinus of Valsalva
	• VSD associated with the following:
	  • Valve abnormality (mitral, tricuspid)
	  • Aortic insufficiency
	  • RVOTO
	  • Stenotic lesions (AoV, RVOT)
	• AoV disease
	• Subaortic stenosis
	• Supra-aortic stenosis
		• Single ventricle lesions and Fontan physiology
		• TA
		• Mitral atresia
		• Eisenmenger physiology
		• Cyanotic CHD
		• Existence of conduits—either with valve or without
		• Presence of intracardiac baffles
		• TGV
		  • Jatene procedure
		  • Mustard procedure
		• Truncus arteriosus/hemitruncus

ACHD, adult congenital heart disease; ASD, adult atrial septal defect; VSD, ventricular septal defect; AV, atrioventricular; AoV, aortic valve; ToF, tetralogy of Fallot; TA, tricuspid atresia; PS, pulmonary stenosis; CHD, congenital heart disease; TGV, transposition of the great vessels; PDA, patent ductus arteriosus; PV, pulmonary valve; LV, left ventricle; RVOTO, right ventricular outflow tract obstruction.
Adapted with permission from Warnes CA, Williams RG, Bashore TM, et al. ACC/AHA 2008 Guidelines for the management of adults with congenital heart disease: executive summary: a report of the American College of Cardiology/American Heart Association Task Force on Practice Guidelines. *Circulation*. 2008;118(23):2395–2451.

cardiac disease. Since the obstetric population is predominantly young and healthy, it makes sense that CHD patients who reach childbearing age would represent a high proportion of obstetric patients with cardiac disease.

3. **Survival data**
   a. It is estimated that 96% of newborns who survive the first year will reach the age of 16 [5].
   b. Median expected survival has increased significantly since 2000, with current estimates placing the median age of death for ACHD at 57 years [5].
   c. Although the outcome of these patients has improved, more patients with complex disease are surviving into adulthood. Their care remains challenging, as death rates in the population from 20 to >70 years of age may be two to seven times higher for the ACHD population than for their peers who lack ACHD [10].

D. **Healthcare system considerations**
   The ACC/AHA 2008 guidelines for ACHD highlight the fact that pediatric cardiology centers have significant infrastructure to support patients with CHD, but that this is largely lacking in adult healthcare system. This includes access to physicians with training in ACHD, as well as advanced practice nursing, case management, and social workers familiar with the needs of these patients [11]. These guidelines echo the recommendations made by the Bethesda conference, as well as the Canadian Cardiovascular Society Consensus Conference statements from 2010 [2,12–17]. Also, adult patients with CHD report difficulties in several areas of daily life, including employment and insurability [18]. Currently, the Affordable Care Act stipulates that no person may be denied coverage based on a pre-existing condition (including heart disease). However, it is critical that patients ensure that a qualified physician with expertise in CHD be covered by whatever insurance plan they choose.

TABLE 16.2   Summary of qualifications for regional centers of excellence in adult congenital heart disease (ACHD)

Cardiologist specializing in ACHD	One or several 24/7
Congenital cardiac surgeon	Two or several 24/7
Nurse/physician assistant/nurse practitioner	One or several
Cardiac anesthesiologist	Several 24/7
Echocardiography[a] • **Includes TEE, intraoperative TEE**	Two or several 24/7
Diagnostic catheterization[a]	Yes, 24/7
Noncoronary interventional catheterization[a]	Yes, 24/7
Electrophysiology/pacing/AICD implantation[a]	One or several
Exercise testing	• Echocardiography • Radionuclide • Cardiopulmonary • Metabolic
Cardiac imaging/radiology[a]	• Cardiac MRI • CT scanning • Nuclear medicine
Multidisciplinary teams including	• High-risk obstetrics • Pulmonary hypertension • Heart failure/transplant • Genetics • Neurology • Nephrology • Cardiac pathology • Rehabilitation services • Social services • Vocational services • Financial counselors
Information technology	• Data collection • Database support • Quality assessment review/protocols

[a]These modalities must be supervised/performed and interpreted by physicians with expertise and training in CHD.
ACHD, adult congenital heart disease; 24/7, availability 24 hr/day, 7 days/wk; TEE, transesophageal echocardiography; AICD, automatic implantable cardioverter defibrillator; MRI, magnetic resonance imaging; CT, computed tomography.
Reprinted with permission from Warnes CA, Williams RG, Bashore TM, et al. ACC/AHA 2008 Guidelines for the management of adults with congenital heart disease: executive summary: a report of the American College of Cardiology/American Heart Association Task Force on Practice Guidelines. *Circulation.* 2008;118(23):2395–2451.

1. Overall recommendations taken from these reports suggest a focus on improvement in ACHD healthcare delivery through the following:
   a. Improved transition clinics for adolescents approaching adulthood
   b. Outreach programs to educate patients and families about key issues related to their disease
   c. Enhanced education of adult caregivers trained in ACHD management
   d. Coordination of healthcare delivery through regional centers of excellence
   e. Development of ready referral pathways from primary care physicians to these regional centers of excellence
2. Centers of excellence
   a. The services and provider requirements for such centers are summarized in Table 16.2, taken from the 2008 ACC/AHA guidelines. Key areas with physicians specializing in ACHD are indicated.

CLINICAL PEARL   Patients with either moderate or great complexity lesions should be managed at centers of excellence for surgical interventions.

III. **What are the key anesthetic considerations in ACHD?**

To evaluate the ACHD patient prior to surgery, the anesthesiologist must gain an understanding of the patient's medical history, current functional status, state of surgical repair, and overall health. Key items are discussed below.

A. History

Obtaining a thorough and accurate surgical and medical history is critical, however challenging, as only half of patients with ACHD are able to correctly describe their diagnosis [19]. Patients with ACHD have varying functional capacities which may make evaluation of true cardiac capacity more challenging. Remember that an adult with CHD has always lived with this disease and does not know anything different. That makes self-reporting of ACHD inaccurate, because the patients routinely underestimate their degree of compromise. Another fact that must be taken into consideration is that the ACHD population is extremely heterogeneous. There are patients who are diagnosed for the first time in adulthood, patients who have had prior palliative repair with recurrent symptomatology, as well as patients who were thought to have "complete" repairs who now have delayed presentation of pathology. Also, the surgical strategies have markedly changed over the last 50 years, necessitating an understanding of the particular (possibly now obsolete) operation the patient has undergone with its associated consequences.

B. Signs and symptoms of ACHD

Some generalized examination findings that may indicate ACHD include the following [20]:

1. Continuous heart murmurs: There are relatively few acquired cardiac diseases producing a continuous type of murmur.
2. Right bundle branch block (RBBB): This can occur in the general population; however, if found in conjunction with a continuous murmur, this may indicate a congenital defect.
3. Evidence of cyanosis without existing pulmonary disease
4. The above findings should trigger an echocardiographic study prior to surgical care.

C. How can you assess the perioperative risk for ACHD patients?

Anesthetic evaluation should focus on predicting risk of surgery in this patient population. Some key prognostic indicators for outcomes in ACHD surgery (both cardiac and noncardiac) include the presence of the factors listed below [8,11,19,21] (Table 16.3):

1. Pulmonary arterial hypertension (PAH)
2. Cyanosis or residual VSD
3. Need for reoperation (cardiac surgery)
4. Arrhythmias
5. Ventricular dysfunction
6. Single ventricle physiology or a systemic right ventricle

TABLE 16.3 Common medical concerns in patients with ACHD [16]

Comorbidities associated with ACHD:	Common non–ACHD-related comorbidities:
• Cardiac arrhythmias	• Systemic hypertension
• Pulmonary hypertension	• Coronary artery disease
• Ventricular dysfunction	• Diabetes mellitus
• Cyanosis	• Renal insufficiency
• Valve abnormalities	• Chronic lung disease
• Aneurysm	• Cholelithiasis
	• Nephrolithiasis
Complications related to ACHD:	**Conditions associated with elevated surgical risk:**
• Erythrocytosis	• PAH
• Developmental delay	• Cyanosis or residual VSD
• Central nervous system defects	• Need for repeat sternotomy
• Previous ischemic/embolic events	• Arrhythmias
• Seizures	• Ventricular dysfunction
• Intracranial abscesses	• Single ventricle physiology or a systemic right ventricle
• Endocarditis	

ACHD, adult congenital heart disease; PAH, pulmonary arterial hypertension; VSD, ventricular septal defect.

TABLE 16.4   Tachyarrhythmias associated with ACHD [4,7,20]

Lesion[a]	VT	IART	AF	WPW
ToF				
• Repaired	++	++	+	−
• Native	+	−	−	−
Ebstein anomaly	+	+	−	++
TGA				
• Mustard/Senning	++	++	−	−
• Jatene	−	−	−	−
• cc	+	−	−	+
Single ventricle Fontan	−	++	+	−
Congenital AV stenosis	+	−	+	−
LVOT obstruction	++	−	+	−
• ASD	−	−	++	−
• Sinus venosus	−	−	+	−
VSD	+	−	−	−
AVSD	+	−	−	−

[a]All lesions listed are considered to have surgical correction or palliation unless noted as native and listed in order of degree of arrhythmia burden. − denotes rare manifestations; + denotes common occurrence; ++ denotes frequent occurrence.
ACHD, adult congenital heart disease; VT, ventricular tachycardia; IART, intra-atrial reentrant tachycardia; AF, atrial fibrillation; WPW, Wolff–Parkinson–White syndrome; TGA, transposition of great arteries; cc, congenitally corrected; AV, aortic valve; LVOT, left ventricular outflow tract; ASD, atrial septal defect; VSD, ventricular septal defect; AVSD, atrioventricular septal defect; ToF, tetralogy of Fallot.

IV.   What common sequelae are associated with ACHD?

In contrast to the neonate with CHD, ACHD patients begin to acquire additional medical comorbidities that should be considered in management planning. Common comorbidities in this patient population are listed in Table 16.3, and preoperative evaluation should take these into account. Cardiac arrhythmias, pulmonary hypertension, ventricular dysfunction, cyanosis (or residual VSD), valve abnormalities, and aneurysms represent some of the key comorbid conditions commonly associated with ACHD that have serious management considerations and result in overall increased perioperative risk [4]. Obtaining a detailed history on the degree of involvement of these issues will enable adequate planning in management. Two of the most common and critical areas (arrhythmias and pulmonary hypertension) will be addressed here.

A.   Arrhythmias

Ventricular and atrial arrhythmias are extremely common in ACHD patients, accounting for nearly 50% of emergency hospitalizations [8]. The type of rhythm disturbance depends primarily on the lesion and method of surgical repair. Tables 16.4 and 16.5 divide the bradyarrhythmias from tachyarrhythmias by lesion type.

CLINICAL PEARL   ACHD patients are at high risk for cardiac arrhythmias, especially patients with moderate or highly complex repairs.

TABLE 16.5   Bradyarrhythmias associated with ACHD [4,7,20]

Sinus node dysfunction	AV block
• Single ventricle lesions (Fontan physiology)	• VSD
• ccTGA	• AVSD
	• LVOT obstruction
	• TGA (Senning/Mustard)

ccTGA, congenitally corrected transposition of the great arteries; LVOT, left ventricular outflow tract; ASD, atrial septal defect; VSD, ventricular septal defect; AVSD, atrioventricular septal defect; TGA, transposition of the great arteries.

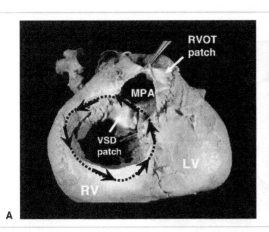
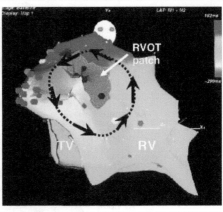

A   B

FIGURE 16.2 Macro-reentrant VT in tetralogy of Fallot. **A:** An autopsy specimen of repaired tetralogy with the anterior RV surface opened to reveal the VSD patch and the patch-augmented RVOT (the outflow patch in this case is transannular). A hypothetical re-entry circuit is traced onto this image (*black arrows*), with the superior portion of the loop traveling through the conal septum (upper rim of the VSD). **B:** Actual electroanatomic map of sustained VT from an adult tetralogy patient, showing a nearly identical circuit. The propagation pattern is shown by the *black arrows* and is reflected by the color scheme (red > yellow > green > blue > purple). A narrow conduction channel was found between the rightward edge of the outflow patch scar (*gray area*) and the superior rim of the tricuspid valve. A cluster of radiofrequency applications at this site (*pink dots*) closed off the channel and permanently eliminated this VT circuit. LV, left ventricle; MPA, main pulmonary artery; RV, right ventricle; RVOT, right ventricular outflow tract; TV, tricuspid valve; VSD, ventricular septal disease; VT, ventricular tachycardia. (Reprinted with permission from Walsh EP, Cecchin F. Congenital heart disease for the adult cardiologist: arrhythmias in adult patients with congenital heart disease. *Circulation*. 2007;115(4):534–545.)

1. In general, patients who fall in the moderate to complex categories are at higher risk for arrhythmias. **ToF** (Fig. 16.2) **and Fontan lesions carry an extremely high arrhythmia burden** [22,23]. **In addition, any patient with a ventricular repair or patch is at high risk for ventricular rhythm disturbances, while those patients with atrial repairs, atrial baffles, etc., are likely to develop atrial arrhythmias** [23].

2. Patients with right-sided lesions have a higher likelihood of developing arrhythmias, although the long-term morbidity/mortality outcomes are similar between right- and left-sided lesions [24].

3. Older patient age at the time of surgical repair seems to be associated with an increased incidence of arrhythmias.

4. Patients with either ASD or VSD can have interruption in the normal conduction pathways or abnormal variants such as duplicate AV nodes (Fig. 16.3), leading to reentrant arrhythmias [23]. The most common arrhythmia seen in older ACHD patients is intra-atrial reentrant tachycardia (IART), a macro-reentrant circuit within atrial tissue, often occurring because of disruption by patches, atriotomy incisions, and scars.

5. **Management**

   a. **Antiarrhythmic** medical therapy remains the mainstay for many patients, although results are often suboptimal in some cases such as IART, despite the use of potent agents such as amiodarone [23].

   b. **Ablative procedures.** Recent advances in electrophysiology have allowed significant improvements in management of these rhythm disturbances. Electrophysiologists are able to map out the conduction pathways in the heart, and ablate malignant tracts (Figs. 16.2 and 16.4). This is most useful for atrial arrhythmias, with short-term success rates nearing 90% [23]. Long-term outcomes following ablation are less promising and not widely reported. de Groot et al. reported a 59% recurrence after the initial ablation, with the location of the recurrent pathway being different for all but one patient. At 5 years, 58% of patients were in sinus rhythm and 33% of the initial population

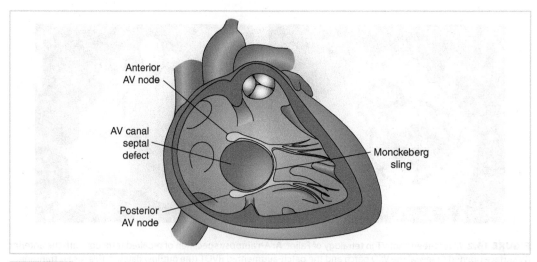

FIGURE 16.3 Representation of twin AV nodes with a Mönckeberg sling. The cardiac anatomy in this sketch includes a large septal defect in the AV canal region, shown in a right anterior oblique projection. Both an anterior and a posterior AV node are depicted (each with its own His bundle) along with a connecting "sling" between the two systems. This conduction arrangement can produce two distinct non–pre-excited QRS morphologies (depending on which AV node is engaged earliest by the atrial activation wave front), and a variety of reentrant tachycardias. AV, atrioventricular. (Redrawn from Walsh EP, Cecchin F. Congenital heart disease for the adult cardiologist: arrhythmias in adult patients with congenital heart disease. *Circulation.* 2007;115(4):534–545.)

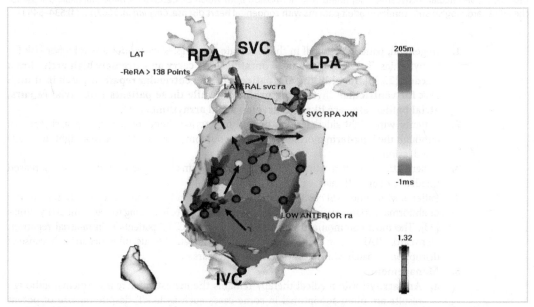

FIGURE 16.4 Electroanatomic map of an IART circuit involving the anterolateral surface of the right atrium in a patient with a previous Fontan operation (cavopulmonary connection). A detailed anatomic shell was generated for the ablation procedure by merging high-resolution computed tomography data with real-time data gathered from the 3D mapping catheter. The propagation pattern for the IART circuit is shown by *black arrows* and is also reflected by the color scheme (red > yellow > green > blue > purple). The critical component of the circuit appeared to be a narrow conduction channel through a region of scar (*central gray area*). A cluster of radiofrequency applications (*maroon dots*) was placed at the entrance zone to this narrow channel and permanently eliminated this IART circuit. IART, intra-atrial reentrant tachycardia; IVC, inferior vena cava; JXN, junction; LAT, lateral; LPA, left pulmonary artery; RA, right atrium; RPA, right pulmonary artery; SVC, superior vena cava. (Reprinted with permission from Walsh EP, Cecchin F. Congenital heart disease for the adult cardiologist: arrhythmias in adult patients with congenital heart disease. *Circulation.* 2007;115(4):534–545.)

were maintained on antiarrhythmic drug therapy [25]. Electrophysiologic testing and ablative procedures are considered a Class I recommendation for patients with known rhythm disturbances [11].

c. **Implantable devices.** For patients at risk for ventricular arrhythmias, automatic implantable cardiac defibrillators (AICDs) can offer a life-saving modality and are a class II recommendation for ACHD patients [11]. **While ventricular tachycardia (VT) is rare in the first and second decades, it becomes increasingly prevalent as the patient ages, with those patients with a history of ventricular intervention being at highest risk** [23]. VT circuits can develop a macro-reentrant characteristic similar to the atrial IART (Fig. 16.4). ToF patients have a high risk, and a careful history should be obtained, inquiring about symptoms and any outpatient studies. Patients at risk for bradyarrhythmias often will have a pacemaker in place, which should be interrogated and sensitivity limits adjusted for the surgical procedure [21].

   1. **Anesthetic management.** A recent practice advisory (2011) for patients with implanted cardiac devices recommends that AICDs be disabled prior to surgery to prevent inadvertent defibrillation due to electrocautery; however, this is specific to procedures where electromagnetic interference is likely [21]. If the AICD is disabled, it is imperative that the patient be placed on continuous monitoring, with external defibrillation pads in place, and that the device be enabled again in the PACU.

   2. **Complex patients.** Actual placement of AICD leads into the heart in patients with complex lesions is often difficult, if not impossible [23]. Presence of abnormal venous return, surgically created shunts or baffles, as well as scarring from previous surgery can make adequate placement challenging. Occasionally, patients will require an open surgical approach to place epicardial pacing/defibrillation leads, although this procedure carries risk as well due to scarring and reoperative concerns (see Section IX below).

B. **Pulmonary arterial hypertension (PAH)**

PAH is defined as a mean pulmonary pressure greater than 25 mm Hg at rest or 30 mm Hg with exercise [26]. ACHD patients have a PAH incidence of up to 10%, with Eisenmenger syndrome (ES) being present in approximately 1% [5]. The etiology of the PAH typically falls in the World Health Organization Group I or II. Group I is PAH due to primary PAH but includes congenital shunts, and group II is due to pulmonary venous hypertension (i.e., disease due to valve disorders, volume excess, and LV dysfunction).

   1. **Surgical risk. PAH patients are high-risk surgical candidates. Published series demonstrate a range of surgical mortalities from a low of 4% to a high of 24% depending on disease severity and surgical procedure** [27]. Surgical and anesthetic risk should be clearly stated to the patient, especially for an elective case. Patients with ES should be considered higher-risk candidates and extreme care should be taken in managing these cases. See Section XII.B.2.

CLINICAL PEARL ACHD patients with concomitant PAH should be considered high risk, and management at a center of excellence is recommended.

   a. **Hemodynamic spiral.** Acute deterioration is possible as RV failure causes reduced pulmonary blood flow, leading to hypoxia which subsequently increases the pulmonary vascular resistance (PVR). The elevated PVR ultimately leads to increased strain on the RV. This initiates a **catastrophic hemodynamic chain of events** in which the decreased RV stroke volume decreases LV preload and output, and coronary blood flow to both the LV and RV decreases. The already failing RV may not be able to recover from this insult, resulting in cardiac arrest. **This "death spiral" is always possible in PAH patients; the anesthesia provider should be aware of it and take steps to prevent it** [26].

> **CLINICAL PEARL** Right coronary perfusion occurs throughout the cardiac cycle, making maintenance of systemic blood pressure important in optimizing right ventricular function.

2. **How do you treat RV failure in the setting of PAH?** Treatment of acute RV failure should focus on reducing PVR (see Section IV.B.3 below), while utilizing β-adrenergic agonist inotropic agents such as dobutamine and/or phosphodiesterase-inhibiting agents such as milrinone, as these provide inotropic support with moderate reductions in PVR (and systemic vascular resistance [SVR]). Consider using a vasopressor such as norepinephrine in the setting of systemic hypotension to increase the coronary perfusion pressure. In severe scenarios, an intra-aortic balloon pump can also be used to increase coronary perfusion pressure, thus supporting the RV [9].

3. **What are some treatment modalities during surgery to reduce PVR acutely** [8,9]?
   a. Consider moderate hyperventilation ($PaCO_2$ low 30s) while administering 100% oxygen.
   b. Use low-pressure ventilation if possible as high-intrathoracic pressure can mechanically compress extra-alveolar vessels and reduce CO.
   c. Utilize nitric oxide for acute reductions in PVR and/or consider inhaled prostanoid (iloprost) if available.
   d. Intravenous (IV) magnesium sulfate may provide temporary reductions in PVR.

> **CLINICAL PEARL** PVR is powerfully influenced by ventilation, so strict attention must be paid to oxygenation, ventilation, and intra-thoracic pressure.

C. **What are some general hemodynamic goals for patients with PAH** [26]?
   Anesthetic and hemodynamic goals for pulmonary hypertension
   1. **Avoid elevations in PVR.** Prevent hypoxemia, acidosis, hypercarbia, and pain. Provide supplemental oxygen at all times. Consider inhaled nitric oxide (iNO) to acutely decrease PVR.
   2. **Maintain SVR.** Decreased SVR can reduce CO dramatically due to the "fixed" PVR. This fixed PVR limits the RV's ability to accommodate the usual increase in CO that ensues from reduced LV afterload. LV and RV ischemia from reduced coronary artery perfusion pressure from the decreased systemic diastolic pressure can also contribute to the decrease in CO and "death spiral." Keep in mind also that right ventricular coronary perfusion occurs during both systole and diastole, which may help explain the right ventricle's dependence on adequate systemic blood pressure.
   3. **Avoid myocardial depressants and maintain myocardial contractility.**
   4. **Maintain chronic prostaglandin therapy without altering dosage.**
   5. **Utilize low-pressure mechanical ventilation (or spontaneous ventilation with normal $PaCO_2$) when possible.**

V. **What laboratory and imaging studies are needed?**
   The overall goal in preoperative laboratory and imaging studies is to assist the physicians in understanding the degree of involvement of any comorbid disease.
   A. **Preoperative laboratory and imaging testing** should be guided by degree of severity of disease. Patients with normal functional status can be treated as any adult presenting for surgery, whereas the patient with severe functional limitation due to cardiac disease warrants additional evaluation. Laboratory evaluation may include complete blood count, coagulation studies, and basic metabolic studies.
   B. **Cardiac catheterization and/or echocardiography** studies are particularly helpful in symptomatic patients by providing information on structural status of the heart, functional status of the ventricles, and degree of PAH. Many patients will also have either magnetic resonance imaging (MRI) or computed tomography (CT) reconstructive imaging as part of standard surveillance, and these can add tremendously to the understanding of the current pathophysiologic state.

C. An **electrocardiogram (ECG)** should be obtained at baseline as there are often abnormalities present. This can also alert the practitioner to the presence of a pacemaker or other abnormal cardiac rhythms.

D. **Chest radiography.** This can be helpful to determine the degree of heart and lung disease at baseline.

VI. **What monitors should be used in ACHD surgery?**

A. **Standard American Society of Anesthesiologists (ASA) monitors** should be employed for every case. In addition, most cases involving moderate to complex ACHD patients will utilize some degree of invasive monitoring. Some key considerations include the following [28]:

1. Location of an arterial line, if needed, should consider previous surgical procedures such as Blalock–Taussig shunts using the subclavian artery, which compromise blood flow to the ipsilateral upper extremity.

2. Central venous catheters (CVCs) should be reserved for the most symptomatic patients, as risk of thrombus and stroke is higher.

3. Pulmonary artery (PA) catheters are often anatomically difficult or impossible to place and are seldom helpful in patients with cyanotic cardiac lesions.

4. **Transesophageal echocardiography (TEE)** may be the most useful real-time monitor of cardiovascular status, especially when using general anesthesia, and should strongly be considered for patients with reduced functional status for all medium- and high-risk procedures.

5. Near-infrared spectroscopy (NIRS) has been suggested as a tool to monitor both cerebral and peripheral oxygenation. The concept is that this technology helps identify changes in oxygen delivery and may be more sensitive to changes in cardiac output. Central nervous system insults associated with cardiac surgery remain an unsolved problem. Brain damage can occur as a result of global hypoxia–ischemia or focal emboli. NIRS may provide data on cerebral oxygenation, and enthusiasm for this technology has increased with hopes of reducing neurologic dysfunction. Many centers have adopted NIRS as a standard of care. Available data suggest that multimodality monitoring, including NIRS, may be a useful adjunct. However, the current literature on the use of NIRS alone does not conclusively demonstrate improvement in neurologic outcome. Data correlating NIRS findings with indirect measures of neurologic outcome or mortality are limited. Although NIRS has promise for measuring regional tissue oxygen saturation, the lack of data demonstrating improved outcomes limits the support for widespread implementation [29].

VII. **What are some general intraoperative anesthetic considerations for patients with ACHD?** While the pathologic categorization (simple, moderate, and complex) of CHD is useful, a more clinically based approach may be more useful in intraoperative planning. One such scheme, as introduced earlier, is to consider patients based on surgical correction such as the following:

A. **Complete surgical correction** (i.e., repaired ASD, VSD, and PDA). Patients with surgically corrected lesions, as well as palliated lesions with good functional results, typically demonstrate hemodynamic stability and normal physiology. As such, these can be assumed to be very low-risk patients and managed as an otherwise healthy adult patient.

B. **Partial surgical correction or palliation** (i.e., Fontan, ToF, and TGA [Mustard or Senning repair]). Palliated patients with complex disease and reduced functional capacity due to the type of lesion should be managed with more concern and will be the main focus below.

C. **Uncorrected lesions** (i.e., minor ASD, minor VSD, and Ebstein anomaly). Uncorrected patients warrant thorough examination into type of lesion and current functional state, as often these are minor lesions if they have not caused any medical or functional issues into adulthood.

D. **General approach.** For both cyanotic lesions (right-to-left shunts) and left-to-right shunts, there are general concepts that will aid in careful anesthetic planning.

1. **Cyanotic lesions** [28]

a. Cyanotic lesions have some element of right-to-left shunt, often even after surgical repair. The degree of this shunt determines the level of cyanosis present. Caution should be taken with sedative medicines, as lowering ventilation can increase PVR and exacerbate cyanosis by increasing right-to-left shunt.

b. Right-to-left shunting reduces the uptake of inhalational anesthetics and can prolong inhalation induction. Conversely, the onset of IV induction may be hastened.

c. Nitrous oxide may elevate PA pressure and should be either avoided or used cautiously.

d. **Air embolus.** Take extreme care to avoid an air embolus. All IV lines should be thoroughly deaired and monitored during medication administration. Epidural catheter placement should use saline for loss of resistance, not air, because air into an epidural vein can cross into the systemic circulation.

e. **SVR.** Changes in SVR disrupt the balance between pulmonary and systemic circulations to change the shunt. All anesthetic medications should be slowly titrated to prevent rapid changes. This holds true for both regional and general anesthetics.

f. Single-shot spinal anesthetic techniques are generally contraindicated, as quick onset of spinal sympathectomy is poorly tolerated.

g. Administration of antibiotics (vancomycin), if given quickly, may reduce SVR and become clinically detrimental.

h. Choice of anesthetic induction drug is not as important as the manner and vigilance used by the anesthesiologist in managing hemodynamics.

i. Clinical endpoints that might decrease PVR, such as increases in mixed venous O_2 (typically via high FiO_2) and modest degrees of respiratory alkalosis, are encouraged.

CLINICAL PEARL Patients with shunt lesions—either cyanotic or left to right, have adapted their physiology to account for this, so anesthetic agents should be titrated carefully to avoid massively disrupting this delicate balance.

---

2. **Chronic left-to-right shunting.** Balance between SVR and PVR determines the shunt fraction and the direction of shunting. Chronic left-to-right shunting causes the following:

a. Excessive pulmonary blood flow leading to pulmonary edema or pulmonary hypertension. The increased pulmonary flow causes PVR to increase over time, reducing left-to-right shunting, leading to eventual equilibration of left and right ventricular pressures. Eventually, this process results in conversion of the left-to-right shunt into a right-to-left shunt, the so-called Eisenmenger physiology or syndrome (ES).

b. Once ES develops, cyanosis ensues along with variable degrees of heart failure which places patients in the **highest-risk** category for surgical procedures.

c. Even without Eisenmenger syndrome, these patients may experience heart failure as a result of the high RV and pulmonary blood flow, which may be as much as four times systemic blood flow.

d. **SVR.** Acute changes in SVR from anesthetic administration or pain can result in alteration or reversal of the shunt, leading to heart failure or cyanosis, depending upon where the patient is in the evolution from large left-to-right shunting into the right-to-left shunting of Eisenmenger physiology. Overall anesthetic goals should be to maintain the balance that the patient has and avoid abrupt alterations.

e. High levels of supplemental oxygen may allow for reduced PVR and worsening of the left-to-right shunt. On the other hand, hypoxemia should be prevented, as this may shift the shunt to right-to-left and result in cyanosis. A fine balance must be struck when managing oxygenation for these patients.

f. **Air embolus.** As in cyanotic lesions, take extreme care to avoid an **air embolus.** Even predominant left-to-right shunts can become bidirectional, putting the patient at risk for a systemic air embolus.

g. **Single-shot spinal anesthesia is** contraindicated for patients who have or are approaching Eisenmenger physiology. Spinal anesthesia is theoretically beneficial for patients with large left-to-right shunts and normal or only slightly elevated PVR that remains far below SVR.

   h. Inhalational agents. Uptake should not be affected by left-to-right shunting. Right-to-left shunting prolongs inhalation inductions, but this is rarely clinically relevant if cardiac output is maintained.

VIII. **What is the ideal approach to postoperative management for ACHD patients?**
Postoperative management should take into account all the risk factors described above in the anesthetic planning, and one should attempt to maintain the patient in the hemodynamic state to which he/she has adapted.

A. Pain management
Patients with palliated lesions often have some degree of residual shunt, or even single ventricle physiology. As such, overall cardiac performance depends to a large degree on the PVR. Attempts should be made to minimize impairment of ventilation in these patients as hypercarbia will increase PVR and potentially worsen cyanosis or increase ventricular failure in susceptible patients.

   1. Regional anesthesia may be ideal for patients with significant anticipated postoperative pain as this can greatly reduce the level of systemic opioid use, thus reducing the risk of respiratory complications. Prior to neuraxial interventions and major plexus blocks, laboratory evaluation of coagulation status should be obtained in any patient with a history of anticoagulant therapy or significant liver dysfunction.

B. Arrhythmias
For patients at elevated risk (Tables 16.4 and 16.5), perioperative monitoring in a telemetry bed may be indicated if there is not an AICD in place. For patients with AICDs or pacemakers, consider postoperative interrogation of the device if there was significant electrical interference during the surgery, or if the device had a magnet applied. Additionally, if the AICD was disabled for the procedure, it is imperative that defibrillation equipment be immediately available until the device is turned back on.

C. Volume considerations
Many ACHD patients with palliated lesions have a narrow margin of error in fluid management. They can easily be pushed into heart failure with overly aggressive fluid management, and conversely may develop significant reductions in cardiac output with a minimalist approach. There is not an ideal volume strategy that fits all patients, but management must be closely tailored to each patient's physiologic status. As discussed above, invasive monitoring may not be possible in many of these patients or may not accurately reflect actual volume status, so management can be complicated. TEE use intraoperatively along with close monitoring of urine output may be the best approach in complex patients.

IX. **What is the approach for patients presenting for repeat sternotomy?**
A. **What are the key surgical considerations in preparation for repeat sternotomy?**
For patients with ACHD, repeat sternotomy is often the initial surgical intervention. Often these patients have had multiple previous chest surgeries, increasing the degree of scarring in the pericardial space and thus making the surgical approach more demanding. Overall mortality increases with repeat sternotomy and is reported to be in the range of 3% to 6%. Reentrant injury has been reported to greatly increase the risk in certain series and may approach 18% to 25%. However, other reports indicate no increase in mortality but a significant increase in duration of surgery [30–33]. **The perioperative mortality risk appears to correlate with increased number of sternotomies, presence of single ventricle physiology, and presence of an RV-to-PA conduit.**

   1. Preoperative preparation. Several preoperative variables are important and can prove valuable in planning a repeat sternotomy. A PA and lateral chest radiograph can be helpful, and should always be examined prior to operative intervention. These radiographs can supply important information such as the number of sternal wires in place and their condition, and the lateral film provides clues about the distance between the posterior sternal table (border) and the heart itself. In addition, many patients have had preoperative cardiac catheterization studies. It is always helpful to the surgeon to assess this study and lateral radiographic images to obtain an anatomic assessment of the level of concern about repeat sternotomy. These pictures can provide much data about what portion of the sternum may be adherent to cardiac structures and which sternal wires are closest to these areas of concern.

2. **Cannulation options.** Should there be any significant concern regarding repeat sternotomy and a high index of suspicion for injury, femoral cannulation should be considered. Preoperative discussions with the perfusion and anesthesia teams are critical to planning alternative strategies for cannulation and the decision to initiate cardiopulmonary bypass (CPB) using extrathoracic cannulation techniques before initiating or completing repeat sternotomy.

3. **Specifics of repeat sternotomy.** Several techniques are important when pursuing a repeat sternotomy. Positional manipulation of the operating table can be critical to visualization of the posterior table of the sternum as the surgeon pursues repeat sternotomy from below (inferiorly). In addition, use of specific retractors (e.g., internal mammary retractor) can also greatly facilitate slow, sequential separation and elevation of the sternum. The goal of this portion of reentry should be to obtain safe removal of previously placed sternal wires while separating the sternum from the heart.

4. **Lysis of adhesions.** Once repeat sternotomy is accomplished, significant lysis of adhesions is undertaken. Good communication with the surgical team is critical during this process. The primary initial surgical goal should be to define and separate areas of cannulation from scar tissue (assuming the patient was not cannulated via femoral or other access before initiating the repeat sternotomy). These areas include the ascending aorta, right atrium (in single venous cannulation), and/or the superior vena cava (SVC) and inferior vena cava (IVC) (in cases of bicaval cannulation). Further dissection of the heart and possible previously placed shunts may be more safely accomplished once cannulae are in place for initiation of CPB.

5. **Initiation of CPB.** It is important to have all systemic-to-PA conduits/shunts adequately isolated and secured prior to initiation of CPB. Once bypass is begun, these connections must be ligated (or clamped) so that the circuit will not induce pulmonary overcirculation and systemic undercirculation.

B. **What are the key anesthetic considerations in preparation for repeat sternotomy?**
The majority of ACHD patients undergoing cardiac surgery will require repeat sternotomy. Often these patients have had multiple prior chest surgeries, increasing the degree of scarring in the pericardial space, thus making the surgical approach more demanding. Key anesthetic considerations for repeat sternotomy revolve around preparation for possible reentrant injury as well as increased transfusion requirements.

1. **Large-bore IV** access is critical in the event of reentrant injury. Consider the patient's vascular anatomy and evaluate any possible central venous clots or strictures, as these patients may have had multiple central lines in the past or unusual anatomic venous connections to the heart. Ultrasound guidance is recommended during central (and possibly peripheral) venous line placement to help evaluate vascular anatomy and patency. A large-bore CVC (8.5-Fr introducer) in addition to one to two large-bore peripheral IV catheters attached to a high-flow fluid warmer may be prudent.

2. **Placement of external defibrillator patches because access to an open chest for internal defibrillation may be delayed.**

3. Crossmatched packed red blood cells (PRBCs) should be available and double checked in a cooler in the OR at incision. Many patients will have had multiple transfusions in the past, and thus may have unique antibody profiles, which can delay the type and cross process. Typically, one should have 2 to 4 units of PRBCs available.

4. Ventilation management during reentry should be discussed with the surgical team. Asghar et al. suggest that slight hyperinflation of the lungs, using a recruitment maneuver during sternal spreading, can actually minimize reentrant injury by reducing venous return through increased intrathoracic pressure, thus decreasing the size of the RV [34].

5. Full discussion of risk should be undertaken with the surgical team before surgery. On the basis of this discussion, the surgical team may elect to cannulate the femoral vessels or perform axillary arterial cannulation to enable emergent institution of cardiopulmonary bypass in the event of reentrant injury.

C. **What is the role of antifibrinolytic therapy?**
Fibrinolysis is known to occur during cardiopulmonary bypass and is associated with increased blood loss and transfusion in cardiac surgery. As a result, antifibrinolytic drugs have been recommended in the 2011 Society of Thoracic Surgeons and Society of Cardiovascular Anesthesiologists (STS/SCA) guidelines [35]. Aprotinin was withdrawn from the market in 2008 due to concerns for increased mortality despite reduction in blood loss which was demonstrated in various trials [35,36]. The STS/SCA recommendations include routine use of either an aminocaproic acid or tranexamic acid infusion for all cardiac surgeries, for which a typical regimen initiates the infusion prior to skin incision and continues it throughout the operation [36–40].

X. **What is the role of heart tranplantation?**

A. **Heart transplantation or combined heart and lung transplantation can be a life-saving measure for the patient who has developed severe heart failure.** ACHD patients most commonly listed for transplant include patients with uncorrectable or partially palliated lesions such as those listed below [11]:

1. Single ventricle physiology with pulmonary vascular disease (heart/lung transplant)
2. Lesions associated with ventricular dysfunction due to pulmonary vascular disease (heart/ lung or isolated lung transplant)
3. Isolated heart failure without significant pulmonary vascular disease (more common in single ventricle physiology, or TGV patients treated by atrial switch procedures) (heart transplant).
4. Patients who clinically meet the metrics for transplant should have a thorough pretransplant evaluation assessing the anatomy of the patient, as well as PVR. Longstanding elevations in PVR can easily lead to right heart failure in the donor heart and must be anticipated in these patients. Sometimes this may tip the scales to a combined heart/lung transplant.
    a. For isolated heart transplant cases in patients with elevated PVR, it is recommended to take steps to avoid acute right heart failure in the transplanted donor heart. This often involves a combination of iNO and vasoactive infusions (dobutamine, milrinone) to provide inotropic support along with pulmonary vasodilation. See Chapter 17 for full discussion.

B. **What are the outcomes of transplant?**
ACHD patients make up nearly 3% of the total number of patients listed for cardiac transplantation [41]. Davies et al. investigated patients listed for transplant from 1995 to 2009. This study indicated that the ACHD patients who went on to heart transplant had a higher early mortality, possibly due to increased repeat sternotomy incidence in this group. They had equivalent long-term mortality to non-CHD heart transplant patients (53% 10-year survival in both groups).

XI. **What are the specific details for managing patients with partially corrected or palliative repairs?**

A. **Fontan repair**
Fontan palliation has been the primary surgical approach for complex lesions such as tricuspid atresia (TA), hypoplastic left heart, double-inlet LV, double-outlet RV, severe AV defects, and heterotaxy syndrome [42]. Management of these lesions in both the neonate and the adult patient present one of the biggest challenges in anesthetic practice [43]. Patient selection is extremely important in determining the success of the Fontan procedure. Ideally, PVR should be low (less than 4 Wood units) and the mean PA pressure less than 15 mm Hg. Adequately sized PAs, the absence of systemic atrioventricular valve dysfunction, reliable sinus rhythm, and preserved LV function are also important. Appropriate patient selection has resulted in survival rates approaching 90% at 10 years following this palliative surgery; thus, more and more Fontan patients may present for adult surgery [44]. Key aspects pertaining to adult management are presented below.

1. **Pathophysiology.** TA creates a situation where blood must pass from the right atrium to the left atrium via an ASD, where it mixes with pulmonary venous return. Blood flow is then directed to both the PA and the aorta by various routes. Regardless of type of repair,

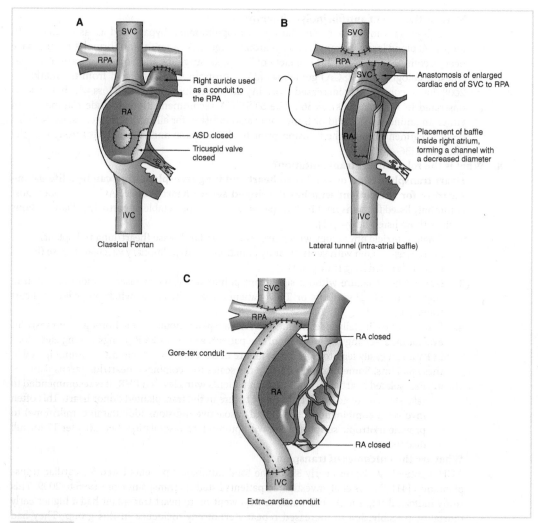

FIGURE 16.5 Fontan surgical techniques: Classical atriopulmonary connection (includes SVC to RPA anastomosis that is not shown) (**A**), lateral tunnel (**B**), and extracardiac conduit (**C**). ASD, atrial septal defect; RPA, right pulmonary artery; SVC, superior vena cava; IVC, inferior vena cava; RA, right atrium. (Redrawn from d'Udekem Y, Iyengar AJ, Cochrane AD, et al. The Fontan procedure: contemporary techniques have improved long-term outcomes. *Circulation.* 2007;116(Suppl I): I157–I164.)

blood flow depends entirely on the left ventricle (LV) for cardiac output [28,42]. For a more detailed review, please see the extensive discussion of adult Fontan physiology provided by Dr. Eagle and Dr. Daves in 2011 [42].

2. **Surgical correction.** The Fontan procedure, which is the definitive palliative surgical approach, creates a univentricular circulation via a cavopulmonary anastomosis. The procedure creates a classical or bidirectional Glenn shunt (SVC to PA connection), closure of the ASD, ligation of the proximal PA, and creation of a right atrial-to-PA or IVC-to-PA connection. Multiple variations of the Fontan procedure exist (Fig. 16.5); however, the same general physiologic principles most often apply [28].

3. **What are the key physiologic and anesthetic management considerations?**

   a. **Blood flow to the PAs is passive.** Elevations in PVR will therefore reduce pulmonary flow, and hence decrease cardiac output, by reducing the gradient between the vena cava and the PA.

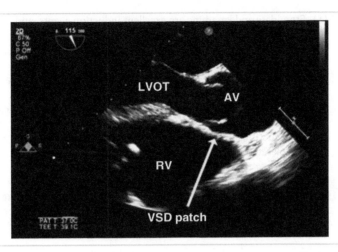

FIGURE 16.6 Transesophageal echocardiographic image of the VSD patch repair typically visualized in adult patients with previous ToF repair. This is the midesophageal long-axis view demonstrating the over-riding aorta with the in situ patch. AV, atrioventricular (mitral) valve; LVOT, left ventricular outflow tract; RV, right ventricle; ToF, tetralogy of Fallot; VSD, ventricular septal defect. (Image courtesy of Bryan Ahlgren DO, University of Colorado Denver.)

b. **Hemodynamic stability is highly dependent upon maintaining appropriately high systemic venous pressures and right atrial preload.** Decreased right atrial preload causes dramatic declines in pulmonary blood flow and cardiac output. Peripheral edema often results from the high systemic venous pressures, hence the margin of error differentiating adequate and excessive systemic venous preload can be perilously small.

c. Spontaneous respiration assists forward flow by keeping PVR low. Any compromise in pulmonary function can be detrimental by increasing PVR. Preoperative sedation should be used carefully due to risk of hypercapnia and resultant elevation in PVR. **If positive pressure ventilation is necessary, use the lowest pressure possible to achieve adequate ventilation.**

d. The single ventricle is prone to failure leading to pulmonary edema. The atrial contribution to flow is significant, yet arrhythmias that compromise its contribution are common. As expected, such arrhythmias are poorly tolerated.

e. Progressive hepatic failure is widely prevalent due to altered hepatic circulation from increased systemic venous pressures. This can present as a bleeding tendency, a clotting tendency, or as a mixed picture. Pulmonary embolism and stroke are common late complications.

f. **Invasive monitoring** can be problematic and may be unnecessary except for hemodynamically unstable patients.

   (1) CVC placement probably carries a higher risk of thromboembolic events but may nevertheless be appropriate for short-term use. The decision to place a CVC should not be taken lightly, as thrombosis of the SVC in this setting would be deadly. CVPs as high as 25 to 30 mm Hg are not unexpected and may be essential to drive blood through the pulmonary circulation. A PA catheter is unnecessary as the CVP reflects PA pressures.

   (2) Arterial line monitoring is advised, but its location must take surgical shunts into account.

   (3) TEE should be strongly considered for intraoperative monitoring during general anesthesia.

g. **General anesthesia.** A careful selection of induction agents that will provide a smooth hemodynamic profile is preferred.

(1) Etomidate and ketamine are excellent induction agents, and moderate doses of an opioid such as fentanyl, sufentanil, or remifentanil will reduce the stress response.

(2) A muscle relaxant with minimal hemodynamic effects (e.g., succinylcholine or rocuronium) is desirable.

(3) The particular choice of anesthetic agent is not as important as understanding the hemodynamic goals and administering the agents carefully.

h. **Regional anesthesia** may be employed for appropriate surgical cases. However, titrated epidural anesthesia may be preferable to single-injection spinal anesthesia, as abrupt reductions in sympathetic tone may precipitously reduce SVR, which will not be well tolerated.

> **CLINICAL PEARL**   During anesthesia, patients with Fontan physiology require extreme emphasis on appropriate preload, minimizing PVR via adequate ventilation strategies, and inotropic support of the single ventricle.

4. **Anesthetic and hemodynamic goals for patients with Fontan physiology**
   a. **Maintain preload.** Avoid aortocaval compression.
   b. **Avoid elevation in PVR** by preventing acidosis, hypoxemia, and hypercarbia.
   c. **Maintain sinus rhythm.**
   d. **Maintain spontaneous respiration when possible,** which can pose a major challenge in the context of providing adequate anesthesia and analgesia.
   e. **Avoid myocardial depressants.**

B. **Tetralogy of Fallot (ToF)—"Blue baby syndrome"**

ToF is characterized by existence of a VSD, pulmonic stenosis/right ventricular outflow tract obstruction (RVOTO), overriding aorta, and right ventricular hypertrophy. There is great variability in the extent of these defects ranging from small VSD and overriding aorta with minimal pulmonary stenosis (PS) to severe PS and large VSD. Outcomes with current surgical repair techniques are excellent, and there is a 36-year survival of nearly 86% [45].

1. **Palliative shunts** (Blalock–Taussig, Waterston, or Potts), which involve systemic arterial (aorta or subclavian artery) to PA anastomoses, were the initial solution. These palliative shunts provided temporary relief of symptoms, but often at the expense of significant long-term sequelae [28].

2. **Definitive surgical repair** involves closure of the VSD and relief of RVOTO using resection and reconstruction with Gore-Tex patch grafting across the RVOTO or conduits to bypass the RVOTO (Fig. 16.6).

3. Common reasons for reoperation include residual VSD or recurrence of the VSD (10% to 20%), residual RVOTO or stenosis (10%) leading to right heart failure, and progressive RV dilation/dysfunction caused by pulmonic insufficiency (PI) from the RVOT patch.

4. Additional concerns include a higher risk of sudden cardiac death compared with age-matched controls, elevated risk of arrhythmias (especially atrial fibrillation), RBBB, pulmonary regurgitation, and right ventricular aneurysms.

5. Patients with either PS or significant pulmonic valvular regurgitation are more likely to develop right heart failure. Avoidance of elevated PVR and maintenance of high-normal filling pressures are critical in patients with pulmonic valvular regurgitation [43]. See discussion for RV–PA conduits below.

6. **General anesthesia.** Choice of induction agents should be tailored to achieve the hemodynamic goals below and based on underlying cardiac function.
   a. If an arterial catheter is placed, patients with Blalock–Taussig shunts will require cannulation in the contralateral arm or in either leg.
   b. TEE should be considered during general anesthesia.

7. **Regional anesthesia** may be employed for appropriate surgical cases. However, titrated epidural anesthesia may be preferable to single-shot spinal anesthesia for certain ToF patients depending on the degree of palliation and current symptoms.

8. **Anesthetic and hemodynamic goals in ToF**
   a. **Avoid changes (especially decreases) in SVR** to prevent altering any existing shunt.
   b. **Avoid increases in PVR** by preventing hypoxia, hypercarbia, acidosis, and providing supplemental oxygen.
   c. Maintain normal to elevated cardiac filling pressures, especially in patients with right ventricular impairment. Avoid aortocaval compression.
   d. Continuous ECG monitoring is particularly important due to the high incidence of both atrial and ventricular arrhythmias.
   e. Tachycardia and increases in myocardial contractility should be avoided in situations where there is residual RVOTO, as this may exacerbate the obstruction and cause right-to-left shunting.

C. **Right (pulmonary) ventricle to pulmonary artery conduits**
The RV–PA conduit is a surgical technique used in the palliation of multiple lesions including pulmonary atresia, ToF, truncus arteriosus, TGA with VSD, PS, and forms of double-outlet RV [46]. Various types of conduits have been employed for initial repair ranging from aortic homografts (Ross procedure), pulmonary homografts, pericardial patches/reconstructions, to a variety of valved or nonvalved artificial conduits (Dacron, Gore-Tex, etc.). For this section, it is useful to discuss the ventricle as either the pulmonary ventricle (i.e., the ventricle supplying the PA) or the systemic ventricle (i.e., the ventricle supplying the aorta).

1. **Risk factors leading to reoperation:** Conduit failure is thought to occur in roughly 50% of patients at 10 years and 70% of patients at 20 years after placement. Conduit failure, typically, is due to patient growth, thus resulting in a functionally "small" conduit, development of pulmonary valve (PV) insufficiency, and/or various degrees of calcification. Conduit failure is defined by a variety of methods depending on the type of conduit, but in general include the following [45–48]:
   a. Symptomatic patients (dyspnea, fatigue, chest pain, palpitations, presyncope, and decreased exercise tolerance) demonstrating signs of RV failure with elevated pulmonic valve (PV) peak gradients >40 mm Hg.
   b. Asymptomatic patients with pulmonary ventricular pressures approaching systemic pressures, increasing pulmonary ventricular size with increasing PV insufficiency and/or tricuspid insufficiency.
   c. Patients with severe PI and NYHA functional class II or III symptoms should be considered for PV replacement with or without conduit repair [48].
   d. Deterioration in exercise testing or functional capacity.
   e. Patients who are very young at the time of conduit placement, those with small-diameter conduits, those with diagnosis of truncus arteriosus or TGA, and those receiving homografts are at elevated risk of conduit failure.

2. **What are the key anesthetic concerns for pulmonary ventricle–PA conduit replacements?**
   a. These are repeat sternotomy procedures, so all the considerations outlined in Section IX should be followed. The pulmonary ventricle–PA conduit is an anterior structure, so has high risk of injury on reentry sternotomy.
   b. Hemodynamic considerations should take into account the current physiologic and functional status of the patient. The majority of these patients will be suffering from some degree of right heart failure, so careful control of the PVR should be of utmost concern. In addition, PI is common and often in the moderate to severe range. This leads to overdistention of the right (or pulmonary) ventricle with the potential to worsen RV failure.
   c. Patients with residual VSD are at risk for alterations in the shunt fraction if there are significant changes to either PVR or SVR, which can worsen right heart function or create cyanosis.
   d. As with PAH, the right (or pulmonary) ventricle is susceptible to failure, which leads to reduced pulmonary blood flow, hypoxia, and subsequent increases in PVR. This in turn initiates a **catastrophic hemodynamic chain of events** where the decreased RV (or pulmonary) stroke volume decreases LV output and coronary blood flow to both the LV and RV decreases.

> **CLINICAL PEARL** Repeat sternotomy on patients with failed RV–PA conduits are especially high risk for injury during sternotomy.

3. **What are the hemodynamic goals for patients with pulmonary ventricle–PA conduit failure?**

   Management should be based on the etiology of the conduit failure, which usually falls into two basic categories: stenosis or insufficiency. Stenotic lesions are discussed in Section XI.D on PV stenosis. PI is frequently caused by balloon valvuloplasty to treat pulmonic stenosis. It is also common after successful repair of the RVOTO associated with ToF [49]. For patients with PI, there are some basic hemodynamic suggestions that will assist in developing the anesthetic plan.

   a. Overall management goals include to maintain a relative tachycardia (heart rate 80 to 90) and to minimize PVR. This approach will help reduce the regurgitant fraction and promote increased forward flow across the conduit.

   b. In patients with elements of RV (or pulmonary) failure, be careful using agents with direct myocardial depressant effects such as propofol. Etomidate may be an ideal choice.

   c. Consider early inotropic support for patients with RV (or pulmonary) failure. Dobutamine is a good option given the relative tachycardia coupled with reduction in PVR/SVR associated with this β-adrenergic agent. Guidelines provided for PAH also apply to these patients (see Section IV.C).

D. **Pulmonary valve abnormalities**

   PV abnormalities are associated with approximately 12% of ACHD lesions [47]. The causes of PS range from valve-specific abnormalities to problems with the development of the RV itself (see Table 16.6), and derive almost exclusively from congenital lesions. PS may be found in patients with palliated disease (i.e., ToF following repair), or may represent an unrepaired lesion, but is discussed here due to its association with RV–PA conduit abnormalities.

   1. **How is PS diagnosed and what are typical symptoms?** Patients with severe PS generally have exertional dyspnea. The diagnosis is often made via echocardiographic examination. With isolated PV disease, cardiac catheterization is rarely needed.

   2. **How is PS categorized?**

      a. Trivial PS = peak gradient <25 mm Hg.

      b. Mild PS = peak gradient of 25 to 49 mm Hg.

      c. Moderate PS = peak gradient of 50 to 79 mm Hg.

      d. Severe PS = peak gradient >80 mm Hg.

   3. **What are the available therapeutic options for PS?** Patients with trivial or mild PS can expect a 96% and 77% 10-year surgery-free survival, respectively, based on existing outcome studies. These patients are typically followed by echocardiography every 5 to 10 years for progression, or more frequently based on symptom development [48].

      a. **Balloon valvuloplasty** is the treatment of choice (Class I recommendation) for patients with symptomatic PS with gradients >50 mm Hg and <2+ PI, or any patient with exertional dyspnea and gradients in the 30 to 40 mm Hg range. It is not recommended for most patients with dysplastic valve disease (characterized by poorly mobile valve without commissural fusion), for patients with gradients <30 mm Hg or in patients with moderate to severe PI. Both short- and long-term results are quite good with balloon valvuloplasty with restenosis rates <5% [50,51]; results that are essentially equivalent to surgical management with commissurotomy.

      b. **Surgical intervention** is also effective and carried out under direct visualization for patients deemed poor candidates for balloon valvuloplasty. There is typically some residual PI following surgical commissurotomy, and depending on the valve morphology, occasionally PV replacement is required. Bioprosthetic valves carry a long life span in the pulmonic position and are the replacement valve of choice [48,49].

TABLE 16.6 Causes of RVOTO in adult patients

Unoperated
  Valvular
    Dome-shaped PV
    Dysplastic PV
    Unicuspid or bicuspid PV
      Infundibular stenosis, usually associated with ToF
  Hypertrophic infundibular stenosis
    Associated with PS, hypertrophic cardiomyopathy
  Infundibular obstruction
    Tricuspid valve tissue
    Fibrous tags from IVC or coronary sinus
    Aneurysm of the sinus of Valsalva
    Aneurysm of the membranous septum
  Subinfundibular obstruction
    Double-chambered RV
  Supravalvular stenosis
    Hourglass deformity at valve
    PA membrane
    PA stenosis
    PA aneurysm
    Peripheral PA stenosis
      Associations: rubella, Alagille, Williams, Keutel syndromes
Operated
  Valvular
    Native valve restenosis
    Prosthetic valve stenosis
  Conduit stenosis
  Double-chambered RV restenosis
  Peripheral or branch PS
    At insertion site of prior systemic-to-pulmonary shunt
    After other complex surgical repair
  Infundibular stenosis after tunnel repair of double-outlet RV

IVC, inferior vena cava; PV, pulmonary valve; PS, pulmonic stenosis; RV, right ventricle; PA, pulmonary artery; RVOTO, right ventricular outflow tract obstruction; ToF, tetralogy of Fallot.
Reprinted with permission from Bashore TM. Adult congenital heart disease: right ventricular outflow tract lesions. *Circulation.* 2007;115(14):1933–1947, with permission.

4. **What are the key anesthetic management concerns for patients with PS?** The right ventricle in a patient with PS develops a characteristic pathophysiology in a similar fashion to that of the LV in a patient with aortic stenosis, although the resultant symptomatology is different. Over time, the increased RV systolic pressure required to overcome the obstructive lesion leads to RV hypertrophy, and, if left untreated, to RV failure. Ideally, these lesions should be treated before the onset of RV failure for best outcomes.

5. **Hemodynamic considerations** during anesthetic management should follow the guidelines for any stenotic lesion.

   a. Relative bradycardia (heart rate in the 60 to 80 range) is preferred to allow time for complete ventricular ejection. Slower heart rates will also allow for increased coronary perfusion time.

   b. PS represents a fixed obstruction to outflow, so alterations in PVR will not change the obstruction. Preload should be maintained to promote forward flow.

   c. SVR should be maintained in the patient's normal range, as reductions in diastolic pressure will decrease coronary perfusion pressure, leading to RV ischemia. Normally, the RV receives blood flow during both diastole and systole; however, with RV hypertrophy this is shifted primarily to the diastolic phase.

E. **Transposition of great vessels (TGV)**

  TGV is relatively rare, representing 1% to 5% of congenital heart defects. The two main types are congenitally corrected TGV (L-TGV) and complete TGV (D-TGV). Without surgical intervention, survival to 6 months in D-TGV is less than 10% [8,11,28]. L-TGV allows survival, albeit typically at the cost of early adult heart failure.

1. **How is D-TGV palliated and what are the physiologic sequelae?**

   D-TGV is described as blood flow in a parallel system, such that systemic venous return flows to the right atrium and right ventricle, which then ejects blood into the aorta [9,28]. Pulmonary venous blood flow proceeds to the left atrium (LA), LV, and then into the PA. Without additional communication from septal defects or a PDA, there is no connection between blood oxygenated in the lungs and systemic arteries, and therefore survival is impossible.

   a. Atrial switch operations such as the Mustard or Senning procedure create an atrial baffle that causes venous blood to cross at the atrial level into the appropriate ventricle. Since the morphologic right ventricle then continues to eject blood into the aorta, these patients experience a higher risk of heart failure as a result of that ventricle's impaired capacity to chronically pump against systemic arterial pressures [8].

   b. The arterial switch, known as the Jatene procedure, switches the PA and aorta with reimplantation of the coronary vessels. This requires that the LV be sufficiently large to provide systemic flows. These patients often have relatively normal physiology following surgical repair and should be considered in the surgically corrected category [8]. There are **two long-term complications** to be aware of, which include **development of aortic insufficiency on the neoaortic valve (occurring in 25% of patients), and coronary ostial lesions leading to myocardial ischemia** [8].

2. **What are the key anesthetic considerations for patients with TGV?**

   a. Patients with D-TGV who have been treated with the arterial switch (Jatene) will typically have normal cardiac function, so management should focus on any coexisting medical issues. Contrary to this, those patients managed with the Mustard or Senning approach (atrial switch) are at higher risk of developing heart failure due to the systemic right ventricle, as well as the atrial baffle, which occasionally obstructs flow.

   b. As mentioned above, L-TGV patients are also at increased risk of heart failure, so evaluation should focus on determining functional status and symptoms of heart failure.

   c. Arrhythmias are very common in patients treated with Mustard or Senning repairs. VT and IART are the most common (Table 16.4).

   d. Invasive monitors should be used selectively. CVCs may be useful for vascular access and monitoring in patients with heart failure, but PA catheters are probably ill-advised in patients who have undergone atrial switch procedures. Preoperative information from recent echocardiograms can be invaluable for symptomatic patients.

3. **How should induction of general anesthesia be managed?**

   Induction should focus on the degree of heart failure present in the patient. Choose induction agents with minimal myocardial depressant effects; etomidate, ketamine, midazolam, or fentanyl may be ideal choices. Additional effects of inhaled agents in moderate doses are generally well tolerated as the afterload reduction improves forward flow.

4. **Anesthetic and hemodynamic goals for TGV**

   a. Consider an arterial catheter and/or CVC and avoid excessive fluids in patients with evidence of heart failure.

   b. Avoid negative inotropic agents.

   c. Monitor for arrhythmias and treat as indicated.

5. **Should regional anesthesia be utilized in patients with TGV?** As with general anesthesia, the afterload reduction following the sympathetic blockade from neuraxial anesthesia will improve forward flow in patients with mild to moderate degrees of heart failure. Care should be taken in patients with severe heart failure symptoms. Single-shot spinal anesthetic techniques may not be tolerated due to the rapid reduction in preload and SVR. Instead, consider using an epidural catheter with a slow titration of local anesthetic agents.

XII. What are the key details for patients with uncorrected CHD?

Uncorrected lesions presenting in the adult patient represent a group of diagnoses that are typically on the mild end of the spectrum, given that these patients remain largely symptom-free into adulthood. Examples include ASD, VSD, Ebstein anomaly, or undiagnosed ACHD due to limited

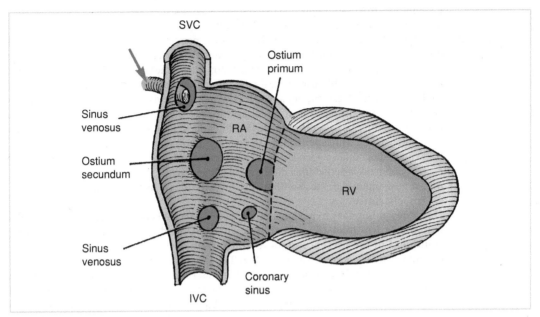

FIGURE 16.7 Location of atrial septal defects (ASDs). IVC, inferior vena cava; RA, right atrium; RV, right ventricle; SVC, superior vena cava. (Reprinted with permission from Rouine-Rapp K, Miller-Hance WC. Transesophageal echocardiography for congenital heart disease in the adult. In: Perrino AC Jr, Reeves ST, eds. *A Practical Approach to Transesophageal Echocardiography*. 2nd ed. Philadelphia, PA: Lippincott Williams & Wilkins; 2008:372.)

healthcare access as child. Patients with more complex disease states that are unrepaired due to limited healthcare access should be managed according to the existing lesion's pathophysiology, and will represent a more complex situation. This section will focus primarily on septal defects presenting in the adult patient.

A. Adult atrial septal defect (ASD)

ASDs account for nearly one-third of adult congenital heart defects and are found in women more commonly than in men [52]. Small defects (less than 5 mm) are hemodynamically insignificant, but large defects (greater than 20 mm) can lead to significant shunting and eventual RV overload or failure [28,53]. ASDs do not typically close spontaneously and are commonly associated with additional cardiac defects. The anatomy of septal defects in the adult is typically the same as that described for the child (Fig. 16.7). Common defects include ostium primum, ostium secundum, sinus venosus, and patent foramen ovale. These defects are often linked to more complex CHD, which should be considered during initial workup. Ostium primum defects are frequently associated with a mitral cleft or other atrioventricular valve abnormalities, while sinus venosus defects are associated with partial anomalous pulmonary venous return. Hemodynamic consequences of ASD follow that of a left-to-right shunt as described above, the severity of which depends on the shunt fraction (pulmonary:systemic or Qp:Qs ratio).

1. **What are the clinical symptoms for adult ASDs?**

   The natural course of unrepaired ASD is that as the patient ages and LV diastolic dysfunction develops, the increased LV end-diastolic pressure tends to worsen the left-to-right shunt. This leads to increased shunt fraction, RV dilation, and development of clinical symptoms, often in the fourth or fifth decade of life [53]. Typical clinical symptoms include the following:

   a. Dyspnea with exertion, possibly due to chronic preload reduction of the LV along with overloaded pulmonary system. This symptom typically is improved with ASD closure.

   b. Cardiac arrhythmias (atrial fibrillation) due to atrial enlargement and stretching of conduction system. Atrial volumes tend to remain elevated in the adult following repair, and thus arrhythmias tend to persist after repair.

    c. Embolic stroke—typically due to paradoxical embolism.

    d. Exercise-induced cyanosis can occur (see below).

2. **What are the indications for repair** [52,53]? A combination of echocardiographic and catheterization-based diagnostic testing is generally used to determine eligibility for repair. Outcomes with repair (either surgical or transcatheter) seem to indicate a benefit in overall survival, as 10-year survival rates for adult patients following repair exceed 95%, while medical management alone has a 10-year 84% survival [54]. Outcomes appear to be better for patients repaired at earlier ages (before the fourth decade), whereas medical management may be better later in life [54,55]. Indications for repair include the following:

    a. Adult patients with a pulmonary-to-systemic shunt (Qp:Qs) ratio >1.5:1.0

    b. Echocardiographic evidence of RV volume overload

    c. Development of arrhythmia due to atrial enlargement

    d. Exercise-induced cyanosis without existing pulmonary hypertension

    e. Embolic stroke

3. **How does pulmonary hypertension relate to ASD? PAH is rarely caused by an ASD, is found in less than 10% of patients with ASD, and if PAH is not diagnosed by adulthood in the presence of an ASD, it rarely develops.** In addition, Eisenmenger physiology rarely develops due to ASD. There is debate regarding the mechanism of PAH associated with ASD, but many consider ASD a marker of PAH, and not a causative agent [53,54]. Regardless, there are important considerations for patients with ASD and moderate to severe PAH. The presence of an ASD allows for blood to flow from right to left, bypassing the high-resistance pulmonary bed in PAH, and thus decompressing the RV. This reduces the classic heart failure symptoms, at the cost of cyanosis, and these patients should not have the ASD closed. Occasionally, creation of an ASD is a temporary measure used to bridge patients with severe PAH to transplant. **In fact, presence of PAH with PVR >4 Wood units may be a contraindication for ASD closure.**

4. **Should surgical repair or transcatheter closure be used to repair the ASD?** Surgical closure of ASD is a safe and effective operation, with mortality rates below 1.5 % and long-term survival >95% as mentioned above [51]. Recent advances in transcatheter approaches have shown excellent outcomes, equivalent to surgical repair, with the obvious avoidance of the morbidity associated with sternotomy [54–58]. Typically, transcatheter closure is associated with shorter hospital stays, less overall complications, and reduced cost.

5. **What characteristics of the lesion increase difficulty with transcatheter repair?** Once the indications for closure listed previously are established, certain anatomic characteristics must be considered for adequate transcatheter closure. Key anatomic features include the following:

    a. **Size of defect.** ASD <26 mm is considered normal size, with >26 mm considered a large defect. Large ASD is not a contraindication for device closure, but there is an elevated risk of dislodgement or erosion when using large devices [54].

    b. **Central lesions**, that is, ostium secundum defects, are the most amenable to treatment. Ostium primum and sinus venosus lesions are often not anatomically suited to transcatheter techniques, so surgical repair is recommended [11].

        (1) **Lesions with deficient anterior-superior rim.** This deficiency is common in large ASDs, and makes placement of the device more technically challenging. Despite this, complications such as dislodgement or erosion are well below 1% in multiple studies [54], and seem to be most related to oversizing of devices. As such, device sizing should be limited to 1.5 times the diameter of the ASD by TEE.

        (2) **Lesions with deficient posterior-inferior rim.** This lesion is even more technically challenging than deficient anterior-superior rim. However, the incidence is also lower and thus there are insufficient data to determine overall complications in these lesions.

    c. **Multiple lesions/fenestrated defects.** This type of abnormality also poses a technical challenge. Approaches vary between balloon atrial septostomy to create a single ASD versus placement of multiple smaller occlusion devices.

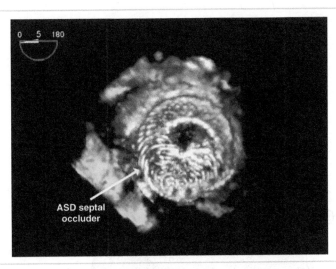

FIGURE 16.8 Three-dimensional (3D) TEE view of an Amplatzer device placed in a large centrally located ASD. ASD, atrial septal defect; TEE, transesophageal echocardiography. (Image by Nathaen Weitzel, MD, University of Colorado Denver.)

    d. Atrial septal aneurysms. The aneurysmal septal wall creates difficulty with device closure using standard devices that rely to some degree on the septal structure. Patch or double disc devices are more appropriate, which are more technically challenging.

6. What are the typical devices used in the catheterization laboratory?
Currently, two main devices have become the standard following multiple studies using many different devices. In the United States, Amplatzer (St. Jude Medical) and Helex (W.L. Gore) are the two devices with current FDA approval. Three-dimensional (3D) TEE imaging of an Amplatzer device in place is seen in Figure 16.8.

7. What are the anesthetic considerations for surgical or device closure in ASD?
General considerations for patients with shunts are discussed in Section VII.D, all of which apply to these patients. Typically, adult patients presenting for ASD closure are hemodynamically stable even in the setting of the clinical symptoms discussed above. On the basis of preoperative evaluation, specifically current functional status, the anesthesiologist can anticipate a relatively normal induction plan aiming for overall smooth hemodynamics. Some key aspects of this procedure to anticipate in anesthetic planning are listed below:

    a. Discuss the device procedure plans with the cardiology team, as many times the interventional cardiologist will want to place right heart catheters while the patient is spontaneously ventilating to obtain catheter-based measurements of RA, RV, and PA pressures. Typically, this portion of the procedure will be carried out under light sedation and on room air to avoid any changes to the PVR due to oxygen supplementation.

    b. Device closure is typically carried out using both echocardiography and x-ray imaging in the catheterization suite. Total procedural time can vary in duration, but typically ranges from 1 to 4 hours. Due to the length of the procedure and the need for prolonged TEE evaluation, general anesthesia is typically employed. Standard ASA monitors are usually all that is needed. However, for patients with severe hemodynamic compromise, invasive blood pressure monitoring may be utilized.

    c. General anesthesia can be safely induced with various approaches in nearly all patients and agents such as propofol or etomidate are acceptable. Heparin is typically given during the device procedure to maintain an Activated Clotting Time (ACT) >250 seconds. Surgical repairs are performed on CPB and require higher ACTs.

    d. Patients with septal defects are at risk for embolic events to the brain. All IV lines should be thoroughly deaired, and extreme care should be taken to avoid any injection of air through IV lines.

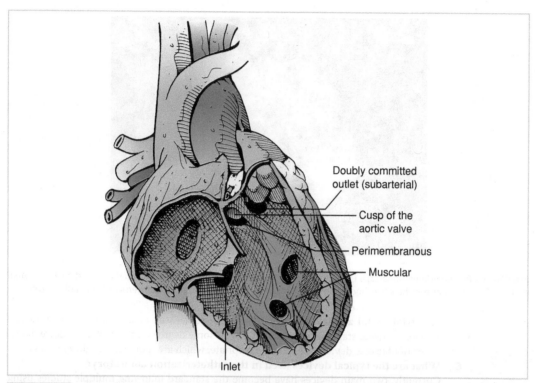

Doubly committed
outlet (subarterial)

Cusp of the
aortic valve

Perimembranous

Muscular

Inlet

FIGURE 16.9 Common locations for ventricular septal defects (VSDs). (Reprinted with permission from Rouine-Rapp K, Miller-Hance WC. Transesophageal echocardiography for congenital heart disease in the adult. In: Perrino AC Jr, Reeves ST, eds. *A Practical Approach to Transesophageal Echocardiography*. 2nd ed. Philadelphia, PA: Lippincott Williams & Wilkins; 2008: 377.)

B. Ventricular septal defects (VSDs)

VSD is the most common congenital heart lesion in children, although nearly 90% close spontaneously by age 10 [52,53]. Those patients with large lesions who are symptomatic at birth will usually be surgically corrected, while asymptomatic patients will often be closely monitored for evidence of spontaneous closure. Surgical closure often involves a right atriotomy or ventricular incision, and this carries a significant risk of interventricular and even atrioventricular conduction abnormalities. VSDs can present in multiple areas of the septum, with 80% being in the perimembranous region (Fig. 16.9), the muscular septum the next highest frequency, and the subarterial or double-committed outlet being rather rare. **In contrast to ASD, unrepaired VSDs can have significant consequences and may lead to development of Eisenmenger physiology if left untreated.**

1. **Can transcatheter closure be utilized to treat VSD?** This question is not as clearly answered as for ASD closure. However, advances over the past decade have led to significant improvements in device closure for VSD. Outcome data seem to favor this approach, with the most common associated complication being arrhythmias. Placement success is more than 95% in multiple studies, and 6-year follow-up demonstrates more than 85% freedom from event rates [59–64]. The considerations for device closure in ASD apply here as well. Establishing good communication with the cardiology team before the procedure to discuss specific diagnostic and therapeutic plans that may impact anesthetic planning is critical.

2. **What if ES is present? ES represents the most common cyanotic cardiac defect in adults** [65]. Chronic left-to-right shunting results in right ventricular hypertrophy, elevated PVR, and significant ventricular and arterial remodeling on the right side. In pregnancy, ES carries a maternal mortality ranging from 30% to 70% along with a high incidence of fetal demise, so patients are usually **counseled against pregnancy** [65],

and are considered extremely high risk for surgery. Sudden death is common and may be due to stroke, arrhythmia, abscess, or heart failure. In the absence of pregnancy, 25-year survival after diagnosis of ES is reported to be 42% [52].

   a. **Pathophysiology.** ES is defined by a PVR greater than 800 dynes $\cdot$ sec/cm^5 along with right-to-left or bidirectional shunt flow. Correction of the shunt may resolve the pulmonary hypertension, but once pulmonary arteriolar remodeling (i.e., medial hypertrophy) develops, the elevated PVR is **irreversible**, differentiating ES from primary pulmonary hypertension.

   b. Symptoms. Fatigue, dyspnea, cyanosis, edema, clubbing, and polycythemia.

   c. The underlying right-to-left shunt, hyperviscosity from polycythemia, and the development of heart failure promote thrombus formation and may elevate stroke risk.

3. **Anesthetic management in ES.** Historically, regional anesthesia was thought to be contraindicated and general anesthesia was the standard. A review of cases of noncardiac surgery including labor and cesarean section in ES indicates that regional anesthesia is indeed safe for these patients [66]. Martin et al. state that mortality is related to a type of surgical procedure, independent of choice of anesthetic. Despite this, anesthetic delivery requires utmost vigilance to maintain hemodynamic goals (see below) with any type of anesthesia.

   a. **Regional anesthesia.** Slow titration of local anesthetic. Aggressive treatment of any reduction in SVR (i.e., systemic hypotension) with phenylephrine is effective. Maintenance of intravascular volume status with careful fluid boluses and phenylephrine for decreased SVR should be used to prevent onset or exacerbation of cyanosis. Single-shot spinal anesthesia is considered contraindicated. Avoidance of elevations in PVR is critical; thus, additional sedative medications should be used cautiously, as reductions in ventilation will lead to hypercarbia and elevation of PVR.

   b. **For general anesthesia**, slow titration of induction agents is preferred, as rapid sequence inductions carry a high risk of SVR alterations and subsequent hemodynamic collapse. This places the patient at increased risk of aspiration, so strict NPO guidelines, use of pharmacologic prophylaxis against aspiration (sodium citrate, H$_2$ blockade, etc.), and mask ventilation using cricoid pressure should be considered. Ketamine and etomidate are probably the best options for induction agents, whereas propofol and thiopental should be avoided due to marked reductions in SVR or cardiac output. Inhalational agents should be used with caution because of their propensity to decrease SVR. Nitrous oxide should be avoided or used with great caution because of its propensity to increase PVR. Maintenance of anesthesia may be accomplished using careful titration of IV agents such as nondepolarizing neuromuscular blockers, opioids, and sedative–hypnotic agents such as midazolam or ketamine, "topping off" with potent inhalational agents at concentrations of less than 0.5 MAC.

   c. **Monitors. Pulse oximetry** may be the most important monitor, as changes in saturation directly correlate with alterations in shunt flow [28]. **Intra-arterial monitoring** is generally employed to closely follow blood pressure. CVCs are controversial. CVC placement carries a risk of air embolus, thrombus, and pneumothorax, which can be devastating in these patients, although information about cardiac filling pressures can be useful. **PA catheters are relatively contraindicated** in patients with ES for a number of reasons [28]. The anatomic abnormality causing ES typically renders flow-directed flotation of PA catheters difficult or impossible, and the risks for arrhythmia, PA rupture, and thromboembolism are elevated. Cardiac output measurements will be inaccurate due to the large shunt. TEE may provide the best real-time monitor of cardiac preload and the status of right-to-left shunting.

4. **Anesthetic and hemodynamic goals for ES**

   a. **Avoid elevations in PVR.** Prevent hypoxemia, acidosis, hypercarbia, and pain. Provide supplemental oxygen at all times.

   b. **Maintain SVR.** Reductions in SVR will increase right-to-left shunting.

   c. **Avoid myocardial depressants and maintain myocardial contractility.**

   d. **Maintain preload and sinus rhythm.**

TABLE 16.7   Cardiac conditions associated with highest risk of adverse outcomes from endocarditis for which prophylaxis with dental procedures is reasonable

Condition	Congenital specific condition[a]
• Previous infective endocarditis • Prosthetic cardiac valve or prosthetic material used for cardiac valve repair	• Unrepaired cyanotic CHD, including palliative shunts and conduits • Completely repaired congenital heart defect with prosthetic material or device, whether placed by surgery or by catheter intervention, during the first 6 mo after the procedure[b] • Repaired CHD with residual defects at the site or adjacent to the site of a prosthetic patch or prosthetic device that inhibit endothelialization • Cardiac transplant recipients who develop cardiac valvulopathy

[a]Except for the conditions listed above, antibiotic prophylaxis is no longer recommended for any other form of CHD.
[b]Prophylaxis is reasonable because endothelialization of prosthetic material occurs within 6 mo after the procedure.
CHD, congenital heart disease.
Modified with permission to include footnotes from Wilson W, Taubert KA, Gewitz M, et al. Prevention of infective endocarditis: Guidelines from the American Heart Association: a guideline from the American Heart Association Rheumatic Fever, Endocarditis, and Kawasaki Disease Committee, Council on Cardiovascular Disease in the Young, and the Council on Clinical Cardiology, Council on Cardiovascular Surgery and Anesthesia, and the Quality of Care and Outcomes Research Interdisciplinary Working Group. *Circulation*. 2007;116:1736–1754.

5. **Can iNO be employed in ES?** iNO is a direct-acting pulmonary vasodilator that avoids systemic vasodilation, thus reducing shunt flow and hypoxia. In general, it is thought that patients with ES are not responsive to most pulmonary vasodilators, including iNO. However, there is some evidence for the use of iNO for labor in Eisenmenger patients, with several case reports indicating improvement in oxygenation and reduced pulmonary pressures [67]. Patients are arriving to the OR on chronic oral pulmonary vasodilators. Therapy with IV pulmonary vasodilators may be required postoperatively to prevent rebound elevation in pulmonary pressures.

XIII. **What are the antibiotic prophylactic considerations for patients with ACHD?**
Infective endocarditis carries high morbidity and mortality, and as such has led to previous recommendations about antibiotic prophylaxis regimens for patients with heart defects. Current recommendations center around the concept that most exposures to infectious agents occur during daily activities, and suggest maintaining a high index of suspicion for signs of endocarditis in susceptible patients [68]. Good oral hygiene is critical to prevent infection in these patients, and antibiotic prophylaxis is recommended only in select lesions listed in Table 16.7.

XIV. **Conclusions**
ACHD encompasses a wide range of patients with variable presentations, symptoms, and degree of illness. Some of the most common and critical presentations have been addressed in this chapter; however, due to the huge range of presentations, variations in all of these lesions are likely to be found, and many other diagnoses have not been covered. The underlying concept found throughout management of ACHD is to obtain as much information as possible about the patient's medical and surgical history, along with current functional capacity. This will give the greatest information about the current level of heart function. On the basis of this information, consider the lesion based on the classifications discussed above, and develop an anesthetic management plan based on individualized physiology for your patient. Consultation with congenital cardiologists or cardiothoracic surgeons can be invaluable. Patients with complicated residual lesions requiring medium- to high-risk surgery should be handled at centers of excellence with physicians and nursing staff trained in adult congenital disease.

REFERENCES

1. Kaemmerer H, Meisner H, Hess J, et al. Surgical treatment of patent ductus arteriosus: a new historical perspective. *Am J Cardiol*. 2004;94(9):1153–1154.
2. Webb GD, Williams RG. 32nd Bethesda Conference: "Care of the adult with congenital heart disease." *J Am Coll Cardiol*. 2001;37(5):1162.
3. Marelli AJ, Ionescu-Ittu R, Mackie AS, et al. Lifetime prevalence of congenital heart disease in the general population from 2000 to 2010. *Circulation*. 2014;130(9):749–756.
4. Mitchell SC, Korones SB, Berendes HW. Congenital heart disease in 56,109 births. Incidence and natural history. *Circulation*. 1971;43(3):323–332.

5. van der Bom T, Zomer AC, Zwinderman AH, et al. The changing epidemiology of congenital heart disease. *Nat Rev Cardiol.* 2011;8(1):50–60.

6. Connelly MS, Webb GD, Somerville J, et al. Canadian Consensus Conference on Congenital Heart Defects in the Adult 1996. *Can J Cardiol.* 1998;14(4):533–597.

7. Connelly MS, Webb GD, Somerville J, et al. Canadian Consensus Conference on Adult Congenital Heart Disease 1996. *Can J Cardiol.* 1998;14(3):395–452.

8. Warnes CA, Williams RG, Bashore TM, et al. ACC/AHA 2008 Guidelines for the management of adults with congenital heart disease: executive summary: a report of the American College of Cardiology/American Heart Association Task Force on Practice Guidelines (writing committee to develop guidelines for the management of adults with congenital heart disease). *Circulation.* 2008;118(23):2395–2451.

9. **Chassot PG, Bettex DA. Anesthesia and adult congenital heart disease. *J Cardiothorac Vasc Anesth.* 2006;20(3):414–437.**

10. Verheugt CL, Uiterwaal CS, van der Velde ET, et al. Mortality in adult congenital heart disease. *Eur Heart J.* 2010;31(10):1220–1229.

11. Williams RG, Pearson GD, Barst RJ, et al. Report of the National Heart, Lung, and Blood Institute Working Group on research in adult congenital heart disease. *J Am Coll Cardiol.* 2006;47(4):701–707.

12. Silversides CK, Dore A, Poirier N, et al. Canadian Cardiovascular Society 2009 Consensus Conference on the management of adults with congenital heart disease: shunt lesions. *Can J Cardiol.* 2010;26(3):e70–e79.

13. Silversides CK, Kiess M, Beauchesne L, et al. Canadian Cardiovascular Society 2009 Consensus Conference on the management of adults with congenital heart disease: outflow tract obstruction, coarctation of the aorta, tetralogy of Fallot, Ebstein anomaly and Marfan's syndrome. *Can J Cardiol.* 2010;26(3):e80–e97.

14. Silversides CK, Marelli A, Beauchesne L, et al. Canadian Cardiovascular Society 2009 Consensus Conference on the management of adults with congenital heart disease: executive summary. *Can J Cardiol.* 2010;26(3):143–150.

15. Silversides CK, Salehian O, Oechslin E, et al. Canadian Cardiovascular Society 2009 Consensus Conference on the management of adults with congenital heart disease: Complex congenital cardiac lesions. *Can J Cardiol.* 2010;26(3):e98–e117.

16. Sable C, Foster E, Uzark K, et al. Best practices in managing transition to adulthood for adolescents with congenital heart disease: the transition process and medical and psychosocial issues: a scientific statement from the American Heart Association. *Circulation.* 2011;123(13):1454–1485.

17. Karamlou T, Diggs BS, Ungerleider RM, et al. Adults or big kids: what is the ideal clinical environment for management of grown-up patients with congenital heart disease? *Ann Thorac Surg.* 2010;90(2):573–579.

18. Ladouceur M, Iserin L, Cohen S, et al. Key issues of daily life in adults with congenital heart disease. *Arch Cardiovasc Dis.* 2013;106(6–7):404–412.

19. Seal R. Adult congenital heart disease. *Paediatr Anaesth.* 2011;21(5):615–622.

20. Ashley EA, Niebauer J. *Cardiology Explained.* London: Remedica Pub Ltd; 2004.

21. Gallagher M, David Hayes M, Jane EH. Practice advisory for the perioperative management of patients with cardiac implantable electronic devices: pacemakers and implantable cardioverter-defibrillators. *Anesthesiology.* 2011;114(2):247–261.

22. Khairy P, Aboulhosn J, Gurvitz MZ, et al. Arrhythmia burden in adults with surgically repaired tetralogy of Fallot: a multi-institutional study. *Circulation.* 2010;122(9):868–875.

23. **Walsh EP, Cecchin F. Arrhythmias in adult patients with congenital heart disease. *Circulation.* 2007;115(4):534–545.**

24. Bernier M, Marelli AJ, Pilote L, et al. Atrial arrhythmias in adult patients with right- versus left-sided congenital heart disease anomalies. *Am J Cardiol.* 2010;106(4):547–551.

25. de Groot NM, Atary JZ, Blom NA, et al. Long-term outcome after ablative therapy of postoperative atrial tachyarrhythmia in patients with congenital heart disease and characteristics of atrial tachyarrhythmia recurrences. *Circ Arrhythm Electrophysiol.* 2010;3(2):148–154.

26. Weitzel N. Pulmonary hypertension. In: Chu L, Fuller A, eds. *Manual of Clinical Anesthesiology.* 1st ed. Philadelphia, PA: Lippincott Williams & Wilkins; 2012:447–452.

27. **Blaise G, Langleben D, Hubert B. Pulmonary arterial hypertension: pathophysiology and anesthetic approach. *Anesthesiology.* 2003;99(6):1415–1432.**

28. Weitzel N, Gravlee G. Cardiac disease in the obstetric patient. In: Bucklin B, Gambling D, Wlody D, eds. *A Practical Approach to Obstetric Anesthesia.* 1st ed. Philadelphia, PA: Lippincott Williams & Wilkins; 2009:403–434.

29. Hirsch JH, Charpie JR, Ohye RG, et al. Near infrared spectroscopy (NIRS) should not be standard of care for postoperative management. *Semin Thorac Cardiovasc Surg Pediatr Card Surg Annu.* 2010;13(1):51–54.

30. Holst KA, Dearani JA, Burkhart HM, et al. Risk factors and early outcomes of multiple reoperations in adults with congenital heart disease. *Ann Thorac Surg.* 2011;92(1):122–138.

31. Kirshbom PM, Myung RJ, Simsic JM, et al. One thousand repeat sternotomies for congenital cardiac surgery: risk factors for reentry injury. *Ann Thorac Surg.* 2009;88(1):158–161.

32. Park CB, Suri RM, Burkhart HM, et al. Identifying patients at particular risk of injury during repeat sternotomy: Analysis of 2555 cardiac reoperations. *J Thorac Cardiovasc Surg.* 2010;140(5):1028–1035.

33. Elahi M, Dhannapuneni R, Firmin R, et al. Direct complications of repeat median sternotomy in adults. *Asian Cardiovasc Thorac Ann.* 2005;13(2):135–138.

34. Asghar Nawaz M, Patni R, Chan KM, et al. Hyperinflation of lungs during redo-sternotomy, a safer technique. *Heart Lung Circ.* 2011;20(11):722–723.

35. Society of Thoracic Surgeons Blood Conservation Guideline Task Force; Ferraris VA, Brown JR, Despotis GJ, et al. 2011 update to the Society of Thoracic Surgeons and the Society of Cardiovascular anesthesiologists blood conservation clinical practice guidelines. *Ann Thorac Surg.* 2011;91(3):944–982.

36. Fergusson DA, Hebert PC, Mazer CD, et al. A comparison of aprotinin and lysine analogues in high-risk cardiac surgery. *N Engl J Med.* 2008;358(22):2319–2331.

37. Henry DA, Carless PA, Moxey AJ, et al. Anti-fibrinolytic use for minimising perioperative allogeneic blood transfusion. *Cochrane Database Syst Rev.* 2011:CD001886.

38. Henry DA, Carless PA, Moxey AJ, et al. Anti-fibrinolytic use for minimising perioperative allogeneic blood transfusion. *Cochrane Database Syst Rev.* 2007:CD001886.
39. Karkouti K, Beattie WS, Dattilo KM, et al. A propensity score case-control comparison of aprotinin and tranexamic acid in high-transfusion-risk cardiac surgery. *Transfusion.* 2006;46(3):327–338.
40. Ranucci M, Castelvecchio S, Romitti F, et al. Living without aprotinin: the results of a 5-year blood saving program in cardiac surgery. *Acta Anaesthesiol Scand.* 2009;53(5):573–580.
41. Davies RR, Russo MJ, Yang J, et al. Listing and transplanting adults with congenital heart disease. *Circulation.* 2011;123(7):759–767.
42. **Eagle SS, Daves SM. The adult with Fontan physiology: systematic approach to perioperative management for non-cardiac surgery.** *J Cardiothorac Vasc Anesth.* **2011;25(2):320–334.**
43. Heggie J, Karski J. The anesthesiologist's role in adults with congenital heart disease. *Cardiol Clin.* 2006;24(4):571–585, vi.
44. d'Udekem Y, Iyengar AJ, Cochrane AD, et al. The Fontan procedure: contemporary techniques have improved long-term outcomes. *Circulation.* 2007;116(11 Suppl):I157–I164.
45. Nollert G, Fischlein T, Bouterwek S, et al. Long-term survival in patients with repair of tetralogy of Fallot: 36-year follow-up of 490 survivors of the first year after surgical repair. *J Am Coll Cardiol.* 1997;30(5):1374–1383.
46. Dearani JA, Danielson GK, Puga FJ, et al. Late follow-up of 1095 patients undergoing operation for complex congenital heart disease utilizing pulmonary ventricle to pulmonary artery conduits. *Ann Thorac Surg.* 2003;75(2):399–410; discussion 410–411.
47. Rodefeld MD, Ruzmetov M, Turrentine MW, et al. Reoperative right ventricular outflow tract conduit reconstruction: risk analyses at follow up. *J Heart Valve Dis.* 2008;17(1):119–126; discussion 126.
48. Bashore TM. Adult congenital heart disease: right ventricular outflow tract lesions. *Circulation.* 2007;115(14):1933–1947.
49. Bonow RO, Carabello BA, Chatterjee K, et al. 2008 Focused update incorporated into the ACC/AHA 2006 guidelines for the management of patients with valvular heart disease: a report of the American College of Cardiology/American Heart Association Task Force on Practice Guidelines (Writing Committee to Revise the 1998 Guidelines for the Management of Patients With Valvular Heart Disease): endorsed by the Society of Cardiovascular Anesthesiologists, Society for Cardiovascular Angiography and Interventions, and Society of Thoracic Surgeons. *Circulation.* 2008;118(15):e523–e661.
50. Jarrar M, Betbout F, Farhat MB, et al. Long-term invasive and noninvasive results of percutaneous balloon pulmonary valvuloplasty in children, adolescents, and adults. *Am Heart J.* 1999;138(5 Pt 1):950–954.
51. Chen CR, Cheng TO, Huang T, et al. Percutaneous balloon valvuloplasty for pulmonic stenosis in adolescents and adults. *N Engl J Med.* 1996;335(1):21–25.
52. **Brickner ME, Hillis LD, Lange RA. Congenital heart disease in adults. First of two parts.** *N Engl J Med.* **2000;342(4): 256–263.**
53. Geva T, Martin JD, Wald RM. Atrial septal defects. *Lancet.* 2014;383(9932):1921–1932.
54. Rao PS. When and how should atrial septal defects be closed in adults? *J Invasive Cardiol.* 2009;21(2):76–82.
55. Calvert PA, Rana BS, Kydd AC, et al. Patent foramen ovale: anatomy, outcomes, and closure. *Nat Rev Cardiol.* 2011;8(3): 148–160.
56. Tomar M, Khatri S, Radhakrishnan S, et al. Intermediate and long-term followup of percutaneous device closure of fossa ovalis atrial septal defect by the Amplatzer septal occluder in a cohort of 529 patients. *Ann Pediatr Cardiol.* 2011;4(1):22–27.
57. Kretschmar O, Sglimbea A, Corti R, et al. Shunt reduction with a fenestrated Amplatzer device. *Catheter Cardiovasc Interv.* 2010;76(4):564–571.
58. Sadiq M, Kazmi T, Rehman AU, et al. Device closure of atrial septal defect: medium-term outcome with special reference to complications. *Cardiol Young.* 2012;22(1):71–78.
59. Zeinaloo A, Macuil B, Zanjani KS, et al. Transcatheter patch occlusion of ventricular septal defect in Down syndrome. *Am J Cardiol.* 2011;107(12):1838–1840.
60. Yang R, Sheng Y, Cao K, et al. Transcatheter closure of perimembranous ventricular septal defect in children: safety and efficiency with symmetric and asymmetric occluders. *Catheter Cardiovasc Interv.* 2011;77(1):84–90.
61. Wei Y, Wang X, Zhang S, et al. Transcatheter closure of perimembranous ventricular septal defects (VSD) with VSD occluder: early and mid-term results. *Heart Vessels.* 2012;27(4):398–404.
62. Ramakrishnan S, Saxena A, Choudhary SK. Residual VSD closure with an ADO II device in an infant. *Congenit Heart Dis.* 2011;6(1):60–63.
63. Li X, Li L, Wang X, et al. Clinical analysis of transcatheter closure of perimembranous ventricular septal defects with occluders made in China. *Chin Med J (Engl).* 2011;124(14):2117–2122.
64. Gu M, You X, Zhao X, et al. Transcatheter device closure of intracristal ventricular septal defects. *Am J Cardiol.* 2011;107(1):110–113.
65. **Lovell AT. Anaesthetic implications of grown-up congenital heart disease.** *Br J Anaesth.* **2004;93(1):129–139.**
66. Martin JT, Tautz TJ, Antognini JF. Safety of regional anesthesia in Eisenmenger's syndrome. *Reg Anesth Pain Med.* 2002; 27(5):509–513.
67. Ray P, Murphy GJ, Shutt LE. Recognition and management of maternal cardiac disease in pregnancy. *Br J Anaesth.* 2004; 93(3):428–439.
68. **Wilson W, Taubert KA, Gewitz M, et al. Prevention of infective endocarditis. Guidelines from the American Heart Association. A guideline from the American Heart Association Rheumatic Fever, Endocarditis, and Kawasaki Disease Committee, Council on Cardiovascular Disease in the Young, and the Council on Clinical Cardiology, Council on Cardiovascular Surgery and Anesthesia, and the Quality of Care and Outcomes Research Interdisciplinary Working Group.** *Circulation.* **2007;116(15):1736–1754.**

17

Anesthetic Management of Cardiac and Pulmonary Transplantation

James M. Anton, Anne L. Rother, Charles D. Collard, and Erin A. Sullivan

PART I: CARDIAC TRANSPLANTATION

KEY POINTS

1. Nonischemic cardiomyopathy (49%) is the most common pretransplant diagnosis worldwide.
2. Nearly 85% of recipients in the United States (US) require some form of life support prior to cardiac transplantation. For example, the number of pretransplant patients with ventricular assist devices (VADs) has risen dramatically (29% in 2008 vs. 45% in 2015).
3. Increased preoperative pulmonary vascular resistance (PVR) in the recipient predicts early graft dysfunction and an increased incidence of right heart dysfunction. Right ventricular (RV) failure accounts for nearly 20% of early mortality after transplantation.
4. During orthotopic cardiac transplantation, the cardiac autonomic plexus is transected leaving the transplanted heart without autonomic innervation. The denervated heart responds to direct-acting agents such as catecholamines, which are utilized frequently in the post-bypass period.
5. In contrast to the nontransplanted patient, where increases in cardiac output (CO) can be quickly achieved through a sympathetically mediated increase in heart rate, the cardiac transplanted patient, whose sympathetic innervation to the heart will be interrupted, tends to require an increase in preload in order to increase CO.

ALTHOUGH "DESTINATION THERAPY" USING MECHANICAL CIRCULATORY SUPPORT (MCS) devices has increasingly become a viable option, and advances in MCS devices have resulted in a significant survival benefit, cardiac transplantation remains the gold standard for the treatment of heart failure (HF) refractory to medical therapy [1]. Since the first human cardiac transplant by Christiaan Barnard in 1967, over 118,000 cardiac transplants have been performed worldwide [2]. Currently, approximately 4,500 cardiac transplants are performed per year, with approximately 2,700 occurring in the United States (US) [2]. Despite an increasingly high-risk patient population, survival rates continue to improve due to advances in immunosuppression, surgical technique, perioperative management, and the diagnosis and treatment of allograft rejection and allograft vasculopathy [3]. In the US, cardiac transplantation is limited to member centers of the United Network for Organ Sharing (UNOS). UNOS, in turn, administers the Organ Procurement and Transplantation Network (OPTN) which maintains the only national patient waiting list in US.

I. Heart failure (HF)

More than 6.5 million American adults carry a diagnosis of HF, with an incidence of 960,000 new cases per year [4]. The American College of Cardiology (ACC) and the American Heart Association (AHA) define HF as a clinical syndrome that can result from any structural or functional cardiac disorder that

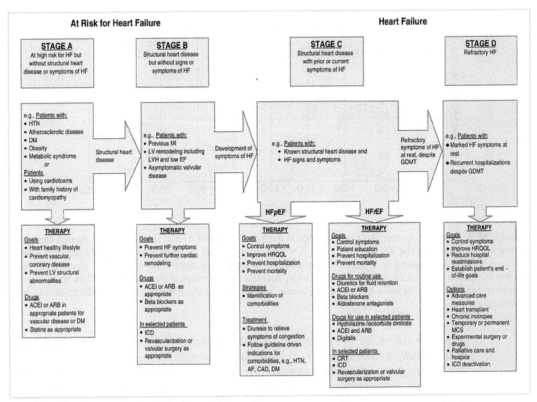

FIGURE 17.1 Stages in the development of heart failure (HF) and recommended therapy. HTN, hypertension; DM, diabetes mellitus; LV, left ventricle; ACEI, angiotensin converting enzyme inhibitor; ARB, angiotensin receptor blocker; MI, myocardial infarction; LVH, left ventricular hypertrophy; EF, ejection fraction; HF, heart failure; HFpEF, heart failure with preserved ejection fraction; HFrEF, heart failure with reduced ejection fraction; HRQOL, health-related quality of life; ICD, implantable cardioverter defibrillator; AF, atrial fibrillation; GDMT, goal-directed medical therapy; MCS, mechanical circulatory support. (From Yancy CW, Jessup M, Bozkurt B, et al. ACCF/AHA guideline for the management of heart failure: executive summary: a report of the American College of Cardiology Foundation/American Heart Association Task Force on practice guidelines. *Circulation.* 2013;128(16):1810–1852.)

impairs the ability of the ventricle to fill with or eject blood. The majority of patients with HF owe their symptoms to impairment of left ventricular (LV) myocardial function [5]. Because volume overload is not necessarily present, the term "HF" is now preferred to the older term "congestive HF."

The New York Heart Association (NYHA) scale is used to quantify the degree of functional limitation imposed by HF. Most patients with HF, however, do not show an uninterrupted and inexorable progression along the NYHA scale [5]. In 2005, the ACC/AHA created a staging scheme reflective of the fact that HF has established risk factors, a clear progression, and specific treatments at each stage that can reduce morbidity and mortality (Fig. 17.1). Patients presenting for heart transplantation invariably present in stage D, refractory HF.

A. Etiology

Nonischemic cardiomyopathy (49%) is the most common pretransplant diagnosis worldwide [2]. Ischemic cardiomyopathy accounts for 35%, with valvular cardiomyopathy, restrictive cardiomyopathy, hypertrophic cardiomyopathy, viral cardiomyopathy, retransplantation, and congenital heart disease accounting for the remaining percentage of adult heart transplant recipients.

B. Pathophysiology

The neurohormonal model portrays HF as a progressive disorder initiated by an index event, which either damages the myocardium directly or disrupts the ability of the myocardium to generate force [6]. HF progression is characterized by declining ventricular function and activation of compensatory adrenergic, and salt and water retention pathways. Ejection fraction (EF)

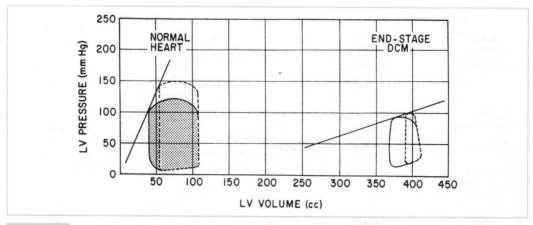

FIGURE 17.2 Pressure–volume (P–V) relationships in a normal heart and a heart with end-stage, dilated cardiomyopathy (DCM). Shown are the left ventricular (LV) P–V loops (*dotted lines*) obtained from a normal heart and a heart with end-stage DCM following an increase in afterload. The slope depicts the LV end-systolic P–V relationship. Note that the myopathic heart stroke volume (SV) is markedly decreased by increases in afterload. (From Clark NJ, Martin RD. Anesthetic considerations for patients undergoing cardiac transplantation. *J Cardiothorac Anesth*. 1988;2:519–542, with permission.)

is initially maintained by increases in LV end-diastolic volume, myocardial fiber length, and adrenergically mediated increases in myocardial contractility. LV remodeling takes place during this time, and while initially adaptive, may independently contribute to HF progression [6]. The chronic overexpression of molecular mediators of compensation (e.g., norepinephrine, angiotensin II, endothelin, natriuretic peptides, aldosterone, and tumor necrosis factor) may lead to deleterious effects on cardiac myocytes and their extracellular matrix [6,7]. The result is progressive LV dilation, as well as decreasing EF and cardiac output (CO). Fatigue, dyspnea, and signs of fluid retention develop. Other organ systems such as the liver and kidneys become compromised by persistent decreases in CO and elevated venous pressures. With continued progression of HF, stroke volume (SV) becomes unresponsive to increases in preload, and increases in afterload are poorly tolerated (Fig. 17.2). Chronic exposure to circulating catecholamines may result in downregulation of myocardial β_1-adrenergic receptors, making the heart less responsive to inotropic therapy.

CLINICAL PEARL   Patients with end-stage HF are chronically exposed to high circulating catecholamine levels and, as a result, are less responsive to inotropic therapy.

C. Medical management of HF
   1. Therapeutic goals
   The therapeutic goal for HF management is to slow or halt the progression from stages A to D. Lifestyle modifications and selected pharmacotherapy are the mainstays of therapy for stages A and B. When stage C is reached, combination pharmacotherapy includes diuresis, interruption of the renin–angiotensin axis, and β-blockade. Selective use of direct vasodilators and inotropes is also indicated. Utilization of cardiac resynchronization therapy (CRT) and/or an implantable defibrillator may be recommended. Despite optimum medical management, some patients will progress to stage D, refractory HF. Chronic intravenous (IV) inotropes, MCS devices, and heart transplantation are the only measures available for palliation or treatment.
      a. Inotropes
      Inotropic agents commonly used to treat cardiac failure include digitalis, catecholamines, and phosphodiesterase-III inhibitors. Digitalis, in combination with β-blockers,

is effective in treating HF complicated by atrial fibrillation, but does not confer increased survival [8]. Similarly, recent evidence indicates that digitalis may have a role in the treatment of HF in patients with normal sinus rhythm, but this remains without documented mortality benefit [9]. Administered orally, digitalis exerts a positive inotropic effect by inhibiting the myocardial cell sodium pump and increasing cytosolic calcium concentrations. Digitalis also prolongs atrioventricular conduction time, leading to PR interval prolongation and possible heart block. Digitalis blood levels should be monitored as significant side effects, including atrial and ventricular arrhythmias, can occur particularly in the presence of hypokalemia.

Myocardial β_1-adrenergic receptor stimulation by IV administration of catecholamines, such as epinephrine, norepinephrine, dobutamine, or dopamine, is often used to improve cardiac performance, diuresis, and clinical stability. Phosphodiesterase-III (PDE) inhibitors, such as milrinone and enoximone, may also be used. PDE inhibitors combine both positive inotropic and vasodilatory activity by inhibiting cyclic AMP (cAMP) metabolism. Occasionally, patients may not be weaned from IV inotropic support despite repeated attempts. At such times, an indwelling IV catheter may be placed to allow for the continuous infusion of an inotrope for patients awaiting transplantation, or to facilitate home palliation. However, chronic inotrope use has not been shown to increase survival [10].

b. Diuretics

Diuretics provide symptomatic relief to HF patients more quickly than any other class of drug, and are the only class of drug used in HF that can adequately control fluid retention. Classes of diuretics used include the loop diuretics (e.g., furosemide, bumetanide, torsemide), the thiazide diuretics (e.g., hydrochlorothiazide), and the thiazide-like drug metolazone. Adverse diuretic effects include electrolyte disturbances (particularly of potassium and magnesium), hypotension, intravascular volume depletion, and azotemia.

c. Renin–angiotensin–aldosterone system inhibitors

Inhibition of the renin–angiotensin–aldosterone system may occur at the level of the angiotensin-converting enzyme inhibitors (ACEIs), the angiotensin receptor blockers (ARBs), or the aldosterone receptor. In combination with β_1-antagonists, ACEIs have been shown to reduce HF progression by interfering with the neurohormonal pathways that modulate LV remodeling. ACEIs alleviate symptoms, enhance the overall sense of well-being, and reduce the risk of hospitalization and death in patients with HF [11,12]. Adverse effects of ACEIs include hypotension, worsening renal function, and hyperkalemia. If the adverse effects of ACEIs cannot be tolerated, ARBs may be considered as an alternative. ARBs have been shown to reduce morbidity and mortality in HF patients [12]. The propensity of ARBs to increase serum potassium levels limits their usage in patients with impaired renal function. A new class of medication, combined angiotensin receptor blocker neprilysin inhibitors (ARNIs), has been associated with significant reductions in hospital admissions and mortality as compared to ACEIs. Guidelines now recommend substituting ARNIs for ACEIs or ARBs in appropriate patients [11,12]. Aldosterone exerts an adverse effect on heart structure and function independent of angiotensin II [13]. Spironolactone is the most widely used aldosterone antagonist in HF patients, although eplerenone has been studied in HF after myocardial infarction.

d. Vasodilators

Vasodilators are used in the acute treatment of HF to reduce myocardial preload and afterload, thereby reducing myocardial work and oxygen demand. By preferentially reducing preload via venodilation, nitroglycerin may be useful for relieving the symptoms of pulmonary edema. β-Type natriuretic peptide (nesiritide) is used effectively for the medical management of decompensated HF [10]. Nesiritide, an arterial and venous dilator, acts by increasing cyclic GMP (cGMP) [10]. In hospitalized patients, a dose-dependent reduction of pulmonary capillary wedge pressure, right atrial pressure, and mean pulmonary artery (PA) pressure was demonstrated, along with improvements in cardiac index and clinical outcome [14]. A recent meta-analysis found reduced readmission rates and in-hospital mortality rates with nesiritide therapy as compared to dobutamine therapy for patients with acute decompensated HF [14].

e. β-Adrenergic receptor blockade

In combination with interruption of the renin–angiotensin–aldosterone axis and diuresis, β-adrenergic receptor blockade is now standard treatment for HF. Carvedilol, bisoprolol, and sustained release metoprolol have been demonstrated to be effective in reducing mortality in patients with chronic HF [11]. Chronic adrenergic stimulation initially supports the failing heart, but may lead to progression of HF through neurohormonal-mediated LV remodeling. β-Blockers likely exert their benefit through attenuation of this influence. Adverse reactions to β-blockers in patients with HF include fluid retention, fatigue, bradycardia, heart block, and hypotension.

f. Anticoagulants

Patients with HF are at increased risk of thromboembolism as a result of low CO and a high incidence of coexistent atrial fibrillation. Long-term prophylactic anticoagulation with agents such as warfarin is common and may contribute to perioperative bleeding at the time of cardiac transplantation.

g. Cardiac implantable electronic devices (CIEDs)

CIEDs broadly consist of devices that seek to manage bradyarrhythmias (pacemakers), tachyarrhythmias (implantable cardiac defibrillators), and ventricular dyssynchrony (biventricular pacing/CRT). These devices are used to reduce the incidence of sudden cardiac death, and to slow HF progression [15]. Their presence may complicate the placement of central venous catheters and require the involvement of the electrophysiology team for interrogation and reprogramming [16].

D. Mechanical circulatory support (MCS) devices

Nearly 85% of recipients in the US require some form of life support prior to heart transplantation [17]. These include IV medications, mechanical ventilation, intra-aortic balloon pump (IABP), extracorporeal life support (ELS), total artificial hearts (TAHs), and ventricular assist devices (VADs). IV medications, IABPs, ELS, and extracorporeal VADs are useful in temporizing a hospitalized patient with cardiogenic shock. Intracorporeal MCS devices offer the potential for discharge to home and may yield the greatest potential improvement in quality of life for patients with class D HF who are awaiting heart transplant surgery.

In the US, the number of patients undergoing heart transplantation with a pre-existent VAD has risen dramatically (29% in 2008 vs. 45% in 2015) [17]. The increased use of VADs has contributed to a decline in the heart transplant waiting list mortality despite increased waiting times secondary to their use as a bridge-to-transplantation [17,18]. One-year survival while being supported on a VAD has risen to 85% [19]. However, the influence of VADs on post–heart-transplant survival remains controversial, with some studies suggesting an increased 6-month mortality after transplant, while others suggest no increase in mortality [19,20].

> **CLINICAL PEARL** The increased use of VADs has resulted in a decline in heart transplant waiting list mortality, however, the influence of VADs on post-heart-transplant survival remains controversial.

II. Cardiac transplant recipient characteristics

The number of active transplant candidates in US has increased by 90% between 2004 and 2015 [17]. In 1999, UNOS modified its listing system to be two-tiered (Table 17.1), and in 2006, UNOS modified the allocation of donor hearts to expand organ sharing within geographic regions. In 2014–2015, the median time to transplantation was 12.4 months. Among adults, there was an increase in the number of candidates >65 years (14% in 2008 vs. 18% in 2015) [17]. Among all age groups, there was an increase in cardiomyopathy as a primary diagnosis (44.7% in 2005 vs. 57.5% in 2015) and a decrease in both congenital heart disease as a primary diagnosis (5.6% in 2005 vs. 3.7%

TABLE 17.1   United Network for Organ Sharing (UNOS) listing criteria for heart transplantation

1A: Admitted to the listing transplant center hospital with *at least one* of the following:
    a. Assisted mechanical circulatory support (MCS) with either:
        Total artificial heart (TAH)
        Intra-aortic balloon pump (IABP)
        Extracorporeal membrane oxygenation (ECMO)
    b. Continuous mechanical ventilation
    c. Continuous infusion of a single high-dose intravenous (IV) inotrope or multiple IV inotropes, and requires continuous hemodynamic monitoring of left ventricular (LV) filling pressures

1A: May or may not be admitted to the listing transplant center hospital with *at least one* of the following:
    a. Has *one* of the following MCS devices in place:
        Left ventricular assist device (LVAD)
        Right ventricular assist device (RVAD)
        Left and right ventricular assist devices (BiVAD)
    b. Assisted MCS with significant device-related complications

1B: Has at least one of the following devices or therapies in place:
    a. Left (LVAD), right (RVAD), or left and right (BiVAD) ventricular assist devices
    b. Continuous infusion of intravenous (IV) inotropes

2: Does not meet the criteria for status 1A or 1B but is suitable for transplant

7: Considered temporarily unsuitable to receive a thoracic organ transplant

From OPTN policy 6.1 at https://optn.transplant.hrsa.gov/media/1200/optn_policies.pdf#nameddest=Policy_06; Accessed 27 May, 2017.

in 2015), and coronary artery disease (CAD) as a primary diagnosis (41% in 2005 vs. 33% in 2015) [17]. Finally, the percentage of patients classified as 1A or 1B has increased dramatically (13.2% in 2005 vs. 53.8% in 2015) [17]. The reduction in waiting list mortality and increases in category 1A and 1B candidates may be in part due to the impact of VADs.

A. Cardiac transplantation indications

Indications for heart transplantation are listed in Table 17.2 [21]. Potential cardiac transplant candidates must have all reversible causes of HF excluded, and their medical management optimized.

B. Cardiac transplantation contraindications

There has been a gradual relaxation in the cardiac transplantation exclusion criteria as experience with increasingly complex cases has grown [2]. Absolute exclusion criteria have been simplified (Table 17.3) [21].

Increased preoperative pulmonary vascular resistance (PVR) predicts early graft dysfunction and increased mortality, due to an increased incidence of right heart dysfunction [21–23]. Methods used to quantify the severity of pulmonary hypertension (HTN) include calculation of PVR and the transpulmonary gradient (mean PA pressure – pulmonary capillary wedge pressure [PCWP]). At most centers, patients are not considered orthotopic cardiac transplant candidates if they demonstrate a PVR >5 Wood units or transpulmonary gradient >15 mm Hg without evidence of pharmacologic reversibility [23]. The reversibility of pulmonary HTN

TABLE 17.2   Indications for heart transplantation

Refractory HF/cardiogenic shock requiring continuous IV inotropic support or MCS

Persistent NYHA class IV HF symptoms refractory to maximal medical therapy (LVEF <20%; peak VO$_2$ <12 mL/kg/min with β-blockade, VO$_2$ <14 mL/kg/min without β-blockade)

Intractable or severe anginal symptoms in patients with CAD not amenable to percutaneous or surgical revascularization

Intractable life-threatening arrhythmias unresponsive to medical therapy, catheter ablation, and/or implantation of a intracardiac defibrillator

From Mancini D, Lietz K. Selection of cardiac transplantation candidates in 2010. *Circulation.* 2010;122:173–183.
HF, heart failure; IV, intravenous; MCS, mechanical circulatory support; NYHA, New York Heart Association; LVEF, LV ejection fraction; VO$_2$, oxygen consumption; CAD, coronary artery disease.

TABLE 17.3 Contraindications to heart transplantation

■ **Absolute contraindications**

Systemic illness with a life expectancy <2 yrs despite transplant, including:
    Active or recent solid organ or blood malignancy within 5 yrs
    AIDS with frequent opportunistic infections
    Systemic lupus erythematosus, sarcoidosis, or amyloidosis that has multisystem involvement and is still active
    Irreversible renal or hepatic dysfunction in patients considered only for heart transplant
    Significant obstructive pulmonary disease (FEV_1 <1 L/min)
Fixed pulmonary hypertension
    PA systolic pressure >60 mm Hg
    Mean transpulmonary gradient >15 mm Hg
    PVR >6 Wood units

■ **Relative contraindications**

Age >72 yrs
An active infection excepting device-related infection in patients with VAD
Severe peripheral vascular or cerebrovascular disease
    Symptomatic carotid stenosis
    Uncorrected abdominal aortic aneurysm >6 cm
    Severe diabetes mellitus with end-organ damage (neuropathy, nephropathy, or retinopathy)
    Peripheral vascular disease not amenable to percutaneous or surgical therapy
Morbid obesity (BMI >35 kg/m²)
Recent pulmonary infarction (6–8 wks)
Irreversible neurologic or neuromuscular disorder
Drug, tobacco, or alcohol abuse within 6 months
Active mental illness or psychosocial instability
Difficult-to-control hypertension
Active peptic ulcer disease
Heparin-induced thrombocytopenia within 100 days
Creatinine >2.5 mg/dL or creatinine clearance <25 mL/min
Bilirubin >2.5 mg/dL, serum transaminases >3× upper limit of normal, INR >1.5 off Coumadin

From Mancini D, Lietz K. Selection of cardiac transplantation candidates in 2010. *Circulation*. 2010;122:173–183.
AIDS, acquired immune deficiency syndrome; FEV1, forced expiratory volume in 1 second; PA, pulmonary artery; PVR, pulmonary vascular resistance; VAD, ventricular assist device; BMI, body mass index; INR, international normalized ratio.

can be evaluated by vasodilator administration, including IV sodium nitroprusside, inhaled nitric oxide (iNO), and inhaled epoprostenol (PGI_2). In patients who receive VADs, "fixed" elevated PVR may be reduced and thus improve posttransplant outcome, or qualify a previously excluded patient for heart transplant [21–23]. The only transplant options for patients with severe irreversible pulmonary HTN include heterotopic cardiac or combined heart–lung transplantation (HLT).

III. The cardiac transplant donor

  A. Donor selection

    The primary factor limiting cardiac transplantation is a shortage of donors. Standard criteria for donors, first outlined in the 1980s, resulted in a paucity of donor organs relative to the number of patients who could benefit from heart transplantation. In an attempt to increase donor numbers, the criteria for cardiac organ donation have been relaxed. So-called "marginal donor" hearts may be transplanted into borderline heart transplant candidates with good results when compared to their expected prognosis without transplantation [24]. Characteristics of marginal donors include older age (>55 years), the presence of CAD, donor/recipient size mismatch, history of donor drug abuse, increased ischemic times, and donor seropositivity for viral hepatitis [24–26]. Nonetheless, the risk of failed transplantation has been shown to increase with increased donor age, LV hypertrophy, and the presence of concomitant disease [26]. In an effort to further expand the donor pool, donation after circulatory death (DCD) for heart transplantation has been described recently using ex vivo perfusion. Early evidence suggests that with strict limitations and the use of ex vivo perfusion systems, DCD donation for heart transplantation may be feasible [25,27]. Contraindications to heart donation are listed in Table 17.4.

TABLE 17.4   Contraindications to heart donation

▦ **Absolute contraindications**
Positive serology for syphilis, HTLV-4 and HIV
Presence of malignancy with extracranial metastatic potential
LVEF of <40%
Significant valvular abnormality
Significant CAD

▦ **Relative contraindications**
Sepsis
Hepatitis B surface antigen positive
Hepatitis C antibody positive
Repeated need for cardiopulmonary resuscitation
High-dose inotropic support exceeding 24 hrs

HTLV-4, human T-lymphotropic virus type 4; HIV, human immunodeficiency virus; LVEF, LV ejection fraction; CAD, coronary artery disease.

Before a donor heart may be harvested, permission for donation must be obtained, the suitability of the heart for donation must be ascertained, and the diagnosis of brain death must be made. Initial functional and structural evaluation of the potential heart donor ought to be done with electrocardiography and transthoracic echocardiography. Normal LV function predicts suitability for heart transplantation, and subsequent management of the donor may be guided by other invasive monitors such as PA catheters or serial echocardiography [24]. Coronary angiography may be performed on patients ≥40 years old [24]. Donor–recipient factors such as size, ABO compatibility, and antihuman leukocyte antigen (HLA)–antibody compatibility are also being assessed. Logistic factors, including ischemic organ time must be considered. Finally, the harvesting surgeon will directly inspect the donor heart [24].

B. Determination of brain death

In the US, The Uniform Determination of Death Act defines death as either (1) the irreversible cessation of circulatory and respiratory functions, or (2) irreversible cessation of all functions of the entire brain, including the brain stem. A determination of death must be made in accordance with accepted medical standards. For the diagnosis of brain death to be made, the patient's core body temperature must be >32.5°C, and no drug with the potential to alter neurologic or neuromuscular function must be present.

C. Pathophysiology of brain death

When brain death results from severe brain injury, increased intracranial pressure results in progressive herniation and ischemia of the brain stem. Subsequent hemodynamic instability, endocrine, and metabolic disturbances disrupt homeostasis, and may render organs unsuitable for transplantation (Table 17.5).

1. Cardiovascular function

   In an attempt to maintain cerebral blood flow to the increasingly ischemic brain stem, blood pressure (BP) and heart rate rise. While usually transient, this adrenergically mediated

TABLE 17.5   Incidence of pathophysiologic changes after brain stem death

Hypotension	80%
Diabetes insipidus (DI)	46–86%
Disseminated intravascular coagulation	28–55%
Cardiac arrhythmias	25–32%
Pulmonary edema	13–18%
Systolic myocardial dysfunction	42%
Thrombocytopenia	56%

From Maciel CB, Greer DM. ICU management of the potential organ donor: state of the art. *Curr Neurol Neurosci Rep.* 2016;16:86.

"sympathetic storm" may precipitate electrocardiographic and echocardiographic findings consistent with myocardial ischemia [28,29]. Occasionally, severe systemic hypertension may persist and require management [28,29]. Hypotension will affect most brain-dead patients and may be refractory to pressors [28,29]. Hypotension may result from hypovolemia caused by traumatic blood loss, central diabetes insipidus (DI), or osmotic therapy for management of elevated intracranial pressure. Loss of sympathetic tone resulting in blunted vasomotor reflexes, vasodilatation, and impaired myocardial contractility also contributes to hypotension [28,29]. Noxious stimuli may induce exaggerated hypertensive responses mediated by intact spinal sympathetic reflexes that are no longer inhibited by descending pathways. Despite optimal donor support, terminal cardiac arrhythmias may occur within 48 to 72 hours of brain death.

2. Endocrine dysfunction

Dysfunction of the posterior pituitary gland occurs in a majority of brain-dead organ donors. The loss of antidiuretic hormone (ADH) results in DI, which is manifested by polyuria, hypovolemia, and hypernatremia [28,29]. Derangements in other electrolytes including potassium, magnesium, and calcium may also occur as a result of DI. Dysfunction of the anterior pituitary gland has been inconsistently described, with hemodynamic and electrolyte disturbances attributable in part to loss of thyroid-stimulating hormone (TSH), growth hormone (GH), and adrenocorticotropic hormone (ACTH) [28–30]. Plasma concentrations of glucose may become variable (most often elevated), due to changes in serum cortisol levels, the use of catecholamine therapy, progressive insulin resistance, and the administration of glucose-containing fluids [29].

3. Pulmonary function

Hypoxemia resulting from lung trauma, infection, or pulmonary edema may occur following brain death. Pulmonary edema in this setting may be neurogenic, cardiogenic, or inflammatory in origin [29].

4. Temperature regulation

Thermoregulation by the hypothalamus is lost after brain death. Increased heat loss occurs because of an inability to vasoconstrict, along with a reduction in metabolic activity, which puts brain-dead organ donors at risk for hypothermia. Adverse consequences of hypothermia include cardiac dysfunction, arrhythmias, decreased tissue oxygen delivery, coagulopathy, and cold-induced diuresis [28].

5. Coagulation

Coagulopathy may result from hypothermia and from dilution of clotting factors following massive transfusion and fluid resuscitation. Disseminated intravascular coagulation occurs in 28% to 55% of brain-dead organ donors due to the release of tissue thromboplastin and activation of the coagulation cascade by the ischemic brain [29].

D. Management of the cardiac transplant donor

Posttransplant graft function is in part dependent on optimal donor management prior to organ harvesting. Strategies for the management of brain-dead organ donors seek to stabilize their physiology through active resuscitation so that the functional integrity of potentially transplantable organs is maintained [28,29].

1. Cardiovascular function

Donor systemic BP and central venous pressure (CVP) should be monitored continuously using arterial and central venous catheters [26]. Goals include a mean arterial pressure >60 to 70 mm Hg, a CVP of 6 to 10 mm Hg, urinary output >1 mL/kg/hr, and an LV ejection fraction (LVEF) >45% [28,29]. The initial treatment step in maintaining hemodynamic stability is maintenance of euvolemia using aggressive replacement of intravascular volume with crystalloids, colloids, and packed red blood cells (pRBCs) if the hemoglobin (Hgb) concentration is <10 g/dL or the hematocrit is <30% [26,28].

If hemodynamic stability is not restored with fluid resuscitation, placement of a PA catheter, use of echocardiography, or continuous CO monitoring should be used to assess right and left-sided intracardiac pressures, CO, and systemic vascular resistance

(SVR) [28,29]. Use of inotropes and pressors should be guided by these additional diagnostics. Dopamine and vasopressin are recommended as first-line agents, with epinephrine, norepinephrine, phenylephrine, and dobutamine utilized for severe shock [29]. However, prolonged use of catecholamines at high doses should be avoided due to potential downregulation of β-receptors on the donor heart, and the negative impact this may have on graft function after cardiac transplant [28]. High-dose α-adrenergic receptor agonists should be used cautiously, as peripheral and splanchnic vasoconstriction may result in decreased perfusion of other potential donor organs and metabolic acidosis. Vasopressin has catecholamine-sparing effects without impairing graft function [26,28].

Hormonal replacement is indicated in brain-dead donors with hemodynamic instability refractory to fluids, catecholamines, and vasopressin; however, its efficacy has not been completely validated [29]. Regimens vary widely, but a combination of thyroid hormone, corticosteroid, ADH, and insulin seem to maximize organ yield [29]. All are part of the UNOS standard donor management protocol.

2. Fluid and electrolytes

Hypernatremia (sodium >155 mEq/L) in the donor has been associated with higher rates of primary graft failure, particularly in liver transplantation [28,29]. Aggressive treatment of DI with 1-desamino-8-D-arginine vasopressin (ddAVP) is indicated. IV fluids should be given to replace urinary losses and to maintain urine output [29]. Normoglycemia (120 to 180 mg/dL) should be achieved through the use of dextrose-containing fluids, and/or an insulin infusion [29]. Metabolic acidosis and respiratory alkalosis should be corrected, with a goal pH of 7.40 to 7.45 [29].

3. Pulmonary function

If lung procurement is also being considered, a lung protective management protocol consisting of lower tidal volumes (6 to 8 mL/kg) and higher positive end-expiratory pressure (PEEP) of 8 to 10 cm H_2O and optimal positioning of the patient (head of bed >30 degrees) should be initiated. Optimal volume management with goal CVP of 6 to 8 mm Hg and PCWP of 6 to 10 mm Hg has been shown to improve donor lung function without increasing other organ (heart/liver/kidney) dysfunction [29].

Efforts to prevent pulmonary aspiration, atelectasis, and infection are warranted. Neurogenic pulmonary edema should be managed with PEEP, careful diuresis, and iNO in appropriate donors [29].

4. Temperature

Monitoring of core temperature is mandatory, as hypothermia adversely affects coagulation, cardiac rhythm, and oxygen delivery. Use of heated IV fluids, blankets, and humidifiers may prevent hypothermia.

5. Coagulation

Different transplant centers have individual guidelines for blood component therapy for management of coagulopathy. In general, component therapy should be guided by repeated donor platelet and clotting factor measurements. Generally accepted goals include an international normalized ratio (INR) of <1.5 and a platelet count of >100,000/mm^3 [29]. Antifibrinolytics to control donor bleeding are not recommended due to the risk of microvascular thrombosis.

E. **Anesthetic management of the donor**

Anesthetic management of the donor during organ harvesting is an extension of preoperative management. If the lungs are to be harvested, a lung protective ventilation strategy should be employed as well as judicious fluid management to keep the CVP <10 cm H_2O [31]. Vasopressors to maintain adequate BP, hormone replacement, and transfusion per institutional protocol to keep Hgb >8 g/dL and to manage coagulopathy should be continued through the intraoperative period [31]. Although intact spinal reflexes may result in hypertension, tachycardia, and muscle movement, these signs do not indicate cerebral function or pain perception. Nondepolarizing muscle relaxants may be used to prevent spinal reflex-mediated muscle contraction.

> **CLINICAL PEARL** Anesthetic management of the organ donor includes the use of vasopressors to maintain adequate BP, lung protective ventilatory strategies, and transfusion per institutional protocol to keep Hgb >8 g/dL.

F. Organ harvest technique

After initial dissection, the patient is fully heparinized. The perfusion-sensitive organs (i.e., kidneys and liver) are removed prior to cardiectomy. The donor heart is excised en bloc via median sternotomy after dissection of the pericardial attachments. The superior and inferior venae cavae are ligated first, allowing exsanguination. The aorta is cross-clamped and cold cardioplegia administered. The aorta and pulmonary arteries are transected, leaving the native donor arterial segments as long as possible. Finally, the pulmonary veins are individually divided after lifting the donor organ out of the thoracic cavity. Most donor hearts are currently preserved with specialized cold colloid solutions (e.g., University of Wisconsin [UW], histidine-tryptophan-ketoglutarate [HTK], or Celsior solution) and placed in cold storage at 4°C [32]. When this technique is used, optimal myocardial function after transplantation is achieved when the donor heart ischemic time is <4 hours [32].

IV. Surgical techniques for cardiac transplantation

A. Orthotopic cardiac transplantation

Over 98% of cardiac transplants performed are orthotopic. The recipient is placed on standard cardiopulmonary bypass (CPB) and, if present, the PA catheter withdrawn into the superior vena cava. The femoral vessels are often selected for arterial and venous CPB cannulation in patients undergoing repeat sternotomy. Otherwise, the distal ascending aorta is cannulated and bicaval cannulae with snares placed, completely excluding the heart from the native circulation. The aorta and pulmonary arteries are then clamped and divided. Depending on the implantation technique (Fig. 17.3), either both native atria or a single left atrial cuff containing

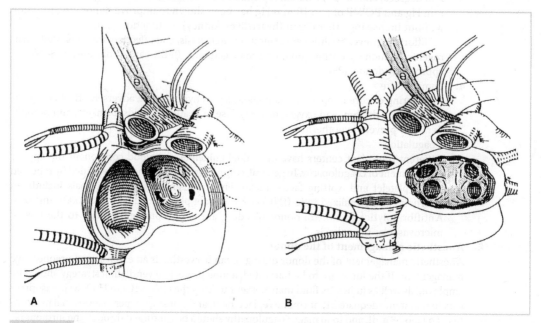

A   **B**

FIGURE 17.3 Surgical techniques for cardiac transplantation. **A:** Biatrial technique. The donor heart is anastomosed to the main bulk of the recipient's native right and left atria. **B:** Bicaval technique. The donor heart left atrium is anastomosed to a single left atrial cuff, including the pulmonary veins, in the recipient. (From Aziz TM, Burgess MI, El Gamel A, et al. Orthotopic cardiac transplantation technique: a survey of current practice. *Ann Thorac Surg.* 1999;68:1242–1246, with permission.)

the pulmonary veins is preserved. The native atrial appendages are discarded because of the risk of postoperative thrombus formation.

The donor heart is inspected for the presence of a patent foramen ovale. If patent, it is surgically closed, as right-to-left interatrial shunting and hypoxemia may occur in the presence of elevated right-sided pressures following transplantation. The donor and recipient left atria are anastomosed first, followed by the right atria, or cavae when a bicaval anastomotic technique is chosen. The subsequent order of anastomoses varies depending on the donor heart ischemic time and the experience of the surgeon. The donor and recipient aortas are joined and the aortic cross-clamp removed with the patient in Trendelenburg position to decrease air embolism. After completion of the PA anastomosis and placement of temporary epicardial pacing wires, the heart is de-aired and the patient weaned from CPB.

1. Biatrial implantation

    Biatrial implantation is the technique originally described by Barnard. It preserves portions of the recipient's native atria to create two atrial anastomoses (Fig. 17.3A). Biatrial orthotopic heart transplantation has been performed successfully for over four decades and has the advantage of being relatively simple and possibly faster to perform [33]. It is, however, falling out of favor. The biatrial technique puts the sinoatrial node at risk of injury, redundant atrial tissue may contribute to atrial dysrhythmias, and distortion of the right atrium may contribute to a higher risk for tricuspid regurgitation [33]. Although patients receiving biatrial transplant experience a higher incidence of permanent pacemakers (2.0% vs. 9.1%) and tricuspid regurgitation, no definitive difference in long-term survival has been demonstrated [33–35].

2. Bicaval implantation

    The bicaval implantation technique is a modification of the biatrial technique. Only a single, small left atrial cuff containing the pulmonary veins is preserved in the recipient. Bicaval and left atrial anastomoses are performed (Fig. 17.3B). The bicaval technique is growing in popularity, particularly at higher volume transplant centers [33]. Demonstrated advantages of the bicaval technique include a higher incidence of postoperative sinus rhythm, lower right atrial pressures, a reduced need for permanent pacemaker, and lower incidence of tricuspid regurgitation [33–35]. A decreased risk of perioperative mortality may exist [33].

B. **Heterotopic cardiac transplantation**

Heterotopic transplantation accounts for less than 1% of cardiac transplantation procedures per annum. In this technique, the recipient's heart is not excised. Instead, the donor heart is placed within the right anterior thorax, and anastomosed to the recipient's native heart such that a parallel circulation is established. The recipient and donor atria are anastomosed, followed by the aortas. An artificial conduit usually joins the pulmonary arteries, with the native and donor right ventricles ejecting into the native PA. Similarly, both the native and donor left ventricles eject into the native aorta. Thus, the recipient's RV, which is conditioned to eject against elevated PA pressures, will provide most of the right-sided ventricular output, whereas the healthy donor LV will make the major contribution to left-sided ventricular output. Situations in which heterotopic cardiac transplantation may be advantageous include recipients with severe pulmonary HTN, a small donor-to-recipient size ratio, and a marginal donor heart [36]. Disadvantages of heterotopic cardiac transplantation include relatively high operative mortality, a requirement for continued medical treatment of the failing native heart, the potential for the native heart to be a thromboembolism source, compromised pulmonary function due to placement of donor heart in the right chest, and possible increased incidence of tachyarrhythmias in both the native and heterotopic hearts [36].

V. **Preoperative management of the cardiac transplant patient**

A. **Timing and coordination**

When planning cardiac transplantation, important considerations include the time required for donor organ transport and potential for failure to complete recipient cannulation in a timely fashion (e.g., repeat sternotomy). Since the timing of heart transplants is dictated by donor availability, transplantation can take place at any hour of the day. Ideally, to minimize ischemic time, anesthetic induction of the recipient should be timed so that the recipient is already on CPB when the donor heart arrives. However, since the attendant risks of general anesthesia are magnified in the recipient, who by definition has advanced HF, induction of anesthesia ought to be delayed until a definitive "go" is received from the harvesting team.

B. Preoperative evaluation

The anesthesiologist usually has limited time for preoperative assessment of the cardiac transplant recipient. The presentation of this patient population varies widely, from a stable outpatient requiring no inotropic or mechanical support to a critically ill inpatient requiring cardiac support ranging from inotropes to IABP to extracorporeal membrane oxygenation (ECMO) [37]. These recipients will have been under the care of a medical team experienced in the management of HF, and their medical therapy is likely to have already been optimized. When the recipient is already admitted to the intensive care unit (ICU), all aspects of their ongoing care should be reviewed, including pulmonary status and ventilation settings, presence of invasive monitors and existing venous access, use of inotropes and/or pressors, and the use of MCS devices. In any case, the preoperative anesthetic evaluation should include a thorough history, physical examination, review of the patient's medical record, and assessment of the patient's functional status [37]. The electrocardiogram (ECG), echocardiogram, chest x-ray, and cardiac catheterization results should be noted, and all hematologic, renal, and liver function tests reviewed.

1. Concomitant organ dysfunction

Chronic systemic hypoperfusion and venous congestion in the recipient may produce reversible hepatic and renal dysfunction. Mild to moderate elevations of hepatic enzymes, bilirubin, and prolongation of prothrombin time are common. Preoperative hepatic dysfunction and anticoagulant medication may also contribute to the abnormal coagulation profile frequently observed in cardiac transplant recipients. Blood urea nitrogen is commonly elevated in patients with end-stage heart disease due to chronic hypoperfusion and the concomitant prerenal effects of high-dose diuretics.

2. Preoperative medications

Preoperative inotropic support should be continued throughout the pre-CPB period. Patients receiving digitalis and diuretics have an increased risk of dysrhythmias in the presence of hypokalemia. Anticoagulants such as warfarin, heparin, and aspirin may increase the need for perioperative blood product administration.

3. Preoperative monitoring

The position, function, and duration of invasive monitoring catheters should be noted. The function and settings of IABPs and VADs should be reviewed. If a CIED is present, it should be interrogated and the antitachyarrhythmia/rate responsiveness functions suspended in the operating room after external defibrillation pads have been applied [37]. Patients with invasive monitoring and/or MCS require extra personnel and vigilance to ensure safe transport from the ICU to the operating room.

4. The combined heart–lung recipient

The combined heart–lung transplant recipient often requires special preoperative evaluation. Cystic fibrosis recipients should first have an otolaryngologic evaluation before being placed on a waiting list. Many of these patients will require endoscopic maxillary antrostomies for sinus access and monthly antibiotic irrigation. This measure has decreased the incidence of serious posttransplant bacterial infections in that patient population. Previous smokers must undergo screening to exclude malignancy. A negative sputum cytology, thoracic CT scan, bronchoscopy, and otolaryngologic evaluation are required. In addition, left heart catheterization, coronary angiography, and a carotid duplex scan may be performed in previous smokers.

VI. Anesthetic management of the cardiac transplant recipient

A. Premedication

The HF patient has elevated levels of circulating catecholamines and is preload dependent. Even a small dose of sedative medication may result in vasodilatation and hemodynamic decompensation. Therefore, sedatives should be avoided or carefully titrated, along with supplemental oxygen.

CLINICAL PEARL The HF patient presenting for heart transplant has high circulating catecholamine levels and is preload dependent, and small doses of sedative medications may cause vasodilatation and hemodynamic decompensation.

Patients presenting for cardiac transplantation should be considered "full stomach," as most present with short notice. If oral cyclosporine or azathioprine is started preoperatively, gastric emptying is slowed. Oral sodium citrate and/or IV metoclopramide may be useful in raising gastric pH and reducing gastric volumes.

B. **Importance of aseptic technique**

Perioperative immunosuppressive therapy places the cardiac transplant recipient at increased risk of infection. All invasive procedures should be done under aseptic or sterile conditions.

C. **Monitoring**

Noninvasive monitoring should include a standard 5-lead ECG, BP measurement, pulse oximetry, capnography, and nasopharyngeal temperature. If not already in situ, large-bore peripheral and central venous access should be obtained. Invasive monitoring should include systemic arterial as well as central venous and/or PA pressures and a urinary catheter. Intraoperative transesophageal echocardiography (TEE) is standard practice [37]. A PA catheter may be helpful in the post-CPB period, allowing monitoring of CO, ventricular filling pressures, and calculation of SVR and PVR. Additional monitors (e.g., cerebral oximetry) may be indicated in selected patients [37]. Traditionally, catheterization of the right internal jugular vein is avoided to preserve this route for the endomyocardial biopsies (EMBs) routinely performed to screen for myocardial rejection. Nonetheless, difficulty with EMB by alternative routes has not been reported in circumstances where the right internal jugular vein was used for central access.

D. **Considerations for repeat sternotomy**

Many cardiac transplant recipients will have undergone previous cardiac surgery and are at increased risk of inadvertent trauma to the great vessels or pre-existing coronary artery bypass grafts during sternotomy. Patients having repeat sternotomy should have external defibrillation pads placed before induction and cross-matched, irradiated pRBCs available in the operating room prior to sternotomy. The potential for a prolonged surgical dissection time in patients with a "redo chest" may necessitate anesthetic induction earlier than usual in order to coordinate with donor heart arrival. Other considerations for repeat sternotomy include the potential for bleeding and the need for femoral or axillary CPB cannulation.

E. **Anesthetic induction**

1. Hemodynamic goals

   Cardiac transplant recipients typically have hypokinetic, noncompliant ventricles sensitive to alterations in myocardial preload and afterload. Hemodynamic priorities for anesthetic induction are to maintain heart rate (HR) and contractility, avoid acute changes in preload and afterload, and prevent increases in PVR. Inotropic support is very often required during anesthetic induction and throughout the pre-CPB period. Owing to afterload sensitivity, epinephrine or norepinephrine infusions are probably preferable to phenylephrine or vasopressin infusions for BP support.

2. Aspiration precautions

   Rapid sequence induction with maintenance of cricoid pressure should be considered.

3. Anesthetic agents

   Due to the slow circulation time in patients with end-stage HF, a delayed response to administered anesthetic agents is common. IV anesthetics commonly used for anesthetic induction of the cardiac transplant recipient include etomidate (0.1 to 0.3 mg/kg) in combination with fentanyl (2.5 to 10 µg/kg) or sufentanil (5 to 8 µg/kg). High-dose narcotic regimens (e.g., fentanyl 25-50 ug/kg) have also been used successfully. Bradycardia occurring in response to high-dose narcotics should be treated promptly, as CO in patients with end-stage heart disease is HR dependent. Small doses of midazolam, ketamine, or scopolamine help ensure amnesia, but should be used cautiously as they may synergistically lower SVR and induce hypotension.

4. Muscle relaxants

Muscle relaxants with minimal cardiovascular effects (e.g., rocuronium, cisatracurium, or vecuronium) are most commonly utilized. As an added advantage, their relatively rapid onset facilitates rapid sequence induction in patients at risk for aspiration [37].

F. Anesthetic maintenance

During the pre-CPB period, anesthetic goals include maintenance of hemodynamic stability and end-organ perfusion. Most anesthetic maintenance regimens are narcotic-based with supplemental inhalational agents and benzodiazepines. Although most inhalational agents have negative inotropic effects, low concentrations of these agents are usually well tolerated and decrease the risk of awareness. Anesthetic depth can be difficult to assess in this patient population, as the sympathetic response to light planes of anesthesia is often blunted. The use of narcotic-based anesthetic regimens may also increase the risk of awareness during anesthesia.

Antifibrinolytics such as tranexamic acid or epsilon-aminocaproic acid may be administered following anesthetic induction to reduce bleeding.

G. Cardiopulmonary bypass (CPB)

CPB for cardiac transplantation is similar to that employed for routine cardiac surgical procedures. Femoral venous and arterial cannulation sites are frequently chosen in patients undergoing repeat sternotomy. Moderate hypothermia (28° to 30°C) is commonly used during CPB to improve myocardial protection. Hemofiltration and/or mannitol administration is common during CPB, as patients with HF often have a large intravascular blood volume and coexistent renal impairment. Although immunosuppressive regimens vary among transplantation centers, high-dose IV glucocorticoids such as methylprednisolone are frequently administered prior to aortic cross-clamp release to reduce the likelihood of hyperacute rejection. Immunosuppressive induction therapy with an interleukin-2 receptor (IL2R) antagonist, or a polyclonal antilymphocyte antibody, has been employed in over 50% of patients between 2009 and 2014 in order to reduce the risk of T-cell rejection. [2]. However, no consensus on the safety and efficacy of induction therapy exists [37,38]. The availability and timing of immunosuppressive medications should be discussed with the transplant team ahead of time.

VII. Postcardiopulmonary bypass (Post-CPB)

Prior to CPB termination, the patient should be normothermic and all electrolyte and acid–base abnormalities corrected. Complete de-airing of the heart prior to aortic cross-clamp removal is essential. TEE may be particularly useful for assessing the efficacy of cardiac de-airing maneuvers. Inotropic agents may be commenced prior to CPB termination. A HR of 90 to 110 beats/min, a mean systemic arterial BP >65 mm Hg, and ventricular filling pressures of approximately 12 to 16 mm Hg (CVP) and 14 to 18 mm Hg (PCWP) are often required in the immediate post-CPB period. Although inotropic support is usually required for several days, patients are often extubated within 24 hours and discharged from the ICU by the third postoperative day. Clinical considerations in the immediate postoperative period include:

A. Autonomic denervation of the transplanted heart

During orthotopic cardiac transplantation, the cardiac autonomic plexus is transected, leaving the transplanted heart without autonomic innervation. The transplanted heart thus does not respond to direct autonomic nervous system stimulation or to drugs that act indirectly through the autonomic nervous system (e.g., atropine). The denervated, transplanted heart responds to direct-acting agents such as catecholamines. Transient bradycardia and slow nodal rhythms are common following aortic cross-clamp release. An infusion of a direct-acting β-adrenergic receptor agonist such as isoproterenol or dobutamine is frequently started prior to CPB termination, and titrated to achieve a HR around 100 beats/min. Newly transplanted hearts unresponsive to pharmacologic stimulation may require temporary epicardial pacing. Although most initial dysrhythmias resolve, some cardiac transplant recipients require placement of a permanent pacemaker.

B. Right ventricular (RV) dysfunction

RV failure is a significant cause of early morbidity and mortality, and is one of the most common causes of failure to wean from CPB [37]. Acute RV failure following cardiac transplantation may be due to prolonged donor heart ischemic time, mechanical obstruction at the level of the PA anastomosis, pulmonary hypertension (both pre-existing and protamine induced), donor-recipient size mismatch, and acute rejection [37]. RV distension and hypokinesis may be diagnosed by TEE or direct observation of the surgical field. Other findings suggesting RV failure include elevations in the CVP, PA pressure, or the transpulmonary gradient (>15 mm Hg).

Goals for managing RV dysfunction include maintaining systemic BP, lowering PVR, and minimizing RV dilation. Maintaining atrioventricular synchrony is especially important in optimizing RV preload. Correction of electrolyte and acid–base disturbances and the use of inotropic support may improve RV function. Optimizing ventilator settings and the use of inhaled pulmonary vasodilators may reduce RV afterload. Useful inotropes include epinephrine, dobutamine, isoproterenol, and milrinone; the latter three agents may also reduce pulmonary vascular resistance [37]. Inhaled pulmonary vasodilators include prostacyclin (PGI_2), prostaglandin E_1 (PGE_1), and nitric oxide (NO) [37]. Nitric oxide selectively reduces PVR by activating guanylate cyclase in vascular smooth muscle cells, producing an increase in cGMP and smooth muscle relaxation. Little systemic effect is seen as it is inactivated by Hgb and has a 6-second half-life. NO administration results in the formation of the toxic metabolites nitrogen dioxide and methemoglobin. In the presence of severe LV dysfunction, selective dilation of the pulmonary vasculature by NO may lead to an increase in PCWP and pulmonary edema. PGI_2 is an arachidonic acid derivative with a half-life of 3 to 6 minutes. It binds to a prostanoid receptor and causes an increase in intracellular cAMP, and consequently vasodilation. PGI_2 has been shown to be efficacious for over 20 years in heart transplant patients [37]. Relative to NO, PGI_2 is less costly, easier to administer and does not create toxic metabolites. It may, however, cause a degree of systemic hypotension due to its longer half-life, and may be implicated in increased bleeding due to inhibition of platelet function [39]. RV failure refractory to medical treatment may require insertion of a right VAD or institution of extracorporeal circulation.

CLINICAL PEARL   RV dysfunction is a significant cause of early morbidity and mortality following heart transplant, and managing RV dysfunction includes maintaining systemic BP, lowering PVR, and minimizing RV dysfunction.

C. **Left ventricular (LV) dysfunction**

Post-CPB LV dysfunction may result from prolonged donor heart ischemic time, inadequate myocardial perfusion, intracoronary embolization of intracavitary air, or surgical manipulation. The incidence of post-CPB LV dysfunction is greater in donors requiring prolonged, high-dose inotropic support prior to organ harvest. Continued postoperative inotropic support with dobutamine, epinephrine, or norepinephrine may be required.

D. **Coagulation**

Coagulopathy following cardiac transplantation is common, and perioperative bleeding should be treated early and aggressively. Potential etiologies include hepatic dysfunction secondary to chronic hepatic venous congestion, preoperative anticoagulation, CPB-induced platelet dysfunction, hypothermia, and hemodilution of clotting factors. After ruling out surgical bleeding, blood product administration should be guided by repeated measurements of platelet count and plasma coagulation. Due to an increased risk of infection and graft versus host disease, all administered blood products should be cytomegalovirus (CMV)-negative and irradiated or leukocyte-depleted. RBCs and platelets should be administered through leukocyte filters. Desmopressin (DDAVP) has been shown to reduce postoperative blood loss in selected surgical patients, but has not been shown to reliably decrease transfusion requirements post-CPB [40].

E. **Renal dysfunction**

Renal dysfunction, as evidenced by increased serum creatinine and oliguria, is common in the immediate postoperative period. Contributing factors include pre-existing renal impairment, cyclosporine-associated renal toxicity, perioperative hypotension, and CPB. Treatment of renal dysfunction includes optimization of CO and systemic BP, as well as judicious use of diuretics to avoid volume overload.

F. Pulmonary dysfunction

Postoperative pulmonary complications such as atelectasis, pleural effusion, and pneumonia are common and may be reduced by ventilation using PEEP, regular endobronchial suctioning, and chest physiotherapy. Bronchoscopy to clear pulmonary secretions is often useful. Pulmonary infection in the immunosuppressed recipient should be treated early and aggressively.

G. Hyperacute allograft rejection

Cardiac allograft hyperacute rejection is caused by preformed HLA antibodies present in the recipient. There are several explanations for the pre-existing antibodies that initiate hyperacute rejection. First, prior recipients of blood transfusions may develop antibodies to major histocompatibility complex (MHC) antigens in the transfused blood. Multiple pregnancies may also expose females to fetal paternal antigens, resulting in antibody formation. Finally, prior transplant recipients may have already formed antibodies to other MHC antigens, so that they may be present at the time of a second transplant. Collectively, these antibodies are formulated into a panel reactive antibody (PRA) score that represents the percentage of the population to which the recipient will likely react. Higher scores are thus associated with longer wait times because it takes longer to find a donor without antibodies. Although extremely rare, hyperacute rejection results in severe cardiac dysfunction and death within hours of transplantation. Assisted MCS until cardiac retransplantation is the only therapeutic option.

VIII. The role of intraoperative transesophageal echocardiography (TEE)

Intraoperative TEE is a valuable tool for the evaluation and management of the cardiac transplant recipient. In addition to monitoring ventricular function, TEE in the pre-CPB period may be used to identify intracavitary thrombus, estimate recipient PA pressures, and evaluate the aortic cannulation and cross-clamp sites for the presence of atherosclerotic disease. TEE may also be used in the post-CPB period to evaluate the efficacy of cardiac de-airing, cardiac function, and surgical anastomoses. The caval veins, left atrium, and pulmonary vein anastomoses should be evaluated for any evidence of obstruction or distortion [41]. Stenosis of the main PA should also be excluded by continuous-wave Doppler measurement of the pressure gradient across the anastomosis. After orthotopic cardiac transplantation, the long axis of the left atrium often appears larger than usual because of joining of the donor and recipient left atria. Occasionally, excess donor atrial tissue may obstruct the mitral valve orifice resulting in pulmonary HTN and RV failure. TEE findings in the immediate post-CPB period frequently include impaired ventricular contractility, decreased diastolic compliance, septal dyskinesis, and acute mild to moderate tricuspid, pulmonic, and mitral valve regurgitation. Although LV size and function is typically normal on long-term echocardiographic follow-up of healthy cardiac transplant recipients, RV enlargement and tricuspid valve regurgitation persist in up to 33% of patients. Persistent tricuspid valve regurgitation may result from geometrical alterations of the right atrium or ventricle, asynchronous contraction of the donor and recipient atria, or valvular damage occurring during EMB.

IX. Cardiac transplantation survival and complications

Survival following cardiac transplantation in the US in 2008–2010 was 89.6%, 82.9%, and 77% at 1, 3, and 5 years, respectively [17]. These figures are consistent across the adult range of ages, except for recipients aged 65 or older (1-year survival of 85%) [17]. Beyond the first-year posttransplant, lower survival was seen in recipients aged 18 to 35, African Americans and in retransplant recipients (5-year survival of 73.8%, 72.2%, and 74.5%, respectively) [17]. Overall, 6-month, 1-, 3-, and 5-year survival after heart transplantation has improved since 2004 (Fig. 17.4). Important causes of morbidity and mortality are infection, acute rejection, graft failure and cardiac allograft vasculopathy (CAV), renal insufficiency (RI) and malignancy. Other causes of long-term morbidity after transplantation include hypertension, diabetes mellitus, and hyperlipidemia.

A. Infection

Infections in the early period (<30 days) are mainly nosocomial and bacterial in nature, and account for 14% of deaths [2]. With the routine use of bacterial and viral prophylaxis, there has been a significant reduction in pneumocystis pneumonia infection and herpesviridae (including CMV) [42]. Beyond 30 days, infection remains an important cause of mortality, reaching its peak as a primary cause of death (32%) from 31 days to 1 year posttransplant [2].

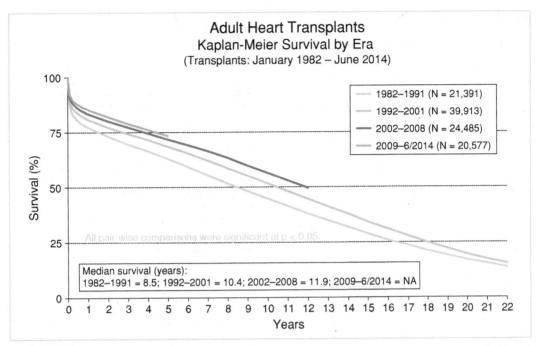

FIGURE 17.4 Survival for adult heart transplants performed between January 1982 and June 2014, stratified by era of transplant. (From Lund LH, Edwards LB, Dipchand AI, et al; International Society for Heart and Lung Transplantation. The registry of the International Society for Heart and Lung Transplantation: thirty-third adult heart transplantation report—2016. *J Heart Lung Transplant*. 2016;35(10):1158–1169.)

B. **Acute rejection**

Improvements in management have rendered acute rejection of the transplanted heart a less common cause of death (9%) between 2009 and 2015 [2]. However, up to 30% of recipients may experience rejection within the first year [17]. Female recipients are at higher risk than males, and the risk of rejection decreases with increasing age of the recipient [17]. EMB remains the gold standard for confirming acute allograft rejection. Repeated EMB is associated with an increased incidence of tricuspid valve regurgitation.

C. **Graft failure and cardiac allograft vasculopathy (CAV)**

Graft failure is the leading cause of death in the first 30 days after transplant (40%), presumably due to primary graft failure [2]. After 30 days, chronic processes such as antibody-mediated rejection and CAV are more likely causes of graft failure. Graft failure continues to be a significant cause of death after 1 year, accounting for 17% of deaths [2]. Graft failure confirmed due to CAV becomes prominent between 1 to 3 years posttransplant, and accounts for 26% of deaths [2]. The prevalence of CAV is 27% at 5 years and 47% at 10 years [2]. Significant CAV is defined angiographically by a stenosis of at least 50%. Unlike atherosclerotic CAD, CAV is characterized by a diffuse intimal hyperplasia [42]. Nonimmune risk factors for CAV include hypertension, hyperlipidemia, diabetes mellitus, explosive etiology of donor brain death, hyperhomocysteinemia, and older donor age. Immune risk factors include HLA donor/recipient mismatch, recurrent cellular rejection, and antibody-mediated rejection (high PRA score). Aggressive management of risk factors is the primary strategy for preventing CAV. The diffuse nature of the vasculopathy defies percutaneous or surgical revascularization strategies.

D. **Renal insufficiency (RI)**

RI is a strong predictor of reduced survival after transplant. Defined as a serum creatinine >2.5 mg/dL, or necessitating dialysis or kidney transplant, severe RI is identified as the primary cause of death in a significant number of patients [43]. Risks for early RI, developing within 1 year of transplant, are increased donor and recipient age, increased recipient

TABLE 17.6 Immunosuppressive agents

Agent	Mechanism of action	Side effects
Cyclosporine	Inhibits T-cell proliferation Inhibits interleukin-2 expression	Nephrotoxicity, hypertension, tremors, headache
Azathioprine	Inhibits DNA synthesis Inhibits lymphocyte proliferation	Leukopenia, thrombocytopenia, anemia, infection, hepatotoxicity, pancreatitis, nausea, vomiting, diarrhea
Corticosteroids	Decreases T-cell activation Inhibit cytokine production Inhibits leukocyte chemotaxis	Infection, hyperglycemia, hypertension, osteoporosis, adrenal suppression, myopathy, peptic ulcer disease, hyperlipidemia, psychological disturbances
Mycophenolate mofetil	Inhibits DNA synthesis Inhibits lymphocyte proliferation	Nausea, abdominal cramps, diarrhea, neutropenia, rarely hepatic and bone marrow toxicity
Tacrolimus (FK506)	Inhibits T-cell activation	Nephrotoxicity, anemia, hyperkalemia, hyperglycemia, hypertension, nausea, vomiting
OKT3	Opsonizes and lyses T cells	Fever, chills, hypotension, bronchospasm, pulmonary edema, aseptic meningitis, seizures, nausea, vomiting, diarrhea
Antilymphocyte globulin	Opsonizes and lyses T cells	Anaphylaxis, leukopenia, thrombocytopenia, hypotension, infection, fever, chills, hepatitis, serum sickness
Rapamycin	Promotes T-cell apoptosis	Abdominal pain; weakness; back pain; headache; upset stomach; swelling of the hands, feet, ankles, or lower legs; joint pain; insomnia; tremor; rash; fever
Basiliximab or Daclizumab	Interleukin-2 receptor (IL2R) blocker inhibits IL-2 dependent T-cell activation	Anaphylaxis, abdominal pain, back pain, fever or chills, loss of energy or weakness, sore throat, vomiting, white patches in the mouth or throat, tremor

serum creatinine at time of transplant, presence of a VAD, female recipient, rapamycin use at discharge, and IL2R-antagonist induction [43]. Fortunately, the incidence of impaired renal function after heart transplant is decreasing, with 86% of patients transplanted between 1994 and 2005 being free of severe renal dysfunction at 5 years [2].

E. **Malignancy**

Presumably as a consequence of long-term immunosuppression, solid-organ transplant recipients experience a higher risk for malignancy than does the general population. Skin cancer is the most common malignancy in heart transplant recipients, with incidence at 1, 5, and 10 years of 1.7%, 9.3%, and 18.1%, respectively [2]. Lymphoproliferative malignancies occur less frequently than do malignancies of the skin, but their treatments are much less likely to be curative. Incidence at 1, 5, and 10 years is 0.5%, 1.1%, and 1.9%, respectively [2]. Mortality attributed to malignancy depends on time after transplant, and is as high as 21% after 10 years [2].

F. **Immunosuppressive drug side effects**

Cardiac transplant recipients require lifelong immunosuppression. Protocols vary among transplant centers; however, most regimens include triple therapy with corticosteroids, a calcineurin inhibitor, and an antiproliferative agent [3]. Immunosuppressants increase the risk of infection and are associated with numerous side effects (Table 17.6) [44]. Furthermore, chronic immunosuppression increases the risk of malignancies including skin cancers; lymphoproliferative malignancies; various adenocarcinomas; cancers of the lung, bladder, kidney, breast, and colon; and Kaposi sarcoma.

X. **Pediatric cardiac transplantation**

In the US in 2015, children accounted for 13% of cardiac transplant recipients [2]. The primary indications for pediatric cardiac transplantation are complex congenital heart disease and idiopathic dilated cardiomyopathy (DCM) [17]. At present, the majority of pediatric heart transplants take place in children >1 year of age at highly specialized pediatric centers [17]. Five-year survival rates for transplant recipients younger than 1 year, ages 1 to 5 years, ages 6 to 10 years, and ages 11 to

17 years are 71.2%, 78.4%, 87.5%, and 77.4%, respectively [17]. Like adult programs, pediatric cardiac transplant programs face a severe donor heart shortage. The use of implantable VADs for bridge-to-transplantation is limited by the small body size of most pediatric transplant candidates, with only 21% of pediatric heart transplant recipients being supported by a VAD [17].

XI. Combined heart–lung transplantation (HLT)

In 2014, only 27 HLTs were done in the US [2]. Donor procurement is of critical importance to the success of the operation, especially with respect to lung preservation. However, current techniques have led to safe procurement with ischemic times up to 6 hours.

The operation is performed using a double- or single-lumen endotracheal tube with the patient in the supine position. The surgical approach is generally through a median sternotomy, with particular emphasis on preservation of the phrenic, vagal, and recurrent laryngeal nerves [45]. After fully heparinizing the recipient, the ascending aorta is cannulated near the base of the innominate artery, and the venae cavae are individually cannulated laterally and snared. CPB with systemic cooling to 28° to 30°C is instituted, and the heart is excised at the midatrial level. The aorta is divided just above the aortic valve, and the PA is divided at its bifurcation. The left atrial remnant is then divided vertically at a point halfway between the right and left pulmonary veins. Following division of the pulmonary ligament, the left lung is moved into the field, allowing full dissection of the posterior aspect of the left hilum, being careful to avoid the vagus nerve posteriorly. After this is completed, the left main PA is divided, and the left main bronchus is stapled and divided. The same technique of hilar dissection and division is repeated on the right side, and both lungs removed from the chest. Meticulous hemostasis of the bronchial vessels is necessary, as this area of dissection is obscured once graft implantation is completed. Once hemostasis is achieved, the trachea is divided at the carina.

The donor heart–lung bloc is removed from its transport container, prepared, and then lowered into the chest, passing the right lung beneath the right phrenic nerve pedicle. The left lung is then gently manipulated under the left phrenic nerve pedicle. The tracheal anastomosis is then performed, and the lungs ventilated with room air at half-normal tidal volumes to inflate the lungs and reduce atelectasis. The heart is then anastomosed as previously described. After separation from CPB, the patient is usually ventilated with a FiO_2 of 40% and PEEP at 3 to 5 cm H_2O, being very careful to avoid high inspiratory pressures that may disrupt the tracheal anastomoses.

XII. Anesthesia for the previously transplanted patient

Many heart transplant recipients will undergo additional surgical procedures in their lifetime. Common surgical procedures following cardiac transplantation are listed in Table 17.7. Many of

TABLE 17.7   Common surgical procedures following cardiac transplantation

Reexploration for mediastinal bleeding
Infectious complications
Laparotomy
Craniotomy
Thoracotomy
Abscess drainage
Bronchoscopy
Steroid-related complications
Hip arthroplasty or pinning
Laparotomy for perforated viscus
Cataract excision
Vitrectomy
Scleral buckle
Aortic or peripheral vascular surgery and amputation
Pancreatic and biliary tract surgery
Retransplantation

these subsequent surgical procedures are attributable to sequelae of the transplant surgery itself, atherosclerosis, and immunosuppression. Optimal anesthetic management of the previous transplant recipient requires full understanding of the patient's ongoing physiology and pharmacology.

A. Physiology of the previously transplanted patient

During orthotopic cardiac transplantation, the cardiac autonomic plexus is transected, leaving the transplanted heart without autonomic innervation [46]. Due to the absence of parasympathetic innervation of the sinoatrial node, the transplanted heart will exhibit a resting HR of 90 to 110 beats/min. In addition, reflex bradycardia does not occur. Increases in HR and SV in response to stress are blunted, as they depend on circulating adrenal hormones. Although most transplanted hearts have near-normal contractility at rest, stress may reveal a reduction in functional reserve. The Starling volume–CO relationship, however, tends to remain intact.

A higher rate of dysrhythmia is seen due to the absence of parasympathetic tone coupled with conduction abnormalities. First-degree atrioventricular block is common, and 30% of patients will have right bundle branch block [46].

B. Pharmacology of the previously transplanted patient

Autonomic denervation of the transplanted heart alters the pharmacodynamic activity of many drugs (Table 17.8). Drugs that mediate their actions through the autonomic nervous system are ineffective in altering HR and contractility. In contrast, drugs that act directly on the heart are effective. The β-adrenergic response of the transplanted heart to direct-acting catecholamines such as epinephrine is often increased. Reflex bradycardia or tachycardia in response to changes in systemic arterial BP is absent. Narcotic-induced decreases in HR are frequently diminished in the transplanted heart. Drugs with mixed activity (e.g., dopamine and ephedrine) will mediate an effect only through their direct actions. Vagolytic drugs such as atropine and glycopyrrolate will not alter HR, although their peripheral anticholinergic activity remains unaffected. Anticholinergic coadministration with reversal of neuromuscular blockade is still warranted to counteract the noncardiac muscarinic effects of neostigmine or edrophonium.

C. Preoperative evaluation

A thorough medical history, physical examination, and review of the medical record should be undertaken. Current medications should be noted. Particular attention should be paid to determining cardiac allograft function, evidence of rejection or infection, complications of immunosuppression, and end-organ disease. Systemic HTN is common and a significant proportion of patients will have CAV within 1 year of cardiac transplantation. The absence of angina pectoris does not exclude significant CAD, because the transplanted heart is denervated. The patient's activity level and exercise tolerance are good indicators of allograft function. Symptoms of dyspnea and HF suggest significant CAD or myocardial rejection.

TABLE 17.8 Drug effects on the denervated heart

Drug	Action	Heart rate	Blood pressure (BP)
Atropine	Indirect	–	–
Digoxin	Direct	–/↓	–
Dopamine	Indirect and Direct	↑	↑
Ephedrine	Indirect and Direct	–/↑	–/↑
Fentanyl	Indirect	–	–
Isoproterenol	Direct	↑	–/↓
Neostigmine	Indirect	–/↓	–
Norepinephrine	Direct	↑	↑
Pancuronium	Indirect	–	–
Phenylephrine	Direct	–	↑
Verapamil	Direct	↓	↓

↑, increased; ↓, decreased; –, no effect.

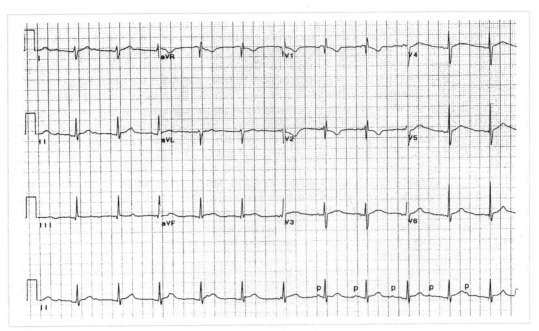

FIGURE 17.5 Transplanted heart electrocardiogram (ECG). The transplanted heart ECG is commonly characterized by two sets of P waves, right-axis deviation, and incomplete right bundle branch block (with biatrial technique). The donor heart P waves are small and precede the QRS complex, whereas P waves originating from the recipient's atria (labeled as *p*) are unrelated to the QRS complex. (From Fowler NO. *Clinical Electrocardiographic Diagnosis*. Philadelphia, PA: Lippincott Williams & Wilkins; 2000:225, with permission.)

The presentation of infection may be atypical in immunosuppressed patients, with fever and leukocytosis often absent. Soft tissue changes in the patient's airway may occur due to lymphoproliferative disease and corticosteroid administration. Cyclosporine may cause gingival hyperplasia and friability. Hematocrit, coagulation profile, electrolytes, and creatinine should be checked, because immunosuppressive therapy is commonly associated with anemia, thrombocytopenia, electrolyte disturbances, and renal dysfunction. Recent chest x-rays, ECGs, and coronary angiograms should be reviewed. More than one P wave may be seen on the ECG in patients in whom cardiac transplantation was performed using a biatrial technique (Fig. 17.5). Although seen on the ECG, the P wave originating in the native atria does not conduct impulses across the anastomotic line.

D. Anesthesia management

1. Clinical implications of immunosuppressive therapy

   All cardiac transplant patients are immunosuppressed and consequently at higher risk of infection. All vascular access procedures should be carried out using aseptic or sterile technique. Antibiotic prophylaxis should be considered for any procedure with the potential to produce bacteremia. Oral immunosuppressive medication should be continued without interruption or given IV to maintain blood levels within the therapeutic range. IV and oral doses of azathioprine are approximately equivalent. Administration of large volumes of IV fluids will decrease blood levels of immunosuppressants, and therefore levels should be checked daily. Immunosuppressant nephrotoxicity may be exacerbated by coadministration of other potentially renal toxic medications such as nonsteroidal anti-inflammatory agents or gentamicin. Chronic corticosteroid therapy to prevent allograft rejection may result in adrenal suppression. Supplemental "stress" steroids should thus be administered to critically ill patients or patients undergoing major surgical procedures.

2. Monitoring

Standard anesthetic monitors should be used, including 5-lead ECG to detect ischemia and dysrhythmias. Cardiac transplant patients frequently have fragile skin and osteoporotic bones secondary to chronic corticosteroid administration. Care with tape, automated BP cuffs, and patient positioning is essential to avoid skin and musculoskeletal trauma. As for all patients undergoing anesthesia, invasive monitoring should only be considered for situations in which the benefits outweigh the risks. Importantly, cardiac transplant patients have an increased risk of developing catheter-related infections with a high associated morbidity and mortality. Intraoperative TEE permits rapid evaluation of volume status, cardiac function and ischemia, and may be a useful substitute for invasive monitoring. Should central venous access be required, alternatives to the right internal jugular vein should be considered to preserve its use for EMB. Careful monitoring of neuromuscular blockade with a peripheral nerve stimulator is recommended in the previously transplanted patient, as cyclosporine may prolong neuromuscular blockade following administration of nondepolarizing neuromuscular blocking agents. In contrast, an attenuated response to nondepolarizing muscle relaxants may be seen in patients receiving azathioprine.

3. Anesthesia techniques

Both general and regional anesthesia techniques have been used safely in cardiac transplant patients. In the absence of significant cardiorespiratory, renal, or hepatic dysfunction, there is no absolute contraindication to any anesthetic technique. For any selected anesthetic technique, maintenance of ventricular filling pressures is essential, as the transplanted heart increases CO primarily by increasing SV.

a. General anesthesia

General anesthesia is frequently preferred over regional anesthesia for cardiac transplant patients, as alterations in myocardial preload and afterload may be more predictable. Cyclosporine and tacrolimus decrease renal blood flow and glomerular filtration via thromboxane-mediated renal vasoconstriction. Thus, renally excreted anesthetics and muscle relaxants should be used with caution in patients receiving these medications. Cyclosporine and tacrolimus also lower the seizure threshold, hence hyperventilation should be avoided. Elevations in the resting HR and a delayed sympathetic response to noxious stimuli in cardiac transplant recipients may make anesthetic depth difficult to assess.

b. Regional anesthesia

Many immunosuppressants cause thrombocytopenia and alter the coagulation profile. Both the platelet count and coagulation profile should be within normal limits if spinal or epidural regional anesthesia is planned. Ventricular filling pressures should be maintained following induction of central neural axis blockade to prevent hypotension caused by the delayed response of the denervated, transplanted heart to a rapid decrease in sympathetic tone. Volume loading, ventricular filling pressure monitoring, and careful titration of local anesthetic agents may avoid hemodynamic instability. Hypotension should be treated with vasopressors that directly stimulate their target receptors.

4. Blood transfusion

The cardiac transplant recipient is at increased risk for blood product transfusion complications. Adverse reactions include infection, graft-versus-host disease, and immunomodulation. Use of irradiated, leukocyte-depleted, CMV-negative blood products and white blood cell filters for blood product administration reduces the incidence of adverse transfusion reactions. The blood bank should receive early notification if the use of blood products is anticipated, because the presence of reactive antibodies delaying cross-match is not infrequent.

E. **Pregnancy following cardiac transplantation**

Despite an increased incidence of preeclampsia and preterm labor, increasing numbers of cardiac transplant recipients are successfully carrying pregnancies to term. In general, the transplanted heart is able to adapt to the physiologic changes of pregnancy. Due to an increased sensitivity to the β-adrenergic effects of tocolytics such as terbutaline and ritodrine, use of alternative drugs such as magnesium and nifedipine may be considered. Although pregnancy does not adversely affect cardiac allografts, the risk of acute cardiac allograft rejection may be increased postpartum. All immunosuppressive drugs used to prevent cardiac allograft rejection cross the placenta, though most are not thought to be teratogenic.

XIII. **Future directions**

As medical management of HF continues to improve, a patient's need for definitive therapy with heart transplantation may become delayed or diminished. Based on trends over the previous decade, it is to be expected that patients who do present for heart transplant will have an increasing number and severity of comorbidities [3]. The emerging role of MCS devices for destination therapy will also affect future developments in heart transplantation [1]. Intensive investigation into the use of stem cells and bioengineered organs may someday obviate the current organ shortage. Continuing advances in our understanding of mechanisms of rejection are likely to improve immunomodulation and delay graft failure. Improvements in surveillance, such as intravascular ultrasound, may eliminate the need for routine EMB. For the immediate future, however, heart transplantation continues to offer patients with advanced HF their best opportunity for a better quality and length of life.

PART II: LUNG TRANSPLANTATION

KEY POINTS

6. End-stage pulmonary disease (ESPD) is one of the five leading causes of mortality and morbidity in adults in the US. ESPD results from destruction of the pulmonary parenchyma and vasculature. Lung transplantation is the definitive treatment for these patients.

7. Due to a severe shortage of suitable donor lungs, other therapeutic options were developed that may offer alternatives to those patients who otherwise might succumb to their disease while awaiting lung transplantation.

8. For those patients with ESPD who develop cardiogenic shock due to right ventricular (RV) failure or worsening respiratory failure (hypoxia, hypercarbia, and acidosis), bridging to transplantation may be a consideration (e.g., extracorporeal membrane oxygenation [ECMO], Novalung, or Decap).

9. Because the number of lung transplant recipients far exceeds the number of suitable lung donors, up to one-third of recipients die while awaiting transplantation. Recently, improvements to the method for allocation of lungs have served to decrease recipient waiting time for transplantation.

10. Depending on the patient's pathophysiology, there are several surgical options: single-lung transplantation (SLT), bilateral sequential lung transplantation (BSLT), en bloc double-lung transplantation (DbLT), heart–lung transplantation (HLT), and living-related lobar transplantation (LRT).

6 End-stage pulmonary disease (ESPD) is one of the five leading causes of mortality and morbidity in adults in US. ESPD results from destruction of the pulmonary parenchyma and vasculature. Lung transplantation is the definitive treatment for these patients. Depending on the patient's pathophysiology, there are several surgical options: single-lung transplantation (SLT), bilateral sequential lung transplantation (BSLT), en bloc double-lung transplantation (DbLT), heart–lung transplantation (HLT), and living-related lobar transplantation (LRT). Prior to 1989, the most common type of lung transplant was combined HLT. Currently BSLT has become the most common approach. Due to a severe shortage of suitable donor lungs, other therapeutic 7 options were developed that may offer alternatives to those patients who otherwise might succumb to their disease while awaiting lung transplantation. Several improvements in the management of a highly selected group of patients with emphysema via lung volume reduction surgery (LVRS), patients with cystic fibrosis (CF) via newer antibiotic agents, and patients with pulmonary hypertension via long-term prostacyclin therapy have been reported as viable options. Likewise, for those patients with ESPD who develop cardiogenic shock due to right ventricular (RV) failure or worsening respiratory failure (hypoxia, hypercarbia, and

8   acidosis), bridging to transplantation may be a consideration (e.g., extracorporeal membrane oxygenation [ECMO], Novalung, or Decap).

XIV. Lung transplantation

A. Epidemiology

1. **Total candidates.** In the US, there are in excess of one million potential lung transplant recipients among those suffering from ESPD.

2. **Survival of candidates.** Because the number of lung transplant recipients far exceeds the number of suitable lung donors, up to one-third of recipients die while awaiting transplantation. Recently, improvements to the method for allocation of lungs have decreased recipient waiting time for transplantation. In May 2005, the lung allocation score (LAS) was adopted in the US [47]. This system is based on the severity of the recipient's disease coupled with medical urgency for transplantation. The LAS attempts to balance the risk of death while awaiting transplantation with posttransplant survival. Since the LAS has been implemented, the total number of recipients on the waiting list has decreased by 50% and the total waiting time has also decreased from a median of 792 days in 2004 to 200 days or less during the time period of 2005 to 2008 [48]. Statistics from August 2017 indicate that there are 1,763 lung recipients and 40 heart–lung recipients awaiting transplantation (Organ Procurement and Transplantation Network, https://optn. transplant.hrsa.gov/data).

3. **Total procedures.** According to the most recent data supplied by the International Society of Heart and Lung Transplant (ISHLT) Registry, a total of 55,795 lung transplants and 3,879 HLT have been performed through June 30, 2015 [49].

B. Pathophysiology of end-stage pulmonary disease (ESPD)

1. **Parenchymal ESPD** is classified as obstructive, restrictive, or infectious.

    a. **Obstructive diseases** are characterized by elevation of airway resistance, diminished expiratory flow rates, severe V/Q mismatching, and pronounced air trapping. The most common cause is smoking-induced emphysema; however, other causes include asthma and several comparatively rare congenital disorders. Among these, α_1-antitrypsin deficiency is associated with severe bullous emphysema that manifests in the fourth or fifth decade of life.

    b. **Restrictive diseases** are characterized by interstitial fibrosis that results in a loss of lung elasticity and compliance. Most fibrotic processes are idiopathic in nature but they may also be caused by an immune mechanism or inhalation injury. Interstitial lung diseases may affect the pulmonary vasculature as well; therefore, pulmonary hypertension is frequently present. Functionally, diseases in this category are associated with diminished lung volumes and diffusion capacities, albeit with preserved airflow rates. Respiratory muscle strength is usually adequate because of the increased work of breathing experienced by this patient population.

    c. The common **infectious etiologic factors** are associated with CF and bronchiectasis.

        (1) CF produces mucous plugging of peripheral airways leading to the development of pneumonia, chronic bronchitis, and bronchiectasis. The incidence of CF is 0.2% of live births in US.

        (2) Smoking, α_1-antitrypsin deficiency, and environmental exposures may lead to the development of bronchiectasis.

2. **Etiologic factors of end-stage pulmonary vascular diseases** are (a) diffuse arteriovenous malformations, (b) congenital heart disease with Eisenmenger syndrome, or (c) pulmonary arterial hypertension (PAH). PAH is rare and most frequently idiopathic. It is characterized by marked elevation of pulmonary vascular resistance (PVR) secondary to hyperplasia of the muscular pulmonary arteries combined with fibrosis and obliteration of the smallest arterioles.

C. Recipient selection criteria: Indications and contraindications

1. **Recipient selection criteria and indications** for lung transplantation are listed in Table 17.9 [50]. Referral and listing of potential candidates are based on the progression of the patient's disease along with their risk of death on the waiting list balanced with the likelihood of survival

TABLE 17.9 Indications and contraindications for lung transplantation[a]

Indications
  High (>50%) risk of death from lung disease within 2 yrs if lung transplantation is not performed
  High (>80%) likelihood of surviving at least 90 days after lung transplantation
  High (>80%) likelihood of 5-year posttransplant survival from a general medical perspective provided that there is
    adequate graft function

Relative contraindications
  Age >65 yrs in association with low physiologic reserve or other contraindication
  Critical or unstable clinical conditions (e.g., shock, mechanical ventilation, or ECMO)
  Progressive or severe malnutrition
  Extensive prior chest surgery with lung resection
  Colonization with highly resistant or virulent bacteria, fungi, or mycobacteria
  Class I obesity defined as a BMI >30 kg/m^2
  Severe or symptomatic osteoporosis
  Atherosclerotic disease burden sufficient to put the candidate at risk for end-organ disease after lung
    transplantation
  Other medical conditions not resulting in end-organ damage (e.g., diabetes mellitus, systemic hypertension,
    epilepsy, central venous obstruction, peptic ulcer disease, or gastroesophageal reflux) should be optimally
    treated prior to transplantation

Absolute contraindications
  Untreatable advanced dysfunction of another major organ system (e.g., heart, liver, kidney, or brain)
  Active malignancy within the previous 2 yrs
  Uncorrected atherosclerotic disease with suspected or confirmed end-organ ischemia or dysfunction and/or CAD
    not amenable to revascularization
  Acute medical instability, including acute sepsis, myocardial infarction, and liver failure
  Uncorrectable bleeding diathesis
  Noncurable chronic extrapulmonary infection
  Chronic active viral hepatitis B, hepatitis C, and HIV
  Significant chest wall/spinal deformity
  Class II or III obesity (BMI ≥35 kg/m^2)
  Documented nonadherence or inability to follow through with medical therapy, office follow-up, or both
  Untreatable psychiatric or psychologic condition associated with inability to cooperate or comply with medical
    therapy
  Absence of a consistent or reliable social support system
  Substance addiction (e.g., alcohol, tobacco, or narcotics) active either currently or within the previous 6 mo

[a]Weill D, Benden C, Corris PA, et al. A consensus document for the selection of lung transplant candidates: 2014-an update from the Pulmonary Transplantation Council of the International Society for Heart and Lung Transplantation. *J Heart Lung Transplant.* 2015;34:1–15.
ECMO, extracorporeal membrane oxygenation; BMI, body mass index; CAD, coronary artery disease; HIV, human immunodeficiency virus.

after transplantation; however, each patient must be considered on an individual basis and subjected to standardized selection criteria.

2. **Relative and absolute contraindications** to lung transplantation are listed in Table 17.9. Although candidates for organ transplantation frequently have abnormal physical or laboratory findings, such information must be distinguished from concurrent primary organ failure or a systemic disease that otherwise might disqualify candidacy. The relative contraindications to lung transplant have changed as improvements in the medical management of potential recipients have evolved. For example, coronary artery disease (CAD), previous CABG and corticosteroid usage, once absolute contraindications, are now not prohibitive, particularly if left ventricular (LV) function is preserved and corticosteroid doses are moderate [51,52]. Another highly controversial and debated issue is the transplantation of patients with multiple or pan-resistant bacteria, in particular, patients with CF who concurrently have been diagnosed with *Burkholderia cepacia* [53]. Although the international guidelines do not regard the presence of *B. cepacia* as an absolute contraindication to lung transplantation, there are multiple transplant centers that limit organ allocation and treatment in these patients. It has been reported in the literature that triple antimicrobial therapy can be bactericidal toward multiresistant *B. cepacia* [54,55]. Ultimately, the decision to transplant

CF patients with this microbe rests with each transplant center, because the previous data indicate a much higher incidence of preoperative and postoperative morbidity and mortality in this population.

D. Medical evaluation of lung transplant candidates

All candidates are systematically evaluated by history, physical examination, and laboratory studies. Additionally, pretransplant evaluation includes chest radiographs, computerized tomography (CT) scans, arterial blood gas (ABG) values, spirometric and respiratory flow studies, ventilation and perfusion scanning, 6-minute walk test, right heart catheterization, and echocardiography. On the basis of studies of the natural history of ESPD, specific laboratory criteria for referral to most lung transplantation programs that depend on the specific underlying disease have been developed (e.g., cardiac index less than 2 L/min/m^2 in patients with PAH and FEV$_1$ less than 30% predicted in patients with COPD or CF). Most centers provide documentation of the evaluation results on a summary sheet that is readily available to the anesthesiology team on short notice.

E. Choice of lung transplant procedure

Choice of lung transplant procedure is based upon (a) the consequences of leaving a native lung in situ; (b) the procedure most likely to yield the best functional outcome for a given pathophysiologic process; and (c) the relative incidence of perioperative complications associated with a particular procedure. Currently, the vast majority of lung transplants are performed using the BSLT technique.

1. **SLT**

   a. SLT can be selected for transplant recipients with noninfectious lung pathophysiology. SLT is a frequent option for older patients with end-stage pulmonary fibrosis or emphysema, as it poses a lower perioperative risk [56]; however, in patients with severe bullous emphysema, SLT may exacerbate native lung hyperinflation and result in severe acute and/or chronic allograft compromise secondary to compression atelectasis. Preoperative measurement of the recipient static lung compliance has been suggested as a screening technique to determine whether SLT alone, SLT plus LVRS, or BSLT is most beneficial.

   b. SLT offers several advantages over the less frequently used en bloc DbLT: (a) SLT may extend the limited supply of donor organs to more patients but has less functional reserve as a buffer for complications. It is also associated with a worse outcome [49]; (b) SLT is feasible in many patients without the use of cardiopulmonary bypass (CPB), so complications arising from coagulopathic states are less frequent; and (c) bronchial anastamoses used in SLT show a decreased rate of dehiscence compared to tracheal anastomosis used for en bloc DbLT.

   c. SLT involves pneumonectomy and implantation of the lung allograft. The choice of the native lung to be extracted is determined preoperatively. The lung with the poorest pulmonary function as delineated by V/Q scanning is generally chosen for replacement by the allograft. If the native lungs are equally impaired and pleural scarring is absent, the left lung is chosen for relative technical simplicity:

      (1) The native left pulmonary veins are more accessible than those on the right.

      (2) The left hemithorax can more easily accommodate an oversized donor lung.

      (3) The recipient's left main stem bronchus is longer.

2. **BSLT**

   a. Since 1996, there has been a proportional increase in adult BSLT for every major indication for lung transplantation except for CF (which remains essentially a 100% indication for BSLT) and in 2015 it accounted for 78% of lung transplant procedures [49].

   b. While SLT is still performed frequently for end-stage IPF and emphysema in older recipients (>65 years of age), BSLT is also increasingly utilized for these conditions. Between 1996 and 2015, the share of BSLT for these conditions almost doubled [50].

   c. BSLT is the procedure of choice for septic lung disease (e.g., generalized bronchiectasis), CF, young patients with COPD, and PAH. In contrast to en bloc DbLT, the BSLT procedure offers several advantages: (a) it permits two lungs to be implanted without CPB; (b) it decreases the incidence of bronchial anastomotic complications; and (c) it is less technically difficult.

    d. In some instances, BSLT may lead to better functional outcomes in the treatment of end-stage pulmonary hypertension.

3. HLT

    a. The indications for HLT are diminishing as experience with isolated lung transplantation evolves. The latter operation will suffice in most cases when it is performed before irreversible heart failure (HF) occurs or in concert with intracardiac repair of simple congenital defects. The total number of centers performing HLT has increased from 37 in 2003 to 177 in 2015 due to the addition of reporting centers to the ISHLT Registry. Participating centers reported a total of 58 adult and pediatric HLT for calendar year 2015 [49].

    b. HLT is **indicated** for patients with ESPD complicated by irreversible HF or end-stage congenital heart disease with secondary pulmonary vascular involvement (Eisenmenger syndrome). Specific pathologic diagnoses in recipients include idiopathic PAH, COPD/emphysema with right heart failure, acquired heart disease, CF, and fibrotic and granulomatous diseases of the lung. Congenital heart disease and PAH remain the main indications for adult HLT [49].

4. Living-related donor lobar transplantation

    a. As of May 2006, 243 living-donor lobar transplants have been performed in US. Although outcomes in adult recipients are similar to cadaveric transplants, results in the pediatric recipient population are reported to be superior to those who receive cadaveric allografts [57,58]. Improved function and a decrease in the incidence of bronchiolitis obliterans have been noted. Despite these findings, LRT is rarely performed.

    b. Although lobar donation is considered to be a relatively safe procedure, one group noted a 61% postoperative complication rate in the living donors. Complications included pleural effusions, bronchial stump fistulas, phrenic nerve injury, and bronchial strictures.

F. Selection criteria for donor lungs

    1. Suitable lung allografts are characterized by **PaO_2 greater than 300 mm Hg during mechanical ventilation with FiO_2 of 1.0 and positive end-expiratory pressure (PEEP) of 5 cm H_2O; ABO compatibility; no chest trauma or cardiopulmonary surgery; no aspiration sepsis; negative Gram stain sputum; no purulent secretions.**

    2. The donor **ideally should be younger than 55 years old with either no smoking history or one of 20 pack-years or less** [59].

    3. **Extended donor criteria:** age >55 years; compatible nonidentical ABO group; chest x-ray with focal or unilateral abnormality; PaO_2 <300 mm Hg during mechanical ventilation with FiO_2 1.0 and PEEP of 5 cm H_2O; smoking history >20 pack-years; absence of extensive chest trauma; prior cardiopulmonary surgery; secretions in upper airways; positive serology (e.g., hepatitis B or C) [60].

    4. In an attempt to provide a larger pool of suitable lung donors, the lungs from **non–heart-beating donors** (donation after cardiac death) have been transplanted and reported to produce a successful recipient outcome [61].

    5. As experience in the field of genetic therapy continues to grow, **cytokine profiling** has become an important method to identify organs suitable for donation and transplantation. Fisher et al. [62] reported that elevated levels of interleukin-8 in donor lungs were associated with early graft failure and decreased recipient survival. These data suggest that cytokine profiles could be an early indicator of recipient outcome.

    6. **Procurement procedure.** Because both the heart and lungs are often harvested from the same donor for different recipients, a method has been developed to perform cardiectomy and reduce the risk of lung injury. During cardiectomy, a residual atrial cuff is left attached to the donor lungs. The trachea is stapled and divided at its midpoint, and the lungs are removed en bloc. Subsequently, the pulmonary vasculature is flushed and immersed in a hypothermic preservative (most commonly Euro-Collins or University of Wisconsin solution ± prostaglandin E1 [PGE1]).

    7. **Lung allograft preservation**

        a. There are several relevant issues surrounding donor lung preservation; however, all focus on methods to provide ready sources of energy and cryoprotection and to prevent vasospasm, cellular swelling, and accumulation of toxic metabolites. For example, free radical scavengers such as superoxide dismutase and catalase can be added to prevent oxygen-derived free radicals from damaging key intracellular constituents after reperfusion, and PGE1 can be added to promote uniform cooling and distribution of preservative solutions.

b. **Standard preservation techniques allow a reported maximum allograft ischemic time of 6 to 8 hours; however, ischemic times of 10 to 12 hours may be tolerated depending on the preservative solution.**

c. Normothermic ex vivo lung perfusion (EVLP) is a newer preservation technique aimed at reconditioning and improving the function of marginal donor lungs. The harvested donor lung is perfused in an ex vivo circuit using an acellular normothermic perfusate while they are ventilated at body temperature to mimic physiologic conditions. Cypel et al. [63] demonstrated that transplantation of high-risk donor lungs that were physiologically stable during 4 hours of EVLP had a lower incidence of primary graft dysfunction 72 hours posttransplant compared with controls.

8. **Clinical immunology of organ matching.** ABO matching is essential before transplantation, because the donor-specific major blood group isoagglutinins have been implicated as a cause of allograft hyperacute rejection. Once procured, the practical matter of a 6- to 8-hour donor lung ischemic time limit severely restricts prospective matching of histocompatibility antigens, panel reactive antibody (PRA) screens, and the geography of organ donation. One study suggests that the total ischemic time alone does not predict a poor outcome after transplantation. Rather, the additive effect of increased donor age (older than 55 years) plus increased ischemic allograft time (more than 6 to 7 hours) is a more reliable indicator of poor posttransplant survival [64].

G. **Preanesthetic considerations**

1. Because of a chronic shortage of suitable lungs available for transplantation, many patients experience long waiting periods ranging from several months to several years. **Interval changes** may occur since completion of the initial medical evaluation. Specifically, reduction in exercise tolerance; new drug regimens or requirements for oxygen and steroids; appearance of purulent sputum; signs or symptoms indicative of right HF (e.g., hepatomegaly, peripheral edema); or presence of fever are among the most common occurrences that should be explored in the immediate preoperative period.

2. Lung transplants are always performed as emergency procedures because of the relatively short safe ischemic time for allografts. As is customary for any emergent surgical procedure, the time of **last oral intake** should be ascertained before induction of general anesthesia.

3. Patients undergoing lung transplantation may exhibit signs and symptoms of anxiety. They usually have not received the benefit of anxiolytic **premedication** before their arrival in the operating room. One should be vigilant when administering anxiolytic agents to these patients so that their impaired respiratory drive is not further compromised.

CLINICAL PEARL One should be vigilant when administering anxiolytic agents to lung transplant recipients so that their impaired respiratory drive is not further compromised.

4. Insertion of a **thoracic epidural catheter** for both intraoperative and postoperative analgesia may be performed before induction of general anesthesia. The catheter should be inserted at a spinal level that provides appropriate anesthesia and analgesia in concordance with the surgical incision site (e.g., T-4 to T-5 or T-5 to T-6) [65]. Alternatively, bilateral paravertebral catheters may be inserted. Placement of a thoracic epidural catheter or bilateral paravertebral catheters when anticoagulation is anticipated for CPB remains controversial.

CLINICAL PEARL Regional anesthesia is an option for perioperative analgesia that may be performed prior to induction of general anesthesia. A thoracic epidural catheter or bilateral paravertebral catheters may be used for this purpose. Placement of these catheters remains controversial when anticoagulation is anticipated for the use of CPB in lung transplantation.

5. Chronically cyanotic patients are frequently severely polycythemic (hematocrit greater than 60%) and may manifest clotting abnormalities. In these instances, phlebotomy and hemodilution may be beneficial in minimizing the occurrence of end-organ infarction.

6. **Size matching** between donor and recipient is facilitated by comparing the vertical and transverse radiologic chest dimensions of the donor and recipient. Organs are also matched on the basis of ABO compatibility, because the value of histocompatibility matching is still unknown and requires time in excess of the tolerable ischemic time for the lung allograft.

7. Some **transfusion practices** are specific for transplantation. For example, CMV seronegative blood products must be available for seronegative recipients if CMV sepsis is to be avoided. When transplantation of CMV-negative donors and recipients occurs, leukocyte filters are used to reduce exposure to CMV during transfusion of blood and blood products. Likewise, if human leukocyte antigen alloimmunization is to be avoided, leukocyte-reduced blood is necessary for transplant candidates, particularly if they require transfusion before organ transplantation.

8. Close **coordination and effective communication** between the transplant team and the organ harvesting team is vital so that excess allograft ischemic time is avoided.

9. Arrangements should be made for intraoperative availability of a multimodality ventilator for patients with the most severe forms of lung disease. Useful **ventilator settings** include the ability to deliver minute volumes greater than 15 L/min (especially helpful if airway leaks are present); adjustable inflation pressure "pop-offs" (to allow high inflation pressures to be delivered to noncompliant lungs); adjustable respiratory cycle waveforms; and availability of high levels of PEEP (e.g., 15 to 20 cm H_2O during reperfusion pulmonary edema).

10. iNO and inhaled nebulized prostacyclin have been proven effective for treatment of pulmonary hypertension and early reperfusion injury in some patients.

CLINICAL PEARL iNO and inhaled nebulized prostacyclin have been proven effective for treatment of pulmonary hypertension and early reperfusion injury in some patients.

H. **Induction and maintenance of anesthesia**

1. **Preoperative laboratory studies.** These studies are useful to predict difficulties during the induction of general anesthesia. For example, air trapping and diminished expiratory flow rates may exacerbate hypercapnia and lead to hemodynamic instability during mask ventilation and after endotracheal intubation. Elevated pulmonary artery (PA) pressures may indicate the likelihood that CPB may be necessary.

2. **Intraoperative monitoring**

   a. Both **systemic and PA pressure monitoring** are essential during lung transplant procedures. Dyspnea, arrhythmias, RV dilation, and pulmonary hypertension may complicate PA catheter insertion before induction of general anesthesia. Oximetric PA catheters are useful in this setting to evaluate tissue oxygen delivery in patients who are subject to sudden cardiac instability. Some suggest that RV ejection fraction catheters may be useful for the diagnosis of right HF. Radial arterial cannulation with or without femoral artery cannulation is appropriate for monitoring of systemic arterial blood pressure. Femoral arterial catheters may interfere with groin cannulation for CPB; however, they can also serve as a means of quick access should VA ECMO be required.

   b. **Pulse oximetry** is especially useful for continuous monitoring of SpO_2 during stressful intervals, such as the onset of one lung ventilation (OLV) or cross-clamping of the PA.

   c. Near infrared reflectance spectroscopy (NIRS) monitoring has proven very useful in monitoring the adequacy of cerebral oxygenation during both ECMO and CPB as well as in detecting lower limb ischemia related to femoral cannulation.

   d. Transesophageal echocardiography (TEE) is perhaps the most useful monitor available. TEE allows for (a) direct visualization of RV and LV wall motion and function as well as assessment of intracardiac valvular function; (b) assessment of PA and pulmonary vein anastomoses and blood flow; (c) assessment of the elimination of intracardiac air that occurs during pulmonary venous anastomosis; and (d) calculation of PA pressure as measured by color Doppler flow velocity.

> **CLINICAL PEARL** TEE is perhaps the most useful monitor available. TEE allows for (a) direct visualization of RV and LV wall motion and function as well as assessment of intracardiac valvular function; (b) assessment of PA and pulmonary vein anastomoses and blood flow; (c) assessment of the elimination of intracardiac air that occurs during pulmonary venous anastomosis; and (d) calculation of PA pressure as measured by color Doppler flow velocity.

3. **Intravenous (IV) access.** Large-caliber IV catheters inserted peripherally and centrally (e.g., 14-gauge peripheral IV; 8.5- to 9.0-Fr central venous introducer), supplemented by a rapid infusion device, are essential for lung transplant operations in which massive transfusion requirements are anticipated (e.g., HLT for congenital heart disease with Eisenmenger syndrome; BSLT for CF with pleural scarring). For patients with significant PAH and RV dysfunction, preinduction femoral vascular access for rapid cannulation for ECMO or CPB should be considered.

4. **Positioning.** Full lateral decubitus position is typically used during SLT, even when CPB is anticipated (e.g., SLT for PPH). One groin is usually prepped into the field to allow for the option of femoral cannula insertion for CPB. The supine position is used for BSLT, facilitating either median sternotomy, clamshell incision, or bilateral anterior thoracotomy incision.

5. **"Pump standby."** This safeguard is prudent for patients with pulmonary hypertension or borderline ABG values, even when SLT is planned.

6. **Selection of anesthetic agents**
   a. Agents that promote hemodynamic homeostasis are preferred for induction of general anesthesia. One example is etomidate and a nondepolarizing neuromuscular blocking agent such as rocuronium, which may be used during a modified rapid sequence induction technique. Modest amounts of fentanyl (5 to 10 μg/kg) administered IV may be used if indicated to control cardiovascular responses to endotracheal intubation.
   b. If early postoperative extubation is not planned, we recommend maintenance of anesthesia using high doses of opioids (e.g., fentanyl 20 to 75 μg/kg) supplemented with low doses of a potent inhaled agent (e.g., isoflurane 0.2% to 0.6%) and a neuromuscular blocking agent. **Thoracic Epidural Anesthesia**, in addition to providing excellent postoperative analgesia, may be used to enhance general anesthesia intraoperatively. Continuous infusion of a local anesthetic, such as 0.2% to 0.5% ropivacaine, provides ideal surgical anesthesia and analgesia and allows for reduced doses of both IV opioids and inhaled agents.
   c. **Nitrous oxide** is generally avoided for the following reasons: (a) 100% oxygen is almost always required to maintain an acceptable arterial saturation during OLV; (b) bullae may expand and compress the residual normal lung parenchyma, thus exacerbating V/Q mismatching; and (c) occult pneumothoraces may occur.

7. **Securing the airway.** Lung isolation is required for optimal surgical exposure. Both double-lumen endobronchial tubes (EBTs) and bronchial blockers are useful for this purpose. A general discussion of these choices is provided in Chapter 15.
   a. Advantages of double-lumen EBTs in the setting of lung transplantation include the following:
      (1) Facilitation of lung isolation
      (2) Ability to suction the nonventilated lung
      (3) Ability to apply CPAP to the nonventilated lung
      (4) Provision for postoperative independent lung ventilation
   b. Left-sided EBTs (e.g., Broncho-Cath) are recommended for both right and left SLTs as well as for BSLT (right-sided DLTs are still used for left SLT in some centers). There is a

higher incidence of right upper lobe obstruction when right-sided double-lumen EBTs are used, because the right upper lobe orifice is relatively close to the right main stem bronchus.

c. **Selecting the correct size of EBT.** In general, the largest-sized EBT that can be placed without causing airway trauma is preferred to facilitate therapeutic flexible bronchoscopy both intraoperatively and postoperatively. This is typically 39 Fr for a male and 37 Fr for a female recipient. CF patients are generally of lesser build and may require a 35-Fr EBT.

d. Many lung transplant recipients have limited pulmonary reserve, and desaturation during intubation may occur rapidly. Therefore, **initial EBT positioning** can be accomplished quickly and accurately with the aid of a flexible FOB.

> **CLINICAL PEARL**   Many lung transplant recipients have limited pulmonary reserve, and desaturation during intubation may occur rapidly. Therefore, initial EBT positioning can be accomplished quickly and accurately with the aid of a flexible FOB.

8. **Management of ventilation**
   a. **Lateral decubitus positioning** may be associated with significant alterations in oxygenation and ventilation, depending on the underlying pulmonary pathophysiology. Positional improvement or deterioration in blood gas values is sometimes predictable on the basis of the patient's preoperative V/Q scan.
   b. General strategies for supporting oxygenation during OLV (i.e., during SLT and BSLT) are discussed in Chapter 15.
   c. Alteration of the inspired to expired ratios during mechanical ventilation may be useful during SLT in patients with emphysema. Increasing the expiratory time during each respiratory cycle allows for adequate exhalation, thus reducing the possibility of overinflation of the native lung (breath stacking) and subsequent compromise of the allograft.
   d. Similarly, **independent or differential ventilation** is often used during SLT for emphysema recipients, particularly those with gross V/Q mismatching.
   e. After allograft implantation, **the lowest possible FiO$_2$** to maintain adequate oxygenation is used in concert with **10 cm H$_2$O PEEP**. In patients with emphysema, independent lung ventilation allows PEEP to be selectively delivered to the allograft and avoid air trapping and overinflation of the native lung.
   f. Frequent **suctioning and lavage** via **flexible FOB** is helpful to maintain airway patency during BSLT for CF or whenever airway bleeding and secretions are sufficient to cause obstruction and impair gas exchange.

I. **Surgical procedures and anesthesia-related interventions**
   1. **Surgical dissection** may be complicated by extensive pleural adhesions, vascular anomalies, vascular collaterals, or previous cardiac or thoracic surgery.
   2. **OLV** is almost always used during lung transplantation to facilitate dissection. With the onset of OLV, acute deterioration in gas exchange and hemodynamics must be anticipated. Strategies for improving oxygenation under these circumstances include the following:
      a. PEEP applied to the nonoperative (ventilated) lung provided that bullous disease or emphysema is absent
      b. CPAP or high-frequency jet ventilation in the operative (nonventilated) lung
      c. Ligation of the branch PA of the operative lung
      d. Initiation of mechanical circulatory support
   3. **Clamping the branch PA** when PA pressures are low is usually well tolerated and improves V/Q matching and ABG values. If elevated PA pressures exacerbate right HF, vasodilators and inotropes may improve systemic hemodynamics; however, gas exchange may be further impaired, depending on the agents that are selected (e.g., sodium nitroprusside may worsen V/Q mismatching). Should the patient's condition deteriorate despite pharmacologic intervention, implementation of CPB or ECMO should be considered.

4. Immediately before implantation of the donor lung, the donor hilar structures are trimmed to match the size of the recipient bronchus, branch PA, and atrial cuff containing the pulmonary venous orifices. While the allograft is kept scrupulously cold, the bronchial anastomoses, atrial cuff, and PA anastomoses are completed in sequence.

5. The **ischemic interval** ends with the removal of vascular clamps, but until ventilation is restored, systemic arterial saturation remains unchanged. Immediately before vascular unclamping, **methylprednisolone** (250 to 500 mg) is administered IV to minimize the potential for hyperacute allograft rejection. Reperfusion may be associated with systemic hypotension due to circulation of vasoactive substances requiring preemptive adjustment of hemodynamic support.

6. **Reinflation of the allograft** follows, sometimes with the aid of a flexible FOB to clear airway secretions. This procedure allows for direct viewing of the airway anastomosis to ensure patency.

7. After SLT for emphysema, independent lung ventilation can be instituted if indicated using the anesthesia ventilator for the native lung (increased expiratory time, low tidal volume, no PEEP) and an intensive care unit–quality ventilator for the allograft (increased respiratory rates, low tidal volumes of 5 to 7 mL/kg, 10 cm H_2O PEEP, and FiO_2 ≤0.3).

8. **Reperfusion injury**, characterized by increasing alveolar–arterial gradients, deteriorating compliance, and gross pulmonary edema, may follow allograft reperfusion within minutes to hours. The most effective treatments are PEEP and strict limitation of volume infusion, both crystalloid and colloid. Rarely, reperfusion injury may be accompanied by pulmonary hypertension. Inhaled NO (40 to 80 ppm) has been the agent of choice in this instance; however, inhaled prostacyclin has also been effective in decreasing PA pressure [39]. If evidence of right HF occurs, continuous IV infusion of norepinephrine (0.05 to 0.2 µg/kg/min), milrinone (0.375 to 0.5 µg/kg/min), or a combination of the two may prove efficacious.

> **CLINICAL PEARL** The most effective treatments for reperfusion injury are PEEP and strict limitation of volume infusion, both crystalloid and colloid. Rarely, reperfusion injury may be accompanied by pulmonary hypertension. Inhaled NO (40 to 80 ppm) has been the agent of choice in this instance; however, inhaled prostacyclin has also been effective in decreasing PA pressure.

9. At the conclusion of surgery, the EBT can be exchanged for a standard single-lumen ETT or retained for independent lung ventilation in the intensive care unit (ICU).

10. **BSLT** is used to treat the same spectrum of patients as those previously treated by the en bloc DbLT procedure. BSLT is the preferred technique in many centers. BSLT can often be accomplished without the use of CPB. Its major disadvantage is that serial implantation prolongs the ischemic time for the second allograft lung.

J. **Postoperative management and complications**

1. The immediate priorities are acute, intensive **respiratory and cardiovascular support**.

   a. Early **respiratory insufficiency** is usually due to reperfusion injury, which is characterized by large alveolar–arterial O_2 gradients, poor pulmonary compliance, and parenchymal infiltrates despite low cardiac filling pressures. Mechanical ventilation with PEEP is essential, but inflation pressures are kept to a minimum in consideration of the new airway anastomoses.

   b. FiO_2 is maintained at the lowest levels compatible with an acceptable arterial oxygen saturation.

   c. Fifteen percent of lung transplant recipients may develop severe lung injury secondary to reperfusion injury and lymphatic disruption during the surgical procedure. This pattern of lung injury can be treated with ECMO, NO, or selective lung ventilation if indicated.

   d. Acute allograft dysfunction can occur and is associated with a mortality rate of up to 60%.

  e. **Cardiovascular deterioration** may be secondary to hemorrhage, PA or pulmonary venous anastomotic obstruction, tension pneumothorax, or pneumopericardium. TEE may be a useful diagnostic tool in the setting of vascular obstructive lesions. Hemorrhage most frequently occurs in patients with pleural disease and Eisenmenger syndrome. Tension pneumothorax occurs more frequently in patients with concomitant end-stage emphysema.

2. **Immunosuppressive drug regimens** (Table 17.6) have been developed to control the recipient's immune response and prevent allograft rejection [66]. Clinical immunosuppression for lung transplant can be considered in several different contexts: (1) induction therapy, (2) maintenance therapy, and (3) antirejection therapy. Most centers use a triple-drug maintenance regimen that includes corticosteroids, a calcineurin inhibitor (e.g., cyclosporine or tacrolimus), and an antiproliferative agent (e.g., azathioprine). Although these regimens may adequately control acute rejection, chronic rejection still accounts for a majority of long-term morbidity and mortality.

  a. **Cyclosporine** is a cyclic polypeptide derived from a soil fungus. Its major actions are to inhibit macrophage and T-cell production of interleukins and to block activation of helper T cells.

  b. **Azathioprine blocks** de novo purine biosynthesis, which is important to both DNA and RNA production, thus inhibiting both T- and B-cell proliferation.

  c. **Prednisone** is an anti-inflammatory drug that suppresses helper T-cell proliferation and interleukin production by T cells.

  d. **Tacrolimus** is a macrolide antibiotic with immunosuppressant properties that blocks interleukin production and proliferation of T lymphocytes. It is used as a substitute for cyclosporine in the setting of acute allograft rejection. Tacrolimus, in comparison to cyclosporine, has been associated with a lower rate of rejection, similar infection rates, and increased incidence of new-onset diabetes mellitus. It is effective in slowing progression of bronchiolitis obliterans. Some suggest using tacrolimus as a primary immunosuppressive agent for these reasons.

  e. Approximately 50% of lung transplant centers also utilize induction therapy with polyclonal antibody (antithymocyte globulin), interleukin-2 receptor antagonists (daclizumab or basiliximab), or alemtuzumab.

3. The rate of **postoperative infectious complications** is higher in lung transplant patients compared with other solid organ transplant recipients. Therefore, one must be able to differentiate **infection versus allograft rejection.**

  a. Several factors increase the susceptibility of transplanted lungs to infection: (a) exposure to the external environment; (b) pulmonary lymphatic disruption; (c) impairment of mucociliary function; (d) prolonged mechanical ventilation predisposing the patient to nosocomial infection and airway colonization; and (e) presence of airway foreign bodies (e.g., sutures).

  b. Proper diagnosis is crucial to successful outcome and is usually performed via a transbronchial biopsy using flexible FOB. Occasionally, open lung biopsy is necessary.

  c. During the initial 2 postoperative months, **nosocomial gram-negative bacteria are the most frequent causes of pneumonia.** Thereafter, CMV pneumonitis becomes more common and is associated with progression to a state of chronic allograft rejection.

4. The **vagus, phrenic, and recurrent laryngeal nerves are jeopardized during lung transplantation.** Their injury complicates weaning from mechanical ventilation.

5. Postoperative airways complications include bronchial anastamotic dehiscence, bronchial stenosis (most common), obstructive granulomas, bronchomalacia, and bronchial fistula formation [67].

K. Outcome

1. **Survival.** Recent reports from the ISHLT Registry indicate that the median survival is 5.8 years. The unadjusted benchmark survival rate was 89% at 3 months, 80% at 1 year, 65% at 3 years, 54% at 5 years, and 32% at 10 years for the time period of January 1990 through June 2014 [49]. These rates are slightly higher than previously reported.

    a. Categorical risk factors significantly associated with mortality during the first post-transplant year include recipient male gender, type of underlying lung disease (e.g., COPD), pretransplant long-term steroid use, retransplantation, earlier era of transplantation, increased severity of illness at the time of transplantation (mechanical ventilation or dialysis), donor cause of death other than anoxia, CVA or stroke or head trauma, higher mismatching of donor and recipient HLA type, CMV mismatch and nonidentical donor and recipient blood groups.

    b. Continuous risk factors significantly associated with mortality include older recipient and donor age at transplantation, lower transplant center volume, shorter donor height, extremes of donor height minus recipient height difference, lower donor–recipient BMI ratio, higher pretransplantation bilirubin, higher amount of supplemental O_2 at rest, lower percentage predicted value of FVC, increased serum creatinine.

    c. Post–lung-transplant morbidity factors include (a) hypertension, (b) renal dysfunction, (c) hyperlipidemia, (d) diabetes mellitus, (e) bronchiolitis obliterans, and (f) coronary artery vasculopathy.

  2. **Exercise tolerance has** been shown to improve after lung transplantation, as have the quality-of-life factors for survivors.

L. **Special considerations for pediatric lung transplantation**

  1. **Epidemiology**

    a. Since 1986, there have been 2,229 lung transplant procedures reported in children 17 years old and younger [68].

    b. CF, idiopathic PAH, interstitial lung disease, and proliferative bronchiolitis obliterans account for almost all diagnoses in pediatric lung recipients. BSLT is the most frequent procedure.

  2. **Outcome.** One-year survival is currently comparable with that reported for adults [68].

  3. **Pathophysiology.** In children with severe developmental anomalies of the lung (e.g., congenital diaphragmatic hernia with pulmonary hypoplasia, cystadenomatous malformations), isolated lung transplantation may offer the only chance for survival. Rarely, HLT may be indicated during childhood for PPH, CF, or Eisenmenger syndrome.

  4. **Donor lungs.** Size considerations place additional limitations on organ matching for pediatric recipients and thereby exacerbate shortages. The scarcity of suitable donor organs has propagated living-related lung lobe donation; however, the success of this approach is somewhat uncertain. In addition, donor and recipient morbidity and mortality inherent to this operation have sparked considerable controversy.

  5. **Intubation.** In smaller children, using DLTs is not feasible; instead, **selective endobronchial intubation** with a conventional cuffed single-lumen tube is the most frequent choice.

M. **Anesthesia for the post–lung-transplant patient**

In addition to certain specific considerations, several general principles apply to all patients who have undergone successful lung transplantation, including the toxicity of immunosuppressants, potential for infectious and malignant complications, and interactions between immunosuppressants and other pharmacologic agents (including anesthetics).

  1. **Cardiac denervation** may result after en bloc DbLT because extensive retrocardiac dissection is often necessary.

  2. Airway anastomoses may be associated with chronic strictures and **inadequate clearance of secretions**.

  3. **Toxic systemic effects of immunosuppressants**

    a. **Cyclosporine** is a potent nephrotoxin. Blood urea nitrogen and creatinine levels increase and most patients develop systemic hypertension. Cyclosporine can produce hepatocellular injury, hyperuricemia, gingival hypertrophy, hirsutism, and tremors or seizures (at high serum levels).

    b. **Azathioprine** suppresses all formed elements in the bone marrow. Anemia, thrombocytopenia, and occasionally aplastic anemia may result. Azathioprine is associated with hepatocellular and pancreatic impairment, alopecia, and gastrointestinal distress. There may be an increased requirement in the dosage of nondepolarizing neuromuscular blocking agents in this patient population.

    c. **Prednisone** produces adrenal suppression, glucose intolerance, peptic ulceration, aseptic osteonecrosis, and integument fragility. Controversy surrounds the need to administer intraoperative "stress doses" of glucocorticoids to patients with chronic adrenal suppression.

    d. **Tacrolimus** exhibits a spectrum of toxicities (including nephrotoxicity) similar to those for cyclosporine.

4. Infections

    a. Early posttransplant bacterial infections are typically related to **pneumonia** (*Streptococcus pneumoniae;* gram-negative bacilli), **wound infection** (*Staphylococcus aureus*), and use of **urinary catheters** (*Escherichia coli*). Because of the particular susceptibility of pneumonia, early extubation of the trachea after general anesthesia is highly recommended.

    b. CMV is the most frequent viral pathogen in lung transplant recipients and results either from primary infection (after contaminated allograft implantation or blood transfusion in seronegative recipients) or secondary to reactivated infection in a seropositive patient.

    c. After the first few months of immunosuppression, vulnerability to **opportunistic pathogens** increases (CMV, *Pneumocystis carinii,* herpes zoster). If diagnosis is rapid and treatment decisive, survival prevails. Prophylactic antibiotic regimens are available and have been successful in reducing the prevalence of some of these infections (e.g., trimethoprim-sulfamethoxazole for *P. carinii*).

5. Posttransplant lymphoproliferative disorders are more likely to develop in immunosuppressed patients. Posttransplant lymphoproliferative disorder is the third leading cause of death outside the perioperative period, with an incidence ranging from 1.8% to 20%. Other neoplasms have been associated with immunosuppression, including (a) non-Hodgkin lymphoma; (b) squamous cell carcinoma of the skin and lip; (c) Kaposi sarcoma; and (d) carcinoma of the vulva, perineum, kidney, and hepatobiliary tree.

6. Drug interactions

    a. Both cyclosporine and prednisone are metabolized by the cytochrome P450 enzyme system in hepatocytes. Drugs that inhibit those enzymes (e.g., calcium channel blockers) may increase their serum concentrations and promote toxic side effects.

    b. Other drugs (e.g., barbiturates and phenytoin) may induce the P450 enzymes and decrease cyclosporine levels below therapeutic range.

N. The future of lung transplantation

Lung transplantation is a viable therapeutic option for many patients with ESPD. Although advances in surgical techniques, organ preservation, and perioperative care have led to improved recipient survival and quality of life, a limited availability of suitable donor organs remains an obstacle. Efforts to expand the donor organ pool through the use of allografts from older donors and nonbeating heart donation are continuing. These efforts, coupled with refinement of the organ allocation and prioritization criteria, should ideally expedite transplantation for the most critically ill patients. Development of perioperative optimization protocols and a more widespread use of mechanical life support such as ECMO have been instrumental in improving patient survival in both the pre- and posttransplantation periods. Ongoing research about mechanisms, prevention, and treatment of bronchiolitis obliterans offers hope that this devastating complication can be reduced or eliminated.

REFERENCES

1. Mohamed A, Mehta N, Eisen HJ. New role of mechanical assist device as bridge to transplant: USA perspective. *Curr Opin Organ Transplant.* 2017;22(3):231–235.
2. Lund LH, Edwards LB, Dipchand AI, et al; International Society for Heart and Lung Transplantation. The Registry of the International Society for Heart and Lung Transplantation: thirty-third adult heart transplantation report-2016; Focus theme: primary diagnostic indications for transplant. *J Heart Lung Transplant.* 2016;35:1158–1169.
3. Andrew J, Macdonald P. Latest developments in heart transplantation: a review. *Curr Opin Organ Transplant.* 2017;22(3):231–235.
4. Benjamin EJ, Blaha MJ, Chiuve SE, et al; American Heart Association Statistics Committee and Stroke Statistics Subcommittee. Heart Disease and Stroke Statistics-2017 Update: a report from the American Heart Association. *Circulation.* 2017;135(10): e146–e603.

5. **Yancy CW, Jessup M, Bozkurt B, et al. 2013 ACCF/AHA guideline for the management of heart failure: executive summary: a report of the American College of Cardiology Foundation/American Heart Association Task Force on practice guidelines.** *Circulation.* 2013;128(16):1810–1852.

6. Mann DL, Bristow MR. Mechanisms and models in heart failure: the biomechanical model and beyond. *Circulation.* 2005; 111:2837–2849.

7. Neubauer S. The failing heart—an engine out of fuel. *N Engl J Med.* 2007;356:1140–1151.

8. Ziff OJ, Kotecha D. Digoxin: the good and the bad. *Trends Cardiovasc Med.* 2016;26(7):585–595.

9. Hood WB Jr, Dans AL, Guyatt GH, et al. Digitalis for treatment of heart failure in patients in sinus rhythm. *Cochrane Database Syst Rev.* 2014;(4):CD002901.

10. Yandrapalli S, Tariq S, Aronow WS. Advances in chemical pharmacotherapy for managing acute decompensated heart failure. *Expert Opin Pharmacother.* 2017;18(5):471–485.

11. Metra M, Teerlink JR. Heart failure. *Lancet.* 2017;390(10106):1981–1995.

12. Yancy CW, Jessup M, Bozkurt B, et al. 2016 ACC/AHA/HFSA focused update on new pharmacological therapy for heart failure: an update of the 2013 ACCF/AHA guideline for the management of heart failure: a report of the American College of Cardiology/American Heart Association Task Force on Clinical Practice Guidelines and the Heart Failure Society of America. *Circulation.* 2016;134(13):e282–e293.

13. Murphy KM, Rosenthal JL. Progress in the presence of failure: updates in chronic systolic heart failure management. *Curr Treat Options Cardiovasc Med.* 2017;19(7):50.

14. Kong LG, Wang CL, Zhao D, et al. Nesiritide therapy is associated with better clinical outcomes than dobutamine therapy in heart failure. *Am J Ther.* 2017;24(2):e181–e188.

15. Choi AJ, Thomas SS, Singh JP. Cardiac resynchronization therapy and implantable cardioverter defibrillator therapy in advanced heart failure. *Heart Fail Clin.* 2016;12(3):423–436.

16. Epstein AE, DiMarco JP, Ellenbogen KA, et al; American College of Cardiology Foundation; American Heart Association Task Force on Practice Guidelines; Heart Rhythm Society. 2012 ACCF/AHA/HRS focused update incorporated into the ACCF/AHA/HRS 2008 guidelines for device-based therapy of cardiac rhythm abnormalities: a report of the American College of Cardiology Foundation/American Heart Association Task Force on Practice Guidelines and the Heart Rhythm Society. *Circulation.* 2013;127(3):e283–e352.

17. **Colvin M, Smith JM, Skeans MA, et al. OPTN/SRTR 2015 annual data report: heart.** *Am J Transplant.* **2017;17(Suppl 1): 286–356.**

18. Taghavi S, Jayarajan SN, Komaroff E, et al. Continuous flow left ventricular assist device technology has influenced wait times and affected donor allocation in cardiac transplantation. *J Thorac Cardiovasc Surg.* 2014;147(6):1966–1971.

19. Holley CT, Harvey L, John R. Left ventricular assist devices as a bridge to cardiac transplantation. *J Thorac Dis.* 2014;6(8): 1110–1119.

20. Kamdar F, John R, Eckman P, et al. Postcardiac transplant survival in the current era in patients receiving continuous-flow left ventricular assist devices. *J Thorac Cardiovasc Surg.* 2013;145:575–581.

21. Mancini D, Lietz K. Selection of cardiac transplantation candidates in 2010. *Circulation.* 2010;122:173–183.

22. **Kanwar M, Raina A, Aponte MP, et al. Pulmonary hypertension in potential heart transplant recipients: current treatment strategies.** *Curr Opin Organ Transplant.* **2015;20(5):570–576.**

23. Fang JC, DeMarco T, Givertz MM, et al. World Health Organization Pulmonary Hypertension group 2: pulmonary hypertension due to left heart disease in the adult—a summary statement from the Pulmonary Hypertension Council of the International Society for Heart and Lung Transplantation. *J Heart Lung Transplant.* 2012;31(9):913–933.

24. Toyoda Y, Guy TS, Kashem A. Present status and future perspectives of heart transplantation. *Circ J.* 2013;77(5):1097–1110.

25. Andrew J, Macdonald P. Latest developments in heart transplantation: a review. *Clin Ther.* 2015;37(10):2234–2241.

26. DePasquale EC, Schweiger M, Ross HJ. A contemporary review of adult heart transplantation: 2012 to 2013. *J Heart Lung Transplant.* 2014;33(8):775–784.

27. Dhital KK, Iyer A, Connellan M, et al. Adult heart transplantation with distant procurement and ex-vivo preservation of donor hearts after circulatory death: a case series. *The Lancet.* 2015;385:2585–2591.

28. Dictus C, Vienenkoetter B, Esmaeilzadeh M, et al. Critical care management of potential organ donors: our current standard. *Clin Transplant.* 2009;23(suppl 21):2–9.

29. Maciel CB, Greer DM. ICU management of the potential organ donor: state of the art. *Curr Neurol Neurosci Rep.* 2016;16:86.

30. Floerchinger B, Oberhuber R, Tullius SG. Effects of brain death on organ quality and transplant outcome. *Transplant Rev (Orlando).* 2012;26(2):54–59.

31. Anderson TA, Bekker P, Vagefi PA. Anesthetic considerations in organ procurement surgery: a narrative review. *Can J Anaesth.* 2015;62(5):529–539.

32. Minasian SM, Galagudza MM, Dmitriev YV, et al. Preservation of the donor heart: from basic science to clinical studies. *Interact Cardiovasc Thorac Surg.* 2015;20(4):510–519.

33. Davis RR, Russo MJ, Morgan JA, et al. Standard versus Bicaval techniques for orthotopic heart transplantation: an analysis of the United Network for Organ Sharing database. *J Thorac Cardiovasc Surg.* 2010;140:700–708.

34. Mallidi HR, Bates M. Pacemaker use following heart transplantation. *Ochsner J.* 2017;17(1):20–24.

35. Berger Y, Har Zahav Y, Kassif Y, et al. Tricuspid valve regurgitation after orthotopic heart transplantation: prevalence and etiology. *J Transplant.* 2012;2012:120702.

36. Flécher E, Fouquet O, Ruggieri VG, et al. Heterotopic heart transplantation: where do we stand? *Eur J Cardiothorac Surg.* 2013;44(2):201–206.

37. **Ramakrishna H, Rehfeldt KH, Pajaro OE. Anesthetic pharmacology and perioperative considerations for heart transplantation.** *Curr Clin Pharmacol.* **2015;10(1):3–21.**

38. Penninga L, Møller CH, Gustafsson F, et al. Immunosuppressive T-cell antibody induction for heart transplant recipients. *Cochrane Database Syst Rev*. 2013;(12):CD008842.
39. **Khan TA, Schnickel G, Ross D, et al. A prospective, randomized, crossover pilot study of inhaled nitric oxide versus inhaled prostacyclin in heart transplant and lung transplant recipients. *J Thorac Cardiovasc Surg*. 2009;138:1417–1424.**
40. Wademan BH, Galvin SD. Desmopressin for reducing postoperative blood loss and transfusion requirements following cardiac surgery in adults. *Interact Cardiovasc Thorac Surg*. 2014;18(3):360–370.
41. Asante-Korang A. Echocardiographic evaluation before and after cardiac transplantation. *Cardiol Young*. 2004;14:88–92.
42. Costello JP, Mohanakumar T, Nath DS. Mechanisms of chronic allograft rejection. *Tex Heart Inst J*. 2013;40(4):395–399.
43. Lachance K, White M, de Denus S. Risk factors for chronic renal insufficiency following cardiac transplantation. *Ann Transplant*. 2015;20:576–587.
44. Page RL 2nd, Miller GG, Lindenfeld J. Drug therapy in the heart transplant recipient: part IV: drug-drug interactions. *Circulation*. 2005;111:230–239.
45. Roselli EE, Smedira NG. Surgical advances in heart and lung transplantation. *Anesthesiol Clin North America*. 2004;22:789–807.
46. **Blasco LM, Parameshwar J, Vuylsteke A. Anaesthesia for noncardiac surgery in the heart transplant recipient. *Curr Opin Anaesthesiol*. 2009;22:109–113.**
47. Egan TM, Murray S, Bustami RT, et al. Development of the new lung allocation system in the United States. *Am J Transplant*. 2006;6:1212–1227.
48. Yusen RD, Shearon TH, Qian Y, et al. Lung transplantation in the United States 1999–2008. *Am J Transplant*. 2010;10:1047–1068.
49. **Yusen RD, Edwards LB, Dipchand AI, et al; International Society for Heart and Lung Transplantation. The registry of the International Society for Heart and Lung Transplantation: thirty-third adult lung and heart-lung transplant report—2016; Focus theme: primary diagnostic indications for transplant. *J Heart Lung Transplant*. 2016;35:1170–1184.**
50. Weill D, Benden C, Corris PA, et al. A consensus document for the selection of lung transplant candidates: 2014-an update from the Pulmonary Transplantation Council of the International Society for Heart and Lung Transplantation. *J Heart Lung Transplant*. 2015;34:1–15.
51. Snell GI, Richardson M, Griffiths AP, et al. Coronary artery disease in potential lung transplant recipients greater than 50 years old: the role of coronary intervention. *Chest*. 1999;116:874–879.
52. McKellar SH, Bowen ME, Baird BC, et al. Lung transplantation following coronary artery bypass surgery-improved outcomes following single-lung transplant. *J Heart Lung Transplant*. 2016;35:1289–1294.
53. DeSoyza A, Corris PA. Lung transplantation and the Burkholderia cepacia complex. *J Heart Lung Transplant*. 2003;22:954–958.
54. Aris RM, Gilligan PH, Neuringer IP, et al. The effects of pan-resistant bacteria in cystic fibrosis patients on lung transplant outcome. *Am J Respir Crit Care Med*. 1997;155:1699–1704.
55. Meachery GJ, Archer L, DeSoyza A, et al. Survival outcomes following lung transplantation for cystic fibrosis patients infected with Burkholderia cenocepacia—a UK experience. *J Heart Lung Transplant*. 2007;26(25):S126–S127.
56. Low DE, Trulock EP, Kasier LR, et al. Morbidity, mortality and early results of single versus bilateral lung transplantation for emphysema. *J Thorac Cardiovasc Surg*. 1992;103:1119–1126.
57. Starnes VA, Woo MS, MacLaughlin EF, et al. Comparison of outcomes between living donor and cadaveric lung transplantation in children. *Ann Thorac Surg*. 1999;68:2279–2283.
58. Bowdish ME, Barr ML, Schenkel FA, et al. A decade of living lobar lung transplantation: perioperative complications after 253 donor lobectomies. *Am J Transplant*. 2004;4:1283–1288.
59. Reyes KG, Mason DP, Thuita L, et al. Guidelines for donor lung selection: time for revision? *Ann Thorac Surg*. 2010;89:1756–1764.
60. Bhorade SM, Vigneswaran W, McCabe MA, et al. Liberalization of donor criteria may expand the donor pool without adverse consequence in lung transplantation. *J Heart Lung Transplant*. 2000;19:1199–1204.
61. Snell GI, Levvy BJ, Oto T, et al. Early lung transplantation success utilizing controlled donation after cardiac death donors. *Am J Transplant*. 2008;8:1282–1289.
62. Fisher AJ, Donnelly SC, Hirani N, et al. Elevated levels of interleukin-8 in donor lungs is associated with early graft failure after lung transplantation. *Am J Respir Crit Care Med*. 2001;163:259–265.
63. **Cypel M, Yeung JC, Liu M, et al. Normothermic ex vivo lung perfusion in clinical lung transplantation. *N Engl J Med*. 2011;364:1431–1440.**
64. Novick RJ, Bennett LE, Meyer DM, et al. Influence of graft ischemic time and donor age on survival after lung transplantation. *J Heart Lung Transplant*. 1999;18:425–431.
65. **Feltracco P, Barbieri S, Milefoy M, et al. Thoracic epidural analgesia in lung transplantation. *Transplant Proc*. 2010; 42:1265–1269.**
66. Scheffert JL, Raza K. Immunosuppression in lung transplantation. *J Thorac Dis*. 2014;6(8):1039–1053.
67. Dutau H, Vandemoortele T, Laroumagne S, et al. A new endoscopic grading system for macroscopic central airways complications following lung transplantation: the MDS classification. *Eur J Cardiothorac Surg*. 2014;45(2):e33–e38.
68. Goldfarb SB, Levvey BJ, Edwards LB, et al; International Society for Heart and Lung Transplantation. The Registry of the International Society for Heart and Lung Transplantation: nineteenth pediatric lung and heart-lung transplantation report—2016; Focus theme: primary diagnostic indications for transplant. *J Heart Lung Transplant*. 2016;35(10):1196–1205.

18

Arrhythmia, Rhythm Management Devices, and Catheter and Surgical Ablation

Soraya M. Samii and Jerry C. Luck, Jr.

KEY POINTS

1. Patients with moderate-to-severe left ventricular dysfunction are at a higher risk for sustained monomorphic ventricular tachycardia (VT) than those with preserved left ventricular function.

2. VT commonly causes syncope, and when it is associated with structural heart disease, it is also associated with a high risk of sudden cardiac death.

3. Symptomatic patients with sinus node dysfunction (SND) or evidence of other conduction disease such as second- or third-degree atrioventricular (AV) block almost always need a permanent pacemaker preoperatively.

4. For VT, intravenous (IV) amiodarone is the initial drug of choice, but lidocaine may also be considered, especially if there is concern for ongoing ischemia. For torsades de pointes, management includes eliminating offending drugs in the setting of the long QT syndromes.

5. Bifascicular block with periodic third-degree AV block and syncope is associated with an increased incidence of sudden death. Prophylactic permanent pacing is indicated in this circumstance.

6. The requirement for temporary pacing with acute MI by itself does not constitute an indication for permanent pacing.

7. Sensor-driven tachycardia may occur with adaptive-rate devices that sense vibration and impedance changes. Thus, we advise disabling rate responsiveness in the perioperative period. Placing a magnet on the pacemaker will usually deactivate the rate–responsiveness feature and program the device to asynchronous pacing.

8. Most contemporary pacemaker devices respond to magnet application by a device-specific single- or dual-chamber asynchronous pacing mode. Adaptive-rate response is generally suspended with magnet mode as well. With asynchronous pacing, the pacemaker will no longer be inhibited by sensed activity and will instead pace at a fixed rate regardless of underlying rhythm.

9. Some manufacturers, e.g., Biotronik, St. Jude Medical, and Boston Scientific devices, have a programmable magnet mode that may make response to magnet application different than anticipated. Although rarely used, this feature may be programmed to save patient-activated rhythm recordings with magnet application, rather than revert the pacemaker to asynchronous pacing.

10. Electromagnetic interference (EMI) signals between 5 and 100 Hz are not filtered because these overlap the frequency range of intracardiac signals. Therefore, EMI in this frequency range may be interpreted as intracardiac signals, giving rise to abnormal behavior. Possible responses include (i) inappropriate inhibition or triggering of stimulation, (ii) asynchronous pacing (Fig. 18.5), (iii) mode resetting, (iv) direct damage to the pulse generator circuitry, and (v) triggering of unnecessary ICD shocks.

11. Treatment options for VT include antitachycardia pacing, cardioversion, or defibrillation. Up to 90% of monomorphic VTs can be terminated by a critical pacing sequence, reducing the need for painful shocks and conserving battery life. With antitachycardia pacing, trains of stimuli are delivered at a fixed percentage of the VT cycle length.

12. Acute MI, severe acute acid–base or electrolyte imbalance, or hypoxia may increase defibrillation thresholds, leading to ineffective shocks. Any of these also could affect the rate or morphology of VT and the ability to diagnose VT.

13. Magnet application does not interfere with bradycardia pacing and does not trigger asynchronous pacing in an ICD. Magnet application in contemporary ICDs causes inhibition of tachycardia sensing and delivery of shock only. All current ICDs remain inhibited as long as the magnet remains in stable contact with the ICD. Once the magnet is removed, the ICD reverts to the programmed tachyarrhythmia settings.

14. Baseline information about the surgery is needed by the CIED team (cardiologist, electrophysiologist, and pacemaker clinic staff managing the device) such as (i) type and location of the procedure, (ii) body position at surgery, (iii) electrosurgery needed and site of use, (iv) potential need for DC cardioversion or defibrillation, and (v) other EMI sources.

15. Pacemaker-dependent patients are at particular risk of asystole in the presence of EMI. If EMI is likely (e.g., unipolar cautery in the vicinity of the pulse generator or leads and surgery above the umbilicus), then the device should be programmed to an asynchronous mode. In most situations, this can be done with magnet application, which will also inactivate the rate-responsive pacing.

16. In cases where the pacemaker-dependent patient has an ICD or the location of surgery precludes placement of a magnet, programming the device to an asynchronous mode is recommended.

17. Use of a magnet eliminates the complexity of reprogramming the CIED in the operating room. The magnet can be easily removed when an underlying rhythm competes with asynchronous pacing.

I. Introduction

Any disturbance of rhythm or conduction or arrhythmia that destabilizes hemodynamics perioperatively will need to be addressed. Treatment with antiarrhythmic agents has been the standard approach to manage symptomatic arrhythmias acutely. Device therapy indications have expanded for long-term rhythm management. The emphasis in this chapter is on perioperative management of patients with implanted devices. Concepts of arrhythmogenesis, antiarrhythmic action, and drug selection are discussed only briefly.

II. Concepts of arrhythmogenesis

A. **Basic electrophysiology**

1. **Action potential (AP).** A ventricular muscle cell's AP has five phases caused by changes in the cell membrane's permeability to sodium, potassium, and calcium (Fig. 18.1). Phase 0 represents depolarization and is characterized by a rapid upstroke, as sodium rapidly enters the cell. There is a rapid drop in the cell's impedance from a resting state at −80 to −85 mV. Phase 1 is an early rapid repolarization period caused by potassium egress from the cell. Phase 2 is a plateau phase representing a slow recovery phase: The slow inward calcium current is counterbalanced by outward potassium current. Phase 3 is a rapid repolarization phase as a result of accelerated potassium efflux. The diastolic interval between APs is termed phase 4 and is a cell's resting membrane state in atrial and ventricular muscle.

2. **Ion channels.** Electrical activation of cardiac cells is the result of membrane currents crossing the hydrophobic lipid membranes through their specific protein channel. Opening and closing of gates in these channels are determined by the membrane potential (voltage dependence) and by the time elapsed after changes in potential (time dependence). Membrane channels cycle through the "activated," "inactivated," and "recovery" stages with each AP. Inward currents of sodium and calcium ions enter the cell using this gating mechanism. On the surface electrocardiogram (ECG), rapid-acting sodium currents contribute to the "P" and the "QRS" complexes. Depolarization of the sinoatrial (SA) node and the atrioventricular (AV) node, in contrast, occurs as a result of the slower-opening calcium-dependent channels. The slowly conducting calcium channel in the AV node creates the delay in the node and is responsible for nearly two-thirds of the PR interval during normal conduction. A group of potassium channels is responsible for repolarization and the "T" wave on the ECG.

    Cardiac arrhythmias occur when abnormal channel proteins are substituted for the normal protein and the ion channel is altered. For example, QT prolongation may be inherited as a result of encoding an altered gene or it may be acquired as a consequence of an antiarrhythmic agent inhibiting a specific ion channel [1].

3. **Excitability.** Reducing the cell's transmembrane potential to a critical level will initiate a propagated response, and this level is termed the threshold potential. There are two mechanisms by which a propagated AP is developed: (i) a natural electrical stimulus and (ii) an applied electrical current. For an applied stimulus, threshold of a tissue is defined as the minimum amount of energy that will elicit a response. When external electrodes are used, only that part of the stimulus which penetrates the cell membrane contributes to excitation. The size of the stimulating electrode is critical to threshold. Reducing the size of the stimulating electrode (from 3 to 0.5 mm) will increase the current density over a smaller area and decrease the amount of energy needed to achieve threshold. It is common practice in pacing to use a small stimulating electrode and a larger indifferent electrode to reduce threshold and facilitate excitation.

4. **Conduction.** There are regions of cells with specialized conduction characteristics within the heart that propagate conduction in a preferential direction, spreading to adjacent areas faster though the preferential sites. This allows for a more organized direction of conduction so that, for example, both atria are depolarized prior to the stimulus reaching the AV node to depolarize the ventricles. In the sinus and AV nodes, L- and T-type calcium channels are the source of the propagated current [2]. In the Purkinje fiber, the sodium channel is the source of the conducted current. Conduction velocity is much slower at about 0.2 m/sec in the node versus 2 m/sec in the Purkinje cells. These different characteristics explain the effects of certain antiarrhythmic medications. For instance, blocking the sodium channel with a class I antiarrhythmic agent will preferentially reduce the conduction velocity in the Purkinje cells compared to the AV node because of this agent's primary effect on sodium channels.

B. **Mechanism of arrhythmia** (Table 18.1)

1. **Automaticity.** Automaticity is a unique property of an excitable cell allowing spontaneous depolarization and initiation of electrical impulse in the absence of external electrical stimulation. The SA node serves as the primary automatic pacemaker for the heart.

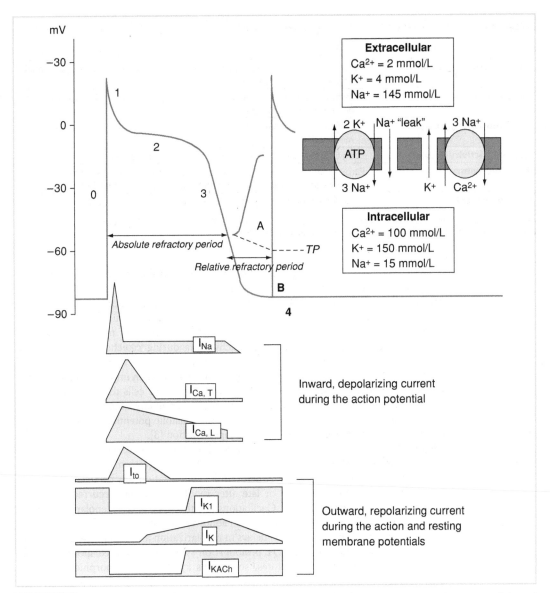

FIGURE 18.1 Action potential (AP) and resting membrane potential (RMP) of a quiescent Purkinje fiber. Extracellular and intracellular ion concentrations during phase 4 and the active and passive ion exchangers that restore intracellular ion concentrations during phase 4 are shown to the right of the AP. The inward currents include the sodium current (I_{Na}); the Calcium current (I_{Ca}) from both the T and L type channels, and the transient outward potassium current (I_{to}). The outward currents are all potassium currents from the inward rectifier channel (Ik1), potassium channels (IK) and the G-protein coupled acetylcholine channel (IKach). Inward depolarizing and outward repolarizing currents are shown below the AP. The adenosine triphosphate (ATP)-dependent Na/K pump maintains steep outwardly and inwardly directed gradients (*arrows*) for K^+ and Na^+, respectively, and generates small net outward current. The passive Na/Ca exchanger generates small net inward current. A small, inward "leak" of Na^+ keeps the RMP slightly positive to the K equilibrium potential (−96 mV). AP phase 0 is the upstroke, phase 1 is initial rapid repolarization, phase 2 is the plateau, and phase 3 is final repolarization. The cell is unresponsive to propagating AP or external stimuli during the absolute refractory period. A small electronic potential (**A**) occurs in response to a propagating AP or external stimulus during the relative refractory period (RRP). It is incapable of self-propagation. A normal AP is generated at the end of the RRP (**B**), when the Na channels have fully recovered from inactivation. It is capable of propagation. Note that threshold potential (TP) for excitation is more positive during the RRP.

TABLE 18.1 Confirmed or postulated electrophysiologic mechanisms for clinical arrhythmias

Mechanism	Arrhythmias
Altered normal automaticity	Sinus bradycardia and tachycardia, wandering atrial pacemaker, AV junctional and ventricular escape rhythms
Abnormal automaticity	Slow monomorphic VT, junctional or idioventricular rhythms in acute MI; some ectopic atrial tachycardia
Triggered activity (DAD)	VT in first 24 hrs of acute MI, atrial or VT with digitalis toxicity, catecholamine-mediated VT
Triggered activity (EAD)	Long QT interval with polymorphic VT (i.e., torsades de pointes)
Anatomic reentry	Paroxysmal SVT due to reentry involving the SA node, atria, AV node, or accessory AV pathways; VT with healed infarction; atrial flutter
Functional reentry	Atrial fibrillation, monomorphic or polymorphic VT with acute MI, VF

AV, atrioventricular; DAD, delayed afterdepolarization; VT, ventricular tachycardia; MI, myocardial infarction; EAD, early afterdepolarization; SA, sinoatrial; SVT, supraventricular tachycardia; VF, ventricular fibrillation.

Subsidiary pacemakers exhibiting automaticity are also found along the crista terminalis, the coronary sinus ostium, within the AV junction, and in the ventricular His–Purkinje system. They may assume control of the heart if the SA node falters. Automaticity is either normal or abnormal. Alterations in automaticity due to changes in the ionic currents normally involved in impulse initiation are considered normal. Examples of normal automaticity include sinus tachycardia and junctional tachycardia during catecholamine states that increase current through the T-type calcium channels in the nodal cells. Abnormal automaticity occurs when ionic currents not normally involved in impulse initiation cause spontaneous depolarizations in atrial and ventricular muscle cells that normally do not have pacemaker activity. An example of abnormal automaticity occurs during ischemic injury, causing muscle cells to shift their maximum diastolic potential to a more positive resting level and thus facilitate spontaneous depolarization [3].

2. **Triggered activity.** Triggered activity is the result of abnormal oscillations in membrane potential reaching the threshold to induce another AP, following a normal AP depolarization. These afterdepolarizations can occur before full repolarization has occurred, known as early afterdepolarizations (EADs), or late after repolarization has occurred, known as delayed afterdepolarization (DAD). Oscillations of either type of afterdepolarizations that exceed the threshold potential may trigger an abnormal tachycardia.

EADs occur most frequently with delays in repolarization and prolongation of the QT interval. Acquired and congenital QT prolongation syndromes are predisposed to EADs and can result in torsades de pointes, sometimes known as polymorphic ventricular tachycardia (VT) and sudden death. The torsades de pointes, triggered in prolonged QT syndromes, is facilitated by bradycardia and adrenaline. Examples of inherited predisposition to triggered initiation include defects in genes encoding Na and K ion channels that produce a net reduction in outward positive current during repolarization, resulting in prolongation of the QT interval. Acquired prolongation of the QT interval from hypokalemia, pharmacologic agents including class IA and III antiarrhythmics, antibiotics such as erythromycin and antifungal agents, antihistamines, and the phenothiazine piperidine class can cause EADs.

DAD potentials cause arrhythmias related to calcium overload. Digoxin toxicity is the most common agent causing DAD, and triggered activity is the common mechanism for digitalis-induced accelerated junctional rhythm and bidirectional VT. Catecholamines facilitate calcium loading and the development of DADs.

3. **Reentry.** For either anatomical or functional reentrant excitation to occur, the electrical wave front must circle around a core of inexcitable tissue at a rate that preserves an excitable gap. For initiation, there must be (i) an area of unidirectional conduction block, (ii) two conduction pathways that are connected at each end, and (iii) an area of

slow conduction. Anatomical reentrant circuits are common to several supraventricular tachycardias (SVTs), including Wolff–Parkinson–White syndrome, with an accessory AV pathway and typical and atypical AV nodal reentrant tachycardia. Classic atrial flutter has an anatomical right atrial loop classically involving the area of slow conduction known as the cavotricuspid isthmus. Pathologic sustained monomorphic VT is commonly due to scar or fibrosis. This creates a mechanism for anatomic reentry.

A functional reentrant loop involves a small circuit around an area of tissue with an inexcitable core. Functional reentry may occur with some forms of atrial tachycardia and is a mechanism for the multiple wavelet theory of atrial fibrillation.

C. Anatomical substrates and triggers

1. **Supraventricular.** The highly complex atria have a heterogeneous branching network of subendocardial muscle bundles that create functional areas of block as well as preferential planes of excitation. Longitudinal connected myocardial fibers conduct faster than fibers connected along transverse or parallel lines (the so-called anisotropic conduction). In the right atrium, the crista terminalis and eustachian ridge tend to act as anatomical barriers that help to facilitate a single reentrant loop during atrial flutter. An area of slow conduction can usually be found in the isthmus of atrial tissue between the tricuspid annulus and the inferior vena cava. This is a frequent anatomical area for ablation of both clockwise and counterclockwise atrial flutter. The ostia of the pulmonary veins are frequently the sites of the initiation of atrial fibrillation. This chaotic atrial rhythm can be triggered by a single focus, frequently localized to a pulmonary vein. Once initiated by a premature depolarization, the multiple wavelets are facilitated by the complex nature of the atria.

2. **Ventricular.** Myocardial ischemia and infarction can create both acute and chronic substrates for VT and fibrillation. As mentioned above, scar from previous infarction can create an anatomic reentrant circuit, providing the substrate for reentrant VT. In the acute events such as acute coronary occlusion, metabolic derangements occur including local hyperkalemia, hypoxia, acidosis, and an increase in adrenergic tone, increasing the likelihood for automaticity, triggered activity, and functional reentry. With acute coronary occlusion, ventricular fibrillation (VF) is common and is directly related to an increase in sympathetic tone. Accelerated idiopathic ventricular rhythm is frequently seen with acute myocardial infarction and is attributed to abnormal automaticity. In the chronic phase, the infarct becomes mottled, and over several weeks, islands of viable muscle cells are surrounded by electrically inert barriers of scar tissue. Slow conduction is present and allows for unidirectional block. These factors are conducive to reentry, which is the mechanism for sustained monomorphic VT in about 6% to 8% of survivors of myocardial infarction. Myocardial remodeling as a consequence of infarction provides a classic substrate for arrhythmias. Patients with moderate-to-severe left ventricular dysfunction are at a higher risk for sustained monomorphic VT than those with preserved left ventricular function.

D. Neural control of arrhythmias

1. **β-Adrenergic modulation.** Increased sympathetic tone increases the susceptibility to VF in the early stage of myocardial infarction. In the chronic phase, it facilitates initiation of sustained monomorphic VT. β-Adrenergic blocking drugs (e.g., propranolol, metoprolol, and nadolol), significantly reduce the incidence of VF during acute infarction and reduce the risk of sudden death later. Also, β-blockers do not prevent reperfusion arrhythmias.

2. **Parasympathetic activation.** During acute infarction, vagal activation exerts a protective effect against VF. Bradycardia appears necessary for this protective effect. Increasing heart rate by pacing will negate this protective effect. Vagal stimulation does little to protect against reperfusion arrhythmias.

E. Clinical approach to arrhythmias

1. **Syncope** is defined as the loss of consciousness and muscle tone with spontaneous resolution. It may occur in up to 40% of the general population. The most common type is vasovagal or neurally mediated syncope, which is quite common in the young. This type of syncope is not associated with increased risk of death. Syncope occurs at an annual rate of 6% in patients 75 years or older but in only 0.7% of those below age 45. The goal

is to determine if syncope is of the benign vasovagal variety or of the more dangerous cardiac type [4]. The 1-year mortality from syncope of a cardiac cause can range from 18% to 33%, while the noncardiac group has 0% to 6% mortality. Patients with vasovagal-mediated syncope do not die from syncope. The anatomical cardiac causes of syncope result in obstruction to cardiac output, such as aortic stenosis and outflow obstruction in hypertrophic cardiomyopathy. Arrhythmias that suddenly reduce cardiac output and profoundly affect blood pressure can cause syncope. Sinus node dysfunction (SND) and AV block are common causes of bradyarrhythmias that can cause syncope. SVT causes syncope less often. VT more commonly causes syncope, and when it is associated with structural heart disease, it is also associated with a high risk of sudden cardiac death. In patients with syncope, check the ECG for arrhythmias such as atrial fibrillation, evidence of myocardial infarction, or conduction disease such as bundle branch block. Other important features to evaluate include preexcitation (delta waves), the QT interval, and ectopy. Any of these abnormalities may predict a greater risk of mortality and a need for further evaluation.

2. **Bradycardia.** Heart rates less than 60 bpm are considered bradycardic. Slow heart rhythms become an issue generally in older patients, who may be asymptomatic. Resting slow heart rates in young patients are most likely a result of high vagal tone and are not pathologic. Heart rates greater than 50 bpm tend to be hemodynamically stable, while those less than 40 bpm while the patient is awake often are not. If the asymptomatic bradycardic patient has no evidence of conduction disease (normal QRS morphology) and a chronotropic response to exercise, atropine, or isoproterenol, a pacemaker is rarely indicated. On the other hand, symptomatic patients with SND or evidence of conduction disease such as second- or third-degree AV block almost always need a permanent pacemaker preoperatively. Bradycardia secondary to neurocardiogenic syncope, medications, or increased vagal tone will not generally require a pacemaker. Simply removing the offending medicine or treating the inciting condition will be sufficient.

3. **Tachycardia.** Heart rates above 100 bpm are termed "tachycardia." These can be sinus, a pathologic SVT, or VT. Sinus tachycardia rarely exceeds 140 bpm at rest, unless the patient is in distress, shock, acute respiratory failure, or thyroid storm. In adults not in distress, a narrow, regular QRS tachycardia at rates above 150 bpm is rarely sinus. Regular and narrow QRS tachycardia at these rapid rates is frequently paroxysmal supraventricular tachycardia (PSVT) or atrial flutter with 2:1 conduction. Irregular SVTs are either the more common atrial fibrillation or multifocal atrial tachycardia. The latter is seen in elderly patients with severe chronic pulmonary disease.

Wide QRS tachycardia may be ventricular or supraventricular in origin. In general, if the patient has underlying heart disease, the mechanism of the wide complex tachycardia is VT until proven otherwise. However, there are several conditions in which the mechanism may be SVT, including (i) SVT with an underlying or functional bundle branch block, (ii) SVT with nonspecific intraventricular conduction delay, or (iii) preexcitation syndrome. The ECG diagnosis of VT hinges on seeing AV dissociation or fusion or capture beats. Intraventricular conduction delay can occur with the use of class I antiarrhythmic agents or in the setting of extreme hyperkalemia. Wolff–Parkinson–White syndrome should be considered in a young healthy individual presenting with atrial fibrillation and a wide QRS rhythm. Functional bundle branch block is seen in the young but rarely in the elderly.

III. **Treatment modalities**

A. **Pharmacologic treatment**

Algorithms are in place for acute treatment of SVTs. SVT is usually treated with intravenous (IV) adenosine acutely in the symptomatic patient. For atrial fibrillation, the initial focus is on rate control. Agents that are effective acutely include IV diltiazem and the β-blockers metoprolol and esmolol. Esmolol has an extremely short half-life. Digoxin is of little use acutely and is very unpredictable. IV amiodarone is now being used more frequently in the acute management of patients with poor ventricular function and atrial fibrillation with rapid ventricular rates. This medication should ideally be infused through a central line, given the risk for tissue necrosis with extravasation. The pharmacologic treatment of ventricular arrhythmias in the hemodynamically stable patient involves treating the underlying causes. For VT, IV amiodarone is the initial drug of choice, but lidocaine is also considered, especially if there is concern for ongoing ischemia. For torsades de pointes, management includes eliminating offending drugs in the setting of the long QT syndromes. Correcting electrolyte deficiencies with IV magnesium and potassium is particularly helpful in correcting the prolonged QT interval, as is possibly stopping medications contributing to bradycardia. Amiodarone in the setting of torsades de pointes can prolong the QT interval and make the problem worse. For the hemodynamically unstable patient with sustained ventricular arrhythmias, pharmacologic management would follow the current advanced cardiac life support (ACLS) protocols.

Proarrhythmia. Although drugs have proved safe and effective in the normal heart, their safety and efficacy have proved worrisome in the structurally abnormal heart. Chronic drug therapy for arrhythmias in patients with structural heart disease is associated with increased mortality due to proarrhythmic effects. Class IA antiarrhythmic agents are contraindicated in individuals with congestive heart failure and poor left ventricular function (ejection fraction below 0.30). Class IC agents should be avoided in individuals with a prior myocardial infarction because of the increased risk of sudden death [5]. Class III agents will prolong the QT interval and increase the risk of torsades de pointes.

B. **Nonpharmacologic treatments**

The emphasis on the chronic treatment for arrhythmias, especially ventricular arrhythmias in patients with structural heart disease, has moved from drugs to electricity. Because of technologic advances, cardiac implantable electrical devices (CIEDs) have become smaller and increasingly complex. This complexity has greatly expanded therapeutic options, but it has greatly increased the potential for unexpected medical device interference and, in rare cases, malfunction in the perioperative setting. Except in infants and small children, a formal thoracotomy is no longer used for implantation of a CIED.

1. **External cardioversion and defibrillation.** External direct-current (DC) cardioversion differs from defibrillation, only in that the former incorporates a time delay circuit for shock synchronization to the QRS complex of the surface ECG. Current devices employ universal use of biphasic shocks, which lower shock current requirements for DC cardioversion and defibrillation. Automated external defibrillators self-analyze and give instructions for defibrillation.

   a. **Indications.** Synchronized shocks are used for most pathologic hemodynamically unstable tachycardias, except VF or VT when the QRS complex cannot be distinguished from T waves. Automatic rhythm disturbances (e.g., accelerated AV junctional or accelerated idioventricular rhythms) are not amenable to DC cardioversion.

   b. **Procedure.** Synchronizing **cardioversion** with the largest R or S wave on the ECG will prevent inadvertent triggering of VF. Improper synchronization may occur when there is bundle branch block with a wide R wave, when the T wave is highly peaked, and with pacing artifacts from a malfunctioning pacemaker (i.e., failure to capture). Synchronization should be checked after each discharge. Electrodes are placed in an anterior–lateral, posterior–lateral, or an anteroposterior (AP) position. Current should pass though the heart's long axis, depolarize the bulk of myocardium, and minimize flow through high-impedance bony tissue. Standard electrode pads with adhesive gel are usually used to ensure effective skin contact and electrode stability. The electrode paste or gel is used to reduce transthoracic impedance. Bridging of the electrodes by conductive paste or gel should be avoided because this will reduce the amount of energy delivered to the heart. Present-day units automatically boot to an energy setting of 200 J. This is the starting energy dosage for defibrillating adults. For cardioversion, energy titration (initially use only the lowest possible energies) reduces both energy use and complications. Initial settings of 20 to 50 J may be successful for terminating typical atrial flutter or stable monomorphic VT. DC cardioversion is extremely painful. Patients must be deeply sedated for DC cardioversion at any power setting. In general, an anesthesiologist or nurse anesthetist will administer a short-acting sedative such as IV propofol or etomidate. The combination of midazolam and fentanyl can be an alternative but is not ideal due to the longer duration of action.

c. **Cardiac implantable electrical devices and cardioversion.** External cardioversion has been shown to be safe in the presence of CIEDs with proper electrode positioning [6]. Using the anterior–posterior pads position and the anterior pad location at least 8 cm from the CIED will prevent malfunction or damage to the device. Directly applied currents on the CIED could cause a power-on-reset phenomenon. Directly applied currents to the ventricles during open cardiac surgery on occasion can also cause reset of the pulse generator. In general, interrogation of the CIED system is recommended after cardioversion to confirm that no circuitry has been damaged.

2. **Temporary pacing.** Compared to drugs for treating cardiac rhythm disturbances, temporary pacing has several advantages. The effect is immediate, control is precise, and there is reduced risk of untoward effects and proarrhythmia. The risks of temporary pacing involve placement of the pacemaker electrode and ensuring pacemaker position stability.

a. **Indications.** Temporary pacing is indicated for rate support in patients with symptomatic bradycardia or escape rhythms, usually with heart rates less than 40 bpm. Prophylactic or stand-by pacing is indicated for patients at increased risk for sudden high-degree AV heart block. Temporary pacing can be used to overdrive or terminate atrial flutter and some sustained monomorphic VT. More specific established and emerging indications for temporary pacing are shown in Table 18.2. The endpoint for temporary pacing is resolution of the indication or implantation of a permanent pacemaker for a continuing indication.

b. **Technology.** Transvenous endocardial or epicardial leads are usually used for temporary pacing. Transvenous (endocardial) leads are passed from above using the internal jugular or subclavian approaches or from below using a femoral vein. Epicardial leads are routinely used in patients having cardiac surgery. The noninvasive transcutaneous and transesophageal routes are also available. Transcutaneous pacing is uncomfortable and used in emergency situations, and capture is sometimes difficult to obtain. In the operating room, it is for transient backup pacing only. It produces ventricular capture and does not preserve optimal hemodynamics in patients with intact AV conduction. With available technology for transesophageal pacing, only atrial pacing is reliable. Thus, the method is not suitable for patients with advanced AV block or atrial fibrillation.

3. **Permanent pacing.** Permanent pacemakers are no longer prescribed simply for rate support. They have become an integral part of treatment, along with drugs and other measures, to prevent arrhythmias and improve quality of life in patients with conduction disease and heart failure [7].

TABLE 18.2 Usual and less-established indications for temporary cardiac pacing

Usual indications	Less-established indications
• Sinus bradycardia or escape rhythm with symptoms or hemodynamic compromise	• During AMI: New or age-indeterminate right BBB with LAFB, LPFB, or first-degree AV heart block, or with left BBB; recurrent sinus pauses refractory to atropine; overdrive pacing for incessant VT
• As bridge to permanent pacing with advanced second- or third-degree AV heart block, regardless of etiology	
• During AMI: Asystole; new bifascicular block with first-degree AV heart block; alternating BBB with disadvantageous bradycardia not responsive to drugs; or type II, second-degree AV heart block	• During AMI: New or age-indeterminate bifascicular block or isolated right BBB
• Bradycardia-dependent tachyarrhythmias (e.g., torsades de pointes with LQTS)	• Heart surgery: (i) to overdrive hemodynamically disadvantageous AV junctional and ventricular rhythms, (ii) to terminate reentrant SVT or VT, (iii) to prevent pause- or bradycardia-dependent tachydysrhythmias, (iv) insertion of pulmonary artery catheter with left BBB

AMI, acute myocardial infarction; AV, atrioventricular; BBB, bundle branch block; LAFB, left anterior fascicular block; LPFB, left posterior fascicular block; LQTS, long QT syndrome; SVT, supraventricular tachycardia; VT, ventricular tachycardia.

a. **Indications.** The presence or absence of symptoms directly attributable to bradycardia has an important influence on the decision to implant a permanent pacemaker. There is increasing interest in multisite pacing as part of the management for patients with structural heart disease and heart failure. In the past, pacemakers were also prescribed to treat reentrant tachyarrhythmias. Today, this capability can be programmed for either the atrium or ventricle as part of "tiered therapies" with an **internal cardioverter–defibrillator** (ICD) and in only a few pacemakers.

(1) **AV block.** Patients may be asymptomatic or have symptoms related to bradycardia, ventricular arrhythmias, or both. There is little evidence that pacing improves survival with isolated first-degree AV block. With type I second-degree AV block due to AV nodal conduction delay, progression to higher-degree block is unlikely. Pacing is usually not indicated unless the patient has symptoms. With type II second-degree AV block within or below the His bundle, symptoms are frequent, prognosis is poor, and progression to third-degree AV block is common. Pacing is recommended for chronic type II second-degree AV block. It is recommended for type I second-degree AV block in the presence of symptoms such as syncope. Pacing improves survival in both types of second-degree AV blocks. Nonrandomized studies strongly suggest that pacing improves survival in patients with third-degree AV block [7].

(2) **Bifascicular and trifascicular block.** Although third-degree AV block is commonly preceded by bifascicular block, the rate of progression is slow (years) [8]. Further, there is no credible evidence for acute progression to third-degree AV block during anesthesia and surgery. Bifascicular block with periodic third-degree AV block and syncope is associated with an increased incidence of sudden death. Prophylactic permanent pacing is indicated in this circumstance.

(3) **AV block after acute MI.** The requirement for temporary pacing with acute MI by itself does not constitute an indication for permanent pacing. The long-term prognosis for survivors of acute MI is related primarily to the extent of myocardial injury and nature of intraventricular conduction defects, rather than to AV block itself. Acute MI patients with intraventricular conduction disturbances have unfavorable short- and long-term prognoses, with increased risk of sudden death. This prognosis is not necessarily due to the development of high-grade AV block, although the incidence of such block is higher in these patients.

(4) **SND.** SND may manifest as sinus bradycardia, pause or arrest, or SA block, with or without escape rhythms. It often occurs in association with atrial fibrillation or atrial flutter (tachycardia–bradycardia syndrome). Patients with SND may have symptoms due to bradycardia, tachycardia, or both. Correlation of symptoms with arrhythmias is essential and is established by ambulatory monitoring. SND also presents as chronotropic incompetence (inability to increase rate appropriately). An adaptive-rate pacemaker may benefit these patients by restoring more physiologic heart rates. Although symptomatic SND is the primary indication for a pacemaker, pacing does not necessarily improve survival, but it can improve the quality of life.

(5) **Hypersensitive carotid sinus syndrome or neurally mediated syndrome.** Hypersensitive carotid sinus syndrome is manifest by syncope due to an exaggerated response to carotid sinus stimulation. It is an uncommon cause of syncope. If purely cardioinhibitory (asystole, heart block) and without vasodepressor components (vasodilatation), then a pacemaker can be prescribed. A hyperactive response is defined as asystole for longer than 3 seconds due to sinus arrest or heart block and an abrupt decrease in blood pressure. With the more common neurally mediated mixed response, attention to both components is essential for effective therapy. Neurally mediated (vasovagal) syncope accounts for nearly 25% of all syncope. The role of permanent pacing is controversial but probably limited.

(6) **Pacing in children and adolescents.** Indications for pacing are similar in children and adults, but there are additional considerations. For example, what is the

optimal heart rate for the patient's age? Further, what is optimal given ventricular dysfunction or altered circulatory physiology? Hence, pacing indications are based more on correlation of symptoms with bradycardia, rather than arbitrary rate criteria, and include the following:

(a) Bradycardia only after other causes (e.g., seizures, breath holding, apnea, or neurally mediated mechanisms) are excluded.

(b) Symptomatic congenital third-degree AV block

(c) Persistent, advanced second- or third-degree AV block after cardiac surgery. However, for patients with residual bifascicular block and intermittent AV block, the need is less certain.

(d) Use along with β-blockers in patients with congenital long QT syndrome, especially with pause-dependent VT.

(7) Miscellaneous pacing indications

(a) In **obstructive hypertrophic cardiomyopathy,** a dual-chamber pacemaker with short AV delay reduces left ventricular outflow tract obstruction, alleviates symptoms in some cases, and may improve functional status. Permanent pacing does not reduce mortality or prevent sudden death in this disease.

(b) **Bradyarrhythmias after cardiac transplantation** are mostly due to SND. Cardiac transplantation today preserves the sinus node, so SND is much less likely. Most patients with bradycardia show improvement by 1 year, so that long-term pacing is unnecessary.

(c) A combination of pacing and β-blockers may be used for **prophylaxis for tachyarrhythmias** in congenital long QT syndrome. Pacing therapy alone is not recommended. Backup dual-chamber defibrillator therapy is now preferred.

b. **Technology.** Current single- and dual-chamber and cardiac resynchronization therapy (CRT) pacemakers are sophisticated devices with multiple programmable features, including automatic mode switching, rate-adaptive pacing, automatic threshold pacing, and programmable lead configuration. Current pacemakers also allow for remote monitoring technology, so that regular device follow-up can be done from home via a dedicated cellular line. Older pacemaker systems may not have this updated technology and still require in-office and from-home magnet checks for routine follow-up of these devices. Pacemakers are powered by lithium iodide batteries, with an expected service life of 5 to 12 years, depending on device capabilities, need for pacing, and programmed stimulus parameters. Most systems use transvenous leads. Lead configuration is programmable. With the unipolar configuration, the pacemaker housing (can) serves as anode (+) and the distal electrode of the bipolar pacing lead as cathode (−). With the bipolar configuration, proximal and distal lead electrodes serve as anode and cathode, respectively. The ability to program unipolar pacing is necessary if lead insulation or conductor failure occurs in a bipolar lead system. Also, it permits exploitation of either configuration while minimizing its disadvantages (e.g., oversensing with unipolar leads). A dual-chamber pacemaker with automatic mode switching is optimal for patients with AV block and susceptibility to paroxysmal atrial fibrillation. Algorithms detect fast, non-physiologic atrial rates and automatically switch the pacing mode to one that excludes atrial tracking and the associated risk of upper-rate ventricular pacing. There is also the recently Food and Drug Administration (FDA)-approved leadless intracardiac pacing technology that currently is only available for single-chamber ventricular pacing but does provide rate-response therapy [9]. This is a rapidly expanding technology that will likely grow with expanding indications and sophistication in the next few years.

4. **Implantable cardioverter–defibrillator.** Current ICDs are multiprogrammable, mainly involving transvenous leads, and may incorporate **all** capabilities of a modern dual-chamber pacemaker and CRT pacemakers. ICDs are powered by a combination of both batteries and capacitors. All current models also have remote monitoring technology that allows patients to have remote follow-up via dedicated cellular lines for routine ICD evaluations. This limits the required in-person visits to the device clinic or doctor's office to annual or biannual evaluations. In addition, ICDs have multiple tachycardia detection zones, with programmable detection criteria and "tiered therapy" for each (antitachycardia pacing → cardioversion shocks → defibrillatory shocks, if necessary). ICDs also store arrhythmia event records and treatment results. In addition, ICDs have undergone significant downsizing (50 mL or smaller) and nearly all are prepectoral implants. The exception to this location is now the completely subcutaneous ICD with essentially no pacing function [10]. The subcutaneous positioning of this device generator is the left lateral chest, with the lead positioned subcutaneously to the lower sternum and just lateral and parallel to the sternum.

    a. Indications. ICDs are used for **secondary or primary prevention** of sudden death.

        (1) Secondary prevention. ICDs are used for **secondary prevention** in patients who have survived a cardiac arrest from sustained ventricular arrhythmias. Most commonly, these are patients with heart failure and reduced left ventricular systolic function. Of this population, coronary artery disease and ischemic cardiomyopathy are the most common etiologies of the heart failure. Secondary prevention indications for ICDs also include individuals with structural heart disease, who have documented sustained ventricular tachyarrhythmias or inducible sustained ventricular tachyarrhythmias by electrophysiologic testing. ICDs are widely accepted for improving outcomes in these patients by preventing sudden cardiac death. Other indications for secondary prevention include patients with long QT syndrome and recurrent syncope, sustained ventricular arrhythmias, or sudden cardiac arrest despite drug therapy. ICD plus class IA drugs are prescribed for patients with idiopathic VF and Brugada syndrome with recurrent ventricular arrhythmias. Other indications are (i) sudden death survivors with hypertrophic cardiomyopathy; (ii) prophylaxis for syncope and sudden death with arrhythmogenic right ventricular dysplasia; and (iii) children with malignant tachyarrhythmias or sudden death and congenital heart disease, cardiomyopathies, or primary electrical disease (e.g., long QT syndrome) [7].

        (2) Primary prevention. ICDs are used for **primary prevention** of sudden death in patients who are at high risk for sudden cardiac death. This population mainly includes those with systolic heart failure (with ejection fractions ≤35%) that has not improved despite medical therapy. The cause of heart failure may be from coronary artery disease or of nonischemic origin. Other indications for primary prevention ICDs include patients with high-risk features with inherited or acquired conditions that place them at increased risk for life-threatening ventricular arrhythmias, including long QT syndrome, hypertrophic cardiomyopathy, arrhythmogenic right ventricular dysplasia, cardiac sarcoidosis, Brugada syndrome, and congenital heart disease [7].

    b. Technology. The ICD pulse generator is a self-powered minicomputer with one or two (in series) batteries that power the pulse generator, circuitry, and aluminum electrolytic capacitors. The batteries may be lithium–silver vanadium oxide or evolving hybrid technology, and they vary among the manufacturers. A major challenge in ICD design is the large range of voltages within a very small package. Intracardiac signals may be as low as 100 μV, and therapeutic shocks approach 750 V. Further, ICD batteries contain up to 20,000 J, and a potential hazard exists if the charging and firing circuits were to electrically or thermally unload all this energy into the patient in a brief time period. The number of shocks delivered during treatment is usually limited to five or six per arrhythmia. The expected service life is 5 to 12 years.

IV. Device function, malfunction, and interference [11]

    A. Pacemakers

    A single-chamber pacemaker stimulates the atria or ventricles at programmed timing intervals. Sensing spontaneous atrial or ventricular depolarizations inhibits the device from delivering unnecessary or inappropriate stimuli. Dual-chamber devices time the delivery of ventricular stimuli relative to sensed atrial depolarizations to maintain proper AV synchrony. Figure 18.2

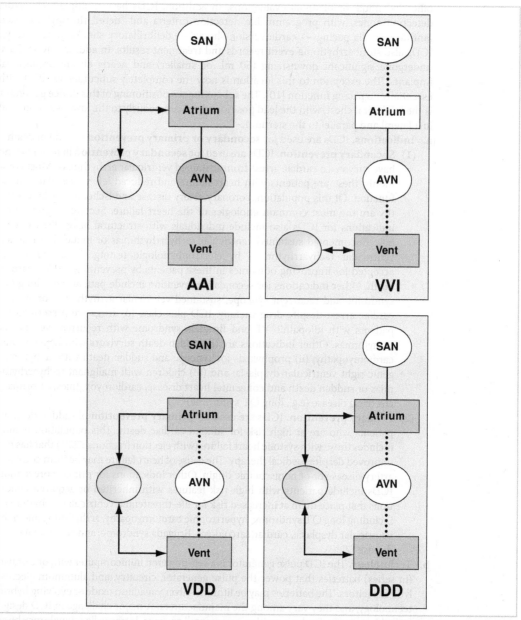

FIGURE 18.2 Bradycardia pacing modes. A dysfunctional sinoatrial node (SAN), atrium, or atrioventricular node (AVN) is indicated by *white circles* or *rectangles*. Normal impulse transmission between these structures and the ventricles (Vent) is indicated by *solid lines,* with blocked or ineffective conduction indicated by *hashed lines.* An *arrow* pointing toward the pulse generator (*blue*) indicates sensing, whereas one pointing toward the atrium or ventricle indicates pacing in that chamber. **Top left:** AAI pacing for sinus arrest or bradycardia. There is a single atrial lead for both sensing and pacing. Atrial pacing occurs unless inhibited by a sensed spontaneous atrial depolarization. **Top right:** VVI pacing for AV heart block with atrial fibrillation. There is a single ventricular lead for both sensing and pacing. Ventricular pacing occurs unless inhibited by a sensed spontaneous ventricular depolarization. **Bottom left:** VDD pacing for AV heart block with normal SAN and atrial function. The atrial lead is for sensing only, and the ventricular lead is for both pacing and sensing. After a sensed atrial depolarization, the ventricle is paced after the programmed AV interval (i.e., atrial-triggered ventricular pacing [VAT]), unless first inhibited by a sensed ventricular depolarization (i.e., the VVI component of the VDD mode). **Bottom right:** Dual-chamber sequential or AV universal (DDD) pacing for sinus bradycardia with AV heart block. Both atrial and ventricular leads are for sensing and pacing. This mode incorporates all of the preceding pacing capabilities (AAI, VVI, and VAT).

TABLE 18.3 NASPE/BPEG (NBG) pacemaker code used as shorthand to designate pacing modes

I	II	III	IV	V
Chamber paced	Chamber sensed	Response to sensed event	Programmability/rate response[a]	Antitachycardia functions[b]
O = none	O = none	O = none	O = none	O = none
A = atrium	A = atrium	I = inhibit	R = adaptive rate	P = Antitachycardia pacing
V = ventricle	V = ventricle	T = triggered		S = shock
D = dual (A & V)	D = dual (A & V)	D = dual (I & T)		D = dual (P + S)
S = single[c]	S = single[c]			

[a]In current terminology, only the adaptive rate response (R) is indicated by the fourth position. All current pacemakers have full programming and communicating capability; therefore, the letters P (programmable), M (multiprogrammable), and C (communicating) are no longer used.
[b]Implantable cardioverter–defibrillator (ICD) with antibradycardia and antitachycardia pacing capabilities.
[c]Single-chamber device that paces either the atrium or ventricle.
From Bernstein AD, Daubert JC, Fletcher RD, et al. The revised NASPE/BPEG generic code for antibradycardia, adaptive-rate, and multisite pacing. North American Society of Pacing and Electrophysiology/British Pacing and Electrophysiology Group. *Pacing Clin Electrophysiol.* 2002;25(2):260–264.

illustrates how a pacemaker might be configured to pace in patients with SND or AV heart block (AVHB).

In Figure 18.2 and throughout this chapter, the North American Society for Pacing and Electrophysiology–British Pacing and Electrophysiology Group (NASPE/BPEG) pacemaker code (also known as the NBG code) is used as a shorthand to describe pacing modes (Table 18.3).

1. **Function.** Today, most US pacemakers are dual-chamber (DDD or DDDR) devices with rate-adaptive features (rate response) that can be activated if clinically indicated. Single-chamber pacemakers may pace either the atrium or ventricle depending on lead placement and also may have rate-adaptive features turned on. Dual-chamber pacemakers may also be programmed to act like a single-chamber pacer, activating either the atrial or ventricular lead through the use of the proprietary programmer. For example, in individuals with normal conduction and sinus node function, dual-chamber pacemakers may operate as a single-chamber device in the AAI (AAIR, AAI) or VVI (VVIR) modes (Fig. 18.2). There are also expanding indications for CRT pacing systems to improve cardiac resynchronizations in both heart failure and pacer-dependent patients [12].

   a. **Single-chamber pacemaker.** These devices have a single timing interval, the atrial or ventricular escape interval, between successive stimuli in the absence of sensed depolarization. In the AAI or VVI mode (Fig. 18.3), pacing occurs at the end of the programmed atrial or ventricular escape interval, unless a spontaneous atrial or ventricular depolarization is sensed first, resetting these intervals. If the device has rate hysteresis as a programmable option, then the atrial or ventricular escape interval after a sensed depolarization is programmed longer than that after a paced depolarization to encourage emergence of intrinsic rhythm and prolong battery life.

   b. **Dual-chamber pacemaker.** A DDD ("AV universal") pacemaker can pace and sense in both the atrium and the ventricle. It has two basic timing intervals whose sum is the pacing cycle duration (Fig. 18.4). The first is the AV interval, which is the programmed interval from a paced or sensed atrial depolarization to ensuing ventricular stimulation. Some devices offer the option of programmable AV interval hysteresis. If so, the AV interval after paced atrial depolarization is longer than that after sensed depolarization to maintain greater uniformity between atrial and ventricular depolarizations. The second interval is the VA interval, the interval between sensed or paced ventricular depolarization and the next atrial stimulus. During atrial and ventricular refractory periods (Fig. 18.4), sensed events do not reset the device escape timing. During the ventricular channel blanking period (Fig. 18.4), ventricular sensing is disabled to avoid overloading of the

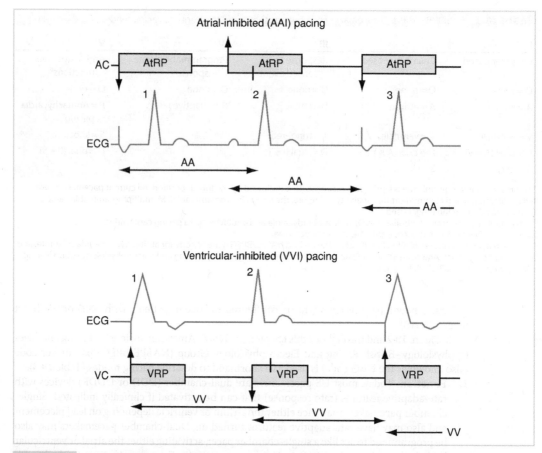

FIGURE 18.3 **Top:** AAI pacing, as for a patient with sinus bradycardia and intact AV conduction. The atrium is paced (beats 1 and 3)—*arrow* pointing toward the electrocardiogram (ECG) in the atrial channel (AC) timing diagram—unless inhibited by sensed spontaneous atrial depolarization (beat 2)—*arrow* pointing away from the ECG in the AC timing diagram. The atrial refractory period (AtRP) prevents R and T waves from being sensed by the AC and inappropriately resetting the atrial escape timing (AA interval). Note that spontaneous atrial depolarization (beat 2) occurs before the AA interval times out, resetting the AA interval. The *short vertical line* in the AC timing diagram above beat 2 shows where the stimulus would have occurred had the previous AA interval timed out. In the absence of subsequent spontaneous atrial depolarization (beat 3), the AA interval times out with delivery of a stimulus. **Bottom:** VVI pacing, as for a patient with atrial fibrillation and AV heart block. Beats 1 and 3 are paced and beat 2 is spontaneous. The latter resets the ventricular escape interval (VV), which otherwise would have timed out with delivery of a stimulus, indicated by the *short vertical line* in the ventricular channel (VC) timing diagram above beat 2. The new VV interval times out with stimulus delivery (beat 3) because there is no sensed ventricular depolarization to reset the timing. VRP, ventricular refractory period.

ventricular sense amplifier by voltage generated by the atrial stimulus, thereby inappropriately resetting the VA interval. Sensing during the alert periods outside the ventricular blanking and postventricular atrial and ventricular refractory periods initiates new AV or VA intervals (Fig. 18.4). Operationally, depending on sensing patterns, a DDD pacemaker can provide atrial, ventricular, dual-chamber sequential, or no pacing (Fig. 18.4). There is also proprietary software in most dual-chamber pacemakers that promotes intrinsic ventricular conduction (if appropriate) or minimizes unnecessary right ventricular pacing. This programming can appear abnormal and may be misinterpreted as pacemaker malfunction [13]. On rhythm strips or ECGs, this pacemaker programming may result in variable and prolonged AV delays with resumption of ventricular pacing and shortening of paced AV delay when the intrinsic AV delay becomes too long.

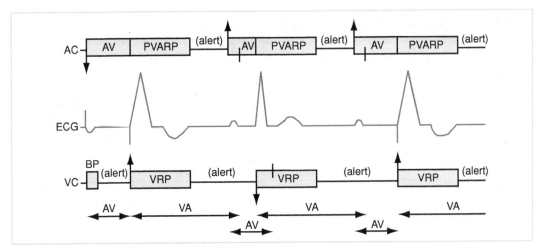

FIGURE 18.4 AV universal (DDD) pacing, as for a patient with sinus node dysfunction (SND) and atrioventricular (AV) heart block. The atrium is paced (beat 1)—*arrow* pointing toward the electrocardiogram (ECG) in the atrial channel (AC) timing diagram above beat 1—unless inhibited by sensed atrial depolarization (beats 2 and 3)—*arrows* pointing away from the ECG in the AC timing diagram. The AC is refractory during the AV interval and from delivery of the ventricular stimulus until the end of the postventricular atrial refractory period (PVARP). This prevents atrial sensing from resetting the escape timing (i.e., AV interval). The ventricular channel (VC) blanking period (BP) prevents sensing of the atrial pacing stimulus, thereby resetting the AV interval and delaying ventricular stimulus delivery. However, sensed ventricular depolarization or noise (e.g., electrocautery) in the alert period (VC) after the blanking period also could inhibit ventricular stimulation. As shown, this does not occur, so the AV interval times out with delivery of a ventricular stimulus. The ventricular refractory period (VRP) prevents sensed T waves from inappropriately resetting the ventriculoatrial (VA) interval. However, sensing during the alert periods after the PVARP or VRP will reset basic timing, initiating new AV and VA intervals, respectively. Since the first beat is fully paced, it is an example of asynchronous AV sequential pacing (i.e., DOO). With the second beat, a sensed spontaneous atrial depolarization initiates a new AV interval, inhibiting the atrial stimulus that would have occurred, indicated by the *short vertical line* in the AC timing diagram. Subsequently, there is spontaneous ventricular depolarization before the AV interval times out. The ventricular stimulus that otherwise would have occurred at the end of the AV interval is indicated by the *short vertical line* in the VC timing diagram below beat 2. The third beat begins with a sensed atrial depolarization. As with beat 2, this also occurs before the VA interval times out. In the absence of sensed ventricular depolarization (beat 3), the new AV interval times out with ventricular stimulus delivery. Beat 3 is an example of atrial-inhibited, ventricular-triggered pacing (i.e., VDD).

c. **Cardiac resynchronization therapy pacemakers.** CRT pacemakers are indicated in patients with systolic heart failure and conduction disease. These devices have an additional lead pacing the left ventricle. They may be programmed to AV sequentially pace in the case of sinus rhythm or just pace the ventricle in the case of permanent atrial fibrillation. With CRT pacing, there is simultaneous pacing of both the right and left ventricles to improve the intraventricular depolarization time. Multipoint pacing, which paces at multiple sites in the left ventricle, has proved to further enhance the heart failure response to this therapy [14].

d. **Adaptive-rate pacing (ARP).** ARP is a programmable feature in nearly all implanted devices (both pacemakers and ICDs) in service today. In patients with chronotropic incompetence, ARP has been shown to improve exercise capacity and quality of life. Activity-based sensors are used most commonly to determine the paced heart rate. These are piezoelectric crystals that sense vibration (up-and-down motion) or acceleration (forward–backward movement) as an index of physical activity. Minute ventilation sensors measure changes in transthoracic impedance with respiration (i.e., increase with inspiration and decrease with expiration) and provide an estimate of metabolic need that is more proportional to exercise. Some pacemaker algorithms detect changes in contractility in determining the ARP response. ARP sensors may have a disproportionate response time at the beginning of exercise versus steady-state

TABLE 18.4 Categories of pacemaker malfunction, electrocardiogram (ECG) appearance, and likely cause for malfunction

Category of malfunction	ECG appearance	Cause for malfunction
Failure to pace	For one or both chambers, either no pacing artifacts will be present on the ECG or artifacts will be present for one but not the other chamber	Oversensing, battery failure, open circuit due to mechanical problems with leads or system component malfunction, fibrosis at electrode–tissue interface; lead dislodgment, recording artifact
Failure to capture	Atrial and/or ventricular pacing stimuli are present, with persistent or intermittent failure to capture	Fibrosis at electrode–tissue interface, drugs or conditions that increase pacing thresholds (Table 18.5)
Pacing at abnormal rates	I. Rapid pacing rate (upper rate behavior) II. Slow pacing rate (below lower rate interval) III. No stimulus artifact, intrinsic rate below lower rate interval	I. Adaptive-rate pacing (ARP), tracking atrial tachycardia, pacemaker-mediated tachycardia (PMT), oversensing II. Programmed rate hysteresis, or rest or sleep rates; oversensing III. Power source failure, lead disruption, oversensing
Failure to sense	Pacing artifacts in middle of normal P waves or QRS complexes	Inadequate intracardiac signal strength, component malfunction, battery depletion, misinterpretation of normal device function
Oversensing	Abnormal pacing rates with pauses (regular or random)	Far-field sensing with inappropriate device inhibition or triggering, intermittent contact between pacing system conducting elements
Malfunction unique to dual-chamber devices	Rapid pacing rate (i.e., upper rate behavior)	Cross-talk inhibition, pacemaker-mediated tachycardia (see text)

exercise; a dual-sensor ARP or physiologic sensor device may provide a more proportional response. Obviously, such complexity and the use of multiple physiologic sensors increase the potential for unexpected device interactions in the perioperative setting. For example, simple manipulation of the generator may inappropriately activate the ARP sensor, resulting in increased pacing heart rate. In addition, changes in breathing may result in changes in ARP if minute ventilation sensors are activated.

2. **Malfunction.** Primary pacemaker malfunction is rare (less than 2% of all device-related problems). Pacing malfunction can occur with ICDs because all ICDs today include a pacing function which can pace at least the ventricle. Some devices have programmed behavior that simulates malfunction, termed pseudomalfunction. For example, failure to pace may be misdiagnosed with programmed rate hysteresis. Also, apparent device malfunction in response to electromagnetic interference (EMI) may be normal device operation, as described later in this chapter.

Pacemaker malfunction is classified as failure to pace, failure to capture, pacing at abnormal rates, failure to sense, oversensing, and malfunction unique to dual-chamber devices (Table 18.4). Among the causes for failure to capture are drugs or conditions that affect pacing thresholds (Table 18.5). To diagnose malfunction, it is necessary to obtain a 12-lead ECG and chest x-ray film and to interrogate the device for pacing and sensing thresholds, lead impedances, battery voltage, and magnet rate.

Malfunctions unique to dual-chamber devices are crosstalk inhibition and pacemaker-mediated tachycardia (PMT).

a. **Crosstalk inhibition.** Crosstalk refers to the oversensing of atrial signals from atrial stimulation on the ventricular sense channel or circuit of a dual-chamber pacemaker. This oversensing has the potential to inhibit ventricular output. Crosstalk is prevented by increasing the ventricular sensing threshold, decreasing atrial stimulus output, or programming a longer ventricular blanking period (Fig. 18.4), so long as these provide adequate safety margins for atrial capture and ventricular sensing. If crosstalk cannot

TABLE 18.5 Drugs and conditions that affect or have no proven effect on pacing thresholds

Effect	Drugs	Conditions
Increase pacing threshold	Bretylium, encainide, flecainide, moricizine, propafenone, sotalol	Myocardial ischemia and infarction, progression of cardiomyopathy, hyperkalemia, severe acidosis or alkalosis, hypoxemia, hypothermia, irradiation, after cardioversion or defibrillation (implantable cardioverter–defibrillator or external)
Possibly increase pacing threshold	β-Blockers, lidocaine, procainamide, quinidine, verapamil	Myxedema, hyperglycemia
Possibly decrease pacing threshold	Atropine, catecholamines, glucocorticoids	Pheochromocytoma, hyperthyroid or other hypermetabolic states
No proven effect on pacing threshold	Amiodarone; anesthetic drugs, both inhalation and intravenous	Hyperthermia

be prevented, many dual-chamber devices have a feature referred to as nonphysiologic AV delay or ventricular safety pacing. Whenever the ventricular channel senses anything early during the AV interval, a ventricular stimulus is triggered after an abbreviated AV interval. This either will depolarize ventricular myocardium or will fail to do so if myocardium is refractory due to spontaneous depolarization. The premature timing of the triggered ventricular stimulus prevents it from occurring during the vulnerable period of the T wave.

    b. Pacemaker-mediated tachycardia (PMT). PMT is undesired rapid pacing caused by the device or its interaction with the patient. PMT includes sensor-driven tachycardia, tachycardia due to tracking of myopotentials or atrial tachyarrhythmias, pacemaker reentrant tachycardia, and runaway pacemaker.

        Sensor-driven tachycardia may occur with adaptive-rate devices that sense vibration, impedance changes, or the QT interval if they sense mechanical or physiologic interference, which leads to inappropriate high-rate pacing. Thus, it is advised that ARP be disabled in perioperative settings.

        Pacemaker reentrant tachycardia can occur in a device programmed to an atrial tracking mode. Up to 50% of patients with dual-chamber devices are susceptible to PRT because they have retrograde (VA) conduction via the AVN. PRT occurs when spontaneous or paced ventricular beats are conducted back to the atria to trigger ventricular pacing. To prevent PRT, a longer postventricular atrial refractory period is programmed (Fig. 18.4). Also, placing a magnet over the pulse generator will terminate PRT in most devices by disabling sensing. However, PRT may recur after the magnet is removed.

   3. Response of pacemaker to magnet application. Most contemporary pacemaker devices respond to magnet application by a device-specific single- or dual-chamber asynchronous pacing mode. Adaptive-rate response is generally suspended with magnet mode as well. With asynchronous pacing, the pacemaker will no longer be inhibited by sensed activity and instead will pace at a fixed rate regardless of underlying rhythm. The first few magnet-triggered beats may occur at a rate and output other than that seen later. Pacing amplitudes remain constant at the programmed output in Biotronik, Boston Scientific, and Medtronic pacemakers. The pacing amplitude with magnet application in ELA/Sorin and St. Jude pacemakers may be higher than the programmed output settings. The response to a magnet should be determined prior to an anticipated surgical procedure and is predicted by the brand of the pacemaker in most circumstances. However, some manufacturers, Biotronik, St. Jude Medical, and Boston Scientific devices, have a programmable magnet mode that may make response to magnet application different than anticipated. Although rarely used, this feature may be programmed to save patient-activated rhythm recordings with magnet application, rather than revert the pacemaker to asynchronous pacing. Discussion or documentation with the providers that follow the device can confirm that

TABLE 18.6	Elective replacement indicators (ERI) that may affect the nominal rate of pacing

- **Stepwise change in pacing rate:** Pacing rate changes to some predetermined fixed rate or some percentage decrease from the programmed rate
- **Stepwise change in magnet rate:** Magnet pacing rate decreases in a stepwise fashion related to the remaining battery life
- **Pacing mode change:** DDD and DDDR pulse generators may automatically revert to another mode, such as VVI or VOO, to reduce current drain and extend battery life

the typical magnet response is "on." Alternatively, if this communication is not possible, a magnet can be placed on the device to evaluate if there is a change to asynchronous pacing on telemetry. The magnet-triggered rate and the duration of pacing do vary based on manufacturer and battery status. For example, Biotronik pacemakers have a magnet rate at 90 bpm for 10 beats only, while all other manufacturers pace asynchronously as long as the magnet is in contact with the pacemaker. The fixed magnet rate for Boston Scientific pacemakers is 100 bpm; St. Jude is 98.6 bpm; ELA/Sorin is 96 bpm. Medtronic pacemakers are triggered for three beats at 100 bpm, then default to 85 bpm. However, with impending power source depletion, the magnet rate will approach the programmed rate of the end-of-life (EOL) or elective replacement indicator (ERI) and is usually a slower pacing interval than the standard magnet rate (Table 18.6).

In a patient whose intrinsic rhythm inhibits the device, magnet application may serve to identify the programmed mode when the correct programmer is not available for telemetry. Also, with device malfunction due to improper sensing, magnet-initiated asynchronous pacing may temporarily correct the problem, confirming the presence of far-field sensing, crosstalk inhibition, T-wave sensing, or PMT. Finally, in pacemaker-dependent patients, magnet application may ensure pacing if EMI inhibits output (e.g., surgical electrocautery).

4. **Interference.** CIEDs are subject to interference from nonbiologic electromagnetic sources. In general, devices in service today are effectively shielded against many forms of EMI. However, with the continued advances and changes in technology with medical procedures as well as CIEDs, it is recommended that a CIED management plan be established for the patient based on both the planned medical procedure and type and indication for the CIED [11]. This process is recommended for elective procedures. The following describes some scenarios where the programming may not be predictable, supporting the practice of establishing a perioperative CIED management plan. EMI frequencies above 10^9 Hz (i.e., infrared, visible light, ultraviolet, x-rays, and gamma rays) do not typically interfere with pacemakers or ICDs because the wavelengths are much shorter than the device or lead dimensions. High-intensity therapeutic x-rays and irradiation can directly damage circuitry. A management plan is often required in individuals who require therapeutic radiation near their CIED. In general, EMI enters a device by conduction (direct contact) or radiation (leads acting as an antenna). Devices are protected from EMI by (i) shielding the circuitry, (ii) using a bipolar (versus unipolar) lead configuration for sensing to minimize the antenna, and (iii) filtering incoming signals to exclude noncardiac signals. If EMI does enter the pulse generator, noise protection algorithms in the timing circuit help reduce its effect on the patient. However, EMI signals between 5 and 100 Hz are not filtered because these overlap the frequency range of intracardiac signals. Therefore, EMI in this frequency range may be interpreted as intracardiac signals, giving rise to abnormal behavior. Possible responses include (i) inappropriate inhibition or triggering of stimulation, (ii) asynchronous pacing (Fig. 18.5), (iii) mode resetting, (iv) direct damage to the pulse generator circuitry, and (v) triggering of unnecessary ICD shocks (Table 18.7).

Finally, with EMI and inappropriate device behavior, it is widely assumed that placing a magnet over a pulse generator invariably will cause asynchronous pacing as long as the magnet remains in place. However, this is not always the case. Although used rarely, some devices (see Section IV.A.3) may have programmed magnet response off.

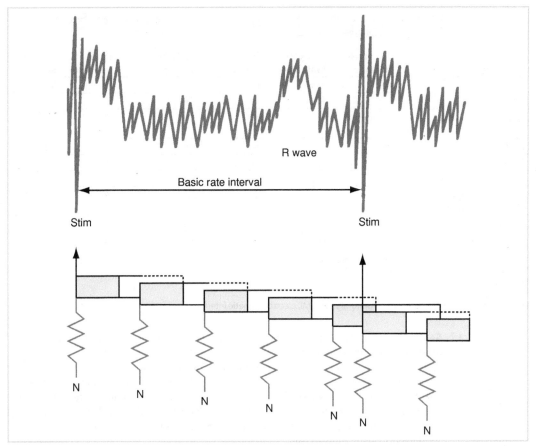

FIGURE 18.5 VVI pacemaker response to continuous electromagnetic interference (EMI). Temporary asynchronous pacing stimulation (Stim) occurs at the programmed basic rate interval. The ventricular refractory period (*rectangles*) begins with the noise (N) sampling period (*blue rectangles*), during which time there is no sensing. During the remainder of this refractory period, repeated noise (N) sensing above a specified minimal frequency (e.g., 7 Hz) is interpreted as EMI. This restarts the ventricular refractory period. Portions of the previous refractory period preempted by the newly initiated ventricular refractory period are indicated by *hashed rectangles*. Therefore, so long as interference persists, the pacemaker remains refractory and escape timing is determined entirely by the programmed basic rate interval. In this example, the second paced R wave falls in the noise sampling period. It is not sensed, but it initiates a new ventricular refractory period. The spontaneous R wave is not sensed and does not affect escape timing.

In contrast to pacemakers, magnet application on ICDs will not alter the pacing mode and will not change the mode to asynchronous pacing (see IV.B.7). Thus, if possible, one should determine before EMI exposure what pulse generator is present and what must be done to provide protection. If this is not possible preoperatively, then one must observe the magnet response during EMI to ascertain whether there is protection from EMI sensing. For example, if a pacemaker-dependent patient has inappropriate inhibition or triggering of output during electrosurgery even with magnet application, then electrosurgery must be limited to short bursts.

B. Internal cardioverter–defibrillator (ICD)

An ICD consists of a pulse generator and leads for tachyarrhythmia detection and therapy. Modern ICDs use transvenous lead systems for sensing, pacing, and biphasic shock delivery. Epicardial leads are still used in infants and small children and occasionally in adult patients. Use of biphasic compared to monophasic shocks has greatly lowered defibrillation energy requirements and has led to development of smaller ICDs.

TABLE 18.7   Perioperative EMI sources and their potential effects on implanted pacemakers or implantable cardioverter–defibrillators

EMI source	Generator damage	Complete inhibition	One-beat inhibition	Asynchronous pacing	Rate increase	Spurious shocks
Electrocautery	Yes	Yes	Yes	Yes	Yes[a,b]	Yes
External DC/DF	Yes	No	No	Yes	Yes	No
Magnetic resonance imaging scanner	Possible	No	Yes	Yes	Yes	Yes
Lithotripsy	Yes[b]	Yes[c]	Yes[c]	Yes[c]	Yes[d]	Yes
Radiofrequency ablation	Yes	Yes	No	No	Yes	Yes
Electroconvulsive therapy	No	Yes	Yes	Yes	Yes[b]	Yes
Transcutaneous electrical nerve stimulation	No	Yes	No	Yes	Yes	Unlikely
Radiation therapy	Yes	No	No	No	Yes	Yes
Diagnostic radiation	No	No	No	No	Yes	No

[a]Impedance-based adaptive-rate (AR) pulse generators.
[b]Piezoelectric crystal-based AR pulse generators.
[c]Potential for interference.
[d]DDD mode only.
DC/DF, direct-current cardioversion or defibrillation; EMI, electromagnetic interference.

1. **Sensing ventricular depolarizations.** Reliable sensing is essential. The sense amplifier must respond quickly and accurately to rates of 30 to 360 bpm or greater and to the varying amplitude and morphology of intracardiac signals during VT or VF. Unfiltered intracardiac electrograms are sent to the sense amplifier. This has a band-pass filter to reject low-frequency T waves and high-frequency noise. There is automatic gain control (auto-gain), a rectifier to eliminate polarity dependency, and a fixed or auto-adjusting threshold event detector. The sense amplifier produces a set of R–R intervals for the VT/VF detection algorithms to use.

2. **VF detection.** ICDs use rate criteria as the sole method for detecting VF. Due to the circumstances of VF, the detection algorithms must have high sensitivity and low specificity. If criteria for detection are too aggressive, the ICD likely will oversense T waves during sinus rhythm, leading to spurious shocks. If too conservative, it likely will undersense some VF but work very well during sinus rhythm. An ICD X/Y detector triggers when X of the previous Y-sensed ventricular intervals are shorter than the VF detection interval. Typically, this is 70% to 80% of intervals in a sliding window of 10 to 24. This approach is very good at ignoring the effect of a small number of undersensed events due to the small amplitude of VF intracardiac signals. Any tachycardia with a cycle length less than the VF detection interval will initiate VF therapy. After capacitor charging but before shock delivery, an algorithm confirms the presence of VF. After shock delivery, redetection and episode termination algorithms determine whether VF has terminated, continued, or changed.

3. **Tachycardia detection and discrimination (single-chamber ICD).** Most VT algorithms require a programmable number of consecutive R–R intervals shorter than the VT detection interval. A longer R–R interval, as might occur during atrial fibrillation, would reset the VT counters. In patients with both supraventricular and ventricular tachyarrhythmias, up to 45% of ICD discharges may be inappropriate if rate is used as the sole criterion for VT therapy.

    To increase specificity, VT detection algorithm enhancements are programmed for one or more VT zones in single-chamber ICDs, including criteria for stability of rate, suddenness of onset, and intracardiac QRS morphology.

    a. The **rate-stability criterion** is used to distinguish sustained monomorphic VT with little cycle length variation from atrial fibrillation with much greater cycle length variation. Such enhancement criteria are not available in the VF zone, where maximum sensitivity is required. Also, they are programmed only in rate zones that correspond to VT hemodynamically tolerated by the patient.

   b. The **suddenness of onset criterion** is used to distinguish sinus tachycardia from VT because VT has a more sudden rate increase.

   c. Finally, **morphology algorithms** discriminate VT from SVT based on morphology of intracardiac electrograms.

4. **Tachycardia detection and discrimination (dual-chamber ICD).** Inadequate specificity of VT detection algorithms, despite enhancements, has been a significant problem with single-chamber ICDs. Dual-chamber ICDs use an atrial lead, which is used for bradycardia pacing and sensing for tachycardia discrimination. Detection algorithms use atrial and ventricular timing data to discriminate SVT from VT. For example, the algorithm in devices of one manufacturer has several key elements: (i) the pattern of atrial and ventricular events; (ii) atrial and ventricular rates; (iii) regularity of R–R intervals; (iv) presence or absence of AV dissociation; and (v) atrial and ventricular pattern analysis.

5. **Tiered therapy.** Treatment options for VT include antitachycardia pacing, cardioversion, or defibrillation. More than 80% of monomorphic VTs can be terminated by a critical pacing sequence, reducing the need for painful shocks and improving quality of life [15]. With antitachycardia pacing, trains of stimuli are delivered at a fixed percentage of the VT cycle length. Repeated and more aggressive trains result either in termination of VT or progression to cardioversion or defibrillation.

6. **ICD malfunction.** Malfunctions specific to ICD include inappropriate shock delivery, failure to deliver therapy, ineffective shocks, and interactions with drugs or devices affecting the efficacy of therapy. There is potential for pacing malfunction as well, since all ICDs have a pacemaker function.

   a. **Inappropriate delivery of shocks.** Artifacts created by lead-related malfunction may be interpreted as tachycardia, with inappropriate shock delivery. Electrocautery artifact may be similarly misinterpreted. Rapid SVT or nonsustained VT may be misdiagnosed as sustained VT or VF, especially if rate-only criteria are used for diagnosis. R- and T-wave oversensing, causing double counting during bradycardia pacing, has led to inappropriate shocks.

   b. **Failure to deliver therapy or ineffective shocks.**

CLINICAL PEARL   Having a magnet placed over the ICD generator will usually turn off detections and will result in no delivery of shocks regardless of the arrhythmia. For this reason, it is recommended that patients be on monitored cardiac telemetry prior to magnet placement.

ICDs can stop delivering therapies after about six shocks for a single episode. If a patient requires repeated shocks for VF, therapy may be exhausted or the tachyarrhythmias may be undersensed, with failure to deliver therapy. Exposure to diagnostic x-rays or computed tomographic scans does not adversely affect shock delivery. Acute MI, severe acute acid–base or electrolyte imbalance, or hypoxia may increase defibrillation thresholds, leading to ineffective shocks. Any of these also could affect the rate or morphology of VT and the ability to diagnose VT. Finally, isoflurane and propofol do not affect defibrillation thresholds. The effect of other anesthetics or drugs used to supplement anesthesia is unknown.

   c. **Drug–device interactions affecting efficacy of ICD therapy.** Antiarrhythmic drugs may be used along with an ICD to suppress (i) recurrent sustained VT and the need for shocks, (ii) nonsustained VT that triggers unnecessary shocks, and (iii) atrial fibrillation with inappropriate shocks to excessive ventricular heart rates. Also, they may be used to slow VT to make it better tolerated or more amenable to termination by antitachycardia pacing and to slow AV nodal conduction with atrial fibrillation.

   Possible adverse effects of combined drug and ICD therapy are (i) slowing of VT to below the programmed rate-detection threshold; (ii) proarrhythmia, increasing the need for shocks; (iii) increased defibrillation thresholds; (iv) reduced hemodynamic tolerance of VT; (v) increase in PR, QRS, or QT intervals, causing multiple counting and spurious shocks; and (vi) altered morphology or reduced amplitude of intracardiac electrograms and failure to detect VT/VF. Lidocaine, chronic amiodarone, class IC drugs (e.g., flecainide), and phenytoin can increase defibrillation thresholds. Class IA drugs (e.g., quinidine) generally do not affect defibrillation thresholds.

   d. **Device–device interactions affecting efficacy of therapy.** In the past, pacemakers were used for bradycardia and antitachycardia pacing in ICD patients. Today, ICDs incorporate both pacing capabilities, but still there may be occasional patients with an ICD and a pacemaker. In a patient with an ICD or pacemaker, the presence of a brain or nerve stimulator may be more common today. Regardless of the type of pulse stimulators, possible adverse interactions between two devices include (i) sensed pacing artifacts or depolarizations that may lead to multiple counting, misdiagnosis as VT/VF, and spurious shocks and (ii) ICD shocks that may reprogram a pacemaker or cause failure to capture or sense. The use of only bipolar pacing from the other device will minimize such interference but must be fully evaluated prior to permanent implantation.

7. **Response of an ICD to magnet application** [8]. Magnet application does not interfere with bradycardia pacing and does not trigger asynchronous pacing in an ICD. Magnet application in current ICDs causes inhibition of tachycardia sensing and delivery of shock only. All current ICDs remain inhibited as long as the magnet remains in stable contact with the ICD. Once the magnet is removed, the ICD reverts to the programmed tachyarrhythmia settings. One deviation from this is in some Biotronik ICD platforms, in which a magnet placed in direct contact with the ICD will inhibit continuously up to 8 hours. After 8 hours, the programmed tachycardia therapy will be reactivated, even if the magnet is still in contact. This universal magnet response across all manufacturers has not always been the case, and has caused confusion about intraoperative ICD management. Older platforms manufactured by Boston Scientific/Guidant Corp. had a programmable response to magnet application, most commonly programmed to Magnet Use Enable, but there were exceptions. Most of these device platforms are no longer in service.

   With an appropriately placed magnet, Boston Scientific (Guidant) ICDs have R-synchronous beeping followed by a continuous sound that indicates inactivation of tachyarrhythmia function. Medtronic devices emit a continuous sound for 20 to 30 seconds to indicate inactivation of tachyarrhythmia sensing. ICDs by St. Jude Medical, Biotronik, and ELA/Sorin do not emit sounds in the presence of a magnet. These different audible responses to magnets may continue to be a source of confusion. Regardless of the audible response, all ICDs turn off tachycardia sensing and therapy when a magnet remains applied to the generator.

8. **Interference and ICD.** Reports of inappropriate ICD shocks due to EMI oversensing are infrequent. EMI initially might be misinterpreted as VF, but spurious shocks will not occur unless it continues beyond the capacitor charging period (see Section IV.B.2 and Table 18.7). **Magnet application does not interfere with bradycardia pacing and does not trigger asynchronous pacing in an ICD.**

V. Perioperative considerations for a patient with a cardiac implantable electrical device (CIED) [11]

   A. Preoperative patient evaluation

   Patients with pacemakers or ICDs, especially the latter, often have serious cardiac functional impairment. Many have debilitating coexisting systemic disease as well. Special attention must be paid to progression of disease and functional status, current medications, and compliance with treatment. No special testing is required just because the patient has an implanted device. However, identifying whether the device is an ICD versus pacemaker and documenting compliance with device follow-up is important in the perioperative management. It is now recommended that a plan of perioperative CIED management be developed prior to elective procedures [11]. This plan is usually scripted by the CIED team after they have been advised about the nature of the planned procedure. Baseline information about the surgery is needed by the CIED team (cardiologist, electrophysiologist, and pacemaker clinic staff managing the device) such as (i) type and location of the procedure, (ii) body position at surgery, (iii) electrosurgery needed and site of use, (iv) potential need for DC cardioversion or defibrillation, and (v) other EMI sources. In some centers, anesthesiologists with additional training in device management fulfill the cardiologist's role on this team in many of these situations.

B. **Cardiac implantable electrical device team evaluation**

Patients are usually regularly followed by a CIED team. Frequently, the management plan for perioperative procedures can be determined by the team that follows the patient's device regularly. If that information or approach is not available, most surgical facilities today have an onsite CIED clinic or service (or access to one) that should be consulted to provide preoperative consultation on the management of the device. All patients should carry a card that identifies the model and serial numbers of the device, the date of implantation, and the implanting physician or clinic. Unless the planned surgery is truly emergent or poses little risk of EMI-related device malfunction (e.g., bipolar cautery will be used; the surgical field is far removed from the device, leads, and grounding plate), it is imperative to (i) identify the device (manufacturer, model, leads, battery status), (ii) determine the date and indication(s) for its implantation, and (iii) check its function. If a recent device check (for pacemakers <12 months and for ICDs <6 months) is not available, then the CIED team should perform a check. The data to be provided by this interrogation are (i) type of device (single, dual, biventricular); (ii) programmed mode; (iii) programmed rates, energy, sensing, tachyarrhythmia settings for an ICD; (iv) pacemaker-dependent status; (v) underlying rhythm; (vi) specifics about magnet response; and (vii) pacing safety margin and battery longevity. If the CIED has no recent device check data and it cannot be interrogated, then obtain (i) a 12-lead ECG (for pacemakers, with and without a magnet) and (ii) an x-ray film of the pulse generator area which **may** reveal a unique radiopaque code ("signature") that identifies the manufacturer and model of the device (Table 18.8). **If the surgery is truly emergent and it is not possible to identify the device, then placing the patient on cardiac telemetry and then placing a magnet on the device to deactivate VT/VF detections in case the device is a defibrillator is recommended.** This may result in asynchronous pacing if the device is a pacemaker.

C. **Device management**

A qualified physician with device expertise must supervise the recommended preoperative prescription for device management. The prescription should not be provided by industry-employed representatives.

TABLE 18.8 North American manufacturers of pacemakers and implantable cardioverter–defibrillators

Biotronik, Inc.	Medtronic Corporation
6024 Jean Road	7000 Central Avenue NE
Lake Oswego, OR 97035–5369	Minneapolis, MN 55432
1-800-547-9001 (24-hr hotline)	1-800-328-2518 (24-hr hotline)
1-503-635-9936 (fax)	1-800-824-2362 (fax)
www.biotronik.com	*www.medtronic.com*
	Abbott[a]
Boston Scientific CRM	(St. Jude Medical)
(Guidant, CPI, Intermedics)[a]	Cardiac Rhythm Management
4100 Hamline Avenue North	Division (Pacesetter, Ventritex)[a]
St. Paul, MN 55112–5798	15900 Valley View Court
(CPI, Intermedics)	Sylmar, CA 91342
1-800-227-3422 (24-hr hotline)	1-800-777-2237 (24-hr hotline)
1-800-582-4166 (fax)	1-800-756-7223 (fax)
www.bostonscientific.com	*www.sjm.com*

[a]Recently acquired or merged companies by parent company.

> **CLINICAL PEARL**   For pacemaker-dependent patients: These patients are at particular risk of asystole in the presence of EMI. If EMI is likely (e.g., unipolar cautery in the vicinity of the pulse generator or leads and surgery above the umbilicus) and short bursts of electrocautery cannot be guaranteed, then the device should be programmed to an asynchronous mode. In the case of pacemakers, this can be done with magnet application in most situations, which will also inactivate the rate-responsive pacing. However, it is best to confirm the magnet response prior to the surgical procedure.

> **CLINICAL PEARL**   In cases where the pacemaker-dependent patient has an ICD or the location of surgery precludes placement of a magnet, consideration of programming the device to an asynchronous mode with the proprietary programmer is recommended. If reprogramming is not an option, the alternative is to limit EMI to short bursts while closely watching the pacing response to minimize episodes of asystole.

For patients with adaptive-rate pacemakers (including some ICDs), this capability should be programmed off if EMI causes inappropriate rate response. As stated above, for pacemakers, magnet application will inactivate this feature, but ICDs will need to be reprogrammed (Table 18.7). In ICDs, tachycardia sensing and therapy should be turned off. This can be accomplished with magnet application or with reprogramming. If any reprogramming is planned, then patients must stay on monitored telemetry until the CIED is reprogrammed back to baseline settings. If the magnet is applied, then the patient must remain on monitored telemetry until the magnet is removed.

In an emergency, obtain a rhythm strip or ECG to determine if there is pacing. If the device is determined to be a pacemaker and the patient is pacing, then the assumption is that the patient is pacemaker dependent. In this situation, there needs to be continuous hemodynamic monitoring that will not be distorted with EMI, such as a pulse waveform from an arterial line or plethysmography. A form of backup pacing should also be considered such as anterior–posterior transcutaneous pacing pads. A magnet should be placed on the device to force asynchronous pacing if the surgery is above the umbilicus or use of extensive electrosurgery is likely. If the procedure is performed below the umbilicus, then have the magnet available if pacing inhibition is seen. Use of short electrosurgical bursts will reduce the likelihood of pacemaker inhibition.

If intrinsic conduction (i.e., no pacing) is seen on the 12-lead ECG and the device is found to be a pacemaker, then proceed with surgery and have a magnet available. Please note that if the patient has an ICD rather than a pacemaker in either the situation of pacing or not pacing, deactivation of VT/VF detections with a magnet is recommended. In the case of an ICD, the magnet will not affect the pacing programming, and the electrosurgery could result in pacing inhibition. Short bursts of electrocautery are recommended to reduce the risk of pacing inhibition.

> **CLINICAL PEARL**   Magnet versus reprogramming: If the CIED is reprogrammed, then continuous monitoring is mandated. In the operating room, it is difficult to reverse reprogramming. If spontaneous heart rates exceed the asynchronous programmed pacing rate, then both deleterious hemodynamic and arrhythmia events may develop. The ICD antitachyarrhythmia therapies must be reactivated immediately after the procedure. This does not always occur, and is a possible source of medical error. Use of a magnet eliminates the complexity of reprogramming the CIED in the operating room. The magnet can be easily removed when competing rhythms develop with asynchronous pacing. However, the magnet behavior of the specific CIED needs to be known preoperatively.

D. **Precautions: Surgery unrelated to device**

The chief concern is to reduce risk of hemodynamic instability due to inappropriate inhibition or triggering of output (pacing stimuli or shocks) or upper-rate pacing behavior (adaptive-rate devices). If EMI is likely to cause device malfunction and the patient does not have an adequate intrinsic rhythm, the pacemaker should be programmed to an asynchronous mode and tachy-cardia sensing disabled for ICD. If the device features ARP, this should be programmed off. If ICD sensing is disabled, continuous cardiac monitoring must be maintained and an external cardioverter–defibrillator must be available.

1. **Surgical sources for EMI.** Technology has provided a variety of new surgical tools to assist in a variety of procedures. Many of these new technologies create EMI. It is this EMI that can cause erratic behavior in pacemakers and ICDs. Any tool that uses electricity or uses a magnetic field can emit interfering signals when close to the device or heart. Locating the grounding plate as far as possible from the cautery tool reduces EMI from unipolar cautery. The pulse generator and leads should not be between the Bovie tool and grounding plate (i.e., in the current pathway). Pacing function is confirmed by monitoring heart sounds or the pulse waveform. Only the lowest possible energies and brief bursts of electrocautery or other sources of EMI such as RF should be used, especially with instability due to device malfunction. Bipolar electrocautery also greatly reduces the risk for EMI. If cautery must be used in the vicinity (less than 15 cm) of the pulse generator or leads and there is significant hemodynamic instability due to EMI, then it is reasonable to place a magnet directly over the pulse generator of a pacemaker. This will cause most devices to pace asynchronously until the magnet is removed, unless the magnet mode has been programmed off. In a situation with an ICD and no device information, a magnet should **not** be placed over the ICD pulse generator unless EMI is unavoidable. If EMI is unavoidable, then the patient needs to be placed on cardiac monitor, and a magnet will need to be placed on (and kept on) the ICD generator during cautery or RF therapy. In this case, EMI has a potential to trigger antitachycardia pacing or shocks that may destabilize the patient. By placing the magnet over the generator, the device will no longer sense or treat tachyarrhythmias. It will not react to EMI or to a real tachyarrhythmia. However, as discussed above, the magnet will not affect the pacing programming, including rate response of the ICD.

2. **External cardioversion or defibrillation.** Shocks probably will not cause temporary inhibition or transient loss of capture. Today's devices are better shielded, and nearly all have a backup bradycardia pacing capability and a reset mode. Pulse generator damage is related to the distance of the external paddles or electrode pads from the pulse generator. All device manufacturers recommend the AP paddle configuration, with the paddles located at least 8 cm from the pulse generator. Further, it is advised that the lowest possible energies be used for cardioversion or defibrillation. After cardioversion or defibrillation, the device must be interrogated to assure proper function.

E. **Management for system implantation or revision**
Except in infants and small children, in whom epicardial leads are widely used, most CIED systems use transvenous leads. The pulse generator and leads are often implanted using local anesthesia and sedation. For epicardial lead placement with a thoracotomy, general anesthesia is needed. General anesthesia or monitored anesthesia care with heavy sedation may be requested for some pacer and ICD system implants, especially if the patient has significant advanced comorbidities.

1. Lead extraction [16]—general anesthesia is often recommended for cases involving lead extractions, especially in leads that are more than 10 years old. Cases involving lead extraction are often more prolonged procedures and carry additional procedural risk, the most concerning being catastrophic bleeding. Indications for lead extraction have expanded with recent updates in the HRS Guidelines. Class I indications for lead extraction mainly involve infected pacemaker and ICD systems and symptomatic occlusion of central veins. Other important indications involve removing nonfunctional leads to avoid future complications of superior vena cava syndrome, especially in young patients. In the case of device infection, these patients may have sepsis and are certainly at risk of becoming septic during the lead extraction. The potential bleeding sites include tearing of the superior vena cava and intracardiac perforation or avulsion. This type of procedure also involves the use of large-bore central venous sheaths up to 18 Fr in size that may be used from

both the subclavian and femoral venous sites. The prolonged procedure time involving large sheaths also places the patients at risk for pulmonary embolism or stroke caused by either air or clot. Fortunately, enhanced tools have been devised that improve patient safety and ease of extraction, including Excimer laser tools and cutting sheaths. Even with these enhanced tools, the risk of life-threatening bleeding is real and requires immediate recognition and action. Cardiothoracic surgeons and facilities need to be available within minutes if there are complications. In these situations, there is an emergent need for thoracotomy and surgical repair. Tools for pericardiocentesis and chest tube insertion must be in arm's reach. In addition, these cases may be further complicated by the patient being pacemaker dependent. This situation will require the use of temporary pacing that may become dislodged during the intracardiac manipulation of the leads. Because of the potential complications that can occur in lead extraction, it is imperative to have continuous hemodynamic monitoring. A sudden drop in blood pressure may be the only warning sign to alert clinicians of pending circulatory collapse due to a complication from lead extraction.

2. For all procedures requiring general anesthesia or monitored anesthesia care, consider the following:

   a. Most patients with symptomatic bradycardia will have temporary pacing. Otherwise, chronotropic drugs with backup external pacing should be available. By potentially suppressing an escape rhythm, sedation may worsen the situation.

   b. Have reliable plethysmography waveform or direct arterial blood pressure monitoring.

   c. Select the best surface ECG leads for P waves (II, V1) and for ischemia diagnosis (V5).

   d. Pulmonary artery catheters are seldom used or needed today. They may interfere with ICD lead positioning.

   e. An external cardioverter–defibrillator must be available and functioning. Defibrillator patches should be applied to the patient in the anterior–posterior configuration and more than 8 cm away from the CIED.

   f. With an ICD, tachycardia sensing should be disabled by a magnet or with reprogramming when unipolar electrosurgery is used.

   g. Contemporary inhalation and IV anesthetics are not known to increase defibrillation thresholds and are selected more with a view to hemodynamic tolerance. Inhalation agents and propofol may affect the morphology of sensed intracardiac electrograms and inducibility of tachyarrhythmias, which is a consideration during EP testing. Contemporary inhalation anesthetics (e.g., isoflurane, sevoflurane, desflurane) and small amounts of lidocaine for vascular access are not known to affect defibrillation thresholds.

   h. Paralytic agents must be used with caution during lead implant procedures. It is customary to assure that lead placement does not cause diaphragmatic or chest wall stimulation during pacing. This avoidable extracardiac stimulation will be inhibited by paralytic agents. If extracardiac stimulation occurs, the pacemaker lead usually requires repositioning.

VI. Catheter or surgical modification of arrhythmia substrates

RF catheter ablation has replaced antiarrhythmic drug therapy for the treatment of many types of chronic or recurring cardiac tachyarrhythmias. Tachyarrhythmias amenable to this form of treatment include those shown at EP study to have a focal origin (triggered or automatic) or are sustained by fixed, defined reentry circuits. Surgical ablation may be performed for these same arrhythmias if catheter ablation has failed or is not feasible. In addition, a catheter or surgical maze procedure may be used to interrupt multiple reentry circuits associated with atrial fibrillation [17].

A. **Radiofrequency catheter ablation** [18]

RF catheter ablation procedures are often performed in an EP laboratory using light to moderate sedation (generally with midazolam, fentanyl, dexmedetomidine, and/or propofol). Usually, both tachyarrhythmia diagnosis and RF ablation can be performed in a single session. Three to five electrode catheters are inserted percutaneously into the femoral, internal jugular, or subclavian vein, or via a retrograde aortic or transseptal approach, and positioned within the heart to allow pacing and recording at key sites. The efficacy of RF catheter ablation depends on accurate identification of the site of origin of the arrhythmia. Once this site has been identified and the electrode catheter is positioned in direct contact with the site, RF energy is delivered through the catheter to eliminate the source or circuit of the arrhythmia. After AV nodal ablation, all patients require a permanent pacemaker because of AV block. Pulmonary vein isolation with RF energy or cryo-ablation with transvenous catheters is used generally for symptomatic patients with recurrent paroxysmal and persistent atrial fibrillation [19]. Owing partly to lengthy procedures, atrial fibrillation ablations are often performed with general endotracheal anesthesia.

For CIED patients undergoing RF catheter ablation, RF energy may cause electrical reset, reprogramming, over- or undersensing, and inappropriate inhibition. Rarely does RF energy lead to reset or damage at the lead–tissue interface.

B. **Arrhythmia surgery** [20]

The potential morbidity of open chest surgery, as well as associated high costs, length of hospitalization, and delayed functional recovery, fostered the development of percutaneous catheter ablation. Nonetheless, direct surgical approaches and hybrid approaches continue to have an important role for patients with arrhythmogenic conditions refractory to catheter ablation or with associated surgical abnormalities [21].

ACKNOWLEDGMENTS

Jerry Luck, Jr., MD, has been a contributing author to this book since the first edition. His passion for education and his wealth of knowledge has been legendary. Dr. Luck was my mentor, colleague, and friend. Following his passing in 2015, I am honored to continue the updates in this chapter.

REFERENCES

1. Yang P, Kanki H, Drolet B, et al. Allelic variants in long-QT disease genes in patients with drug-associated torsades de pointes. *Circulation.* 2002;105(16):1943–1948.
2. Schram G, Pourrier M, Melnyk P, et al. Differential distribution of cardiac ion channels as a basis for regional specialization in electrical function. *Circ Res.* 2002;90(9):939–950.
3. Janse MJ, Wit AL. Electrophysiological mechanisms of ventricular arrhythmias resulting from myocardial ischemia and infarction. *Physiol Rev.* 1989;69(4):1049–1169.
4. Moya A, Sutton R, Ammirati F, et al. Guidelines for the diagnosis and management of syncope (version 2009). *Eur Heart J.* 2009;30(21):2631–2671.
5. Echt DS, Liebson PR, Mitchell LB, et al. Mortality and morbidity in patients receiving encainide, flecainide, or placebo. The Cardiac Arrhythmia Suppression Trial. *N Engl J Med.* 1991;324(12):781–788.
6. Manegold JC, Israel CW, Ehrlich JR, et al. External cardioversion of atrial fibrillation in patients with implanted pacemaker or cardioverter–defibrillator system: a randomized comparison of monophasic and biphasic shock energy application. *Eur Heart J.* 2007;28(14):1731–1738.
7. **Epstein AE, DiMarco JP, Ellenbogen KA, et al. ACC/AHA/HRS 2008 Guidelines for device-based therapy of cardiac rhythm abnormalities: a report of the American College of Cardiology/American Heart Association Task Force on Practice Guidelines (Writing Committee to Revise the ACC/AHA/NASPE 2002 Guideline Update for Implantation of Cardiac Pacemakers and Antiarrhythmia Devices) developed in collaboration with the American Association for Thoracic Surgery and Society of Thoracic Surgeons. *J Am Coll Cardiol.* 2008;51(21):e1–e62.**
8. McAnulty JH, Rahimtoola SH, Murphy E, et al. Natural history of "high-risk" bundle branch block: final report of a prospective study. *N Engl J Med.* 1982;307(3):137–143.
9. Reynolds D, Duray GZ, Omar R, et al. A leadless intracardiac transcatheter pacing system. *N Engl J Med.* 2016;374(6):533–541.
10. Lambiase PD, Barr C, Theuns DA, et al. Worldwide experience with a totally subcutaneous implantable defibrillator: early results from the effortless S-ICD Registry. *Eur Heart J.* 2014;35(25):1657–1665.
11. **Crossley GH, Poole JE, Rozner MA, et al. The Heart Rhythm Society (HRS)/American Society of Anesthesiologists (ASA) Expert consensus statement on the perioperative management of patients with implantable defibrillators, pacemakers and arrhythmia monitors: facilities and patient management. *Heart Rhythm.* 2011;8(7):1114–1154.**
12. **Russo AM, Stainback RF, Bailey SR, et al. ACCF/HRS/AHA/ASE/HFSA/SCAI/SCCT/SCMR 2013 Appropriate use criteria of implantable cardioverter-defibrillators and cardiac resynchronization therapy: a report of the American College of Cardiology Foundation appropriate use criteria task force, Heart Rhythm Society, American Heart Association, American Society of Echocardiography, Heart Failure Society of America, Society for Cardiovascular Angiography and Interventions, Society of Cardiovascular Computed Tomography, and Society for Cardiovascular Magnetic Resonance. *Heart Rhythm.* 2013;10(4):e11–e58.**

13. Lloyd MS, El Chami MF, Langberg JJ, et al. Pacing features that mimic malfunction: a review of current programmable and automated device functions that cause confusion in the clinical setting. *J Cardiovasc Electrophysiol.* 2009;20(4):453–460.
14. Pappone C, Calovic Z, Vicedomini G, et al. Improving cardiac resynchronization therapy response with multipoint left ventricular pacing: twelve month follow-up study. *Heart Rhythm.* 2015;12(6):1250–1258.
15. Wathen MS, DeGroot PJ, Sweeney MO, et al. Prospective randomized multicenter trial of empirical antitachycardia pacing versus shocks for spontaneous rapid ventricular tachycardia in patients with implantable cardioverter–defibrillators: Pacing Fast Ventricular Tachycardia Reduces Shock Therapies (PainFREE Rx II) trial results. *Circulation.* 2004;110(17):2591–2596.
16. Wilkoff BL, Love CJ, Byrd CL, et al. Transvenous lead extraction: Heart Rhythm Society expert consensus on facilities, training, indications and patient management. *Heart Rhythm.* 2009;6(7):1085–1104.
17. Pappone C, Oreto G, Lamberti F, et al. Catheter ablation of paroxysmal atrial fibrillation using a 3D mapping system. *Circulation.* 1999;100(11):1203–1208.
18. Morady F. Radio-frequency ablation as treatment for cardiac arrhythmia. *N Engl J Med.* 1999;340(7):534–544.
19. Falk RH. Atrial fibrillation. *N Engl J Med.* 2001;344(14):1067–1078.
20. Page PL. Surgery for atrial fibrillation and other supraventricular tachyarrhythmias. In: Zipes DP, Jalife J, eds. *Cardiac Electrophysiology.* 2nd ed. Philadelphia, PA: WB Saunders; 2000:1065–1077.
21. Cox JL, Schussler RB, D'Agostino HJ Jr, et al. The surgical treatment of atrial fibrillation. III. Development of a definitive surgical procedure. *J Thorac Cardiovasc Surg.* 1991;101(4):569–583.

19

Anesthetic Considerations for Patients with Pericardial Disease

Matthew S. Hull and Matthew M. Townsley

KEY POINTS

1. Although the etiology of pericardial disorders is quite variable, the manifestations of pericardial disease are primarily expressed as pericardial effusion, inflammation, and constriction. The common theme is impaired cardiac filling, with the severity of symptoms dependent upon the degree to which filling is impaired.

2. A relatively small amount of fluid (50 to 100 mL) that accumulates rapidly within the closed pericardial space is sufficient to dramatically increase intrapericardial pressure and interfere with cardiac filling. Conversely, a chronic increase in pericardial fluid will result in hemodynamic instability only after a large volume of fluid accumulation, perhaps as great as a liter.

3. The right heart is most vulnerable to pericardial compression due to its thinner walls and lower chamber pressures as compared to the left heart.

4. Cardiac tamponade is often described with Beck triad: muffled heart sounds, jugular venous distention (JVD), and hypotension.

5. Pulsus paradoxus (an abnormally high drop in systolic pressure >20 mm Hg during inspiration) occurs secondary to ventricular septal shift crowding the left ventricle (LV) during right ventricular (RV) filling. The opposite occurs during expiration. This phenomenon is described as enhanced ventricular interdependence.

6. Electrical alternans is due to swinging of the heart within the fluid of the pericardial sac, leading to beat-to-beat changes in the electrical axis as seen on electrocardiogram (ECG).

7. Diastolic collapse lasting more than one-third of diastole, as demonstrated with echocardiography, is fairly specific for tamponade.

8. Cardiovascular collapse may quickly ensue with induction of general anesthesia in a patient with cardiac tamponade. If pericardiocentesis cannot be performed in a hemodynamically compromised patient prior to surgical intervention, the patient should be prepped and draped prior to anesthetic induction so that surgery may proceed immediately following intubation. Volume loading prior to general anesthetic induction, as well as inotropic and vasopressor support, is often required. Expect further deterioration after positive pressure ventilation is initiated.

(continued)

9. Constrictive pericarditis (CP) is a diagnosis that encompasses a wide spectrum of disease, from acute and subacute cases that may resolve spontaneously, or with medical therapy, to the classic chronically progressive form of CP.

10. Although manifestations of hemodynamic instability are less with chronic pericarditis than with tamponade, induction and maintenance of anesthesia must encompass the same concerns and principles for hemodynamic management.

I. Introduction

Pericardial disease is common throughout the world and is frequently encountered in the cardiac operating room. Clinical significance varies from asymptomatic incidental findings to life-threatening emergencies. Associated morbidity and mortality can be significant and the altered physiology of these disease states presents numerous challenges to safe perioperative management. Although the etiology of pericardial disorders is quite variable—including infectious, inflammatory, autoimmune, and malignant states—common themes arise allowing the anesthesiologist to safely approach the patient presenting with pericardial disease. Regardless of the underlying cause, the effects of pericardial disease on cardiac function most often present as **impaired cardiac filling**, with the severity of symptoms dependent upon the degree to which filling is impaired. This filling impairment is usually represented by pericardial effusion or constriction.

Although imaging modalities such as computed tomography (CT) and cardiac magnetic resonance imaging (MRI) are increasingly used to characterize pericardial disease, echocardiography has become the first-line diagnostic tool given its noninvasive and relatively inexpensive nature [1]. In addition, echocardiography allows for rapid recognition of life-threatening pericardial tamponade in the perioperative setting.

This chapter will review the normal structure and function of the pericardium, as well as the most common causes of pericardial disease. The two most clinically relevant pericardial disorders—**cardiac tamponade** and **constrictive pericarditis (CP)**—will be discussed in detail, focusing on pertinent anesthetic management considerations. Additionally, online supplemental content provides specific echocardiographic examples of tamponade, chronic pericardial effusion, and CP.

II. Pericardial anatomy and physiology

A. The normal pericardium is a dual-enveloped sac surrounding the heart and great vessels. It is comprised of two layers: the parietal pericardium and the visceral pericardium. The **parietal pericardium** is a thick, fibrous outer layer comprised primarily of collagen and elastin. It attaches to the adventitia of the great vessels, diaphragm, sternum, and the vertebral bodies. The inner **visceral pericardium** rests on the surface of the heart. It is composed of a single layer of mesothelial cells, which adhere to the pericardium. Normal pericardial thickness is 1 to 2 mm.

B. Two distinct sinuses are formed at points where the pericardium appears to fold onto itself (Fig. 19.1). The **oblique sinus** forms posteriorly, between the left atrium and pulmonary veins, and is a common location for blood to collect after cardiac surgery (Supplemental Video 19.1). The **transverse sinus** also forms posteriorly behind the left atrium, situated behind the aorta and pulmonary artery (Supplemental Video 19.2).

C. Normal cardiac function can still occur in the absence of the pericardium, making it nonessential for survival. However, it does provide several useful physiologic functions. It aids in the reducing friction between the heart and surrounding structures, limits acute dilatation of cardiac chambers, provides a barrier to infection, optimizes coupling of left and right ventricular (RV) filling and function, and limits excessive motion of the heart within the chest cavity. The pericardium is also metabolically active, secreting prostaglandins that affect coronary artery tone and cardiac reflexes [2].

D. The pericardium is a highly innervated structure. Pericardial inflammation or manipulation may produce severe pain or vagally mediated reflexes.

III. Causes of pericardial disease

The etiologies of pericardial disease are numerous and can lead to pericardial inflammation, effusion, or both. Often, the care of these patients must not only consider the underlying pericardial

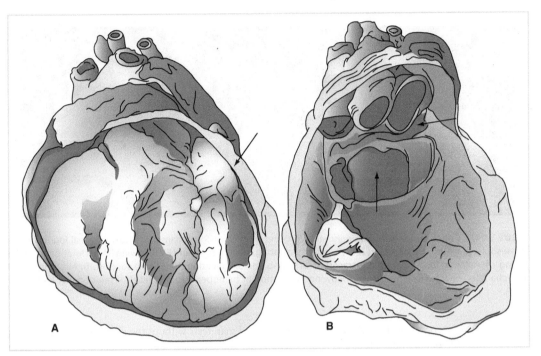

FIGURE 19.1 Anatomy of the pericardium and pericardial sinuses. The left image (**A**) demonstrates the heart in situ with a section of the parietal pericardium cut away. The right image (**B**), with the heart cut away, demonstrates the oblique sinus (*arrow at ~6 o'clock*) and the transverse sinus (*arrow at ~3 o'clock*). (Reprinted with permission from Lachman N, Syed FF, Habib A, et al. Correlative anatomy for the electrophysiologist, part I: The pericardial space, oblique sinus, transverse sinus. *J Cardiovasc Electrophysiol.* 2010;21(12):1421–1426.)

pathology, but the manifestations and complications of the underlying condition as well. Pericardial disease can be caused by infection (i.e., viral, bacterial, fungal, tuberculosis), connective tissue disorders (i.e., systemic lupus erythematosus, sarcoidosis, rheumatoid arthritis), trauma, uremia, malignancy, postmyocardial infarction (Dressler syndrome), or following cardiac surgery and other invasive cardiac procedures.

IV. Pericardial tamponade

    A. Natural history

        1. Etiology. The visceral pericardium is responsible for the production of pericardial fluid, which is an ultrafiltrate of plasma. This fluid provides lubrication to decrease friction between the pericardial layers. The pericardial space normally contains **10 to 50 mL** of fluid, which is drained by the lymphatic system. As previously discussed, many conditions can cause fluid (serous, serosanguineous, and purulent) and/or blood to accumulate within the pericardial space. The majority of pericardial effusions are not hemodynamically significant and do not progress to tamponade. Tamponade occurs when extrinsic pericardial compression of the heart leads to diminished venous filling and, ultimately, reduced cardiac output. In addition to fluid collection within the pericardium, tamponade may also be caused by the accumulation of clot or air in the pericardial space. Acute, life-threatening tamponade most frequently results from bleeding into the pericardial space after cardiac surgery or other invasive cardiac procedures, following blunt chest trauma, or due to a ruptured ascending aortic aneurysm or aortic dissection [3] (Fig. 19.2). Tamponade may occur in as many as 8.8% of patients presenting for cardiac surgery, although it is more commonly seen after valve surgery than coronary artery bypass grafting (CABG). The onset is typically in the immediate postoperative period, but may potentially occur several days following surgery. Frequently there is localized clot or effusion, which causes nonuniform

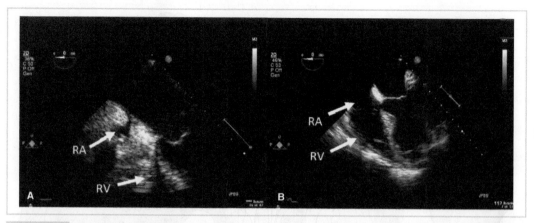

FIGURE 19.2 Critical tamponade with right atrial (RA) and ventricular (RV) collapse. **A:** Midesophageal four-chamber transesophageal echocardiography (TEE) view demonstrating collapse of RA and RV following RA perforation by J-wire during cannulation for venoarterial extracorporeal membrane oxygenation (VA ECMO) support. **B:** Midesophageal four-chamber view from same patient following evacuation of hemopericardium, relief of tamponade, and repair of RA.

compression of the cardiac chambers and manifests without the classical clinical features of tamponade (Supplemental Video 19.3). The diagnosis of postcardiac surgery tamponade can therefore be challenging, especially when considering the many potential causes of hemodynamic instability during this time period. Unfortunately, morbidity and mortality increases significantly the longer the diagnosis is delayed [4].

2. **Symptomatology.** Symptoms of cardiac tamponade are usually rapid in onset, but depend upon the rate at which pericardial fluid accumulates. A relatively small amount of fluid (50 to 100 mL) that rapidly accumulates within the closed pericardial space is sufficient to dramatically increase intrapericardial pressure and interfere with cardiac filling. However, a chronic increase in pericardial fluid will produce tamponade only after a large volume (>1 L) is present. A gradual accumulation of fluid stretches the parietal pericardium, allowing larger volumes to be tolerated before symptoms occur (Supplemental Videos 19.4 and 19.5). Lack of this pericardial stretch explains the abrupt onset of symptoms and clinical deterioration in the setting of acute tamponade. The primary symptoms of cardiac tamponade include dyspnea, orthopnea, diaphoresis, and chest pain. Dyspnea is often the first and most sensitive symptom [5].

B. **Pathophysiology**

The primary abnormality in cardiac tamponade is impaired diastolic filling of the heart, caused by elevated intrapericardial pressure that leads to compression of the atria and ventricles. The right heart is most vulnerable to the compression due to its thinner walls and lower chamber pressures as compared to the left heart (Supplemental Video 19.6). Diastolic filling pressures (i.e., central venous pressure [CVP], left atrial pressure, pulmonary capillary wedge pressure, left and right ventricular end-diastolic pressures [LVEDP and RVEDP]) become elevated and began to equilibrate with one another, as well as the intrapericardial pressure. Physiologic manifestations of pericardial fluid, as previously discussed, are contingent upon the rate and amount of fluid accumulation, with a continuum ranging from clinical insignificance to severe hemodynamic collapse (Fig. 19.3). Cardiac filling is critically reduced, which translates into decreased stroke volume, cardiac output, and systemic blood pressure. Compensatory sympathetic responses attempt to offset this reduction in stroke volume, with elevated levels of plasma catecholamines resulting in systemic vasoconstriction and tachycardia. This may temporarily maintain cardiac output and systemic perfusion; however, sudden hemodynamic collapse may rapidly occur with depletion of catecholamines and/or continued elevation of intrapericardial pressure.

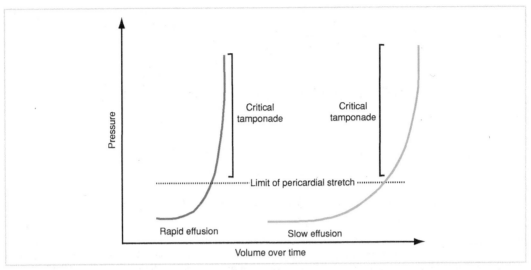

FIGURE 19.3 Pressure–volume relationship in acute versus chronic pericardial effusions. Intrapericardial pressure is contingent upon the change in intrapericardial volume. Pressure is relatively stable until a critical volume occurs. At this point, minimal increases in volume will lead to significant changes in intrapericardial pressure. With chronic effusions, pericardial stretch allows for a greater amount of volume to accumulate before critical increases in pressure occur. The lack of pericardial stretch explains the significant elevations in pressures seen with only small amounts of rapidly accumulating intrapericardial fluid. (Reprinted with permission from Avery EG, Shernan SK. Echocardiographic evaluation of pericardial disease. In: Savage RM, Aronson SA, Shernan SK, eds. *Comprehensive Textbook of Perioperative Transesophageal Echocardiography*. 2nd ed. Philadelphia, PA: Lippincott Williams & Wilkins; 2011:726—this figure is originally from Spodick DH. Acute cardiac tamponade. *N Engl J Med*. 2003;349(7):684–690.)

C. **Diagnostic evaluation and assessment**
   1. Clinical evaluation
      a. Acute tamponade is often described by **Beck triad:** muffled heart sounds, jugular venous distention (JVD) (due to increased venous pressure), and hypotension. Other common findings include tachypnea and tachycardia.
      b. Pulsus paradoxus, although not specific for tamponade, may be present. While a modest decrease of systolic arterial blood pressure during inspiration is physiologic, and exaggerated decrease in blood pressure is pathologic. Pulsus paradoxus is defined as a decrease of more than 10 mm Hg in systolic arterial pressure that occurs with inspiration. Tamponade physiology leads to respiratory variability in ventricular diastolic filling, in which the negative intrathoracic pressure accompanying inspiration leads to enhanced right-sided filling. Since total intracardiac volume is fixed by the pericardial compression, as the RV fills it will lead to a shift of the interventricular septum toward the left ventricle (LV). This crowding of the LV impedes its filling, decreasing LV stroke volume and resulting in an exaggerated decline in systolic blood pressure seen with inspiration. The opposite is true during expiration, with diminished RV and enhanced LV filling. Pulsus paradoxus is also seen in patients with chronic lung disease, large pleural effusions, RV dysfunction, and CP.
      c. The chest x-ray may show an enlarged, globular, and bottle-shaped cardiac silhouette. The right costophrenic angle is reduced to less than 90 degrees and the lung fields are typically clear. Pericardial fat lines in a lateral film are an uncommon, but highly specific, finding.
      d. The ECG is nonspecific, but may demonstrate sinus tachycardia, low-voltage QRS, nonspecific ST-T wave abnormalities, and electrical alternans. **Electrical alternans** (Fig. 19.4) is due to swinging of the heart within the fluid of the pericardial sac, leading to beat-to-beat changes in the electrical axis.

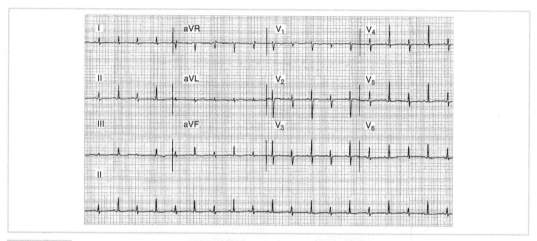

FIGURE 19.4 Electrical alternans with cardiac tamponade. Note that this phenomenon is not seen in all electrocardiographic leads. (Reprinted with permission from Badescu GC, Sherman BM, Zaidan JR, Barash PB. Appendix 2: Atlas of Electrocardiography. In: Barash PB, Cullen BF, Stoelting RK, et al, eds. Clinical Anesthesia. 8th ed. Philadelphia: Wolters Kluwer, 2017:1718.)

    e. Table 19.1 summarizes the classic clinical manifestations most commonly described in cardiac tamponade.

  2. Catheterization data. Cardiac tamponade is a clinical diagnosis that cannot be made with catheterization data alone; however, common patterns of intracardiac pressures are usually seen. There is elevation and near equalization of the CVP, RVEDP, pulmonary capillary wedge pressure, left atrial pressure, and LVEDP. Increased CVP and right atrial (RA) pressures are seen with a prominent x-descent and a diminished or absent y-descent (Fig. 19.5).

CLINICAL PEARL   When hemodynamic instability occurs within the setting of elevated filling pressures (as demonstrated by CVP and/or pulmonary artery pressure measurements), cardiac tamponade must be immediately included in the differential diagnosis (especially in the postcardiac surgery patient).

---

  3. Echocardiography. Echocardiography is the diagnostic modality of choice in evaluating cardiac tamponade. It is the most sensitive tool for making the diagnosis of pericardial effusion. Initial evaluation should focus on the presence, size, and extent (circumferential vs. localized/loculated) of the pericardial effusion, which is seen as an echo-free space

TABLE 19.1   Cardiac tamponade—clinical manifestations
Hypotension
Tachycardia
Widened mediastinum (on chest x-ray)
Elevation and near-equalization of filling pressures
Increasing inotrope requirements
Pulsus paradoxus
Electrical alternans
Initial high-output chest tube drainage that abruptly subsides

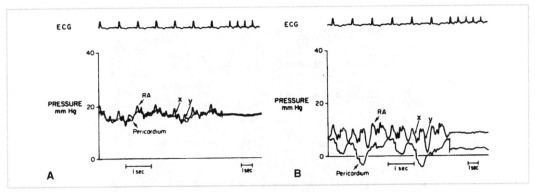

FIGURE 19.5 Right atrial (RA) and pericardial pressures in cardiac tamponade. **A:** Note equal RA and pericardial pressures and the diminished y-descent of the RA waveform. **B:** After removal of 100 mL of fluid, the pericardial pressure is lower than RA pressure, and the normal large descent has returned. (Reprinted with permission from Hensley FA, Martin DE, Gravlee GP. *A Practical Approach to Cardiac Anesthesia*. 3rd ed. Philadelphia, PA: Lippincott Williams & Wilkins; 2003:475.)

surrounding the heart. The effusion should be measured to estimate its severity (Table 19.2; Fig. 19.6).

Although echocardiography alone cannot definitively diagnose tamponade, in the presence of a pericardial effusion there are several echocardiographic features consistently associated with tamponade physiology (Figs. 19.7 and 19.8). With tamponade, RA collapse is a sensitive sign, typically beginning in end diastole and continuing through systole (Supplemental Video 19.7). Systolic RA collapse persisting for more than one-third of the cardiac cycle is specific for tamponade. Diastolic RV collapse is also observed and, when lasting for more than one-third of diastole, is even more specific than systolic RA collapse for the identification of tamponade. End-diastolic dimensions of the RV will be reduced, reflective of diminished ventricular filling. Paradoxical motion of the interventricular septum is a frequent finding, reflecting the reciprocal respiratory variability in diastolic filling. These changes are also reflected with Doppler transmitral and transtricuspid inflow velocity profiles.

CLINICAL PEARL   If tamponade is suspected, bedside echocardiography can provide immediate information to assist/confirm clinical suspicion by allowing for visualization of pericardial effusion and/or compression leading to cardiac chamber collapse.

D. Treatment

Definitive treatment of cardiac tamponade is emergent drainage and/or relief of pericardial compression, which may be accomplished through either pericardiocentesis or surgical decompression.

1. **Pericardiocentesis.** Pericardiocentesis may be performed with or without imaging guidance (i.e., echocardiography, fluoroscopy). Imaging is often preferred to assist in safely

TABLE 19.2 Estimation of effusion severity	
	Size of effusion (mm)
Minimal effusion (50–100 mL)	<5
Small effusion (100–250 mL)	5–10
Moderate effusion (250–500 mL)	11–20
Large effusion (>500 mL)	>20

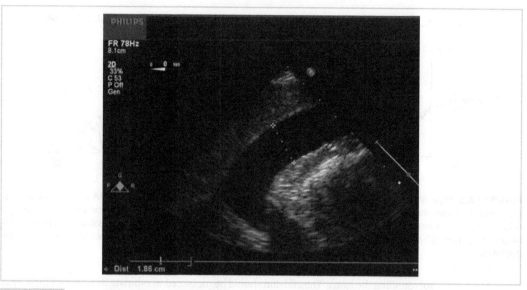

FIGURE 19.6 Measurement of pericardial effusion volume with echocardiography. Transgastric transesophageal echocardiography (TEE) view showing caliper measurement to estimate the size of pericardial effusion. As shown in Table 19.2, caliper measurement of 1.86 cm is indicative of a 250- to 500-mL pericardial effusion volume.

guiding the needle tip through the pericardium to the most optimal location for drainage, as well as assessing the adequacy of fluid removal. Without imaging there is a significantly higher risk of complications, such as cardiac perforation, puncture of coronary or internal mammary arteries, and pneumothorax. In the setting of severe hemodynamic instability, however, it may be necessary to proceed without imaging due to the significant risk of rapid and profound clinical deterioration. A catheter is frequently left in the pericardial space to allow for continuous drainage (Fig. 19.9).

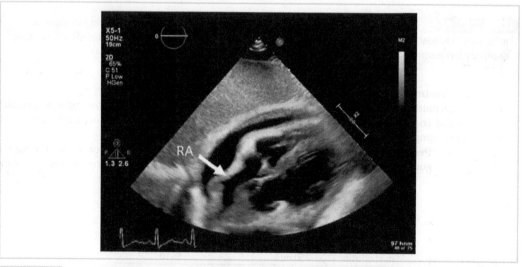

FIGURE 19.7 Right atrial (RA) systolic collapse in a patient with cardiac tamponade. Transthoracic subcostal four-chamber view demonstrating RA bowing and collapse during systole. Pericardial effusion can be seen surrounding the RA right ventricle. ECG monitoring is helpful in identifying systolic RA collapse in tamponade.

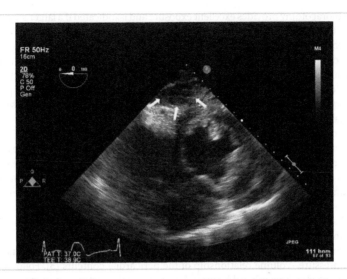

FIGURE 19.8 The pericardial space is occupied by a large amount of clot (marked by the white *arrows*), seen posterior to the inferior wall of the left ventricle (LV) in a transgastric short-axis midpapillary transesophageal echocardiography (TEE) view.

2. **Surgical drainage.** Indications for surgical drainage include unsuccessful pericardiocentesis, localized/loculated effusions, removal of clot, and ongoing intrapericardial bleeding (i.e., acute aortic dissection, trauma, following cardiac surgery or percutaneous cardiac procedures). The surgical approach is primarily via subxyphoid pericardial window or a small anterior thoracotomy. The subxyphoid approach is easier to perform but offers a limited exposure, while

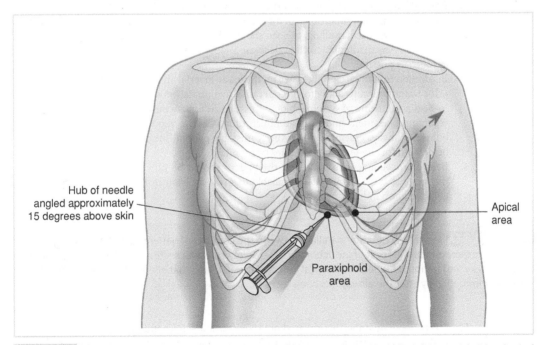

FIGURE 19.9 The most common needle insertion points for pericardiocentesis, including the paraxiphoid and apical approaches. When using the paraxiphoid approach, the needle tip should be directed toward the left shoulder. With the apical approach, the needle tip is aimed internally. (Reprinted with permission from Spodick DH. Acute cardiac tamponade. *N Engl J Med.* 2003;349(7):684–690.)

a thoracotomy provides excellent exposure and is indicated if a larger surgical field is required. Both approaches allow for open exploration, facilitating the removal of clot and fibrinous debris. With hemorrhagic tamponade following cardiac surgery, full mediastinal exploration is often needed to localize the source of bleeding and stabilize the patient. In the setting of malignant effusions, diagnostic pericardial biopsies can be obtained with a surgical approach to drainage [3]. Some patients may continue to experience recurrent pericardial effusions, requiring consideration of pericardiectomy. This is most commonly seen in patients with malignant effusions or uremia [6].

E. Goals of perioperative management

8

The hemodynamic state of the patient will dictate the sequence of anesthesia and surgery. While general anesthesia is frequently used, it may likely contribute to clinical decompensation in the severely compromised patient. Direct myocardial depression, systemic vasodilation, and diminished preload accompanying the induction of general anesthesia can lead to a profound decrease in cardiac output. Potentially life-threatening cardiac collapse may ensue. In this scenario, pericardiocentesis or subxyphoid pericardial window can be performed under local anesthesia to avoid these complications. Frequently, hemodynamic instability is dramatically improved with the removal of only a small amount of fluid. This is due to the steep curve of the pressure–volume relationship of the pericardial contents [3]. Following initial drainage, the patient may become stable enough to tolerate the institution of general anesthesia for the remainder of the procedure.

> **CLINICAL PEARL** In a patient with tamponade, it is important to discuss with the surgeon the feasibility of draining at least a portion of the pericardial effusion prior to induction in order to relieve cardiac compression and minimize the risk of severe cardiac compromise.

1. Premedication with anxiolytics or opioids should be avoided in patients with true cardiac tamponade, as even small doses of these medications can precipitate acute cardiac collapse.
2. To facilitate ventricular filling, preload should be optimized with intravenous fluids prior to induction. Any manipulations that decrease venous return should be avoided or minimized as much as possible.
3. In addition to standard noninvasive monitors, an arterial line should be strongly considered prior to induction to allow for preoperative quantification of pulsus paradoxus and beat-to-beat monitoring of systemic blood pressure. Adequate intravenous access is needed for volume replacement and drug administration. Central venous access may be beneficial, but is not always essential. In a severely unstable patient, surgical intervention should not be delayed for the placement of lines or monitors.
4. Before proceeding with induction the patient should be fully prepped and draped, with the surgical team immediately available to make incision in the event of hemodynamic collapse upon induction.

> **CLINICAL PEARL** Many describe parallels between the conduct of general anesthetic induction for cardiac tamponade with that of induction for emergency cesarean section, in which it is critical to have close coordination between the surgical and anesthesia teams that allows for surgical incision to occur immediately after the airway has been secured.

5. The perioperative anesthetic plan should have the following hemodynamic goals (Table 19.3): Reductions in heart rate should be avoided and contractility optimized to preserve cardiac output, as these patients have both a fixed and reduced stroke volume. Adequate preload is essential to promote RV filling. Decreases in systemic vascular resistance are particularly detrimental, as this will reduce RV filling and systemic perfusion pressure.

TABLE 19.3	Hemodynamic goals in cardiac tamponade			
	Heart rate	**Contractility**	**Preload**	**Systemic vascular resistance**
Tamponade	↑	↑	↑	↑

6. Positive pressure ventilation can cause a dramatic decline in preload and cardiac output. It is therefore suggested that patients with tamponade be allowed to breathe spontaneously until the pericardial sac is opened and drained. If spontaneous ventilation is not possible, ventilation with high respiratory rates and low tidal volumes should be considered to minimize elevation in mean airway pressures.

CLINICAL PEARL Airway management in a patient with tamponade is complicated by the presence of surgical drapes above the patients head, so in the setting of a potentially difficult airway it is crucial to have all preparations and equipment in place prior to induction (i.e., video laryngoscope, additional anesthesia providers to provide help).

7. Careful consideration should be given to the selection of induction drugs, with particular attention aimed at minimizing myocardial depression and peripheral vasodilation. Etomidate is a reasonable induction agent, as it produces minimal decreases in contractility and systemic vascular resistance, although hemodynamic instability may still occur in the setting of tamponade physiology. Benzodiazepines are also a reasonable choice. Many advocate the use of ketamine in this setting, relying on the sympathetic stimulation it provides to minimize hemodynamic compromise. It is important to note, however, that in a catecholamine-depleted state many patients will have a diminished ability to increase their own sympathetic nervous system activity. In these patients, the myocardial depressant properties of ketamine will be unmasked and significant hypotension is likely to occur. Opioids should be given with caution, as vagally mediated bradycardia can significantly diminish cardiac output.

CLINICAL PEARL Vasopressor and inotropic drugs should be immediately available to administer with general anesthetic induction and, in many cases, it is prudent to begin infusions of vasoactive medications (if not already started prior to arrival in the operating room) to support the patient's hemodynamics during and following induction.

8. Inotropes (i.e., epinephrine, norepinephrine) and vasoconstrictors (i.e., phenylephrine, vasopressin) are often needed to maintain cardiac output and peripheral vascular resistance, but serve only as a temporizing measure until tamponade can be definitively treated with drainage.

9. Tamponade is rarely seen in patients presenting for surgical drainage of chronic, recurrent pericardial effusions. In this scenario, however, it is still essential to obtain as much information as possible regarding the clinical significance and severity of the effusion. This should include a review of the preoperative echocardiogram, a thorough discussion with the surgeon, and a detailed history and physical focusing, in particular, on any vital sign abnormalities. A high index of suspicion should be maintained for the potential of perioperative hemodynamic instability.

CLINICAL PEARL While tamponade is not commonly seen in the setting of a chronic pericardial effusion, it is still important to remain vigilant and prepared for the occurrence of hemodynamic instability.

V. **Constrictive pericarditis (CP)**

A. **Natural history**

1. **Etiology.** CP is a diagnosis that encompasses a wide spectrum of disease, from acute or subacute cases that may resolve spontaneously (or with medical therapy) to the classic chronic, progressive CP, which will be the focus of this section. Other entities noted in the literature include effusive CP, in which patients present with cardiac effusion or tamponade but retain characteristics of CP following drainage of the effusion; localized CP, involving only parts of the pericardium with variable hemodynamic sequelae; and occult CP, in which rapid infusion of intravenous fluids can provoke the signs and symptoms of the disease [7]. While many etiologies have been documented, the most common are idiopathic, viral, postcardiac surgery, mediastinal radiation, and, in developing countries, tuberculosis.

2. **Symptomatology.** CP presents most commonly as chronic and progressive fatigue, orthopnea, dyspnea on exertion, peripheral edema, and abdominal distention. Given the nonspecific nature of these findings, care must be taken to differentiate this disease process from other entities such as hepatic failure, RV failure, tricuspid valve disease, and, in particular, restrictive cardiomyopathy. As the pathophysiology underlying these conditions is markedly different, the medical and surgical management varies considerably as well.

B. **Pathophysiology**

The hallmark of CP is a thickened, calcified, and adherent pericardium. This effectively confines the heart inside a rigid shell. From a pathophysiologic perspective, this has three major consequences [8]:

1. **Impaired diastolic filling.** The noncompliant pericardium limits filling of all cardiac chambers, with elevation and near equalization of end-diastolic pressures. Ventricular filling occurs rapidly during early diastole, but ceases abruptly as the volume, and thus pressure, in the ventricle reaches a critical point. This results in the characteristic "dip and plateau," or "square root sign," noted in ventricular pressure tracings. Atrial systole does little to augment LV filling, and cardiac output is maintained by a compensatory increase in heart rate.

2. **Dissociation of intrathoracic pressures.** The rigid pericardium isolates the cardiac chambers from the negative pressure generated during inspiration, resulting in a decreased gradient between the pulmonary veins and the left atrium. Consequently, left heart filling, and thus cardiac output, are decreased.

3. **Ventricular interdependence.** As discussed previously, left and right heart filling are not independent events. Increases in right heart filling may cause a leftward shift in the interventricular septum at the expense of left heart filling. Expiration, as would be expected, reverses this pattern. This phenomenon is known as ventricular interdependence and is exaggerated in CP.

4. One of the most important consequences of pericardial constriction is significant respiratory variation in left and RV filling patterns. This is an important consideration in the diagnosis of CP and provides the foundation for the diagnostic workup to be discussed later. Of note, this respiratory variation is maintained, but reversed, in patients on mechanical ventilation [9].

C. **Diagnostic evaluation and assessment**

1. **Clinical evaluation**

a. The diagnosis of CP is difficult to make on history and physical examination alone, but must be considered in patients presenting with the signs and symptoms of venous congestion mentioned previously. On examination, JVD with Kussmaul sign (an increase in JVD on inspiration) and Friedreich sign (a rapid decrease in JVD during early diastole) may be present. Pulsus paradoxus is variably present. On cardiac auscultation, a "pericardial knock" may be noted. This is a high-pitched sound in early diastole that is caused by the sudden cessation of ventricular filling and is a highly specific, but insensitive, clue to the diagnosis. Pulmonary edema is often absent and pulsatile hepatomegaly may be noted on abdominal examination.

b. Laboratory investigation may reveal organ dysfunction secondary to the disease process (i.e., kidney injury, elevated liver enzymes). Natriuretic peptide levels, which are released in response to myocardial stretch and are increased in many cases of heart failure, are usually normal or only slightly elevated. This is attributed to the rigid pericardium limiting the amount of potential chamber dilatation.

c. ECG findings are nonspecific and may include sinus tachycardia, atrial fibrillation, conduction delays, p mitrale, and ST-segment and T-wave changes.

d. While calcification of the pericardium is not universal, its presence on the lateral chest x-ray may suggest CP. A thickened pericardium (>2 mm) may be appreciated on CT or MRI and other imaging techniques may demonstrate the pericardium being adherent to the myocardium.

2. **Catheterization data.** As in tamponade, cardiac catheterization is not always necessary for the diagnosis of CP. However, it may be helpful in the diagnosis of effusive CP, with some suggesting its routine use during the drainage of pericardial effusions. Certain waveform characteristics may be seen during placement of invasive monitors in the operating room (Fig. 19.10). RA pressure tracings may show "M" or "W" waveforms with

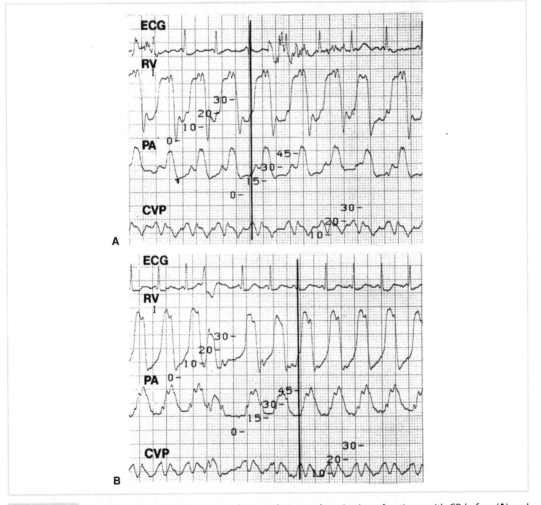

FIGURE 19.10 Waveform characteristics commonly seen during catheterization of patients with CP before (**A**) and after (**B**) pericardiectomy. Note the "square root sign" in the right ventricular (RV) pressure tracing, and the "M" waveform in the central venous pressure (CVP) tracing prior to pericardiectomy. ECG, electrocardiogram; PA, pulmonary artery. (Reprinted with permission from Skubas NJ, Beardslee M, Barzilai B, et al. Constrictive pericarditis: intraoperative hemodynamic and echocardiographic evaluation of cardiac filling dynamics. *Anesth Analg.* 2001;92(6):1424–1426.)

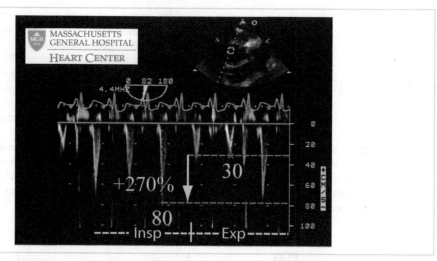

FIGURE 19.11 Transesophageal pulsed wave transmitral Doppler profile in a patient with CP during positive pressure ventilation. Note the preserved, but reversed, respiratory variation as opposed to that which would be seen in a spontaneously ventilating patient. Insp, inspiration; exp, expiration. (Reprinted with permission from Avery EG, Shernan SK. Echocardiographic evaluation of pericardial disease. In: Savage RM, Aronson SA, Shernan SK, eds. *Comprehensive Textbook of Perioperative Transesophageal Echocardiography*. 2nd ed. Philadelphia, PA: Lippincott Williams & Wilkins; 2011:737.)

a prominent y-descent, the diagnostic equivalent of Friedreich sign. Ventricular pressure tracings may show the characteristic "dip and plateau," or "square root sign," as previously described. The end-diastolic pressures in all chambers are elevated and nearly equal (≤5 mm Hg difference). RV systolic pressures are usually <50 mm Hg, with an RV end-diastolic to RV systolic ratio of ≥1:3.

3. **Echocardiography.** Echocardiography is essential to the diagnosis of CP and more advanced techniques have become useful in its differentiation from other disease processes. Two-dimensional and M-mode examination may show a thickened, hyperechoic pericardium; diastolic flattening of the LV posterior wall, reflective of the abrupt cessation of ventricular filling; a ventricular septal "bounce," caused by the sudden changes in the transseptal pressure gradient (Supplemental Video 19.8); atrial tethering (Supplemental Video 19.9); premature closure of the mitral valve and opening of the pulmonic valve, indicative of high chamber pressures; enlarged hepatic veins; and IVC plethora, where the vessel remains dilated and lacks the normal change in diameter during the respiratory cycle. Doppler evaluation of transmitral, transtricuspid, and pulmonary vein flow shows characteristic tracings with profound respiratory variation (often >25%) (Fig. 19.11). Newer techniques, such as tissue Doppler imaging (TDI) of the mitral annulus (Fig. 19.12) and color Doppler M-mode of transmitral flow propagation velocity (Fig. 19.13) allow further characterization and differentiation from restrictive cardiomyopathy [10] (Table 19.4).

D. **Treatment**

As previously mentioned, some cases of acute constriction may resolve spontaneously or with medical management. The definitive management of chronic CP, however, is usually surgical. Pericardiectomy, or pericardial decortication, is often performed via left thoracotomy or midline sternotomy, depending on the extent of resection necessary. The goal of treatment is total resection of both the visceral and parietal pericardium, and while this can often be performed without the use of cardiopulmonary bypass (CPB), its use may be indicated in more difficult dissections. Despite improvements in surgical technique, operative mortality remains as high as 10%, with poor prognostic predictors including prior cardiac surgery, radiation, malignancy, and advanced heart failure on presentation. As opposed to patients with tamponade, where surgical drainage may provide immediate improvement in hemodynamic and clinical status, an immediate improvement in symptoms is not generally observed.

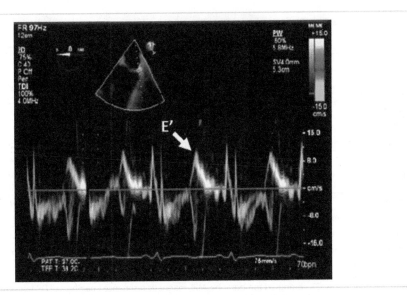

FIGURE 19.12 Lateral Wall Tissue Doppler Imaging (TDI) in a patient with constrictive pericarditis (CP). Note lateral TDI E′ velocity (*arrow*) is greater than 8 cm/s, distinguishing CP from restrictive cardiomyopathy (as outlined in Table 19.3).

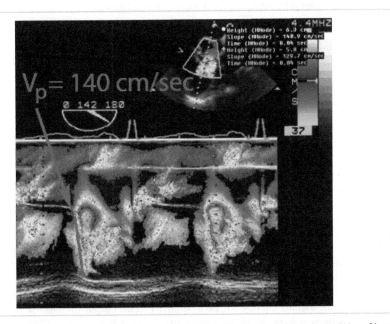

FIGURE 19.13 Transesophageal image of the transmitral color M-mode (propagation velocity, V_p) profile of a patient with CP. The slope of the first aliasing velocity is used in this determination and is depicted by the *pink line*. (Reprinted with permission from Avery EG, Shernan SK. Echocardiographic evaluation of pericardial disease. In: Savage RM, Aronson SA, Shernan SK, eds. *Comprehensive Textbook of Perioperative Transesophageal Echocardiography*. 2nd ed. Philadelphia, PA: Lippincott Williams & Wilkins; 2011:738.)

TABLE 19.4 Clues to the differentiation of CP and restrictive cardiomyopathy

	CP	Restrictive cardiomyopathy
Pulsus paradoxus	Variable	Absent
Kussmaul sign	Common	Absent
Pericardial knock	Common	Absent
Chest x-ray	Pericardial calcification	No pericardial calcification
CT and MRI	Pericardial thickening (>2 mm)	Normal pericardium
B-type natriuretic peptide	Normal to mildly elevated	Significantly elevated
Catheterization data	LVEDP–RVEDP ≤5 mm Hg PASP <40–50 mm Hg RVEDP:RVSP >1:3	LVEDP–RVEDP >5 mm Hg PASP >40–50 mm Hg RVEDP:RVSP < 1:3
Atrial size	Usually normal	Enlarged
Ventricular septal motion	Abnormal: septal "bounce"	Normal
Respiratory variation (Doppler flow patterns)	Exaggerated (often >25%)	Normal/minimal (<10%)
Color M-mode propagation velocity	>100 cm/s	<100 cm/s
Tissue Doppler imaging of mitral annulus	E' >8 cm/s	E' <8 cm/s

CP, constrictive pericarditis; CT, computed tomography; MRI, magnetic resonance imaging; LVEDP, left ventricular end-diastolic pressure; RVEDP, right ventricular end-diastolic pressure; PASP, pulmonary artery systolic pressure; RVSP, right ventricular systolic pressure.

> **CLINICAL PEARL** When pericardiectomy is performed without the use of CPB, it is not uncommon for patients to require significant support with inotropic and/or vasopressor drugs—the anesthetic plan should carefully (and preemptively) plan for the use of these agents.

E. Goals of perioperative management

As the pathophysiologic manifestations of CP generally parallel that of tamponade, the anesthetic management of a patient presenting for pericardiectomy is similar to those mentioned for tamponade.

1. Premedication with benzodiazepines or opioids must be titrated judiciously and according to the patient's preoperative hemodynamic status. The sympathetic nervous system plays an important role in maintaining cardiac output and any inhibition may lead to clinical and hemodynamic deterioration.

2. In addition to standard noninvasive monitors, the intraoperative and postoperative management of patients with CP often requires invasive monitors. An arterial line is beneficial for frequent blood gas analysis (most importantly for cases involving thoracotomy), as well as continuous blood pressure monitoring (especially during cardiac manipulation and when CPB is utilized). The decision to place an arterial line either preoperatively or after induction of anesthesia must take into account the patient's clinical status and the possibility of hemodynamic instability on induction. Adequate intravenous access must be obtained given the possibility of marked and precipitous blood loss (cardiac chamber or coronary artery perforation, myocardial injury due to stripping of the pericardium), with central venous access allowing the rapid infusion of IV fluids/blood products and vasoactive drugs, as well as the monitoring of CVP. Perioperative cardiac output monitoring via a pulmonary artery catheter may be beneficial, especially as low cardiac output syndrome may persist into the postoperative period [4]. Intraoperative transesophageal echocardiography (TEE) provides useful information for both the surgeon and the anesthesiologist, in particular with regard to ventricular filling and function.

3. Pericardiectomy requires general anesthesia and care must be taken to avoid hemodynamic deterioration during induction and maintenance of anesthesia. Preload must be maintained, and often augmented, to ensure cardiac filling, and reductions in either preload or afterload are usually poorly tolerated. An elevated heart rate plays an important role in maintenance

of cardiac output and bradycardia can be particularly detrimental. While the atrial "kick" does little to enhance ventricular filling in patients with CP, extreme tachycardia, such as atrial fibrillation with a rapid ventricular rate, may be poorly tolerated. Contractility should be maintained, as significant myocardial depression will adversely impact cardiac output and systemic flow.

4. Based on these hemodynamic goals, induction and maintenance of anesthesia involve similar considerations as previously described for patients presenting with tamponade. Vasoactive medications must be readily available to offset any perturbations caused by the anesthetic agents or surgical manipulations, most notably decreased preload, afterload, contractility, and heart rate. Surgical blood loss and coagulopathy may be significant, necessitating aggressive resuscitation and correction of the underlying coagulopathy.

CLINICAL PEARL Depending on the extent of surgical dissection, severe surgical bleeding and coagulopathy are common with pericardiectomy.

REFERENCES

1. **Klein AL, Abbara S, Agler DA, et al. American Society of Echocardiography clinical recommendations for multi-modality cardiovascular imaging of patients with pericardial disease: endorsed by the Society for Cardiovascular Magnetic Resonance and Society of Cardiovascular Computed Tomography.** *J Am Soc Echocardiogr.* **2013;26(9): 965–1012.e15.**
2. Little WC, Freeman GL. Contemporary reviews in cardiovascular medicine: pericardial disease. *Circulation.* 2006;113:1622–1632.
3. **O'Connor CJ, Tuman KJ. The intraoperative management of patients with cardiac tamponade.** *Anesthesiol Clin.* **2010;28(1):87–96.**
4. Oliver WC, Mauermann WJ, Nuttall GA. Uncommon cardiac diseases. In: Kaplan JA, Reich DL, Savino JS, eds. *Kaplan's Cardiac Anesthesia: The Echo Era.* 6th ed. St. Louis, MO: Elsevier Saunders; 2011:706–713.
5. Gandhi S, Schneider A, Mohiuddin S, et al. Has the clinical presentation and clinician's index of suspicion of cardiac tamponade changed over the past decade? *Echocardiography.* 2008;25(3):237–241.
6. Dinardo JA, Zvara DA. *Anesthesia for Cardiac Surgery.* 3rd ed. Malden, MA: Blackwell Publishing; 2008.
7. Sagrista-Salueda J. Pericardial constriction: uncommon patterns. *Heart.* 2004;90(3):257–258.
8. **Myers RB, Spodick DH. Constrictive pericarditis: clinical and pathophysiologic characteristics.** *Am Heart J.* **1999; 138(2 Pt 1):219–232.**
9. Abdalla IA, Murray RD, Awad HE, et al. Reversal of the pattern of respiratory variation of Doppler inflow velocities in constrictive pericarditis during mechanical ventilation. *J Am Soc Echocardiogr.* 2000;13(9):827–831.
10. Rajagopalan N, Garcia MJ, Rodriguez L, et al. Comparison of new Doppler echocardiographic methods to differentiate constrictive pericardial heart disease and restrictive cardiomyopathy. *Am J Cardiol.* 2001;87(1):86–94.

Circulatory Support

20

Cardiopulmonary Bypass: Equipment, Circuits, and Pathophysiology

Eugene A. Hessel, II

KEY POINTS

1. All anesthesiologists who care for patients undergoing cardiopulmonary bypass (CPB) should be intimately familiar with the details and function of the heart–lung (H–L) machine (also referred to as the extracorporeal circuit [ECC]) and be involved in the establishment of protocols and the conduct of CPB during cardiac surgery.

2. The goal of CPB is to provide adequate gas exchange, oxygen delivery, and systemic blood flow with adequate perfusion pressure while minimizing the detrimental effects of bypass.

3. Roller pumps may cause more damage to blood elements than centrifugal pumps and can result in massive air embolism if the venous reservoir becomes empty.

4. Although centrifugal pumps pose less risk for massive air emboli, they can pump potentially lethal quantities of smaller bubbles. When a centrifugal pump is connected to the patient's arterial system but is not rotating, blood will flow backward through the pump and out of the patient *unless* the CPB systemic arterial line is clamped or a one-way valve is incorporated into the arterial line.

5. Membrane oxygenators (MOs) function similarly to natural lungs, imposing a membrane between the ventilating gas and the flowing blood, thereby eliminating direct contact between blood and gas.

6. An important limitation of polymethyl pentene (PMP) diffusion MOs is that they do not appear to allow transfer of volatile anesthetics and therefore intravenous anesthetics must be employed during CPB.

7. During bypass, excessive and rapid warming of blood with the bypass heat exchanger must be avoided (1) to prevent gas coming out of solution risking embolism and (2) excessive heating of the brain with potential neurologic damage.

8. Cardiotomy suction should be minimized or cell salvage techniques used to process the aspirated cardiotomy blood, as it contains microaggregates and is thought to be a major source of hemolysis and microemboli during CPB.

9. Adequate venting of the left ventricle (LV) requires constant monitoring, and several methods of venting the LV are available.

10. Adverse events during CPB are not uncommon. Risk containment requires the attention of anesthesiologists in addition to perfusionists and surgeons.

11. CPB introduces major physiologic abnormalities and contributes to the systemic inflammatory response (SIR) and organ dysfunction associated with cardiac surgery. However, CPB is not the only nor necessarily even the major cause of these adverse events.

PART I. THE CARDIOPULMONARY BYPASS CIRCUIT

I. Introduction

A. Cardiopulmonary bypass (CPB), introduced in 1953 to facilitate open heart surgery, is considered one of the major advances in medicine. **All anesthesiologists who care for these patients should be intimately familiar with the details and function of the heart–lung (H–L) machine (also referred to as the extracorporeal circuit [ECC]) and be involved in the establishment of protocols and the conduct of CPB during cardiac surgery.** In this chapter, the components of the H–L machine, the physiologic principles and pathophysiologic consequences of CPB, and the important role the anesthesiologist should play in its optimal and safe conduct are described. In Chapter 7, the medical management of patients during CPB is described.

B. The primary goal and function of CPB is to divert blood away from the heart and lungs and return it to the systemic arterial system, thereby permitting surgery on the nonfunctioning heart. In doing so, it must replace the function of both the heart and the lungs. **The CPB circuit must provide adequate gas exchange, oxygen delivery, systemic blood flow, and arterial pressure while minimizing adverse effects.** This is accomplished by the two principal components of the H–L machine: The **artificial lung** (blood gas–exchanging device or

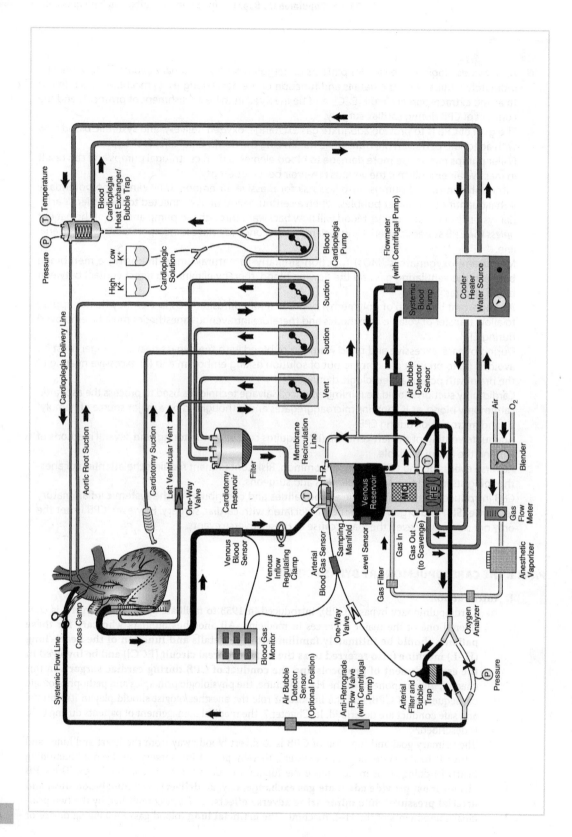

2

"oxygenator") and the **arterial pump**. The "oxygenator" removes carbon dioxide and adds oxygen to provide the desired $PaCO_2$ and PaO_2, while the arterial pump returns the blood to the patient's arterial system to maintain adequate systemic arterial pressure and organ perfusion.

C. Because the proximal ascending aorta is often cross-clamped to arrest the heart to facilitate surgery, a **cardioplegia delivery system** is added to minimize myocardial ischemia. **Other components** of the ECC include cannulae that connect to the systemic venous and arterial systems, a venous reservoir, a heat exchanger to control body temperature, surgical field and cardiotomy suction, and various safety and monitoring devices.

D. The components listed above will all be described in this chapter. The interested reader may find further details on CPB components in other texts [1–4].

II. Components of the circuit

A. Overview

The essential components of the H–L machine include the CPB console, oxygenator, venous reservoir, arterial pump, cardioplegia circuit, ventilating circuit, monitoring and safety systems, and various filters. These components can be assembled in myriad configurations depending on perfusionist/surgeon preference and patient need. Figure 20.1 shows a detailed schematic of a typical CPB circuit. Desaturated blood exits the patient through a right atrium **(RA)/inferior vena cava (IVC) venous ("cavoatrial" or "two-stage") cannula** and is diverted to the **venous reservoir** by **gravity siphon drainage** through large-bore polyvinyl chloride (PVC) tubing. Blood is then drawn from the **venous reservoir** by the **systemic blood pump**, which can be either roller or centrifugal (kinetic), and pumped through a **heat exchanger** (integral to the membrane oxygenator [MO]). Blood then passes through the **oxygenator**, through an **arterial filter**, and back into the patient through the **arterial cannula** inserted into the ascending aorta. Additional parts of the circuit include a **recirculation line** between the arterial side of the oxygenator and the venous reservoir that is used to facilitate priming the system and as a blood source for cardioplegia. A **purge line** is located on the housing of the arterial filter and is kept open during CPB to vent any air from the circuit back to either the venous reservoir or a second reservoir called **cardiotomy reservoir**.

Other roller pumps on the H–L machine are used for various functions including delivery of cardioplegia solution, return of shed blood in the surgical field via aspiration, venting of blood from intracardiac sources, or the removal of air from the venous reservoir when collapsible venous reservoir "bag" systems are used. Additional components of the CPB system include **microprocessors** for console control and electronic data recording, a **cooler/heater** which serves as an adjustable temperature water source used in conjunction with the **circuit heat exchangers**, an **anesthetic vaporizer** for the administration of volatile anesthetic

---

FIGURE 20.1 Detailed schematic diagram of arrangement of a typical cardiopulmonary bypass (CPB) circuit using a membrane oxygenator (**MO**) with integral **hardshell venous reservoir** and **heat exchanger** (HE) (lower center) and external **cardiotomy reservoir**. Venous cannulation is by a **cavoatrial** cannula and **arterial cannulation** is in the ascending aorta. Some circuits do not incorporate an MO **recirculation line**; in these cases the cardioplegia blood source is a separate outlet connector built-in to the oxygenator near the arterial outlet. The systemic blood pump may be either a roller or centrifugal type. The **cardioplegia delivery system** (right) is a one-pass combination blood/crystalloid type. The **heater–cooler water source** may be operated to supply water separately to both the oxygenator heat exchanger and cardioplegia delivery system. The **air bubble detector sensor** may be placed on the line between the venous reservoir and systemic pump, between the pump and MO inlet or between the oxygenator outlet and arterial filter (neither shown) or on the line after the arterial filter (optional position on drawing). **One-way valves** prevent retrograde flow (some circuits with a centrifugal pump also incorporate a one-way valve after the pump and within the systemic flow line). Other safety devices include an **oxygen analyzer** placed between the **anesthetic vaporizer** (if used) and the oxygenator gas inlet and a **venous reservoir-level sensor** attached to the housing of the hardshell venous reservoir (on the left). *Arrows*, directions of flow; *X*, placement of tubing clamps; *P* and *T*, pressure and temperature sensors, respectively. Hemoconcentrator (described in text) not shown. (From Figure 2.2 in Hessel EA, Shann KG. Blood pumps, circuitry and cannulation techniques in cardiopulmonary bypass. In: Gravlee GP, Davis RF, Hammon J, eds. *Cardiopulmonary Bypass and Mechanical Support: Principles and Practice*. 4th ed. Philadelphia, PA: Wolters Kluwer; 2016:21, with permission.)

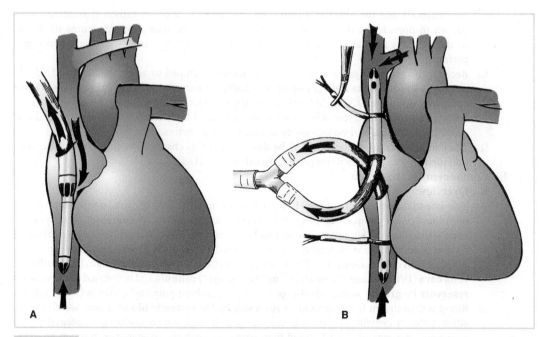

FIGURE 20.2 Venous cannulation (central, intrathoracic). Methods of venous cannulation: **A:** Single cannulation of right atrium (RA) with a "two-stage" cavoatrial cannula. This is typically inserted through the RA appendage. Note that the narrower tip of the cannula is in the inferior vena cava (IVC), where it drains this vein. The wider portion, with additional drainage holes, resides in the RA, where blood is received from the coronary sinus and superior vena cava (SVC). The SVC must drain via the RA when a cavoatrial cannula is used. **B:** Separate cannulation of the SVC and IVC. Note that there are loops placed around the cavae and venous cannulae and passed through tubing to act as tourniquets or snares. The tourniquet on the SVC has been tightened to divert all SVC flow into the SVC cannula and prevent communication with the RA. (From Figure 2.5 in Hessel EA, Shann KG. Blood pumps, circuitry and cannulation techniques in cardiopulmonary bypass. In: Gravlee GP, Davis RF, Hammon J, eds. *Cardiopulmonary Bypass and Mechanical Support: Principles and Practice.* 4th ed. Philadelphia, PA: Wolters Kluwer; 2016:25, with permission.)

agents, **cardioplegia delivery system**, various **sensors** for monitoring arterial and venous blood parameters as well as oxygen concentrations in the ventilating circuit, and various **safety devices**. Most of the components through which the blood passes are disposable and commercially custom-prepared to meet the specific requirements of individual cardiac teams.

B. **Venous cannulation and drainage**

1. **Overview.** Blood must be diverted into the H–L machine to keep it from passing through the heart and lungs, which permits access to the heart by the surgeon.

2. **Central venous cannulation** (Fig. 20.2)

   a. **Single simple cannula** in RA. Inserted through a purse-string suture in the RA free wall or atrial appendage. This type of cannulation tends to be unstable, does not reliably divert flow away from the right ventricle (RV), and is rarely used in adult CPB.

   b. **Cavoatrial or "two-stage" single cannula.** A single-lumen cannula with a wide proximal portion with drainage slits situated in the RA, and a narrower distal end placed into the IVC. The tip in the IVC makes this cannula more stable. It is usually inserted through a purse-string suture in the atrial appendage. Insertion may be difficult in the presence of RA masses, hardware, or a prominent Eustachian valve or Chiari network, and tears of the IVC in this region are difficult to manage. This is the most common type of cannulation for coronary artery and aortic valve surgery. It may not reliably prevent blood from entering the RV, and may not provide optimal myocardial cooling (especially the RA and RV). Superior vena cava (SVC) drainage and hence venous return to the H–L machine can be compromised if the junction of the SVC to the RA is kinked, which can occur when the heart is lifted up for grafting of vessels on the back of the heart.

c. **Bicaval cannulation.** Separate cannulae are placed into the SVC and IVC either directly or indirectly through the RA through purse-string sutures. **Bicaval cannulation is most effective at totally diverting blood away from the heart.** When the right heart must be opened, additional large ligatures or tapes are placed around the SVC and the IVC surrounding the indwelling venous cannulae to prevent any caval blood from entering the atrium (and any air getting from the atrium into the venous drainage). When the caval tapes are tightened, this is termed "complete bypass." When these tapes are tightened, it is critical to avoid obstruction of the cannulae to avoid venous hypertension (congestion). This is of particular concern in the SVC because of the potential adverse impact on cerebral perfusion; pressure in the SVC cephalad to the tip of the SVC cannula should be monitored. **Bicaval cannulation is necessary** whenever the surgeon plans to open the right heart (for surgery involving the tricuspid valve, RA masses, transatrial septal approaches to left heart, and for some congenital heart surgery) and for mitral valve (MV) surgery. Viewing the MV requires either RA retraction (which may kink the cavoatrial junction) or direct (transseptal) access via the RA. Bicaval cannulation, by diverting blood away from the right heart, minimizes cardiac warming, especially of the RA and RV during cold cardioplegia. However, when the caval tapes are tightened and the RA remains closed, there is no place for coronary sinus blood to drain both prior to aortic cross-clamping and when giving antegrade cardioplegia, so the RA and RV will distend. In that case, either one of the caval tapes must be released or the RA opened or vented.

CLINICAL PEARL When bicaval venous drainage cannulation is employed during CPB, it is important to monitor central venous pressure cephalad to the tip of the venous drainage cannula.

d. **Impact of persistent left superior vena cava (LSVC)** on venous cannulation: About 0.3% to 0.5% of the general population and about 3% to 10% of patients with congenital heart disease have a persistent LSVC. This remnant of fetal development drains blood from the junction of the left internal jugular (IJ) and left subclavian veins into the coronary sinus, and thence into the RA. A dilated coronary sinus (≥~11 mm) seen on echocardiography may be a clue to its presence. In the presence an LSVC, placing cannulae in the right SVC and IVC will not divert all systemic venous drainage away from the RA. One solution is for the surgeon to temporarily occlude (snare) the LSVC. However, in about two-thirds of these patients, the left innominate vein is absent or small, so this maneuver may result in cerebral venous hypertension. In these cases, the surgeon may place a third venous cannula in the LSVC either retrograde via the coronary sinus or directly into the LSVC through a purse-string suture.

CLINICAL PEARL A dilated coronary sinus may suggest the presence of a persistent LSVC, which can adversely impact the conduct of CPB and administration of retrograde cardioplegia.

3. **Peripheral venous cannulation** is used for minimally invasive "port-access" approaches, heart surgery via left thoracotomy, or for cannulation before entering the chest (electively or emergently when bleeding is anticipated or encountered). Most commonly, these venous cannulae are placed via the femoral vein (and rarely the IJ vein). If the femoral vein is used, the cannula is usually positioned with the tip at the SVC–RA junction. Positioning the cannula is often guided by transesophageal echocardiography (TEE). Bicaval cannulation is possible with a special IVC cannula designed for this purpose. If a separate IJ venous cannula is placed, it is often inserted by the anesthesiologist shortly after induction. As peripheral venous cannulae are smaller and longer than directly placed

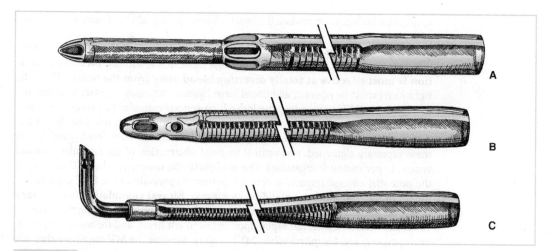

FIGURE 20.3 Venous cannulae. Drawings of commonly used venous cannulae. **A:** Tapered, "two-stage" right atrium (RA)–inferior vena cava (IVC) cannula. **B:** Straight, wire-reinforced "lighthouse"-tipped cannula for RA or separate cannulation of the superior vena cava (SVC) or IVC. **C:** Right-angled, metal-tipped cannula for cannulation of the SVC or IVC. (From Figure 2.3 in Hessel EA, Shann KG. Blood pumps, circuitry and cannulation techniques in cardiopulmonary bypass. In: Gravlee GP, Davis RF, Hammon J, eds. *Cardiopulmonary Bypass and Mechanical Support: Principles and Practice*. 4th ed. Philadelphia, PA: Wolters Kluwer; 2016:22, with permission.)

cannulae, resistance to drainage is greater, which may require use of augmented venous drainage (see Section II.B.5.b).

4. **Venous cannulae** are plastic (Fig. 20.3). Some are wire-reinforced to minimize kinking. Others designed for direct caval cannulation have curved thin metal or plastic tips for a favorable internal diameter to external diameter (ID:OD) ratio.

5. **Types of venous drainage**
   a. **Gravity.** Venous drainage is usually accomplished by gravity (siphon effect). This requires that the venous drainage tubing is full of fluid (blood). Drainage is based upon the pressure difference of the column of fluid between the level of the patient and that of the H–L machine (venous reservoir). Flow is influenced by central venous pressure (intravascular volume and venous tone), height differential between the patient and the H–L machine, and resistance in the venous cannula and tubing (length, ID, mechanical obstruction, or malposition of cannulae). "Chattering" of the venous lines suggest excessive drainage or inadequate venous return. Since drainage depends on a siphon, this will be interrupted if the venous line becomes filled with air.
   b. **Augmented venous drainage** is used when long or smaller venous cannulae are employed and to permit elevation of the H–L machine to the level of the patients (all designed to decrease the prime volume or for peripheral or port-access cannulation). Two classes of systems are utilized: vacuum-assisted and kinetic.
      (1) **Vacuum-assisted drainage** is accomplished by attaching the venous line to a closed "hardshell" venous reservoir (see Section II.D.1.a) to which vacuum (usually negative 20 to 50 mm Hg) is applied. Whenever augmented venous drainage is employed, there is increased risk of aspirating air from around the venous cannulae, and application of a second purse-string suture around them is recommended. There is also additional risk of developing positive pressure in the closed reservoir, which can lead to retrograde venous air embolism. This requires inclusion of a positive pressure release valve and heightened perfusionist attention.
      (2) **Kinetic-assisted drainage** is accomplished by inserting a pump, which is usually a centrifugal pump and rarely a roller pump). Centrifugal pumps are easier to control and minimize collapse of the cavae or atrium around the tip of the cannulae. As

with vacuum-assisted drainage, this technique requires close perfusionist attention to avoid air aspiration into the ECC.

(3) Studies have not found that use of augmented venous return increases blood trauma or aggravates the inflammatory response to CPB.

C. Arterial cannulation

1. Overview. The blood from the H–L machine must be returned to the systemic arterial system through an arterial cannula. These cannulae must carry the entire systemic blood flow ("cardiac output") through the narrowest part of the circuit. Cannula size selection balances the desired blood flow (mainly influenced by patient size) and a desire to keep blood velocity below 200 cm/sec and pressure gradients below 100 mm Hg. Higher flows and pressures may traumatize blood elements and the arterial wall (via "sandblasting" to potentially induce intimal dissection and/or atheroembolism) and reduce flow into critical side branches (e.g., right brachiocephalic artery) via high-velocity streaming effects. To maximize the ID:OD ratio, cannula tips are often constructed of metal or hard plastic. To minimize both pressure gradient and the size of the aortic incision, this narrowest part of the arterial line is kept as short as possible. Some special tips have been designed to minimize the exit velocities and jet effects (Fig. 20.4). Most commonly the arterial cannula is inserted into the distal ascending aorta, but other sites are also used. Special arterial

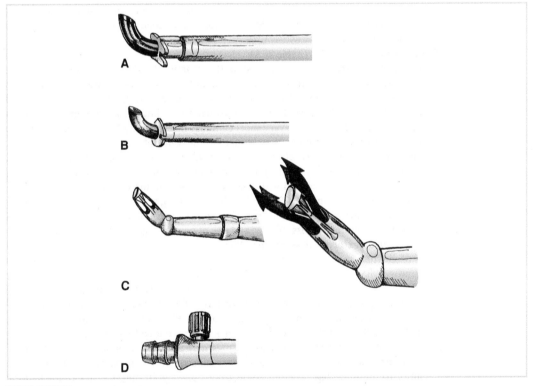

FIGURE 20.4 Arterial cannulae. Drawings of commonly used arterial cannulae. **A:** Thin metal–tipped, right-angled cannula with a plastic molded flange for securing cannula to the aorta. **B:** Similar design to (**A**) but with plastic right-angled tip. **C:** Angled, diffusion-tipped cannula designed to direct systemic flow in four directions (**right**) to avoid a "jetting effect" that may occur with conventional single-lumen arterial cannulae. **D:** Integral cannula/tubing connector and luer port (for deairing) incorporated onto some newer arterial cannulae. (From Figure 2.8 in Hessel EA, Shann KG. Blood pumps, circuitry and cannulation techniques in cardiopulmonary bypass. In: Gravlee GP, Davis RF, Hammon J, eds. *Cardiopulmonary Bypass and Mechanical Support: Principles and Practice.* 4th ed. Philadelphia, PA: Wolters Kluwer; 2016:30, with permission.)

TABLE 20.1 Arterial cannulation sites

	Indications and advantages	Limitations and hazards
Ascending aorta	Convenient Lowest risk of dissection (~0.08%)	Atheroembolism May not be available due to ascending aortic pathology (e.g., atherosclerotic, "porcelain aorta," aneurysm, dissection)
Femoral/Iliac	Ease of access Peripheral site During reentry, especially if bleeding occurs Preincision if severe heart failure For minimal-access surgery	Retrograde dissection (~0.5%) Unavailable if peripheral vascular disease (PVD) Ischemia of cannulated extremity Compartment syndrome Postrelease emboli Risk of malperfusion when used in patients with aortic dissection
Axillary/subclavian	Perhaps best for patients with aortic dissection Permits selective cerebral perfusion (SCP) Lowest risk of atheroemboli	More difficult and time consuming Not risk-free Dissection (~0.5%)

cannulae (e.g., Soft-Flow™ [Medtronic, Minneapolis, Minnesota], Optiflow™ [LivaNova, London, England] Embol-X™ [Edwards Lifesciences, Irvine, CA], and Cardiogard™ [Cardiogard Medical ltd, Hertzliya Pituach, Israel]) have been developed to minimize risk of embolization, but are not widely used.

2. **Cannulation site options** (Table 20.1)

a. **Ascending aorta.** The surgeon inserts the cannula through one or two concentric purse-string sutures in the distal ascending aorta and directs it toward the transverse arch to avoid preferential streaming to any of the three arch branches. Some surgeons place a long cannula directed into the proximal descending aorta to minimize jet effects in the arch, while others use very short cannulae inserted only 1 to 2 cm into the aorta. Dislodgement of atheromatous material from the cannulation site is a primary concern. Because palpation of the aorta may not detect atheroma and this site is hidden from TEE imaging, many advocate imaging of the intended cannulation site using epiaortic ultrasound. Dissection associated with ascending aortic cannulation occurs in about 0.08% (1 per 1,250 cases, range 0.02% to 0.2%). The ascending aorta may not be a suitable cannulation site for various reasons including severe atherosclerotic disease, aortic dissection, use of minimal-access surgery, and risk of hemorrhage during repeat sternotomy.

b. **Femoral or external iliac artery.** This is the second most common approach and is used when ascending aortic cannulation is not desirable or feasible. However, this approach has a number of limitations, including risk of dissection (0.3% to 0.8% or ~1/200 cases), atheroembolism (especially into brain and heart), malperfusion of the brain and other organs in the presence of aortic dissection or atherosclerosis, and ischemia of the cannulated limb. Upon initiation of CPB and intermittently throughout it, TEE surveillance of the descending aorta is recommended to detect retrograde dissection. Prolonged femoral cannulation times may release emboli and acid metabolites from the limb upon reperfusion and cause subsequent compartment syndrome in the limb. To minimize leg ischemia, some groups sew a graft onto the side of the femoral artery and insert the arterial cannula into this graft so that blood flows both retrograde and antegrade, while others insert a supplemental arterial cannula into the distal femoral artery.

CLINICAL PEARL Cannulation of the femoral artery for arterial inflow carries substantial risk of iatrogenic retrograde aortic dissection, which should be monitored via TEE intermittently during CPB.

    c. Axillary/subclavian artery cannulation is often advocated in the presence of aortic dissection or severe atherosclerosis. These vessels are usually free of significant atherosclerosis, and may pose less risk of malperfusion, but risk of iatrogenic dissection is similar (~0.7% or ~1/140 cases) to that with femoral cannulation. The artery is approached through an infraclavicular incision, and the cannula can be placed either directly into the vessel or via a graft sewn onto the side of the artery. The right side is favored since it permits selective cerebral perfusion (SCP) if circulatory arrest is required (see Section III.D.3). If the vessel is cannulated directly (i.e., not through a side-arm graft), then the artery in the contralateral upper extremity (radial or brachial) must be used for systemic arterial pressure monitoring during CPB.

    d. Innominate (brachiocephalic) artery cannulation is uncommonly used, because the presence of the cannula (flow directed toward the aortic arch) may restrict flow around it into the right carotid artery and hence the brain.

D. Venous reservoir

    1. Overview. Venous drainage from the patient flows into a reservoir placed immediately before the systemic arterial pump to serve as a "holding tank" and act as a buffer for imbalances between venous return and arterial flow. As a high capacitance (i.e., low pressure) receiving chamber for venous return, it facilitates gravity drainage of venous blood. As much as 3 L of blood may need to be translocated from the patient to the ECC when full CPB begins. This reservoir may also serve as a gross bubble trap for air that enters the venous line and as a site for adding blood, fluids, or drugs to the circulation. One of its most important functions is to provide a source (reservoir) of blood if venous drainage is sharply reduced or stopped, hence providing the perfusionist with a **reaction time** in order to avoid "pumping the CPB system dry" and risking massive air embolism. These reservoirs usually include various filtering devices. There are two classes of reservoirs:

    a. Rigid hardshell plastic, "open" venous canisters. Advantages include ability to handle venous air more effectively, simplicity of priming, larger capacity, and ease of applying suction for vacuum-assisted venous return. Most hardshell venous reservoirs incorporate macro- and microfilters (usually coated with defoaming agents), and can also serve as the cardiotomy reservoir (see Section II.I.1) by directly receiving suctioned and vented blood. Their ability to remove gaseous microemboli (GME) varies.

    b. Softshell, collapsible plastic bag, "closed" venous reservoirs. These reservoirs eliminate the gas–blood interface and reduce the risk of massive air embolism because they will collapse when emptied and do not permit air to enter the systemic pump. Closed collapsible reservoirs also make the aspiration of air by the venous cannulae more obvious to the perfusionist, but require a way of emptying the air out of the reservoir. When softshell reservoirs are used, a separate cardiotomy reservoir is required (see Section II.I.1). Because of reduction of the gas–blood interface, their use may be associated with less inflammatory activation. Data comparing clinical outcome with use of the two types of venous reservoirs are conflicting and inconclusive [5].

E. Systemic (arterial) pump

There are currently two types of blood pumps used in the CPB circuit: roller and kinetic (most commonly called centrifugal) (Table 20.2). In the United States, kinetic pumps are used in approximately 50% of all procedures.

    1. Roller pump (Fig. 20.5)

    a. Principles of operation. Blood is moved through this pump by sequential compression of tubing by a roller against a horseshoe-shaped backing plate or raceway. A typical pump has two roller heads configured 180 degrees apart to maintain continuous roller head contact with the tubing. The output is determined by the stroke volume of each revolution (the volume within the tubing, which is dependent upon the tubing size and the length of the compressed pathway) times the revolutions per minute (rpm). Flow from a systemic roller pump increases or decreases linearly with rpm. With larger ID tubing (e.g., 1/2-in ID), lower rpm are required to achieve the same output compared to smaller ID tubing. The total pump output is displayed in milliliters

TABLE 20.2 Comparison of roller versus centrifugal pumps

Centrifugal	Roller
Output inversely proportional to afterload (i.e., arterial pressure)	Output independent of afterload
Output not directly related to revolutions per minute (rpm) Require flowmeter to determine output Will allow retrograde flow out of aorta when turned off if line not clamped	Output = rpm × volume per revolution Minimal retrograde flow risk
Will not blow out arterial line	Will blow out arterial line if line clamped
No need to adjust occlusiveness	Must adjust occlusiveness
Won't pump massive air (but can pass amounts of air that can harm the patient)	Can pump massive air Wear (release particles of plastic ["spallation"]); can rupture with prolonged use
Perhaps less blood trauma Perhaps safer Requires constant attention to adapt to available venous return	Requires constant attention to adapt to available venous return.

or liters per minute on the pump control panel. Roller pumps are also used to deliver cardioplegia solution, remove blood and air from heart chambers or great vessels, and suction shed blood from the operative field.

    b. Adjustment of occlusion. To minimize hemolysis, the occlusion must be properly set. Occlusion describes the degree to which the tubing is compressed between the rollers and the backing plate. An underocclusive pump will allow retrograde movement of fluid when the pressure in the downstream location exceeds that generated by the pump, thereby reducing forward flow. Conversely, an overocclusive pump will create cellular damage (red blood cell [RBC] hemolysis, white blood cell [WBC], and platelet activation) and excessive wear on the tubing with release of microparticles ("spallation"). Occlusion is set by the perfusionist by adjusting the distance between the raceway and each of the roller heads. Typically, occlusion is adjusted to be barely nonocclusive.

    c. Advantages and disadvantages. Roller pumps offer the advantages of being simple, effective, inexpensive, having a low priming volume, and producing a reliable output that is afterload independent. The drawback to afterload independence is that, in the presence of downstream obstruction, high pressure will develop which may cause rupture of connections in the arterial line. If upstream inflow is obstructed, roller pumps can generate high negative pressures creating microbubbles ("cavitation") and RBC damage. **Roller pumps may cause more damage to blood components and can result in massive air embolism if the venous reservoir becomes empty.** They do not adjust to changes in venous return and require more careful attention by the perfusionist.

  2. Centrifugal pumps (Fig. 20.6)

    a. Principles of operation. Centrifugal pumps consist of a nest of smooth plastic cones or a vaned impeller located inside a plastic housing. When rotated rapidly (2,000 to 3,000 rpm), these pumps generate a pressure differential that causes fluid movement. Vaned, impeller-type rotary (centrifugal) pumps are predominantly being used rather than the traditional cone-type centrifugal pumps, because they have smaller prime volumes and may cause less hemolysis.

    b. Advantages and disadvantages. Unlike roller pumps, these devices are totally nonocclusive and afterload dependent (an increase in downstream resistance or pressure decreases forward flow). Flow is not determined by rotational rate alone, and therefore a **flowmeter** *must* be incorporated in the outflow line to quantify pump flow. **Furthermore, when the pump is connected to the patient's arterial system but is not rotating, blood will flow backward through the pump and out of the patient**

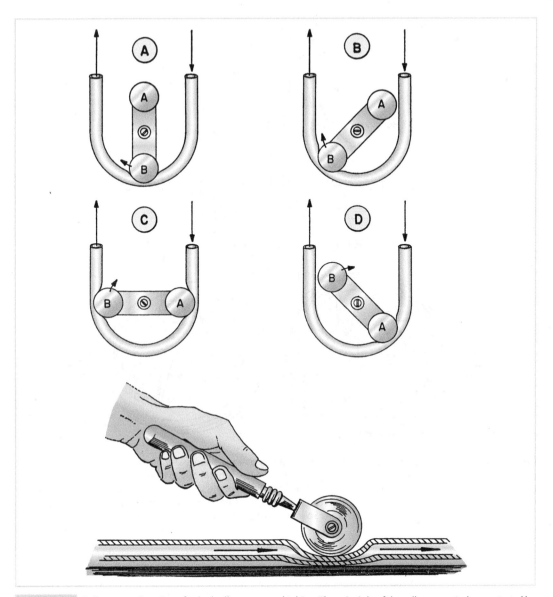

FIGURE 20.5 Roller pump. Drawing of a dual roller pump and tubing. The principle of the roller pump is demonstrated by the hand roller in the lower drawing moving along a section of tubing pushing fluid ahead of it and suctioning fluid behind it. The upper four drawings in sequence (**A–D**) show how roller B first moves fluid ahead of it and suctions fluid behind it (**A**). As the pump rotates clockwise, the second roller A begins to engage the tubing (**B**). As the rotation continues there is a very brief period with volume trapped between the two rollers (**C**) and no forward flow, which imparts some pulsatility. In position (**D**), roller B leaves the tubing, while the second roller A continues to move fluid in the same direction. Not shown are the roller pump backing plate, tubing holders, and tube guides for maintaining the tubing within the raceway. *Large arrows* in and out of tubing indicate direction of fluid flow, and *small arrows* near roller B indicate direction of roller arm rotation. (From Stofer RC. *A Technic for Extracorporeal Circulation*. Springfield, IL: Charles C. Thomas; 1968:22, with permission.)

4   *unless* the CPB systemic arterial line is clamped or a one-way valve is incorporated into the arterial line. This can cause exsanguination of the patient or aspiration of air into the arterial line around the purse-string sutures. On the other hand, if the arterial line becomes occluded, these pumps will not generate excessive pressure and will not rupture the systemic flow line. Likewise, they will not generate as much

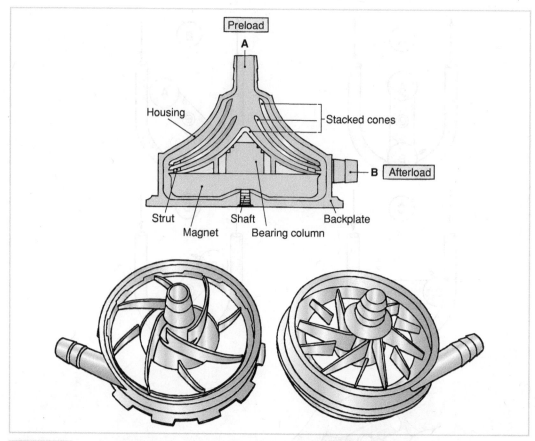

FIGURE 20.6 Centrifugal pumps. Drawings of centrifugal pump heads. A cross-sectional view of a smooth, cone-type pump is shown on the top. Blood enters at *A* and is expelled on the right (*B*) due to kinetic forces created by the three rapidly spinning cones. Impeller-type pumps with vanes are shown in the bottom drawings. (Modified from Trocchio CR, Sketel JO. Mechanical pumps for extracorporeal circulation. In: Mora CT, ed. *Cardiopulmonary Bypass: Principles and Techniques of Extracorporeal Circulation*. New York: Springer-Verlag; 1995:222, 223, with permission.)

negative pressure and hence as much cavitation and microembolus production as a roller pump if inflow becomes occluded.

A reputed advantage of centrifugal pumps over roller pumps is less risk of pumping massive air emboli into the arterial line; centrifugal pumps will become deprimed and stop pumping if more than approximately 50 mL of air is introduced into the circuit. **However, they will pass smaller but still potentially lethal quantities of smaller bubbles.** A number of studies have demonstrated that centrifugal pumps cause less trauma to blood elements, less activation of coagulation, produce fewer microemboli, and may be associated with better clinical outcomes than roller pumps [5].

3. **Pulsatile flow and pulsatile pumps**

   a. **Overview.** Most roller pumps produce only a low-amplitude, high-frequency pulsatile flow of little physiologic relevance, while centrifugal pumps produce a nonpulsatile flow. The necessity and importance of pulsatile flow has long been debated [5].

   b. **How pulsatile flow is generated during CPB.** Several methods are commonly used to achieve arterial pulsations during CPB:

      (1) If partial CPB is being used, venous drainage can be reduced to permit some cardiac ejection.

      (2) If an intra-aortic balloon is in place, it can be used to impart pulsatility to the flow.

(3) Pulsations can be produced by roller pumps, and to a lesser degree by centrifugal pumps, designed to rotate at varying speeds.

c. **Damping effects of the aortic cannula.** The first two methods of producing pulsations are more effective because they generate the pulse in the aorta itself. Although many pumps can generate a pulsatile outflow, the amount of pulsatile energy transmitted into the aorta is limited by the damping effects caused by the narrow aortic cannula, MOs, and arterial microfilters. Calculations show that very little of the pulsatile energy generated is actually delivered into the patient's arterial system [6].

d. **Liabilities of attempting to generate pulsatile flow inside the ECC**
   (1) Increased cost and complexity
   (2) Requires use of larger arterial cannulae
   (3) Associated with higher peak nozzle velocities out of the arterial cannula (risking vascular injury and atheroembolism)

F. **The oxygenator (artificial lung or gas-exchanging device)**

1. Although numerous **types of oxygenators** have been used in the past, currently only MOs are used in most parts of the world. These produce less blood trauma and microemboli, permit more precise control of arterial blood gases, and likely improve patient outcomes as compared with bubble oxygenators. Virtually all current MOs are positioned after the arterial pump because the resistance in the blood path requires blood to be pumped through them, and to minimize the risk of pulling air through the membrane and producing GME. Most oxygenators also include an integral heat exchanger (see Section II.G.1).

   MOs function similarly to natural lungs, **imposing a membrane between the ventilating gas and the flowing blood and eliminating direct contact between the blood and the gas**. At least three types of membranes are used:

   a. **Silicone membranes.** Rarely used today, these true membranes usually consist of thin sheets of silicone rubber wrapped circumferentially over a spool.

   b. **Microporous polypropylene (PPL) membranes.** Usually configured in longitudinal bundles of narrow hollow fibers, but occasionally as folded sheets of membrane. The pores fill with autologous plasma which serves as the "membrane" through which gas exchange occurs. With excessive pressure in the blood path or over prolonged time, plasma may leak through the membrane (which degrades gas transfer), while excessive negative pressure can lead to entrainment of air emboli. In hollow fiber MOs, the blood typically flows outside the hollow fibers, while ventilating gases flow through the hollow fibers (in a countercurrent direction).

   c. **Polymethyl pentene (PMP) diffusion membranes.** Hollow fiber MOs made of a nonporous plastic, PMP, are true membranes. This has the advantage of minimizing the risk of plasma leak and microair aspiration and permits prolonged oxygenation (days). Gas exchange occurs by diffusion across this true membrane. **An important limitation is that PMP does not appear to allow adequate transfer of volatile anesthetics, therefore intravenous anesthetics must be employed during CPB.** Because of this limitation and because they are more expensive, PMP "diffusion" MOs are not commonly used for conventional CPB, at least in the United States. Because of their reduced risk of plasma leak ("oxygenator pulmonary edema"), they are commonly used for long-term extracorporeal support (e.g., extracorporeal membrane oxygenation [ECMO]).

2. **Membrane oxygenators (MOs)** were thought to serve as bubble filters and to prevent venous GME from passing into the arterial system, but it is now recognized that the majority of microscopic venous gas emboli do transit through MOs. The effectiveness of GME removal varies among MOs [5]. Because of this limitation, teams must make every effort to minimize the entrainment and administration of air into the venous drainage system.

3. **Control of gas exchange and gas supply to the MO.** Gas exchange by MO is controlled similarly to that in normal lungs. Arterial carbon dioxide levels are controlled by flow of fresh gas (commonly called "sweep gas flow") through the oxygenator (analogous to alveolar minute ventilation), and arterial PO_2 is controlled by varying fractional inspired

oxygen (FiO_2). Oxygenators require a **gas supply system**. This typically includes a source of oxygen and air (and occasionally carbon dioxide), which passes through a **blender**. An **oxygen analyzer** should be incorporated in the MO gas supply line after the blender. An **anesthetic vaporizer** may also be placed in the gas supply line near the oxygenator. Volatile anesthetic liquids may destroy plastic components of ECCs; therefore, care must be taken when filling them with volatile agents. A method of **scavenging** waste gas from the oxygenator outlet should be provided (American Society of ExtraCorporeal Technology [AmSECT] standard 6.8.) [7].

4. MOs can fail during CPB. Groom et al. [8] have advocated inserting a shunt (3/8-in tubing) between the inlet and outlet of the MO to facilitate exchange of the defective oxygenator with a new oxygenator using a parallel replacement (PRONTO) procedure.

G. **Heat exchanger**

1. **Overview.** The passage of blood through the ECC results in heat loss and patient cooling. To maintain normothermia, heat must be added to the circuit. This is accomplished with a **heat exchanger**, which may also be used to intentionally cool and rewarm the patient. Heat exchangers consist of heat-exchanging tubes (often metal) through which the blood flows. These tubes are surrounded by water of varying temperatures. As mentioned earlier, heat exchangers are often incorporated in the oxygenator, which is called an integral heat exchanger.

2. **Heater–cooler.** To control the temperature of the water flowing through the heat exchanger, a heater–cooler device adjusts the water temperature and pumps it through the heat exchanger (countercurrent with the blood flow, which is more efficient).

3. Recently sporadic and relatively rare outbreaks of *mycobacterium chimaera* surgical site and prosthetic device infections have been traced to bioaerosols of this agent emanating from contamination of one model of heater–cooler units.

4. Excessive gradients between the blood and water temperature should be avoided. **Excessive warming can lead to gases coming out of solution and causing GME as well as excessive heating of the brain to induce or aggravate injury.** As a result, guidelines for temperature management during CPB have been promulgated [9].

   a. Oxygenator arterial outlet temperature is the recommended surrogate for cerebral temperature (class I recommendation, level C evidence)

   b. Oxygenator arterial outlet temperature is assumed to underestimate cerebral temperature (class I, level C)

   c. Nasopharyngeal or pulmonary arterial (PA) temperatures are reasonable estimates of core temperature after weaning from CPB (class IIa, level C)

   d. Arterial outlet temperature should be no higher than 37°C during CPB to prevent cerebral hyperthermia (class I, level C)

   e. Peak cooling temperature gradient between the oxygenator arterial outlet and venous inlet should not exceed 10°C to prevent the generation of gaseous emboli (class I, level C)

   f. Peak warming temperature gradient between the oxygenator arterial outlet and venous inlet should not exceed 10°C to prevent outgassing (microemboli formation) (class I, level C)

   g. During warming, when oxygenator arterial outlet temperature ≥30°C, the warming gradient between the oxygenator arterial outlet and venous inlet should be ≤4°C and/or warming rate ≤0.5°C/min

5. Separate heat exchangers are also used in the cardioplegia circuits (see Section II.H.3).

H. **Cardioplegia delivery system or circuit**

1. **Overview.** When the aorta is cross-clamped (distal to the aortic valve but proximal to the arterial inflow cannula) to provide a quiet operative field or access to the aortic valve, the heart is deprived of coronary perfusion and becomes ischemic. This is usually managed by perfusing the heart with cardioplegia solutions. See also Chapter 23 for further discussion on myocardial protection.

2. **Routes of delivery of cardioplegia solutions**

   a. **Aortic root.** A cannula is inserted in the aortic root (proximal to the cross-clamp). Typically this has a "Y" configuration: one limb is connected to the cardioplegia delivery system and the other to suction (to vent the left ventricle [LV] or aspirate air). The cardioplegia solution is delivered into the aortic root and thence into the coronary arteries. **This is not effective in the presence of severe aortic regurgitation or when the aortic root is open;** it is also less effective in the presence of severe proximal coronary artery stenosis. Ideally, pressure in the aortic root should be measured during administration of the cardioplegia to assure adequate coronary flow and maintained at about 70 to 100 mm Hg.

b. **Directly into the coronary ostia.** Special handheld cannulae are placed directly into the right and left main coronary arteries after the aortic root is opened for delivery of the cardioplegia solutions. This is commonly done in the presence of aortic regurgitation and during open aortic valve procedures.

c. **Retrograde into the coronary sinus.** Balloon-tipped cannulae are inserted blindly (or under direct vision if the RA is opened) into the coronary sinus through a purse-string suture in the low lateral wall of the RA. TEE may be helpful in guiding and assessing placement. Many of these cannulae have a pressure port near the tip so that the pressure in the coronary sinus can be monitored during perfusion (ideally maintained between 30 and 50 mm Hg). Retrograde administration of cardioplegia may be advantageous in the presence of severe coronary artery stenosis or aortic regurgitation and during aortic valve surgery. **However, it may provide inferior protection of the RV,** because the cannula may exclude some veins draining RV myocardium into the coronary sinus or directly into the RA (Thebesian veins). The presence of a persistent LSVC compromises retrograde cardioplegia efficacy.

3. **Delivery systems.** These vary in their complexity. If blood cardioplegia is being used, blood is taken out of the arterial perfusion line following oxygenation and mixed with the crystalloid cardioplegia solution (at various blood–crystalloid ratios). This may be accomplished by using two separate roller pumps, or with a single roller pump which drives two tubes of different sizes (to produce the proper flow ratio). The mixture is then passed through a dedicated heat exchanger. Microfiltration may be added and pressures and temperatures are monitored. Some use more complex delivery systems which permit rapid change of the concentration of various components in the cardioplegia solution.

I. **Cardiotomy, field suction, cell salvage processors, and cell (RBC) savers**

1. **Overview.** During CPB there is often considerable bleeding into the surgical field due to systemic heparinization and persistent pulmonary and coronary venous drainage. It is usually not desirable to discard this large volume of blood via conventional discard suction. Traditionally, this blood is removed from the field by roller pumps on the H–L machine (**"cardiotomy suckers"**) and returned to the H–L machine via the **cardiotomy reservoir** (which includes filters and, as noted above, is commonly incorporated into the hardshell venous reservoir, but must be added separately when a softshell reservoir is used). The cardiotomy suction should not be used until the patient is adequately anticoagulated and should be discontinued as soon as heparin neutralization with protamine commences (to avoid clotting of blood in the ECC).

2. **Hazards of cardiotomy blood.** Cardiotomy blood contains microaggregates of cells, fat, foreign debris, and thrombogenic and fibrinolytic factors, and is thought to be a major source of microemboli and hemolysis during CPB. **For these reasons cardiotomy suction should be used sparingly.**

3. **An alternative strategy** is to suction the field blood into a **cell salvage washer/processor/ saver system** (or to process the blood that has been suctioned into a standalone cardiotomy reservoir with this cell salvage system before returning it to the H–L machine). These devices wash the blood with saline, and separate the red cells from the plasma and saline by centrifugation with the intent of reducing the microemboli, fat, etc. They also remove plasma proteins, platelets, heparin, and some of the WBCs while retaining concentrated RBCs (hematocrit about 70%). Not all processors are equally effective at removing fat, and the salvaged blood may have to be specially filtered before administration. Some of the problems associated with the use of cell processors include delayed availability and turnover time (not adequate in the face of rapid hemorrhage) and loss of platelets and

coagulation factors (resulting in a consumptive coagulopathy if >6 bowls or 1,500 mL of blood is processed). Comparative studies of cardiotomy suction versus cell processors have produced conflicting results [5].

J. **Venting**

1. **Overview.** Both the RV and LV must be decompressed during CPB to improve surgical exposure, reduce myocardial oxygen demand, and attenuate mechanical damage to the heart from overdistention.

2. The RV is readily visible to the surgeon, and decompression depends on adequacy of venous drainage. The LV is more difficult to observe, has more adverse consequences if distended, and requires various strategies for venting.

3. **Consequences of distention of the left heart:**
   a. Stretches myocardium causing ventricular dysfunction
   b. Myocardial ischemia: impairs subendocardial perfusion and increases myocardial oxygen needs
   c. Increases left atrial pressure, leading to pulmonary edema and hemorrhage
   d. Interferes with surgical exposure

4. **Distention of the left heart is likely to occur** when the LV is unable to empty (e.g., on initiation of CPB, especially in the presence of aortic regurgitation; during cardiac arrest, aortic cross-clamping, and administration of antegrade cardioplegia; during ventricular fibrillation; and following aortic cross-clamp release).

5. Sources of blood coming into the left heart during CPB:
   a. Bronchial venous drainage (normal ~100 mL/min)
   b. Systemic venous blood that bypasses venous cannulae and passes through right heart and lungs
   c. Aortic regurgitation
   d. Thebesian veins draining into the left heart (but these are not common)
   e. Patent ductus arteriosus (PDA) (~1/3,500 adults)
   f. Atrial septal defect (ASD), ventricular septal defect (VSD)

6. **Assessment of adequacy of decompression of the left heart** by inspection or palpation is difficult because of its position and thick walls of the LV. Elevation of the pulmonary artery pressure if a pulmonary artery catheter (PAC) is in place may suggest distention of the left heart, but the best method of evaluating the adequacy of LV decompression is TEE.

CLINICAL PEARL Distention of the LV can be difficult to detect clinically during CPB, and is best diagnosed by use of TEE.

7. **Methods of venting or decompressing the left heart** (see Fig. 20.7 and Table 20.3): Cannulae are inserted in various locations and attached to tubing connected to roller pumps which transmits the blood to the venous or cardiotomy reservoirs. **The end of the suction tubing from the H–L machine should first be placed into fluid to assure that it is sucking and not emitting air before it is connected to any intracardiac or aorta venting cannula.** The amount of suction must be constantly adjusted by the perfusionist to avoid excessive (risk of damage to heart or aspirating air) or inadequate (over distention) venting.

   a. **Aortic root vent** (one limb of the antegrade cardioplegia cannula): This is the most common technique used during coronary artery bypass graft (CABG) surgery. Suction is applied to the antegrade cardioplegia cannula (directly or via a side limb). Aortic root venting of the LV is only effective when the aorta is cross-clamped, when antegrade cardioplegia is not being administered, and when the aortic root is not opened.

   b. **LV vent placed via the right superior pulmonary vein.** A cannula is inserted at the junction of the right superior pulmonary vein with the left atrium and then threaded through the left atrium and MV into the LV. This method is used during aortic valve and MV surgery (especially in the presence of aortic regurgitation) and for patients with poor LV function undergoing CABG.

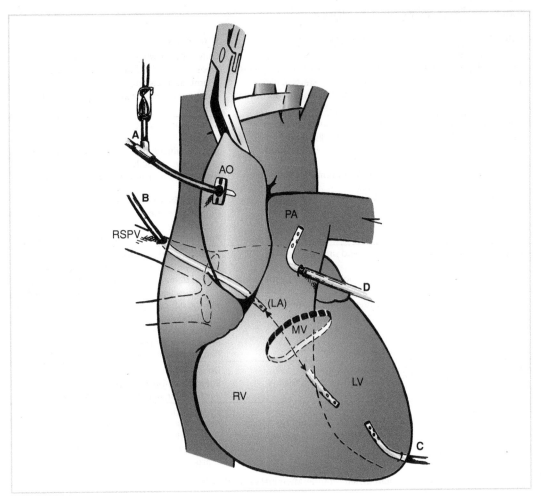

FIGURE 20.7 Sites for venting the left heart. **A:** Aortic root cannula; one limb of the "Y" is connected to the cardioplegia delivery system and the other limb to suction (siphon or roller pump) for venting the aortic root and hence the left ventricle (LV). **B:** Cannula inserted at the junction of the right superior pulmonary vein (RSPV) with the left atrium and then threaded through the left atrium and mitral valve (MV) and into the LV. **C:** Cannula inserted directly into the apex of the LV. **D:** Cannula is inserted into the pulmonary artery. AO, aorta; PA pulmonary artery; LA, left atrium; RV, right ventricle. (From Figure 2.25 in Hessel EA, Shann KG. Blood pumps, circuitry and cannulation techniques in cardiopulmonary bypass. In: Gravlee GP, Davis RF, Hammon J, eds. *Cardiopulmonary Bypass and Mechanical Support: Principles and Practice.* 4th ed. Philadelphia, PA: Wolters Kluwer; 2016:69, with permission.)

    c. **LV vent placed directly through the LV apex.** This is rarely used today because of difficulty in positioning, control of bleeding after removal, and the possibility of forming late apical LV aneurysms.

    d. **Vent placed through the left atrial appendage or the top of the left atrium** (into either the left atrium or LV). This is rarely used.

    e. **Vent placed in the main pulmonary artery.** This method minimizes the risk of air entry into the left heart (although it can still occur). It does **not** provide reliable decompression of the LV in the presence of aortic regurgitation, and closure of the incision in the pulmonary artery can be problematic in patients with pulmonary hypertension.

  8. **Complications of venting the left heart** include systemic air embolism, bleeding, damage to cardiac structures, dislodgement of thrombi, calcium, tumor, etc., and MV

TABLE 20.3 Methods of venting the left heart

Method	Advantages	Disadvantages
Ascending aortic (cardioplegia cannula)	Simple; no additional cannula Also vents air when unclamp aorta and when LV starts to eject Can be used to monitor aortic root infusion pressure	Only vents LV when aorta is cross-clamped Does not vent LV during administration of antegrade cardioplegia Can permit air to be aspirated into the aortic root
Indirect LV (via stab incision in RSPV, through LA and MV)	Handles all sources of blood causing LV distention Best for aortic regurgitation Provides optimal decompression of LV Avoids problems of direct LV vent	Somewhat difficult exposure of insertion site May be difficult to thread cannula into LV and position correctly Risk of bleeding and tears at insertion site in RSPV Potential for air entry into left heart Potential problem if mechanical prosthesis in MV Potential embolism if tumor or clots in LA or LV
Direct LV (through stab incision in apex)	Direct and simple Avoids going across prosthetic MV Handles all sources of blood causing LV distention	Positioning may be a problem—tip becomes easily obstructed by LV wall or MV apparatus Risk of damage to LV and injury to coronary arteries and collaterals (myocardial ischemia) May be difficult to control bleeding from stab wound Late LV aneurysm Potential embolism if clots in LV Potential for air entry into the left heart
Direct LA (via LA appendage, roof of LA, or RSPV)	Relatively simple Avoids going across the MV	Does not handle AR Potential embolism if clots in LA Potential for air entry into the left heart
Pulmonary artery	Simple, easy access Reduces risk of admitting air into the left heart (but still can occur)	Does not handle AR Renders use of PA pressure as a monitor of LV distention invalid Risk of damage and bleeding from pulmonary artery

AR, aortic regurgitation; LA, left atrium; LV, left ventricle; MV, mitral valve; PA, pulmonary artery; RSPV, right superior pulmonary vein; AR, aortic regurgitation.
Modified from Table 2.14 in Hessel EA, Shann KG. Blood pumps, circuitry and cannulation techniques in cardiopulmonary bypass. In: Gravlee GP, Davis RF, Hammon J, eds. *Cardiopulmonary Bypass and Mechanical Support: Principles and Practice*. 4th edition. Philadelphia, PA: Wolters Kluwer; 2016:68.

incompetence. A critical complication is inadvertent pumping of air into the heart via these vent lines. This occurs if tubing is misaligned in the roller pump-head or if the pump is in reverse mode. Air can also enter the left heart when these lines are inserted or removed; therefore, **the volume and pressure in the left heart should be elevated at these times and ventilation interrupted.**

9. Any time the heart is opened, even by simply placing a catheter in a chamber, air may collect in the heart. If not removed, this air will embolize with resumption of cardiac contractions. Even right-heart air has the potential to pass into the left heart via septal defects or through the lungs. In addition to vigorous attempts at removal of all air before closing the left heart, **the use of venting at the highest point of the aorta is considered the final safety maneuver against systemic air embolism.** This is most commonly accomplished using the **antegrade cardioplegia cannula** (see Section II.H.2.a) which is placed on suction. TEE is particularly useful in assessing the adequacy of deairing. Because of carbon dioxide's increased solubility and its potential for reducing the size of microemboli, **some surgical teams flood the surgical field with carbon dioxide during open cardiac procedures.**

K. **Ultrafiltration/hemoconcentrators**

A hemofiltration device (also referred to as an ultrafilter) consists of a semipermeable membrane which separates blood flowing on one side (under pressure) and air (sometimes under vacuum) on the other side. **Water and small molecules (sodium, potassium, water-soluble non–protein-bound anesthetic agents) can pass through it and be removed from the blood, but protein and cellular blood components do not.** Hemoconcentrators are used to eliminate excess crystalloid and potassium, and to raise hematocrit (hemoconcentrate). They may also remove inflammatory mediators and hence reduce the systemic inflammatory response syndrome (SIRS). The device is usually placed distal to the arterial pump with drainage into the venous limb or reservoir. It can also be placed in the venous limb of the circuit, which requires a separate pump. Five hundred to 2,000 mL or more of fluid may be removed during an adult case. When used postbypass (but before reversing heparin) it is referred to as **"modified ultrafiltration" or "MUF."** MUF is commonly used in pediatric cases but less so in adult cases [3,10].

L. **Filters and bubble traps**

1. **Overview.** CPB generates macro- and microemboli of gas, lipids, and other particles (WBCs, platelets, foreign debris) which must be filtered out.

2. **Types and location.** Many different types of filters (screen and packed fibers ["in-depth"], made of various materials) with various pore sizes are employed in multiple locations in the ECC. These sites include the venous and cardiotomy reservoirs, "built" into the MO, in the arterial and cardioplegia lines, blood administration sets such as the cell processor, and the gas line supplying the oxygenator. The "in-depth filters" mainly work by adsorption. The clinical importance of the various types of filters remains controversial [5].

3. **Arterial line filter/bubble trap.** Most centers employ a microfilter/bubble trap on the arterial line, especially to reduce air embolization [5]. If used, often a clamped bypass line is placed around the filter in case the filter becomes obstructed and a vent line with a one-way valve runs from the filter/bubble trap to the venous reservoir to vent any trapped air. The inclusion of a microfilter in some commercial MOs may eliminate the need for a separate arterial line microfilter.

4. Some advocate the employment of **leukocyte-depleting filters** in various ECC locations, but their benefit remains to be proven.

M. **Safety devices and monitors on the heart–lung (H–L) machine**
See Table 20.4 and the 2017 American Society of Extracorporeal Technology standards and guidelines for perfusion practice [7].

III. **Special topics**

A. **Surface coating**

Many commercial circuits coat all of the surfaces that come in contact with blood (tubing, reservoirs, oxygenators) with various proprietary substances designed to minimize activation of blood components. Many of these coatings include heparin, which should be avoided in patients with heparin-induced thrombocytopenia (HIT). The clinical benefits of any or of one type of coating over another remain controversial [5].

B. **Miniaturized or minimized circuits**

By reducing the surface area and prime volume, miniaturized circuits reduce the amount of hemodilution (resulting in less blood transfusions) and are purported to reduce the inflammatory response to CPB and contribute to improved clinical outcomes [11]. They often feature a closed venoarterial circuit (i.e., no venous reservoir or cardiotomy suction) and kinetic-assisted venous drainage. A sophisticated air detection and elimination system is required, as well as stringent avoidance of air entrance into the venous line. Concerns about safety (especially air embolization), inability to handle fluctuations in venous return (especially if the patient has a large blood volume or experiences exsanguination), and lack of cardiotomy and field suction require careful consideration. These systems require close communication among all team members. Miniaturized circuits are less commonly used in the United States compared with Europe. Their use is usually limited to uncomplicated CABG and aortic valve surgery and cases associated with minimal intravascular volume shifts or need to scavenge blood from the surgical field.

TABLE 20.4   Monitors and safety devices

A. Monitors
1. Pressure in arterial line[a]
2. Level sensor in hardshell venous reservoir[a]
3. Bubble/air detector[a]
4. Microprocessor/console monitor and control
5. Inline venous[a] and/or arterial oxygen saturation or PO_2 monitor ± of other gases, electrolytes, glucose, lactates, and hematocrit/hemoglobin
6. Arterial line flowmeter[a]
7. Temperature of systemic blood coming out of and going into the patient[a], and of water going into the heat exchangers, and of the cardioplegia solution[a]
8. Oxygen analyzer of gas going into the oxygenator[a]
9. Expired concentration of carbon dioxide and anesthetic vapors from the MO

B. Safety devices
1. High arterial line pressure alarm + servo control or turn off of arterial pump[a]
2. Low level in venous reservoir alarm + servo control or turn off of arterial pump[a]
3. Air/bubble detector alarm + servo control or turn off of arterial pump[a]
4. One-way check valves in arterial line,[a] cardiac vents,[a] and arterial line filter/bubble-trap purge line
5. Arterial line filter[a]
6. Bypass line around arterial line filter/bubble trap
7. Purge line off of the arterial line filter/bubble trap

C. Emergency personnel, supplies, and equipment
1. Second perfusionist (NOT a standard of care)
2. Battery backup for H–L machine including the pumps and monitors[a]
3. Portable lighting and flashlights
4. Backup oxygen supply[a] (cylinders with regulators)
5. Hand cranks to drive arterial and other pumps[a]
6. Spare oxygenator[a]

[a]Per American Society of ExtraCorporeal Technology Standards and Guidelines for Perfusion Practice [7].

C.   Pediatric circuits

The major challenges of pediatric CPB are (1) the small blood volume of the patient compared with the prime volume of the ECC, and (2) the small venous and arterial cannulae required. Pediatric cardiac surgery groups and industry have made great strides in miniaturization and reduction of priming volumes (some as little at 100 to 200 mL) by including augmented venous return to allow narrower tubing and elevation of the H–L machine to keep it closer to the patient and shorten the tubing. Most pediatric cardiac surgery centers in North America include albumin in the priming fluids; packed RBCs and fresh-frozen plasma or whole blood are often used for infants [10]. Some groups exclude arterial microfilters and others use an oxygenator which has an integrated arterial-side microfilter. In contradistinction to adult CPB, inline arterial blood gas monitoring is employed by the vast majority of North American pediatric centers. See additional discussion in Chapter 16.

D.   Cerebral perfusion during circulatory arrest

1.   **Overview.** Circulatory arrest is often required for conduct of surgery involving the aortic arch and in congenital heart surgery. Deep hypothermia (<18°C) can be used to minimize cerebral injury. For periods of circulatory arrest exceeding 30 minutes, two strategies for cerebral perfusion listed below are commonly employed. The benefits and preference of one over the other remain controversial.

2.   **Retrograde cerebral perfusion (RCP).** The arterial line from the H–L machine is connected to the SVC cannula (in the case of bicaval cannulation), or to a separate cannula inserted through a purse-string suture in the SVC. The SVC is occluded between the entrance of the catheter and the junction with the RA. Cold blood (15° to 18°C) is then pumped at flow rates of 250 to 500 mL/min and pressures maintained between 20 and 40 mm Hg. It may be desirable to measure the pressure via a catheter placed directly into the right IJ vein, since valves may reduce the amount of delivered flow and pressure. If pressure is measured in this location, it is probably prudent to keep the pressure <25 mm Hg to

minimize cerebral edema. Although RCP provides minimal nutritional flow to the brain, it helps limit rewarming and likely washes out atheroemboli and air in the cerebral arteries.

3. **Antegrade cerebral perfusion (ACP) or selective cerebral perfusion (SCP).** Catheter(s) (sometimes with balloon cuffs) connected to the arterial line are inserted into the right innominate or carotid arteries or the left carotid and subclavian arteries. Cold blood is then infused at a rate of about 10 mL/kg/min at a pressure of 30 to 70 mm Hg. This technique provides more cerebral blood flow than RCP but adds a risk of arterial trauma and embolization. If the systemic arterial cannula has been inserted into the right subclavian artery (see Section II.C.2.c), then selective perfusion of the right carotid artery can be accomplished by occluding the proximal innominate artery. If a subclavian arterial cannula has been placed via a graft sewn onto the side of the artery, the pressure in the right radial or brachial artery also represents the right carotid cerebral arterial perfusion pressure. Obviously this provides only unilateral perfusion and relies on an adequate circle of Willis to perfuse the left side of the brain. Monitoring hemispheric oxygenation with bilateral cerebral oximetry may identify the need to add left-sided arterial perfusion.

E. **Less common cannulation**
   1. **Minimally invasive or port access CPB** involves use of smaller incision and often smaller or specially designed venous and arterial cannulae for transthoracic placement or peripheral cannulation. This may require augmented venous drainage and increase the risk of aortic dissection (e.g., femoral artery cannulation). Peripherally placed retrograde coronary sinus catheters (placed via the right IJ vein often by the anesthesiologist), and aortic balloon occlusion catheters and antegrade cardioplegia cannulae (passed via the femoral artery) are used. These require TEE and/or fluoroscopic guidance for proper placement.
   2. **Right thoracotomy.** This approach gives excellent views of the MV and RA, but aortic cannulation, occlusion of the ascending aorta, administration of antegrade cardioplegia, and deairing of the LV are problematic. Often some of the minimally invasive cannulation techniques mentioned above are employed.
   3. **Left thoracotomy.** This approach is used for surgery on the descending thoracic aorta and occasionally for reoperative MV surgery and CABG surgery for revascularization of the lateral or posterior heart. Venous cannulation is problematic. Peripheral RA cannulation via the femoral vein is commonly employed (see Section II.B.3). For descending thoracic aortic surgery, **isolated partial left heart bypass (LHB)** can be accomplished by cannulating the left atrium or ventricle directly or via purse-string guarded incisions in the left superior pulmonary vein or left atrial appendage for venous outflow and into the distal aorta or femoral artery for arterial return. Partial LHB presumes adequate RV output and pulmonary perfusion, hence it does not require an oxygenator or venous reservoir and may not include a heat exchanger. LHB typically employs a centrifugal pump and use heparin-coated tubing, permitting minimal systemic heparinization. This technique only supplies oxygenated blood to the lower half of the body, as the LV supplies the upper half via the intact ascending aorta and transverse aortic arch. LHB flows are typically 1 to 1.5 L/min/m^2 and are adjusted to adequately decompress the left heart and maintain adequate pressures in the lower (via LHB) and upper (via native circulation) parts of the body. Management of partial LHB is quite challenging and requires excellent communication between the anesthesiologist and perfusionist. TEE assessment of LV filling is extremely valuable [12].

IV. **Priming**
   A. **Overview**
   The ECC (including venous and arterial lines) must be filled with fluid ("primed") before use and all air in the circuit eliminated. Circuits are usually primed with asanguinous (clear) fluids. To minimize hemodilution, much effort has recently been directed at reducing the priming volume of ECCs to as low as 1,000 to 1,250 mL for adults.

   B. **Consequence of asanguinous primes**
   Priming results in hemodilution with reduction of hematocrit, plasma proteins, and coagulation factors. Controversy surrounds the acceptable lower level of hematocrit [5]. However, prior to initiation of CPB, the predicted hematocrit should be estimated to determine if the team wishes to add RBCs to the prime.

$$\text{Predicted hematocrit} = (\text{Baseline hematocrit} \times \text{estimated blood volume [EBV]})/(\text{EBV} + \text{prime volume} + \text{first dose of crystalloid in the cardioplegia solution})$$

Baseline hematocrit used for this calculation should be obtained immediately prior to CPB to account for any crystalloids administered prior to CPB and is expressed as a fraction (e.g., hematocrit of 33 = 0.33) in this formula.

C. **Retrograde autologous priming (RAP)**

RAP is a method of reducing hemodilution. Before commencing CPB, arterial blood is drained retrograde to displace asanguineous prime in the arterial line (which is sequestered in a collection bag). Immediately before going onto CPB, venous blood may also be allowed to drain out of the patient through the venous line into the collection bag (**"antegrade autologous priming"**). With this method 500 to 1,000 mL of asanguineous prime may be eliminated. However, it is associated with a reduction of the patient's blood volume and may result in hypotension. Placing the patient in Trendelenburg position and administering a vasopressor are often required. The majority of randomized trials have demonstrated that RAP reduces perioperative packed RBC transfusions and is usually safe. However, this technique can be dangerous in certain high-risk patients, leading to hypotension and immediate initiation of CPB because of loss of cardiac preload. Further studies are needed to determine the effect of retrograde priming on major morbidity and mortality. Another method of reducing asanguineous prime is to remove fluid from the venous line and initiate CPB with a "dry" venous line. The use of this technique presumes the presence of sufficient pre-CPB intravascular blood volume to sustain adequate CPB perfusion flows once CPB commences.

D. **Composition of the prime**

Many formulations are used. Most comprise a balanced electrolyte solution without glucose. Much controversy surrounds the need to add colloid, and the use of albumin has been recommended. Many add mannitol to the prime and most include heparin (about 5,000 to 10,000 units).

E. **Priming of the circuit**

The perfusionist fills the circuit with the priming fluid and circulates it employing various maneuvers to remove all air. Often before introducing the prime the circuit is flushed with carbon dioxide, which is more easily removed from the prime than air bubbles. Usually, a **prebypass microfilter** is temporarily included in the circuit during this recirculation process to remove any foreign particles.

F. **Final disposition of prime at the end of cardiopulmonary bypass (CPB)**

Usually, as much of this volume as possible is returned to the patient before removing the arterial line. That which is left may either be pumped directly (sometimes through a hemoconcentrator) via a pre-existing IV line into the patient or placed into an IV bag for administration by the anesthesiologist (preserving platelets and protein but also containing heparin which may require neutralization), or first processed by a cell-washing device and hemoconcentrated, which eliminates heparin.

V. **Complications, safety, and risk containment**

A. **Incidence of adverse events**

Four surveys covering practice between 1994 and 2007 have reported CPB-associated rates of adverse events of 1/16, 1/35, 1/138, and 1/199 (average 2.6%), with severe injury or death rates of 1/1,236, 1/1,288, 1/1,453, and 1/3,220 (average 0.065%) [13–16].

B. **Specific complications and their diagnosis and management**

These are discussed in Chapter 7.

CLINICAL PEARL Cardiac anesthesiologists should be prepared to diagnose and help manage serious complications that can occur during CPB.

C. **Risk containment**

This requires the active and continuing participation of all members of the team (surgeons, perfusionists, anesthesiologists, and nurses).

1. **Vigilance** on the part of all members of the team is required.
2. **Special monitoring** of the adequacy of global and specific organ perfusion is discussed in Chapter 7 and by Murphy et al. [5]. Two issues deserve special attention:
   a. **Central nervous system (CNS).** Many advocate the use of cerebral near-infrared spectroscopy (NIRS) (i.e., cerebral oximetry) or other monitors of cerebral perfusion/function (e.g., transcranial Doppler, processed electroencephalography) to detect problems with venous drainage and arterial cannulation and malperfusion (e.g., dissection) [17].
   b. **TEE** is useful not only to diagnose cardiac abnormalities pre-CPB and evaluate surgical repairs, but also **to assist with the conduct of CPB.** Some of these applications include the following:
      (1) Evaluating atherosclerosis in the aorta (typically requiring epiaortic scanning) as it relates to cannulation and placement of clamps
      (2) Detect abnormal-size coronary sinus or presence of patent foramen ovale
      (3) Evaluating placement of cannulae, especially retrograde coronary sinus cannula, LV vents, and transfemorally placed IVC cannulae, and intra-aortic balloon pump (IABP)
      (4) Detect devices, masses (thrombi and tumors), and anatomic abnormalities that could affect cannulation
      (5) Assess adequacy of decompression of the LV
      (6) Detect and evaluate deairing of left heart
      (7) Detect aortic dissection and malperfusion of arch vessels

> **CLINICAL PEARL** TEE and epiaortic scanning contribute to the safe conduct and monitoring of CPB.

3. Education, practice, experience, retraining, certification, and recertification of perfusionists and other team members.
4. Communication between surgeon, perfusionist, and anesthesiologist. Each must warn team members of actions that could impact all the others, and of any variance with normal course of CPB or deviations in expected parameters. Commands must be positively and verbally acknowledged.
5. **The "two-minute drill":** Although serious complications are uncommon, **it is prudent to wait about 2 minutes after going on "full bypass"** *before arresting the heart,* **to assure that all is going well and to rule out serious complications which can be most easily managed by discontinuing CPB and resuming normal circulation.** One should confirm the following endpoints:
   a. Able to achieve targeted systemic ("pump") flow
   b. Adequate venous return and not losing volume
   c. Adequate oxygenation of arterial blood (i.e., function of the MO)
   d. Acceptable arterial pressure and exclusion of arterial dissection as a cause of hypotension
   e. RV and LV are decompressed
   f. Acceptable systemic venous pressure
   g. Acceptable arterial line pressure
   h. Acceptable venous oxygen saturation

> **CLINICAL PEARL** The aorta should not be cross-clamped nor cardioplegia administered until sufficient time (about 2 minutes) has elapsed to assure satisfactory and stable function of the H–L machine and conduct of CPB.

6. Planning, development of, and adherence to **protocols** for routine as well as unusual types of CPB and of complications

7. Use of prebypass **checklists** and for other key times during CPB and for adverse events
8. Use of safety equipment and alarms
9. Appropriate preventive maintenance program, replacement of old equipment, and familiarity and testing of new equipment
10. Team practice at diagnosing and management of major complications
11. Periodic audit, team meetings, quality assurance, and quality improvement. Use of a registry to measure variation and for benchmarking
12. Automated control and regulation of the H–L machine

D. **Key role of the anesthesiologist in the conduct of CPB**

Anesthesiologists are in a unique position to assist with the conduct and management of CPB. Their detailed knowledge about the patient's medical history and the patient's course prior to arrival in the operation room and prior to CPB gives them a unique perspective. They are able to observe both the surgical field and the H–L machine, and can facilitate communication between the perfusionist and surgeon. Anesthesiologists should oversee the anesthetic and vasoactive drug management and patient monitoring during CPB and make recommendations concerning the safe and appropriate conduct of CPB. They should be vigilant for any adverse events and assist with the management of the complications discussed in Chapter 7. Finally, anesthesiologists should collaborate with surgeons and perfusionists in the development of protocols for the conduct of safe CPB, participate in practice sessions for handling emergency situations and complications, and be involved in education, and quality assessment and improvement activities related to perfusion.

> **CLINICAL PEARL** Cardiac anesthesiologists should participate in the conduct and monitoring of CPB and manage anesthesia during CPB.

> **CLINICAL PEARL** Cardiac anesthesiologists should participate with surgeons and perfusionists in developing protocols for conduct of CPB and in the quality assessment and improvement activities associated with it.

PART II. PATHOPHYSIOLOGY OF CARDIOPULMONARY BYPASS

I. Introduction

Improvements in the design of the CPB circuit and greater understanding of the physiologic insult of CPB have contributed to the relative safety of modern cardiac surgery [18]. Despite advancements in technology and knowledge during the past several decades, a variety of minor and major complications are observed following CPB.

Major physiologic trespasses introduced by CPB include:

A. Alterations of pulsatility, blood flow patterns, and pressure
B. Exposure of blood to nonphysiologic surfaces and shear stresses
C. Hemodilution
D. Systemic stress response and inflammation
E. Varying degrees of hypothermia (or hyperthermia during rewarming).

Improving the safety of CPB depends on greater understanding of these aberrations [19].

II. CPB as a perfusion system

A. **Circulatory control during CPB**

"Cardiac output" during CPB is the pump flow rate, which can be set at any level desired, but is limited by the amount of venous return. Systemic and venous blood pressures are partially dependent on the patient's autonomic tone, but can be manipulated by increasing or decreasing venous drainage and by administering various fluids, vasopressors or vasodilators. Thus, the circulation during CPB is controlled in large part by the perfusionist and the anesthesiologist. The management of systemic blood flow, systemic arterial pressure, and venous pressure are discussed in Chapter 7.

Distribution of blood flow. In addition to total blood flow, one must be concerned about flow in each organ. Studies have noted a **hierarchy** of distribution of blood flow during normothermia and hypothermia as total flow is reduced [20]. Even at "normal flow" (i.e., 2.4 L/min/m^2), muscle blood flow is significantly reduced during CPB. **As flow is progressively reduced, first splanchnic, then renal, and eventually (only at extremely low flows) cerebral flows are reduced.**

B. **Circulatory changes during CPB**

1. **Changes at onset of CPB.** At commencement of CPB, there is usually a fall in systemic blood pressure due to reduced intravascular blood volume or to a decrease in systemic vascular resistance (SVR). The latter may result from the following:

    a. Decreased blood viscosity secondary to hemodilution by the pump-priming fluid

    b. Decreased vascular tone secondary to:

       (1) Dilution of circulating catecholamines

       (2) Temporary hypoxemia. Hypoxemia from initial circulation of pump asanguineous priming fluid may lead to decreased vascular tone

       (3) Low pH, calcium, and magnesium levels in the priming fluid

2. **Circulatory changes during hypothermic CPB**

    a. **Increased SVR.** There is considerable patient-to-patient variation in SVR during CPB. However, as CPB progresses, there will generally be a steady increase in systemic pressure due to increasing SVR if flow rates are kept constant. The observed increase in SVR during the course of CPB is due to several factors:

       (1) Decreased vascular cross-sectional area from closure of portions of the microvasculature

       (2) Vasoconstriction brought on by the following factors:

          (a) Hypothermia

          (b) Increasing levels of circulating catecholamines, arginine vasopressin (AVP), endothelin, and angiotensin II

       (3) Increase in blood viscosity secondary to hypothermia and rising hematocrit (due to urine output or translocation of fluid into the interstitial compartment or hemoconcentrator)

    b. **Decreased SVR.** Transient decreases in SVR and systemic pressure may be observed shortly after infusion of cardioplegic solutions, especially if the solutions contain nitroglycerin

3. **Circulatory changes during the rewarming phase of CPB**

    a. As the perfusate temperature is increased to rewarm the patient, variable circulatory responses are observed depending on the anesthetics used, patient hematocrit, underlying disease, and other factors. SVR and mean arterial pressure (MAP) increase frequently during initial rewarming from 25° to 32°C, but then usually decrease as temperature increases above 32°C.

    b. A more consistent decrease in SVR and MAP usually occurs with release of the aortic cross-clamp and reperfusion of the heart. Despite cardioplegia and hypothermia, there is some degree of ongoing metabolic activity and utilization of myocardial energy stores during the ischemic period. This results in coronary vasodilation and a marked increase in coronary blood flow and decrease in arterial pressure. In addition, when the heart is reperfused, accumulated metabolites are washed out of the heart into the general circulation. Some of these metabolites, most notably **adenosine**, are potent vasodilators which decrease SVR.

4. **Changes in the microcirculation and adequacy of tissue perfusion during CPB**

    a. During CPB, cardiac output and arterial pressure can be easily maintained at "normal" values. However, decreases in oxygen consumption and increases in serum lactate concentrations during CPB as well as evidence of organ dysfunction post-CPB suggest that tissue perfusion may be impaired.

    b. Factors contributing to this may include:

       (1) Constriction of precapillary arteriolar sphincters caused by catecholamines, angiotensin, vasopressin, thromboxane, endothelin, and decreased release of nitric oxide (NO)

(2) Increased interstitial fluid volume (edema)

(3) Decreased lymphatic drainage

(4) Loss of pulsatile flow

(5) "Sludging" in the capillaries due to hypothermia

(6) Altered deformability of RBCs

(7) Microaggregation and adhesion of white cells, platelets, and fibrin onto the endothelium related to the SIR

(8) Microemboli (gas, lipids, cellular aggregates), primarily from the cardiotomy suction

c. Suggested ways to optimize microcirculatory function during CPB include administration of vasodilators, use of pulsatile perfusion techniques, hemodilution to a hematocrit between 20% and 30%, use of microfiltration, minimizing return of unprocessed cardiotomy suction blood directly into the H–L machine, and anti-inflammatory strategies.

5. **Pulsatile versus nonpulsatile flow during CPB.** One of the major physiologic derangements introduced by CPB is loss of pulsatile arterial blood flow. Intuitively, it seems desirable to reproduce normal flow patterns as closely as possible during CPB. Ways of generating pulsatile flow and their limitations were presented earlier (see Section II.E.3). There is considerable controversy about the merits of and need for pulsatile perfusion as compared to conventional nonpulsatile perfusion [5,21].

a. Putative benefits of pulsatile flow

(1) Transmission of more energy to the microcirculation, which improves tissue perfusion, lymphatic flow, and cellular metabolism

(2) Reduction of adverse neuroendocrine responses (mainly vasoconstrictive) to nonpulsatile flow that emanate from baroreceptors, the kidneys, and the endothelium

b. Clinical outcome. Clinical outcome data have been conflicting. A recent evidence-based review concluded that existing data were insufficient to support recommendations for or against pulsatile perfusion to reduce the incidence of complications following CPB [5].

III. Adequacy of perfusion

A. How to define

No widely accepted definition of *optimal* perfusion during CPB exists. Perfusion can be considered *acceptable* if the patient survives without evidence of organ dysfunction. However, optimal CPB perfusion should be followed by a healthy, productive, and long life after cardiac surgery. To support this goal, perfusion during CPB should ideally achieve the following goals:

1. **Maintain adequate oxygen delivery, blood flow, and perfusion pressure to all organs**
2. **Avoid activation of undesirable reactions, for example, neuroendocrine stress response and inflammation**
3. **Minimize microembolization and disturbance of the coagulation system**

B. Monitoring

Monitoring adequacy of perfusion is discussed in Chapter 7.

IV. Hypothermia and CPB

A. Effects of hypothermia on biochemical reactions

The Q_{10} for **chemical reactions** is a measure of **changes in rate of reaction** for each 10°C increase in temperature. **For human tissues, Q_{10} is approximately 2**. As a result, for each 10°C decrease in body temperature, the rate of reaction (i.e., metabolic rate or oxygen consumption) is roughly halved.

B. Effects of hypothermia on blood viscosity

Hypothermia increases blood viscosity. In contemporary CPB practice, patients are typically hemodiluted to hematocrits of 20% to 30% during CPB due to asanguineous pump-priming. Although oxygen-carrying capacity is decreased from hemodilution, oxygen delivery may paradoxically increase as a result of decreased viscosity and enhanced microcirculatory flow. Experimental data suggest that viscosity remains stable if hematocrit (%) matches temperature (in °C) during hypothermia. The optimal degree of hemodilution during hypothermic CPB has not been determined. Recent studies have demonstrated an association between substantial

CPB hemodilution (hematocrits below 20% to 24%, depending upon the study) and morbidity and mortality. Clinicians should avoid both excessively high (increased blood viscosity and decreased microcirculatory flow) and low (inadequate oxygen content) hematocrits during CPB.

C. **Changes in blood gases associated with hypothermia**

1. **Changes in oxygen–hemoglobin dissociation curve.** As temperature decreases, the affinity of oxygen for hemoglobin increases, that is, the oxygen–hemoglobin dissociation curve shifts to the left. Consequently, a lower partial pressure of oxygen in the tissues is required to remove the same amount of oxygen from the hemoglobin molecule.

2. **Changes in solubility of O_2 and CO_2.** As temperature decreases, gases become more soluble in liquid. For a given partial pressure, more gas will be dissolved in the plasma. This is more significant for CO_2 due to a higher solubility in plasma at any given temperature. The higher solubility of oxygen partially offsets the left shift in the oxygen–hemoglobin dissociation curve.

3. **Neutrality of water.** Neutral water is water in which the [H+] is equal to the [OH–]. At 37°C, the pH of neutral water is 6.8. At 25°C the pH of neutral water is 7. The neutral pH of water increases linearly 0.017 units for each degree Celsius decrease in temperature. This impacts optimal management of pH and $PaCO_2$ during CPB.

4. **Differing strategies for measuring and managing blood gases during CPB** are discussed in Chapters 7 and 26.

V. **Systemic effects of the CPB**

CPB triggers an "explosion" of highly unphysiologic events that may cause or contribute to complications (Fig. 20.8) [21,22].

A. **Causes and contributors of adverse systemic effects of CPB**

1. Microemboli (gas and particulate matter)
2. Activation of the inflammatory and coagulation systems
3. Altered temperature with active or passive cooling followed by active warming
4. Exposure of blood to foreign surfaces
5. Reinfusion of shed blood and transfusion of blood products
6. Hemodynamic alterations (abnormal flow rate and pattern, abnormal arterial and venous pressures)
7. Ischemia and reperfusion (especially of heart, lungs, and gut)
8. Hyperoxia
9. Hemodilution (with anemia and reduced oncotic pressure)

B. **Blood**

1. **Coagulation and fibrinolytic systems and tissue factor (TF).** Changes in the coagulation cascade, platelets, and the fibrinolytic cascade are discussed in Chapter 21.

2. Changes in formed elements

   a. RBCs

      (1) RBCs become stiffer and less deformable during CPB, which may interfere with microcirculatory blood flow and increase susceptibility to hemolysis.

      (2) During CPB, RBCs are exposed to foreign surfaces and shear stresses which may cause their destruction. The degree of hemolysis is increased by both higher flow rates and the accompanying increase in rate of shear, and by gas–fluid interfaces in the ECC. As red cells are lysed, the free hemoglobin produced binds to haptoglobin. When the amount of free hemoglobin generated exceeds the binding capacity of haptoglobin, serum-free hemoglobin concentrations increase and hemoglobin is then filtered by the kidney, resulting in hemoglobinuria. Cardiotomy suction contributes importantly to hemolysis during CPB.

   b. **Leukocytes.** CPB affects primarily neutrophils (polymorphonuclear leukocytes [PMNs]) and, to a lesser degree, monocytes. Shortly after the onset of CPB, circulating PMNs decrease markedly. This results from sequestration in various vascular beds. Blockage of vessels by PMN clumping or microcirculatory derangements induced by substances released from PMNs may contribute to organ dysfunction after CPB.

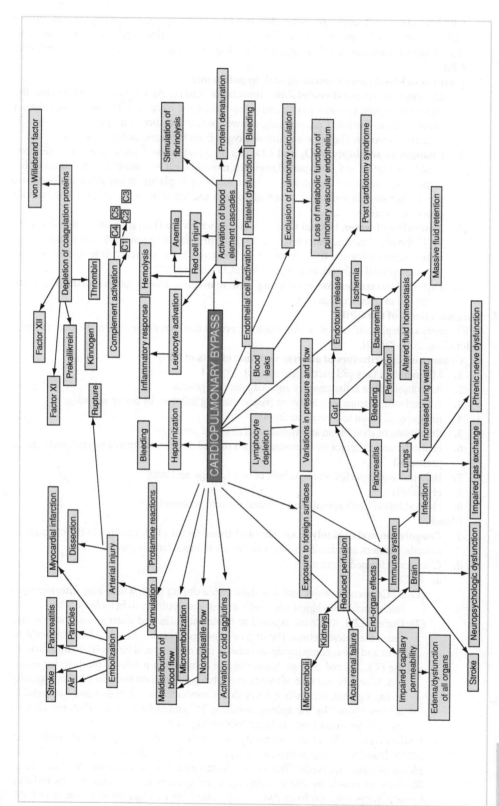

FIGURE 20.8 The "explosion" of adverse events triggered by cardiopulmonary bypass. (From Elefteriades JA. Mini-CABG. A step forward or backward? The "pro" point of view. *J Cardiothorac Vasc Anesth.* 1997;11:661, with permission.)

Circulating PMN levels increase dramatically with rewarming. Neutrophils released from the pulmonary circulation and younger cells released from the bone marrow contribute to this neutrophilia.

Effects of CPB on the host defense functions of PMNs remain controversial. Studies demonstrating decreased responsiveness of PMNs to chemotactic and aggregating stimuli indicate impaired defense mechanisms. However, other studies show that the bactericidal activity of PMNs increases for up to 3 days after CPB.

3. Changes in plasma proteins

a. Denaturation. Exposure of proteins to gas–liquid interfaces causes denaturation. Protein denaturation leads to altered enzymatic function, altered solubility, lipid release into the blood stream, and RBC membrane alteration that promotes capillary sludging and microcirculatory dysfunction.

b. Reduced colloid osmotic (oncotic) pressure (COP). Because of hemodilution, plasma protein concentration and hence COP fall with onset of CPB if no colloids are added to the CPB circuit. There is controversy about the need for and benefits of avoiding the fall in COP by using albumin or artificial colloids (e.g., dextrans, starches) in the priming solution.

4. Activation of humoral cascade systems, for example, complement, coagulation, and fibrinolytic systems (see Sections V.D.1 and V.D.2).

C. Fluid balance and interstitial fluid accumulation ("capillary leak syndrome") during CPB

Increased interstitial fluid in many tissues and organs is common during and following CPB. If extreme, this can cause pathologic capillary leak syndrome (e.g., adult respiratory distress syndrome [ARDS], cerebral edema). Until recently, fluid fluxes at the microcirculatory level were attributed mainly to the factors described by Starling:

$$\text{Tissue fluid accumulation} = K[(P_c - P_{is}) - \delta(\pi_c - \pi_{is}c)] - Q_{lymph}$$

where K is the filtration coefficient ("permeability") of capillary membrane, P_c the mean intracapillary hydrostatic pressure, P_{is} the mean interstitial hydrostatic pressure, δ the reflection coefficient to macromolecules, π_c the intracapillary oncotic pressure, π_{is} the interstitial oncotic pressure, Q_{lymph} the lymph flow out of interstitium.

CPB shifts this balance toward accumulation of interstitial fluid by affecting several of these variables. Membrane permeability is increased by activation of a systemic inflammatory response (SIR) and intermittent ischemia/reperfusion potentially leading to organ injury. Plasma oncotic pressure falls from the use of asanguineous priming fluids. Inadequate venous drainage may increase mean capillary hydrostatic pressure, whereas immobility, lack of pulsatile flow, and loss of negative intrathoracic pressure impede lymphatic flow. The **endothelial glycocalyx (EG)** is now recognized as playing an important role in modifying the effect of these Starling factors [23]. Shredding of the EG has been demonstrated during CPB in infants and adults, and even following off-pump CABG [24]. This likely increases capillary permeability and perhaps induces capillary leak syndrome.

D. Inflammation

All patients undergoing cardiac surgery will experience a systemic inflammatory response (SIR) to the procedure [25]. Although the trauma of major surgery per se induces inflammation, CPB accentuates this response.

SIR represents unphysiologic activation of the innate immune system resulting in a whole-body response resembling that associated with sepsis and trauma. This presents as a spectrum of responses ranging from near-universal evidence of mild inflammation (fever, leukocytosis), to more significant clinical signs (tachycardia, increased cardiac output, decreased SVR, increased oxygen consumption, increased capillary permeability) to frank organ dysfunction (cardiac, renal, pulmonary, GI, hepatic, CNS) and potentially to the multiple organ dysfunction syndrome (MODS) and death.

Normal inflammation is a localized protective response composed of cellular and humoral components. When the localized inflammatory response becomes excessive, it may spill over to the rest of the body. The same response occurs when the injury is systemically widespread (e.g., CPB), in which case a generalized inflammatory response leads to diffuse end-organ damage [25].

1. **Activation.** Nonspecific activators of the inflammatory response include surgical trauma and tissue injury, blood loss or transfusion, and hypothermia. However, CPB may independently activate the inflammatory response by several unique mechanisms:

   a. **Contact activation** occurs when blood comes into contact with the foreign surface of the ECC. This activates the complement, coagulation, kallikrein–bradykinin and fibrinolytic systems as well as WBCs and platelets. **The use of cardiotomy suction contributes importantly to this response.** Blood aspirated via cardiotomy suction becomes contaminated with TF, TF activator, and fibrin degradation products.

   b. **Ischemia–reperfusion.** Reperfusion injury refers to damage to tissue caused when blood supply returns to the tissue after a period of ischemia. The absence of oxygen and nutrients from blood creates a condition in which the restoration of circulation results in inflammation and oxidative damage from the oxygen rather than reestablishment of normal function. The reintroduction of oxygen via restored blood flow promotes the formation of oxygen-free radicals, which damage cellular proteins, DNA, and plasma membranes. WBCs carried to the area also release a host of inflammatory substances such as interleukins (IL). As noted above, these activated leukocytes can build up in small capillaries to cause obstruction and more ischemia.

   c. **Endotoxemia related to splanchnic hypoperfusion/ischemia.** Transient splanchnic hypoperfusion (see below) during CPB damages GI mucosa to induce endotoxemia. Endotoxin, which is a lipopolysaccharide in the cell wall of gram-negative bacteria, binds with lipopolysaccharide-binding protein to stimulate the release of tumor necrosis factor (TNF) from macrophages, thus potentially triggering SIR (see below).

   d. **Gaseous and particulate microemboli** also induce an inflammatory response.

2. **Propagation.** Once the inflammatory response is triggered, components of the immune and coagulation systems and various cells are activated which propagate the SIR. These components include the following:

   a. **Complement.** The complement system is activated by exposure of blood to foreign surfaces, endotoxin released from the GI tract, and heparin–protamine complexes. Its activation leads to the release of various substances (e.g., C3a, C3b, and C5a) which increase production of cytokines and leukotrienes as well as capillary permeability and leukocyte–endothelial adhesion.

   b. **Cytokines** are released **from** activated monocytes, macrophages, lymphocytes, and the endothelium leading to both pro- and antiinflammatory effects.

   c. **Nitric oxide** production is upregulated, contributing to vasodilation, increased vascular permeability, and potential end-organ dysfunction.

   d. **Leukotrienes** are potent vasoconstrictors.

   e. **Platelet-activating factor (PAF)** contributes to activation of clotting as well as inflammation (see "Platelets" below).

   f. **TF** is expressed by many cells and initiates coagulation and release of cytokines.

   g. The **kallikrein–bradykinin** system amplifies the inflammatory response and increases vascular permeability.

   h. **Metalloproteinases (collagenases, gelatinases)** rise following CPB. They are released from activated neutrophils and degrade collagen in basement membrane. They facilitate migration of neutrophils into tissues and may contribute to the inflammatory response and organ injury.

   i. **Endothelins** are released by endothelial cell and are potent vasoconstrictors.

   j. **Coagulation and fibrinolysis.** The coagulation–fibrinolysis cascade is closely intertwined with the inflammatory response and are activated by cardiac surgery and CPB. These lead to both bleeding and thrombotic–embolic complications.

   k. **The endothelium.** The endothelium is an active participant in a variety of physiologic and pathologic processes. It plays a major role in regulating vascular tone, membrane permeability, coagulation and thrombosis, fibrinolysis, and inflammation. It attracts and directs the passage of leukocytes into areas of inflammation through the expression of adhesion molecules. CPB causes extensive activation and dysfunction of the endothelium due to ischemia/reperfusion, exposure to inflammatory mediators, surgical manipulation, and hemodynamic shear stresses. Expression of adhesion molecules mediates the binding of neutrophils to the endothelium and translocation into the interstitium. Resultant neutrophil degranulation attacks the endothelial barrier function to induce capillary leak and edema.

l. **Neutrophils, monocytes, macrophages, and lymphocytes.** Interaction of activated endothelium and neutrophils with the endothelium leads to tissue damage and endorgan dysfunction via microvascular occlusion or release of toxic metabolites and enzymes. B and T lymphocytes decrease in number and function following CPB, which may cause immunosuppression and increase the risk for infections.

m. **Platelets.** Through the production and release of leukotrienes, serotonin, chemokines, PF4, and other substances, platelets contribute to the inflammatory response.

3. Although some studies have found that modifying the ECC and practice of CPB (e.g., surface coating, minimizing circuit size, leukofiltration, eliminating or reducing cardiotomy suction, and shortening duration) and even elimination of CPB (e.g., off-pump CABG) reduce inflammatory markers, they do not eliminate the SIR to cardiac surgery and may not improve clinical outcomes.

4. **Consequences of the inflammatory response to CPB.** The inflammatory response to major surgery per se and to CPB likely contributes to multiple organ injuries, coagulopathy and disseminated intravascular coagulation (DIC), infection risk, and death. In most patients, the early SIR resolves without significant injury as a result of discontinuation of the stimulus, dissipation of mediators, or the action of naturally occurring antagonists (e.g., IL-10). The variability in the expression, consequences, and outcome of the inflammatory response to CPB is the subject of much speculation. Factors likely to influence this variability include the preoperative condition of the patient, type and complexity of the surgery, and, perhaps most importantly, underlying genetic polymorphism.

5. **Strategies to minimize the inflammatory response to CPB** are discussed in Chapter 7.

E. **Stress response**

1. **Endocrine, metabolic, and electrolyte effects.** CPB is associated with a marked exaggeration of the **stress response** associated with all types of surgery. This is manifested by large increases in epinephrine, norepinephrine, AVP, adrenocorticotropic hormone, cortisol, growth hormone, and glucagon. Elevated catecholamines may adversely affect regional and organ blood flow patterns. Catecholamines also increase myocardial oxygen consumption, which may adversely affect the balance of myocardial oxygen supply and demand at the time of reperfusion. Other stress hormones also increase catabolic reactions to increase energy consumption and potentially cause tissue breakdown and impaired wound healing.

2. **Hyperglycemia** is invariably encountered during CPB, especially in patients with diabetes mellitus. Contributors to hyperglycemia include decreased insulin production, insulin resistance (enhanced by stress hormones and hypothermia), decreased consumption (related to insulin resistance and hypothermia), increased glycogenolysis and gluconeogenesis (related to stress hormones), increased reabsorption of glucose by the kidney, and administration of glucose in cardioplegia solutions. Observational studies have demonstrated an association between post-CPB hyperglycemia and increased morbidity and mortality. Although measurement and control of blood glucose values during and following CPB is strongly recommended, the optimal "target range" for serum glucose concentrations remains controversial.

3. **Renin, angiotensin II, and aldosterone** levels all tend to rise during CPB. Some patients display the so-called **sick euthyroid syndrome** with reduced tri-iodothyronine (T3), thyroxine (T4), and free thyroxin levels but normal thyroid-stimulating hormone levels. The etiology of this phenomenon is unclear, but it provides the rationale for administration of thyroid hormone in some patients with low cardiac output syndrome postoperatively.

4. **Calcium, magnesium, and potassium.** Both ionized calcium and total and unfilterable fractions of magnesium commonly fall, whereas potassium levels may fluctuate widely during CPB. The latter may be related to diuretics, catecholamines, preoperative spironolactone (aldactone) and β-blockers, potassium-containing cardioplegia, and renal dysfunction. The importance of maintaining normal levels of these ions to preserve normal muscle and cardiac function and prevent dysrhythmias is apparent.

VI. **Effect of CPB on various organs**

A. **Heart**

Some degree of myocardial injury and cell necrosis, as evidenced by release of troponin, occurs during CPB, which may result in myocardial stunning and dysfunction. However, frank myocardial infarction is relatively uncommon, although the ECG and cardiac enzyme changes which identify myocardial infarction have not been precisely defined. The effects of cardiac surgery on the heart and myocardial protection are reviewed in Chapter 23.

B. **Central nervous system (CNS)**

Cerebral dysfunction (ranging from subtle neurocognitive dysfunction to frank stroke or coma) is not infrequent following CPB. Its etiology is multifactorial and includes hypoperfusion, macroemboli, microemboli, and the inflammatory response to CPB. For further discussion, see Chapters 7 and 26.

C. **Kidneys**

1. Renal dysfunction or acute kidney injury (AKI), which ranges from a rise in creatinine and release of renal tubular proteins to severe renal failure requiring renal replacement therapy (RRT), remains a persistent and prevalent problem following cardiac surgery involving CPB (15% to 30%) and is associated with increased morbidity and short- and long-term mortality [21,26,27]. Even mild elevations of serum creatinine are associated with increased morbidity and mortality, and RRT is associated with a mortality of as high as 60%. Features of CPB thought to contribute to AKI include the inflammatory response, ischemia/reperfusion, and embolization (microparticles, air, and atheroma).

2. An increase in renal vasoconstriction (~20%), decrease in percent of systemic flow to the kidney (~28%) and renal oxygen delivery (~20%), an increase in renal oxygen extraction (~40%), and release of a protein marker of tubular injury were found in humans undergoing CPB [28]. All of these changes suggest impaired renal oxygenation (ischemia) during conventional CPB [28].

3. AKI has been associated with the severity of atherosclerosis of the ascending aorta [29], the magnitude duration of MAP below the lower limit of autoregulation in the *brain* [30], and a critically low systemic oxygen delivery (<272 mL/min/m^2) during CPB [31]. Intravascular hemolysis and hemoglobinuria can also cause acute tubular necrosis.

4. Urine output is a crude indicator of renal function, but there is no correlation between the amount of urine output during CPB and the incidence of postoperative renal failure. Urine output is greater when MAP is higher, when pulsatile perfusion is used, and when mannitol is added to pump-priming fluids.

5. Although CPB per se may contribute to AKI after cardiac surgery, other preoperative and intraoperative surgical factors (e.g., low hematocrit and transfusion of RBCs) and postoperative course and care contribute to it [21,26]. Some studies comparing off-pump with on-pump CABG have found less renal dysfunction but most have not observed less renal failure or RRT by avoiding the use of CPB [32]. Thus the development of renal failure appears to depend more on the preoperative renal function and postoperative hemodynamic status than on various manipulations during CPB.

6. Methods of renal protection during CPB are discussed in Chapter 7.

D. **Splanchnic, gastrointestinal (GI), and hepatic effects**

1. GI complications are relatively uncommon (~1.2%, range 0.3% to 6.1%) following cardiac surgery but are associated with morbidity and high mortality (~34%, range 9% to 87%) [33,34]. These complications include GI bleeding (~31% of GI complications and ~0.4% of all cardiac surgery cases), mesenteric ischemia (18% and 0.2%), pancreatitis (11% and 0.1%), cholecystitis (11% and 0.1%), peptic ulcer (4% and 0.05%), diverticulitis (3% and 0.03%), liver failure (4% and 0.05%), and others (18%) [33].

2. Multiple risk factors have been identified, but the most prominent preoperative factors include age >70, low cardiac output, peripheral vascular disease (PVD), chronic renal failure, reoperative procedures, and CABG plus valve procedures. The most prominent intraoperative factors include duration of CPB, transfusion and administration of vasopressors. A complicated postoperative course (e.g., sepsis, mediastinitis, bleeding, and prolonged mechanical ventilation [>24 to 48 hours]) is frequently associated with GI complications.

3. The presumed cause of these complications is splanchnic ischemia, which may be related to abnormal systemic hemodynamics (low flow, low MAP, lack of pulsatility), SIR, and athero- and other microemboli.

4. Clinical and animal studies suggest that, although global splanchnic blood flow appears to be preserved during high-flow CPB, splanchnic flow will be compromised early in the hierarchy of regional blood flow whenever systemic flow is reduced [20]. Administration of vasoconstrictors, such as phenylephrine, norepinephrine, and AVP likely further reduce splanchnic blood flow. Furthermore, many subjects exhibit increased intestinal permeability, decreased gastric or intestinal mucosal pH and increased mucosal Pco_2, decreased mucosal blood flow, and endotoxemia, all of which suggest that mucosal ischemia occurs frequently during CPB. Although SIR likely contributes to GI ischemia, conversely GI ischemia may play a primary role in the development of SIR syndrome and injury of other organs. **Thus, the GI tract is both the cause and a target of SIR in cardiac surgery.**

5. Hyperbilirubinemia (>2.50 to 3.0 mg/dL) is encountered in ~25% (range 9% to 40%) of cardiac surgery patients, with an associated mortality of ~4%. Liver failure occurs in 0.03% to 0.1% of cardiac surgery patients with an extremely high associated mortality of 56% to 78%. As with renal failure, hepatic dysfunction appears to be more dependent on hemodynamic status before and after CPB than on any direct effect of CPB. The risk of postoperative jaundice increases in the setting of high RA pressures, persistent hypotension after CPB, or significant transfusion.

6. As with other adverse effects attributed to CPB following cardiac surgery, most studies have not found a reduced incidence of GI complications when CABG is done off-pump (OPCAB) nor that use of CPB was an independent risk factor for GI complications in studies comparing on- and off-pump CABG.

7. Strategies to prevent GI complications are discussed in Chapter 7.

E. **Lungs**
1. Since the dawn of CPB, the lungs have been the unfortunate target of post-CPB organ injury. Although less frequent (at ~25% of patients) than in the past, postoperative pulmonary complications remain a leading cause of morbidity and mortality [35,36]. Manifestations range from the nearly ubiquitous decline in PaO_2/FiO_2 ratio to ARDS (incidence 0.4% to 3%, mortality 15% to 70%). Other pulmonary complications include pulmonary effusions, pulmonary edema, pneumonia (incidence 2% to 10%, mortality up to 43%), diaphragmatic dysfunction, and phrenic nerve paralysis. The pathophysiology is likely multifactorial [21,36] and is thought to include the aforementioned inflammatory response as well as activation of coagulation, pulmonary ischemia and reperfusion (I/R) (as well as I/R in other organs), left heart failure, atelectasis from absent ventilation during CPB, mechanical injury from entering the pleural cavities, blood transfusion, and perioperative lung management. Preoperative lung disease, poor LV function, age, and probably genetic makeup comprise some of risk factors. Lung ischemia during CPB is likely an important cause. This probably derives from loss of pulmonary artery flow as well as marked reduction in bronchial artery flow during CPB, leading in turn to inflammation, increased capillary permeability, increased pulmonary vascular resistance, reduced pulmonary compliance and gas exchange, and perhaps vulnerability to infection.

2. **Methods to reduce lung injury associated with CPB** are discussed in Chapter 7.

VII. **Role of CPB on adverse effects of cardiac surgery**
A popular hypothesis has been that CPB principally causes the adverse consequences of cardiac surgery as a result of amplification of the inflammatory response, embolization, ischemia/reperfusion, and lack of pulsatility, among other things. This hypothesis has largely been dispelled

[11] based upon multiple studies comparing CABG surgery with versus without CPB. Although often more evidence of inflammation has been found with CPB, recent large randomized controlled trials (RCTs) and meta-analyses incorporating over 50 RCT studies including over 16,000 patients have found no difference in the usual composite endpoints of 30-day mortality plus major complications. These comparisons have found conflicting results for the individual complications of renal dysfunction, lung dysfunction, and strokes. Nevertheless, avoiding CPB was associated with reductions in RBC transfusion along with small reductions in duration of mechanical ventilation (~3 to 4 hours), intensive care unit (ICU) stay (~0.35 day), and hospital stay (~1 day). The most recent and largest meta-analysis also detected a decrease in strokes (1.34% vs. 2.0%, odds ratio 0.72) [37].

VIII. Summary

CPB is performed safely and effectively in most patients throughout the world. This results from a combination of sophisticated equipment and well-trained and educated perfusionists. The responsibility for safe CPB is shared by surgeons, anesthesiologists, and perfusionists in order to manage cardiac surgery with the lowest possible patient risk. Despite technologic advances in circuit design over the past several decades, CPB imposes physiologic aberrations that may cause postoperative organ dysfunction. Post-CPB organ dysfunction comprises a spectrum ranging from mild dysfunction in one organ system to death from multiorgan failure. **One should remember that, despite myriad improvements to CPB over many decades, placing a patient on CPB still constitutes a physiologic trespass.** Absence of significant damage caused by CPB depends primarily on a particular patient's ability to compensate for the derangements introduced by that trespass.

ACKNOWLEDGMENT

The author gratefully acknowledges the contributions of other authors to a previous version of this chapter which appeared in the 4th edition of this text: Glenn S. Murphy, Robert C. Groom, and Joseph N. Ghansah.

REFERENCES

1. Ghosh S, Falter F, Perrino AC Jr. *Cardiopulmonary Bypass*. 2nd ed. Cambridge, United Kingdom: Cambridge University Press; 2015.
2. Schell RM, Hessel, EA II, Reves JG. Chapter 10: Cardiopulmonary bypass. In: Reves JG, Reeves S, Abernathy JH III, eds. *Atlas of Cardiothoracic Anesthesia*. 2nd ed. New York: Springer; 2009.
3. Groom RC, Fitgerald D. Chapter 32: Extracorporeal devises and related technologies. In: Kaplan JA, Augoustides JGT, Manecke GR Jr, et al., eds. *Kaplan's Cardiac Anesthesia for Cardiac and Noncardiac Surgery*. 7th ed. Philadelphia, PA: Elsevier; 2017:1162–1213.
4. **Hessel EA, Shann KG. Blood pumps, circuitry and cannulation techniques in cardiopulmonary bypass. Chapter 2. In: Gravlee GP, Davis RF, Hammon J, eds. *Cardiopulmonary Bypass and Mechanical Support: Principles and Practice*. 4th ed. Philadelphia, PA: Wolters Kluwer; 2016:22.**
5. **Murphy GS, Hessel EA, Groom RC. Optimal perfusion during cardiopulmonary bypass: an evidence-based approach. *Anesth Analg*. 2009;108:1394–1417.**
6. Wright G. Mechanical simulation of cardiac function by means of pulsatile blood pumps. *J Cardiothorac Vasc Anesth*. 1997; 11:299–309.
7. **Baker RA, Bronson SL, Dickinson TA, et al; International Consortium for Evidence-Based Perfusion for the American Society of ExtraCorporeal Technology. Report from AmSECT's international consortium for evidence-based perfusion: American society of extracorporeal technology standards and guidelines for perfusion practice: 2013. *J Extra Corpor Technol*. 2013;45(3):156–166. For the May 2017 Update of the American Society of ExtraCorporeal Technology standards and guidelines for perfusion practice see: http.//www.amsect.org/page/perfusion-practice-guidelines. Accessed April 5, 2018.**
8. Groom RC, Forest RJ, Cormack JE, et al. Parallel replacement of the oxygenator that is not transferring oxygen: the PRONTO procedure. *Perfusion*. 2002;17:447–450.
9. Engelman R, Baker RA, Likosky DS, et al. The society of thoracic surgeons, the society of cardiovascular anesthesiologists, and the American society of extracorporeal technology: clinical practice guidelines for cardiopulmonary bypass—temperature management during cardiopulmonary bypass. *J Cardiothorac Vasc Anesth*. 2015;29(4):1104–1113.
10. Groom RC, Froebe S, Martin J, et al. Update on pediatric perfusion practice in North America: 2005 survey. *J Extra Corpor Technol*. 2005;37:343–350.
11. Zangrillo A, Garozzo FA, Biondi-Zoccai G, et al. Miniaturized cardiopulmonary bypass improves short-term outcome in cardiac surgery: a meta-analysis of randomized controlled studies. *J Thorac Cardiovasc Surg*. 2010;139:1162–1169.
12. **Hessel EA. Bypass techniques for descending thoracic aortic surgery. *Semin Cardiothoracic Vasc Anesth*. 2001;5: 293–320.**

13. Jenkins OF, Morris R, Simpson JM. Australasian perfusion incident survey. *Perfusion.* 1997;12:279–288.
14. Mejak BL, Stammers A, Rauch E, et al. A retrospective study on perfusion incidents and safety devices. *Perfusion.* 2000;15: 51–61.
15. Charrière JM, Pélissié J, Verd C, et al. Survey: retrospective survey of monitoring/safety devices and incidents of cardiopulmonary bypass for cardiac surgery in France. *J Extra Corpor Technol.* 2007;39:142–157.
16. Groenenberg I, Weerwind PW, Everts PA, et al. Dutch perfusion incident survey. *Perfusion.* 2010;25:329–336.
17. Edmonds HL Jr. 2010 Standard of care for central nervous system monitoring during cardiac surgery. *J Cardiothorac Vasc Anesth.* 2010;24:541–543.
18. Hessel EA 2nd. History of cardiopulmonary bypass (CPB). *Best Pract Res Clin Anaesthesiol.* 2015;29:99–111.
19. **Gravlee GP, Davis RF, Hammon JW, et al., eds. *Cardiopulmonary Bypass and Mechanical Support: Principles and Practice.* 4th ed. Philadelphia, PA: Wolters Kluwer; 2016.**
20. Slater JM, Orszulak TA, Cook DJ. Distribution and hierarchy of regional blood flow during hypothermic cardiopulmonary bypass. *Ann Thorac Surg.* 2001;72:542–547.
21. **Grocott HP, Stafford-Smith M, Mora-Mangano CT. Chapter 31: Cardiopulmonary bypass management and organ protection. In: Kaplan JA, Augoustides JGT, Manecke GR Jr, et al., eds. *Kaplan's Cardiac Anesthesia for Cardiac and Noncardiac Surgery.* 7th ed. Philadelphia, PA: Elsevier; 2017:1111–1161.**
22. Murphy GJ, Angelini GD. Side effects of cardiopulmonary bypass: what is the reality? *J Card Surg.* 2004;19:481–488.
23. Woodcock TE, Woodcock TM. Revised starling equation and the glycocalyx model of transvascular fluid exchange: an improved paradigm for prescribing intravenous fluid therapy. *Br J Anaesth.* 2012;108(3):384–394.
24. Bruegger D, Brettner F, Rossberg I, et al. Acute degradation of the endothelial glycocalyx in infants undergoing cardiac surgical procedures. *Ann Thorac Surg.* 2015;99:926–931.
25. Whitlock R, Bennett-Guerrero E. Chapter 9: Systemic inflammation. In: Kaplan JA, Augoustides JGT, Manecke GR Jr, et al., eds. *Kaplan's Cardiac Anesthesia for Cardiac and Noncardiac Surgery.* 7th ed. Philadelphia, PA: Elsevier; 2017:231–246.
26. **Stafford-Smith M, Patel UD, Phillips-Bute BG, et al. Acute kidney injury and chronic kidney disease after cardiac surgery. *Adv Chronic Kidney Dis.* 2008;15:257–277.**
27. Heringlake M, Knappe M, Vargas Hein O, et al. Renal dysfunction according to the ADQI-RIFLE system and clinical practice patterns after cardiac surgery in Germany. *Minerva Anestesiol.* 2006;72(7–8):645–654.
28. Lannemyr L, Bragadottir G, Krumbholz V, et al. Effects of cardiopulmonary bypass on renal perfusion, filtration, and oxygenation in patients undergoing cardiac surgery. *Anesthesiology.* 2017;126:205–213.
29. Dávila-Román VG, Kouchoukos NT, Schechtman KB, et al. Atherosclerosis of the ascending aorta is a predictor of renal dysfunction after cardiac operations. *J Thorac Cardiovasc Surg.* 1999;117:111–116.
30. Ono M, Arnaoutakis GJ, Fine DM, et al. Blood pressure excursions below the cerebral autoregulation threshold during cardiac surgery are associated with acute kidney injury. *Crit Care Med.* 2013;41:464–471.
31. Ranucci M, Romitti F, Isgro G, et al. Oxygen delivery during cardiopulmonary bypass and acute renal failure after coronary operations. *Ann Thorac Surg.* 2005;80:2213–2220.
32. **Deppe AC, Arbash W, Kuhn EW, et al. Current evidence of coronary artery bypass grafting off-pump versus on-pump: a systematic review with meta-analysis of over 16,900 patients investigated in randomized controlled trials. *Eur J Cardiothorac Surg.* 2016;49:1031–1041.**
33. Hessel EA 2nd. Abdominal organ injury after cardiac surgery. *Semin Cardiothorac Vasc Anesth.* 2004;8:243–263.
34. Allen SJ. Gastrointestinal complications and cardiac surgery. *J Extra Corpor Technol.* 2014;46:142–149.
35. Bignami E, Guarnieri M, Saglietti F, et al. Mechanical ventilation during cardiopulmonary bypass. *J Cardiothorac Vasc Anesth.* 2016;30:1668–1675.
36. Huffmyer JL, Groves DS. Pulmonary complications of cardiopulmonary bypass. *Best Pract Res Clin Anaesthesiol.* 2015;29: 163–175.
37. **Kowalewski M, Pawliszak W, Malvindi PG, et al. Off-pump coronary artery bypass grafting improves short-term outcomes in high-risk patients compared with on-pump coronary artery bypass grafting: meta-analysis. *J Thorac Cardiovasc Surg.* 2016;151:60–77.**

21 Coagulation Management During and After Cardiopulmonary Bypass

*Jacob Raphael, Alan Finley, S. Nini Malayaman, Jay C. Horrow,
Glenn P. Gravlee, and Linda Shore-Lesserson*

KEY POINTS

1. Previous concepts of independent intrinsic and extrinsic plasma coagulation pathways, a cell-free final common pathway, and platelet clotting have given way to an integrated concept of cell-based coagulation occurring on the platelet surface as depicted in Figure 21.2.

2. In the absence of a history suggesting a preoperative bleeding disorder (e.g., von Willebrand disease, warfarin therapy), routine hemostatic screening for patients undergoing cardiac surgery is not cost-effective at predicting excessive perioperative bleeding.

3. Unfractionated heparin (UFH) is a hydrophilic macromolecular glycosaminoglycan of varying chain lengths which anticoagulates principally by potentiating antithrombin III (ATIII)–induced inactivation of factors IIa (thrombin) and Xa.

4. Intravenously administered heparin typically peaks within 1 minute, redistributes only slightly, and has a dose-related half-life that reaches approximately 2 hours in the large doses used for cardiopulmonary bypass (CPB). Heparin bolus administration decreases systemic vascular resistance by 10% to 20%.

5. The usual initial heparin dose is 300 to 400 units/kg to achieve an activated clotting time (ACT) exceeding 400 seconds for safe initiation and maintenance of CPB. Heparin 5,000 to 10,000 units should be added to the CPB priming solution.

6. Heparin is most often monitored using ACT, but ACT precision is suboptimal at the heparin concentrations required for CPB, and it is also subject to prolongation from hemodilution and hypothermia. As a result, some practitioners choose to monitor and maintain a target whole blood heparin concentration (typically 3 to 4 units/mL), in addition to exceeding a target ACT during CPB.

7. Resistance to heparin-induced anticoagulation is multifactorial. Treatment most commonly consists of either administration of additional heparin or ATIII supplementation with ATIII concentrates or FFP.

8. Heparin-induced thrombocytopenia (HIT) produces a severe procoagulant state that may occur after 5 or more continuous days of heparin administration. Diagnosis requires the combination of an appropriate clinical context and a complex variety of laboratory tests.

9. Documented presence of HIT in a patient who must urgently undergo cardiac surgery requiring CPB is possibly best managed by using bivalirudin for anticoagulation.

10. Protamine neutralizes heparin stoichiometrically as a result of a strong cation (protamine)-to-anion (heparin) interaction.

11. A variety of protamine dosing methods are used clinically. Most often 60 to 80 mg of protamine per 100 units of heparin administered prior to CPB (including heparin placed in the CPB priming solution if residual CPB volume is to be reinfused unaltered by hemoconcentration or cell washing) suffices to neutralize heparin. Excessive protamine administration impairs blood clotting.

12. In order to avoid hypotension, protamine should be administered slowly, ideally by a continuous intravenous infusion over 5 to 10 minutes.

13. Protamine can induce severe anaphylactic or anaphylactoid reactions.

14. Post-CPB clotting abnormalities are best managed using a systematic approach. Post-CPB bleeding algorithms reduce bleeding and transfusion.

I. Introduction

In essence, CPB creates a blood "detour" to permit surgery on the heart. This detour must route the blood through an artificial heart and lung while maintaining its fluidity. Historically, fluidity represented the final frontier in the development of cardiac surgery because effective mechanisms for blood gas exchange and for propelling the blood had been established more than a decade before surmounting the fluidity challenge. The challenge was to find a therapeutic approach that would inhibit blood's natural propensity to clot when it contacts foreign surfaces. Since the restoration of normal coagulation was desirable at the end of the surgical procedure, this clotting inhibition needed to be reversible, like turning a spigot on and off. The long-awaited solution was monumental: **anticoagulation with heparin followed by neutralization with protamine. This fundamental approach to establishing and reversing blood fluidity remains unchanged after over 60 years**, although much fine-tuning has occurred. This chapter reviews anticoagulation and the restoration of coagulation in the patients undergoing CPB.

II. Physiology of coagulation

A. Mechanisms of hemostasis

1. Plasma coagulation. Figure 21.1 depicts the plasma coagulation pathway. Blood contact with foreign surfaces classically was thought to activate the intrinsic pathway, whereas vascular injury or disruption was thought to activate the extrinsic pathway. These definitions seem counterintuitive because vascular disruption should be intrinsic and foreign bodies extrinsic, but logic has held little sway in coagulation pathway nomenclature. Thankfully, distinctions between the intrinsic and extrinsic pathways have become less important because both the activators and the pathways overlap (e.g., connection between VIIa and IXa).

   a. Intrinsic pathway. Contact activation involves binding of factor XII to negatively charged surfaces, which leads to the common pathway through factors XI, IX, platelet factor 3, cofactor VIII, and calcium. Kallikrein is also formed in this reaction and serves as a positive feedback mechanism and as an initiator of fibrinolysis (a negative feedback mechanism) and inflammation. For cardiac surgery, this pathway's clinical importance lies more in the access it provides for heparin monitoring and neutralization than in its role in normal hemostasis.

   b. Extrinsic pathway. Tissue factor (TF) initiates the extrinsic pathway, which proceeds to activate factor IX and rapidly stimulates the common pathway with the aid of factor VII and calcium.

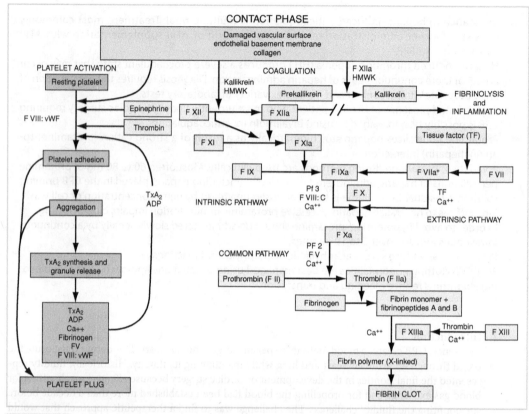

FIGURE 21.1 Schematic representation of the hemostatic system depicting the vascular, platelet, and coagulation components. F, factor; HMWK, high–molecular-weight kininogen; vWF, von Willebrand factor; Ca^{++}; ionized calcium; VIII:C, factor VIII coagulation component; TxA_2, thromboxane A_2; ADP, adenosine diphosphate.

    c. Common pathway. Beginning with the assisted activation of factor X, this pathway proceeds to convert prothrombin (factor II) to thrombin and fibrinogen (factor I) to fibrin monomer, which initiates the actual substance of the clot. Fibrin monomer then crosslinks to form a more stable clot with the aid of calcium and factor XIII. **Rather than thinking of the common pathway as the result of activation of two independent paths, the concept of cell-based coagulation has been adopted to better explain the hemostatic mechanisms that occur simultaneously in the body (Fig. 21.2).**

    When tissue injury occurs, TF is expressed on the surface of TF-bearing cells. Presentation of TF to its ligand factor VII causes the activation of factors IX and X on the TF-bearing cell. This is called "initiation." The activation of factor X causes thrombin formation, which then incites further protease activation. These reactions occur on the phospholipid surface of the platelet and are called "amplification." The final stage of clot formation is known as "propagation."

    Activated factor X also initiates platelet-surface clotting activity, as depicted in Figure 21.2. This platelet-surface activity greatly speeds the overall formation of clot and should be considered as a vital component of the clotting cascade.

    d. Thrombin is the most important enzyme in the pathway because (in addition to activating fibrinogen) it

    (1) Provides positive feedback by activating cofactors V and VIII

    (2) Accelerates crosslinking of fibrinogen by activating factor XIII

    (3) Strongly stimulates platelet adhesion and aggregation

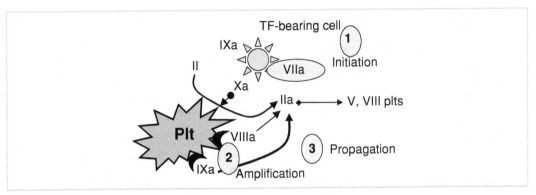

FIGURE 21.2 Cell-based model of hemostasis. Cellular hemostasis is thought to occur in three stages: initiation, amplification, and propagation. The initiation stage (1) takes place on tissue factor (TF)-bearing cells (cells such as monocytes that can bind TF and present it to a ligand), which come into play when endothelial injury occurs and TF is exposed. The initiation stage is characterized by presentation of TF to its ligand factor VII and the subsequent activation of factors IX and X on the TF-bearing cell. The activation of factor X to Xa causes thrombin production and activation. Once generated, thrombin feeds back to activate factors VIII, V, and platelets (Plt, plts). The amplification stage (2) then occurs on the surface of the activated platelet, which exposes surface phospholipids that act as receptors for the activated factors VIIIa and IXa. The platelet surface allows for further thrombin formation and hence the amplification of coagulation. Continued generation and activation of thrombin causes further positive feedback mechanisms (3) to occur that ultimately ensure the formation of a stable clot, including cleavage of fibrinogen to fibrin, release and activation of factor XIII for fibrin cross-linkage, and the release of a thrombin-activatable fibrinolysis inhibitor.

        (4) Facilitates clot resorption by releasing tissue plasminogen activator (tPA) from endothelial cells

        (5) Activates protein C, which provides negative feedback by inactivating factors Va and VIIIa

  2. Platelet activation. As shown in Figure 21.1, a variety of stimuli initiate platelet activation, and thrombin is an especially potent one. This sets off a cascade of events that initiates platelet adhesion to endogenous or extracorporeal surfaces, followed by platelet aggregation and formation of a primary platelet plug. Fibrin clots and platelet plugs form simultaneously and mesh together, yielding a product more tenacious and difficult to dissolve than either alone. Whereas formerly plasma-based and platelet-based clotting were often thought to represent independent pathways, more recent accounts show that **the plasma coagulation pathway evolves mainly on the platelet surface**, such that the plasma and platelet clotting processes are more interdependent than independent.

    a. von Willebrand factor (vWF) is an important ligand for platelet adhesion at low shear stress and for aggregation at higher shear rates. Fibrinogen is the major ligand for platelet aggregation.

    b. Products released from platelet storage granules (adenosine diphosphate [ADP], epinephrine, calcium, thromboxane A_2, factor V, and vWF) serve to perpetuate platelet activation and the plasma coagulation cascade.

  3. Nature's system of checks and balances demands counterbalancing forces to discourage runaway clot formation and to dissolve clots. These counterbalances include the following:

    a. Proteins C and S, which inactivate factors Va and VIIIa

    b. Antithrombin III (ATIII), antithrombin, or AT, which inhibits thrombin as well as factors XIa, IXa, XIIa, and Xa

    c. TF inhibitor, which inhibits the initiation of the extrinsic pathway

    d. tPA, which is released from endothelium and converts plasminogen to plasmin, which in turn breaks down fibrin. Plasminogen activator inhibitor 1 in turn inhibits tPA to prevent uncontrolled fibrinolysis.

TABLE 21.1 Common clinical tests of hemostatic function

Test	Normal values	Comment
Platelets		
Platelet count	150,000–400,000/μL	
Bleeding time (Ivy)	<8 min	Controversial clinical test of platelet function; inconvenient; arms must be exposed
Coagulation system		
Whole blood clotting time (WBCT, Lee–White CT)	2.5–6 min	Prolonged by marked deficiencies in intrinsic system or final common pathway; formerly used to monitor heparin therapy
Activated clotting time (ACT)	Manual = 90–110 sec Automated = 90–130 sec[a] = 100–140 sec[b]	Modified WBCT: Commonly performed to monitor heparin in the operating room because of convenience
Prothrombin time (PT)	12–15 sec, compare to control INR 1.0–1.5	Tests extrinsic system and final common pathway; used to monitor warfarin anticoagulation
Activated partial thromboplastin time (aPTT)	35–45 sec, compare to control	Tests intrinsic system and final common pathway; used to monitor heparin anticoagulation
Thrombin time	<14 sec, compare to control	Tests final common pathway; prolonged by heparin, fibrinogen ≤100 mg/dL, abnormal fibrinogen, and increased fibrin split products
Fibrinogen	250–500 mg/dL	Decreased in disseminated intravascular coagulation (DIC)
Fibrinolytic system		
Fibrin(ogen) split (degradation) products	<10 μg/mL	Increased during fibrinolysis (normal clot lysis process) or fibrinogenolysis (pathologic process that compromises clotting)
D-dimer	<0.5 μg/mL	Increased during fibrinolysis; specific assay of cross-linked fibrin degradation

[a]Hemochron, International Technidyne, Edison, NJ, USA.
[b]Medtronic, HemoTec, Fridley, MN, USA.
INR, international normalized ratio.

B. Tests of hemostatic function

1. Table 21.1 lists commonly used laboratory tests of hemostatic function [1]. These tests may be used to detect hemostatic abnormalities preoperatively or after CPB. With the exception of the ACT, typically they are not commonly used during CPB except under extenuating circumstances, because most of them will be abnormal as a result of hemodilution, anticoagulation, and sometimes hypothermia.

   a. **Most studies suggest that routine preoperative hemostatic screening is not helpful in predicting patients who will bleed excessively during surgery.** If the patient's clinical history (e.g., nosebleeds; prolonged bleeding with small cuts, dental work, or surgery; easy bruising; strong family history of pathologic bleeding) suggests the need for hemostatic screening, selective use of these and other tests is appropriate. Similarly, when the patient is taking medications that alter hemostatic function, specific hemostatic function tests may be indicated. Examples include the following:

   CLINICAL PEARL Even in cardiac surgery, neither *routine* preoperative nor postbypass routine hemostatic laboratory testing has proven helpful in predicting patients who will bleed excessively.

   (1) Heparin: Activated partial thromboplastin time (aPTT) or ACT
   (2) Low–molecular-weight heparin (LMWH), including the pentasaccharide fondaparinux: No test or anti-Xa plasma activity

      (3) Warfarin: Prothrombin time (PT) and/or international normalized ratio (INR)

      (4) Platelet inhibitors including aspirin: No testing, bleeding time, or specific platelet function tests. Preliminary data suggest that specific platelet function tests in patients taking thienopyridine agents may correlate with postoperative bleeding risk.

III. **Anticoagulation for cardiopulmonary bypass (CPB)**

Heparin is the drug of choice for anticoagulation, unless there is a contraindication such as ongoing HIT.

A. **Heparin pharmacology** [2]

Structure. As drugs go, unfractionated heparin (UFH) might be described as impure. Heparin resides physiologically in mast cells, and it is commercially derived most often from the lungs of cattle (bovine lung heparin) or the intestines of pigs (porcine mucosal heparin). Commercial preparations used for CPB typically include a range of molecular weights from 3,000 to 40,000 Da, with a mean molecular weight of approximately 15,000 Da. Each molecule is a heavily sulfated glycosaminoglycan polymer, so heparin is a strong biologic acid that is negatively charged at physiologic pH. Porcine mucosal and bovine lung heparin historically provided satisfactory conditions for CPB but currently only porcine UFH is commercially available.

1. Action. A specific pentasaccharide sequence that binds to ATIII is present on approximately 30% of heparin molecules. This binding potentiates the action of ATIII more than 1,000-fold, thereby allowing heparin to inhibit thrombin and factor Xa most importantly, but also factors IXa, XIa, and XIIa.

    a. **Inhibition of thrombin requires simultaneous binding of heparin to both ATIII and thrombin, whereas inhibition of factor Xa requires only that heparin binds to ATIII.** The former reaction limits thrombin inhibition to longer saccharide chains (18 or more saccharide units); hence, shorter chains can selectively inhibit Xa. This is the primary principle underlying therapy with LMWH and with the "ultimate" LMWH fondaparinux, which contains just the critical pentasaccharide sequence needed for binding ATIII; hence, it induces virtually exclusive Xa inhibition.

      (1) Because thrombin inhibition appears pivotal for CPB anticoagulation and also because LMWH and heparinoids have a long half-life and are poorly neutralized by protamine, LMWH (including fondaparinux) is inadvisable as a CPB anticoagulant.

    b. Heparin binds and activates cofactor II, a non–ATIII-dependent thrombin inhibitor. This may explain why heparin-induced anticoagulation can be effective even in the presence of marked ATIII deficiency, although the primary mechanism of anticoagulant action is potentiation of the ATIII-mediated inhibition of thrombin.

2. Potency. Heparin potency is tested by measuring the anticoagulation effect in animal plasma. The United States Pharmacopoeia (USP) defines 1 unit of activity as the amount of heparin that maintains the fluidity of 1 mL of citrated sheep plasma for 1 hour after recalcification.

    a. Heparin dosing is best recorded in USP units because commercial preparations vary in the number of USP units per milligram. The most common concentration is 100 units/mg (1,000 units/mL) and is standardized to have a variation in potency of no more than 10% [3].

3. Pharmacokinetics. **After central venous administration, heparin's effect peaks within 1 minute, and there is a small rapid redistribution that most often is clinically insignificant** [4,5].

    a. Heparin's large molecular size and its polarity restrict its distribution mainly to the intravascular space and endothelial cells.

    b. The onset of CPB increases circulating blood volume by approximately 1,000 to 1,500 mL; hence, plasma heparin concentration drops proportionately with the onset of CPB, unless heparin is added to the CPB priming solution.

    c. Heparin is eliminated by the kidneys or by metabolism in the reticuloendothelial system.

     d. Elimination half-life has been determined only by bioassay—that is, by the time course of clotting time prolongation. By this standard, heparin's elimination time is dose dependent [6]. At lower doses, such as 100 to 150 USP units/kg, elimination half-time is approximately 1 hour. At CPB doses of 300 to 400 USP units/kg, elimination half-time is 2 or more hours; hence, clinically significant anticoagulation might persist for 4 to 6 hours in the absence of neutralization by protamine. Hypothermia and probably CPB itself prolong elimination.

> **CLINICAL PEARL**   The half-life of heparin is dose dependent.

  4. Side effects. Heparin's actions on the hemostatic system extend beyond its primary anticoagulant mechanism to include activation of tPA, platelet activation, and enhancement of TF pathway inhibitor.

     a. Lipoprotein lipase activation influences plasma lipid concentrations, which indirectly affects the plasma concentrations of lipid-soluble drugs.

     b. Heparin boluses decrease systemic vascular resistance. Typically this effect is small (10% to 20%), but rarely it can be more impressive and may merit treatment with a vasopressor or calcium chloride.

     c. Anaphylaxis rarely occurs.

     d. HIT is covered elsewhere in this chapter.

B. **Dosing and monitoring**

  1. Dosing. The initial loading dose of heparin varies among centers and most commonly ranges from 300 to 400 USP U/kg. Still other centers base the initial dose on a bedside ex vivo heparin dose–response titration.

     a. Since heparin distributes primarily into the plasma compartment, increasing the dose with increasing body weight assumes that plasma volume increases in direct proportion to body weight. This is not the case because fat does not increase blood volume in proportion to weight. Consequently, there is seldom reason to exceed an initial dose of 35,000 to 40,000 units, even in patients weighing more than 100 kg, as lean body mass tends to peak at 90 kg for females and 110 kg for males.

     b. Heparin dosing for coronary revascularization procedures performed without CPB is controversial. Published doses range from 100 to 300 U/kg, but most centers use 100 to 150 units/kg and set minimum acceptable ACT values at 200 to 300 seconds.

     c. The CPB priming solution should contain heparin at approximately the same concentration as that of the patient's bloodstream at the onset of CPB. Since this most often would be 3 to 4 U/mL, a priming volume of 1,500 mL should contain at least 5,000 units of heparin. CPB priming solutions commonly contain 5,000 to 10,000 units of heparin.

     d. Supplemental heparin doses typically are guided by monitoring of anticoagulation.

  2. Monitoring. Until the late 1970s, heparin dosing was guided by experiential practices and varied a great deal from hospital to hospital. Using ACT, a variation on the Lee–White clotting time, **Bull et al.** [7] **identified rather staggering variations in the approach to heparin dosing and in both the initial anticoagulant response and the time course of anticoagulation in response to a fixed dose of heparin.** This landmark work rapidly led to the realization that the anticoagulant response to heparin should be monitored.

  3. Approaches to anticoagulation monitoring for CPB. **The ACT is the most widely used test**, although some centers monitor blood heparin concentration as well.

     a. ACT uses an activant such as celite or kaolin to activate clotting, then measures the clotting time in a test tube. Heparin prolongs ACT with a roughly linear dose–response pattern (Fig. 21.3). Normal ACT depends upon such factors as the specific activant and device, prewarming (vs. room temperature) of test tubes, and operator technique but generally falls between 110 and 140 seconds.

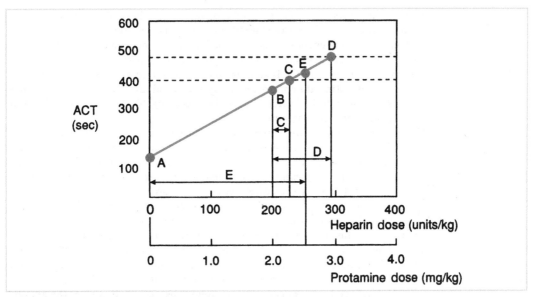

FIGURE 21.3 Graph of a heparin (and protamine) dosing algorithm. In the graph, the control activated clotting time (ACT) is shown as point A, and the ACT resulting from an initial heparin bolus of 200 units/kg is shown in point B. The line connecting A and B then is extrapolated and a desired ACT is selected. Point C represents the intersection between this line and a target ACT of 400 seconds, theoretically requiring an additional heparin dose represented by the difference between points C and B on the horizontal axis (*arrow C*). Similarly, to achieve an ACT of 480 seconds (*higher horizontal dotted line* intersecting the ACT vs. heparin dose line at point D), one would administer the additional heparin dose represented by *arrow D*. To estimate heparin concentration and calculate protamine dose at the time of heparin neutralization, the most recently measured ACT value is plotted on the dose–response line (point E in the example). The whole blood heparin concentration present theoretically is represented by the difference between point E and point A on the horizontal axis (*arrow E*). The protamine dose required to neutralize the remaining heparin then may be calculated. Protamine 1 mg/kg is administered for every 100 units/kg of heparin present. (Modified from Bull BS, Huse WM, Brauer FS, et al. Heparin therapy during extracorporeal circulation: II. The use of a dose-response curve to individualize heparin and protamine dosage. *J Thorac Cardiovasc Surg*. 1975;69:686 by Gravlee GP. Anticoagulation for cardiopulmonary bypass. In: Gravlee GP, Davis RF, Kurusz M, et al., eds. *Cardiopulmonary Bypass: Principles and Practice*. 2nd ed. Philadelphia, PA: Lippincott Williams & Wilkins; 2000:435–472, with permission.)

Although originally described as a manual test, most centers use one of the two automated approaches to ACT (International Technidyne, Edison, NJ, USA or Medtronic HemoTec, Fridley, MN, USA). These two automated approaches yield slightly different values, both at baseline and with anticoagulation, because of different activators and endpoint detection techniques.

ACT is prolonged by hypothermia and hemodilution; hence, conditions often imposed by CPB alter the ACT–heparin dose–response relationship [8]. Some see this as risking underanticoagulation, although hemodilution and hypothermia legitimately enhance anticoagulation. Overreliance on hypothermic enhancement of ACT prolongation risks underanticoagulation upon rewarming. Also, at temperatures below 25°C, ACT prolongation becomes so profound that alternative tests such as whole blood heparin concentration measurement may be advisable.

The minimum ACT acceptable for CPB is the level below which anticoagulation is not optimized. Accepting an ACT below this value will result in activation of the coagulation system and potentially the development of a consumptive coagulopathy or catastrophic thrombus. Although the concept of the minimum ACT is clear, the actual minimum ACT remains controversial. Furthermore, clinicians often choose a target ACT value much higher than the minimum ACT to provide a margin of safety. There are studies supporting the safety of ACT values as low as 300 seconds, with or without extracorporeal surfaces coated with heparin or other anticoagulants, yet most centers accept only values exceeding 400 or 480 seconds. In addition, different devices and tests yield different dose–response relationships for heparin concentration versus ACT, as well as different sensitivities to hypothermia and hemodilution.

(1) **As a clotting test, ACT is somewhat crude and may vary as much as 10% on repeated testing at heparin concentrations used for CPB** [9], **so it seems reasonable to build in a safety margin by accepting 400 seconds as a minimum safe threshold for sustained CPB.**

(2) Aprotinin, which is now used rarely in clinical practice, complicates the use of ACT monitoring, as a result of marked prolongation of celite ACTs in the presence of heparin and aprotinin. This may represent enhanced anticoagulation to some degree, but in the presence of aprotinin, it is probably wise to titrate heparin to a celite ACT level exceeding 750 seconds or to use a kaolin ACT instead. Kaolin ACT minimum levels do not have to be adjusted in the presence of aprotinin.

b. Whole blood heparin concentrations can be measured during CPB. The most commonly used technique is automated protamine titration (Medtronic HemoTec, Fridley, MN). Advocates of this monitoring technique argue that CPB-induced distortion of the ACT–heparin dose–response relationship mandates maintenance of the heparin concentration originally needed before CPB to achieve the target ACT level [10]. **Heparin dosing based upon concentration alone substantially increases the amount of heparin given during CPB**, which enhances suppression of thrombin formation. This benefit may accrue at the expense of heparin rebound, if not monitored, and more profound platelet activation that may aggravate and prolong platelet dysfunction after CPB. The distortion of the ACT–heparin sensitivity relationship can be partly overcome using plasma-modified ACT testing [11] or by maximal activation of the ACT test sample, as is done in a thromboelastograph (TEG) modification of the ACT [12]. Whole blood point-of-care measurement of heparin concentration can also be performed with the HepTest POC-Hi (Americana Diagnostica, Stamford, CT). This test correlates well with heparin concentrations during CPB and more closely approximates the trend in plasma anti-Xa levels than does the standard ACT [13].

(1) **Whole blood heparin concentrations of 3 to 4 U/mL most often are sufficient for CPB.** Plasma heparin concentrations (typically anti-Xa concentrations) are higher because circulating heparin only resides in the plasma compartment.

(2) Patients can vary widely in their sensitivity to heparin-induced anticoagulation; therefore, **isolated use of heparin concentration could lead to dangerous underanticoagulation**. If this technique is chosen, simultaneous use of ACT or another clotting time is strongly advised.

(3) Heparin concentration monitoring may be a useful adjunct to ACT monitoring both in the presence of aprotinin and during periods of hypothermia below 25°C.

(4) Heparin concentration monitoring may be advantageous in selecting a protamine dose because the dose will be chosen in relation to approximate actual blood heparin concentration. The weakness of this technique is its dependence on a calculated blood volume determination at a time when blood volume may vary substantially.

c. **Other monitors of anticoagulation.** Neither ACT nor heparin concentration is perfect, so other tests have been evaluated or are under investigation. The aPTT and traditional thrombin time are typically so sensitive to heparin that those tests are not useful at the heparin concentrations needed for CPB. The high-dose thrombin time (HiTT, International Technidyne) offers a linear dose–response in the usual heparin concentration range used for CPB. The heparin management test (HMT, Helena, Beaumont, TX) offers another platform for ACT monitoring and can be used to monitor heparin at high (cardiac surgery) and low (vascular surgery) concentration ranges. Clotting times have also been successfully monitored using viscoelastic tests—the Sonoclot (SkACT, Sienco, Arvada, CO) [14] and the TEG.

C. Heparin resistance

No universal definition of heparin resistance exists, but it can be loosely defined as the need for greater-than-expected heparin doses to achieve the target ACT for CPB. As noted earlier, ACT prolongation in response to heparin varies greatly. A number of factors that may decrease the ACT response to heparin are listed in Table 21.2 [2]. ATIII deficiency is cited most often for heparin resistance, but overall, the correlation between ATIII concentrations and anticoagulant response to a bolus of heparin has been weak and inconsistent, perhaps because heparin resistance often is multifactorial [15].

Clinical approach. When faced with heparin resistance, four treatment options exist: (1) Administer additional heparin, (2) ATIII supplementation with fresh frozen plasma (FFP), (3) ATIII supplementation with ATIII concentrate, and (4) proceed with CPB with the current ACT.

1. **Most often heparin resistance can be managed by simply giving more heparin to account for the potential that an adequate heparin concentration has not been achieved.** If heparin concentrations are being monitored, then achieving a heparin concentration of 4 U/mL should be adequate, as there is likely no improvement in anticoagulation at higher heparin concentrations. When using higher-than-normal doses of heparin, clinicians should consider monitoring and potentially treating heparin rebound, as the risk of its development increases with higher heparin doses.

2. When higher doses of heparin have failed to increase the ACT sufficiently (i.e., >600 USP units/kg), ATIII supplementation should be considered, as it has been shown to increase the ACT. Traditionally, this was achieved with FFP. The concentration of ATIII in FFP is ~1 U/mL, which translates to a standard dose of 2 units of FFP to achieve 500 units of ATIII. Although FFP is known to increase the ACT by providing ATIII supplementation, it is no longer considered a first-line therapy due to the risk of allogeneic transfusion and limited data supporting its use. Furthermore, FFP is only recommended for single-factor deficiencies when a concentrate is not available for that factor.

TABLE 21.2 Potential causes of heparin resistance

Hypercoagulable states
Antithrombin III (ATIII) deficiency
Familial
Acquired
Arteriosclerotic disease
Unstable angina pectoris
Septicemia
Bacterial endocarditis
Pregnancy
HIT
Thrombocytosis
Drugs
Heparin
Nitroglycerin[a]
Protein binding
Acid glycoprotein
Histidine-rich glycoprotein
Immunoglobulins
Others
Neonates
Elderly patients

[a]Controversial cause. Probably not clinically significant.
HIT, heparin-induced thrombocytopenia.

3. Because of these issues, **ATIII supplementation with ATIII concentrate has become standard therapy**. In addition to limiting the negative sequelae of transfusing FFP, multiple studies exist showing a consistent increase in the ACT after ATIII supplementation. The Society of Thoracic Surgeons/Society of Cardiovascular Anesthesiologists (STS/SCA) blood conservation guidelines recommend ATIII concentrate as a class I recommendation for use in patients with ATIII-mediated heparin resistance immediately before cardiopulmonary bypass [16]. The increase in ACT abates concerns about subtherapeutic anticoagulation, although evidence showing an improvement in clinical outcomes is lacking.

4. Occasionally, a fourth option can be chosen, which is to accept the achieved ACT and commence CPB. Although the minimum ACT value for safely commencing CPB remains unclear, the wide variation in target ACT values across institutions indicates that the acceptable safe range for target ACT may be very large.

   a. Prediction of heparin resistance. Medtronic HemoTec's HMS Plus Hemostasis Management System and International Technidyne's Hemochron RxDx system each provide an in vitro opportunity to titrate the patient's whole blood to predetermined heparin concentrations and hence predict the initial heparin dose required to achieve a particular target ACT. Some centers use one of these devices to predict heparin resistance prior to heparin administration. This approach allows "customization" of initial heparin dosing as well as advance preparation for anticipated heparin resistance—for example, ordering ATIII concentrate or FFP.

D. **Heparin-induced thrombocytopenia (HIT)**

1. **Benign thrombocytopenia** from heparin's proaggregatory effect on platelets develops in 5% to 28% of patients.

   a. This mild decrease in platelet count typically occurs within 1 to 2 days of heparin administration without thrombosis or immune response. This response was formerly called HIT type I, and it is not considered pathologic. However, thrombocytopenia occurring within 1 to 2 days of heparin administration can be pathologic immune-mediated HIT if the patient's plasma retains heparin antibodies from a previous exposure. This latter situation is most likely to occur in a patient who has experienced clinical HIT within the past several weeks.

   b. **HIT is a severe condition that most often occurs after 5 continuous days of heparin administration** (average onset time, 9 days) and is immune mediated. Antibody binding to the complex formed between heparin and platelet factor 4 (PF4) is responsible for the syndrome. Antibody binding to platelets and endothelial cells causes platelet activation, endothelial injury, and complement activation. This syndrome is highly morbid and can be fatal as a result of thromboembolic phenomena.

      (1) **Among patients who develop HIT, the incidence of thrombosis approximates 20%, the mortality of which can be as high as 40%.**

      (2) Diagnosis. Thrombocytopenia (usually defined as platelet count <100,000/uL, but this is complicated for several days by post-CPB hemodilution), demonstration of heparin/PF4 antibody plus (ideally) documentation of heparin-induced aggregation of platelets.

         (a) Heparin-induced serotonin release assay: A functional test, often considered the gold standard.

         (b) Heparin-induced platelet activation assay (HIPAA): A functional test, may be nonspecific.

         (c) Enzyme-linked immunosorbent assay (ELISA) specific for the heparin/PF4 complex or for PF4 alone: Patients with a positive antibody test do *not* always develop thrombosis. Antibodies to the heparin/PF4 complex are associated with adverse outcomes after cardiac surgery [17]. Whether the antibody causes these outcomes or merely serves as a marker for a more critically ill patient has not been determined. Antibodies associated with HIT often become undetectable 50 to 85 days after discontinuing heparin. After 100 days of heparin discontinuation, one can be confident that short-term reexposure to heparin (as for CPB) will not result in antibody formation [18]. Continued heparin reexposure is not recommended, even though the clinical syndrome does not always recur upon reexposure to the drug. Sometimes the syndrome resolves despite continued heparin therapy. HIT can be associated with heparin resistance and thus should be part of the differential diagnosis.

CLINICAL PEARL The antibodies that cause HIT typically disappear from plasma 50 to 85 days after the most recent exposure to heparin. Once that occurs, it is safe to administer heparin for short periods such as those required for surgical cardiopulmonary bypass.

      (3) Treatments for HIT and alternative anticoagulant sources:
          (a) In HIT, changing the heparin formulation or using LMWH or heparinoids is no longer recommended, because cross-reactivity with other heparins exists (see Section III.E).
          (b) Plasmapheresis can be used to remove the antibody but may be insufficient therapy by itself.
          (c) Heparin can be combined with platelet inhibitors (e.g., iloprost) to reduce the aggregability of platelets.
          (d) Hirudin, bivalirudin, and argatroban are direct thrombin inhibitors.
  E. **Alternatives to unfractionated heparin (UFH)**
     1. LMWH (shorter-chain heparin molecules, including fondaparinux). Intravenously administered LMWH has a half-life at least twice as long as that of UFH and possibly several times as long for some LMWH compounds. Problems in CPB arise from the fact that protamine neutralization only reverses the factor IIa inhibition and leaves the predominant factor Xa inhibition intact. LMWH therapy also complicates heparin monitoring because aPTT (and presumably ACT) is much less sensitive to Xa inhibition and will not accurately measure the full anticoagulant effect. Factor Xa inhibition can be measured directly in plasma and with a plasma-modified whole blood test, but there is no simple point-of-care test available. LMWHs are not recommended for use in HIT patients because of cross-reactivity of the antibody, although some reports suggest that fondaparinux may be safe because it is too small to bind to antibodies.
     2. Bivalirudin
        a. Synthetic polypeptide that directly inhibits thrombin by binding simultaneously to its active catalytic site and its substrate recognition site. Shown to be a safe and effective alternative to heparin anticoagulation in patients undergoing cardiac surgery requiring CPB [19].
        b. Half-life is 24 minutes. Elimination is primarily by proteolysis and, to a smaller degree, renal elimination. **Even though this half-life is shorter than heparin's, the absence of a reversal agent and the profound degree of anticoagulation used for CPB may cause coagulopathy for 2 or more hours following CPB.**
        c. Dose during interventional procedures: 0.75 mg/kg bolus followed by a 1.75 mg/kg/hr infusion, yielding a median ACT of 346 seconds [20].
        d. Dose for CPB: 1 mg/kg bolus followed by a 2.5 mg/kg/hr infusion. **A recirculation limb and avoidance of circuit (and saphenous vein graft) stasis is necessary.**
        e. Studies in interventional procedures suggest lower bleeding rates than UFH and similar efficacy.
     3. Argatroban. A direct thrombin inhibitor that is approved by the U.S. Food and Drug Administration (FDA) for anticoagulation in HIT patients but not yet approved for use in CPB. Argatroban undergoes hepatic metabolism with a half-life of 39 to 51 minutes.

CLINICAL PEARL Although drugs such as bivalirudin may be theoretically superior to heparin for anticoagulation for cardiopulmonary bypass, the absence of effective reversal agents makes them impractical for routine use.

IV. Neutralization of heparin

A. **Proof of concept**

Protamine, commercially prepared from fish sperm, first found clinical utility in its combination with insulin to delay insulin's absorption and prolong its effect. Combination of protamine with heparin, intended to achieve a similar prolongation of heparin's effect, resulted instead in inactivation of heparin. Combining the strongly cationic protamine with strongly anionic heparin produces a stable complex devoid of anticoagulant activity.

1. **Heparin and protamine combine in proportion to weight. One milligram of protamine neutralizes 1 mg (typically 100 U) of heparin** [21].

B. **Protamine dose**

Since protamine appears to distribute within the circulatory system as heparin does, the protamine dose required to neutralize a given dose of heparin equals the number of milligrams of heparin remaining in the patient's circulation at the time of neutralization. Thus, clinical protocols to determine the initial dose of protamine first estimate the blood heparin concentration and blood volume. Direct assay of heparin concentration is difficult and unnecessary. Indirect assay using protamine effect in vitro is more accurate than ratio-based estimates and is easily performed. Three different methods of choosing an initial protamine dose are commonly used:

1. Empiric ratio. Most clinicians choose a dose of protamine based on the total number of units of heparin administered, giving between 0.6 and 1.3 mg of protamine for every 100 units of heparin administered.

2. **Clinical efficacy has been documented using a ratio as low as 0.6 mg of protamine to 100 units of heparin administered.** Initial doses using this ratio result in a mild-to-moderate protamine excess relative to heparin that ensures total neutralization and minimizes the likelihood of subsequent heparin rebound. Ratios exceeding 1 mg/100 units tend to be excessive.

    Example: A patient receives 25,000 units of heparin before CPB, with no subsequent heparin required, and 5,000 units in the bypass pump prime. A ratio of 1 mg:100 units yields a 300-mg protamine neutralizing dose. A ratio of 0.6 mg:100 units would result in 180 mg of protamine as the neutralizing dose. The former dose applies best when the patient receives all residual extracorporeal circuit blood, unwashed, prior to protamine administration; the latter dose makes most sense for CPB durations of 1 to 2 hours, during which heparin has ample opportunity for metabolism and excretion.

3. Estimated from a heparin dose–response curve. This method depends upon construction of a heparin dose–response curve prior to or during bypass (see Fig. 21.3). The technique then estimates the blood concentration of heparin at the time of neutralization (see Fig. 21.3 legend for details). Assumptions include (i) linearity of the heparin dose–ACT response relationship, (ii) potential extrapolation beyond actual data collected, and (iii) constancy of the volume of distribution of heparin and protamine. Most often, clinicians choose the arbitrary ratio of 1 mg of protamine to 100 units of heparin to calculate the protamine dose.

4. Calculated from in vitro protamine effect, by measuring ACT both with and without protamine added to blood at the time of neutralization. The HMS system from Medtronic HemoTec automates this technique to calculate protamine dose. These curves assume a linear dose–response and extrapolate to a baseline ACT in calculating the initial protamine dose. These devices also calculate blood volume based on patient's height and weight rather than on any definitive measurement, which can be a source of error. The same protamine titration curve can be performed using the TEG, but this assay has not become fully automated.

C. **Protamine administration. Always administer protamine slowly**

The rate of administration is more important than the route of administration in preventing adverse hemodynamic effects (see Section IV.E.1). One can either use a syringe or dilute the drug in a small volume of intravenous fluid and infuse by gravity or calibrated pump. Because the syringe technique results in multiple boluses, restricting its use to doses less than 1 mg/kg, or 20 mg in any 60-second period, appears advisable. **We recommend a continuous infusion technique rather than hand-operated syringe administration**, because this reduces the natural tendency to administer the protamine too quickly and it frees our hands for other important patient care activities (e.g., vasoactive drug titration, echocardiography examination) that coincide with protamine administration.

1. The injected dose of protamine cannot neutralize heparin bound to plasma proteins or within endothelial cells. Release of heparin from these stored areas after initial protamine administration may result in reappearance of heparin anticoagulant effect (heparin rebound). Small additional doses of protamine will provide neutralization when repeat testing (e.g., ACT initially normalizes to 110 seconds but 30 minutes later is 140 seconds) shows a heparin effect in a bleeding patient.

2. Protamine does not remain long in the vascular system following administration. Therefore, administration of heparinized blood, such as that remaining in the CPB machine without washing, following completion of the neutralizing protamine infusion, will likely result in renewed anticoagulation to a small extent. An additional small dose of protamine, about 1 mg/20 mL of transfused pump blood, should address this contingency.

D. **Monitoring heparin neutralization**
1. ACT. After protamine administration, the ACT test should return a value no more than 10% above the value before heparin administration. If more prolonged, residual heparin activity is likely. An ACT value that remains prolonged despite additional protamine suggests a technical error or, less commonly, some other hemostatic abnormality.

2. Protamine titration. This test utilizes a series of tubes with increasing amounts of added protamine, beginning with none. One adds patient blood to each tube and determines which tube clots first. Because protamine has anticoagulant properties in vitro, it prolongs the coagulation time of normal blood in test tubes. Knowing which tube clots first allows identification of unneutralized heparin as well as estimation of the additional amount of protamine needed to achieve complete neutralization. This test can be performed manually or by using an automated device (Medtronic HemoTec).

E. **Adverse effects** [22]
1. **Hypotension from rapid administration. Administration of a neutralizing dose of protamine (about 3 mg/kg) over 3 or fewer minutes decreases both systemic and pulmonary arterial pressures as well as venous return.** This predictable response may be blunted, but not predictably avoided, by volume loading. Release of vasoactive compounds from mast cells or other sites may be responsible for this adverse response.

2. Anaphylactoid reactions. Although protamine is a foreign protein, immune responses occur infrequently following exposure so that true allergy to protamine is uncommon. Table 21.3 lists those patients at potential risk.

3. Pulmonary vasoconstriction. Occasionally protamine increases pulmonary arterial pressure, resulting in right ventricular failure, decreased cardiac output, and systemic hypotension. Formation of large heparin–protamine complexes may stimulate production of thromboxane by pulmonary macrophages, causing vasoconstriction. In some animal models, the probability of experiencing this response is increased by faster rates of protamine administration.

4. Antihemostatic effects. Protamine activates thrombin receptors on platelets, causing partial activation and subsequent impairment of platelet aggregation. Transient thrombocytopenia

TABLE 21.3 Patients at potential risk for true allergy to protamine

Condition	Risk increase
Prior reaction to protamine	189-fold
Allergy to true (vertebrate) fish	24.5-fold
Exposure to neutral protamine Hagedorn (NPH) insulin	8.2-fold
Allergy to any drug	3.0-fold
Prior exposure to protamine	No increase!

Adapted from Kimmel SE, Sekeres MA, Berlin JA, et al. Risk factors for clinically important adverse events after protamine administration following cardiopulmonary bypass. *J Am Coll Cardiol*. 1998;32(7):1916–1922.

also occurs in the first hour after a full neutralizing dose of protamine. Inhibition of plasma coagulation can also occur.

5. **Treatment of adverse protamine reactions.** Systemic hypotension during or within 10 minutes after protamine administration suggests protamine as the cause but other causes such as hypovolemia and left ventricular dysfunction should be considered. Specific treatment depends on other hemodynamic events.

   a. Normal or low pulmonary artery pressures suggest either rapid administration or an anaphylactoid reaction. Rapid fluid administration alone often suffices to treat the former, whereas the latter cause usually requires aggressive volume resuscitation, large doses of epinephrine, and possibly other vasoactive compounds and inhaled bronchodilators. Refer to other sources for the treatment of acute anaphylaxis, including use of systemic corticosteroids.

   b. High pulmonary artery pressures suggest a pulmonary vasoconstriction reaction. Inotropes with pulmonary dilating properties, such as isoproterenol or milrinone, will support the failing heart while facilitating movement of blood across the pulmonary circulation. Inhaled nitric oxide may also be useful. With extreme hemodynamic deterioration, reinstitution of CPB may be necessary. In this case, give a full heparin dose (at least 300 U/kg). Occasionally, heparin alone will correct the pulmonary hypertension (presumably by breaking up large heparin–protamine complexes, the putative stimulant to thromboxane production) such that reinstitution of CPB no longer becomes necessary, although neutralization of heparin becomes an even bigger problem.

6. **Prevention of adverse responses**

   a. **Rate of administration. Always administer fully neutralizing doses of protamine slowly (minimum duration 3 minutes, with a target of 10 minutes recommended).** Rather than depend on volume loading to prevent hypotension, simply dilute the drug and give it slowly. Place the calculated dose in 50 mL or more of clear fluid and connect a small-drop (approximately 60 drops/mL) administration set to limit the infusion rate or use an infusion pump connected either to a 50-mL syringe or a 50-mL (or greater) fluid bag containing protamine. Some clinicians advocate a protamine "test dose," such as 1 mg intravenously, prior to protamine administration. Our view is that slow initiation of a continuous protamine infusion accomplishes the same end, after which the infusion rate can be increased as tolerated down to a minimum infusion time as above.

CLINICAL PEARL The most common cause of hypotension during protamine administration is overly rapid administration.

   b. Route of administration. The preponderance of evidence suggests that peripheral vein infusion offers no benefit over central venous infusion as long as the infusion is dilute and not rapid. Injection directly into the aorta provides no reliable protection and risks introduction of embolic material, such as small bubbles, pieces of rubber stopper, or glass.

   c. High-risk subgroups. Patients without previous exposure to protamine, including those with diabetes or prior vasectomy, require no special measures before initial exposure. **Even patients who have received protamine-containing insulin preparations rarely develop an adverse response; however, the presence of antibodies to the heparin/protamine complex has been demonstrated** [23]. Only patients with a prior history of an adverse response to protamine warrant special treatment. See Table 21.3 for the relative risks of protamine administration to these subgroups.

   d. Prior protamine reaction. Prepare a special, dilute protamine solution of about 1 mg in 100 mL and administer over 10 minutes. If no adverse response occurs, administer the fully neutralizing dose as described earlier. Skin tests taken before giving protamine provide little predictive value and frequently are falsely positive. Special immunologic tests for protamine allergy, such as radioallergosorbent test (RAST) and ELISA, also demonstrate many false-positive results.

F. **Alternatives to protamine administration**
1. Allow heparin's effect to dissipate. This approach results in continued hemorrhage with substantial transfusion requirements, bouts of hypovolemia, and the potential for consumptive coagulopathy. Although this may be the only option available, ideally it should be avoided.
2. Platelet concentrates. PF4 is released from activated platelets. It combines with and neutralizes heparin. However, platelet concentrates do not effectively restore coagulation following CPB. A recombinant form of PF4 failed in clinical trials as a protamine alternative.
3. Hexadimethrine. This synthetic polycation, no longer readily available in the United States because of renal toxicity, can avoid true allergic reactions to protamine. However, like protamine, it forms complexes with heparin that can incite pulmonary vasoconstriction if administered quickly.
4. Methylene blue. Even large doses do not effectively restore the ACT. However, inhibition of nitric oxide synthetase can incite pulmonary hypertension, making this approach potentially hazardous.
5. Investigational substances. Heparinase I, an enzyme produced by harmless soil bacteria, failed in clinical trials as a protamine alternative. Virus-like particles, engineered from bacteriophage Qβ coat protein, have shown consistent neutralization of heparin with less variability than protamine in plasma from heparin-treated patients [24]. Cationically modified chitosan binds to heparin to form complexes similar to those formed by protamine [25].
6. With no alternative to protamine immediately available, or even under active clinical investigation, alternatives to heparin (see Section III.E) assume greater importance in the management of patients with demonstrated severe adverse responses to protamine.

V. Hemostatic abnormalities in the cardiac surgical patient [1,26]
A. **Management of the patient taking preoperative antithrombotic drugs**
Table 21.4 lists commonly used antithrombotic drugs and their mechanisms of action.
1. Anticoagulant therapy. Patients receiving warfarin anticoagulant medications should be advised to discontinue the medication 3 to 5 days before the anticipated cardiac surgery. In general, an INR value less than 2 reflects an acceptable recovery of vitamin K–dependent clotting factors. In fact, some residual inhibition of the extrinsic coagulation pathway advantageously accentuates anticoagulation for CPB. If anticoagulation is so vitally important that it must be maintained until the time of surgery, an intravenous infusion of heparin may be started preoperatively. Heparin may be discontinued a few hours before surgery or continued into the operative period.
    a. In urgent or semi-urgent surgery, the effects of warfarin may need rapid reversal, which can be accomplished by giving FFP until INR correction occurs [30]. Concomitant administration of vitamin K may accelerate warfarin reversal.
    b. In clinical studies, prothrombin complex concentrate (PCC) was found more effective with quicker time to INR correction and no volume overload observed compared to FFP [27].

> **CLINICAL PEARL**   When available, **PCC**, and not FFP, should be used for the emergency reversal of warfarin effect.

2. The use of novel direct oral anticoagulants (DOACs) (dabigatran and the Xa inhibitors, apixaban, rivaroxaban, and edoxaban) for treatment of venous thromboembolism and prevention of thromboembolic complications in patients with nonvalvular atrial fibrillation has increased over the last several years. In patients with atrial fibrillation, when compared with warfarin, DOACs have a similar efficacy in preventing stroke but a lower risk for intracranial bleeding [28,29].
    a. Recommendations are to discontinue dabigatran 24 hours prior to cardiac surgery and the factor Xa inhibitors 3 to 5 days prior to surgery. Patients with renal failure (dabigatran) or liver failure (factor Xa inhibitors) metabolize and clear these drugs more slowly.

TABLE 21.4   Common antithrombotic drugs

Drug	Mechanism	Clinical uses
Plasma coagulation inhibitors	All are parenteral agents unless otherwise stated	
Heparin	ATIII agonist, anti-Xa, and anti-IIa	Deep vein thrombosis, atrial fibrillation, unstable angina, surgical, extracorporeal circulation, bridging anticoagulants
Low–molecular-weight heparin (includes fondaparinux)	ATIII agonist, anti-Xa primarily	Deep vein thrombosis, pulmonary embolus, unstable angina
Bivalirudin	Direct thrombin inhibitor (two-site inhibition)	Percutaneous coronary intervention, acute coronary syndrome, CPB in patients with contraindication for heparin or protamine
Warfarin	Inhibit production of vitamin K–dependent coagulation factors	Deep vein thrombosis, atrial fibrillation, heart valve
Dabigatran	Oral direct thrombin inhibitor	Thromboembolic prophylaxis in patients with atrial fibrillation
Apixaban, rivaroxaban, and edoxaban	Oral anti-Xa agents	Thromboembolic prophylaxis in patients with atrial fibrillation
Platelet inhibitors	All are oral agents	
Acetylsalicylic acid (aspirin)	Inhibit cyclooxygenase, inhibit thromboxane, prevent platelet activation	Atherosclerotic cardiovascular disease, cerebrovascular disease, percutaneous coronary intervention
Dipyridamole	Adenosine enhancing, inhibit thromboxane	Peripheral vascular disease
Abciximab	GPIIb/IIIa receptor antagonist (monoclonal antibody)	Percutaneous coronary intervention/stent
Eptifibatide	GPIIb/IIIa receptor antagonist (small peptide)	Percutaneous coronary intervention/stent
Tirofiban	GPIIb/IIIa receptor antagonist (nonpeptide)	Percutaneous coronary intervention/stent
Ticlopidine	Thienopyridine, ADP receptor antagonist	Percutaneous coronary intervention/stent, cerebrovascular disease
Clopidogrel	Thienopyridine, ADP receptor antagonist	Percutaneous coronary intervention/stent, acute coronary syndrome, acute myocardial infarction
Prasugrel and Ticagrelor	Thienopyridine, P2Y12 ADP receptor inhibitors	Percutaneous coronary intervention/stent, acute coronary syndrome

ATIII, antithrombin III; ADP, adenosine diphosphate; GPIIb, Glycoprotein IIb; CPB, cardiopulmonary bypass.

    b. DOACs present special management challenges when rapid reversal in bleeding patients or prior to emergency surgery is required. Routine laboratory coagulation tests (PT and aPTT) are unreliable in assessing residual anticoagulant effect, and specific quantitative assays may not be widely available in every medical center.

    c. For patients treated with dabigatran, the humanized monoclonal antibody idarucizumab was approved in 2015 for reversal in cases of serious bleeding or prior to emergency surgery [30].

    d. Currently, there is no approved specific reversal agent for factor Xa inhibitors. Case reports and human volunteer studies suggest that PCC can be used to reverse the effect of factor Xa inhibitors. Andexanet alfa, a specific reversal agent for factor Xa inhibitors and LMWH, is currently undergoing clinical trials for emergency reversal of these agents.

3. Antiplatelet therapy

   a. Aspirin. Many studies support the use of aspirin in the prevention of thrombosis in coronary and cerebral vascular disease. Patients taking aspirin who undergo cardiac surgery have a propensity for increased bleeding postoperatively; however, the benefits of aspirin therapy, weighed against a potential for bleeding, often lead to preoperative continuation of aspirin therapy. Most patients do not bleed excessively with this approach. An increase in bleeding, if it exists, is not necessarily accompanied by an increase in transfusion requirements due to blood conservation strategies in use.

   b. Glycoprotein IIb/IIIa (GPIIb/IIIa) inhibitors. The GPIIb/IIIa receptor is the platelet fibrinogen receptor, which causes fibrinogen bridging of adjacent platelets and subsequent platelet aggregation. GPIIb/IIIa inhibitors inhibit platelet aggregation and have been increasingly used during interventional cardiology procedures. Their beneficial effects include reductions in mortality and cardiac events after angioplasty and stent procedures. However, there is strong potential for hemorrhagic complications if these patients present for emergent cardiac surgery. Currently, the three intravenous GPIIb/IIIa inhibitors in clinical use are abciximab, tirofiban, and eptifibatide. Abciximab is a monoclonal antibody to the GPIIb/IIIa receptor that inhibits fibrinogen binding and covalently alters the GPIIb/IIIa receptor. Tirofiban and eptifibatide are smaller competitive receptor blockers whose effects are reversible after discontinuation of therapy. Their short duration of action may mitigate some perioperative bleeding complications [31] and may actually provide some platelet protection during CPB.

   c. ADP receptor inhibitors. The thienopyridine derivatives ticlopidine, clopidogrel, and prasugrel noncompetitively antagonize at a platelet ADP receptor known as the P2Y12 receptor. Blockade of this receptor by one of these agents elevates cyclic adenosine monophosphate levels to induce profound and rapid platelet disaggregation. Clopidogrel use in conjunction with percutaneous coronary intervention or in acute coronary syndromes reduces the occurrence of adverse ischemic events [32]. Antiplatelet activity is permanent for the life span of the platelet because the P2Y12 receptor is permanently altered. Clopidogrel is a prodrug that is metabolized by cytochrome P450 (2C19 and 3A4) to its active metabolite. The combination of clopidogrel and aspirin is synergistic. Meta-analyses demonstrate that clopidogrel pretreatment before cardiac surgery is associated with more bleeding than that observed in nonexposed patients [33].

B. Abnormalities acquired during cardiac surgery

1. Endothelial dysfunction. Contact of blood with extracorporeal surfaces initiates a "total body inflammatory response" characterized by activation of coagulation, fibrinolysis, and inflammation. This leads to an abnormal cellular–endothelial interaction.

2. Persistent heparin effect. This is uncommon because most clinicians fully neutralize the administered heparin, although **heparin rebound (resumption of heparin effect after complete neutralization) is relatively common within the first 2 hours following CPB and usually responds well to small (e.g., 25 mg), incremental doses of protamine.**

3. Platelet abnormalities (Table 21.5)

   a. Thrombocytopenia occurs frequently after CPB due to dilution of the blood volume with extracorporeal circuit volume and platelet consumption or sequestration. This thrombocytopenia can be severe (<50,000/µL) but, in the absence of other hemostasis abnormalities, often does not lead to excessive bleeding. With modern techniques, platelet counts after CPB most often exceed 100,000/µL.

   b. Platelet dysfunction. **The most prevalent yet elusive cause of hemostatic abnormalities after CPB is platelet dysfunction.** Platelets are rendered inactive by contact activation from the extracorporeal surfaces, hypothermia, receptor downregulation, and by heparin and protamine. Heparin activates platelets to render them less functional after CPB, and protamine also depresses platelet function. The use of antithrombotic drugs preoperatively leads to an even greater degree of platelet dysfunction after CPB.

4. Coagulopathy. Hemodilution and consumption of coagulation factors by microvascular coagulation combine to cause the deficiencies of coagulation seen after CPB. Despite the

TABLE 21.5 Causes of platelet dysfunction in cardiac surgery

CPB-related causes

Hypothermia
Materials-induced activation
Trauma-induced activation (cardiotomy suction)
Fibrinolysis
Glycoprotein Ib receptor downregulation
Glycoprotein IIb/IIIa receptor downregulation/destruction
Thrombin receptor downregulation/destruction

Drug-related causes

Heparin
Nitrates
Phosphodiesterase inhibitors
Protamine
Platelet antagonists preoperatively

use of large doses of heparin, contact activation causes microvascular activation of factor XII and initiates the intrinsic pathway of coagulation.

5. Fibrinolysis. Fibrinolysis can be primary or secondary during CPB (Fig. 21.4). Primary fibrinolysis occurs from release of endothelial plasminogen activators. Secondary fibrinolysis describes activation of plasmin as a result of a feedback response to fibrin formation. Circulating plasmin degradation products adversely affect platelet function.

6. Pharmacology. As noted earlier, heparin and protamine impair platelet function. Other drugs commonly used during CPB (milrinone, nitroglycerin, nitroprusside) adversely affect platelet function in vitro, but in vivo their effects appear to be clinically undetectable.

7. Hypothermia. Hypothermia impairs the enzymatic cascades of the coagulation pathway. Platelets are activated during mild hypothermia and are depressed during moderate to severe hypothermia.

C. **Pharmacologic and protective prophylaxis**

1. Platelet protection

   a. Antifibrinolytic agents. See Section V.C.2.

   b. Coated surfaces. Heparin-bonded circuits attenuate the inflammatory response to CPB and may confer some platelet protective properties.

   c. Antiplatelet agents that are active during CPB may confer platelet protection so long as they are short acting. Patients who have emergency surgery after having been exposed to tirofiban or eptifibatide do not experience excessive postoperative bleeding and receive equivalent or reduced transfusion volumes.

2. Antifibrinolytic agents [34]

   a. Synthetic antifibrinolytic agents: ε-aminocaproic acid (EACA) and tranexamic acid (TA). EACA and TA act as lysine analogs that bind to the lysine-binding sites of plasmin and plasminogen (Fig. 21.4). TA is a more potent analog of EACA that has a higher affinity for plasminogen than does EACA. Fibrin degradation products inhibit platelet function. Thus, plasmin inhibition may protect platelets. **The benefits of EACA and TA have been demonstrated in multiple meta-analyses to reduce bleeding in cardiac surgery, when these agents are used prophylactically (i.e., initiated before CPB and maintained throughout CPB) rather than as rescue agents** [35]. *Dosing:* **EACA:** 100 to 150 mg/kg bolus, 10 to 15 mg/kg/hr *or* 4- to 10-g bolus, 1 g/hr. Reports suggest constant plasma activity may be best achieved with smaller initial boluses (approximately 50 mg/kg) followed by higher maintenance doses (20 to 25 mg/kg/hr). **TA:** Low dose: 10 to 20 mg/kg bolus, 1 to 2 mg/kg/hr; moderate dose: 30 to 50 mg/kg bolus, 15 to 30 mg/kg/hr; *or* high dose: 5-g bolus, repeat bolus to total 15 g. The latter dosing scheme probably is much higher than necessary, and there is concern that high-dose TA may be associated with seizures and other central nervous system adverse events [36,37].

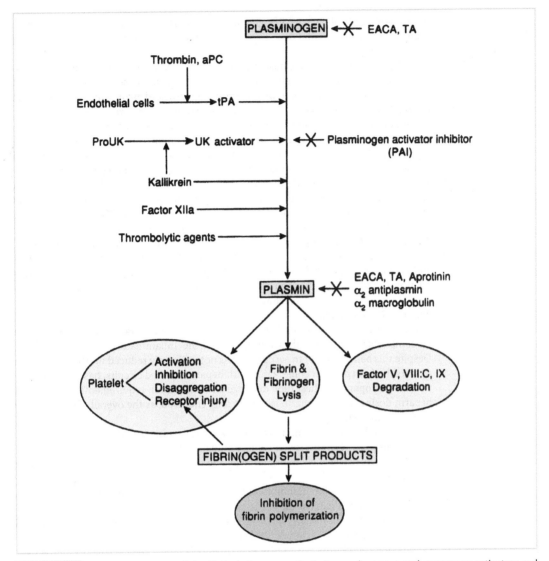

FIGURE 21.4 Schematic diagram of the fibrinolytic system displaying endogenous and exogenous activators and inhibitors of fibrinolysis. The antihemostatic actions of plasmin and fibrin(ogen) split products (FSPs) are illustrated. aPC, activated protein C; EACA, ε-aminocaproic acid; TA, tranexamic acid; tPA, tissue plasminogen activator; UK, urokinase.

    b. Aprotinin, a high–molecular-weight proteinase inhibitor of bovine origin, inhibits plasmin, kallikrein, and other serine proteases. Aprotinin decreases activation of the hematologic system during CPB and subsequent fibrinolysis, resulting in significant decrease in postoperative bleeding. It is the only agent found to be successful in reducing the rate of reoperation for bleeding in meta-analyses. However, an increased rate of mortality and renal morbidity has been reported with aprotinin that caused the drug to be removed from commercial use [38–40]. Recently, the drug has been reapproved for use in cardiac surgery patients in Canada and several European countries, but it is still not available in the United States. Newer protease inhibitors are currently under investigation for use in cardiac surgery.

    c. Investigational substances: Carbon monoxide–releasing molecule-2 (CORM-2) significantly improved velocity of clot formation and clot strength in plasma in patients, both before and following CPB. Pending further trials, CORM-2 may be of use in improving coagulation and decreasing fibrinolysis in patients with persistent bleeding after CPB [41].

3. Accurate heparin and protamine dosing. Attempts to individualize heparin and protamine doses in order to minimize bleeding rely on patient-specific doses of each drug based on patient sensitivity. **A number of different heparin and protamine management strategies have been reported to result in reduced perioperative bleeding.**

   a. Higher heparin concentrations during CPB have been associated with increased mediastinal tube bleeding postoperatively. Higher doses might predispose to greater bleeding as a result of heparin rebound or platelet dysfunction. This leads to the practice of giving just enough heparin to maintain a "threshold" minimum acceptable ACT.

   b. Some investigators postulate that higher heparin levels allow for reduced activation of the coagulation cascade and may blunt the consumptive coagulopathy that occurs with microvascular coagulation. This leads to the practice of maintaining heparin at a specific concentration in the blood, which leads to large doses of heparin and higher ACTs. Heparin management strategies are still highly variable and institution specific.

   c. Lower protamine doses have been used successfully to neutralize heparin after CPB and have been associated with reduced bleeding and transfusion requirements. This relationship between higher heparin and lower protamine doses has been suggested to result in less postoperative bleeding.

4. Inhibition of inflammation

   a. Coated surfaces. Heparin-bonded CPB circuits make the extracorporeal circuit more biocompatible and thus effectively attenuate the inflammatory response to CPB. Despite this benefit, use of these circuits has not uniformly reduced morbidity. Use of a reduced heparin dose, in conjunction with heparin-bonded circuits, has shown reductions in postoperative chest tube drainage and transfusion requirements, but reduced heparin dosing in this scenario is not yet fully endorsed, as the overall effect on safety for CPB is unclear.

   b. Steroids. Methylprednisolone and dexamethasone have been used to reduce the inflammatory response, but improved clinical outcomes have not been demonstrated. The use of steroids has also fallen out of favor due to risks of hyperglycemia and immune suppression [42,43].

   c. Aprotinin acts by kallikrein inhibition to reduce the inflammatory response; however, it is not in common clinical use at this time.

   d. Modified ultrafiltration has a beneficial effect of reducing postoperative morbidity and improving organ function after CPB in pediatric patients.

   e. Complement inhibitors are mostly experimental agents. They act to prevent activation of complement by kallikrein inhibition or direct complement antagonism. Reduction of the inflammatory response theoretically should reduce morbidity. Clinical trials have demonstrated marginal effects that did not reach clinical endpoints; thus, these agents have not become mainstream therapy in CPB.

VI. **Management of postbypass bleeding** [1]

CLINICAL PEARL Treatment of any abnormal laboratory value should not take place unless warranted by the clinical situation—that is, observation of clinical coagulopathy. Treat the patient, not the number!

A. **Evaluation of hemostasis**

1. Achieve surgical hemostasis.

2. Confirm adequate heparin neutralization. Tests of heparin neutralization: heparinase ACT, protamine titration test, heparinase TEG/rotational thromboelastometry (ROTEM).

   Note: The standard ACT is not a specific test for complete heparin neutralization—that is, it is possible to have ACT return to normal while some residual heparin effect remains.

If the ACT has returned to baseline and residual heparin effect is either suspected or identified using a protamine titration technique, treat this by titrating in additional protamine. Most often protamine, 25 mg, completes the neutralization.

> **CLINICAL PEARL** Even if ACT has returned to baseline, its insensitivity to low concentrations of heparin makes it reasonable to administer a small additional dose of protamine if coagulopathic bleeding continues.

  3. Point-of-care testing to diagnose and treat bleeding. Point-of-care tests, preferably viscoelastic tests (TEG/ROTEM), should be used appropriately in order to accurately and rapidly pinpoint the cause of a hemostasis defect. Etiologies of post-CPB bleeding should be prioritized by the clinician and should be tested in logical order. These tests should include heparin neutralization (see Section VI.A.2), platelet function, platelet number, coagulation, fibrinogen, and fibrinolysis (Table 21.6).
      a. Tests of platelet function: TEG/ROTEM, Sonoclot, Plateletworks, Platelet Function Analyzer-100, VerifyNow, and whole blood aggregometry to name a few. **Treatment of platelet dysfunction may include administration of desmopressin acetate (DDAVP) 0.3 µg/kg slowly (over approximately 15 to 20 minutes, as vasodilation may occur). If platelet number is less than 50,000/µL or platelet dysfunction persists after DDAVP, a transfusion of platelet concentrates is recommended.** Since some platelet dysfunction routinely exists after CPB, some clinicians transfuse platelets in the presence of coagulopathic bleeding if platelet count is below 100,000/µL. This approach appears reasonable if tests of platelet function are not readily available.
      b. Coagulation tests. Standard coagulation tests are usually not helpful in directing treatment for the bleeding surgical patient, as they have a prolonged turnaround time, do not correlate with surgical bleeding, and do not measure indices such as platelet function and fibrinolysis. Yet, if viscoelastic coagulation tests are unavailable, standard coagulation tests (PT, aPTT, thrombin time) should be used. Treating abnormalities in coagulation factors usually includes transfusion of FFP. Recent clinical studies have reported that administration of 3- or 4-factor PCC is as effective as FFP transfusion, especially in the context of preoperative warfarin therapy [44–46] and avoids FFP-related complications such as transfusion-related acute lung injury (TRALI) and transfusion-associated circulatory overload (TACO). For massive bleeding when hemostasis cannot be achieved with conventional therapies, administration of recombinant factor VIIa (rVIIa) has been used as rescue therapy [47]. Administration of rVIIa will also treat CPB- or drug-induced platelet dysfunction by creating a thrombin burst; however, its safety has not been fully established, and risks of thromboembolic complications need to be considered [48].

TABLE 21.6 Point-of-care tests of platelet function

Test/monitor	Mechanism
Bleeding time	Collagen-activated in vivo adhesion
TEG/Sonoclot/ROTEM	Viscoelastic clot strength
Platelet function analyzer (PFA-100)	In vitro activated bleeding time
Plateletworks	Platelet count ratio
Standard aggregometry (PRP)	Optical density–light transmittance
Whole blood aggregometry	Electrical impedance
Ultegra/VerifyNow	Activated fibrinogen bead agglutination
Clot Signature Analyzer (research)	High shear and collagen activation
Hemodyne (PRP/whole blood) (research)	Platelet-mediated force transduction

PRP, platelet-rich plasma; TEG, thromboelastography; ROTEM, rotational thromboelastometry.

    c. Tests of hypofibrinogenemia and fibrinolysis. TEG/ROTEM, euglobulin lysis time, fibrin degradation products, D-dimers. Low fibrinogen levels are common after CPB and may need to be replaced with cryoprecipitate or fibrinogen concentrate (where available). The FIBTEM assay of ROTEM or functional fibrinogen of TEG are the primary assays performed to assess fibrinogen-related clot firmness. Quantification of fibrinogen levels is also reasonable, but this takes more time. Treatment of primary increased fibrinolysis includes administration of an antifibrinolytic agent. If an antifibrinolytic agent has already been administered and discontinued, the same agent should be restarted. Starting a different class of antifibrinolytic drug in the same patient is not recommended. Secondary fibrinolysis should be treated by replacement of consumed coagulation factors (FFP or cryoprecipitate).

B. **Treatment of postbypass hemostatic disorders**

Follow the steps below in order. They reflect the causes of postoperative bleeding in decreasing frequency of occurrence. Remember to maintain intravascular volume to avoid generating or exacerbating a consumptive coagulopathy. These steps are designed to address the situation where urgency dictates that one must treat a presumed cause before obtaining laboratory results. Do not embrace any one presumed cause; rather, constantly reevaluate and question your assumptions. **Instead of bedside empiricism, however, we encourage the development and use of transfusion algorithms based on evaluation of multiple possible etiologies for bleeding, preferably using viscoelastic-based point-of-care coagulation testing** (see Section VI.C).

    1. Rule out a surgical cause. Excessive intraoperative bleeding or postoperative chest tube drainage usually results from surgical bleeding. A generalized slower ooze suggests a nonsurgical cause. Keep the blood pressure in the low normal range to facilitate surgical repair and optimally for some time thereafter to maximize the potential for clot formation.

    2. Maintain normothermia. Surface warming devices or raising the operating room temperature may be appropriate. In the effort to restore intravascular volume rapidly, clinicians must infuse refrigerated blood products only with adequate warming, lest they cause or accentuate hypothermia, thereby decreasing platelet function and enzymatic activity of clotting proteins.

    3. Heparin reversal. Confirm complete heparin neutralization with an ACT or by viscoelastic testing. If viscoelastic tests are unavailable, aPTT should be evaluated.

    4. Administer more protamine if the ACT exceeds its baseline (pre-heparin) value by >10 seconds (or other tests suggest residual heparin effect). A dose of 25 to 50 mg usually suffices. Remember that transfusion of large volumes of unwashed RBCs directly from the CPB machine ("pump blood") may expose the patients to additional heparin and thus may require administration of additional protamine.

    5. In the absence of hypovolemia, consider application of 5 cm of positive end-expiratory pressure (PEEP) to help tamponade open blood vessels in the chest. This maneuver may be most effective after the sternum is closed because of limitations in the ability of PEEP to effectively increase mediastinal end-expiratory pressure while the chest remains open.

    6. Platelet transfusion and/or DDAVP. If testing uncovers platelet dysfunction, or if it is highly suspected, give platelet concentrates for platelet count below 100,000/μL. While awaiting platelet concentrates from the blood bank, consider administration of DDAVP 0.3 μg/kg, especially if there is laboratory evidence of platelet dysfunction (e.g., decreased maximum amplitude on TEG or ROTEM). This may resolve the coagulopathy and avoid the need for platelet concentrates.

    7. FFP. Administer 15 mL/kg of FFP for evidence of clotting factors deficiency on TEG or ROTEM (prolonged R time or CT index, respectively), PT in excess of 1.5 times control, or an INR in excess of 2. Administration of PCC may be an alternative to FFP, especially when volume overload is of concern [49].

    8. Administer an antifibrinolytic agent. Although these agents work best when administered prophylactically before and during CPB, about half of their benefit occurs if given (or continued) in the post-CPB period. An increased D-dimer value or the TEG/ROTEM tracings and assays may indicate active fibrinolysis that would warrant antifibrinolytic agent administration or higher doses if antifibrinolytic agents are already being administered.

9. Consider measuring fibrinogen concentration, D-dimer, and thrombin time, the last of which is prolonged only by residual heparin, inadequate amount or functionality of fibrinogen, and fibrin degradation products. Cryoprecipitate or fibrinogen concentrate: Cryoprecipitate 1 unit/4 kg body weight (generally 15 to 20 units in adults) will correct fibrinogen deficiency (<100 mg/dL). Its use is best reserved for situations where hypofibrinogenemia has been documented (by viscoelastic testing or direct quantification of fibrinogen level). Fibrinogen concentrate is an alternative for cryoprecipitate and is in wide use in Europe. Initial clinical studies demonstrated favorable outcomes of reduced bleeding and less transfusions in high-risk patients treated with fibrinogen concentrate [50]; however, recent prospective randomized trials have failed to demonstrate a similar result [51,52].

10. Administration of rVIIa. rVIIa has been frequently used as "off-label" rescue medication for massive bleeding situations when conventional hemostatic therapy failed. In cardiac surgery, reductions in bleeding have clearly been documented; however, a dose of 80 μg/kg has been associated with thromboembolic complications [48,53]. Administration of rVIIa probably makes the most sense when given as a secondary intervention when two "rounds" of FFP 10 to 15 mL/kg and platelet concentrates 1 unit/10 kg have not resolved the coagulopathy. Overwhelming coagulopathy may at times call for earlier use of this potentially lifesaving agent, for which an initial dose of 30 to 40 μg/kg is recommended. Remember that optimization of fibrinogen level prior to administration of rVIIa is crucial for an optimal hemostatic effect.

C. **Transfusion medicine and the use of point-of-care (POC)–based algorithms**
Allogeneic transfusions after CPB are common because of the wide range of hemostatic insults incurred. The lack of adequate testing of hemostasis and the subjectivity of a diagnosis of microvascular bleeding lead to indiscriminate transfusion practices.

1. Excessive bleeding leading to massive transfusion of red blood cells, platelets, cryoprecipitate, and plasma is associated with increased morbidity and mortality [54]. Numerous clinical trials and meta-analyses demonstrate that the use of point-of-care–based transfusion algorithms is associated with less bleeding and transfusion requirements in cardiac surgery patients [55]; therefore, the rational use of transfusion algorithms should create an approach to transfusion medicine that is stepwise, logical, and based on the hemostatic defects that are most common and easily treated [56–58].

   This usually starts with a specific test of heparin neutralization. After residual heparin is ruled out, other point-of-care coagulation tests (preferably viscoelastic assays) are measured.

CLINICAL PEARL Standardized point-of-care algorithms for diagnosis and management of post-bypass coagulopathy reduce both bleeding and transfusion, and the specific diagnostic device(s) used are likely less important than local accessibility and rapid results.

2. **One of the most critical tests that should be measured "early" in a transfusion algorithm is an accurate point-of-care test of platelet function.**

3. Aside from confirming neutralization of heparin, the routine use of coagulation tests after CPB has not proven beneficial in the absence of a clinical coagulopathy. In patients who are suspected to have microvascular coagulopathic bleeding, an individualized goal-directed hemostatic approach that is based on POC-guided algorithms has been associated with improved patient outcomes when compared to standard laboratory-based or empiric transfusion therapy.

REFERENCES

1. Horrow JC, Mueksch JN, Weber N, et al. Coagulation testing. In: Gravlee GP, Davis RF, Hammon JW, et al., eds. *Cardiopulmonary Bypass and Mechanical Support: Principles and Practice.* 4th ed. Philadelphia, PA: Wolters Kluwer; 2016;449–462.
2. Shore-Lesserson L, Finley A, Murphy GS, et al. Anticoagulation for cardiopulmonary bypass. In: Gravlee GP, Davis RF, Hammon JW, et al., eds. *Cardiopulmonary Bypass and Mechanical Support: Principles and Practice.* 4th ed. Philadelphia, PA: Wolters Kluwer; 2016;463–496.

3. Merton RE, Curtis AD, Thomas DP. A comparison of heparin potency estimates obtained by activated partial thromboplastin time and British pharmacopoeial assays. *Thromb Haemost.* 1985;53(1):116–117.

4. Gravlee GP, Angert KC, Tucker WY, et al. Early anticoagulation peak and rapid distribution after intravenous heparin. *Anesthesiology.* 1988;68(1):126–129.

5. Heres EK, Speight K, Benckart D, et al. The clinical onset of heparin is rapid. *Anesth Analg.* 2001;92(6):1391–1395.

6. Olsson P, Lagergren H, Ek S. The elimination from plasma of intravenous heparin. An experimental study on dogs and humans. *Acta Med Scand.* 1963;173:619–630.

7. **Bull BS, Korpman RA, Huse WM, et al. Heparin therapy during extracorporeal circulation. I. Problems inherent in existing heparin protocols. *J Thorac Cardiovasc Surg.* 1975;69(5):674–684.**

8. Cohen EJ, Camerlengo LJ, Dearing JP. Activated clotting times and cardiopulmonary bypass I: the effect of hemodilution and hypothermia upon activated clotting time. *J Extracorp Technol.* 1980;12:139–141.

9. Gravlee GP, Case LD, Angert KC, et al. Variability of the activated coagulation time. *Anesth Analg.* 1988;67(5):469–472.

10. **Despotis GJ, Summerfield AL, Joist JH, et al. Comparison of activated coagulation time and whole blood heparin measurements with laboratory plasma anti-Xa heparin concentration in patients having cardiac operations. *J Thorac Cardiovasc Surg.* 1994;108(6):1076–1082.**

11. Koster A, Despotis G, Gruendel M, et al. The plasma supplemented modified activated clotting time for monitoring of heparinization during cardiopulmonary bypass: a pilot investigation. *Anesth Analg.* 2002;95(1):26–30.

12. Chavez JJ, Foley DE, Snider CC, et al. A novel thromboelastograph tissue factor/kaolin assay of activated clotting times for monitoring heparin anticoagulation during cardiopulmonary bypass. *Anesth Analg.* 2004;99(5):1290–1294.

13. Hellstern P, Bach J, Simon M, et al. Heparin monitoring during cardiopulmonary bypass surgery using the one-step point-of-care whole blood anti-factor-Xa clotting assay Heptest-POC-Hi. *J Extra Corpor Technol.* 2007;39(2):81–86.

14. Ganter MT, Monn A, Tavakoli R, et al. Kaolin-based activated coagulation time measured by Sonoclot in patients undergoing cardiopulmonary bypass. *J Cardiothorac Vasc Anesth.* 2007;21(4):524–528.

15. Garvin S, Fitzgerald D, Muehlschlegel JD, et al. Heparin dose response is independent of preoperative antithrombin activity in patients undergoing coronary artery bypass graft surgery using low heparin concentrations. *Anesth Analg.* 2010;111(4):856–861.

16. Society of Thoracic Surgeons Blood Conservation Guideline Task Force, Ferraris VA, Brown JR, Despotis GJ, et al. 2011 update to the Society of Thoracic Surgeons and the Society of Cardiovascular Anesthesiologists blood conservation clinical practice guidelines. *Ann Thorac Surg.* 2011;91(3):944–982.

17. Bennett-Guerrero E, Slaughter TF, White WD, et al. Preoperative anti-PF4/heparin antibody level predicts adverse outcome after cardiac surgery. *J Thorac Cardiovasc Surg.* 2005;130(6):1567–1572.

18. **Warkentin TE, Kelton JG. Temporal aspects of heparin-induced thrombocytopenia. *N Engl J Med.* 2001;344(17): 1286–1292.**

19. Dyke CM, Smedira NG, Koster A, et al. A comparison of bivalirudin to heparin with protamine reversal in patients undergoing cardiac surgery with cardiopulmonary bypass: the EVOLUTION-ON study. *J Thorac Cardiovasc Surg.* 2006;131(3):533–539.

20. Koster A, Hansen R, Grauhan O, et al. Hirudin monitoring using the TAS ecarin clotting time in patients with heparin-induced thrombocytopenia type II. *J Cardiothorac Vasc Anesth.* 2000;14(3):249–252.

21. Metz S, Horrow JC. Pharmacologic manipulation of coagulation: protamine and other heparin antagonists. In: Lake CL, Moore RA, eds. *Blood: Hemostasis, Transfusion, and Alternatives in the Perioperative Period.* New York: Raven Press; 1995:119–130.

22. **Horrow JC. Protamine: a review of its toxicity. *Anesth Analg.* 1985;64(3):348–361.**

23. Bakchoul T, Zollner H, Amiral J, et al. Anti-protamine–heparin antibodies: incidence, clinical relevance, and pathogenesis. *Blood.* 2013;121(15):2821–2827.

24. Gale AJ, Elias DJ, Averell PM, et al. Engineered virus-like nanoparticles reverse heparin anticoagulation more consistently than protamine in plasma from heparin-treated patients. *Thromb Res.* 2011;128(4):e9–e13.

25. Kamiński K, Szczubiałka K, Zazakowny K, et al. Chitosan derivatives as novel potential heparin reversal agents. *J Med Chem.* 2010;53(10):4141–4147.

26. Spiess BD, Armour S, Horrow J, et al. Transfusion medicine and coagulation disorders. In: Kaplan JA, Augoustides JGT, Manecke Jr., GR, et al., eds. *Kaplan's Cardiac Anesthesia in Cardiac and Noncardiac Surgery.* 7th ed. Philadelphia, PA: Elsevier; 2017;1248–1290.

27. Goldstein JN, Refaai MA, Milling TJ Jr, et al. Four-factor prothrombin complex concentrate versus plasma for rapid vitamin K antagonist reversal in patients needing urgent surgical or invasive interventions: a phase 3b, open-label, noninferiority, randomised trial. *Lancet.* 2015;385(9982):2077–2087.

28. Connolly SJ, Ezekowitz MD, Yusuf S, et al. Dabigatran versus warfarin in patients with atrial fibrillation. *N Engl J Med.* 2009; 361(12):1139–1151.

29. **Ruff CT, Giugliano RP, Braunwald E, et al. Comparison of the efficacy and safety of new oral anticoagulants with warfarin in patients with atrial fibrillation: a meta-analysis of randomised trials. *Lancet.* 2014;383(9921):955–962.**

30. Pollack CV Jr, Reilly PA, Eikelboom J, et al. Idarucizumab for dabigatran reversal. *N Engl J Med.* 2015;373(6):511–520.

31. Brown DL, Fann CS, Chang CJ. Meta-analysis of effectiveness and safety of abciximab versus eptifibatide or tirofiban in percutaneous coronary intervention. *Am J Cardiol.* 2001;87(5):537–541.

32. Bertrand ME, Rupprecht HJ, Urban P, et al. Double-blind study of the safety of clopidogrel with and without a loading dose in combination with aspirin compared with ticlopidine in combination with aspirin after coronary stenting: the clopidogrel aspirin stent international cooperative study (CLASSICS). *Circulation.* 2000;102(6):624–629.

33. Purkayastha S, Athanasiou T, Malinovski V, et al. Does clopidogrel affect outcome after coronary artery bypass grafting? A meta-analysis. *Heart.* 2006;92(4):531–532.

34. Levi M, Cromheecke ME, de Jonge E, et al. Pharmacologic strategies to decrease excessive blood loss in cardiac surgery: a meta-analysis of clinically relevant endpoints. *Lancet.* 1999;354(9194):1940–1947.

35. Brown JR, Birkmeyer NJ, O'Connor GT. Meta-analysis comparing the effectiveness and adverse outcomes of antifibrinolytic agents in cardiac surgery. *Circulation.* 2007;115(22):2801–2813.
36. Murkin JM, Falter F, Granton J, et al. High-dose tranexamic acid is associated with nonischemic clinical seizures in cardiac surgical patients. *Anesth Analg.* 2010;110(2):350–353.
37. Myles PS, Smith JA, Forbes A, et al. Tranexamic acid in patients undergoing coronary artery surgery. *N Engl J Med.* 2017;376(2):136–148.
38. Mangano DT, Tudor IC, Dietzel C. The risk associated with aprotinin in cardiac surgery. *N Engl J Med.* 2006;354(4):353–365.
39. Fergusson DA, Hebert PC, Mazer CD, et al. A comparison of aprotinin and lysine analogues in high-risk cardiac surgery. *N Engl J Med.* 2008;358(22):2319–2331.
40. Henry D, Carless P, Fergusson D, et al. The safety of aprotinin and lysine-derived antifibrinolytic drugs in cardiac surgery: a meta-analysis. *CMAJ.* 2009;180(2):183–193.
41. Malayaman SN, Entwistle JW 3rd, Boateng P, et al. Carbon monoxide releasing molecule-2 improves coagulation in patient plasma in vitro following cardiopulmonary bypass. *Blood Coagul Fibrinolysis.* 2011;22(5):362–368.
42. Dieleman JM, Nierich AP, Rosseel PM, et al. Intraoperative high-dose dexamethasone for cardiac surgery: a randomized controlled trial. *JAMA.* 2012;308(17):1761–1767.
43. Bunge JJ, van Osch D, Dieleman JM, et al. Dexamethasone for the prevention of postpericardiotomy syndrome: a Dexamethasone for Cardiac Surgery substudy. *Am Heart J.* 2014;168(1):126–131.
44. Demeyere R, Gillardin S, Arnout J, et al. Comparison of fresh frozen plasma and prothrombin complex concentrate for the reversal of oral anticoagulants in patients undergoing cardiopulmonary bypass surgery: a randomized study. *Vox Sang.* 2010;99(3):251–260.
45. Ortmann E, Besser MW, Sharples LD, et al. An exploratory cohort study comparing prothrombin complex concentrate and fresh frozen plasma for the treatment of coagulopathy after complex cardiac surgery. *Anesth Analg.* 2015;121(1):26–33.
46. Arnekian V, Camous J, Fattal S, et al. Use of prothrombin complex concentrate for excessive bleeding after cardiac surgery. *Interact Cardiovasc Thorac Surg.* 2012;15(3):382–389.
47. Karkouti K, Arellano R, Aye T, et al. Off-label use of recombinant activated factor VII in surgical and non-surgical patients at 16 Canadian hospitals from 2007 to 2010. *Can J Anaesth.* 2014;61(8):727–735.
48. Levi M, Levy JH, Andersen HF, et al. Safety of recombinant activated factor VII in randomized clinical trials. *N Engl J Med.* 2010;363(19):1791–1800.
49. Tanaka KA, Mazzeffi M, Durila M. Role of prothrombin complex concentrate in perioperative coagulation therapy. *J Intensive Care.* 2014;2(1):60.
50. Rahe-Meyer N, Solomon C, Hanke A, et al. Effects of fibrinogen concentrate as first-line therapy during major aortic replacement surgery: a randomized placebo-controlled trial. *Anesthesiology.* 2013;118(1):40–50.
51. Rahe-Meyer N, Levy JH, Mazer CD, et al. Randomized evaluation of fibrinogen vs. placebo in complex cardiovascular surgery (REPLACE): a double-blind phase III study of haemostatic therapy. *Br J Anaesth.* 2016;117(1):41–51.
52. Bilecen S, de Groot JA, Kalkman CJ, et al. Effect of fibrinogen concentrate on intraoperative blood loss among patients with intraoperative bleeding during high-risk cardiac surgery. *JAMA.* 2017;317(7):738–747.
53. Gill R, Herbertson M, Vuylsteke A, et al. Safety and efficacy of recombinant activated factor VII: a randomized placebocontrolled trial in the setting of bleeding after cardiac surgery. *Circulation.* 2009;120:21–27.
54. Murphy GJ, Reeves BC, Rogers CA, et al. Increased mortality, postoperative morbidity, and cost after red blood cell transfusion in patients having cardiac surgery. *Circulation.* 2007;116(22):2544–2552.
55. Karkouti K, Callum J, Wijeysundera DN, et al. Point-of-care hemostatic testing in cardiac surgery: a stepped-wedge clustered randomized controlled trial. *Circulation.* 2016;134(16):1152–1162.
56. Shore-Lesserson L, Manspeizer HE, DePerio M, et al. Thromboelastography-guided transfusion algorithm reduces transfusions in complex cardiac surgery. *Anesth Analg.* 1999;88(2):312–319.
57. Nuttall GA, Oliver WC, Santrach PJ, et al. Efficacy of a simple intraoperative transfusion algorithm for nonerythrocyte component utilization after cardiopulmonary bypass. *Anesthesiology.* 2001;94(5):773–781.
58. Chen L, Bracey AW, Radovancevic R, et al. Clopidogrel and bleeding in patients undergoing elective coronary artery bypass grafting. *J Thorac Cardiovasc Surg.* 2004;128(3):425–431.

22

Devices for Cardiac Support and Replacement

Jordan R. H. Hoffman, Jay D. Pal, and Joseph C. Cleveland, Jr.

KEY POINTS

1. Mechanical circulatory support (MCS) devices most often are ventricular assist devices (VADs), which are indicated for bridging to myocardial recovery, cardiac transplantation, or as a permanent assist device (destination therapy).

2. The principal growth area for VADs in recent years has been destination therapy. The predominant device used for this indication is the Abbott HeartMate II, although the HeartMate 3 and HeartWare HVAD are likely to receive this indication in the near future.

3. In New York Heart Association class IV heart failure (minimal activity–induced symptoms), VADs provide better survival and quality of life than medical therapy.

4. A variety of nonpulsatile right ventricular assist devices (RVADs) and a pulsatile total artificial heart (TAH) are Food and Drug Administration (FDA) approved for bridging to recovery or to transplantation. RVADs are sometimes needed as a bridge to right ventricle (RV) recovery for patients undergoing destination left ventricular assist device (LVAD) placement.

5. Newer short-term bridging VADs include the CentriMag, Tandem Heart, and Impella pumps, all of which are continuous-flow pumps that implant and operate in separate and distinct ways.

6. Separation from cardiopulmonary bypass (CPB) after LVAD placement may be complicated by RV failure, which may require various combinations of pulmonary arterial vasodilators (e.g., milrinone, nitric oxide), inotropes (e.g., dobutamine, epinephrine), and systemic arterial vasoconstrictors (e.g., vasopressin).

7. Common early postoperative problems include bleeding and RV dysfunction. Late postoperative problems include device thrombosis and infection.

8. Continuous-flow VAD patients presenting for noncardiac surgery pose a variety of clinical problems, which include obtaining accurate measurements of blood pressure (BP) and pulse oximetry, maintaining VAD blood flow, as well as challenges with hemostasis.

9. Intra-aortic balloon pumps (IABPs) are most often used to provide temporary left ventricle (LV) support to patients undergoing interventional cardiology or cardiac surgical procedures. IABPs augment diastolic blood flow to increase coronary artery blood flow and reduce LV afterload.

10. IABP inflation and deflation must be synchronized to the cardiac cycle, which can be done using either electrocardiography (ECG) or an intra-arterial waveform. Inflation should commence just after systole ends, and deflation should end just before systole begins.

I. Introduction

The use of mechanical circulatory support (MCS) devices, most commonly left ventricular assist devices (LVADs) have grown significantly in recent years. As the population ages and the incidence of heart failure rises, the supply of donor hearts for transplantation remains constant. Therefore, a larger percentage of patients are undergoing LVAD surgery as a bridge to heart transplantation. In addition, a significant number of patients who are not eligible for transplantation are undergoing LVAD implantation as permanent, or destination, therapy. This group of patients is the fastest growing group of MCS patients, and are living longer with durable LVADs. In addition, the development of newer, short-term MCS devices has led increased growth of patients being supported for interventional cardiology and cardiac surgery procedures, as well as for bridging strategies for myocardial recovery after infarction or myocarditis.

CLINICAL PEARL   Relatively small intracardiac shunts can enlarge when the left-sided filling pressures are reduced after LVAD implantation.

CLINICAL PEARL   Right ventricular (RV) function will typically deteriorate after LVAD implantation and will often require significant inotropic support.

Devices are getting smaller, easier to implant, and more durable. This chapter will discuss the current state of MCS, including available devices and therapies.

II. History

Dr. Michael DeBakey performed the first successful clinical implant of a ventricular assist device (VAD) for postcardiotomy cardiac failure in 1966 [1]. The patient was mechanically supported for 4 days. The first successful use of MCS as a "bridge" to transplantation occurred by Dr. Denton Cooley in 1978 at the Texas Heart Institute [2]. That patient was supported for 5 days by a pneumatically actuated paracorporeal device. The first implant of a total artificial heart (TAH) was performed on Dr. Barney Clarke, a retired dentist, by Dr. William DeVries in 1982 at the University of Utah [3]. The pump was a Jarvik-7 TAH designed by Dr. Robert Jarvik. Dr. Clarke lived for 112 days; unfortunately, the world watched him slowly and courageously die over the ensuing months from sepsis and embolic events. As with the pioneering experience with cardiac transplantation in the 1960s, there was public criticism of TAH as an "advancement" that was not worthwhile. Nevertheless, development of more sophisticated devices for short- and long-term use quietly persisted. Successful recovery of patients in acute cardiogenic shock using short-term

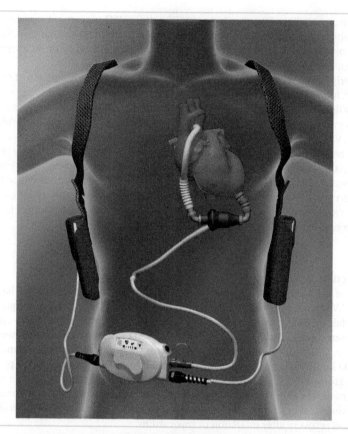

FIGURE 22.1 Diagram of a patient with an implanted HM II continuous-flow LVAD including driveline and portable power source. (Reproduced with permission from Thoratec, Inc., Pleasanton, CA, USA.)

VADs occurred and the data improved. The first pump to receive Food and Drug Administration (FDA) approval in the United States was the Abiomed BVS 5000 (Abiomed, Danvers, MA, USA) in November, 1992. Two implantable pumps were then approved for inpatient long-term use, the HeartMate IP system (Thoratec Corp., Pleasanton, CA, USA) and the Novacor system (Worldheart, Ontario, Canada). In 1995, both the HeartMate vented electric (VE) system and the Novacor system were subsequently approved for outpatient use. This was followed by the Thoratec VAD system (Thoratec Corp., Pleasanton, CA, USA), which was approved as a long-term support system in 1996. In 2001, the landmark REMATCH (Randomized Evaluation of Mechanical Assistance for the Treatment of Congestive Heart Failure) trial led to the approval of the Thoratec VE for destination therapy [4].

The TAH also evolved during this time. The SynCardia Systems Inc. CardioWest TAH represented the evolution of the Jarvik TAH and has had over 1,700 implants worldwide. It is currently the only TAH system approved for bridge to transplantation, and is in a clinical study for the use as destination therapy.

The period of 2007 to 2012 has marked an exciting and exponential rise in the use of newer, smaller rotary and centrifugal LVADs. The HeartMate II (HM II) LVAD (Abbott, Abbott Park, USA) received FDA approval for bridge to transplantation in 2008 and destination therapy in 2010 (Fig. 22.1). The HeartMate 3 (HM 3) (Fig. 22.2), the successor to the HM II, is currently only available for use in clinical trials in the United States for bridge to transplantation and destination therapy. Its touted benefits include less blood trauma, a frictionless magnetically suspended rotor, and fully intrapericardial implantation. The Heartware HVAD (Medtronic, Minneapolis, USA) is a centrifugal pump which also has the advantage of implantation directly into the left ventricle (LV)

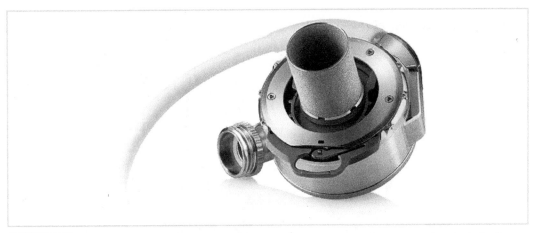

FIGURE 22.2 HeartMate 3 magnetically levitated centrifugal LVAD. (Reprinted with permission from SJMedical.)

apex without requiring an additional extrapericardial pocket (Fig. 22.3). Since an additional pump pocket is not required, alternate approaches for implantation are possible, reserving sternotomy for future cardiac procedures. The Heartware HVAD is currently approved for bridge to transplantation and likely to be approved for destination shortly.

Concurrent with the development of long-term, implantable LVADs, a number of short-term devices have been brought to market and are seeing increasing use. The Centrimag (Abbott, Abbott Park, USA) and TandemHeart (CardiacAssist Technologies, Pittsburgh, USA) both use centrifugal, paracorporeal pumps to provide short-term mechanical support in a variety of configurations. The Impella temporary VAD (Abiomed, Danvers, USA) is a system of catheter-based pumps which can be inserted percutaneously or via a surgical cutdown, and is approved for use in protected percutaneous coronary interventions (Impella 2.5, CP), as well as for circulatory support (Impella 5.0) (Fig. 22.4). An RV support device (Impella RP) is currently in trials in the United States.

III. Indications

There are three commonly described indications for the use of mechanical circulatory support devices (MCSDs): bridge to myocardial recovery, bridge to cardiac transplantation, and destination therapy.

A. Bridge to recovery

The use of an MCSD as a recovery system has focused on short-term use. **Traditionally, this has been thought of as support for days to weeks.** Clinical indications for this use include cardiogenic shock in the following settings:

1. Postcardiotomy
2. Acute myocardial infarction (MI)
3. Viral cardiomyopathies
4. Primary graft failure after cardiac transplantation

The postcardiotomy use of these pumps has declined over the past several years. This likely derives from improved perfusion and preservation techniques. Nevertheless, in this patient population the anticipated recovery time was 3 to 5 days. Animal data for support to recovery supported this timeline, as recovery was seen quite early [5]. **We now recognize that there may be substantial variability in the time it may take for patients' hearts to recover while on support, dependent on the etiology of cardiac failure.** Data from the Abiomed voluntary registry showed that mean support time to successful recovery may exceed 30 days. Several devices are now employed as short-term bridge-to-recovery devices: the Abiomed Impella 2.5, CP, 5.0, and RP (for right heart dysfunction), the Centrimag system, and the TandemHeart systems. The goal of a short-term bridge-to-recovery device is to provide end-organ perfusion while the heart is recovering. These short-term devices are especially useful in catastrophic, sudden presentations of cardiogenic shock (e.g., prolonged cardiac arrest during high-risk percutaneous coronary interventions) situations in which the likelihood of intact neurologic

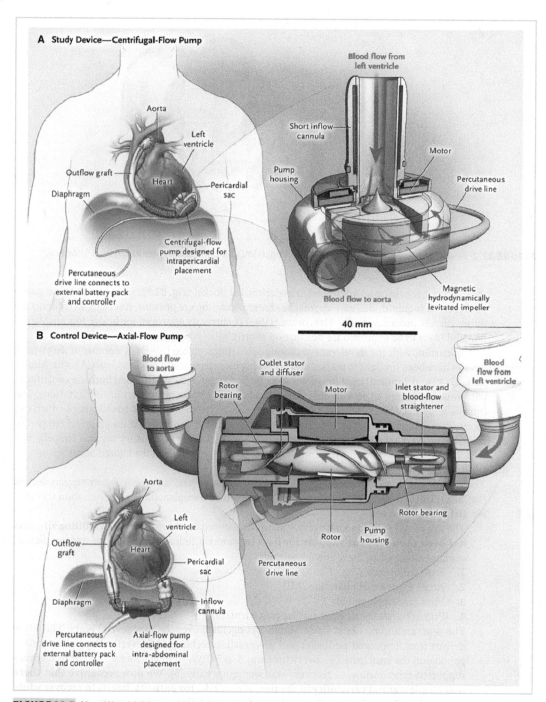

A Study Device—Centrifugal-Flow Pump

Blood flow from
left ventricle

Aorta

Left
ventricle

Short inflow
cannula

Motor

Outflow graft

Heart

Pump
housing

Percutaneous
drive line

Diaphragm

Pericardial
sac

Centrifugal-flow
pump designed for
intrapericardial
placement

Magnetic
hydrodynamically
levitated impeller

Percutaneous
drive line connects to
external battery pack
and controller

Blood flow to aorta

40 mm

B Control Device—Axial-Flow Pump

Blood flow
to aorta

Outlet stator
and diffuser

Blood
flow from
left ventricle

Rotor
bearing

Motor

Inlet stator and
blood-flow
straightener

Aorta

Left
ventricle

Rotor bearing

Outflow
graft

Heart

Rotor

Pump
housing

Percutaneous
drive line

Pericardial
sac

Diaphragm

Inflow
cannula

Percutaneous
drive line connects to
external battery pack
and controller

Axial-flow pump
designed for
intra-abdominal
placement

FIGURE 22.3 HeartWare HVAD intrapericardial centrifugal LVAD. (Reprinted with permission from Rogers JG, Pagani FD, Tatooles AJ, et al. Intrapericardial left ventricular assist device for advanced heart failure. *N Engl J Med*. 2017;376:451–460.)

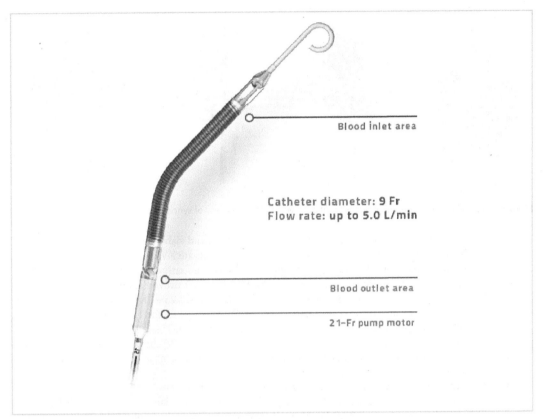

Blood inlet area

Catheter diameter: **9 Fr**
Flow rate: **up to 5.0 L/min**

Blood outlet area

21-Fr pump motor

FIGURE 22.4 Impella catheter-based LVAD. (Reprinted with permission from Abiomed.)

recovery remains unknown. These devices allow time to determine whether an irreversible neurologic injury would determine the patient's ultimate outcome.

B. Bridge to transplantation

The use of MCSDs as a bridge to cardiac transplantation constituted the early human laboratory to understand the long-term effects of support on many physiologic parameters as well as on quality-of-life measures. The therapy was instituted in individuals who were listed for cardiac transplantation, but failing conventional or inotropic therapy. **The MCSD would be employed to support the patient and improve the physiologic condition until a donor heart became available.** The MCSD would then be explanted at the time of cardiac transplantation.

The most commonly used VADs in the United States are the Thoratec Corp. HM II and the HeartWare Inc. HVAD. The SynCardia Systems TAH is also approved for this indication but is used much less commonly. The Thoratec HM II pump has become the mainstay of pumps implanted for a bridge-to-transplantation indication. The Thoratec Corp. HM 3 is the successor to the HM II and remains limited to use in clinical trial. Both the HM II and HVAD are approved for use as bridge-to-transplant due to randomized clinical trials demonstrating survival benefit relative to other bridging strategies [6,7].

C. Destination therapy

As experience with long-term use of MCSD led to successful outpatient use of this therapy, the concept of using MCSD as another option for patients with end-stage heart failure who were not transplant candidates emerged.

A landmark study called REMATCH concluded that **end-stage heart failure patients who received a Thoratec Heartmate VE LVAD experienced improved survival and quality of life when compared to optimal medical therapy.** The use of MCSD as permanent

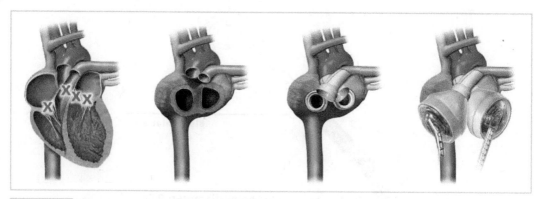

FIGURE 22.5 TAH implant requires resection of both ventricles. (Courtesy of syncardia.com.)

support for end-stage heart failure is now an accepted and viable therapy that is also supported by the Center for Medicare Services (CMS). The Heartmate XVE was the first LVAD approved for this indication. In a subsequent randomized trial comparing the Heartmate XVE with the HM II LVAD (continuous-flow pump), the HM II LVAD proved superior to the Heartmate XVE, with 2-year survival in the HM II cohort of 58% versus 25% in the XVE group. The HM II received FDA approval for destination therapy in 2009. While the HeartWare HVAD has not yet received FDA approval for use as destination therapy, the HeartWare ENDURANCE clinical trial has recently concluded demonstrating noninferior 2-year outcomes when compared to the HM II LVAD in patients ineligible for cardiac transplant and will likely result in FDA approval for this indication [8].

IV. **Classification and attachment sites of ventricular assist devices (VADs)**

VADs can be used as an isolated LVAD, an isolated right ventricular assist device (RVAD), or as a biventricular assist device (BIVAD). These devices can be surgically implanted, or inserted percutaneously. TAHs differ from VADs in that a TAH is inserted by resecting both ventricles, and anastomosing the sewing cuffs of the TAH to the mitral and tricuspid annuli (Fig. 22.5). In contrast, if a BIVAD is implanted, the LV and RV remain in place, but the pulmonary and systemic circulations are redirected through the VADs.

A. **Left ventricular assist device (LVAD)**

For left-sided circulatory support, the inflow for all of the approved devices resides in the LV, with the exception of TandemHeart, which has a cannula in the left atrium. **The LV apex is the preferred site of LVAD attachment for most of the long-term devices.** The Impella platform is placed across the aortic valve, with the inflow in the LV. The left atrium is not the ideal cannulation site for long-term support as the LV may then form large thrombi as a result of blood stasis. In addition, flows through the LVAD are generally higher with LV versus LA cannulation for VAD inflow. For cardiogenic shock where short-term LVAD support is anticipated, left atrial cannulation is a reasonable option. **The LVAD outflow graft is routinely anastomosed to the aorta**, usually the ascending aorta. The Impella outflow is immediately distal to the aortic valve and the TandemHeart outflow is in the femoral artery for retrograde flow into the aorta.

B. **Right ventricular assist device (RVAD)**

For right-sided support, either **right atrial or RV cannulation can be used successfully**. Substantial thrombus formation in the RV does not appear to result from right atrial cannulation even in long-term support, although this experience is limited. **The RVAD outflow graft is anastomosed to the pulmonary artery.** VADs can be implanted without the support of cardiopulmonary bypass (CPB), but CPB is generally used to maintain patient stability [8].

C. **Biventricular assist device (BIVAD)**

A BIVAD (Fig. 22.6) consists of the simultaneous use of RVAD and LVAD with connections as noted earlier for the individual assist devices. A combination of short- and long-term devices can be used in a BIVAD configuration if required.

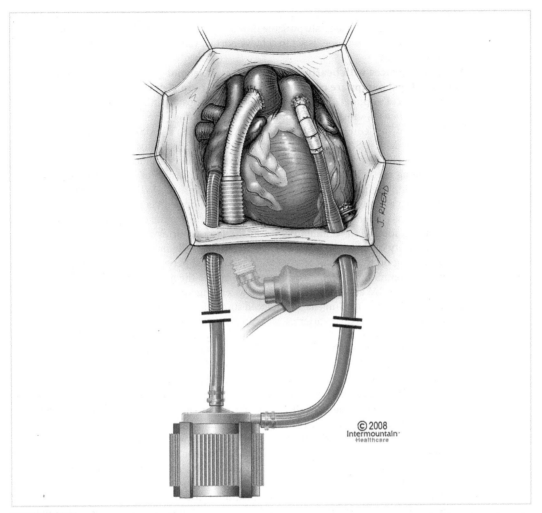

FIGURE 22.6 Illustration of the Centrimag continuous-flow VAD positioned as an RVAD with inflow from the right atrium and outflow into the pulmonary artery. Also pictured is an HM II LVAD with inflow from the LV apex and outflow into the ascending aorta. (Reproduced with permission from Thoratec, Inc., Pleasanton, CA, USA.)

D. Total artificial heart (TAH)

Placement of a TAH requires excision of the native ventricle. The SynCardia TAH requires removal of the ventricles, preserving the tricuspid and mitral annulus for securing the device. Valves are located in both the inlet (atrioventricular) and the outlet (aortic or pulmonary) positions. Separate graft conduits connect the two pumping chambers to the aorta and main pulmonary artery.

V. Mechanical assistance systems

A variety of mechanical support systems are used to treat patients with end-stage heart failure. While early-generation pumps were pulsatile, all currently available devices (with the exception of the Syncardia TAH) are continuous-flow devices. The current technologies include axial flow (HM II, Impella) and centrifugal designs (HeartMate3, HVAD, TandemHeart).

A. Pulsatile

Pulsatile pumps are generally volume displacement pumps that work like the native heart. These are often called first-generation pumps. The pumping chamber fills for a set duration of time, and this volume of blood is ejected into the aorta. Pulsatile pumps all have inflow and outflow valves mimicking the native mitral and aortic valves. The Syncardia TAH is pneumatically driven to generate pulsatile flow similar to the native heart. The device rate and percent systole (ejection time) is set to achieve normal values for cardiac output.

B. Continuous flow

Axial flow devices with bearings are considered "second-generation" devices, whereas the centrifugal pumps are considered "third-generation" devices.

1. **Short-term support.** Three continuous-flow pumps are currently being utilized in the United States as short-term support devices: CentriMag (Thoratec Corp., Pleasanton, CA, USA), the TandemHeart (TandemLife, Inc., Pittsburgh, PA, USA), and Impella (Abiomed, Danvers, MA, USA). The CentriMag pump (Fig. 22.5) is most commonly utilized with an open chest implantation with left atrial or LV inflow cannulation for the LVAD, and ascending aortic cannulation for outflow. The right atrium or RV can be cannulated for inflow and the pulmonary artery as outflow for an RVAD. The TandemHeart pump is attractive as a percutaneous LVAD. The inflow is placed via the right common femoral vein, across the intra-atrial septum into the left atrium. The outflow is in the descending thoracic aorta via a cannula placed in the femoral artery. The Impella system comes in a variety of sizes and can be placed percutaneously or via cutdown through a graft, depending on the goals of treatment. When placed percutaneously, typically it is placed via the common femoral artery, retrograde across the aortic valve into the LV. Inflow is through the LV and outflow is into the ascending aorta—the VAD is placed across the aortic valve. A larger Impella 5.0 is placed surgically through a cutdown and vascular graft in the femoral or axillary arteries, and can provide up to 5 L/min of flow.

2. **Long-term support.** The two most commonly used continuous-flow LVADs are the Thoratec HM II LVAD and the Heartware HVAD. The HM II was FDA approved as a bridge to transplantation in 2008 and received FDA approval for use as destination therapy in January 2010. While the HeartWare HVAD has received FDA approval for the indication of bridge-to-transplant, its use as a destination therapy is not yet approved in the United States. The ENDURANCE trial is a randomized controlled trial comparing Heartware HVAD to the HM II LVAD for destination therapy [8]. The authors found that the HVAD was noninferior to the HM II at 2 years with respect to stroke-free survival, and device malfunction or removal. The HM3 has completed enrollment and is currently available only via the continued access protocol. Early results have been favorable relative to the HM II [9].

3. **Advantages and disadvantages. Continuous-flow devices offer the advantage of being much smaller than their pulsatile counterparts, as no "blood chamber" is needed.** Their smaller size often leads to easier implantation with less intraoperative dissection. This can reduce blood loss, shorten operative times, reduce infection rates, and provide the potential for more rapid patient recovery. The data generated from the outcomes with utilization of continuous-flow devices as a bridge-to-transplant indication show excellent 1-year survival, approaching 90%. The 2-year survival for the cohort that received the HM II for destination therapy was 58%, and continues to improve with recent experience [10–12].

4. Continuous-flow devices pose inherent challenges. These devices do not have valves and need to flow a minimum rate to prevent stasis and thrombus formation. In addition, as patients are managed with long-term devices, certain complications that are device related have emerged. The HM II LVAD universally cleaves von Willebrand factor (vWF). Nearly all patients with an HM II LVAD acquire a deficiency in vWF and are prone to mucosal bleeding events—particularly in the gastrointestinal tract [13]. The recently available HeartMate3 is a magnetically levitated centrifugal pump, and recent studies have demonstrated a decrease in the rate of pump thrombus, while providing full circulatory support [9]. The mag-lev design allows for a bearingless design, which reduces friction, heat, and wear, which are responsible for thrombus formation and device malfunction. **Many patients have minimal arterial pulsatility when on full support.** This is not generally problematic when arterial pressure is monitored with an indwelling arterial

catheter, but may become so when the patient leaves the intensive care unit (ICU) or leaves the hospital for home or an extended care facility. In most cases, an automated blood pressure (BP) cuff is inaccurate, and manual Doppler monitoring of BP is required.

VI. Intraoperative considerations

A. Anesthetic considerations

1. **Monitoring:** Standard American Society of Anesthesiologists monitors (electrocardiography [ECG], pulse oximetry, temperature) are used with the possible exception of a noninvasive BP cuff. As noted earlier, an arterial catheter is essential and consideration might be given to its placement in a larger central artery such as the femoral artery, in order to minimize the potential problem of central-to-peripheral BP discrepancies at separation from CPB or thereafter. Monitoring cerebral oxygenation using near-infrared spectroscopy (NIRS) technology is recommended, especially since the absence of pulsatile blood flow will render conventional pulse oximetry unreliable. Pulmonary artery catheters can be very helpful for the assessment of RV function and pulmonary vascular resistance (PVR), but they may be mechanically infeasible after initiation of therapy with RVAD, BIVAD, or TAH. **Intraoperative transesophageal echocardiography is essential** for the assessment of aortic valve competency, patent foramen ovale (PFO), LV thrombus, adequacy of VAD inflow and outflow, cardiac preload assessment, and RV function (for isolated LVADs).

> **CLINICAL PEARL** Intraoperative transesophageal echocardiography should focus on aortic valve competence, intracardiac shunts, LV thrombus, positioning of LVAD inflow cannula, cardiac preload, and RV function.

2. **Cardiac rhythm management device:** Many of these patients will have an implanted cardiac rhythm management device (automatic implantable cardioverter-defibrillator and/or pacemaker) that requires a management plan prior to proceeding with induction of anesthesia. The antiarrhythmia functions will need to be turned off so they are not triggered by electrocautery during surgery. As soon as such deactivation occurs, patients require continuous ECG monitoring and external cardioversion capability needs to be immediately available. Management of the pacemaker function is dependent on the patient's underlying rhythm, the device's current settings, and its pacing activity. Please see Chapter 18 for these considerations. Once the surgery is completed, it is critical to reinstate antiarrhythmia functions and interrogate the device.

> **CLINICAL PEARL** Dysrhythmias can be particularly detrimental in the setting of depressed ventricular function. External defibrillator pads should be placed on the patient prior to induction of anesthesia.

3. **Vascular access: Large-bore vascular access is required** because blood loss and coagulopathy can be substantial. This can be achieved with one large-bore (16 gauge or larger) peripheral intravenous catheter and a large-lumen (e.g., 9-Fr) central-access introducer or with its equivalent via central venous access (e.g., a pulmonary artery catheter introducer with additional double-lumen large-bore integral ports).

4. **Anesthetic techniques. General endotracheal anesthesia is used, and most practitioners probably place emphasis on use of drugs that minimize hemodynamic impact.** Anesthetic drugs should be titrated carefully, accounting for slower circulation time and a lower volume of distribution for drugs in heart failure patients. Hypoxia and hypercarbia can further impair myocardial function and increase PVR. Hence, periods of apnea should be avoided and ventilation continued even when performing a rapid sequence induction.

    Pre-existing inotropic and vasoactive drugs should be continued. Patients often present with high levels of intrinsic sympathetic tone to the operating room and induction of anesthesia frequently is followed by marked hypotension. In addition to careful titration of anesthetic drugs, starting a low-dose vasoactive infusion, such as norepinephrine, prior to induction may preempt such effects.

Secondary organ dysfunction should be considered in the choice of anesthetic drugs, for example, cisatracurium would be appropriate as a muscle relaxant in a patient with impaired liver function. Nitrous oxide probably should be avoided because of its potential to increase PVR and the high risk of intravascular air.

> **CLINICAL PEARL** Arrhythmia can be detrimental to an already marginal cardiac output and the anesthesiologist should be prepared for immediate cardioversion if needed. Therefore, external pacing pads should be placed on the patient and connected to a defibrillator prior to induction.

  B. Surgical techniques
  1. **Cannulation techniques**
     a. **VADs: VAD implantation is most commonly performed using CPB without myocardial arrest.** Atrial cannulation is the most common approach to gain inflow for short-term support when using either a right- or left-sided VAD system. The atria are easily accessed and the low pressures in these chambers facilitate hemostasis upon decannulation when the heart has recovered. The right atrial appendage is used for right-sided support. For left-sided support, the interatrial groove at the junction of the right superior pulmonary vein or the left atrial appendage are the most common sites for cannulation. Other cannulation options for left-sided support include the dome of the left atrium (between the aorta and superior vena cava), or through the apex of the LV. Cannulation of the LV apex for inflow minimizes blood stasis in the ventricle and provides the best decompression of the heart, which may aid in myocardial recovery in short-term usage. However, decannulation and repair of this high-pressure chamber can be difficult and often requires placement back onto CPB. LV apex cannulation is highly recommended when a prosthetic mitral valve is present to maintain blood flow through the valve and prevent thrombus formation. **The LV apex is the sole acceptable inflow cannulation site for most long-term LVADs.**
     b. **TAH.** For implantation of a TAH, excision of the native ventricles must be performed while preserving the atria. After initiation of CPB with bicaval cannulation, the surgeon attaches sewing cuffs that will connect the atria to the TAH pumping chambers, after which the surgeon sews grafts to both the aorta and the main pulmonary artery. After these grafts and cuffs are sewn, leak testing with pressurized saline (tinged with methylene blue) is used. Leak testing is imperative as the suture lines are often inaccessible if bleeding occurs once the TAH is in place. The TAH is then attached to the atrial cuffs followed by the arterial grafts.
  C. Initiation of support for LVAD
  1. **Initial considerations.** Techniques for the initiation of support are similar in all of the pulsatile systems. Ventilation is reestablished and the heart is gradually filled. The assist device is started at a slow rate until adequate preload and afterload are established. **If the ventricle(s) are not decompressed with the initiation of support, inflow obstruction (into the VAD) must be considered.** Pulmonary edema may also develop as the blood backs up into the pulmonary vasculature. If appropriate inflow and outflow cannula placement and decompression of the LV are achieved, transesophageal echocardiography (TEE) should be utilized to identify interventricular septal position. Displacement toward the LV may compromise right heart function by impairing the septal component of RV contraction, and the physical distortion may also induce tricuspid regurgitation. Treatment is by reducing LVAD speed, and increasing medical therapy for RV function, such as inotropes and inhaled pulmonary vasodilators. **Right-sided function may be further compromised by increased** PVR caused by thromboxane A2 and transfusion-induced cytokine activation as a result of CPB [14].

2. **Role of TEE.** Use of TEE to separate from CPB is essential. TEE is used to assess the presence of air in the ventricle or ejecting from the LVAD into the ascending aorta. The chamber that has been cannulated for the inflow of the MCSD should be decompressed. **If the chamber is full, and there is poor device flow, there is a technical issue that needs to be identified and corrected.** If the LV is empty and there is poor flow through the VAD, then there is either inadequate RV preload or right heart failure (which may be primary or secondary to high PVR). As the LV is decompressed and global cardiac output increases, there may be some tolerable physiologic right heart dilation, which may at times be difficult to distinguish from right heart failure. The apical interventricular septum can occasionally deflect leftward and obstruct inflow into the LVAD. This phenomenon is known as a suction event, and results in decreased pump speed and output. When this occurs, it is easily identified by TEE. TEE is also used to identify aortic insufficiency and the presence of intracardiac shunts, either of which may arise at the time of VAD support even if absent before that time.

3. **Aortic insufficiency. Aortic valve insufficiency (AI) can be challenging, and TEE is essential to identify its presence or absence and severity.** Even mild preoperative AI can be problematic since patients in cardiogenic shock will have a low mean arterial pressure (MAP) and a high LV end-diastolic pressure (LVEDP) to produce a relatively low aortic transvalvular diastolic gradient. With implementation of LVAD support, the LVEDP will become very low and the MAP will be higher, so the aortic transvalvular gradient (MAP–LVEDP) will be much greater. Mild preoperative AI, therefore, can become severe AI with LVAD support. This induces high LVAD flows as the insufficient valve fills the LV and subsequently the VAD. The resulting high LVAD flow rates are deceptive, because much of the flow is "circular" from LV to LVAD to ascending aorta and back via the incompetent aortic valve to the LV, so the net forward flow will be low. The aortic valve incompetence must be eliminated in this situation, but the approach is controversial depending on the indications for device implant and expected duration of support (valve replacement vs. permanent valve closure) [15–19].

CLINICAL PEARL Aortic insufficiency in a patient being supported with a continuous-flow LVAD will typically be underestimated due to the continuous nature of the regurgitant jet.

4. **Intracardiac shunts. Quiescent intracardiac shunts may become clinically apparent and significant as a result of changes in chamber pressures when VAD support is initiated.** A PFO is present in up to 20% of the population, but is clinically quiescent in the vast majority of these patients. Upon unloading the LV and left atrium with LVAD support, right atrial pressure will become higher than left atrial pressure. Under these circumstances, even a small PFO can produce a large right-to-left shunt manifested by arterial desaturation and potential paradoxical air embolism. These shunts should be closed when identified and should be assessed by TEE both before and after initiation of VAD support. If identified preoperatively, cannulation techniques for CPB may be altered to facilitate repair.

5. **Pharmacologic support. Inotropic agents (e.g., dobutamine, milrinone, epinephrine) are important to support the right heart when only left-sided support is used. Inhaled nitric oxide or epoprostenol may be invaluable in the early management of these patients because of its capacity to vasodilate the pulmonary vasculature without the systemic hypotensive effects seen with other pulmonary artery vasodilators.** Alternative approaches include the use of a phosphodiesterase inhibitor (e.g., milrinone, which decreases pulmonary and systemic vascular resistances) in combination with a systemic vasoconstrictor such as vasopressin. **Vasopressin offers an advantage over α-adrenergic agonists because it possesses minimal vasoconstrictive effects on the pulmonary arterial vasculature.**

For a variety of reasons, systemic arterial vasodilation commonly occurs after initiation of LVAD support, so need for a systemic vasoconstrictor is common. Antiarrhythmics are initiated as required before weaning from bypass onto device support.

D. Initiation of support for BIVAD

1. **Initial considerations.** When initiating biventricular support, **the left system should be actuated first** to prevent LV overdistention and resultant pulmonary edema. Inotropic support can be totally discontinued, but vasopressor support is often required. Biventricular support allows more complete resting of the heart and usually allows total decompression of the venous system as well. This minimizes hepatic and other end-organ congestion. The PA catheter should not be withdrawn as it will be difficult to reinsert it. Thermodilution cardiac outputs are not calculable when an RVAD is functioning. All available temporary RVADs have accurate flow measurement tools that can replace the need for Swan–Ganz cardiac output monitoring.

2. **Flow rates.** The RVAD and LVAD should both have similar flow rates. The LVAD often has higher flow rates due to physiologic shunts (bronchial arterial return). RVAD flow that exceeds LVAD flow early after initiating BIVAD support is worrisome. This can occur with two common scenarios:

   One or both left-sided cannulae are malpositioned to impede inflow to or from the device. If the obstruction is not corrected, the lungs can become flooded with the increased blood flow from the RVAD.

   The LV is beginning to recover and is ejecting some blood over and above the LVAD flow. This can be identified by the appearance of an arterial pressure waveform corresponding to the QRS complex of the ECG (see weaning from device support).

E. Initiation of support for RVAD

1. **Initial considerations.** Isolated RVAD support is less common than LVAD or BIVAD support, but when used, the essential considerations are similar to LVAD. CPB is weaned rapidly as RVAD support is increased. All currently available devices can overcome elevated PVR, however, significantly elevated pulmonary artery pressures may lead to pulmonary edema.

2. **Pharmacologic support.** In many instances, some inotropic support of the LV will be necessary to handle the increased RV output.

VII. Postoperative management and complications

7

A. Right-sided circulatory failure

Right-sided circulatory management is the key to perioperative care for LVAD patients. Attention to right heart management and PVR is critical. Strategies include pacing (chronotropy), inotropes, and pulmonary vasodilators to increase flow through the pulmonary vascular bed. For additional considerations, see LVAD initiation.

B. Hemorrhage

Postoperative hemorrhage is common in this patient population. Heart failure often leads to hepatic congestion and renal insufficiency. Both of these processes lead to imbalances in platelet function and the coagulation cascade. The addition of CPB and the consumptive coagulopathy that can be initiated can exacerbate postoperative bleeding. In addition, exposing the blood to the foreign surfaces of the extracorporeal circuit and of the conduit cannulae can also lead to a consumptive coagulopathy. It should not be a surprise that postoperative hemorrhage and reexploration for bleeding is a common occurrence. Reexploration for bleeding/tamponade can then be performed when the patient is adequately resuscitated. Use of a thromboelastogram (TEG) and thromboelastometry to help target the deficiency in the clotting process is gaining popularity. Transfused platelets and red blood cells (packed cells or whole blood) in transplant candidates should ideally be leukoreduced, because exogenous leukocytes induce alloimmunization that can develop antibodies against future potential donated organs. High levels of these preformed antibodies reduce the pool of otherwise-suitable donor organs for these patients. Fresh frozen plasma and cryoprecipitate do not have high leukocyte content and do not need filtration.

C. Thromboembolism

Thromboembolism is associated with all current assist systems. The unique design characteristics of each system as well as the patient's underlying pathology establish the overall risk.

Anticoagulation with heparin is required for short-term devices and warfarin and aspirin are required with all long-term assist devices.

D. Infection

Device-related infection is the most common cause of morbidity in the chronically supported patient. Driveline and device "pocket" infections occur in up to 40% of these patients. The vast majority of these infections may be managed with chronic antibiotic therapy until transplantation. Device exchange for infection has not been demonstrated to be universally effective due to necessary replacement of the new pump into an infected field.

E. Device malfunction

Catastrophic device malfunctions occur infrequently but can be life threatening. These include mechanical device failure, device separation or fracture, graft or valve rupture, and console failure. Minor device malfunctions occur more frequently and are usually addressed at the bedside. These include driveline damage and controller malfunctions. All of these malfunctions are becoming increasingly rare as yearly device modifications and software upgrades are introduced.

VIII. Weaning from VAD support

A minority of patients will experience myocardia recovery sufficient for device explantation [20]. For patients in whom the heart recovers, the heart will be able to eject and the arterial waveform will begin to display pulses corresponding to the QRS complex [21]. When the device flows are weaned downward and cardiac preload conditions move toward normal, these ejections will become more prominent. **If the device can be weaned to 1 L/min flow and the patient can maintain adequate perfusion with reasonable inotropic support, explantation can be considered.** This evaluation can be performed in the ICU. TEE can once again be very helpful in assessing cardiac function as the heart is loaded. **Final weaning from the device is accomplished in the operating room, as CPB or surgical cutdown on the access site needed for device explantation.**

IX. Management of the VAD patient for noncardiac surgery

These patients can be very ill if surgery is contemplated early after MCSD implantation. However, patients will often recover physiologically over the ensuing weeks and months. Patients who are stable on support may safely undergo noncardiac surgical procedures [22,23]. The optimal approach involves asking some basic questions:

A. What chamber(s) are being assisted (LVAD, RVAD, BIVAD, or TAH)?

B. What type of pump is being used? All continuous-flow pumps are preload dependent and afterload sensitive, with centrifugal designs in particular impacted by systemic hypertension. Percutaneous and peripherally inserted pumps are also positional and patient movement may impact device functionality.

C. Is technical support personnel available to help manage and troubleshoot the pump? This is critical for transport as well as intraoperative management.

D. **How does one determine flow through the pump?** This can be quantitative or qualitative, depending upon the pump, but knowledge of pump flow clearly assists in determining systemic vascular resistance and PVR, which in turn guide anesthetic drug selection, pharmacologic support, and volume management.

E. Will TEE be helpful? If major volume shifts are anticipated, use of TEE can be very helpful in assessing preload, valvular function, and intracardiac shunts.

F. What is the patient's clotting status? For most pumps, anticoagulation and antiplatelet medications are required. This has major implications for reversal of anticoagulation (if safely possible) and blood component use. Reversal of warfarin and conversion to intravenous heparin may be indicated. In general, be prepared for transfusion of RBCs and other components.

G. What is the patient's intravenous access? Central venous access is desirable in most situations, but large-bore peripheral access is acceptable for minor surgical procedures.

H. What pharmacologic support is the patient receiving? This will vary from no support to multiple inotropes, antiarrhythmics, vasoconstrictors, and pulmonary vasodilators. If nitric oxide is in use, this will require planning for transport and operating room use.

I. Will electrocautery affect the assist device? For most devices, this will not be a problem, but excessive electrocautery can intermittently interfere with the function of coexisting pacemakers or defibrillators. If electrocautery poses a problem, either short bursts may suffice or the use of an ultrasonic scalpel can be considered.

J. Does the patient have a cardiac rhythm management device? If yes, what is the management plan?

K. If defibrillation or electrical cardioversion is needed, how will it be most safely applied?

L. If the patient does not have pulsatile blood flow, consider the use of NIRS technology to monitor cerebral oxygenation as conventional pulse oximetry relies on pulsatile blood flow.

X. Future considerations

A. Totally implantable LVAD

The totally implantable LVAD will need to employ a replenishable source of power with an internal battery reserve. A transcutaneous energy transfer system (TETS) has been employed in the now discontinued AbioCor device as well as LionHeart (Arrow International, Inc., Reading, PA, USA). This has the potential advantage of improved infection risk, as it obviates the percutaneous driveline. This technology is currently limited by the size of the internal battery and skin injury from transcutaneous charging.

B. Miniaturization of LVADs

Continuous evolution of LVAD therapy will result in smaller devices more amenable to minimally invasive surgical approaches, resulting in less physiologic stress to patients and faster recovery.

C. TAH

Use of a TAH has gained traction in the field of MCSD, however, the vast majority of patients can be managed with isolated LV devices. Many patients with biventricular failure can be managed with a long-term LVAD and short-term RVAD. For those patients not suitable for this strategy, TAH therapy is the only option. Outcomes have not yet approached those of isolated LVAD therapy in general use.

XI. Intra-aortic balloon pump (IABP) circulatory assistance

A. Indications for placement

Thought by some to be reserved for placement after one or more failed attempts at separation from CPB, the number of IABPs placed in the cardiac catheterization laboratory approaches or exceeds the number placed intraoperatively. Interventional cardiologists often place IABPs when high-grade lesions of proximal coronary vessels supplying large regions of myocardium are diagnosed, or when myocardial ischemia persists or MI occurs after an intervention such as coronary stent placement. Retrospective outcome studies for preoperative versus intraoperative placement of IABP for coronary artery bypass graft (CABG) patients suggest that preoperative IABP placement improves outcome and shortens hospital stay, especially for patients with low ejection fractions or those undergoing urgent or emergent CABG [24]. Indications for intraoperative IABP placement vary widely among centers and even among or within surgical teams. LV failure despite moderate- to high-dose inotropic support and/or evidence of ongoing regional myocardial ischemia that is not amenable to surgical revascularization constitutes the primary intraoperative indications. Moderately severe LV failure despite reasonable inotropic support that is thought to derive from an injury that will resolve (or greatly improve) within 24 to 48 hours (e.g., LV stunning) constitutes the most common intraoperative indication. The definitions of "LV failure," "maximal inotropic support," and "ongoing regional myocardial ischemia" may vary widely among surgeons and anesthesiologists. Independent predictors of death among patients with intraoperative IABP insertion include New York Heart Association class III or IV symptom level, mitral valve replacement or repair, prolonged CPB, urgent or emergent operation, emergent reinstitution of CPB, preoperative renal dysfunction, diabetes mellitus, RV failure, complex ventricular ectopy, pacer dependence, and IABP placement via the ascending aorta. IABP assistance can be used during high-risk off-pump CABG as well, where the support of coronary perfusion pressure may be especially helpful while the heart is placed in positions that compromise cardiac filling or emptying. Rarely, prophylactic IABP placement may be appropriate for high-risk urgent noncardiac surgery.

B. **Contraindications to placement**

1. **Aortic insufficiency.** Use of the IABP is relatively contraindicated in patients with AI. As the IABP inflates in the descending aorta during diastole to promote retrograde flow into the ascending aorta, this potentially increases aortic valvular regurgitation, further distending the LV at the expense of coronary perfusion.

2. **Sepsis.** As with any prosthetic intravascular device, bacteremic infections are difficult to treat if the prosthetic surfaces become seeded with bacteria.

3. **Severe vascular disease.** Placement of an IABP may be technically difficult in patients with atherosclerosis or other vascular pathologies. Such patients are more prone to arterial thrombosis during use of an IABP. Patients with abdominal aortic aneurysms are at increased risk for aortic rupture, although balloons have been successfully passed and used in such patients. For patients with severe aortoiliac or femoral arterial disease, another option is to place the balloon directly into the descending thoracic aorta. Alternatively, placement may be performed through a small vascular graft sewn to the subclavian artery. These options require a subsequent trip to the operating room to remove the device when such support becomes unnecessary.

C. **Functional design**

The IABP consists of an inflatable balloon at the end of a catheter that is typically advanced into the descending thoracic aorta percutaneously from the groin (Fig. 22.4). The balloon inflates during diastole, displacing blood from the thoracic aorta and increasing aortic diastolic pressure. Balloon inflation improves coronary perfusion pressure, increasing coronary blood flow to both the LV and the RV. During early systole, rapid balloon deflation reduces LV afterload and wall tension. IABP can improve myocardial energy balance at most by 15%. The IABP drive console consists of a pressurized gas reservoir that is connected to the balloon supply line through an electronically controlled solenoid valve. The gas used to inflate the balloon is either CO_2 or helium. The advantage of CO_2 is its high blood solubility, which reduces the consequences of balloon rupture with potential gas embolization. The advantage of helium is its low density, which thereby decreases the Reynolds number and allows the same flow through a smaller driveline. A tube with a smaller diameter decreases the potential for injury to the artery.

D. **IABP placement**

Insertion of the IABP is usually accomplished either percutaneously or by surgical cutdown into the femoral artery using the Seldinger technique for placement of a large-diameter introducer. Accurate placement of the Seldinger wire is often confirmed intraoperatively using TEE.

The balloon is passed through the introducer.

The balloon is ideally positioned so that its tip is at the junction of the descending aorta and the aortic arch, just distal to the origin of the subclavian artery, as shown in Figure 22.6. This positioning minimizes the risk of subclavian or renal artery injury or occlusion. Radiographically, the tip should lie between the anterior portion of the second intercostal space and the first lumbar vertebra.

When the IABP is placed intraoperatively, transesophageal echocardiography can confirm proper tip location before initiation of balloon assistance. Fluoroscopy, if available, can also facilitate positioning.

CLINICAL PEARL Intraoperative placement of an IABP will typically require TEE guidance for positioning: the tip of the catheter should be approximately 2 cm from the subclavian artery.

E. **IABP control**

Several parameters are important during the setup and operation of an IABP.

1. **Synchronization of the IABP.** Synchronization of the IABP with the cardiac rhythm is accomplished by using either the electrocardiographic QRS complex or the arterial pressure waveform. If there is a natural pulse pressure greater than 40 mm Hg, use of the arterial waveform for synchronization is often preferred in the operating room because

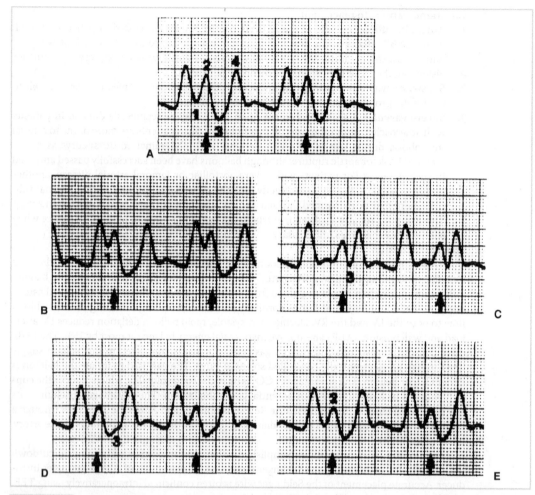

FIGURE 22.7 Manipulation of the timing of inflation and deflation of IABP. Tracings illustrate 1:2 support for the sake of clarity. **A:** Normal tracing. Augmentation commences after the dicrotic notch (*1*) augments diastolic pressure (*2*), and reaches its nadir just before the next contraction (*3*). Peak systolic pressure in the next (nonaugmented) beat is decreased (*4*). **B:** Early inflation. Augmentation commences before aortic valve closure (*1*), thereby increasing afterload and possibly inducing aortic regurgitation. **C:** Late inflation. Diastolic augmentation is inadequate, and end-diastolic pressure is not different from that in the unassisted cycle (*3*). **D:** Early deflation. Diastolic augmentation and afterload reduction are impaired. **E:** Inadequate filling time. Timing is satisfactory, but diastolic augmentation is impaired. (From Sladen RN. Management of the adult cardiac patient in the intensive care unit. In: Ream AK, Fogdall RP, eds. *Acute Cardiovascular Management in Anesthesia and Intensive Care.* Philadelphia, PA: Lippincott; 1982:509.)

the electrical artifact produced by electrocautery inhibits ECG-triggered IABP control units. Recent monitoring systems have advanced suppression circuitry designed to reduce electrical noise from electrocautery. Most current consoles can differentiate pacer spikes from a QRS complex, allowing proper timing of IABP inflation even when atrial or atrioventricular pacing is in use, but pacer interference should be considered in the differential diagnosis of faulty IABP timing.

2. **Timing of balloon inflation and deflation.** When setting the timing of IABP inflation (Fig. 22.7), it is important to time the onset of the pressure rise caused by balloon inflation with the dicrotic notch of the arterial waveform, which signifies aortic valve closure and the start of diastole. If inflation begins sooner, the IABP will impede ventricular ejection. If it begins later, the effectiveness of the balloon in augmenting coronary perfusion and

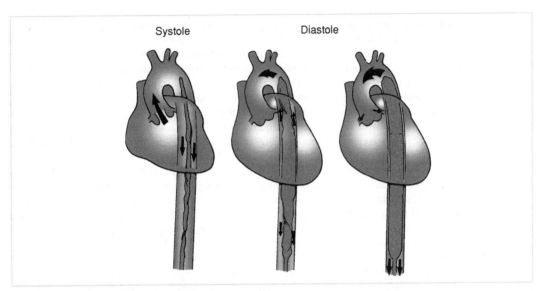

Systole   Diastole

FIGURE 22.8 Placement of the IABP in the aorta. The IABP is shown in the descending aorta, with the tip at the distal aortic arch. During systole the balloon is deflated to enhance ventricular ejection. During diastole the balloon inflates, forcing blood from the proximal aorta into the coronary and peripheral vessels.

reducing afterload will be limited. Deflation should be timed so that the arterial pressure just reaches its minimum level at the onset of the next ventricular pulse. If it deflates too soon, the aorta will not be maximally evacuated before ventricular contraction, and coronary perfusion will not be optimized. If the balloon deflates too late, it will impede LV ejection. Most modern balloon devices use an intra-aortic arterial waveform obtained from the tip of the balloon catheter. If this mechanism should fail and synchronization should be monitored from another site, subtle differences in optimal timing may occur (e.g., balloon inflation and deflation as judged by a femoral arterial waveform are delayed in comparison to an intra-aortic or radial arterial waveform) (Fig. 22.8).

3. **Ratio of native ventricle pulsations to IABP pulsation.** Pumping is frequently initiated at a ratio of 1:2 (one IABP beat for every two cardiac beats), so the natural ventricular beats and augmented beats can be compared to determine IABP timing and efficacy. Depending on the patient's condition, the ratio will often be increased to 1:1 to obtain maximal benefit.

4. **Stroke volume of the balloon.** The volume of gas used to inflate the balloon is determined by the balloon used and the patient's size. Exceeding the volume for which the balloon was designed risks rupture with arterial gas embolization. Typically, balloon volume is set to 50% to 60% of the patient's ideal stroke volume [25].

5. **Balloon filling.** The time required for the balloon to fill and empty is determined by the density of the gas used, gas pressure, the length and diameter of the gas line, and balloon volume. These values are usually constant for any particular balloon. At high heart rates, the time required for balloon filling may limit balloon stroke volume.

F. **IABP weaning**

Weaning the patient from IABP circulatory assistance should be considered when inotropic support has been reduced substantially, allowing "room" to increase inotropic support as IABP support is reduced. Weaning is done primarily by gradually (over 6 to 12 hours) decreasing the ratio of augmented to native heartbeats (from 1:1 to 1:2 to 1:4 or less) and/or decreasing balloon inflation volume while maintaining acceptable hemodynamics, which often necessitates a concomitant increase in inotropic support. The balloon is never turned off while it remains in the aorta except when the patient is anticoagulated, as during CPB, because of the risk of thrombus formation on the balloon or balloon catheter. Comparison of intra-arterial pressure tracings of augmented ventricular pulsations to native pulsations can serve as an indicator of ventricular performance. As ventricular performance improves, the amplitude of the native pressure tracing will increase relative to the augmented pressure tracing. By comparing the magnitude of these two pulses over time, one can obtain a qualitative assessment of ventricular performance. Once the IABP is removed, it is important to continue close examination of the distal ipsilateral leg because partial or total femoral arterial occlusion may occur.

G. Management of anticoagulation during IABP assistance

During extended IABP use, anticoagulation is generally indicated. In the immediate post-CPB period, anticoagulants are not to be required for the first few hours or until drainage from the chest tubes is acceptable (less than 100 to 150 mL/hr). Heparin can prevent IABP-related thrombosis and its ready reversibility offers appeal. Evidence suggests a no-heparin IABP protocol provides acceptable low rates of thrombus formation with less bleeding complications than when anticoagulation is used. The surgeon should weigh the risks of thrombus formation with prolonged heparin-free IABP use against the risk of excessive bleeding when using anticoagulation [24]. If heparin is used, adequate anticoagulation should be confirmed every 4 to 6 hours with activated clotting time (ACT) or activated partial thromboplastin time (aPTT) maintained at 1.5 to 2 times normal values.

H. Complications

The incidence of IABP complications has decreased significantly from its early use, but significant morbidities persist. The most frequent complications are vascular in nature, with a reported incidence of 6% to 33% [25]. These complications include events such as limb ischemia, compartment syndrome, mesenteric infarction, aortic perforation, and aortic dissection. Risk factors for these complications include a history of peripheral vascular disease, female gender, tobacco smoking, diabetes mellitus, and postoperative IABP placement. Because of small femoral artery size and the likelihood of concurrent peripheral vascular disease, a common expression among cardiac surgeons is "little old ladies and balloon pumps don't mix." Other complications include infection, primarily at the groin site of a transcutaneous introducer, and coagulopathies (especially thrombocytopenia). Neurologic complications include paresthesia, ischemic neuritis, neuralgia, footdrop, and rarely paraplegia [26]. Balloon rupture with gas embolus can occur presumably as a result of severe aortic atherosclerotic calcifications. When this occurs, blood is usually seen in the gas driveline and the arterial pressure deflection caused by the IABP is lost. Most pumps have an alarm that indicates low balloon pressure. Air embolism from the pressure monitoring line to the brain is a larger risk from the IABP than from a radial artery catheter, because the monitoring port is located at the tip of the balloon catheter, which is close to the origin of the carotid arteries. Arterial blood gases should be drawn through the IABP pressure monitoring line only if no other locations are available, paying meticulous attention to ensure that no air bubbles or other debris are flushed through the tubing.

I. Limitations

The ability of the IABP to augment cardiac output and unload the LV is limited, because the IABP does not directly affect LV function. With severe LV failure, an IABP will not provide sufficient flow to sustain the circulation. When the LV cannot eject blood into the aorta, the IABP will simply cause pulsations in the arterial waveform without increasing blood flow. In this situation, a VAD must be considered, although readily correctable technical problems with the IABP, such as malpositioning, kinking of the gas line, or improper inflation–deflation timing, should be considered. Early IABPs were not effective during rapid cardiac rhythms. Improvements in the pneumatic circuitry and compressor response time now permit some IABP models to provide hemodynamic improvement at rates up to 190 beats/min. Irregular heart rhythms persist as a limitation to IABP efficacy, because optimal timing of inflation and deflation cannot be achieved with large variations in the R–R interval.

REFERENCES

1. Ross JN Jr, Akers WW, O'Bannon W, et al. Problems encountered during the development and implantation of the Baylor-Rice orthotopic cardiac prosthesis. *Trans Am Soc Artif Intern Organs.* 1972;18(0):168–175, 179.

2. Norman JC, Brook MI, Cooley DA, et al. Total support of the circulation of a patient with post-cardiotomy stone-heart syndrome by a partial artificial heart (ALVAD) for 5 days followed by heart and kidney transplantation. *Lancet.* 1978;1(8074): 1125–1127.

3. Joyce LD, DeVries WC, Hastings WL, et al. Response of the human body to the first permanent implant of the Jarvik-7 total artificial heart. *Trans Am Soc Artif Intern Organs.* 1983;29:81–87.

4. **Rose E, Gelijns A, Moskowitz AJ, et al. Long-term use of a left ventricular assist device for end-stage heart failure. *N Engl J Med.* 2001;345(20):1435–1443.**

5. Konstantinov BA, Dzemeshkevich SL, Rogov KA, et al. Extracorporeal mechanical pulsatile pump and its significance for myocardial function recovery and circulatory support. *Artif Organs.* 1991;15(5):363–368.

6. **Miller LW, Pagani FD, Russell SD, et al. Use of a continuous-flow device in patients awaiting heart transplantation. *N Engl J Med.* 2007;357(9):885–896.**

7. **Aaronson KD, Slaughter MS, Miller LW, et al. Use of an intrapericardial, continuous-flow, centrifugal pump in patients awaiting heart transplantation. *Circulation.* 2012;125(25):3191–3200.**

8. **Rogers JG, Pagani FD, Tatooles AJ, et al. Intrapericardial left ventricular assist device for advanced heart failure. *N Engl J Med.* 2017;376(5):451–460.**

9. **Mehra MR, Naka Y, Uriel N, et al. A fully magnetically levitated circulatory pump for advanced heart failure. *N Engl J Med.* 2017;376(5):440–450.**

10. John R, Naka Y, Smedira NG, et al. Continuous flow left ventricular assist device outcomes in commercial use compared with the prior clinical trial. *Ann Thorac Surg.* 2011;92(4):1406–1413.

11. **John R, Kamdar F, Eckman P, et al. Lessons learned from experience with over 100 consecutive HeartMate II left ventricular assist devices. *Ann Thorac Surg.* 2011;92(5):1593–1599; discussion 1599–1600.**

12. **Schmitto JD, Zimpfer D, Fiane AE, et al. Long-term support of patients receiving a left ventricular assist device for advanced heart failure: a follow-up analysis of the registry to evaluate the HeartWare left ventricular assist system. *Eur J Cardiothorac Surg.* 2016;50(5):834–838.**

13. **Crow S, Chen D, Milano C, et al. Acquired von Willebrand syndrome in continuous-flow ventricular assist device recipients. *Ann Thorac Surg.* 2010;90(4):1263–1269; discussion 1269.**

14. Shenkar R, Coulson WF, Abraham E. Hemorrhage and resuscitation induce alterations in cytokine expression and the development of acute lung injury. *Am J Respir Cell Mol Biol.* 1994;10(3):290–297.

15. Atkins B, Hashmi ZA, Ganapathi AM, et al. Surgical correction of aortic valve insufficiency after left ventricular assist device implantation. *J Thorac Cardiovasc Surg.* 2013;146(5):1247–1252.

16. Bryant AS, Holman WL, Nanda NC, et al. Native aortic valve insufficiency in patients with left ventricular assist devices. *Ann Thorac Surg.* 2006;81(2):e6–e8.

17. **Rajagopal K, Daneshmand MA, Patel CB, et al. Natural history and clinical effect of aortic valve regurgitation after left ventricular assist device implantation. *J Thorac Cardiovasc Surg.* 2013;145(5):1373–1379.**

18. Savage EB, d'Amato TA, Magovern JA. Aortic valve patch closure: an alternative to replacement with HeartMate LVAS insertion. *Eur J Cardiothorac Surg.* 1999;16(3):359–361.

19. Pal JD, McCabe JM, Dardas T, et al. Transcatheter aortic valve repair for management of aortic insufficiency in patients supported with left ventricular assist devices. *J Card Surg.* 2016;31(10):654–657.

20. Helman DN, Maybaum SW, Morales DL, et al. Recurrent remodeling after ventricular assistance: is long-term myocardial recovery attainable? *Ann Thorac Surg.* 2000;70(4):1255–1258.

21. Birks EJ, Tansley PD, Hardy J, et al. Left ventricular assist device and drug therapy for the reversal of heart failure. *N Engl J Med.* 2006;355(18):1873–1884.

22. Garatti A, Bruschi G, Colombo T, et al. Noncardiac surgical procedures in patient supported with long-term implantable left ventricular assist device. *Am J Surg.* 2009;197(6):710–714.

23. Goldstein DJ, Mullis SL, Delphin ES, et al. Noncardiac surgery in long-term implantable left ventricular assist-device recipients. *Ann Surg.* 1995;222(2):203–207.

24. Kogan A, Preisman S, Sternik L, et al. Heparin-free management of intra-aortic balloon pump after cardiac surgery. *J Card Surg.* 2012;27(4):434–437.

25. **Webb CA, Weyker PD, Flynn BC. Management of intra-aortic balloon pumps. *Semin Cardiothorac Vasc Anesth.* 2015;19(2):106–121.**

26. Hurlé A, Llamas P, Meseguer J, et al. Paraplegia complicating intraaortic balloon pumping. *Ann Thorac Surg.* 1997;63(4): 1217–1218.

23

Intraoperative Myocardial Protection

Pedro Catarino, David Philip Jenkins, and Kamen Valchanov

KEY POINTS

1. Aortic cross-clamping is a key step in the vast majority of cardiac surgical procedures, initiating a period of global ischemia of the myocardium.
2. Inadequate myocardial protection remains one of the main causes of postoperative low cardiac output syndrome.
3. Removal of the aortic cross-clamp results in reperfusion of the myocardium and resumption of electromechanical activity but produces a variable ischemia–reperfusion injury, attenuation of which remains the subject of research.
4. Cardioplegia is the predominant technique of intraoperative myocardial protection.
5. The key components of most forms of cardioplegia are hyperkalemia and hypothermia. The hyperkalemia produces electromechanical arrest of the myocardium in diastole, and the hypothermia lengthens the arrest time and further reduces myocardial metabolic activity.
6. Cardioplegia exists in numerous different recipes and various forms of delivery are possible, with little hard evidence to favor any particular strategy.
7. With appropriate intraoperative myocardial protection, the heart will generally comfortably tolerate 120 minutes of ischemia time, after which additional time will come at a cost of increased risk of low cardiac output syndrome.

I. Introduction

Operations on the heart are best performed in a still and bloodless field. This necessitates interruption of blood flow to the heart, at least intermittently. Minimization of injury resulting from this ischemic challenge is the objective of intraoperative myocardial protection. Since the interruption of blood flow is a deliberate sequenced event, there exists the opportunity to set up optimal conditions in which this can occur.

Optimal intraoperative myocardial protection results from a collaboration between surgeon, anesthesiologist, and perfusionist. However, with the surgeon focused on the technical aspect of the procedure and the perfusionist on the conduct of cardiopulmonary bypass (CPB), the anesthesiologist has a particular responsibility to pick up subtle changes in monitoring which might herald inadequate protection.

> **CLINICAL PEARL**   Teamwork, the hallmark of high-functioning cardiac surgery teams, is especially important during cardioplegia administration, as this is perhaps the most important determinant of post-bypass cardiac function.

The context of the myocardial protection is important; for example, the setting of acute myocardial infarction might represent a different challenge to that of the chronically hypertrophied left ventricle. *Integration of general anesthetic principles, conduct of CPB, type of cardioplegia, and nature of delivery are keys to a successful outcome to the procedure.*

II. History

A. The field of intraoperative myocardial protection has evolved from and with the development of CPB in 1953. Although CPB kept the patient's organs perfused while the heart was arrested and decompressed, the requirement for a bloodless field almost invariably necessitated cross-clamping of the aorta with consequent global ischemia of the myocardium.

B. The early years of cardiac surgery involved little attention to myocardial ischemia with surgeons attempting to operate expeditiously during periods of normothermic ischemia. In 1955, Melrose introduced hyperkalemic arrest primarily to provide a still heart for surgery rather than to provide protection from ischemia. This approach frequently proved inadequate with increasingly recognized low cardiac output syndrome and occasionally the development of *"stone heart."*[1] However, the idea that cessation of electromechanical activity was important to myocardial protection had been established, and Lam first used the term cardioplegia (*Greek cardio, heart; plegia, paralysis*) in 1957.

C. In 1956, Lillehei maintained perfusion of the heart during cross-clamping with retrograde perfusion via a catheter in the coronary sinus.

D. Topical cooling was used for myocardial protection in the form of iced slush by Hufnagel in 1961 and iced saline by Shumway in 1964.

E. Continuous coronary perfusion by cannulae placed in the coronary ostia was championed by McGoon in 1965 and remains in use today. In practice it is cumbersome, with leaking cannulae and the risk of coronary ostial damage limiting its use.

F. The first pharmacologic interventions to deliberately address intraoperative myocardial protection did not come until later in the 1960s. There were two relatively distinct forms of cardioplegia, which both used hyperkalemia to produce a depolarization of the myocyte resting potential, arresting the heart in diastole.

   1. Bretschneider (1964) solution was a sodium-poor, calcium-free, procaine-containing solution which, apart from potassium of 10 mmol/L, resembled the intracellular electrolyte milieu.

   2. Hearse and Braimbridge (1975) developed St. Thomas solution, which was hyperkalemic (initially 20 mmol/L, now 16 mmol/L) with an otherwise extracellular electrolyte milieu.

G. Buckberg (1970s) introduced the use of blood as a vehicle for cardioplegia, and this has become the most widely used format worldwide.

H. Substrate enhancement, variation in the temperature of administration, and mode and route of delivery together have produced an enormous variety of options for hyperkalemic depolarizing intraoperative myocardial protection.

I. Alternative forms of pharmacologic cardioplegia seeking to avoid hyperkalemia and depolarization remain under investigation and are largely the preserve of special interest groups.

> **CLINICAL PEARL**   Over the past 75 years, the field of myocardial protection has evolved to the point where it is now used routinely, safely, and effectively.

III. Myocardial energetics

A. The heart has a very high basal oxygen consumption (8 to 10 mL O_2/min/100 g) and the highest oxygen extraction of a major organ (10 to 13 mL O_2/100 mL or 70% of the oxygen content). Basal coronary blood flow is 1 mL/min/100 g or about 250 mL/min—5% of the cardiac output.

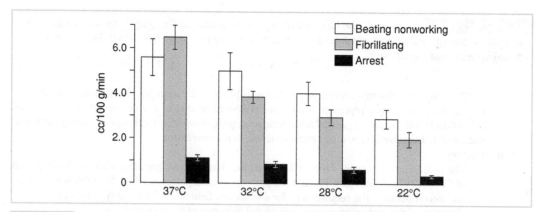

FIGURE 23.1 Oxygen consumption under different conditions in the canine heart. (From Buckberg GD, Brazier JR, Nelson RL, et al. Studies of the effects of hypothermia on regional myocardial blood flow and metabolism during cardiopulmonary bypass. I. The adequately perfused beating, fibrillating, and arrested heart. *J Thorac Cardiovasc Surg.* 1977;73:87–94, with permission.)

In normal coronary arteries, autoregulation between a mean systemic pressure of 60 mm Hg and 140 mm Hg matches coronary blood flow to oxygen demand with up to fivefold increases in coronary blood flow—25% of the cardiac output.

B. In the aerobic state, the heart can use a variety of energy substrates. In the fasting state, 70% is from free fatty acids with the remainder from glucose, but after a meal, this can change to 100% glucose and other carbohydrates. During exercise, lactate can be utilized. Ketone bodies, acetate, pyruvate, and amino acids are other potential sources.

C. Despite this variety of energy substrates, oxidative phosphorylation is responsible for nearly all the production of adenosine triphosphate (ATP), making the heart highly dependent on a continuous supply of oxygen. Thirty-eight moles of ATP will be produced by aerobic metabolism of 1 mole of glucose. Anaerobic enzymes are not present in sufficient concentration to make a significant contribution and under anaerobic conditions ATP production is just 2 moles per mole of glucose.

D. The rate of myocardial oxygen consumption (MvO_2) is therefore indicative of the metabolic demand of the heart and has been commonly used to estimate the energy requirement of the heart under different conditions. The well-known results from Buckberg's work shown in Figure 23.1 [1] demonstrate the reduction in energy requirement by one-third when work is not performed, such as on CPB (i.e., 5.6 mL O_2/min/100 g) and by 90% when the heart is electromechanically arrested (1.1 mL O_2/min/100 g). Further stepwise reductions in energy expenditure result from cooling, with 50% reduction for every 10°C.

CLINICAL PEARL Electromechanical cardioplegic arrest brings a 90% reduction in myocardial energy requirements.

E. Under ischemic conditions, the ATP reserves in the heart diminish markedly within 5 to 10 minutes as shown in Figure 23.2 [2]. The three main reactions requiring ATP are myosin ATPase responsible for actomyosin contraction, Ca^{2+}/Mg^{2+}-ATPase responsible for removal of Ca^{2+} from the myocyte cytosol, and Na^+/K^+-ATPase responsible for removal of Na^+ from the myocyte cytosol. Therefore, ischemia results in a rapid cessation of contractile function and loss of the membrane potential with accumulation of Ca^{2+} and Na^+. Anaerobic glycolysis produces intracellular acidosis, further depressing cellular function. It is likely that increased mitochondrial membrane permeability occurs early. Eventually, loss of cellular membrane integrity results in irreversible necrosis. Complement activation occurs with this injury and there is a wider damaging inflammatory response.

F. The objective of intraoperative myocardial protection is therefore the avoidance of this sequence of events, which can lead to low cardiac output syndrome after CPB, and has focused on the rapid induction and maintenance of cardiac arrest with or without hypothermia as the best strategies to prevent ATP depletion and so to preserve cellular integrity.

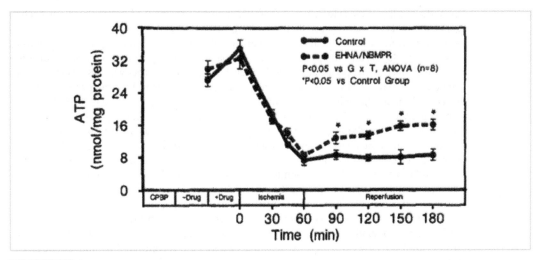

FIGURE 23.2 Effect of 60 minutes of warm global ischemia on myocardial ATP in dogs. Prior to ischemia, one group received a nucleoside transport blocker (NBMPR) and an adenosine deaminase inhibitor (EHNA). (From Anwar S, Ding M, Wechsler AS. Intermittent aortic cross clamping prevents cumulative adenosine triphosphate depletion, ventricular fibrillation, and dysfunction (stunning): is it preconditioning? *J Thorac Cardiovasc Surg.* 1995;110(2):328–339, with permission.)

CLINICAL PEARL   The fundamental goal of any cardioplegia solution is to prevent myocyte ATP depletion and preserve cellular well-being.

IV. Ischemia–reperfusion injury

   A. While physiologic reperfusion of myocytes is key to restarting oxidative phosphorylation, replenishment of ATP, and restoration of ion balance within the cells, it has long been recognized that there is an initial paradoxical reoxygenation-dependent enhancement of tissue injury on reperfusion, known as the ischemia–reperfusion injury [3].

   B. Two main molecular mechanisms are thought to be involved:

   1. Reactive oxygen species [4], particularly superoxide ($\cdot O_2^-$) and hydrogen peroxide (H_2O_2), are generated in the first few minutes of reperfusion by a combination of mitochondrial electron transport chain dysfunction, xanthine oxidase effect, and activated neutrophils. These reactive oxygen species then cause peroxidation of cellular phospholipid layers leading to loss of cellular integrity and function.

   2. Calcium accumulation [5] in the myocyte and within mitochondria during ischemia is exacerbated on reperfusion by activation of the mitochondrial Ca^{2+} uniporter and the sarcolemmal Ca^{2+} channel. Calcium-dependent phospholipases and proteases are activated and induce membrane and other injuries.

   3. Despite substantial research into the field of ischemia–reperfusion injury, almost none of the experimental strategies have been translated into clinical practice. Many units do practice "controlled reperfusion" which usually indicates a period of reduced pressure of reperfusion during the first few minutes. The practice of "terminal hot shot" is more commonly used (see Section VII).

V. Interventions before aortic cross-clamping

   A. Avoidance of ischemia prior to institution of CPB by proper attention to anesthetic technique is recommended, particularly at induction, with avoidance of either hypotension or hypertension. This may include appropriate use of preoperative intra-aortic balloon pump placement.

   B. Inhalational anesthetics and myocardial protection
   Extensive evidence from experimental studies has shown that inhalational anesthetics protect the heart from ischemic injury in animal models and in vitro human myocardium, an effect demonstrated on both myocytes and endothelial cells [6]. While the use of inhalational anesthetics in the clinical setting has been linked to reductions in various markers of myocardial

injury, the totality of the evidence falls short of supporting their use as specific cardioprotective agents. It is a likely useful by-product of these agents, however.

C. Systemic cooling is used to varying degrees by different centers and surgeons and, indeed, may be individualized to the procedure and the patient. Cooling is not invariable, with some surgeons preferring to operate at normothermia, but temperatures between 28°C and 33°C are widely used for standard surgeries. Systemic cooling may be primarily a strategy for neurologic protection, and it is known that each reduction of 10°C (Q_{10}) reduces the MvO_2 by 50% in myocytes as in other tissues (Fig. 23.1). Furthermore, the degree of systemic hypothermia will affect rewarming of the cardioplegia-cooled heart, both via direct contact and through the return of systemic blood to the heart via noncoronary collateral channels [7].

D. Institution of CPB results in immediate unloading of the heart and, therefore, reduction in energy requirement, so long as significant aortic regurgitation is not present. This can be achieved within a couple of minutes if a bypass circuit is ready and primed.

E. Avoidance of ventricular distention is critical. Ventricular distention produces increased wall tension with greater energy consumption and decreased subendocardial perfusion. Aortic regurgitation is usually an issue in regard to this during delivery of cardioplegia (i.e., after cross-clamping). However, there are instances where CPB is continued without aortic cross-clamping—for example, profound systemic cooling or technical difficulties in isolating the aorta (e.g., revision surgery, where aortic regurgitation requires additional precautions). Furthermore, aortic regurgitation may be produced by ventricular fibrillation (VF) or manipulation of the heart. In these circumstances, adequate venting of the left ventricle, typically by a right superior pulmonary vein vent or a left ventricular apical vent, is essential for adequate intraoperative myocardial protection.

> **CLINICAL PEARL** With severe aortic regurgitation is important to prevent the heart from slowing down and distending. It should be allowed to vent itself (by contracting) until deliberately stopped by the surgeon via administration of cardioplegia.

F. Myocardial ischemic preconditioning
Ischemic preconditioning [8] is a phenomenon whereby the heart can be "conditioned" by brief cycles (3 to 5 minutes) of nonlethal myocardial ischemia and reperfusion, such that infarct size is reduced after a subsequent period of sustained ischemia. Other parameters such as ATP levels, intracellular pH, and ultrastructural features are also preserved. This effect has been replicated in a large variety of animal species including humans, and indeed in in vitro cultures of human myocytes. The protective effect has two windows. The first (classical or early preconditioning) lasts between 4 hours and 6 hours with a second window beginning at 24 hours and lasting up to 72 hours. No single pathway explains the ischemic preconditioning, leaving a variety of potential mediators such as adenosine, bradykinin, protein kinase C, and the mitochondrial permeability transition pore. Numerous pharmacologic interventions aiming to replicate the preconditioning effect have been assessed but as yet there is insufficient evidence to support the use of any agent clinically.

G. The discovery that a "conditioning" stimulus could be applied to an organ or tissue away from the heart is termed remote ischemic preconditioning. This phenomenon is more easily translatable into the clinical setting, and indeed has been applied noninvasively using a standard blood pressure cuff placed on the upper or lower limb but without demonstrating a significant clinical effect [9].

VI. Interventions after aortic cross-clamping

A. **Forms of cardioplegia**

1. The primary strategy for intraoperative myocardial protection is through the delivery of cardioplegia solutions to the myocardium to produce a diastolic electromechanical arrest. Although a recent study showed that over 160 different recipes of cardioplegia were in use in the United States, these solutions all share some basic principles.

TABLE 23.1 Composition of various forms of cardioplegia

| | Depolarizing—Crystalloid | | del Nido^a | Depolarizing—Blood | | | Nondepolarizing | |
	St. Thomas II	Bretschneider		Buckberg^b induction/terminal hot shot	Buckberg^b maintenance	Buckberg^b rescue reperfusion	Adenocaine	St. Thomas nondep
K+	16	9	24	16–20	8–10	20–25		
Na+	110	15						
Ca^{2+}	1.2	0		0.2–0.4	0.5–0.6	0.1–0.25		
Mg^{2+}	16	4	8					16
HCO_3^{-}	10	12						
pH	7.8	7.1		7.5–7.7	7.6–7.8	7.5–7.6		
Other		Histidine 198 Tryptophan 2 Ketoglutarate 1 Mannitol 30	Mannitol Lidocaine	THAM Aspartate 13 Glutamate 13		THAM Aspartate 13 Glutamate 13 Diltiazem	Adenosine Lidocaine	Esmolol Adenosine

^a When diluted 1:4 with blood (1 part blood, 4 parts crystalloid).
^b When diluted 4:1 with blood (4 parts blood, 1 part crystalloid).
All values given in mmol/L. Nondep, nondepolarizing.

2. The most common method for rapid induction of diastolic arrest is through elevation of myocardial extracellular potassium resulting in depolarization of the resting membrane potential. At a K^+ concentration of around 10 mmol/L, this reaches around −65 mV and the voltage-dependent fast Na^+ channel crucial for initiation of the action potential is inactivated, arresting the heart in diastole. Of course, given the numerous ion channels and pumps, this does not occur in isolation, and there is a concomitant increase in intracellular Na^+ and Ca^{2+}. Also, the abnormal ion gradients leave ion pumps functioning and thus consuming ATP.

3. The simplest forms of cardioplegia are crystalloid solutions, of which there are two types that produce depolarization: extracellular and intracellular.

   Extracellular types contain relatively higher concentration of Na^+, Ca^{2+}, and Mg^{2+}, whereas intracellular types contain no or low concentrations of Na^+ and Ca^{2+}. All contain K^+ in ranges from 10 to 40 mmol/L (Table 23.1).

4. The prototype of an extracellular cardioplegia is St. Thomas solution [10] (also Plegisol [Pfizer, Inc.]).

5. The characteristic intracellular cardioplegia is Bretschneider solution (also HTK or Custodiol HTK Solution [Essential Pharmaceuticals, LLC]) [11]. The low Na^+ concentration reduces intracellular Na^+ buildup and also intracellular Ca^{2+} levels. Thus at least theoretically, there is a reduced tendency to intracellular edema and reperfusion injury due to Ca^{2+}. The hypocalcemia within the myocardium prolongs the arrest period and reduces the need for maintenance dosing. Bretschneider's and St. Thomas's solutions also have different volumes of administration and induction times.

6. Since the late 1970s, crystalloid solutions have been increasingly replaced by blood cardioplegia [12]. There are several advantages of using blood as the main vehicle for delivery of the active elements of cardioplegia—that is, replacing crystalloid. Blood has a much higher oxygen-carrying potential, better rheologic properties potentially improving microcirculatory perfusion, contains substrates for metabolism (fatty acids and glucose), has strong acid-buffering capacity, contains endogenous antioxidants, and has a natural oncotic force, thereby reducing the tendency for myocardial edema.

7. Blood cardioplegia is primarily produced in a 4:1 ratio of blood to cardioplegia (extracellular type) aimed at producing the same final concentration of K^+ as would be present in the crystalloid infusate. In practical terms, higher concentration (say 84 mmol/L K^+) solutions in commercially produced bags of crystalloid are used to spike blood diverted from the CPB circuit, which passes through a dedicated heat exchanger to determine the cardioplegia temperature.

8. Efforts to reduce hemodilution further have produced a strategy of microplegia [13], where the volume of crystalloid is even further reduced using even more concentrated solutions delivered via syringe drivers. These are probably only really advantageous for strategies of continuous and warm cardioplegia delivery.

9. A more recently developed depolarizing formulation is del Nido cardioplegia which was initially developed for pediatric and infant patients but is increasingly widely used in adults, particularly in the United States. It is a four-part crystalloid to one-part whole blood formulation. The main components are potassium and lidocaine (Table 23.1), but emphasis is given to the presence of bicarbonate, mannitol, and magnesium. It is typically used as a single shot of 1,000 mL in adults and provides arrest maintenance of around 90 minutes [14].

10. Some centers use different solutions, temperatures, and routes of delivery for induction of cardioplegia, for maintenance of cardioplegia, and for reperfusion before cross-clamp removal ("hot shot") [15] (see Table 23.1). This is by no means as widespread as the dominance of blood cardioplegia for reasons of simplicity and the very good results already achieved with a single formulation.

11. There are other forms of cardioplegia which seek to *avoid* depolarization of the myocyte resting potential in order to avoid intracellular Na^+ and Ca^{2+} loading with consequent maintained energy utilization [16]. There are also concerns over the effect of relatively high K^+ causing endothelial injury, local inflammation, arrhythmias, and coronary vasoconstriction [17]. A number of methods of inducing a so-called "polarized" arrest (in which the membrane potential is maintained close to the resting potential) have been put forward including local anesthetics like lidocaine, adenosine, esmolol, and K^+ channel openers such as pinacidil. These forms of cardioplegia are delivered as one-shot crystalloid solutions.

12. Lidocaine blocks fast-acting Na^+ channels to prevent depolarization. Adenosine opens K^+ channels, which increases the outward K^+ current resulting in hyperpolarization via A_1 receptor stimulation [18]. Esmolol is an ultra–short-acting cardioselective β-blocker which has been shown to arrest the heart in diastole due mainly to its negatively inotropic effect, but also blocks Ca^{2+} and Na^+ channels [19]. K^+ ATP channel openers produce hyperpolarization, although they have not been widely adopted in the clinical setting. Two commercially available solutions are adenocaine, combining adenosine and lidocaine, and St. Thomas polarizing cardioplegia, combining esmolol, adenosine, and magnesium (Table 23.1).

CLINICAL PEARL   The majority of adult surgical teams use multiple doses of depolarizing blood cardioplegia solution based on the principle of hyperkalemic diastolic arrest supplemented by hypothermia (local and/or systemic).

B. **Temperature of cardioplegia**
1. The myocardium may have been cooled by systemic cooling in the 30–33°C range achieved through CPB. However, most intraoperative myocardial protection historically (and indeed in clinical practice) involves cooling the myocardium to a temperature of around 15°C. Although a degree of topical cooling can be achieved through iced slush or saline or a cooling jacket, this is primarily effective for the thin-walled right ventricle. Adequate cooling of the left ventricle is achieved by delivery of cardioplegia at 4° to 10°C.

2. The increasing use of blood cardioplegia combined with the realization that leftward shift of the oxygen dissociation curve at low temperatures might reduce oxygen uptake in the cooled myocardium stimulated the use of warm blood cardioplegia.

3. The use of warm (37°C) oxygenated blood cardioplegia for induction is thought to allow for induction of electromechanical arrest while maximizing oxygen and other substrate uptake during the delivery period and therefore minimizing ATP depletion [20]. It has been particularly proposed in cases where there might be evolving myocardial infarction as a technique to rescue these areas at the time of induction.

4. Warm blood cardioplegia may also be used for maintenance, especially if CPB is being conducted at normothermia. Numerous studies have compared it to cold blood cardioplegia, and several studies report lower incidence of perioperative myocardial infarction and a lower incidence of low cardiac output syndromes [21].

5. Infusion of terminal warm blood cardioplegia ("hot shot") may be used as an adjunct to cold cardioplegia to replenish substrates (see Section VII).

6. Tepid cardioplegia (29°C) has also been described [22] and appears to be safe and effective, although it remains to be determined whether it confers better myocardial protection than other temperatures.

C. **Route of delivery**

1. Just as there are many solutions of cardioplegia, there are multiple forms of delivery: antegrade into the aortic root, antegrade down individual coronary ostia, antegrade down vein grafts, and retrograde; and each can be continuous or intermittent.

2. Antegrade cardioplegia may be delivered by a cannula placed in the ascending aorta proximal to the aortic cross-clamp. The cardioplegia is delivered at 200 to 300 mL/min at a pressure of 70 to 100 mm Hg while observing pressure in the aortic root and the myocardium for evenness of cooling, absence of distention, and electromechanical arrest. A 1,000-mL (14 mL/kg) induction dose of blood cardioplegia is typically supplemented at 20-minute intervals with 200- to 400-mL doses. For extracellular crystalloid cardioplegia, 1,000 mL is given at induction and then supplemented at 40-minute intervals with 500-mL doses. Intracellular crystalloid is often one shot with a 2,000-mL induction dose lasting around 120 minutes, when it can then be supplemented if necessary. This makes it quite suitable for minimally invasive procedures, where the ease of supplementation is less.

3. Maintenance of cardioplegic arrest may require supplementation of cardioplegia. This becomes necessary due to rewarming and reperfusion of the myocardium by direct contact with systemically perfused tissues such as the diaphragm, varying amounts of blood returned to the heart from the pulmonary veins, and noncoronary collateral flow—small pericardial and mediastinal vessels communicating with the coronary circulation. All of these vary from case to case and can be difficult to predict. The principle behind maintenance dosing of cardioplegia is that electromechanical quiescence should be maintained and both the ECG and myocardium should be observed. Some centers place a temperature probe in the left ventricular myocardium and use this measurement to determine the adequacy of cardioplegia and thus the need for supplementation. The composition of the cardioplegia will also influence the need for supplementation. Blood cardioplegia typically requires more frequent supplementation than crystalloid as do extracellular formulations compared to intracellular. Temperature is important with warmer systemic temperature and warmer cardioplegia both necessitating more frequent dosage.

4. In the setting of aortic regurgitation, delivery of cardioplegia into the aortic root can produce left ventricular distention. Even where the left ventricle is vented, the cardioplegia may not adequately pressurize the aortic root and it is unclear how much cardioplegia is actually delivered down the coronary arteries. Therefore, it is preferable to open the aorta and deliver the cardioplegia directly down the coronary ostia using cannulae specifically designed for this purpose. The cannulae can be in a Y to perfuse both ostia simultaneously, or each ostium can be perfused sequentially with a volume proportionate to the amount of myocardium it perfuses. Some ostial cannulae can be fixed in place and used for continuous perfusion of cardioplegia.

5. In the setting of a precarious coronary anatomy, severe coronary artery disease may result in uneven distribution of cardioplegia by an antegrade route. A free conduit grafted to a diseased coronary artery can be used for delivery of cardioplegia. Some surgeons use this more generally as a method of checking adequacy of flow in each graft. Supplementary cardioplegia may also be administered retrogradely. This is particularly indicated in redo coronary artery bypass procedures [23].

6. Retrograde cardioplegia [24] is delivered by a purpose-made balloon-tipped cannula placed in the coronary sinus. This is mostly placed blind, via the right atrial free wall,

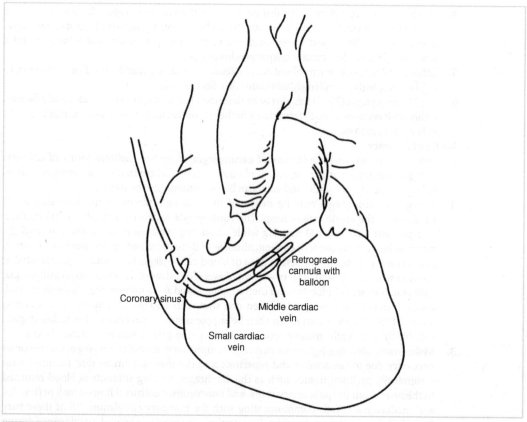

Coronary sinus

Retrograde cannula with balloon

Middle cardiac vein

Small cardiac vein

FIGURE 23.3 Placement of the retrograde cannula in the coronary sinus beyond the veins draining the right ventricle.

but can also be placed directly with the right atrium opened. The perfusion passes via the coronary venous system into the capillary bed and subsequently into the arterial tree and comes out of both coronary ostia. Pressure is limited to <40 mm Hg to avoid edema and this typically produces a flow of 150 to 200 mL/min. Correct placement of the cannula should be confirmed by one or more of: visualization on TEE, digital palpation of the cannula tip, ventricularization of the pressure trace of the cannula, observation of an increase in pressure with flow down the cannula, and observation of perfusate coming out of the coronary ostia when the aorta is open.

7. The right ventricle is drained by the Thebesian veins, which empty directly into the right ventricle. Furthermore, those epicardial veins which do drain the right ventricle enter the coronary sinus near the ostium, near the site of a retrograde cannula balloon (Fig. 23.3). Therefore, there are some concerns that there can be relatively less perfusion of the right ventricle by the retrograde route.

CLINICAL PEARL   Do not rely on retrograde cardioplegia alone to protect the right heart because its venous drainage is predominantly via Thebesian veins; those cardiac veins which do drain to the coronary sinus often do so proximal to the typical location of a retrograde cannula balloon.

8. In valvular surgery, the use of retrograde cardioplegia facilitates the surgical steps. In aortic valve surgery, repeat doses of cardioplegia can be given without interrupting the procedure to cannulate the coronary ostia in antegrade fashion (but note Clinical Pearl above). In mitral valve surgery, retraction of the heart can distort the aortic root and produce

aortic regurgitation if cardioplegia is administered antegradely without letting down the retraction. Retrograde cardioplegia may be administered without changing the exposure.

9. Antegrade and retrograde cardioplegia may be used together [25] either simultaneously or alternatingly. Most commonly, the antegrade route used to arrest the heart (induction) and the retrograde route is used for repeat dosing (maintenance). Retrograde cardioplegia used for induction takes much longer to achieve arrest, which may exacerbate ATP depletion. On the other hand, the use of retrograde cardioplegia for reperfusion prior to cross-clamp removal (hot shot) permits substrate replenishment at a warm temperature and low pressure, achieving several of the principles of controlled reperfusion.

VII. **Interventions around cross-clamp removal**

A. The term "hot shot" refers to the delivery of warm blood [26], frequently with hyperkalemia prior to the removal of the cross-clamp. This is thought to enhance substrate replenishment while maintaining electromechanical arrest—that is, during a period of low substrate utilization.

B. In the 1980s, Buckberg performed a series of experimental studies investigating how altering the conditions of reperfusion affected myocardial recovery. The description "gentle" reperfusion as a cardioprotective strategy arose from this work and is currently practiced as "controlled reperfusion." This involves reducing the systemic pressure when the cross-clamp is removed for a period of a couple of minutes, maintaining a mean pressure of around 40 mm Hg.

C. In this early period of reperfusion, the contractile function of the heart is depressed and the myocardium is particularly susceptible to distention. Due attention is necessary to avoid ventricular distention and to address it by venting if required. The importance of VF in the decompressed heart at this stage is less clear, but the presence of VF certainly makes assessment of distention difficult and usually stimulates the clinicians to reverse it by electrical and/or pharmacologic measures.

D. Immediately prior to removal of the aortic cross-clamp, the left side of the heart should be thoroughly de-aired. This typically involves pushing blood flow through the right side of the heart and then lungs to push air out through the left side, either through an LV or aortic vent. To do this, the perfusionist partially occludes the venous return, filling the right atrium and right ventricle and pushing blood into the lungs. The anesthesiologist ventilates the lungs which helps to push blood and air from the pulmonary circulation into the left heart. Only when this air has been expelled can the cross-clamp be removed to avoid left ventricular ejection of air into the systemic circulation. Even with these measures, it is likely that some pockets of air remain in the most uppermost areas of the circulation. Since the right coronary artery is anterior in the aortic root, any air is most likely to embolize here and could cause malperfusion at this delicate time. Attention to this possibility should be maintained until all this air has been eliminated, which may be several minutes after cross-clamp removal. Some surgeons use insufflation of CO_2 into the operative field which, being denser than air, displaces this during the procedure. Any gaseous emboli at the end are, therefore, composed of highly soluble CO_2 rather than relatively insoluble air.

E. Many years after the description of controlled reperfusion and ischemic preconditioning, the phenomenon of ischemic postconditioning was demonstrated. This is the reduction of ischemic injury by interrupting periods of reperfusion with brief periods of reocclusion. Although initially described in a canine model, this technique has been reported as beneficial in the clinical setting, although its clinical merit remains to be determined [27].

VIII. **Alternatives to cardioplegia**

A. **Cross-clamp fibrillation**

1. This is essentially a historical technique for coronary artery bypass [28]. The heart was deliberately fibrillated and the aortic cross-clamp applied. The specific coronary artery was exposed and grafted. The cross-clamp was then removed and the heart defibrillated. For free grafts, the proximal anastomosis was completed with the heart perfused and beating, using a side-biting clamp on the ascending aorta, allowing immediate reperfusion of that coronary territory. Then the next graft was performed under a further period of cross-clamp fibrillation and so on, until all the grafts were completed. Usually, systemic hypothermia of 28° to 30°C and a pulmonary artery vent were used to provide some protection and avoid distention.

B. **Off-pump coronary artery bypass**

   1. Off-pump coronary revascularization accounts for around 20% of all cases, varying according to institutional and surgeon preferences. As far as intraoperative myocardial protection, attention to general anesthetic principles is all the more critical and this is addressed in Chapter 10. Coronary perfusion must remain adequate and various maneuvers are employed to optimize this including operative table positioning, cardiac positioning, pacing, and judicious use of vasopressors [29].

   2. The left internal mammary artery to left anterior descending artery anastomosis is performed first to provide the greatest territory of revascularization with a minimum of cardiac displacement. As in cross-clamp fibrillation, proximal anastomoses may be performed immediately after the distal anastomosis in order to achieve immediate revascularization. Although some surgeons place intracoronary shunts while performing distal anastomoses, these introduce a degree of stenosis and distal flow is reduced compared to a patent vessel.

C. **Beating heart on cardiopulmonary bypass (CPB)**

   1. In the presence of a competent aortic valve, the myocardium can be perfused from the bypass circuit allowing the heart to beat throughout the procedure.

   2. This is a very common approach for operations on the right side of the heart, particularly tricuspid or pulmonary valve operations, since the right side is bypassed. Attention to entraining air to the left side of the heart is critical.

   3. In mitral valve surgery, this technique is also used with venting of the left ventricle via the mitral valve, both to facilitate exposure and to prevent air embolism, since in this case the left ventricle is full of air [30]. A resurgence in this strategy coincides with an interest in minimal access and transcatheter approaches to the mitral valve.

   4. Aortic arch procedures are typically prolonged and require long periods of cooling and rewarming. If the aortic valve is competent, the ascending aorta can be cross-clamped and the heart perfused by normothermic blood flow at 500 to 700 mL/min proximal to the clamp, essentially separating cardiac and systemic perfusion circuits [31]. Adequacy of cardiac perfusion is assessed by observation of a pressurized aortic root alongside a comfortable and flaccid beating heart with a normal electrocardiogram. Of course, in most cases of aortic arch surgery, concomitant procedures are required on the heart itself and the aortic root. These can be performed with standard cardioplegia techniques during systemic cooling, and then the heart restarted and maintained beating with this normothermic perfusion technique, while the surgeon tackles the aortic arch.

IX. **Conclusion**

   A. An enormous array of formulations and strategies exist for intraoperative myocardial protection. Contemporary results of cardiac surgery produce mortality rates of less than 2% and myocardial infarction rates of less than 4%. The evidence for any particular strategy is usually based on laboratory experiments, which have proved difficult to translate into significant clinical differences in the clinical arena. For this reason, many units and surgeons choose to simplify their approach to provide a practiced and reproducible technique with as universal an application as possible.

   B. With appropriate intraoperative myocardial protection, the heart will generally comfortably tolerate 120 minutes of ischemia time, after which additional time will come at a cost of increased risk of low cardiac output syndrome.

   C. As our understanding of the mechanisms underlying global ischemia–reperfusion injury in the heart improves, so no doubt will our techniques for tolerating and reversing longer and longer periods of myocardial ischemia.

REFERENCES

1. **Buckberg GD, Brazier JR, Nelson RL, et al. Studies of the effects of hypothermia on regional myocardial blood flow and metabolism during cardiopulmonary bypass. I. The adequately perfused beating, fibrillating, and arrested heart. *J Thorac Cardiovasc Surg*. 1977;73:87–94.**

2. Ali AA, White P, Xiang B, et al. Hearts from DCD donors display acceptable biventricular function after heart transplantation in pigs. *Am J Transplant*. 2011;11(8):1621–1632.

3. Piper HM, Garcia-Dorado D. Prime causes of rapid cardiomyocyte death during reperfusion. *Ann Thorac Surg.* 1999;68:1913–1919.
4. Raedschelders K, Ansley DM, Chen DD. The cellular and molecular origin of reactive oxygen species generation during myocardial ischemia and reperfusion. *Pharmacol Ther.* 2012;133:230–255.
5. **Piper HM, Meuter K, Schafer C. Cellular mechanisms of ischemia-reperfusion injury.** *Ann Thorac Surg.* **2003;75:S644–S648.**
6. **Kunst G, Klein AA. Peri-operative anaesthetic myocardial preconditioning and protection—cellular mechanisms and clinical relevance in cardiac anaesthesia.** *Anaesthesia.* **2015;70:467–482.**
7. The Warm Heart Investigators. Randomized trial of normothermic versus hypothermic coronary bypass surgery. *Lancet.* 1994;343:559–563.
8. **Hausenloy DJ, Yellon DM. Ischaemic conditioning and reperfusion injury.** *Nat Rev Cardiol.* **2016;13(4):193–209.**
9. Hausenloy DJ, Candilio L, Evans R, et al. Remote ischemic preconditioning and outcomes of cardiac surgery. *N Engl J Med.* 2015;373:1408–1417.
10. Hearse DJ, Stewart DA, Braimbridge MV. Cellular protection during myocardial ischemia. The development and characterization of a procedure for the induction of reversible ischemic arrest. *Circulation.* 1976;54:193–202.
11. Edelman JJ, Seco M, Dunne B, et al. Custodiol for myocardial protection and preservation: a systematic review. *Ann Cardiothorac Surg.* 2013;2(6):717–728.
12. Buckberg GD. A proposed "solution" to the cardioplegic controversy. *J Thorac Cardiovasc Surg.* 1979;77:803–815.
13. Algarni KD, Weisel RD, Caldarone CA, et al. Microplegia during coronary artery bypass grafting was associated with less low cardiac output syndrome: a propensity-matched comparison. *Ann Thorac Surg.* 2013;95:1532–1538.
14. Matte GS, del Nido PJ. History and use of del Nido cardioplegia solution at Boston Children's Hospital. *J Extra Corpor Technol.* 2012;44:98–103.
15. Kim KK, Ball C, Grady P, et al. Use of del Nido cardioplegia for adult cardiac surgery at the Cleveland Clinic: perfusion implications. *J Extra Corpor Technol.* 2014;46(4):317–323.
16. **Chambers DJ, Fallouh HB. Cardioplegia and cardiac surgery: pharmacological arrest and cardioprotection during global ischemia and reperfusion.** *Pharmacol Ther.* **2010;127:41–52.**
17. Aass T, Stangeland L, Moen CA, et al. Myocardial function after polarizing versus depolarizing cardiac arrest with blood cardioplegia in a porcine model of cardiopulmonary bypass. *Eur J Cardiothorac Surg.* 2016;50:130–139.
18. Corvera JS, Kin H, Dobson GP, et al. Polarized arrest with warm or cold adenosine-lidocaine blood cardioplegia is equivalent to hypothermic potassium blood cardioplegia. *J Thorac Cardiovasc Surg.* 2005;129:599–606.
19. Fallouh HB, Bardswell SC, McLatchie LM, et al. Esmolol cardioplegia: the cellular mechanism of diastolic arrest. *Cardiovasc Res.* 2010;87:552–560.
20. **Rosenkranz ER, Vinten-Johansen J, Buckberg G, et al. Benefits of normothermic induction of blood cardioplegia in energy-depleted hearts, with maintenance of arrest by multidose cold blood cardioplegic infusions.** *J Thorac Cardiovasc Surg.* **1982;84:667–677.**
21. Lichtenstein SV, Ashe KA, el Dalati H, et al. Warm heart surgery. *J Thorac Cardiovasc Surg.* 1991;101:269–274.
22. Hayashida N, Ikonomidis JS, Weisel RD, et al. The optimal cardioplegic temperature. *Ann Thorac Surg.* 1994;58:961–971.
23. Borger MA, Rao V, Weisel RD, et al. Reoperative coronary bypass surgery: effect of patent grafts and retrograde cardioplegia. *J Thorac Cardiovasc Surg.* 2001;121:83–90.
24. Schaper J, Walter P, Scheld H, et al. The effects of retrograde perfusion of cardioplegic solution in cardiac operations. *J Thorac Cardiovasc Surg.* 1985;90:882–887.
25. **Ihnken K, Morita K, Buckberg G, et al. The safety of simultaneous arterial and coronary sinus perfusion: experimental background and initial clinical results.** *J Card Surg.* **1994;9:15–25.**
26. Teoh KH, Christakis GT, Weisel RD, et al. Accelerated myocardial metabolic recovery with terminal warm blood cardioplegia. *J Thorac Cardiovasc Surg.* 1986;91:888–895.
27. Tsang A, Hausenloy DJ, Yellon DM. Myocardial postconditioning: reperfusion injury revisited. *Am J Physiol Heart Circ Physiol.* 2005;289:H2–H7.
28. Akins CW. Noncardioplegic myocardial preservation for coronary revascularization. *J Thorac Cardiovasc Surg.* 1984;88:174–181.
29. Hett DA. Anaesthesia for off-pump coronary artery surgery. *Br J Anaesth.* 2006;6:60–62.
30. Pasic M, Sündermann S, Unbehaun A, et al. Beating heart mitral valve surgery: results in 120 consecutive patients considered unsuitable for conventional mitral valve surgery. *Interact Cardiovasc Thorac Surg.* 2017;25:541–547.
31. Abu-Omar Y, Ali JM, Colah S, et al. Aortic arch replacement with a beating heart: a simple method using continuous 3-way perfusion. *Perfusion.* 2014;29:6–9.

Extracorporeal Membrane Oxygenation for Pulmonary or Cardiac Support

Darryl Abrams, Jonathan Hastie, and Daniel Brodie

KEY POINTS

1. Venovenous extracorporeal membrane oxygenation (ECMO) provides for gas exchange without cardiac support, whereas venoarterial ECMO provides support for both impaired gas exchange and impaired cardiac function.

2. Because carbon dioxide can be removed efficiently at low blood flow rates, extracorporeal carbon dioxide removal ($ECCO_2R$) has the potential to alter the paradigm of the management of respiratory failure through the use of minimization and avoidance of mechanical ventilation.

3. In femoral–femoral venoarterial ECMO, delivery of oxygenated blood to the aortic arch and great vessels may be compromised when native gas exchange is impaired and there is residual native cardiac output. Hybrid, upper-body, or central cannulation strategies may mitigate this problem.

4. Temporary venoarterial ECMO is used in cardiac failure patients as part of several potential strategies or bridges; the endpoints of these bridges may include recovery, heart transplantation, long-term mechanical circulatory support, or, when outcomes are uncertain, a decision. However, ECMO for respiratory failure can only be used as bridge to recovery or transplantation because no other bridge or destination device is currently in existence.

5. Extracorporeal cardiopulmonary resuscitation (ECPR) has the potential to significantly improve neurologically intact survival from cardiac arrest. However, appropriate patient selection is essential in optimizing outcomes and avoiding the widespread application of this resource-intensive strategy.

THE USE OF EXTRACORPOREAL MEMBRANE OXYGENATION (ECMO) for severe respiratory and cardiac failure has grown rapidly over the last several years in the context of both technologic advances in extracorporeal circuitry and a growing body of literature demonstrating favorable outcomes. As cannulation techniques and management strategies evolve, ECMO has the potential to transform the approach to severe cardiopulmonary failure. This chapter addresses the rationale for ECMO use, its potential indications and contraindications, management approaches to the circuit and patient, and common complications. Lastly, because ECMO is a resource-intensive technology that profoundly affects the ability to support critically ill patients, economic impact and ethically challenging situations are discussed.

I. **History of ECMO**

  A. ECMO was first devised as an extension of cardiopulmonary bypass, with the idea that respiratory and cardiac function could be supported through extracorporeal circuitry beyond the operating room setting.

  B. The first successful application of ECMO for acute severe respiratory failure was in 1971.

  C. Although such success held great promise for the future development of the field and expanding use in severe respiratory failure, prospective randomized trials in 1979 and 1994 failed to demonstrate a survival benefit from ECMO compared to conventional management. Much of the failure of ECMO was attributed to high complication rates, particularly bleeding and thrombosis. These complications fundamentally relate to the circuitry components available at the time and limited practitioner experience with the technology.

  D. Over the last 20 years, substantial advances in extracorporeal technology include the following components:

  1. Novel cannula designs that optimize drainage and reinfusion of blood

  2. Biocompatible circuits which decrease the risk of thrombus formation and reduce the requirement for anticoagulation

  3. Oxygenators that improve efficiency through the use of semipermeable membranes to selectively allow for diffusion of gas

  4. Centrifugal pumps that reduce trauma to blood components and decrease the risk of damage to the circuit

  E. The combination of improved technology, with a more favorable risk profile, and concurrent advances in the overall critical care management of patients with severe cardiopulmonary failure have led to a growing body of literature that suggests improving survival in patients supported with ECMO. However, this literature largely comprises nonrandomized observational trials with their inherent limitations in study design.

II. **ECMO physiology**

  A. ECMO provides for gas exchange during severe respiratory failure by directly oxygenating and removing carbon dioxide from blood [1].

  B. Deoxygenated blood is drained from a central vein and pumped through a gas exchange device called a membrane oxygenator. The blood passes along one side of a semipermeable membrane, while gas, referred to as sweep gas, passes along the other side. The gas is typically a mixture of oxygen and air, the proportions of which (i.e., the fraction of delivered oxygen, FDO_2) are controlled by a blender.

  C. The membrane allows for diffusion of oxygen down a gradient from high concentration in the sweep gas to low concentration in the blood compartment. Carbon dioxide also diffuses from high to low concentration (from the blood compartment to the gas compartment).

  D. Well-oxygenated blood leaving the membrane oxygenator is then reinfused back to the patient. The carbon dioxide removed by the membrane oxygenator is vented to the environment.

  E. When blood is drained from a vein and reinfused into a vein, the configuration is called venovenous ECMO. This configuration provides only gas exchange and relies upon the native cardiac function to circulate the reinfused, oxygenated blood.

> **CLINICAL PEARL**   Venovenous ECMO provides gas exchange support, whereas venoarterial ECMO provides both gas exchange and hemodynamic support.

  F. Venoarterial ECMO describes the configuration in which blood is drained from a vein and reinfused into an artery. This provides both gas exchange and hemodynamic support by reinfusing blood under pressure directly into the systemic arterial circulation.

> **CLINICAL PEARL**   In cases of acute right ventricular failure due to severe hypoxemia or hypercapnia, venovenous ECMO may be sufficient to improve right heart function without the need for venoarterial support.

2

G. Extracorporeal oxygen delivery is proportional to extracorporeal blood flow; large cannulae are often required to achieve adequate flow rates. Extracorporeal carbon dioxide removal (ECCO$_2$R) is predominantly determined by the sweep gas flow rate and can be achieved at much lower blood flow rates. This allows for the use of smaller cannulae which may be associated with fewer complications.

CLINICAL PEARL   The main determinant of oxygenation through the ECMO circuit is blood flow rate. The main determinant of carbon dioxide removal through the ECMO circuit, during full-flow ECMO, is the sweep gas flow rate.

III. Cannulation strategies

A. **Venovenous**

ECMO traditionally involves the insertion of two separate cannulae, one for drainage and one for reinfusion. Venous drainage commonly occurs from the inferior vena cava (IVC), which is accessed through a femoral vein, while reinfused blood is delivered to the superior vena cava (SVC) through an internal jugular vein (Fig. 24.1).

1. A two-site venovenous configuration has the advantage of ease of bedside insertion without the need for advanced imaging techniques (although ultrasound guidance is recommended). However, the orientation of the drainage and reinfusion cannulae may result in drainage of reinfused, well-oxygenated blood back into the circuit without first having passed through the systemic circulation. This phenomenon, known as recirculation, limits the efficiency of the circuit's gas exchange.

2. An alternative single-site configuration may minimize recirculation through the use of a bicaval, dual-lumen cannula.

   a. This cannula is inserted into an internal jugular vein with its tip in the IVC. It is positioned so that SVC and IVC drainage ports drain blood into one lumen. After passing through the membrane oxygenator, reinfused blood passes through a second lumen whose port is directed toward the tricuspid valve (Fig. 24.2).

   b. Recirculation is minimized both by separating drainage and reinfusion ports and directing the reinfusion jet toward the tricuspid valve.

   c. By avoiding the cannulation of a femoral vein, this configuration may minimize infectious risks and allow for increased mobility.

   d. In order to ensure correct placement and orientation, this cannula should ideally be placed with guidance from both transesophageal echocardiography and fluoroscopy.

CLINICAL PEARL   Two-site venovenous ECMO is the most common configuration when ECMO is used for respiratory failure; its downsides include femoral cannulation and tendency for recirculation. Single-site cannulation with a dual-lumen cannula avoids femoral cannulation and minimizes recirculation; however, such an approach requires advanced imaging techniques to ensure satisfactory placement.

B. **Venoarterial**

ECMO is most commonly performed with peripheral insertion of cannulae into the femoral vein and artery. This approach, much like two-site venovenous ECMO, can be performed rapidly at the bedside, which is particularly useful for supporting hemodynamically unstable patients. Such an approach is usually adequate to provide sufficient circulatory support to maintain adequate end-organ perfusion.

3

1. **Hybrid configurations.** Femoral venoarterial ECMO creates retrograde flow of reinfused blood in the aorta. In patients receiving venoarterial ECMO for cardiac failure, who have concomitant severe respiratory failure, residual native cardiac function may pump

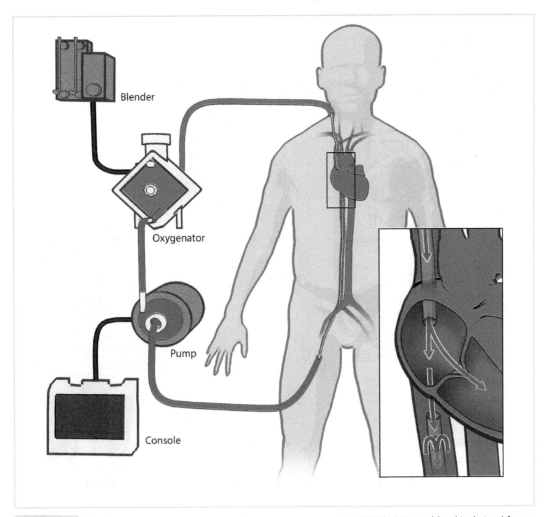

FIGURE 24.1 Two-site venovenous extracorporeal membrane oxygenation (ECMO). Venous blood is drained from a central vein via a drainage cannula, pumped through an oxygenator, and returned to a central vein through a separate reinfusion cannula. *Inset:* Some reinfused blood may be taken back up by the drainage cannula (*purple arrow*) without passing through the systemic circulation, which is referred to as recirculation. (Reprinted with permission from Clinics in Chest Medicine. Abrams D, Brodie D. Extracorporeal circulatory approaches to treat ARDS. *Clin Chest Med.* 2014;35(4): 765–779. Figure 2, also reprinted with permission from www.collectedmed.com)

deoxygenated blood into the ascending aorta. These competing blood flows can lead to the delivery of poorly oxygenated blood to the coronary and cerebral circulations (Fig. 24.3). One remedy to this problem involves the addition of a second reinfusion limb into the internal jugular vein, which will improve the oxygenation of blood passing through the native cardiac circulation. This configuration is referred to as venoarterial venous ECMO (Fig. 24.4).

2. In circumstances in which sufficient circulatory support cannot be provided by the cannulation of peripheral vessels, central cannulation may be necessary, with the use of shorter, larger-bore cannulae. This configuration, which is analogous to typical cardiopulmonary bypass cannulation for open heart surgery, varies based on the patient's needs and may include, for example, right atrial drainage with either aortic or pulmonary venous reinfusion.

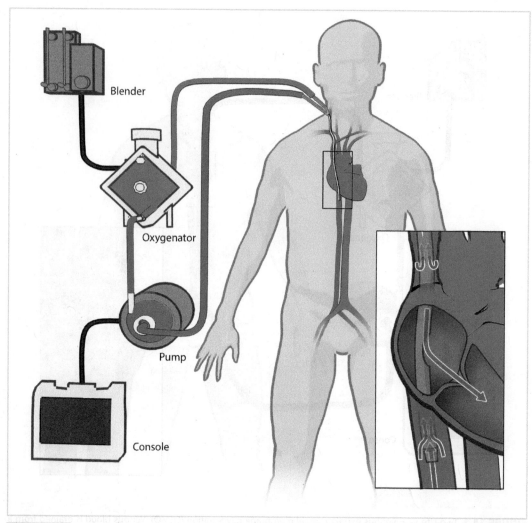

FIGURE 24.2 Single-site venovenous extracorporeal membrane oxygenation (ECMO). Dual-lumen cannula insertion allows for venovenous ECMO through a single venous access point and may minimize recirculation when properly positioned. (Reprinted with permission from Clinics in Chest Medicine. Abrams D, Brodie D. Extracorporeal circulatory approaches to treat ARDS. *Clin Chest Med.* 2014;35(4):765–779. Figure 4, also reprinted with permission from www.collectedmed.com)

3. **Left ventricular venting.** The retrograde flow of reinfused blood in the aorta in femoral venoarterial ECMO may result in several adverse physiologic consequences related to an increase in left ventricular afterload. Increased left ventricular afterload increases wall stress, which both increases myocardial oxygen demand and decreases coronary artery perfusion. Increased left ventricular afterload also leads to an increase in the end-diastolic volume, which is associated with stasis and intracardiac thrombus formation, particularly when the aortic valve is not opening. Left ventricular venting, performed either percutaneously or surgically, mitigates each of these effects by decompressing the ventricle. Left ventricular venting (drainage) into the ECMO circuit also reduces the likelihood of upper-body hypoxemia in patients with impaired lung function.

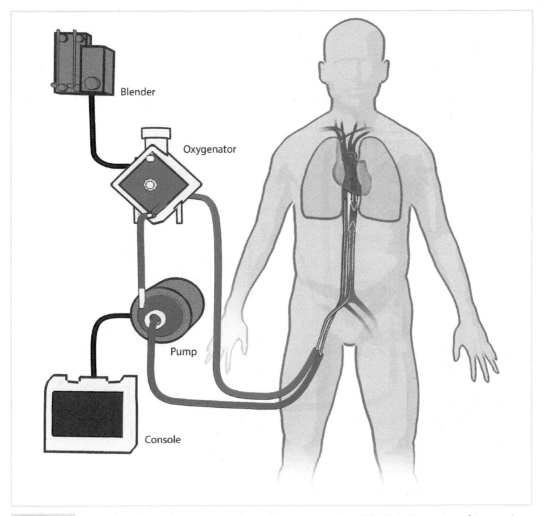

FIGURE 24.3 Femoral venoarterial extracorporeal membrane oxygenation (ECMO) in the setting of impaired gas exchange. Reinfused oxygenated blood flows retrograde up the aorta (*red arrow*) and may meet resistance from antegrade flow from the native cardiac output (*purple arrow*), which, in the context of impaired native gas exchange, may lead to poor upper body oxygenation. (Reprinted with permission from Clinics in Chest Medicine. Abrams D, Brodie D. Novel uses of extracorporeal membrane oxygenation in adults. *Clin Chest Med*. 2015;36(3):373–384. Figure 4, also reprinted with permission from www.collectedmed.com)

CLINICAL PEARL The most common approach for venoarterial ECMO utilizes femoral venous drainage and femoral arterial reinfusion. However, this configuration may be associated with upper-body hypoxia in the setting of impaired native gas exchange and residual native left ventricular function.

IV. **Indications and evidence for ECMO in respiratory failure**

  A. **Bridge to recovery**

   1. **Severe acute respiratory distress syndrome (ARDS).** The most common indication for venovenous ECMO is severe ARDS, defined by the acute onset of severe hypoxemia with bilateral infiltrates on chest imaging that cannot be fully explained by elevated left atrial pressure.

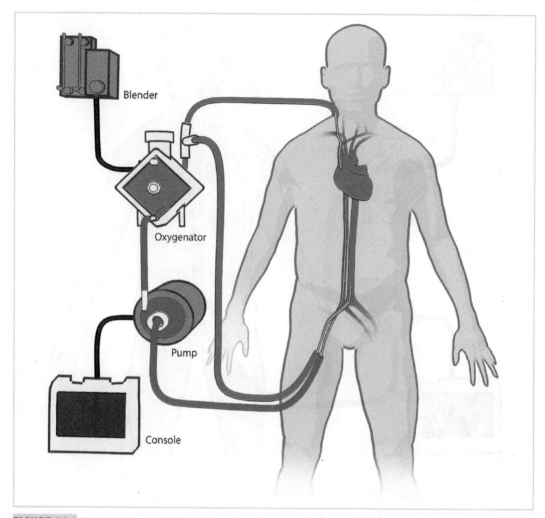

FIGURE 24.4 Venoarterial venous extracorporeal membrane oxygenation (ECMO). Inadequate upper body oxygenation due to a combination of femoral venoarterial ECMO and impaired native gas exchange may be partially overcome by the addition of a second reinfusion limb into an internal jugular vein. (Reprinted with permission from Clinics in Chest Medicine. Abrams D, Brodie D. Novel uses of extracorporeal membrane oxygenation in adults. *Clin Chest Med.* 2015;36(3):373–384. Figure 5, also reprinted with permission from www.collectedmed.com)

a. A volume- and pressure-limited ventilation strategy is standard of care in ARDS, with a proven mortality benefit over conventional higher volumes and plateau airway pressures [2]. Other strategies that confer a mortality benefit in ARDS include prone positioning and possibly the early use of neuromuscular blockade or high levels of positive end-expiratory pressure (PEEP).

b. Propensity analyses of patients with and without ECMO support for severe ARDS in the context of the influenza A (H1N1) pandemic in 2009 showed conflicting results as to the effect of ECMO on survival. One observational study in the United Kingdom demonstrated a significant reduction in mortality (24% vs. 47%, relative risk 0.51; 95% CI 0.31–0.84, $p = 0.008$), whereas a comparable study in a French cohort demonstrated no survival benefit from ECMO.

c. The only prospective randomized trial in which ECMO was performed with relatively modern technology and in the era of standard-of-care low–tidal-volume ventilation for severe acute respiratory failure was the Conventional Ventilation or ECMO for Severe Adult Respiratory Failure (CESAR) trial, which demonstrated an improved rate of 6-month survival without severe disability when a strategy of referral to an ECMO-capable center was compared with usual care management (relative risk 0.69; 95% CI 0.05–0.97, $p = 0.03$) [3]. Of note:

(1) Only 76% of subjects referred for ECMO ever received ECMO. The other 24% either improved with standard of care conventional mechanical ventilation, worsened prior to being able to receive ECMO, or died prior to arrival at the ECMO center.

(2) Only 70% of subjects in the control arm were managed with standard-of-care lung-protective mechanical ventilation at any time during the study.

(3) These methodologic flaws limit the conclusions that can be drawn regarding the effect of ECMO itself on survival in severe acute respiratory failure and rather suggest the benefits associated with adherence to standard of care and referral to a center with the capacity to initiate ECMO. Additional randomized controlled studies are needed to elucidate the role of ECMO in this patient population.

d. A prospective randomized controlled trial of ECMO versus standard-of-care conventional management in severe refractory ARDS is currently ongoing and may help elucidate the role of ECMO in these patients (ClinicalTrials.gov Identifier: NCT01470703).

e. Proposed thresholds to initiate ECMO in ARDS [1]:

(1) Ratio of partial pressure of oxygen in arterial blood (PaO_2) to fraction of inspired oxygen (FiO_2) less than 80 mm Hg with the use of high FiO_2 and PEEP

(2) Respiratory acidosis with pH less than 7.15 despite optimal ventilator management

(3) Excessively high plateau airway pressures (>35 to 45 cm H_2O, depending on patient's body habitus) despite optimal ventilator management

2. **Primary graft dysfunction (PGD) after lung transplantation.** Clinically similar to ARDS, though etiologically thought to be a consequence of ischemia–reperfusion injury, PGD manifests as acute hypoxemic respiratory failure and radiographic infiltrates in the allograft within 72 hours of lung transplantation. ECMO should be considered early in PGD to support severe gas exchange impairment and minimize harm from aggressive ventilator settings. In select patients, particularly those with pretransplantation pulmonary hypertension or right ventricular dysfunction, venoarterial ECMO may be considered intraoperatively as a means of accomplishing two ends: providing intraoperative hemodynamic support and controlling reperfusion to the allograft to minimize the risk of PGD. In some patients with severe pulmonary hypertension, venoarterial ECMO may be instituted preoperatively for respiratory failure associated with hemodynamic instability.

3. **Acute hypercapnic respiratory failure.** $ECCO_2R$ may be used in the management of hypercapnic respiratory failure with a favorable risk–benefit profile while minimizing or eliminating the need for invasive mechanical ventilation. The relatively low risk is rooted in the ability to achieve carbon dioxide removal at low blood flow rates with smaller cannulae as compared to cannulae used for hypoxemic respiratory failure.

a. Potential benefits of this strategy include:

(1) Minimization of dynamic hyperinflation and auto-PEEP

(2) Minimization of ventilator-associated lung injury (VALI)

(3) Avoidance of ventilator-associated pneumonia

(4) Improved delivery of aerosolized medications

(5) Facilitation of early mobilization through better control of dyspnea and work of breathing

b. The feasibility of such a strategy has been demonstrated in small studies of subjects with acute exacerbations of chronic obstructive pulmonary disease [4]. Prospective randomized studies comparing $ECCO_2R$ to conventional management are needed before this approach can be recommended for clinical use.

c. A similar approach may be considered in severe cases of status asthmaticus in which patients have marked ventilatory impairment, often as a consequence of positive pressure ventilation and dynamic hyperinflation.

B. Bridge to transplant

1. ECMO support for end-stage respiratory failure as a bridging therapy to lung transplantation has traditionally been associated with poor posttransplant outcomes, mostly due to poor patient selection and device-associated complications. However, there have recently been improvements in posttransplant outcomes for patients supported with ECMO pretransplant. These improvements are at least in part attributable to:

   a. Careful patient selection and earlier initiation, thereby avoiding patients too moribund to successfully undergo lung transplantation

   b. Increased experience at high-volume centers with an associated reduction in complications

   c. Strategies that optimize physical conditioning and minimize ICU complications. These strategies include avoidance of sedation, endotracheal extubation, and early mobilization

2. Because there is no destination device for respiratory failure equivalent to the left ventricular assist device (LVAD) in advanced cardiac failure, patients with end-stage respiratory failure should be selected for ECMO support only when they are candidates for lung transplantation.

CLINICAL PEARL   Indications for venovenous ECMO include bridge to recovery for severe ARDS and bridge to lung transplantation for end-stage respiratory failure. The use of $ECCO_2R$ for acute hypercapnic respiratory failure is a promising area of ongoing research.

V. Indications and evidence for ECMO in cardiac failure

A. Bridge to recovery

1. **Cardiogenic shock.** Venoarterial ECMO is one of several mechanical circulatory support systems that have the ability to support severe cardiogenic shock, with the advantages that it can be initiated rapidly at the bedside and offers gas exchange support. The success of ECMO support as a bridge to recovery largely depends on the etiology, with cardiac failure due to acute myocardial infarction and fulminant myocarditis having the most favorable outcomes. The data for ECMO in cardiogenic shock are largely limited to case series, small cohort studies, and retrospective propensity analyses [5]. Pre-ECMO prognostication scores have been proposed to help maximize patient outcomes by identifying those most likely to benefit from ECMO support.

   a. Postcardiotomy cardiogenic shock is an uncommon complication of cardiac surgery that is associated with significant mortality. ECMO may be considered as temporary postoperative support when a patient cannot be weaned from cardiopulmonary bypass in the operating room.

   b. Primary graft failure (PGF), a rare complication of heart transplantation that is associated with a high rate of mortality, may be supported with venoarterial ECMO. Patients with PGF who are supported on ECMO and who survive beyond the early posttransplant period have comparable long-term survival to transplant recipients who never developed PGF.

2. **Extracorporeal cardiopulmonary resuscitation (ECPR).** ECPR (the use of ECMO in refractory cardiac arrest) is a rapidly expanding indication for venoarterial ECMO. There are no prospective randomized controlled trials of ECPR compared to conventional CPR; however, propensity analyses suggest significantly higher neurologically intact survival with ECPR compared to conventional CPR in both in-hospital and out-of-hospital cardiac arrests. Younger age, shorter duration of CPR prior to ECMO initiation, and subsequent cardiac interventions have all been associated with more favorable outcomes.

3. **Pulmonary vascular disease**

   a. Decompensated pulmonary hypertension with right ventricular failure, a condition associated with high mortality, is emerging as a potential target for ECMO support [6]. Traditionally a venoarterial configuration is needed to decompress the right ventricle and bypass the high resistance of the pulmonary vasculature. However, such an approach may be inadequate to oxygenate the upper body when femoral vessels are used for venoarterial ECMO. Alternative strategies include the following approaches:

(1) Upper-body venoarterial ECMO with right internal jugular venous drainage and subclavian or innominate arterial reinfusion via an end-to-side graft

(2) Single-site, dual-lumen cannulation (with bicaval drainage) via the internal jugular vein with reinfusion directed across a pre-existing atrial septal defect or intentionally created septostomy

(3) Pumpless arteriovenous ECMO between the main pulmonary artery and the left atrium

(4) Right atrial to left atrial ECMO. This configuration provides right ventricular support and gas exchange but uses the native left ventricle for the systemic circulation. Like venoarterial ECMO, it is associated with increased risk of stroke.

b. Pulmonary embolism, when associated with severe right ventricular dysfunction with or without hemodynamic collapse, may be appropriate for venoarterial ECMO support. Nonrandomized studies have demonstrated favorable survival rates when this strategy has been employed with concomitant consideration of systemic thrombolysis, catheter-directed therapies, or surgical embolectomy.

B. Bridge to left ventricular assist device (LVAD) or transplantation

1. ECMO has been reported as a viable bridging strategy for both LVAD and heart transplantation. LVAD themselves are used as either a longer-term bridge to transplantation or as destination therapy for patients who are not eligible for transplantation. Because venoarterial ECMO is associated with significant morbidity, the duration of support is typically limited to 1 to 2 weeks. During this time, assessment of neurologic function and organ system recovery are significant factors in determining the timing of LVAD insertion. Pre-ECMO patient characteristics that have been associated with poor outcomes for ECMO as bridge to VAD or transplant include age greater than 50, CPR prior to ECMO initiation, and high pre-ECMO severity of illness scores.

2. In cases where it is unclear whether cardiac function will recover (e.g., post-acute myocardial infarction complicated by cardiogenic shock), ECMO may be considered as a bridge to decision, where serial assessments of myocardial recovery are needed to determine whether a patient will proceed to recovery, VAD, or transplantation. Preservation of noncardiac end-organ function is of particular importance if destination device therapy or transplantation is being considered.

> **CLINICAL PEARL** Indications for venoarterial ECMO include bridge to recovery for potentially reversible cardiogenic shock or cardiac arrest and bridge to VAD or heart transplantation for irreversible cardiac failure. An emerging strategy is the use of venoarterial ECMO in patients with decompensated pulmonary hypertension as a bridge to either transplant or recovery.

VI. ECMO management

A. Invasive mechanical ventilation practices

1. VALI is believed to be the main determinant of poor outcomes in ARDS, explaining why a volume- and pressure-limited ventilation strategy has such a significant impact on survival.

2. Several studies have demonstrated that tidal volumes and plateau pressures below the current standard of care could further reduce VALI. However, reductions in tidal volumes, airway pressures, and respiratory rates with conventional invasive mechanical ventilation are often limited by intolerable levels of respiratory acidosis that come with marked reductions in minute ventilation.

3. The presence of extracorporeal ventilation can facilitate even lower tidal volumes and airway pressures by managing the concomitant hypercapnia and acidemia, to the point where in select cases mechanical ventilation may be discontinued and patients could be extubated while on ECMO.

4. In cases of severe ARDS in which ECMO is initiated for refractory gas exchange abnormalities or excess plateau airway pressures, many ECMO centers utilize a strategy of very low tidal volumes and respiratory rates while maintaining a moderate amount of PEEP to minimize alveolar collapse. Occasionally, in select patients, mechanical ventilation can be discontinued altogether.

5. A very lung-protective ventilation strategy may ultimately prove beneficial in less severe forms of ARDS, where oxygenation is better preserved and an approach targeting CO_2 removal alone with lower blood flows and smaller cannulae (i.e., $ECCO_2R$) is sufficient. Prospective randomized controlled trials are in progress, seeking to determine if there is a clinical benefit that outweighs the potential risks of extracorporeal support.

CLINICAL PEARL   The use of ECMO for respiratory failure in mechanically ventilated patients can reduce the incidence of VALI by permitting the use of very low tidal volumes and plateau airway pressures.

B. **Anticoagulation strategies**

1. Continuous systemic anticoagulation is generally needed to maintain ECMO circuit patency and minimize thrombotic risk to the patient. The degree of anticoagulation has to be balanced with the risk of hemorrhagic complications. There are no universally accepted anticoagulation standards for ECMO nor is there a consensus on how anticoagulation should be monitored, with activated clotting time, activated partial thromboplastin time (aPTT), and thromboelastography, among others, having been reported.

2. For VV ECMO, a strategy that combines lower-level anticoagulation, restrictive transfusion thresholds, and reinfusion of circuit blood at the time of decannulation has been shown to be associated with favorable outcomes with minimal transfusion requirements [7].

3. Prolonged heparin infusions may reduce available antithrombin III and thereby impair the efficacy of heparin. Antithrombin III is available in the recombinant form and may be considered to restore the efficacy of heparin in the context of low antithrombin III levels.

4. If heparin cannot be used, for example, in the setting of heparin-induced thrombocytopenia (HIT), alternative anticoagulants include argatroban and bivalirudin.

CLINICAL PEARL   Low levels of systemic anticoagulation appear to be effective at maintaining ECMO circuit patency while minimizing the risk of significant bleeding.

C. **Early mobilization**

1. Early mobilization of critically ill patients has repeatedly been demonstrated to be not only safe but also effective in reducing ICU-associated complications.

2. Extubation and cessation of mechanical ventilation, if feasible while receiving ECMO therapy, may aid in early patient mobilization.

3. Through the use of more compact circuitry and the avoidance of femoral cannulation, it has become feasible for patient supported with ECMO to undergo early mobilization, including ambulation [8].

4. Physical rehabilitation, including early mobilization, is of critical importance in the bridge-to-transplant population in order to maintain transplant candidacy. Whether there is a benefit in the bridge-to-recovery population comparable to that seen in other critically ill patients has yet to be determined and is an area of active research.

D. **Weaning ECMO**

1. *Venovenous.* Patients should be evaluated for their readiness to wean from ECMO support after the underlying cause of respiratory failure is treated and the patient's native gas exchange and respiratory system mechanics improve. There are several approaches to weaning venovenous ECMO. An approach of incremental reductions in sweep gas flow rate and FDO_2 while monitoring the ability to maintain adequate gas exchange with native lung function is most commonly employed. Blood flow rate may also be reduced as a means

of weaning (although very low blood flow rates should be avoided, as the risk of circuit thrombosis increases). A trial with sweep gas flow turned off for a prespecified period of time (e.g., 30 minutes) with acceptable gas exchange, no excess work of breathing, and acceptable ventilator settings (if applicable) should be performed in most patients prior to consideration of decannulation and may be used as the sole determinant of weaning readiness.

2. *Venoarterial.* Weaning from venoarterial ECMO differs significantly from venovenous ECMO. Because venoarterial ECMO provides hemodynamic support, weaning can be performed with incremental reductions in extracorporeal blood flow with serial assessments of vasopressor and inotrope requirements, cardiac function, and end-organ perfusion. Ideally, vasopressors will be able to be minimized or discontinued entirely prior to decannulation from venoarterial ECMO, while it is more common to maintain some pharmacologic inotropic support. During weaning trials, a minimum extracorporeal blood flow rate of 2 L/min should be maintained through the circuit to avoid circuit thrombosis. Sweep gas FDO_2 is typically not weaned in order to avoid the creation of a right-to-left shunt. If a patient appears ready for decannulation from a hemodynamic perspective but continues to require extracorporeal gas exchange support, conversion from venoarterial to venovenous ECMO (with its lower risk of systemic embolization) should be considered.

> **CLINICAL PEARL** When weaning venovenous ECMO, sweep gas flow is typically discontinued to assess adequacy of native gas exchange and readiness for decannulation. In venoarterial ECMO, extracorporeal blood flow is typically reduced to assess hemodynamic readiness for decannulation. In venoarterial ECMO, sweep gas flow should always be maintained; discontinuation of sweep gas flow would lead to hypoxemia from a right-to-left shunt.

VII. ECMO transport

A. Patients with severe refractory respiratory or cardiac failure who would otherwise benefit from ECMO support may be at facilities without ECMO capabilities and yet be too unstable to transport to an ECMO-capable center. Under such circumstances, mobile ECMO transport teams may improve these patients' outcomes by performing ECMO cannulation at the origin hospital and transporting them to specialized centers capable of providing ongoing ECMO management.

B. ECMO transport has been demonstrated to be safe and feasible. This highlights the potential role of regionalization of ECMO in order to maximize outcomes by referring patients to high-volume centers with greater experience [9].

VIII. Complications

A. Potential complications are inherent with any invasive intervention, especially among patients with severe underlying critical illness, and must be weighed against the potential benefit of the intervention. Complication rates for ECMO vary greatly based on center experience, management strategies, devices used, and patient characteristics.

1. Commonly encountered hematologic complications include hemorrhage and thrombotic/thromboembolic events, the severities of which are heavily influenced by center-specific anticoagulation practices and patient-specific factors. Less common hematologic complications include hemolysis, thrombocytopenia, disseminated intravascular coagulation, acquired von Willebrand disease, and HIT.

   a. The diagnosis of HIT during ECMO should be made based on appropriate clinical criteria (e.g., 4T score). If HIT is suspected, a heparin antibody test should be performed as an initial screening test, followed by a serotonin release assay if the heparin antibody test is positive. Alternate anticoagulants (e.g., direct thrombin inhibitors) may be used for anticoagulation while awaiting the results of serologic testing.

2. Infectious complication rates vary substantially by center and by the manner in which ECMO-related infections are defined. Standardized infection control practices should be used for ECMO insertion, maintenance, and removal.

3. Other complications such as limb ischemia, limb engorgement, and vascular perforation may be a consequence of certain ECMO cannulation approaches and techniques and will be influenced by the experience of the provider performing the procedure and the use of radiographic guidance. Prompt Doppler examination in the ICU will guide interventions.

IX. Economic considerations

A. The implementation across a health system of any novel technology, particularly for commonly encountered diseases, has to take into consideration the resources it may require, including financial resources that will vary greatly by region. There are limited data on the economic impact of ECMO use in ARDS and even less in ECMO for cardiac failure. The CESAR trial, conducted within the United Kingdom's National Health Service, estimated that referral for consideration of ECMO led to a gain of 0.03 quality-adjusted life-years (QALYs) at 6-month follow-up, with the predicted cost per QALY of ECMO to be £19,252 (95% CI £7,622–59,200).

B. Any prospective randomized studies assessing the role of ECMO in cardiopulmonary failure would benefit from describing the economic impact in addition to the clinical outcomes, so that hospitals and healthcare systems can best decide how to allocate the resources appropriately.

X. Ethical considerations

With the advent of technology that is able to entirely support the respiratory or cardiac system, and to do so for prolonged periods of time, the creation of ethically challenging situations is inevitable [10].

A. The ability of ECPR to improve survival beyond conventional CPR opens up the potential for ECPR to be used indiscriminately among patients suffering cardiac arrest, a practice that has the capacity to prolong suffering for many patients without changing the ultimate outcome. Whenever possible, evidence-based criteria ought to be used to identify patients most likely to benefit from ECPR.

B. The lack of destination device therapy in end-stage respiratory failure creates its own unique dilemma. Patients supported with ECMO as bridge to transplant who are no longer deemed transplant candidates and yet are dependent on ECMO for respiratory function have no viable long-term solution, often referred to as a "bridge to nowhere." Whether to continue supporting these patients and for how long, particularly those patients who are sentient, is a fraught situation that often requires ethics and palliative care consultations and extensive discussions with the patient and family. Potential bridge-to-transplant candidates ought to be carefully selected so as to *avoid* the "bridge-to-nowhere" scenario whenever possible.

C. Because venoarterial ECMO may adequately support end-organ perfusion in the absence of native cardiac function, the relevance of CPR, and thus a "Do Not Resuscitate" (DNR) order, may be murky. This highlights the need to understand goals of care and not only the procedures to be performed. Even in the absence of a physiologic benefit of CPR, a DNR order may still help convey the overall goals of care for the patient, particularly if it is deemed that meaningful recovery cannot be achieved. At that point, the conversation should focus on limiting or withdrawing life-sustaining treatments.

REFERENCES

1. **Brodie D, Bacchetta M. Extracorporeal membrane oxygenation for ARDS in adults.** *N Engl J Med.* **2011;365(20): 1905–1914.**
2. Acute Respiratory Distress Syndrome Network, Brower RG, Matthay MA, Morris A, et al. Ventilation with lower tidal volumes as compared with traditional tidal volumes for acute lung injury and the acute respiratory distress syndrome. *N Engl J Med.* 2000;342(18):1301–1308.
3. Peek GJ, Mugford M, Tiruvoipati R, et al. Efficacy and economic assessment of conventional ventilatory support versus extracorporeal membrane oxygenation for severe adult respiratory failure (CESAR): a multicentre randomised controlled trial. *Lancet.* 2009;374(9698):1351–1363.
4. Abrams DC, Brenner K, Burkart KM, et al. Pilot study of extracorporeal carbon dioxide removal to facilitate extubation and ambulation in exacerbations of chronic obstructive pulmonary disease. *Ann Am Thorac Soc.* 2013;10(4):307–314.
5. **Abrams D, Combes A, Brodie D. Extracorporeal membrane oxygenation in cardiopulmonary disease in adults.** *J Am Coll Cardiol.* **2014;63(25 Pt A):2769–2778.**

6. **Abrams DC, Brodie D, Rosenzweig EB, et al. Upper-body extracorporeal membrane oxygenation as a strategy in decompensated pulmonary arterial hypertension.** *Pulm Circ.* **2013;3(2):432–435.**

7. Agerstrand CL, Burkart KM, Abrams DC, et al. Blood conservation in extracorporeal membrane oxygenation for acute respiratory distress syndrome. *Ann Thorac Surg.* 2015;99(2):590–595.

8. **Abrams D, Javidfar J, Farrand E, et al. Early mobilization of patients receiving extracorporeal membrane oxygenation: a retrospective cohort study.** *Crit Care.* **2014;18(1):R38.**

9. Combes A, Brodie D, Bartlett R, et al. Position paper for the organization of extracorporeal membrane oxygenation programs for acute respiratory failure in adult patients. *Am J Respir Crit Care Med.* 2014;190(5):488–496.

10. Abrams DC, Prager K, Blinderman CD, et al. Ethical dilemmas encountered with the use of extracorporeal membrane oxygenation in adults. *Chest.* 2014;145(4):876–882.

Perioperative Management

25

Postoperative Care of the Cardiac Surgical Patient

Breandan L. Sullivan and Michael H. Wall

KEY POINTS

1. Transport from the operating room (OR) to the intensive care unit (ICU) is a critical period for patient monitoring or vigilance. Emergency drugs and airway equipment should be present, and adequate transportation personnel (typically three people) should accompany the patient during transport.

2. Patient "handoff" to the ICU should be consistent, careful, and structured and should not distract caregivers from continuous assessment of hemodynamics, oxygenation, and ventilation.

3. Early postoperative respiratory support ranges from full mechanical ventilation to immediate extubation in the OR, depending upon institutional practice patterns, anesthetic techniques, and patient stability. There is no "best" ventilation mode for cardiac surgery patients.

4. Weaning from mechanical ventilation involves assessment of oxygenation adequacy (typically PaO_2/FiO_2 >100 on positive end-expiratory pressure [PEEP] 5 cm H_2O or less), hemodynamic stability, patient responsiveness to commands, and measured ventilatory parameters such as vital capacity and the rapid shallow breathing index (RSBI).

5. Fast-tracking protocols designed to extubate cardiac surgery patients within several hours of completion of surgery are common. With such protocols, early postoperative continuous infusions of propofol or dexmedetomidine may be helpful.

6. Enhanced recovery after cardiac surgery involves a multidisciplinary approach with physical therapists, occupational therapists, dieticians, and pharmacists, with the combined goal of shortening the convalescent time after cardiac surgery.

7. Early postoperative differential diagnosis of hypotension is often challenging and includes hypovolemia, heart valve dysfunction, left ventricular (LV) and/or right ventricular (RV) dysfunction, cardiac tamponade, cardiac dysrhythmia, and vasodilation. Once a diagnosis has been made, optimal therapy usually becomes clear.

8. Hypertension is not uncommon and must be acutely and effectively managed to minimize bleeding and other complications such as LV failure and aortic dissection. The differential diagnoses include pain, hypothermia, hypercarbia, hypoxemia, intravascular volume excess, anxiety, and pre-existing essential hypertension, among others.

9. Acute poststernotomy pain most often is managed by administering intravenous (IV) opioids, but other potentially helpful modalities include nonsteroidal anti-inflammatory drugs (NSAIDs), intrathecal opioids, and central neuraxial or peripheral nerve blocks.

10. Early postoperative acid–base, electrolyte, and glucose disturbances are common. They should be diagnosed and treated promptly.

11. Postoperative bleeding may be surgical, coagulopathic, or both. Aggressive diagnosis and treatment of coagulation disturbances facilitates early diagnosis and treatment of surgical bleeding (i.e., return to OR for reexploration) and avoidance of cardiac tamponade.

12. Discharge from the ICU typically occurs in 1 to 2 days. Criteria vary with cardiac surgical procedures and with institutional capabilities for post-ICU patient care (e.g., stepdown ICU beds vs. traditional floor nursing care).

13. Adequate communication with patients' family members and adequate family visitation and support greatly facilitate postoperative recovery.

THE PURPOSE OF THIS CHAPTER is to briefly discuss the transport of the cardiac surgery patient from the OR to the ICU, the handoff of care from the OR team to the ICU team, and an approach to common problems that occur in the first 24 hours in the ICU. The reader is referred to standard critical care text books for discussion of more chronic ICU problems such as nutrition, infectious disease, sepsis, and multiple organ failure.

I. **Transition from operating room (OR) to intensive care unit (ICU)**
   A. **General principles**
      1. Movement of a critically ill patient in the immediate postoperative period to the ICU or to an intermediate-level postcardiac surgical recovery area is a risky business. Inter- or

intrahospital transport of critically ill patients is associated with increased morbidity and mortality [1].

2. The American College of Critical Care Medicine (ACCM) guidelines state that "during transport, there is no hiatus in the monitoring or maintenance of a patient's vital signs" [2].

3. The ACCM guidelines state that there are four major areas to optimize efficiency and safety of patient transport: communication (or handoffs), personnel, equipment, and monitoring. Each of these areas will be discussed.

B. The transport process

1. **Prior to movement of the patient from OR table to ICU bed**

    a. **Airway/breathing.** If patients are suitable candidates for rapid extubation (see Section IV) and meet standard extubation criteria, they can be extubated in the OR, or within 6 to 8 hours of arrival in the ICU. If the patient is to remain intubated, the endotracheal tube should be checked for position and patency and should be securely attached to the patient. In addition, all chest tubes and drains should be checked for ongoing bleeding to ensure that immediate transport from the OR is appropriate and for proper functioning to avoid hemothorax or pneumothorax during transport.

    b. **Circulation.** The patient should be hemodynamically stable prior to transport. In general, if the patient requires frequent bolus doses or increasing doses of vasoactive drugs, it is better to stabilize prior to transport.

        (1) **Pacemaker.** Proper settings and functioning of the pacemaker should be checked at this point.

    c. **Coagulation.** Bleeding should be controlled, and a plan for correction of ongoing coagulopathy should be made prior to transport.

    d. **Metabolic.** Metabolic abnormalities (glucose, electrolyte, and acid–base) should be identified and corrected as much as possible prior to the transport.

    e. **Brief telephone report.** A brief verbal report to the ICU team should be provided prior to transport (see Section IV).

    f. **Special bed.** Patients at high risk for development of pressure ulcers (pre-existing pressure ulcers, poor nutritional status, elderly, poor ventricular function, etc.) should be placed on special beds/mattresses in the OR.

2. **Patient movement from the OR table to the transport bed.** Movement can cause hemodynamic instability, fluid shifts, and arrhythmias. Movement can also cause inadvertent loss of airway, vascular access, and interruption of intravenous (IV) infusions. Residual intracardiac air is a complication of many procedures (e.g., valve replacement) and this air may be easily dislodged when moving the patient. In addition, the position of a pulmonary artery catheter (PAC) can be altered during patient movement. Confirmation of the PAC position (i.e., pulmonary artery waveform rather than pulmonary artery occluded or right ventricular [RV] waveform) before and after patient movement should be done. Sudden onset of dysrhythmia should trigger examination of the PAC. Ready access to a large-bore IV infusion port and to any ongoing or continuous infusions of medications is critical to managing this period safely and being able to respond promptly.

CLINICAL PEARL Although it is difficult to stop a "moving train," if hemodynamic deterioration occurs in the OR even after transfer from the OR table to the ICU bed, it is better to stop, reassess, and stabilize the patient than to proceed with transport.

3. **Transport from the OR to the ICU**

    a. **Personnel.** Generally, at least three members of the operative team should transport the patient from the OR to the ICU. This should include a member of the anesthesia care team, surgical team, and a nurse or technician. Additional team members (perfusionists, respiratory therapists, etc.) may be needed for patients on mechanical assist devices, inhaled pulmonary vasodilators, or those with acute lung injury (ALI) who require a transport ventilator.

b. **Equipment.** ACCM guidelines recommend a minimum of a blood pressure monitor, pulse oximeter, and cardiac monitor/defibrillator for all transports of critically ill patients [1]. An additional monitor to consider is continuous end-tidal CO_2 for intubated patients. Equipment and drugs for emergency airway management should be immediately available. An oxygen (O_2) source with enough O_2 for the duration of transport plus 30 minutes must be available. Basic emergency advanced cardiac life support (ACLS) drugs should be immediately available. All infusions should be checked and all pumps should be fully charged prior to transport. Supplemental O_2 should be provided to all extubated patients. Ambu bag ventilation (with or without positive end-expiratory pressure [PEEP] valves) can be used for most patients. Transport ventilators may be needed for patients with ALI or acute respiratory distress syndrome (ARDS). Mechanical support device batteries should be immediately available.

c. **Monitoring.** ACCM guidelines state that critically ill patients should "…receive the same level of basic physiologic monitoring and transport as they had in the ICU…." The same concept applies to patients leaving the OR [1].

d. **IV access.** Every effort must be made to avoid a "tangle" of IV tubing. In general, it is best to have one large-bore IV identified for rapid administration of fluids or emergency medications. This line should be easily identified and immediately accessible. Bolus medications should ideally be given via a central venous site for faster onset. Finally, all IV fluid bags should be full enough to give fluid boluses as needed.

e. **Sedation/analgesia.** In extubated patients, it is best *not* to give boluses of narcotics during transport. It is probably better and safer to give analgesics prior to transport and then give additional medications after arrival in the ICU. In intubated patients, it is best to start the postoperative sedation and analgesia plan prior to transport to minimize the need to give bolus medications during transport.

II. Transfer of care to the ICU team

A. **Importance of handoffs**

The handoff of care from the OR team to the ICU team is a surprisingly hazardous and dangerous event. The Joint Commission identified that communication failure was the root cause of 65% of sentinel events in 2006 [2]. Numerous studies have shown that the best handoffs occur when they are structured, standardized, and use checklists [3–6]. Recently, many centers are developing handoff tools from the electronic medical record (EMR) [7].

B. **Logistics**

Ideally, each member of the OR and ICU teams should have specific tasks and the handoff should occur in a standardized sequence [3,4]. One simple sequence would be transition from transport to ICU monitor, then initial ventilator settings, and then formal structured handoff.

C. **Transition to ICU monitors**

The patient must be continuously monitored during this process. Ideally, each parameter (ECG, O_2 saturation, etc.) should be transferred from the transport monitor to the ICU monitor in series, as opposed to unhooking all of them at once and then hooking them up one at a time. Some systems allow for all the monitors to be almost instantly switched over by removing the entire "brick" at once. In any event, based on local monitors, there should be an orderly transition between both sets of monitors.

CLINICAL PEARL Amidst the flurry of activity upon arrival in the ICU, the anesthesiologist must keep a "10,000-feet" oversight perspective and intervene as needed to ensure optimal patient management during this transition.

D. **Initial ventilator settings**

Intubated patients must have their endotracheal tube evaluated for patency, security, and position. This can be accomplished with a chest x-ray or with a bedside bronchoscopy. Ventilator parameters including ventilator mode, rate, fraction of inspired oxygen (FiO_2), PEEP, and pressure support must be selected. The patients who have no respiratory effort can be placed on assist-control (AC) or synchronized intermittent mandatory ventilation (SIMV) with an adequate rate, tidal volume, and PEEP. The patients who have regained spontaneous respiratory effort can be placed on SIMV or **pressure support ventilation (PSV)**. PSV and SIMV modes can be combined. Excessive use of PEEP impedes venous return and may impair RV performance. The application of PEEP may decrease mediastinal bleeding, although the literature on this topic is inconsistent and this technique must be used with caution, as PEEP's adverse effects on hemodynamics are well established.

E. The actual handoff

Once the monitors have been transferred to the ICU bedside monitor and oxygenation and ventilation have been confirmed, a structured handoff should occur. This should include the patient's name, age, allergies, medical history, all significant intraoperative events, and the immediate postoperative plan. One structured handoff form generated from the EMR is shown (see Fig. 25.1). Time should be allowed for questions and answers from all members of OR and ICU teams.

1. The **initial review** of the patient upon his or her arrival to the recovery area includes the patient's history, age, height, weight, pre-existing medical conditions, any allergies, a list of preoperative medications, and review of the most current laboratory findings (with special emphasis on potassium and hematocrit [Hct]). The report should include a detailed review of the patient's cardiac status, including ventricular dysfunction, valvular disease, coronary anatomy, and details of the surgical procedure.

2. An **anesthetic review** should be presented, which includes types and location of IV catheters and invasive monitors, along with any complications that occurred during their placement. A brief description of the anesthetic technique should be discussed to help plan for a smooth emergence. Any difficulties with airway management should be emphasized, particularly when weaning and extubation protocols are utilized. The presence or absence of obstructive sleep apnea should be discussed and the need for continuing patient's home continuous positive airway pressure (CPAP) or bilevel positive airway pressure (BiPAP) should be addressed. A post-cardiopulmonary bypass (CPB) synopsis should be reported, including the use of vasoactive, inotropic, and antiarrhythmic drugs, as well as any untoward events such as arrhythmias and presumed drug reactions. This should also include an update on the presence or absence of bleeding prior to chest closure.

3. Early upon arrival to the ICU, the patient's **heart rate, rhythm, and blood pressure** should be determined. If the heart is being paced, the settings should be reviewed and all electrodes identified and secured, as the patient may be dependent on the device.

   a. If the patient has a permanent pacemaker or defibrillator, the settings should also be reviewed. The devices should be interrogated in the ICU and antitachycardia treatment should be activated. While waiting for the device to be activated, external defibrillator pads should be placed on the patient and a defibrillator should be immediately available [8].

   b. If the patient has a ventricular assist device (VAD), the monitor should be attached to a wall-based energy supply and the output of the device should be attached to the display module. The settings of the device and the position and location of the cannula should be reviewed.

   c. For patients on extracorporal membrane oxygenation (ECMO), the O_2 and air supplies should be attached to the wall outlet supplies, and backup tanks should be available (see Chapter 24).

F. Laboratory tests/electrocardiogram (ECG)/chest radiograph (CXR)

After the handoff is complete and questions are answered, baseline ECG, CXR, and laboratory tests should be obtained. An initial arterial blood gas (ABG) should be drawn to ensure the adequacy of oxygenation and ventilation, whether the patient is on a mechanical ventilator or breathing spontaneously. Potassium, blood glucose, and Hct levels should be obtained. Acid–base status should be reviewed from ABGs. Baseline coagulation parameters, including prothrombin time (PT), activated partial thromboplastin time (aPTT), and platelet count should be acquired if the patient is bleeding excessively.

HI-LIGHTED AREAS ARE TO BE COMMUNICATED
DURING THE FIRST PHONE CALL
OR/ICU/PACUICU TRANSFER REPORT
☐ OR→ICU   ☐ ICU→OR   ☐ OR→PACU→ICU

Patient Name_____

Pertinent preop info:

Procedure: Date:

Anesthesiologist: Surgeon:

Allergies (confirm per BJ protocol):

Patient Identification Band On? Y / N

Lines

☐ Arterial line   ☐ PA   ☐ CORDIS + DLIC   ☐ CVP   ☐ Femoral Art line   ☐ IABP   ☐ Lumbar drain   ☐ Chest Tube

☐ Epidural → Level Placed T__ L __   Drug: _____ Dose: _____ Time Given:_____

Cardiovascular

☐ Hemodynamically Unstable → _____   ☐ Rhythm Disturbance → _____

Vasoactive drips: _____ / _____ / _____ / _____

Notable Intra operative: ☐ Hypotension ☐ Hypertension   Notable Events on Transport: _____
Cross Clamp Time: _____ CPB Time: _____

Respiratory

☐ Anticipated Difficult Airway ☐ Unanticipated Difficult Airway   Describe
☐ Extubated   ☐ Face Mask/NC 0₃%   ☐ Transferred Intubated → Why
Notable Airway Events: _____   ☐ Inhaled NO or PGI₂
VENTILATOR: TV   Rate   FiO₂   PEEP   PSV
Notable events during transfer_____

Neurologic

☐ Ventriculostomy   ☐ ICP Monitor   ☐ Post OP CT ☐ Burst Suppression ☐ C-Collar
☐ IntraOperative Vessel Occlusion
Spinal Cord: Notable events on IntraOperative Electrophysiologic monitoring ?

Mental Status: awake/follows commands / comatose/other _____
Pupils: _____ GAG: _____ Cough: _____
Motor Response: (circle) Follows Commands – Purposeful – Localizes to Pain – Postures to Pain – Unresponsive to Pain
Focal Deficits: **N Y**   RUE/RLE   LUE/LLE

Fluids

PRBC's _____ PLT's _____ FFP _____ Cell Saver_____ Cryo ____ Colloids:_____ Crystalloids _____

Other _____ EBL: _____ Urine Output: _____
Any Reactions? Y N

IntraOp MEDS

Antibiotics: _____ Time: _____ ☐ Lasix/Mannitol → Time: _____ DDAVP_____

Last Narcotic: Drug_____ Dose _____   Time _____ Narcotic TOTAL: _____
Last Neuromuscular: Drug_____ Dose _____   Time _____ Neuromuscular TOTAL: _____
Last Benzodiazepine Dose:_____   Time:_____
Steroids   Drug_____ Dose _____   Time _____ Steroid TOTAL: _____
Reversal given N Y → Time:_____ for: ☐ Paralytics ☐ Narcotics ☐ Benzodiazepines
Other:

Laboratory

LAST
ABG: pH   pCO2   PO2   HCO3   K⁺   Glucose   HCT   Plts   PT/PTT/INR

Pertinent abnormal laboratory values:

OTHER Pertinent/IntraOperative Events/Information:

Special Request/Needs:

☐Blood Warmer ☐Bair Hugger ☐Rapid Transfusers ☐Propofol IMED Pump ☐ SCD ☐ Isolation & Reason_____

PACU UPDATES: Given By:_____
                                                                      Taken By:_____

Recorded by:_____   Recorders contact Number/Beeper: _____

Information Provided by: _____   Information Providers contact Number/Beeper _____

CALLS: 56ICU Ext: 2-5812   84ICU Ext: 2-8493   104ICU 450-0741

FIGURE 25.1 Structured handoff form generated from electronic medical records (EMRs).

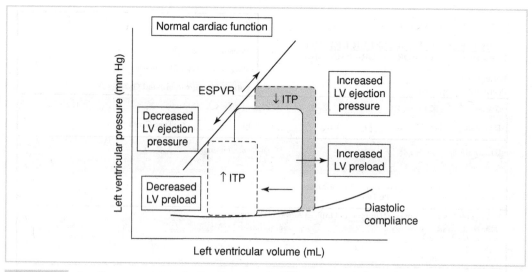

FIGURE 25.2 The effect of increasing and decreasing intrathoracic pressure (ITP) on the pressure–volume loop of the cardiac cycle. The slope of the left ventricular (LV) end-systolic pressure–volume relationship (ESPVR) is proportional to contractility. The slope of the diastolic LV pressure–volume relationship defines diastolic compliance [10].

III. **Mechanical ventilation after cardiac surgery**

    A. **Hemodynamic response to positive-pressure ventilation (PPV)**

        Heart–lung interactions with PPV are complex [9,10]. In patients with normal left ventricular (LV) function, PPV increases intrathoracic pressure (ITP), which reduces venous return, afterload, and stroke volume (SV) and cardiac output (CO) (see Fig. 25.2). On the other hand, in patients with LV dysfunction, decreased preload and afterload actually can *improve* LV performance and CO (see Fig. 25.3). PEEP further increases ITP and decreases venous return.

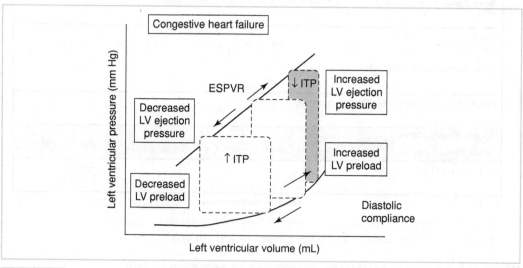

FIGURE 25.3 The effect of increasing and decreasing intrathoracic pressure (ITP) on the left ventricular (LV) pressure–volume loop of the cardiac cycle in congestive heart failure when LV contractility is reduced and intravascular volume is expanded. The slope of the left ventricular end-systolic pressure–volume relationship (LV ESPVR) is proportional to contractility. The slope of the diastolic LV pressure–volume relationship defines diastolic compliance [10].

> **CLINICAL PEARL** During transport and transition from OR to ICU, always consider acute changes in ventilation (e.g., tidal volume, mean airway pressure, PEEP) as the explanation for new-onset hypotension.

B. **Pulmonary changes after sternotomy and thoracotomy**
Cardiac surgery requires either a midline sternotomy or a thoracotomy. Both of these approaches temporarily compromise the function of the thoracic cage, which acts as a respiratory pump. One week after cardiac surgery, there is a significant reduction in total lung capacity, inspiratory vital capacity, forced expiratory volumes, and functional residual capacity compared to preoperative values [11]. Even at 6 weeks postoperatively, total lung capacity, inspiratory vital capacity, and forced expiratory volume remained significantly below preoperative values. These findings suggest a marked tendency toward postoperative atelectasis and the possibility of hypoxemia from increased physiologic shunting. These changes in chest wall function can increase physiologic shunt to as much as 13% (compared to a baseline normal value of 5%).

In addition to these changes in mechanics and volumes, there are also abnormalities in gas exchange, compliance, and work of breathing [12]. The cause of these abnormalities is multifactorial and may include inflammation, reperfusion, and other mechanisms.

C. **Choosing modes of ventilation**
1. **Extubated patient.** If the patient was **extubated in the OR**, supplemental oxygen may be all that is necessary postoperatively. Following a general anesthetic, patients will exhibit a mild increase in the $PaCO_2$. Aggressive pulmonary toilet and frequent incentive spirometry must be performed to prevent the atelectasis and hypoxemia that may develop from changes in chest wall function.

2. **Noninvasive ventilation (NIV).** NIV can be used to treat or prevent postoperative respiratory failure and has been shown to prevent reintubation, decrease ventilator-associated pneumonia, and improve outcomes [13,14]. A sample protocol for the use of NIV is shown in Figure 25.4. Contraindications are shown in Table 25.1. Two types of NIV are commonly used:
   a. **Continuous positive airway pressure (CPAP)**, where constant airway pressure is applied during both inspiration and expiration.
   b. **Bilevel positive airway pressure (BiPAP)**, where PSV is applied during inspiration and PEEP is applied during expiration.

3. **Intubated patient**
   a. If a patient returns from the OR with an **endotracheal tube in place**, an individualized plan of care should be developed for that patient. The choice of mechanical ventilation mode is based on the patient's inherent respiratory effort. If a patient demonstrates an inspiratory effort, PSV or SIMV can be used.
   If a patient is not demonstrating spontaneous respiratory effort, AC or SIMV should be selected. In AC, a set respiratory rate (RR) is delivered regardless of the patient's respiratory effort. If a spontaneous breath is initiated, the ventilator detects the trigger and delivers a set tidal volume (or pressure if on pressure control ventilation). In SIMV, a set RR is also delivered, but spontaneous breaths over the set rate are not fully supported (like they are in AC) but are dependent on the patient's effort.
   b. Patients with severe hypoxemia, respiratory failure, or (mild, moderate, or severe) ARDS will need to be ventilated in a way that minimizes or avoids further "ventilator-induced lung injury" [15]. There have been several recent reviews on the ICU management of ARDS [16–20]. In the early stages of ARDS, complete control over a patient's oxygenation and ventilation is needed. This often involves deep sedation with aggressive titration of PEEP and often neuromuscular blockade as well.
   Initial ventilator settings in patients with ARDS would include (ardsnet.org):
   (1) Any ventilator mode
   (2) Tidal volume (V_T) 6 mL/kg of predicted (i.e., ideal) body weight
   (3) Set RR, so minute ventilation is adequate, 18 to 22 breaths/min
   (4) Adjust V_T and RR to achieve a goal pH of 7.30 to 7.40 and plateau pressure <30 cm H_2O.

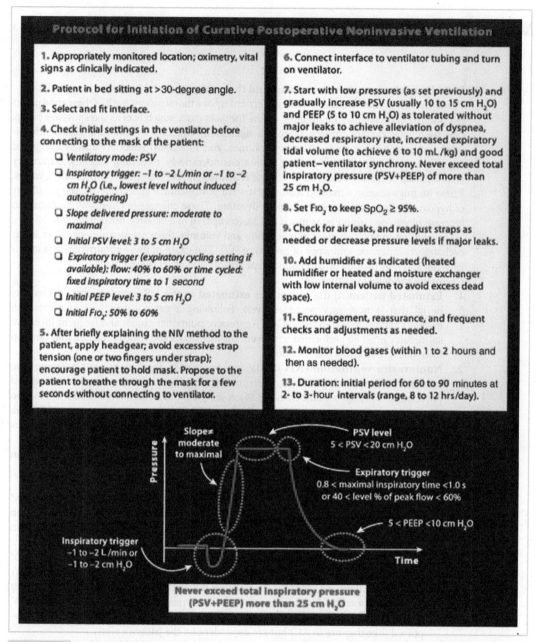

FIGURE 25.4 Protocol for initiation of curative postoperative noninvasive ventilation (NIV). PSV, pressure support ventilation; PEEP, positive end-expiratory pressure; FiO₂, fraction of inspired oxygen; SpO₂, pulse oximetry saturation [13].

4. **Weaning from mechanical ventilation is multifactorial.** In many postoperative environments, this can best be accomplished by using an algorithm so that weaning can proceed methodically and without interruption. Figure 25.5 shows an algorithm that could facilitate efficient weaning. Prior to attempts at weaning, the following parameters must be met:

   a. Normothermia
   b. Hemodynamically stable

TABLE 25.1 Contraindications to noninvasive positive-pressure ventilation

■ **Absolute**
Cardiac or respiratory arrest

Nonrespiratory organ failure
    Severe encephalopathy (e.g., Glasgow Coma Score <10)
    Severe upper gastrointestinal bleeding
    Hemodynamic instability or unstable cardiac dysrhythmia

Facial surgery, trauma, or deformity
Upper airway obstruction
Inability to cooperate
Inability to clear respiratory secretions
High risk for aspiration
Postoperative esophageal or gastric surgery
■ **Relative**
Mildly decreased level of consciousness
Progressive severe respiratory failure
Patient who cannot be calmed or comforted

Modified from Jaber SD, Chanques G, Jung B. Postoperative noninvasive ventilation. *Anesthesiology*. 2010;112:453–461.

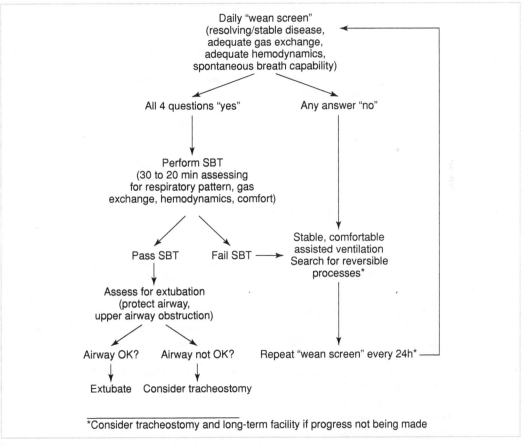

FIGURE 25.5 Protocolized flow chart for ventilator discontinuation [22]. SBT, spontaneous breathing trial.

(1) Stable vasoactive drug requirements

(2) Not requiring increasing doses (infusion rates) or boluses of inotropes or vasopressors

c. Stable heart rate and rhythm

d. Normal acid–base and metabolic state

e. Not bleeding excessively (criteria vary, but generally <150 mL/hr chest tube drainage) If these criteria are met, the patient is ready to be liberated from mechanical ventilation.

D. **Liberation from mechanical ventilation**

1. Current recommendations are that patients should be liberated from mechanical ventilation as quickly as possible, and an attempt should be made at least daily [21,22].

2. The first step is to assess the following to determine "readiness to wean":

   a. PaO_2/FiO_2 >200 mm Hg with PEEP ≤5 cm H_2O

   b. Hemodynamically stable

   c. Awake, alert, and following commands

   d. Able to cough effectively

   e. Adequate reversal of neuromuscular blockade (negative inspiratory force [NIF] of 30 cm H_2O or more, able to lift head off bed >5 seconds, no fade on train-of-four, vital capacity >15 mL/kg, etc.)

   f. A rapid shallow breathing index (RSBI), defined as RR divided by tidal volume in liters (RR/V_T) <80 to 100 breaths/min/L after a 2- to 3-minute spontaneous breathing trial (SBT)

3. If the patient passes the readiness to wean screen, a trial of spontaneous ventilation via T-piece or with low levels of PSV (5 to 7 cm H_2O) and PEEP (≤5 cm H_2O) for 30 to 120 minutes is done. At the end of the trial, if the RSBI is <80 to 100, the patient should be considered for extubation if they meet the following final criteria:

   a. Awake and alert

   b. Able to cough and clear secretions

      (1) Patients who require suctioning more often than every 2 hours are at a higher risk for reintubation.

   c. No airway edema (as judged crudely by edema of tongue and presence of leak when endotracheal tube cuff is deflated)

   d. Hemodynamically stable

      (1) Less than 20% change in HR, BP, pulmonary artery pressures, cardiac index, etc., during the trial.

   e. Normal oxygenation and ventilation

4. If the patient meets the criteria, extubation can be performed.

5. If the patient does not meet the criteria, correctable causes need to be identified and optimized prior to another attempt.

6. Patients who repeatedly fail SBTs may require more long-term weaning from mechanical ventilation [21].

CLINICAL PEARL   Although specific protocols for weaning and extubation can vary, it is critical to establish a checklist for this process and to routinely apply it to every patient.

E. **Incentive spirometry, deep breathing, and coughing maneuvers**

Patients must be encouraged to use **incentive spirometry** and to do **deep breathing** and coughing maneuvers after extubation to reduce atelectasis. There are numerous physiologic causes of hypoxemia. Diffusion abnormality, low FiO_2, hypoventilation, and V/Q mismatch along with shunt comprise the list of possibilities, with atelectasis (causing shunt) being the most common. If hypoxemia persists and atelectasis is the presumed cause, NIV can be used to improve oxygenation and decrease shunt.

IV. **Principles of fast tracking**

A. **Goals of fast tracking**

Fast-track (FT) cardiac surgery was introduced to speed recovery and increase efficiency of limited resources (ICUs). Early extubation, ambulation, cardiac rehabilitation, and discharge are key goals of an FT program. Numerous randomized controlled trials have shown that FT cardiac surgery is safe and less expensive than conventional cardiac anesthesia [23]. Initially, FT protocols were limited to young, low-risk patients; however, it can be used safely in older and higher-risk patients as well [24].

B. **Methods of fast tracking**

A variety of anesthetic techniques can be used to facilitate fast tracking. Shorter-acting IV narcotics can be combined with intrathecal opioids to enhance postoperative analgesia [25,26]. Propofol infusions are often used because of a predictable and rapid recovery profile that is almost independent of the duration of infusion, assuming use of targeted propofol infusions or a processed EEG endpoint. This property makes propofol a very good sedative agent in the early postoperative management of FT cardiac surgery patients, assuming that hemodynamic stability is not compromised by its use. Caution is needed when short-acting agents are used intraoperatively to set the stage for early extubation, as the incidence of intraoperative awareness may be as high as 0.3% [27]. Dexmedetomidine is an IV α_2-adrenergic agonist that may facilitate fast tracking in cardiac surgical patients. Dexmedetomidine possesses both sedative and analgesic properties and allows patients to follow commands despite adequate sedation, and it most often does not require weaning prior to extubation. Dexmedetomidine does not possess reliable amnestic properties.

Dexmedetomidine has been evaluated in a number of trials in the ICU in both cardiac surgery and noncardiac surgery patients. When compared to propofol, midazolam, and morphine in separate trials, dexmedetomidine has been shown to provide adjunctive analgesia, induce less delirium, and decrease the duration of mechanical ventilation [28–31].

C. **Fast tracking in the postanesthesia care unit (PACU)**

Many institutions prepare for the postoperative management of cardiac surgery patients by developing enhanced stepdown or PACUs, where postoperative management can occur safely and efficiently. These units require nurses who understand fast-tracking techniques, so that patients who have undergone cardiac surgery can move smoothly through early extubation in preparation for early transfer to a regular nursing unit. These specialized PACUs can be very effective in providing FT techniques because of their focused effort in caring for FT cardiac surgery patients [32]. Some investigators have even implemented *ambulatory* cardiac surgery programs [33]!

D. **Utilizing protocols**

Developing and utilizing institution-specific FT protocols revolves around systematic plans for weaning patients from ventilators and managing routine postoperative issues to facilitate the progression toward early ICU and hospital discharge. Protocols ideally address most issues before they occur. Fast-tracking protocol development should involve all members of the perioperative care team before implementation.

V. **Enhanced recovery after cardiac surgery**

A. **Goals of enhanced recovery after cardiac surgery**

Abdominal surgery protocols have successfully adopted enhanced recovery protocols with the goals of decreasing surgical stress response, decreasing length of stay and minimizing iatrogenic injury, and ultimately improving patient outcomes [34]. In the United States, cardiac surgical practice has been slower to adopt enhanced recovery practices. Many cardiac surgery patients undergo similar recovery and monitoring protocols regardless of their degree of illness and complexity of surgery [35].

B. **Team approach**

Modern ICUs treat patients with an intensivist-based, multidisciplinary approach that incorporates the proven benefits of having patients that are awake and are able to participate in early mobilization and rehabilitation. Along with early mobilization, multidisciplinary teams strive for early postoperative enteral nutrition and rapid deescalation of invasive monitors in order to prevent hospital-acquired infections. This is in sharp contrast to previous models of patients on mechanical ventilation that were frequently heavily sedated and often paralyzed until their critical illness resolved.

C. **Engaged, empowered team**

This approach involves an engaged and empowered team of physicians, intensive care nurses, physical therapists, dieticians, and pharmacists. Survival at discharge is no longer the main focus of critical care physicians. Retrospective data have suggested that patients who survive critical illness suffer from problems that may be preventable in the ICU. A transition in critical care research in the past 15 years has challenged previous beliefs. Recent research addresses morbidities associated with bed rest, oversedation, iatrogenically induced delirium, posttraumatic stress disorder, and weakness associated with critical illness. In this evolving practice, patients are awake despite mechanical ventilation, ambulated despite advanced therapies like ECMO, and are participating in family meetings and major clinical decisions [36].

VI. Hemodynamic management in the postoperative period

A. Monitoring for ischemia

Ischemia can be detected by utilizing a continuous ECG with ST-segment analysis, although there is a slight delay in diagnosis of ischemia using this method. Many bedside ECG monitoring systems have ST-segment analysis built into their software algorithms, which is a cost-effective method of monitoring for ischemic events. It is important to ensure that the ECG is in diagnostic mode when evaluating potentially ischemic ECG changes. In monitor mode, the ECG filters out some electrical input (to decrease artifact) and may not accurately reflect ischemic changes. If continuous ST-segment analysis is chosen, leads II and V4 or V5 should be monitored, and sensitivity improves if three leads are used (leads I, II, and V4 or V5; or leads II, V4, and V5). When in doubt, proceed to a 12-lead ECG, which, despite limitations, is always more definitive than an electronic monitor. Other indicators of myocardial ischemia include pulmonary artery pressures and CO, which tend to be less reliable (and oftentimes late) markers of myocardial ischemia. Transesophageal echocardiogram (TEE) segmental wall-motion abnormalities represent the most sensitive early detector of myocardial ischemia, but continuous monitoring usually is not done because the TEE probe (if used) typically is removed at the end of surgery. It is important for the intensivist to recognize the changes in ECG and hemodynamics that can result from temporary epicardial ventricular pacing. Epicardial ventricular pacing can mimic septal wall dyskinesis that actually represents a pacemaker-induced change in the ventricular depolarization sequence.

Intraoperative and ongoing postoperative ischemia can be detected as soon as 6 hours after the event begins by examining some specific cardiac markers. The earliest and most useful marker is cardiac troponin I (cTnI). The ability to measure cTnI is particularly useful in cases where ECG monitoring is difficult to interpret, such as with left bundle branch block or LV hypertrophy. Elevated plasma levels of this biologic marker provide clear evidence of ischemia and may suggest a diagnosis of myocardial infarction.

In postoperative cardiac surgical patients, all of the above methods have significant problems. Most often, myocardial ischemia is suspected by ECG changes or unexpected increases in vasoactive drug requirements. The diagnosis is best confirmed by transthoracic echocardiography (TTE) or TEE. Diagnosis may require cardiac catheterization. Treatment options include returning to the OR or medical management.

CLINICAL PEARL Since traditional diagnostic markers for myocardial ischemia often lack sensitivity or specificity after cardiac surgery, TTE or TEE should be used liberally to assess for new wall-motion disturbances when ischemia is suspected.

B. Ventricular dysfunction after cardiac surgery

1. **Causes.** In addition to pre-existing ventricular dysfunction, postoperative causes of ventricular dysfunction include inadequate **myocardial protection, myocardial stunning, incomplete revascularization, and reperfusion injury**. Preoperative predictors of postoperative ventricular dysfunction include cardiac enlargement, advanced age, diabetes mellitus, female gender, high LV end-diastolic pressures at cardiac catheterization, small coronary arteries (for coronary revascularization procedures), and LV ejection fraction less than 0.4. Intraoperative predictors include longer CPB and aortic cross-clamp times. These factors increase the likelihood of needing inotropic support in the postoperative period. The patients who have normal preoperative cardiac performance and short periods of CPB have a much lower likelihood of requiring postoperative inotropic support. The patients who fail to achieve adequate hemodynamics even with pharmacologic support will require mechanical cardiac

assistance such as an intra-aortic balloon pump (IABP) or VAD. Recently, Hollenberg has written an excellent review article on **vasoactive drugs** in circulatory shock [34].

The myocardium has both β_1- and β_2-adrenergic receptors, which contribute to inotropy and lusitropy (enhanced diastolic relaxation). β-Adrenergic agonists (β-agonists) are often the first-line agents used when there is a need to improve ventricular function after CPB. Depletion of endogenous catecholamines and the resulting β-receptor downregulation can blunt the response to β-agonists. Increased G-inhibitory proteins, reperfusion injury, tachycardia, incomplete revascularization, nonviable myocardium, preoperative use of β-agonists, and acute or chronic heart failure also may attenuate the response to β-agonists.

2. **Treatment**
   a. **Catecholamines.** The inotropic response to β_1/β_2-adrenergic receptor stimulation occurs via activation of the G_s protein and adenylyl cyclase leading to increased intracellular cyclic adenosine monophosphate (cAMP). It is important to recognize that lusitropy is an active, energy-consuming process; impaired ventricular relaxation (diastolic dysfunction) can cause heart failure alone or in combination with systolic dysfunction. Until recently, there have been no head-to-head clinical trials comparing the clinical outcomes of inotropes and vasopressors. In a trial of 30 patients with dopamine-resistant cardiogenic shock, the patients were randomized to receive either epinephrine alone or dobutamine in combination with norepinephrine. Both groups experienced an increase in cardiac index and a decrease in their plasma creatinine concentrations. The group receiving epinephrine experienced more arrhythmias, transient lactic acidosis, and a decrease in splanchnic perfusion [37].

   b. **Phosphodiesterase type III inhibitors** (amrinone and milrinone) augment β-adrenergic–mediated stimulation by inhibiting the breakdown of cAMP. Phosphodiesterase inhibitors (PDEIs) act either additively or synergistically with β-adrenergic agonists. PDEIs appear to have anti-ischemic effects and may favorably alter myocardial oxygen consumption [38]. PDEIs can be added to β-agonist therapy or employed as a first-line inotrope. Because PDEIs also induce systemic and pulmonary vasodilation (sometimes they are termed inodilators), clinical paradigms that favor their use include pulmonary hypertension, RV failure, aortic or mitral valvular regurgitation, and acute/chronic β_1/β_2-adrenergic receptor desensitization (long-standing congestive heart failure [CHF], use of β-agonist therapy preoperatively).

   c. **Levosimendan** is a novel inotrope that, at this time, is neither FDA-approved nor available in North America. Levosimendan is a myofilament "calcium sensitizer," which results in increased inotropy by improving the efficiency of the coupling of force-generating myocyte proteins in response to a given level of calcium [39]. Like PDEIs, levosimendan may augment inotropy without significantly increasing myocardial oxygen consumption, thus improving the myocardial oxygen supply/demand balance. In a recent meta-analysis in postoperative coronary artery bypass grafting (CABG), levosimendan was associated with improved mortality and morbidity [40].

   d. **B-type natriuretic peptide** (nesiritide) has been favored by some for the medical management of CHF [41–45], although some work also associates the use of this agent with increased mortality in that setting. The role of nesiritide in the cardiac surgical population remains ill-defined.

   In patients with severely impaired cardiac performance, additional monitoring may be required to ascertain if the patient has optimal myocardial function. Oximetric PACs can provide real-time determinations of mixed venous oxygen saturation (SvO_2). A normal SvO_2 value of 75% corresponds to a PaO_2 of approximately 40 mm Hg. Reductions in SvO_2 result from either decreased oxygen delivery (decreased CO, decreased hemoglobin concentration, or decreased arterial oxygen saturation) or increased oxygen consumption. A sustained SvO_2 below 40% is associated with increased morbidity and mortality. Similarly, some practitioners choose to use PACs with continuous cardiac output (CCO) determination in such patients or with both SvO_2 and CCO.

C. **Fluid management**

Managing postoperative fluids after cardiac surgery can be challenging [41]. The effects of hypothermia (vasoconstriction) and hyperthermia (vasodilation) commonly complicate fluid management, especially in the first few hours after cardiac surgery. Central venous pressure (CVP) and PAC are frequently utilized in the cardiac surgical population; however, it is imperative to recognize that these monitors measure pressure as a surrogate estimate of volume and/or cardiac performance. Filling pressures (CVP, pulmonary artery occlusion pressure [PAOP], and pulmonary artery diastolic pressure [PADP]) poorly assess total blood volume and volume responsiveness [46]. Volume responsiveness is defined by an increase in cardiac index of >15%, in response to a fluid challenge. For mechanically ventilated patients who have a regular respiratory pattern, the pulse pressure variation on an arterial pressure waveform can be a highly useful tool in predicting a hypotensive patient's response to a fluid challenge [47–49].

Cardiac surgical procedures, especially those involving CPB, typically result in fluid sequestration into the interstitial compartment. In addition to the changes in circulating blood volume from blood loss and other factors, fluid shifts into or out of the interstitial or the intracellular compartments can be anticipated in the hours following cardiac surgery. Most cardiac surgery patients reach the recovery area with excess total-body fluids present that must eventually be mobilized. Healthy patients who have adequate cardiac and renal function typically diurese these fluids over the first two postoperative days without assistance. Other cardiac surgery patients, such as the elderly or those with renal or cardiac dysfunction, may require diuretic drugs (or possibly dialysis or hemofiltration) to remove excess body water.

Management of blood components, particularly packed red blood cells (PRBCs), in the cardiac surgical population is controversial [50,51]. Both transfusion of blood products and anemia are associated with increased perioperative morbidity and mortality. Even though cardiac surgical patients frequently require allogeneic blood products, establishing a transfusion trigger is difficult. Most patients probably require transfusion of PRBC at an Hct less than or equal to 21% (hemoglobin concentration [Hgb] less than or equal to 7 g/dL), and few or none require transfusion when Hct is greater than or equal to 30% (Hgb greater than or equal to 10 g/dL).

CLINICAL PEARL   Hemodynamic measurements such as cardiac output, stroke volume, and pulse pressure variation more reliably assess the potential need for additional IV fluids than measurement of cardiac filling pressures.

D. Managing hypotension

Systematic evaluation of preload, afterload, contractility, and heart rate and rhythm should be performed in the hypotensive patient. If preload is adequate and an acceptable heart rate and a normal cardiac rhythm are present, hypotension represents either inadequate myocardial function or vasodilation. Inadequate cardiac function is managed with inotropes. Vasodilation is managed with vasoconstrictors.

1. **Vasodilatory shock.** Eight percent of cardiac surgery patients experience refractory vasodilatory shock after CPB. This refractory shock is associated with increased mortality (as high as 25%). These patients do not respond to traditional treatments, vasopressors, or volume expansion. The causes of the problem are usually multifactorial: long CPB duration, preoperative use of angiotensin-converting enzyme inhibitors (or angiotensin-receptor blockers) or calcium channel blockers, heart transplantation, VAD placement, and myocardial dysfunction. Small clinical trials have shown improved morbidity and mortality in this patient population with the use of an IV bolus of methylene blue followed by a continuous infusion [52]. Arginine vasopressin and high-dose hydroxocobalamin [53] may also be useful.

2. Two other causes of hypotension that are difficult to diagnose without the aid of transesophageal echocardiography are systolic anterior motion (SAM) of the mitral valve and cardiac tamponade.

3. **SAM** of the mitral valve should be assessed in the OR in patients undergoing mitral valve repair or septal myectomy. A c-sept distance (see Fig. 25.6) of 2.5 cm or less is associated with a high risk of SAM [54].

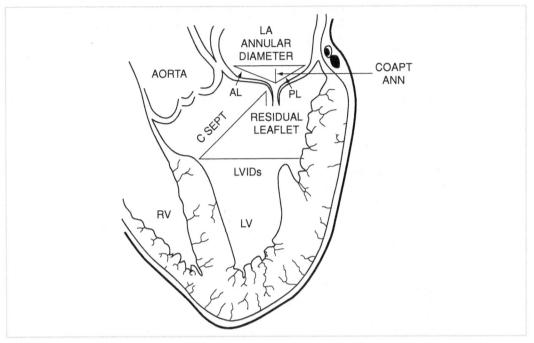

FIGURE 25.6 Schematic demonstrating the transesophageal echocardiographic measurements performed prior to and after mitral valve repair. The biplane image, obtained from the esophageal location at zero degrees, includes the left atrium (LA), left ventricle (LV), mitral valve, and the LV outflow tract. Lengths of the anterior and posterior leaflets were obtained using the middle scallops. AL, anterior leaflet length; Coapt Ann, distance from the mitral coaptation point to the annular plane; C Sept, distance from the mitral coaptation point to the septum; LVIDs, LV internal diameter in systole; PL, posterior leaflet length [50].

4. **Tamponade.** Postcardiac surgery tamponade should be considered, especially if the patient is demonstrating signs of shock from low CO. A large series of patients diagnosed with postcardiac surgery tamponade demonstrated that the classical diagnostic signs such as equalizing filling pressures, increased jugular venous pressure, and pulsus paradoxus are frequently not present. Echocardiography can aid in the diagnosis; however, tamponade is a constellation of symptoms rather than a single echocardiographic finding [55].

CLINICAL PEARL   After cardiac surgery, cardiac tamponade can be localized and is best diagnosed by careful echocardiographic interrogation.

E. **Dysrhythmia management**

Managing postoperative dysrhythmias constitutes an important part of ICU care in cardiac surgery patients. A variety of atrial or ventricular dysrhythmias can occur. Patients with ongoing myocardial ischemia, possibly from incomplete revascularization or myocardial stunning, are predisposed to dysrhythmias. Atrial fibrillation is the most common dysrhythmia to occur after cardiac surgery, and it may occur in as many as half of the patients who undergo myocardial revascularization using CPB. Useful drugs for treating atrial fibrillation include magnesium, digoxin, diltiazem, esmolol, and amiodarone [56].

It has been shown that various preoperative or postoperative pharmacologic prophylactic strategies may reduce the incidence of postoperative atrial fibrillation or other atrial dysrhythmias [57–59]. It is important to identify the patients who are at increased risk for developing perioperative atrial fibrillation. These include patients who have a previous history of atrial fibrillation; have undergone a combination valve and CABG procedure; are receiving inotropic support; or have pre-existing mitral valve disease, lung disease, or congenital heart disease. Prophylaxis against atrial fibrillation may decrease both the number of days spent in the ICU and the total length of stay in the hospital. Administration of a long-acting β-adrenergic receptor antagonist (i.e., atenolol or metoprolol) is frequently initiated on the first postoperative day following cardiac surgery.

The prophylactic use of corticosteroids, and particularly hydrocortisone, has been shown in a recent meta-analysis of randomized controlled trials to be effective in decreasing the incidence of atrial fibrillation in a high-risk patient population [60,61]. It appears that a single dose of steroids during induction of anesthesia is sufficient to provide this benefit.

In the context of arrhythmia prevention, it is particularly important to maintain normal **magnesium** and **potassium** concentrations perioperatively [62,63].

F. Perioperative hypertension

Perioperative hypertension can result from a number of causes:

1. Etiologies of acute postoperative hypertension include **emergence from anesthesia, hypothermia, hypercarbia, hypoxemia, hypoglycemia, intravascular volume excess, pain, and anxiety.** One must consider iatrogenic causes such as administration of the wrong medication or use of a vasoconstrictor when it is not necessary.

2. Another cause of postoperative hypertension is withdrawal from preoperative antihypertensive medications. The β-blockers and centrally acting α_2-agonists (clonidine) are known to elicit rebound hypertension upon withdrawal.

3. Unusual causes include intracranial hypertension (from cerebral edema or massive stroke), bladder distention, hypoglycemia, and withdrawal syndromes (e.g., alcohol withdrawal syndrome, withdrawing from chronic opioid use).

4. Rare causes to consider include endocrine or metabolic disorders such as hyperthyroidism, pheochromocytoma, renin–angiotensin disorders, and malignant hyperthermia.

G. Pulmonary hypertension

Pulmonary hypertension may occur after cardiac surgery, the causes of which can be divided into new-onset acute pulmonary hypertension and continuation of a more chronic pulmonary hypertensive state. A primary consideration in the evaluation of pulmonary hypertension is the effect on RV performance. Echocardiography is critically important in diagnosing right heart failure. Pulmonary artery pressures may decrease, and CVP may increase in the presence of worsening right heart failure. Because of the unique geometry of the RV, traditional echocardiography measurements of LV function cannot be applied to RV performance. Specific validated measurements such as tricuspid annular plane systolic excursion index [64] or Tei index [65,66] should be used to assess the RV function. Pulmonary hypertension and RV failure are particularly problematic following heart or lung transplantation and VAD placement [67].

1. **Chronic pulmonary hypertension** is less responsive than systemic hypertension to traditional therapeutic interventions. Chronic elevation in the pulmonary vascular resistance (PVR) stresses the RV and can lead to RV dysfunction. In addition, the RV hypertrophy associated with chronic pulmonary hypertension enhances susceptibility to inadequate RV oxygen delivery. Chronic pulmonary hypertension is managed by continuing any ongoing medications that the patient has been taking, such as calcium channel blockers, along with utilizing therapeutic agents mentioned below for management of acute pulmonary hypertension.

2. **Acute postoperative pulmonary hypertension** must be managed aggressively to avoid RV failure [68–70]. Parameters that influence pulmonary hypertension (see Table 25.2) should be optimized. There are four major categories of focus in addressing right heart failure associated with acute pulmonary hypertension [71] (Fig. 25.7).

   a. **Volume status of the right ventricle (RV) (echocardiography).** Echocardiography will provide a good understanding of the primary problem: volume versus pressure overload. Chronic pressure overload causes RV hypertrophy, often with normal RV contractility and volume.

   b. **Right ventricular function.** Address the need for inotropic support (dobutamine, PDEIs, epinephrine). In addition, optimize the heart rate and rhythm.

TABLE 25.2   Factors that contribute to pulmonary hypertension

Mitral stenosis
Mitral regurgitation
Clot/thrombus on prosthetic mitral valve
Perivalvular leak around prosthetic mitral valve
Acidosis
Elevated hematocrit (e.g., >16 g/dL)
Hypercarbia
Hypoxemia
Increased mean airway pressure (PEEP, hyperinflation)
Increased pulmonary vascular resistance (PVR)
Mechanical obstruction (e.g., surgical restriction of a main pulmonary artery, pulmonary embolus)
Sympathetic stimulation (pain, inadequate sedation)

    c. Decrease pulmonary vascular resistance (PVR) (and hence RV afterload) by correcting any existing acidosis, hypercarbia, or hypoxemia. Consider adding a pulmonary artery vasodilator (inhaled nitric oxide, inhaled prostacyclin, IV PDEIs, and IV nitroglycerin) and minimize any harmful effects of PPV (high peak airway pressures, excessive tidal volumes, and ventilator-induced lung injury).

    d. Maintain an adequate right coronary artery perfusion pressure by adding a vasopressor (norepinephrine, vasopressin, phenylephrine) or mechanical diastolic pressure support via an IABP [72].

VII. Postoperative pain and sedation management techniques

Managing postoperative pain and agitation are paramount in caring for the postoperative cardiac surgery patient. Pain represents a response to nociceptor stimulation from the surgical intervention. Patients may be agitated after cardiac surgery for a variety of reasons. Table 25.3 lists some

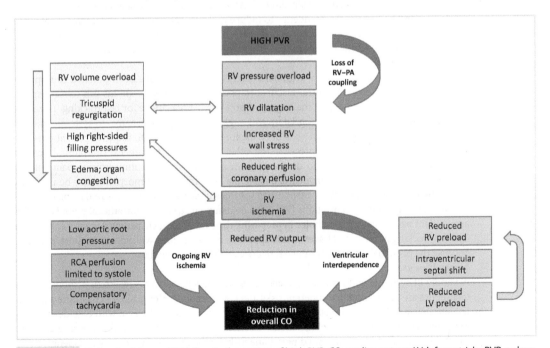

FIGURE 25.7 Pathophysiology of RV failure in the setting of high PVR. CO, cardiac output; LV, left ventricle; PVR, pulmonary vascular resistance; RCA, right coronary artery; RV, right ventricle [68].

TABLE 25.3   Causes of postoperative agitation

Delirium
Alcohol withdrawal syndrome
Electrolyte abnormalities (hyponatremia)
Gastric or urinary retention
Hypercarbia
Hypoxemia
Ischemia or hemorrhage of the central nervous system
Medications (e.g., anticholinergics, benzodiazepines)
Psychological conditions (i.e., anxiety disorder)
Residual anesthetics/emergence from anesthesia
Wernicke encephalopathy
Withdrawal syndrome (i.e., narcotic addiction, chronic benzodiazepine use)

possible causes of agitation that must be considered because they might be "masked" by the administration of a sedative drug or by residual neuromuscular blockade.

A. Systemic opioids

A variety of techniques can be used to manage postoperative pain. It is very useful to initially discern the type, quality, and location of pain before administering an analgesic agent. Commonly used opioids include fentanyl, morphine, and hydromorphone.

B. Nonsteroidal anti-inflammatory drugs (NSAIDs)

NSAIDs can be helpful when managing postoperative pain in cardiac surgery. A small amount of drug can provide analgesia without excessive sedation and other complications (e.g., respiratory depression) associated with opioid use. A concern with NSAIDs is their inhibition of platelet function and the potential for increased bleeding. NSAIDs also have been considered a poor choice after cardiac surgery because of their tendency to induce gastric ulcer formation and impair renal function. Renal insufficiency, active peptic ulcer disease, history of gastrointestinal bleeding, and bleeding diathesis should exclude the use of NSAIDs in the postoperative cardiac surgery patient [73].

C. Intrathecal opioids

In the era of fast tracking, several regional analgesic techniques have been pursued to improve patient comfort. Systemic (IV, intramuscular, transcutaneous, or oral) opioids can cause respiratory depression and somnolence, making them potentially undesirable for fast tracking. Intrathecal opioids (e.g., morphine 5 to 8 μg/kg up to 1 mg) constitute an alternative to systemic opioids for cardiac surgery [74]. This route has been explored in an attempt to improve patient comfort while minimizing respiratory depression and other side effects. Intrathecal or epidural opioids can facilitate early extubation and discharge from an ICU without compromising pain control or increasing the likelihood of myocardial ischemia [75]. Intrathecal morphine may be useful in attenuating the postsurgical stress response in CABG surgery patients as measured by plasma cortisol and epinephrine concentrations [76]. This evidence suggests that intrathecal opioids may be an excellent pain management choice in preparing the cardiac surgical patient for early extubation and fast tracking in the ICU. However, this approach has not gained widespread support, perhaps, because the principal proved advantage is decreased systemic opioid use.

D. Nerve blocks

A variety of systemic and intrathecal analgesic techniques have been suggested. Although these techniques are useful, each has inherent risks and complications. Nerve blocks constitute a potential alternative to these methods. Intercostal nerve blocks can be performed with ease during thoracic surgery procedures, as the intercostal nerves are easily accessible through the surgical field. These blocks can also be performed percutaneously by the anesthesia provider preoperatively or postoperatively. Intercostal nerve blocks do not provide satisfactory analgesia for a median sternotomy. Thoracic epidural analgesia (TEA) for cardiac surgical procedures [74] requiring CPB is

TABLE 25.4   ICU sedation

Sedative	Loading dose	Continuous infusion	Special considerations
Dexmedetomidine	1 mg/kg over 10–15 min	0.2–0.7 µg/kg/hr	Hemodynamic stability; treats withdrawal syndromes; no weaning required for extubation, bradycardia
Propofol	None	15–100 µg/kg/min	Sepsis risk, hypotension
Fentanyl (used with midazolam)	1–3 µg/kg	25–250 µg/hr	Potent analgesic, tolerance
Midazolam (used with fentanyl)	0.02–0.05 mg/kg	0.5–3 mg/hr	Amnestic, treats delirium tremens

considered acceptable by some practitioners and appears to be more accepted in Europe and Asia than in North America. Off-pump coronary artery bypass (OPCAB) procedures may be especially well suited to TEA. TEA decreases the risk of ischemia during cardiac surgery. However, many cardiac anesthesiologists consider the risk of epidural hematoma, however small, to be a deterrent in the face of the hypocoagulable state present during and after CPB. Paravertebral nerve blocks (PVBs) may be an alternative to TEA, which may be associated with less risk of epidural hematoma. PVB and bilateral PVB catheters have been utilized with success in cardiac surgical procedures [77–79]. Recently, parasternal nerve blockade has been described and may prove to be useful [80].

E. Sedation

It is essential to understand the goals of sedation in a critically ill patient. In the ICU, one should titrate sedatives to the desired effect as precisely as one would titrate vasopressors, inotropes, and oxygen. Light sedation with aggressive analgesic techniques shortens ICU stay, decreases delirium, decreases posttraumatic stress disorder, and probably improves mortality. Sedation should be goal directed. The majority of patients in the ICU should be awake and interactive even if they require mechanical ventilation [81]. Not all postoperative cardiac surgery patients require sedation (see Table 25.4).

1. **Benzodiazepines,** when used as sedatives, have been associated with prolonged mechanical ventilation, delirium, and possibly increased mortality when used as continuous infusions [82,83].

2. **Propofol** is commonly administered as a continuous infusion in the ICU for sedation. It is easily titrated to effect but can produce significant vasodilation or myocardial depression with resultant hypotension. Propofol causes a burning pain during peripheral administration, so central venous administration is advisable if possible. In addition, propofol can be a source for sepsis since the lipid mixture can act as a medium for bacterial growth; strict aseptic technique must be used.

3. **Dexmedetomidine** is a potent α_2-adrenergic agonist that provides sedation, hemodynamic stability, decreased cardiac ischemia, improved pulmonary function, and analgesia and can, therefore, be a good choice in cardiac surgical patients [84–86]. Hypotension and bradycardia are occasionally attributed to its use. Dexmedetomidine is unique among sedatives, in that patients remain cooperative yet calm, and it does not require weaning to permit extubation. Dexmedetomidine activates endogenous sleep pathways, which may decrease agitation and confusion. Dexmedetomidine is administered as a continuous IV infusion (0.2 to 0.7 mcg/kg/hr) and is approved for use up to 24 hours. Clinical trials for extended infusion of dexmedetomidine at higher doses (up to 1.5 mcg/kg/hr) in a diverse ICU population have resulted in more ventilator-free days and more delirium-free days when compared to similar sedation end points with lorazepam or midazolam. Withdrawal syndromes (ethanol, chronic pain narcotic use, illicit drugs) can also be managed with the administration of α_2-adrenergic agonists.

CLINICAL PEARL   Postoperative sedation using dexmedetomidine offers several advantages over both propofol and benzodiazepines.

VIII. Metabolic abnormalities

Many metabolic abnormalities can occur in the perioperative period. These irregularities result from the physiologic stress response or from the large fluid and electrolyte shifts that can be derived from IV infusions or from CPB priming or myocardial protectant solutions.

A. Electrolyte abnormalities

1. **Hyperkalemia** can present from cardioplegia, overaggressive replacement, or secondary extracellular shifts associated with respiratory or metabolic acidosis. **Hypokalemia** increases the risk for dysrhythmia following cardiac surgery. Inclusion of mannitol in the CPB priming solution, improved renal perfusion, and aggressive treatment of blood glucose with insulin infusion all contribute to hypokalemia. Hypokalemia is more common than hyperkalemia. Potassium supplementation can be infused at a maximum rate of 20 mEq/hr via a central venous catheter. Rapid potassium infusion can induce lethal arrhythmias. The target serum potassium concentration should be >3.5 mEq/L but not higher than 5 mEq/L.

2. **Hypomagnesemia** is a common perioperative electrolyte abnormality and is associated with postoperative dysrhythmia, myocardial ischemia, and ventricular dysfunction [62,87]. Hypomagnesemia may result from dilution by large CPB priming volumes and from urinary excretion. Renal potassium retention requires adequate magnesium concentration, and thus magnesium administration should always be considered in hypokalemic patients. If magnesium supplementation is required, it can be given in amounts of 2 to 4 g IV over 30 to 45 minutes. An infusion of 1 g/hr of magnesium sulfate can be used as well to assure a slow, steady infusion of this substance. If given too fast, it may cause hypotension or muscle weakness. In refractory dysrhythmias, particularly of the ventricular type, a normal serum magnesium concentration may not exclude the possibility of decreased total-body stores of magnesium. The target serum magnesium concentration should be 2 to 2.5 mEq/L.

3. **Hypocalcemia** may be present and may be related to rapid transfusion of large amounts of citrate-preserved bank blood. Hypocalcemia can be treated with 250- to 1,000-mg IV doses of calcium chloride (or 500 to 2,000 mg of calcium gluconate), while paying careful attention to the potential for development of dysrhythmias. When following the calcium status, it is important to measure ionized calcium and not total calcium because low albumin levels may decrease total calcium levels, whereas ionized calcium remains normal.

4. **Hypophosphatemia** is a common problem encountered in the ICU. Hypophosphatemia can contribute to weakness and poor myocardial function, can change the ability of red blood cells to change shape, and can affect oxyhemoglobin dissociation [88,89].

B. **Shivering.** The exact mechanism of shivering is difficult to discern, but it is thought to be associated with inadequate rewarming and the resulting hypothermic temperature "afterdrop." Many patients are hypothermic when they arrive in the ICU and develop shivering as they emerge from anesthesia. Shivering can result in a 300% to 600% increase in oxygen demand, which potentially places unachievable oxygen delivery demand upon a compromised myocardium. The associated increase in CO_2 production may cause respiratory acidosis. In patients with inadequate end-organ oxygen delivery, sustained shivering frequently will require mechanical ventilation, and consideration should be given to administration of neuromuscular blockers to abolish the increased metabolic demand of shivering. Effective first-line treatments include active rewarming with forced air blankets and prevention of further temperature loss. Pharmacologic interventions that reduce shivering include IV meperidine (12.5 to 25 mg) or dexmedetomidine.

CLINICAL PEARL Patients with tenuous cardiac compensation poorly tolerate the additional oxygen consumption induced by shivering.

C. **Acidosis** can be described as respiratory, metabolic, or mixed. Metabolic acidosis is divided into anion gap and non–anion gap acidosis. A complete discussion of acid–base disorders is beyond the scope of this chapter and can be found in standard critical care textbooks. We will briefly discuss the most common causes of acidosis in the early postoperative period.

1. **Respiratory acidosis** results from hypoventilation or increased CO_2 production. Residual anesthetics or an awakening patient with inadequate analgesia combined with impaired respiratory mechanics may lead to hypoventilation. Treatment consists of support of ventilation while treating the underlying cause.

2. **Metabolic acidosis**, when present, is associated frequently with inadequate systemic perfusion because of compromised cardiac function. Treatment is directed at correcting the underlying cause of the acidosis. Metabolic acidosis in a cardiac surgery patient may require administration of sodium bicarbonate as a temporizing measure, especially in patients who are hemodynamically unstable.

3. **Lactic acidosis**, a frequent finding in cardiac surgery patients, needs to be managed by assuring adequate CO and intravascular volume and avoidance of shivering. There is some evidence that the use of sodium bicarbonate to treat lactic acidosis should be avoided; however, most of the critical care data assessing the effects of buffers in treating acidosis do not include patients with acute pulmonary hypertension or right heart failure. Epinephrine can produce a transient lactic acidosis that does not appear to reflect inadequate perfusion.

D. **Glucose management.** Glycemic control in the critically ill is a highly controversial topic. Data from 2001 indicated that tight glycemic control in cardiac surgery patients (80 to 110 mg/dL) induced a remarkable improvement in mortality [90]; however, subsequent trials have failed to reproduce this dramatic effect. The most recent multicenter, multinational interventional trial of tight glycemic control demonstrated an increase in mortality when hyperglycemia was aggressively managed to maintain a glucose range of 81 to 108 mg/dL [91]. Control of blood glucose levels at less than 150 mg/dL (or some would say less than 180 to 200 mg/dL, as there is no consensus standard) and **avoiding hypoglycemia** with frequent monitoring is a reasonable goal in cardiac surgical patients. Unrecognized hyperglycemia can result in excessive diuresis and the potential for a hyperosmolar or ketoacidotic state. Elevated serum glucose can be managed by using a continuous infusion of regular insulin, often starting at a dose of 0.1 units/kg/hr or less with titration to the desired serum blood glucose level.

CLINICAL PEARL   Overly ambitious glucose control increases mortality.

IX. **Complications in the first 24 hours postoperatively**
A number of life-threatening complications can occur in the first 24 hours after cardiac or thoracic surgery.

A. **Respiratory failure**
Respiratory failure may be the most common postoperative complication of cardiac or thoracic surgery. Pulmonary dysfunction develops from the surgical incision and its attendant disruption of the thoracic cage. Postoperative pain exacerbates this effect. Respiratory failure can present as hypoxemia, hypercarbia, or both. Prompt identification and appropriate treatment is essential. Atelectasis, the most common pulmonary complication following cardiac surgery, can usually be managed with the application of PEEP, BiPAP, or CPAP.

B. **Bleeding**
Postoperative hemorrhage from ongoing surgical bleeding or coagulopathy increases a patient's length of stay and mortality [92]. Bleeding typically is monitored by the amount of blood that drains into the chest tubes after surgery. It is critical to differentiate a bleeding diathesis from a surgical bleeding situation requiring reoperation. Consequently, in bleeding patients, it becomes essential to determine the status of the coagulation system, which is traditionally done by acquiring (at a minimum) PT, aPTT, fibrinogen concentration, and platelet count, in addition to a chest x-ray. This panel of tests does not provide any indication of the functional status of the platelets. A thromboelastogram (TEG) or other platelet functional assays provide useful information about platelet functional status, and the TEG also provides information about plasma clotting function and fibrinolysis. Assessment of platelet function is particularly important in managing the cardiac patients who have received aspirin or other platelet inhibitors (e.g., clopidogrel,

glycoprotein IIb/IIIa inhibitors) preoperatively. Transfusion of **platelet concentrates** may be appropriate when one suspects that the bleeding results from platelet dysfunction.

1. **Fresh frozen plasma (FFP)** should most often be used to correct abnormalities in PT, international normalized ratio (INR), or aPTT, although modest elevations in these tests are often clinically insignificant. When associated with clinical bleeding, elevations of PT or aPTT in excess of 1.3 times the upper limit of normal or of INR in excess of 1.5 should probably be treated. Elevated aPTT may occur from deficiencies of plasma coagulation factors or from residual heparin.

2. **Fibrinogen** deficiency (typically less than 75 mg/dL) is treated with cryoprecipitate. Fibrinogen concentrates are available in some countries.

3. The role of **activated factor VII** in the cardiac surgical population is controversial. A meta-analysis of 35 randomized clinical trials that included both cardiac surgery and noncardiac surgery trials showed no statistically significant difference in venous thrombosis after administration of activated factor VII, including doses up to 80 mcg/kg. However, there was a statistically significant increase in coronary arterial thromboembolic events when compared to placebo [93].

4. **Surgical bleeding** is often considered once coagulopathy has been ruled out, and it may require a return to the OR for mediastinal or thoracic reexploration to identify and control a bleeding site. Surgical reexploration commonly fails to identify a specific source for the bleeding. However, plasminogen (from dissolved blood clots) is removed by irrigation of the pericardium and mediastinum, which may markedly decrease bleeding. In general, chest tube drainage greater than 500 mL/hr (even once), sustained drainage exceeding 200 mL/hr, or increasing chest tube drainage justifies surgical reexploration.

Sudden hemorrhage from a suture line or cannulation site can cause profound hypotension from hypovolemia or tamponade. Rapid infusion of blood products, colloids, or crystalloids is then necessary to maintain intravascular volume. Patients who can be quickly stabilized are transferred to the OR. In some instances, emergency resternotomy must be performed in the ICU to control life-threatening hemorrhage or tamponade.

CLINICAL PEARL Life-threatening hemorrhage or tamponade requires emergency reopening of the sternum at the bedside in the ICU.

C. **Cardiac tamponade**

Excessive mediastinal bleeding with inadequate drainage or sudden massive bleeding can result in cardiac tamponade. Cardiac tamponade after cardiac surgery may seem impossible if the pericardium has been left open, suggesting to the inexperienced observer that tamponade cannot occur. However, this is not true because *tamponade may occur in localized areas*, affecting an area as circumscribed as the right atrium. As discussed above, it is important to recognize that traditionally described equalization of filling pressures is an unreliable sign of postcardiac surgery tamponade. The differential diagnosis includes biventricular failure. TEE or TTE may be important to making the correct diagnosis. At times, cardiac tamponade requires emergent surgical intervention.

D. **Pneumothorax**

Pneumothorax can occur in patients who have undergone sternotomy, thoracotomy, or are undergoing PPV. Most cardiac surgical patients arrive in the recovery or ICU area with one or more chest (intrapleural) tubes in place, in addition to mediastinal tubes. These patients should have a baseline postoperative chest x-ray upon ICU arrival to confirm the adequacy of chest tube placement and the absence of a pneumothorax. Patients who have had a redo sternotomy or who have had an internal mammary artery used for CABG are at particular high risk for pneumothorax and hemothorax. There is increasing evidence that bedside ultrasound is valuable in diagnosing pneumothorax, hemothorax, and lung consolidation. In some studies, it has higher accuracy than portable chest x-ray when compared to CT scan [94]. An intensivist who is skilled in performing the exam can obtain immediate data and perform repeat exams if needed. Pneumothorax can convert to tension pneumothorax when chest tubes function improperly. The resulting shift of mediastinal structures can obstruct the vena cava or distort the heart to cause a low CO state and hypotension.

E. **Hemothorax**

Hemothorax can occur after coronary artery bypass surgery and must be considered in all patients who have undergone internal mammary artery dissection, which most often involves opening the left intrapleural space. These patients may need to be returned to the OR for surgical management.

F. **Acute graft closure**

Acute coronary graft closure, while uncommon, can result in myocardial ischemia or infarction. If cardiac decompensation occurs and graft closure is the suspected cause, reexploration should be performed to evaluate graft patency. However, this may be a diagnosis of exclusion, and reexploration for this reason is uncommon. These patients may need to be taken to the cardiac catheterization laboratory, where emergent cardiac catheterization can be performed to discern the presence of an occluded graft. Controversy continues about whether graft patency is similar or different in off-pump (OPCAB) versus on-pump CABG procedures either acutely or long term [95–97].

G. **Prosthetic valve failure**

Acute prosthetic valve failure should be suspected when sudden hemodynamic changes occur following open heart surgery, particularly if the rhythm is unchanged and intermittent loss of the arterial waveform is noted on the monitor screen. Immediate surgical correction is necessary. Valve dehiscence with a perivalvular leak usually does not present in the early postoperative period. TEE is the diagnostic modality of choice to evaluate prosthetic valve function in this setting. There is increasing experience and success with closing or reducing perivalvular leaks in the interventional cardiology laboratory using percutaneous atrial septal defect (ASD) and ventricular septal defect (VSD) closure devices.

H. **Postoperative neurologic dysfunction**

Neurologic complications are frequently recognized in the postoperative period and remain one of the most important complications following cardiac surgery [98,99], so an early postoperative neurologic examination is very important. Neurologic complications can be divided into three groups: (1) focal ischemic injury (stroke), (2) neurocognitive dysfunction (including diffuse encephalopathy), and (3) peripheral nervous system injury. Central nervous system dysfunction after cardiac surgery is discussed in detail in Chapter 26. Brachial plexus injury resulting from sternal retraction can occur, particularly on the left side during internal mammary arterial dissection. A thorough motor examination of the legs is crucial after descending thoracic aortic or thoracoabdominal aneurysm repairs. A delirium assessment, such as the confusion assessment method for ICU Patients (CAM-ICU), can identify patients with hypoactive delirium [100]. Hypoactive delirium in the ICU carries with it an increased morbidity and mortality. Vanderbilt University ICU physicians have developed an excellent resource about delirium for families and clinicians, which can be found at www.icudelirium.org.

X. **Discharge from the ICU**

Discharge from the ICU historically has occurred 1 to 3 days after cardiothoracic surgery. Reducing the amount of time spent in the ICU after cardiac surgery recently has become a priority. Many patients are now discharged from the ICU on the morning after routine CABG operations without compromise in patient care or safety. Complications such as those noted earlier often delay ICU discharge. Some centers place routine CABG patients in an ICU-level recovery area for several hours before discharging them to a "stepdown" or intermediate care area, or even to a "monitored bed" postoperative nursing unit.

The criteria for ICU discharge vary depending upon the type of surgery. Predicting which patients can leave the ICU in an early FT style can be accomplished by reviewing a variety of preoperative risk factors. Reduced LV ejection fraction is a valid predictor of higher mortality, morbidity, and resource utilization [101]. Other preoperative predictors of prolonged ICU stays include cardiogenic shock, age greater than 80 years, dialysis-dependent renal failure, and surgery performed emergently [102]. These factors and others can be used to predict a patient's length of stay and to plan for resource utilization.

XI. **The transplant patient (see Chapter 17)**

The care of cardiac transplant patients is similar to other cardiac patients with several notable exceptions [103]. Pulmonary hypertension and RV failure are the primary challenges in the early postoperative period following heart or lung transplantation [67]. Heart transplant recipients may have varying degrees of end-organ dysfunction secondary to chronic low CO. Finally, these patients require meticulous attention to medications used to attenuate graft rejection.

XII. **Patients with mechanical assist devices (see also Chapter 22)**

Recent technologic advances have facilitated the development of mechanical assist devices for cardiac surgery patients with severely impaired RV or LV function. The number of assist devices available continues to grow, resulting in options for LV, RV, or biventricular mechanical assistance [104,105]. Postoperative management of patients with mechanical assist devices requires a thorough understanding of the technology underlying any device that may be chosen. The primary risks with mechanical assistance include thrombosis, bleeding from anticoagulation, infection from percutaneous catheters, and failure to wean from assist devices intended for temporary cardiac support.

A. **Intra-aortic balloon pump (IABP)**

An IABP is typically the first mechanical assist device utilized for cardiogenic shock in cardiac surgical patients [106] (see Chapter 22). The goals of IABP therapy are to acutely decrease the LV afterload, thereby improving forward blood flow, and to augment the LV coronary artery perfusion during diastole. Coronary blood flow is only augmented in patients with hypotension associated with their cardiogenic shock [107]. The IABP is most often placed percutaneously via the femoral artery into the descending thoracic aorta. There are two management strategies for weaning IABP support. Some clinicians wean pharmacologic support prior to weaning IABP support; this allows them to resume inotropic support should the patient decompensate after IABP removal. Other clinicians wean IABP support first, due to concerns about lower extremity ischemia from arterial occlusion of the femoral and/or iliac arteries. Despite the clear risk of lower extremity ischemia from arterial occlusion, there is no decrease in embolic or thrombotic complications when the patient undergoes systemic anticoagulation [108]. In either strategy, the IABP is weaned from a 1:1 setting (each cardiac contraction triggers an IABP deflation/inflation cycle) to 1:2, then a brief trial at 1:3 precedes IABP removal.

B. **Ventricular assist device (VAD) (see Chapter 22)**

VAD can be utilized for support of the left (LVAD), right (RVAD), or both (BiVAD) ventricles [104,105]. There are three indications for VAD therapy:

1. Temporary support (less than 14 days) in patients who fail to wean from CPB but are expected to recover sufficient cardiac function for removal of the VAD.
2. Bridge to cardiac transplantation.
3. Destination VAD therapy; patients who require long-term or permanent VAD support with the expectation that they will be discharged from the hospital with the VAD.

   In patients with LVADs, the possibility that LV decompression will result in geometric alterations and precipitation of right heart failure must be considered. Other considerations that must be addressed during the ICU period include adequate oxygenation and ventilation using a mechanical ventilator, along with maintenance of temperature, nutrition, acid–base balance, and electrolyte balance. The patients with mechanical assist devices can be weaned from the ventilator using standard weaning protocols depending upon their hemodynamic status, blood gas exchange, and neurologic stability. If a VAD has been implanted as short-term support with an anticipated return to the OR within a few days to remove the device, this tends to discourage endotracheal extubation.

C. **Extracorporeal membrane oxygenator (ECMO) (see Chapter 24)**

In some circumstances, notably when ARDS coexists with heart failure, temporary support with ECMO is chosen in situations that would otherwise call for LVAD, RVAD, or BiVAD.

XIII. **Family issues in the postoperative period**

Interaction with families is important in communicating any patient's status and in giving appropriate expectations about recovery.

A. **The preoperative discussion**

In the preoperative discussion, it is important for the surgeon and anesthesiologist to give a detailed description of what to anticipate in the postoperative period. This information can be relayed either through preoperative visits or through video or website access describing typical postoperative events. Detailed discussions about planned extubation in the OR or in the ICU may prevent patients from misinterpreting early postoperative intubation as being awake during surgery. It is also important to discuss the goals of general anesthesia versus sedation in the ICU. Caution should be used when assuring the patient that they will have complete amnesia of the OR or being intubated. Family members should be told to expect that the cardiac surgical patient will have invasive monitors and may have significant edema, which alters their appearance. Reassurance that these are temporary cosmetic changes will provide comfort. Preoperative visits allow patients and their families the opportunity to ask questions and to understand the plan of movement through the postoperative course in a more relaxed setting than the preanesthesia holding area. Often anesthesiology preoperative visits may be compromised or precluded by admission day surgery patterns whereby cardiac surgery patients arrive at the hospital on the day of surgery. In these circumstances, opportunities for discussions with anesthesia care providers can be limited and should be anticipated at the preoperative visit with the surgeon, when information can be disseminated and questions can be answered. Some centers compensate for this practice pattern with anesthesia-specific pamphlets or web-based videos, often with a Frequently Asked Questions section.

B. **Family visitation**

Family visitation occurs in the ICU or recovery room for many postoperative cardiac and thoracic surgery patients. This provides reassurance about the patient's clinical course progression as well as encouragement toward subsequent postoperative care. Family members can be very important in encouraging adequate pulmonary toilet, coughing, deep breathing, and early ambulation to improve postoperative outcomes. Most cardiac surgery programs have designated personnel for the liaison between the professional staff caring for postoperative cardiac surgery patients and the family members who need education, encouragement, and the opportunity to assist in postoperative care.

C. **The role of family support**

Family support is a vital link toward the early success of a fast-tracking program. Family members need adequate education by surgical and anesthesia staff, who can outline the expected early postoperative events. The role of family support is heightened when patients spend very short periods in postoperative areas such as the recovery room or ICU. Family members who are educated about the expected postoperative course can facilitate postoperative care and smooth the transition from the ICU to a regular nursing floor and finally to the patient's home.

CLINICAL PEARL   Throughout the perioperative period, close communication with family members enhances patient outcomes.

ACKNOWLEDGMENTS

The authors would like to thank Mark Gerhardt, MD, the author of the previous edition of this chapter, and Jennifer Olin for her editorial assistance.

REFERENCES

1. Warren J, Fromm RE Jr, Orr RA, et al. Guidelines for the inter- and intrahospital transport of critically ill patients. *Crit Care Med.* 2004;32(1):256–262.
2. Commission J. Improving America's hospitals: The Joint Commission's annual report on quality and safety. http://wwwjointcommissionreportorg/pdf/JC_2006_Annual_Reportpdf; 2006.
3. Dunn W, Murphy JG. The patient handoff: medicine's Formula One moment. *Chest.* 2008;134(1):9–12.
4. Saver C. Handoffs: what ORs can learn from Formula One race crews. *OR Manager.* 2011;27(4):1, 11–13.
5. Logio LS, Djuricich AM. Handoffs in teaching hospitals: situation, background, assessment, and recommendation. *Am J Med.* 2010;123(6):563–567.
6. Cohen MD, Hilligoss PB. The published literature on handoffs in hospitals: deficiencies identified in an extensive review. *Qual Saf Health Care.* 2010;19(6):493–497.
7. Raptis DA, Fernandes C, Chua W, et al. Electronic software significantly improves quality of handover in a London teaching hospital. *Health Informatics J.* 2009;15(3):191–198.
8. **American Society of Anesthesiologists. Practice advisory for the perioperative management of patients with cardiac implantable electronic devices: pacemakers and implantable cardioverter-defibrillators: an updated report by the American Society of Anesthesiologists Task Force on Perioperative Management of Patients with Cardiac Implantable Electronic Devices. *Anesthesiology.* 2011;114(2):247–261.**

9. Frazier SK. Cardiovascular effects of mechanical ventilation and weaning. *Nurs Clin North Am.* 2008;43(1):1–15.

10. Singh I, Pinsky MR. *Mechanical Ventilation.* Philadelphia, PA: Saunders Elsevier; 2008.

11. van Belle AF, Wesseling GJ, Penn OC, et al. Postoperative pulmonary function abnormalities after coronary artery bypass surgery. *Respir Med.* 1992;86(3):195–199.

12. Cox CM, Ascione R, Cohen AM, et al. Effect of cardiopulmonary bypass on pulmonary gas exchange: a prospective randomized study. *Ann Thorac Surg.* 2000;69(1):140–145.

13. Jaber S, Chanques G, Jung B. Postoperative noninvasive ventilation. *Anesthesiology.* 2010;112(2):453–461.

14. Burns KE, Adhikari NK, Keenan SP, et al. Use of non-invasive ventilation to wean critically ill adults off invasive ventilation: meta-analysis and systematic review. *BMJ.* 2009;338:b1574.

15. Gattinoni L, Protti A, Caironi P, et al. Ventilator-induced lung injury: the anatomical and physiological framework. *Crit Care Med.* 2010;38(10 Suppl):S539–S548.

16. Diaz JV, Brower R, Calfee CS, et al. Therapeutic strategies for severe acute lung injury. *Crit Care Med.* 2010;38(8):1644–1650.

17. Esan A, Hess DR, Raoof S, et al. Severe hypoxemic respiratory failure: part 1—ventilatory strategies. *Chest.* 2010;137(5):1203–1216.

18. Raoof S, Goulet K, Esan A, et al. Severe hypoxemic respiratory failure: part 2—nonventilatory strategies. *Chest.* 2010; 137(6):1437–1448.

19. Liu LL, Aldrich JM, Shimabukuro DW, et al. Special article: rescue therapies for acute hypoxemic respiratory failure. *Anesth Analg.* 2010;111(3):693–702.

20. Sud S, Sud M, Friedrich JO, et al. High-frequency oscillation in patients with acute lung injury and acute respiratory distress syndrome (ARDS): systematic review and meta-analysis. *BMJ.* 2010;340:c2327.

21. **Brochard L, Thille AW. What is the proper approach to liberating the weak from mechanical ventilation?** *Crit Care Med.* **2009;37(10 Suppl):S410–S415.**

22. MacIntyre N. Discontinuing mechanical ventilatory support. *Chest.* 2007;132(3):1049–1056.

23. Constantinides VA, Tekkis PP, Fazil A, et al. Fast-track failure after cardiac surgery: development of a prediction model. *Crit Care Med.* 2006;34(12):2875–2882.

24. Kogan A, Ghosh P, Preisman S, et al. Risk factors for failed "fast-tracking" after cardiac surgery in patients older than 70 years. *J Cardiothorac Vasc Anesth.* 2008;22(4):530–535.

25. Zarate E, Latham P, White PF, et al. Fast-track cardiac anesthesia: use of remifentanil combined with intrathecal morphine as an alternative to sufentanil during desflurane anesthesia. *Anesth Analg.* 2000;91(2):283–287.

26. Latham P, Zarate E, White PF, et al. Fast-track cardiac anesthesia: a comparison of remifentanil plus intrathecal morphine with sufentanil in a desflurane-based anesthetic. *J Cardiothorac Vasc Anesth.* 2000;14(6):645–651.

27. Dowd NP, Cheng DC, Karski JM, et al. Intraoperative awareness in fast-track cardiac anesthesia. *Anesthesiology.* 1998; 89(5):1068–1073.

28. Maldonado JR, Wysong A, van der Starre PJ, et al. Dexmedetomidine and the reduction of postoperative delirium after cardiac surgery. *Psychosomatics.* 2009;50(3):206–217.

29. Shehabi Y, Grant P, Wolfenden H, et al. Prevalence of delirium with dexmedetomidine compared with morphine based therapy after cardiac surgery: a randomized controlled trial (DEXmedetomidine COmpared to Morphine—DEXCOM study). *Anesthesiology.* 2009;111(5):1075–1084.

30. Herr DL, Sum-Ping ST, England M. ICU sedation after coronary artery bypass graft surgery: dexmedetomidine-based versus propofol-based sedation regimens. *J Cardiothorac Vasc Anesth.* 2003;17(5):576–584.

31. Riker RR, Shehabi Y, Bokesch PM, et al. Dexmedetomidine vs. midazolam for sedation of critically ill patients: a randomized trial. *JAMA.* 2009;301(5):489–499.

32. Novick RJ, Fox SA, Stitt LW, et al. Impact of the opening of a specialized cardiac surgery recovery unit on postoperative outcomes in an academic health sciences centre. *Can J Anesth.* 2007;54(9):737–743.

33. Abeles A, Kwansnicki RM, Darzi A. Enhanced recovery after surgery: current research insights and future direction. *World J Gastrointest Surg.* 2017;9(2):37–45.

34. Yang L, Kaye AD, Venakatesh AG, et al. Enhanced recovery after cardiac surgery: an update on clinical implications. *Int Anesthesiol Clin.* 2017;55(4):148–162.

35. Chavez J, Bortolotto SJ, Paulson M, et al. Promotion of progressive mobility activities with ventricular assist devices and extracorporeal membrane oxygenation devices in a cardiothoracic intensive care unit. *Dimens Crit Care Nurs.* 2015;34(6):348–355.

36. Srivastava AR, Banerjee A, Tempe DK, et al. A comprehensive approach to fast tracking in cardiac surgery: ambulatory low-risk open-heart surgery. *Eur J Cardiothorac Surg.* 2008;33(6):955–960.

37. Hollenberg SM. Vasoactive drugs in circulatory shock. *Am J Respir Crit Care Med.* 2011;183(7):847–855.

38. **Levy B, Perez P, Perny J, et al. Comparison of norepinephrine–dobutamine to epinephrine for hemodynamics, lactate metabolism, and organ function variables in cardiogenic shock. A prospective, randomized pilot study.** *Crit Care Med.* **2011;39(3):450–455.**

39. Prielipp RC, MacGregor DA, Butterworth JF, et al. Pharmacodynamics and pharmacokinetics of milrinone administration to increase oxygen delivery in critically ill patients. *Chest.* 1996;109(5):1291–1301.

40. Toller WG, Stranz C. Levosimendan, a new inotropic and vasodilator agent. *Anesthesiology.* 2006;104(3):556–569.

41. Maharaj R, Metaxa V. Levosimendan and mortality after coronary revascularisation: a meta-analysis of randomised controlled trials. *Crit Care.* 2011;15(3):R140.

42. Arroll B, Doughty R, Andersen V. Investigation and management of congestive heart failure. *BMJ.* 2010;341:C3657.

43. Ezekowitz JA, Hernandez AF, Starling RC, et al. Standardizing care for acute decompensated heart failure in a large megatrial: The approach for the Acute Studies of Clinical Effectiveness of Nesiritide in Subjects with Decompensated Heart Failure (ASCEND-HF). *Am Heart J.* 2009;157(2):219–228.

44. Krum H, Teerlink JR. Medical therapy for chronic heart failure. *Lancet.* 2011;378(9792):713–721.

45. Shah AM, Mann DL. In search of new therapeutic targets and strategies for heart failure: recent advances in basic science. *Lancet.* 2011;378(9792):704–712.

46. Chappell D, Jacob M, Hofmann-Kiefer K, et al. A rational approach to perioperative fluid management. *Anesthesiology.* 2008;109(4):723–740.
47. **Marik PE, Baram M, Vahid B. Does central venous pressure predict fluid responsiveness? A systematic review of the literature and the tale of seven mares. *Chest.* 2008;134(1):172–178.**
48. Michard F, Teboul JL. Using heart–lung interactions to assess fluid responsiveness during mechanical ventilation. *Crit Care.* 2000;4(5):282–289.
49. **Marik PE, Cavallazzi R, Vasu T, et al. Dynamic changes in arterial waveform derived variables and fluid responsiveness in mechanically ventilated patients: a systematic review of the literature. *Crit Care Med.* 2009;37(9):2642–2647.**
50. Society of Thoracic Surgeons Blood Conservation Guideline Task Force, Ferraris VA, Brown JR, Despotis GJ, et al. 2011 update to The Society of Thoracic Surgeons and The Society of Cardiovascular Anesthesiologists blood conservation clinical practice guidelines. *Ann Thorac Surg.* 2011;91(3):944–982.
51. Varghese R, Myers ML. Blood conservation in cardiac surgery: let's get restrictive. *Semin Thorac Cardiovasc Surg.* 2010; 22(2):121–126.
52. Levin RL, Degrange MA, Bruno GF, et al. Methylene blue reduces mortality and morbidity in vasoplegic patients after cardiac surgery. *Ann Thorac Surg.* 2004;77(2):496–499.
53. Burnes ML, Boettcher BT, Woehlck HJ, et al. Hydroxocobalamin as a rescue treatment for refractory vasoplegic syndrome after prolonged cardiopulmonary bypass. *J Cardiothorac Vasc Anesth.* 2017;31(3):1012–1014.
54. Maslow AD, Regan MM, Haering JM, et al. Echocardiographic predictors of left ventricular outflow tract obstruction and systolic anterior motion of the mitral valve after mitral valve reconstruction for myxomatous valve disease. *J Am Coll Cardiol.* 1999;34(7):2096–2104.
55. **Russo AM, O'Connor WH, Waxman HL. Atypical presentations and echocardiographic findings in patients with cardiac tamponade occurring early and late after cardiac surgery. *Chest.* 1993;104(1):71–78.**
56. Rho RW. The management of atrial fibrillation after cardiac surgery. *Heart.* 2009;95(5):422–429.
57. Bradley D, Creswell LL, Hogue CW Jr, et al. Pharmacologic prophylaxis: American College of Chest Physicians guidelines for the prevention and management of postoperative atrial fibrillation after cardiac surgery. *Chest.* 2005;128(2 Suppl):39S–47S.
58. Halonen J, Loponen P, Järvinen O, et al. Metoprolol versus amiodarone in the prevention of atrial fibrillation after cardiac surgery: a randomized trial. *Ann Intern Med.* 2010;153(11):703–709.
59. Chen WT, Krishnan GM, Sood N, et al. Effect of statins on atrial fibrillation after cardiac surgery: a duration– and dose–response meta-analysis. *J Thorac Cardiovasc Surg.* 2010;140(2):364–372.
60. Marik PE, Fromm R. The efficacy and dosage effect of corticosteroids for the prevention of atrial fibrillation after cardiac surgery: a systematic review. *J Crit Care.* 2009;24(3):458–463.
61. Ho KM, Tan JA. Benefits and risks of corticosteroid prophylaxis in adult cardiac surgery: a dose–response meta-analysis. *Circulation.* 2009;119(14):1853–1866.
62. Booth JV, Phillips-Bute B, McCants CB, et al. Low serum magnesium level predicts major adverse cardiac events after coronary artery bypass graft surgery. *Am Heart J.* 2003;145(6):1108–1113.
63. Cook RC, Humphries KH, Gin K, et al. Prophylactic intravenous magnesium sulphate in addition to oral β-blockade does not prevent atrial arrhythmias after coronary artery or valvular heart surgery: a randomized, controlled trial. *Circulation.* 2009;120(11 Suppl):S163–S169.
64. **Forfia PR, Fisher MR, Mathai SC, et al. Tricuspid annular displacement predicts survival in pulmonary hypertension. *Am J Respir Crit Care Med.* 2006;174(9):1034–1041.**
65. Tei C, Dujardin KS, Hodge DO, et al. Doppler echocardiographic index for assessment of global right ventricular function. *J Am Soc Echocardiogr.* 1996;9(6):838–847.
66. Meluzín J, Špinarová L, Bakala J, et al. Pulsed Doppler tissue imaging of the velocity of tricuspid annular systolic motion; a new, rapid, and non-invasive method of evaluating right ventricular systolic function. *Eur Heart J.* 2001;22(4):340–348.
67. Rosenberg AL, Rao M, Benedict PE. Anesthetic implications for lung transplantation. *Anesthesiol Clin North America.* 2004; 22(4):767–788.
68. Taylor MB, Laussen PC. Fundamentals of management of acute postoperative pulmonary hypertension. *Pediatr Crit Care Med.* 2010;11(2 Suppl):S27–S29.
69. **Gordon C, Collard CD, Pan W. Intraoperative management of pulmonary hypertension and associated right heart failure. *Curr Opin Anaesthesiol.* 2010;23(1):49–56.**
70. Yimin H, Xiaoyu L, Yuping H, et al. The effect of vasopressin on the hemodynamics in CABG patients. *J Cardiothorac Surg.* 2013;8:49.
71. Lahm T, McCaslin CA, Wozniak TC, et al. Medical and surgical treatment of acute right ventricular failure. *J Am Coll Cardiol.* 2010;56(18):1435–1446.
72. Price LC, Wort SJ, Finney SJ, et al. Pulmonary vascular and right ventricular dysfunction in adult critical care: current and emerging options for management: a systematic literature review. *Crit Care.* 2010;14(5):R169–R191.
73. Hynninen MS, Cheng DC, Hossain I, et al. Non-steroidal anti-inflammatory drugs in treatment of postoperative pain after cardiac surgery. *Can J Anesth.* 2000;47(12):1182–1187.
74. Chaney MA. Intrathecal and epidural anesthesia and analgesia for cardiac surgery. *Anesth Analg.* 2006;102(1):45–64.
75. Shroff A, Rooke GA, Bishop MJ. Effects of intrathecal opioid on extubation time, analgesia, and intensive care unit stay following coronary artery bypass grafting. *J Clin Anesth.* 1997;9(5):415–419.
76. Hall R, Adderley N, MacLaren C, et al. Does intrathecal morphine alter the stress response following coronary artery bypass grafting surgery? *Can J Anesth.* 2000;47(5):463–466.
77. Ganapathy S, Murkin JM, Boyd DW, et al. Continuous percutaneous paravertebral block for minimally invasive cardiac surgery. *J Cardiothorac Vasc Anesth.* 1999;13(5):594–596.
78. Cantó M, Sánchez MJ, Casas MA, et al. Bilateral paravertebral blockade for conventional cardiac surgery. *Anaesthesia.* 2003;58(4):365–370.

79. Dhole S, Mehta Y, Saxena H, et al. Comparison of continuous thoracic epidural and paravertebral blocks for postoperative analgesia after minimally invasive direct coronary artery bypass surgery. *J Cardiothorac Vasc Anesth.* 2001;15(3):288–292.

80. McDonald SB, Jacobsohn E, Kopacz DJ, et al. Parasternal block and local anesthetic infiltration with levobupivacaine after cardiac surgery with desflurane: the effect on postoperative pain, pulmonary function, and tracheal extubation times. *Anesth Analg.* 2005;100(1):25–32.

81. Jackson DL, Proudfoot CW, Cann KF, et al. A systematic review of the impact of sedation practice in the ICU on resource use, costs and patient safety. *Crit Care.* 2010;14(2):R59.

82. Pandharipande P, Shintani A, Peterson J, et al. Lorazepam is an independent risk factor for transitioning to delirium in intensive care unit patients. *Anesthesiology.* 2006;104(1):21–26.

83. Pandharipande P, Cotton BA, Shintani A, et al. Prevalence and risk factors for development of delirium in surgical and trauma intensive care unit patients. *J Trauma.* 2008;65(1):34–41.

84. Wijeysundera DN, Naik JS, Beattie WS. Alpha-2 adrenergic agonists to prevent perioperative cardiovascular complications: a meta-analysis. *Am J Med.* 2003;114(9):742–752.

85. **Dasta JF, Jacobi J, Sesti AM, et al. Addition of dexmedetomidine to standard sedation regimens after cardiac surgery: an outcomes analysis. *Pharmacotherapy.* 2006;26(6):798–805.**

86. Aantaa R, Jalonen J. Periopertive use of alpha2-adrenoceptor agonists and the cardiac patient. *Eur J Anaesthesiol.* 2006;23(5):361–372.

87. Chakraborti S, Chakraborti T, Mandal M, et al. Protective role of magnesium in cardiovascular diseases: a review. *Mol Cell Biochem.* 2002;238(1–2):163–179.

88. Brown GR, Greenwood JK. Drug- and nutrition-induced hypophosphatemia: mechanisms and relevance in the critically ill. *Ann Pharmacother.* 1994;28(5):626–632.

89. Davis SV, Olichwier KK, Chakko SC. Reversible depression of myocardial performance in hypophosphatemia. *Am J Med Sci.* 1988;295(3):183–187.

90. Van den Berghe G, Wouters P, Weekers F, et al. Intensive insulin therapy in critically ill patients. *N Engl J Med.* 2001;345(19):1359–1367.

91. NICE-SUGAR Study Investigators, Finfer S, Chittock DR, Su SY, et al. Intensive versus conventional glucose control in critically ill patients. *N Engl J Med.* 2009;360(13):1283–1297.

92. Hein OV, Birnbaum J, Wernecke KD, et al. Three-year survival after four major post-cardiac operative complications. *Crit Care Med.* 2006;34(11):2729–2737.

93. Levi M, Levy JH, Andersen HF, et al. Safety of recombinant activated factor VII in randomized clinical trials. *N Engl J Med.* 2010;363(19):1791–1800.

94. Xirouchaki N, Magkanas E, Vaporidi K, et al. Lung ultrasound in critically ill patients: comparison with bedside chest radiography. *Intensive Care Med.* 2011;37(9):1488–1493.

95. Shroyer AL, Hattler B, Wagner TH, et al. Five year outcomes after on-pump and off-pump coronary artery bypass. *N Engl J Med.* 2017;377(7):623–632.

96. Puskas JD, Williams WH, Mahoney EM, et al. Off-pump vs. conventional coronary artery bypass grafting: early and 1-year graft patency, cost, and quality-of-life outcomes: a randomized trial. *JAMA.* 2004;291(15):1841–1849.

97. Parolari A, Alamanni F, Polvani G, et al. Meta-analysis of randomized trials comparing off-pump with on-pump coronary artery bypass graft patency. *Ann Thoracic Surg.* 2005;80(6):2121–2125.

98. Stroobant N, Van Nooten G, Van Belleghem Y, et al. The effect of CABG on neurocognitive functioning. *Acta Cardiol.* 2010;65(5):557–564.

99. Deiner S, Silverstein JH. Postoperative delirium and cognitive dysfunction. *Br J Anaesth.* 2009;103(Suppl 1):i41–i46.

100. **Ely EW, Inouye SK, Bernard GR, et al. Delirium in mechanically ventilated patients: validity and reliability of the confusion assessment method for the intensive care unit (CAM-ICU). *JAMA.* 2001;286(21):2703–2710.**

101. Kay GL, Sun GW, Aoki A, et al. Influence of ejection fraction on hospital mortality, morbidity, and costs for CABG patients. *Ann Thoracic Surg.* 1995;60(6):1640–1650.

102. Doering LV, Esmailian F, Laks H. Perioperative predictors of ICU and hospital costs in coronary artery bypass graft surgery. *Chest.* 2000;118(3):736–743.

103. Sista RR, Wall M. Postoperative care of the patient after heart or lung transplantation. *Postoperative Cardiac Care.* Richmond, VA: Society of Cardiovascular Anesthesiologists; 2011.

104. Thunberg CA, Gaitan BD, Arabia FA, et al. Ventricular assist devices today and tomorrow. *J Cardiothorac Vasc Anesth.* 2010;24(4):656–680.

105. Naidu SS. Novel percutaneous cardiac assist devices: the science of and indications for hemodynamic support. *Circulation.* 2011;123(5):533–543.

106. Trost JC, Hillis LD. Intra-aortic balloon counterpulsation. *Am J Cardiol.* 2006;97(9):1391–1398.

107. Williams DO, Korr KS, Gewirtz H, et al. The effect of intra-aortic balloon counterpulsation on regional myocardial blood flow and oxygen consumption in the presence of coronary artery stenosis in patients with unstable angina. *Circulation.* 1982;66(3):593–597.

108. Jiang CY, Zhao LL, Wang JA, et al. Anticoagulation therapy in intra-aortic balloon counterpulsation: does IABP really need anticoagulation. *J Zhejiang Univ Sci.* 2003;4(5):607–611.

26

Protection of the Brain During Cardiopulmonary Bypass

Satoru Fujii and John M. Murkin

KEY POINTS

1. The incidence of overt stroke is 1.5% to 2.5% for closed-chamber cardiac procedures. For open-chamber, combined and aortic arch procedures, the incidence of stroke ranges from 4.2% to 13%.
2. Risk factors for early stroke include advanced age, duration of cardiopulmonary bypass (CPB), high postoperative creatinine, and extensive aortic atherosclerosis, while delayed stroke was associated with female gender, postoperative atrial fibrillation, cerebrovascular disease, and requirement for inotropic support.

(continued)

3. Within the first postoperative week, a majority of patients undergoing bypass surgery using CPB demonstrate a degree of cognitive dysfunction. This appears to be largely due to underlying patient factors interacting with emboli, inflammation, and blood–brain barrier (BBB) alterations.
4. The incidence of late postoperative cognitive dysfunction appears to be similar to an age- and gender-matched nonsurgical cohort having similar comorbidities, implying progression of underlying disease.
5. A wide variety of autoregulation thresholds occur even with α-stat blood gas management and are likely a consequence of increased age and cerebrovascular disease.
6. α-Stat blood gas management, which maintains a normal transmembrane pH gradient and maintains cerebral autoregulation (CA) of blood flow, should be used in adult patients undergoing bypass. This modality may help reduce cerebral embolization.
7. Cerebral emboli may come from multiple sources that are patient related, procedure related, and equipment related.
8. Watershed lesions are commonly due to profound hypotensive episodes but may also be the result of cerebral embolism. Embolization and hypotension acting together magnify central nervous system (CNS) injury.
9. Leukocytosis is associated with a higher risk for ischemic stroke. The results strongly implicate inflammation and white cell activation as etiologic factors in both the extent and severity of perioperative cerebral events.

I. Central nervous system (CNS) dysfunction associated with cardiac surgery

A. Overview

Despite continuing improvements in surgical and cardiopulmonary bypass (CPB) techniques, stroke remains a devastating postoperative complication for patients and their families. In a randomized study in which 1,800 patients with three-vessel or left mainstem coronary artery disease were assigned to percutaneous coronary intervention (PCI) or conventional coronary artery bypass (CAB) surgery, there was no difference in mortality at 1 year and a significantly lower incidence of primary composite endpoint of major adverse cardiac or cerebrovascular event (MACCE) in CAB versus PCI (12.4% vs. 17.8%; p <0.00) groups [1]. However, while the overall outcome should argue strongly in favor of CAB surgery, the stroke rate was significantly higher in CAB than PCI (2.2% vs. 0.6%; p = 0.003). Given the relatively equivalent risk factors between PCI and CAB patients in this study, the mechanism of perioperative stroke must be better understood if we are to further reduce the risk of CNS morbidity related to cardiac surgery. **This chapter will review the current incidence and risk factors for brain damage in cardiac surgery and will outline strategies aimed at protection of the brain during cardiac surgical procedures.**

B. Stroke incidence

In most series reported to date, the incidence of clinically apparent neurologic injury or overt stroke is 1.5% to 2.5% for closed-chamber cardiac procedures (e.g., CAB surgery). Up to 25% to 65% of strokes after CAB surgeries are bilateral or multiple, suggestive of an embolic etiology [2]. For open-chamber procedures (e.g., valve surgery), the reported incidence of stroke varies from 4.2% to 13%, which could be related to increased risk of particulate embolization, increased hemodynamic instability, or prolonged CPB time [3].

C. Transcatheter aortic valve replacement (TAVR) versus surgical aortic valve replacement (SAVR)

Transcatheter aortic valve replacement (TAVR) is a novel technique and has been available as an alternative to surgical aortic valve replacement (SAVR) for more than a decade. Various types of valves have been commercially available, and their use is dependent on the type of procedure and patients' vascular size and anatomy. Although the initial studies showed increased incidences of stroke post-TAVR compared to medical management, subsequent studies show noninferiority or superiority of TAVR compared with SAVR in terms of neurologic complications. In 2016, 2,032 intermediate-risk patients were recruited and randomly assigned to transfemoral (TF) or transthoracic (TT) TAVR or SAVR. The rate of disabling stroke was 6.2% after TAVR and 6.4% after SAVR at 2 years, while the incidence of new-onset atrial fibrillation was significantly lower in TAVR compared with SAVR (9.1% vs. 26.4%) which may affect the long-term incidence of stroke [4]. While TF approach was formerly associated with higher stroke rates compared with TT—possibly as a consequence of passage through the aortic arch—a recent meta-analysis encompassing seven European national TAVR registries found stroke rates were lower at 3% regardless of TT- or TF-TAVR strategy [5]. Ever improving TAVR devices, improved patient management and expanding indication of TAVR for intermediate-risk patients are thought attributable for the reduced stroke rates.

> **CLINICAL PEARL**   Current stroke rates of TAVR are comparable to SAVR.

D. Early versus delayed stroke

Distinguishing stroke as early (i.e., persistent neurologic deficit apparent within 24 hours of emergence from anesthesia) from delayed (i.e., persistent neurologic deficit developing days after anesthesia recovery) is important to better discriminate etiology and assess potential risk-reduction strategies. Only approximately 50% of perioperative strokes present during the first 24 hours post surgery tend to be more severe with a higher permanent deficit and *early stroke has a higher impact on perioperative mortality* [6,7]. The higher mortality could be related to sicker patients or to stroke being just one manifestation of other concomitant embolic/hypoperfusion-mediated complications. Stroke can also have a long-term effect on mortality (Fig. 26.1). In a prospective study on CAB patients, the adjusted survival rates at 1, 5, and 10 years were 94.1%, 83.3%, and 61.9% among patients free from stroke versus 83%, 58.7%, and 26.9% for those suffering perioperative stroke [8]. Risk factors for early stroke include advanced age, duration of CPB, high preoperative creatinine, and extensive aortic atherosclerosis, while delayed stroke was associated with female gender, postoperative atrial fibrillation, cerebrovascular disease, and requirements for inotropic support [7]. *Delayed but not early stroke was associated with long-term mortality.*

> **CLINICAL PEARL**   Early stroke (persistent neurologic deficit apparent within 24 hours of emergence from anesthesia) has a higher impact on perioperative mortality than late stroke.

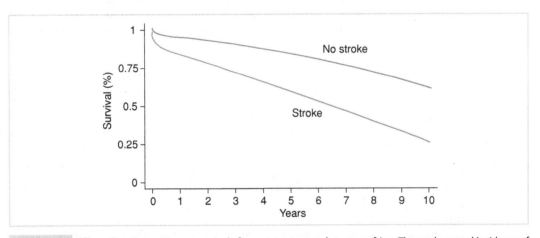

FIGURE 26.1 Effect of stroke on 10-year survival after coronary artery bypass grafting. The crude annual incidence of death was 18.1/100 person-years among patients with strokes and 3.7/100 person-years among patients without strokes ($p < 0.001$). (From Dacey LJ, Likosky DS, Leavitt BJ, et al. Perioperative stroke and long-term survival after coronary bypass graft surgery. *Ann Thorac Surg.* 2005;79(2):532–536, with permission.)

E. **Cognitive dysfunction**

Within the first postoperative week, up to 83% of all patients undergoing CAB surgery using CPB demonstrate a degree of cognitive dysfunction. Of these patients, 38% have symptoms of intellectual impairment and 10% are considered to be overtly disabled. Concentration, retention, and processing of new information and visuospatial organization are the most frequently affected domains [9], and at 5-year follow-up, more than 35% of CAB patients exhibit some degree of neuropsychological dysfunction. Variable definitions, different measurement techniques, and different intervals of postoperative cognitive testing confound this issue, however, giving rise to reported incidences of perioperative cognitive decline that vary from 4% to 90%. Additional confounders include the variability in performance to repeated neuropsychometric testing, even in healthy subjects, and an innate decline in cognitive function associated with both aging and the various comorbidities found in cardiac surgical patients. The challenge lies in discerning whether a specific event—for example, cardiac surgery—is causal or coincidental to deterioration in cognitive function.

CLINICAL PEARL Longer-term cognitive dysfunction has a similar incidence whether patients undergo cardiac surgery with or without the use of CPB, or instead undergo PCI or are managed medically, with the implication that aging and progression of underlying atherosclerosis and related comorbidities are primary risk factors [10].

F. **Comparison groups**

The incidence of new postoperative CNS dysfunction in CAB patients has been compared with that of patients undergoing major abdominal vascular or thoracic surgical procedures. Most of these patients usually have concomitant disease including hypertension, diabetes mellitus, diffuse atherosclerosis, and chronic lung disease. After adjusting for identified risk factors, patients undergoing any surgical procedure have been found more likely to suffer a cerebrovascular accident (CVA) than nonoperated controls, with an odds ratio of 3.9. Even after excluding high-risk surgery (cardiac, vascular, and neurologic), the odds ratio is 2.9, which suggests *the perioperative period itself predisposes patients to stroke*. This observation is of particular relevance in considering the role of inflammatory processes and the salutary effect of statins as discussed below.

Studies on patients undergoing CAB surgery have demonstrated minimal difference in long-term cognitive function between patients undergoing on-pump versus off-pump procedures [11]. However, in general, it does appear that, compared with other noncardiac surgical groups, the incidence *of early postoperative cognitive dysfunction is higher in CAB patients*. Since new ischemic lesions on magnetic resonance imaging (MRI) studies in valve surgery patients correlate with early postoperative cognitive dysfunction [12], as do intraoperative cerebral oxygen desaturation and early postoperative cognitive dysfunction in CAB patients, it appears that *efforts to mitigate early postoperative cognitive dysfunction are warranted, since early postoperative cognitive dysfunction partly reflects subclinical brain injury*.

G. **Risk factors**

Table 26.1 shows risk factors for both stroke and cognitive dysfunction. Risk factors have been pooled into various risk prediction models, which, while useful to compare patient groups, are still not predictive of a particular individual's outcome, although the presence of key risk factors may help in deciding the best procedure for a particular high-risk patient (i.e., surgery vs. angioplasty or valvuloplasty). Specific risk factors (i.e., aortic atherosclerosis, recent stroke) should prompt further preoperative investigations (e.g., carotid scanning, modification of intraoperative management) and may even suggest a change in surgical approach (i.e., off-pump CAB [OPCAB] with no instrumentation of the aorta—anaortic) to minimize the potential for neurologic complications.

H. **Delirium**

The incidence of delirium in cardiac surgery has been reported as 17.5% to 30%, and is associated with increased mortality, pulmonary dysfunction, and longer duration of hospitalization [13,14].

TABLE 26.1   Risk factors for neurologic complications in cardiac surgery

Common risk factors for both stroke and cognitive decline	
Advanced age (>75 yrs)	
Hypertension	
Severe carotid stenosis	
Diabetes mellitus	
Prior cerebrovascular disease	
Aortic atheromatosis	
Postbypass hypotension	
Postoperative arrhythmias	
Hemodynamic instability during CPB	
Risk factors for stroke	**Risk factors for cognitive decline**
Type of surgery (complex procedures)	Cerebral oxygen desaturation during CPB
Emergency surgery	Cerebral hypoperfusion during CPB
Aortic instrumentation (cannulation, cross clamp, side clamp)	Brain hyperthermia during rewarming from CPB
Vascular disease	
CPB longer than 2 hrs	
Elevated preoperative creatinine	
Postoperative atrial fibrillation	

CPB, cardiopulmonary bypass.

Although the exact mechanisms have not been fully elucidated, systemic inflammation, chemokines, cytokines, endothelial dysfunction, and disruption of blood–brain barrier (BBB) have been recognized as potential factors thought to cause neurotransmitter interference, global cognitive disorder, and neuroinflammation [15].

Multiple risk factors have been implicated, including duration of CPB, lowest mean arterial pressure (MAP), hemoglobin level, lowest body temperature, RBC transfusion, and platelet transfusion; however, in multivariate analysis, only platelet transfusion remained as an independent risk factor [16]. Various standardized assessment tools have been employed for detection of delirium, including Confusion Assessment Method for the Intensive Care Unit (CAM-ICU) or Intensive Care Delirium Screening Checklist (ICDSC), which assess level of consciousness, inattention, disorientation, hallucinations/delusions/psychosis, psychomotor agitation or retardation, inappropriate speech or mood, sleep/wake cycle disturbances, and symptom fluctuation [17]. Several studies have compared CAB with OPCAB, but results have been inconclusive, with one study indicating OPCAB was associated with lower incidences of delirium compared to on-pump CAB (7.9% vs. 2.3%) [18]. The incidences of delirium reported by these authors were much lower than those from other reports, and another study found no difference in the incidence of delirium between on-pump and OPCAB [19]. A recent study demonstrated that SAVR-treated patients had a higher incidence of postoperative delirium than TF TAVR (51% vs. 29%) [20]. Also, they demonstrated that delirium was associated with increased mortality at 30 days and 1 year and longer Intensive Care Unit (ICU) and hospital lengths of stay. Delirium is highest with TT compared with TF TAVR, likely reflecting the fact that primarily higher-risk patients with small vascular size or severe aortic tortuosity undergo TT TAVR and that pain from minithoracotomy may play a role in triggering delirium [21].

II. Cerebral physiology

A. Cerebral autoregulation (CA)

In normal subjects, cerebral blood flow (CBF) remains relatively constant at 50 mL/100 g/min over a wide range of MAP from 50 to 150 mm Hg. This ***autoregulatory plateau reflects the tight matching between regional cerebral metabolic rate for O_2 ($CMRO_2$) and CBF.*** With decreased metabolic activity resulting from certain anesthetics or hypothermia, lowered $CMRO_2$ produces a resultant reduction in CBF and establishment of a lower autoregulatory plateau. Rather than a single cerebral autoregulatory curve, there are instead a series of autoregulatory curves, each representing a differing set of metabolic conditions of the brain (e.g., normal metabolic activity at 37°C vs. lowered metabolic activity at 28°C). The autoregulatory

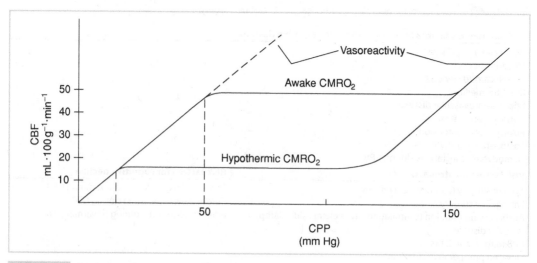

FIGURE 26.2 Cerebral autoregulatory curves during normothermia and hypothermia. The *upper curve* demonstrates a higher cerebral blood flow (CBF) autoregulatory plateau that is appropriate for the higher cerebral metabolic rate for O_2 (CMRO_2) in the awake state versus a lower CBF plateau during hypothermia. With maximal cerebral vasodilation, lower cerebral perfusion pressure (CPP) results in lower CBF that is appropriate at a lower $CMRO_2$ (hypothermia) but not at a higher $CMRO_2$. (From Murkin JM. The pathophysiology of cardiopulmonary bypass. *Can J Anesth*. 1989;36:S41–S44, with permission.)

plateau reflects intact cerebral flow and metabolism coupling, and it varies with metabolic rate (Fig. 26.2).

With intact autoregulation, lowered substrate requirement during conditions of lowered metabolic rate (e.g., anesthesia, hypothermia) requires less blood flow and can be delivered at a lower perfusion pressure—in the absence of direct cerebral vasodilators, such as CO_2. CA is impaired in patients with diabetes mellitus and appears to be lost during deep hypothermia (e.g., less than 20°C) and for several hours after deep hypothermic circulatory arrest (DHCA). This results in pressure-passive CBF; in these instances, hypotension may entail increased risk for cerebral hypoperfusion. Similarly, in patients with chronic hypertension, CA has been reset and higher perfusion pressures are needed during CPB.

B. Lower limit of cerebral autoregulation

An important new area of investigation is detection and monitoring of the lower limit of cerebral autoregulation (LLA). It is relevant that most of the initial studies on CBF and $CMRO_2$ during CPB specifically excluded patients with overt cerebrovascular disease [22], while more recent studies have included both elderly patients and those with previous CVA, and have indicated a striking variability in the LLA threshold (Fig. 26.3) [23,24]. Using transcranial Doppler (TCD) or cerebral near-infrared spectroscopy (NIRS), absent or high LLA ranging from 45 to 80 mm Hg has been demonstrated [23,24]. Several large single-center studies have demonstrated *post hoc* correlations between duration of MAP below LLA and various adverse outcomes including stroke and renal failure [25,26], while MAP above upper limit autoregulation (ULA) has been associated with a higher risk of delirium [27].

CLINICAL PEARL Recent studies have demonstrated a striking interindividual variability in the LLA during CPB.

C. pH management

There is an inverse relationship between solubility of respiratory gases and blood temperature. With cooling of blood in the tissue, CO_2 partial pressure ($PaCO_2$) decreases and arterial pH (pH_a) increases, producing an apparent respiratory alkalosis.

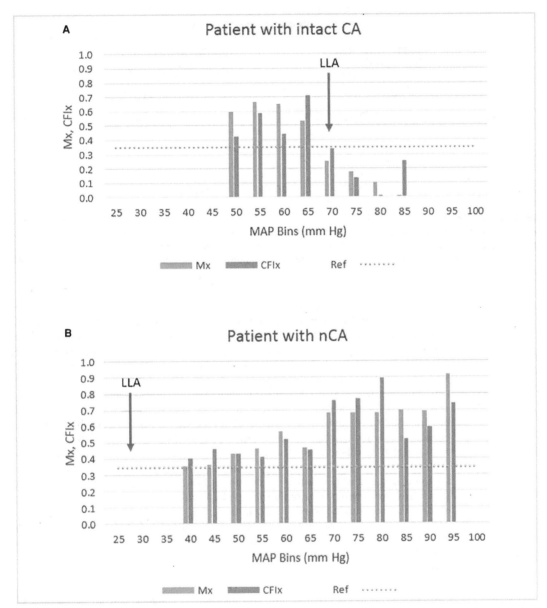

FIGURE 26.3 Example of patients with intact and nonintact CA. CA, cerebral autoregulation; nCA, absent cerebral autoregulation; Mx, mean velocity index; CFIx, cerebral flow index correlation index; LLA, lower limit of CA as shown by vertical arrow (**A**); MAP, mean arterial pressure. *Dotted line* is Mx/CFIx >0.35 indicates pressure passive cerebral blood flow (**B**). (From Murkin JM, Kamar M, Silman Z, et al. Intraoperative cerebral autoregulation assessment using ultrasound-tagged nearinfrared-based cerebral blood flow in comparison to transcranial Doppler cerebral flow velocity: a pilot study. *J Cardiothorac Vasc Anesth.* 2015;29(5):1187–1193 with permission)

1. **α-*Stat maintains* pH_a 7.4 *and* $PaCO_2$ 40 *mm Hg at* 37°C *without addition of exogenous* CO_2.** Intracellular pH is primarily determined by the neutral pH (pH_N) of water. Since pH_N becomes progressively more alkaline with decreasing temperature, intracellular pH becomes correspondingly more alkaline during hypothermia. Since this intracellular alkalosis occurs in parallel with the hypothermia-induced increased solubility of CO_2 and increased blood pH, the normal transmembrane pH gradient of approximately 0.6 units remains

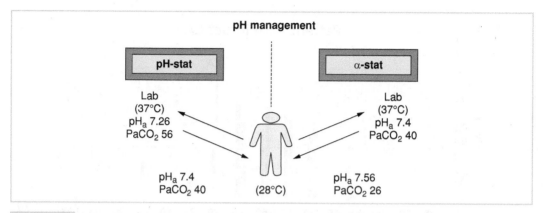

FIGURE 26.4 Contrasting arterial blood gas values as seen in vitro at 37°C or in vivo at 28°C when using α-stat or pH-stat management. Using pH-stat, laboratory values in vitro would be pH_a 7.26 and $PaCO_2$ 56 mm Hg, whereas temperature-corrected values in vivo would be pH_a 7.4 and $PaCO_2$ 40 mm Hg. If α-stat were used, laboratory values in vitro would be pH_a 7.4 and $PaCO_2$ 40 mm Hg, whereas temperature-corrected values in vivo would be pH_a 7.56 and $PaCO_2$ 26 mm Hg.

unchanged, thus preserving optimal function of various intracellular enzyme systems. *The preservation of normal transmembrane pH gradient is the crux of α-stat pH theory,* and, in fact, we function in vivo according to α-stat principles. Since different tissues have differing temperatures (e.g., exercising muscle at 41°C vs. skin at 25°C), they also will have correspondingly different pH_a values (e.g., 7.34 vs. 7.6, respectively), although the net pH_a at 37°C will be 7.4. α-Stat management acknowledges the temperature dependence of normal pH_a and strives to maintain a constant transmembrane pH gradient by maintaining $PaCO_2$ at 40 mm Hg (or at the patient's baseline physiologic $PaCO_2$) and pH_a at 7.4, as measured in vitro at 37°C. For this strategy during CPB, total CO_2 is kept constant by not adding exogenous CO_2 and thus not compensating for increased solubility of CO_2. Blood samples measured at 37°C will show pH_a 7.4 and $PaCO_2$ 40 mm Hg, but those same samples measured at 28°C would have pH_a 7.56 and $PaCO_2$ 26 mm Hg (Fig. 26.4). In recent studies, even with the use of α-stat, a wide variability or absence of LLA autoregulatory threshold has been found, likely as a consequence of the increased age and presence of overt cerebrovascular disease in current surgical populations [23,24].

2. *pH-stat management involves the addition of exogenous CO_2 to maintain $PaCO_2$ 40 mm Hg and pH_a 7.4 when corrected for the patient's body temperature in vivo.* Until the mid-1980s, pH-stat management was generally the most common mode of pH management during moderate hypothermic CPB. Since CO_2 is a potent cerebral vasodilator, such increases in total $PaCO_2$ associated with pH-stat have been shown to produce cerebral vasodilation, impairing cerebral flow and metabolism coupling and producing loss of CA (Fig. 26.5). There is evidence that pH-stat management can increase the incidence of postoperative cognitive dysfunction when CPB duration exceeds 90 minutes [9]. This likely reflects both increased delivery of microemboli into the brain resulting from CO_2-induced vasodilation and impairment of regional CA.

III. Etiology of central nervous system (CNS) damage

A. Embolization

In the context of CPB, focal ischemia is most often a consequence of isolated cerebral arteriolar obstruction by particulate or gaseous emboli. Emboli vary in size, nature (particulate vs. gaseous), and origin (patient vs. equipment). Embolic characteristics influencing tissue distribution include size, solubility, viscosity, and buoyancy relative to blood. Vessel diameter, anatomical location, and inflammatory responsivity influence tissue vulnerability. Open-chamber procedures generally entail greater risk of microgaseous embolizations, which increase BBB permeability and may engender heightened drug toxicity [28]. Calcific or atheromatous

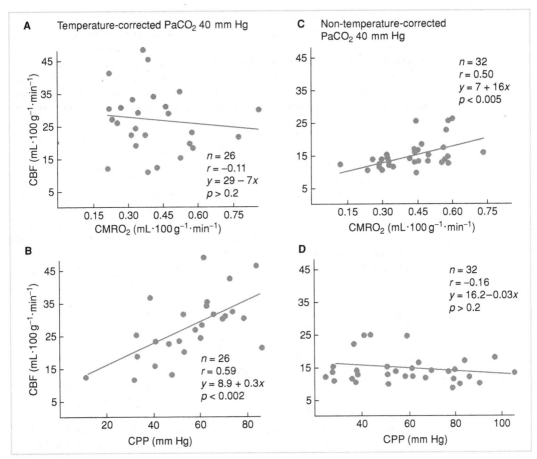

FIGURE 26.5 Linear regression analysis of CBF and $CMRO_2$, or cerebral perfusion pressure (CPP), for patients managed using α-stat (non–temperature-corrected) or pH-stat (temperature-corrected) management during moderate hypothermia (28°C). With pH-stat (**A**), there is no correlation between CBF and $CMRO_2$, demonstrating loss of cerebral flow and metabolism coupling, whereas with α-stat (**C**), there is a highly significant ($p < 0.005$) correlation. CBF significantly ($p < 0.002$) correlates with CPP using pH-stat (**B**) reflecting pressure-passive CBF and loss of autoregulation, whereas with α-stat (**D**), CBF is independent of CPP. (From Murkin JM, Farrar JK, Tweed WA, et al. Cerebral autoregulation and flow/metabolism coupling during cardiopulmonary bypass: the influence of $PaCO_2$. *Anesth Analg.* 1987;66(9):825–832, with permission.)

macroembolic debris from the ascending aorta or aortic arch appears to be a prime factor in the production of clinical stroke syndromes.

1. **Microgaseous emboli.** It was formerly thought that cerebral microgaseous emboli produced cognitive dysfunction. Studies of OPCAB, in which CPB is avoided, appear to have a relatively similar incidence of cognitive dysfunction when compared to CAB. The greatest numbers of microgaseous emboli are found in open-chamber surgery but again this paradoxically does not appear to result in greater incidences of cognitive impairment. Microgaseous emboli thus appear to be relatively less injurious than otherwise predicted, which may reflect a salutary effect of systemic heparinization [29]. However, microgaseous emboli do increase BBB permeability, which has been correlated with cerebral edema, enhanced neurotoxicity and postoperative seizures following high-dose tranexamic acid administration [28].

2. **Detection of emboli**
   a. **Brain histology.** Isolated areas of perivascular and focal subarachnoid hemorrhage, neuronal swelling, and axonal degeneration are seen with higher frequency in the brains

of patients dying after cardiac surgery than after non-CPB major vascular surgery. After surgery using unfiltered CPB circuits, fibrin and platelet emboli and calcific and atheromatous debris were seen frequently in small arterioles and capillary beds. *Small cerebral capillary and arterial dilatations (SCADs)* have been demonstrated histologically, occurring in nonsurvivors after proximal aortic instrumentation after either CPB or coronary angiography. These *SCADs are increasingly believed to be due in part to lipid microemboli from the usage of unprocessed cardiotomy suction blood.*

b. **Intraoperative emboli detection.** Intraoperative fluorescein retinal angiography has demonstrated that extensive retinal microvascular embolization occurs during CPB. The incidence and extent of retinal obstruction are much greater with bubble than with membrane oxygenators, despite the use of 40-μm arterial line filters. Use of TCD insonation enables assessment of blood flow perfusion characteristics through the middle cerebral artery (MCA). TCD insonation permits measurement of blood flow velocity and detection and quantification of emboli, though discrimination of gaseous from particulate emboli remains unreliable. *Proximal aortic instrumentation and initiation of CPB have been identified as particularly embologenic events.* After open-chamber surgery, cerebral emboli are detected as the heart fills and begins to eject, underscoring the importance of meticulous de-airing techniques.

3. **Sources of emboli**
   a. **Patient-related sources**
      (1) **Aortic atheroma.** Atheromatous debris can be embolized during aortic clamping or cannulation. Intraoperative aortic ultrasonography using either transesophageal echocardiography (TEE; high sensitivity, low specificity) or epiaortic scanning (EAS; high sensitivity, high specificity) enables visualization of the aortic wall and can be used to guide cannulation sites. Ultrasonography has demonstrated that plaque may fracture or shear off and embolize during CPB as a consequence of trauma from aortic clamping and cannulation or from blood "jetting" from the aortic cannula, or may result in intimal flap formation with potential for delayed postoperative embolization [30]. Using EAS, Ura et al. compared images before and after CPB in 472 patients undergoing cardiac surgery and noted new lesions in the ascending aortic intima in 16 patients (3.4%) following decannulation [30]. In 10 patients, 3 of whom suffered postoperative CVA, the new lesions were severe with mobile lesions or disruption of the intima, of which 6 were related to aortic clamping and the other 4 to aortic cannulation. Only the maximal thickness of the atheroma near the aortic manipulation site was a predictor of new lesions. As such, embolization of plaque or thrombus from such intimal fractures may explain one mechanism of delayed stroke cited above. *Proximal aortic atherosclerosis is thus a significant risk factor for neurologic injury.*
      (2) **Intraventricular thrombi.** During closed-chamber procedures in patients with recent mural thrombi, manipulation of the heart can dislodge atrial or ventricular thrombi that embolize once the heart begins to fill and eject.
      (3) **Valvular calcifications.** Valve surgery, particularly valve replacement surgery, is associated with increased risk of CVA resulting from embolization of intracavitary valve debris.
      (4) **Postoperative atrial fibrillation.** Early-onset atrial fibrillation is associated with a variety of adverse outcomes, has been strongly linked to increased perioperative stroke risk, and is particularly associated with an increased risk of delayed-onset postoperative stroke [6]. Even transient new-onset atrial fibrillation is associated with an increased risk of 30-day and 1-year major cardiovascular events comprising stroke, cardiac death, and myocardial infarction (MI).

In cardiac surgical patients, a decreased incidence of atrial fibrillation has been associated with perioperative statin therapy as discussed below. *Increased efforts should be aimed at reducing even transient new-onset postoperative atrial fibrillation.*

CLINICAL PEARL   Even transient postoperative atrial fibrillation is associated with an increased risk of 1-year cardiovascular events (stroke, MI, and cardiac death).

  b. **Procedure-related sources**
    (1) While open-chamber procedures (e.g., septal repair, ventricular aneurysmectomy, valve surgery) expose the arterial circulation to air or particulate debris, closed-chamber procedures also can be associated with ventricular air. Use of a ventricular vent, particularly if active suction is applied and the heart is empty, produces localized subatmospheric pressure at the vent tip within the left ventricle (LV) and causes air to be entrained retrograde from the vent insertion site (usually through the superior pulmonary vein) into the LV (Fig. 26.6). In patients with a left ventricular assist device (LVAD), wherein blood is drawn from the ventricular cavity causing a low-pressure gradient, even surgical microtears in fibrotic myocardial tissue can become a rapidly-accruing source of intraventricular air. Inadvertent opening of the left atrium (LA) or LV while the heart is beating also causes rapid air entrainment and increased potential for massive cerebral air embolization, necessitating emergency de-airing techniques [31]. Immediate flooding of the pericardial site is recommended. TEE can assist in visualization and guide the removal of residual intracavitary air.
    (2) Aortic cannulation and clamping are associated with cerebral embolization, particularly in the presence of extensive aortic atherosclerosis.
    (3) After 90 minutes of CPB, the incidence of cognitive dysfunction increases compared to CPB of shorter duration [9]. It is important to note that duration of CPB may be increased by factors (e.g., extensive atherosclerotic disease) that may independently contribute to neurologic injury [2,3]. *Duration of CPB is an independent risk factor for postoperative brain dysfunction.*
  c. **Equipment-related sources**
    (1) Incorporation of a 25-μm filter into the aortic inflow line effectively reduces cerebral embolic load and has been shown to decrease the incidence of postoperative cognitive dysfunction.

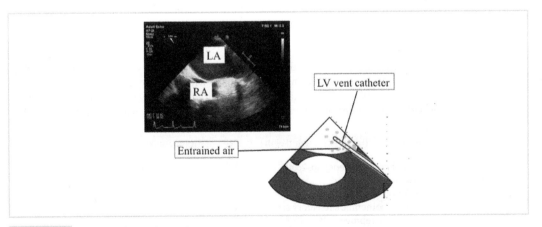

FIGURE 26.6 Diagram of vent air entrainment.

(2) Membrane oxygenators give rise to markedly fewer gaseous microemboli than bubble oxygenators, but do not entirely eliminate the risk of air emboli. Similarly, air entrained into the venous side of a membrane oxygenator (or gaseous emboli resulting from drug administration via injection directly into the CPB circuitry) can transit the membrane and appear in the arterial inflow line despite the use of arterial line filters.

(3) Use of 20- to 40-μm filters in the cardiotomy return line prevents particulate debris from the operative site from entering the CPB circuit. Use of cardiotomy blood washing techniques (Cell Saver) is associated with reduced amounts of cerebral lipid microemboli, but has not been consistently shown to improve CNS outcomes.

(4) Use of nitrous oxide (N_2O) before commencement of CPB has been associated with increased evidence of ischemic damage, likely because residual N_2O increases the size of any microgaseous emboli in the cerebral circulation. This especially applies to the first few hours after CPB, when high fractional inspired oxygen (FiO_2) should be used to minimize the size of residual gaseous microemboli.

B. Hypoperfusion

1. Watershed areas. Areas of brain localized at the boundary limits of major cerebral arteries (e.g., anterior and middle, middle and posterior cerebral arteries, or superior and posteroinferior cerebellar arteries) are known as ***arterial boundary zones or watershed zones***. Rapid severe hypoperfusion can produce ischemic lesions within these boundary zones found at the territorial limits of the major cerebral arteries. The most frequently affected area is the parieto-occipital sulcus located at the limits of the anterior, middle, and posterior cerebral arteries. Despite global ischemic stress, these watershed lesions may be focal and asymmetrical. Although commonly due to profoundly hypotensive episodes, watershed lesions are not pathognomonic of a hypotensive episode, and may result from cerebral emboli.

CLINICAL PEARL Embolization and hypoperfusion acting together can play a synergistic role and either cause or magnify CNS injury in cardiac surgical patients.

2. Cerebral perfusion pressure (CPP). During moderate hypothermia (28° to 30°C) using α-stat pH management, autoregulation is preserved in certain patients over CPP ranging from 20 to 100 mm Hg. However, studies in older cardiac surgical patients and those with cerebrovascular disease indicate a wide variability of LLA between 45 and 80 mm Hg, including some in whom autoregulation could not be shown [23,24]. Additionally, there are several conditions in which autoregulation may be lost (Table 26.2), including during profound hypothermia (15° to 20°C), where there is evidence of hypothermia-induced vasoparesis. Diabetic patients have impaired CA even at moderate hypothermia.

During CPB, there may be dissociation between MAP and CPP as a result of unrecognized cerebral venous hypertension. Particularly with the use of a single two-stage venous cannula, cerebral venous drainage may be impaired, especially during cardiac dislocation for performing posterior distal anastomoses. Consequently, jugular venous pressure (JVP)

TABLE 26.2 Factors associated with loss of cerebral autoregulation (CA)

- pH-stat management (Fig. 26.4)
- Diabetes mellitus
- Profound hypothermia (<20°C)
- Deep hypothermic circulatory arrest (DHCA)
- Previous cerebrovascular accident (CVA)
- Advanced age

should be measured proximally within the superior vena cava (SVC) (e.g., via introducer port of pulmonary artery [PA] or a central venous pressure [CVP]) catheter. CPP can also be compromised during OPCAB surgery, especially while performing multiple-graft procedures. During these operations, the patient is often placed in steep head-down tilt and the heart is lifted to expose the distal targets, two factors which can increase CVP and thus decrease CPP. Concurrent systemic arterial hypotension and low cardiac output may often occur, thereby compounding cerebral hypoperfusion.

3. **Circulatory arrest.** During circulatory arrest under normothermic conditions, O_2 levels are depleted within a few seconds of onset of ischemia, EEG activity is lost (isoelectric EEG) within 30 seconds, high-energy phosphates are exhausted within 1 minute, and ischemic neuronal damage is found after periods of anoxia as brief as 5 minutes. During surgical circulatory arrest, profound hypothermia (16° to 18°C) is used to minimize $CMRO_2$ and increase the tolerance for ischemia.

   For certain cardiac electrophysiologic (EP) procedures (e.g., mapping and ablation of certain refractory arrhythmias and deployment of implantable defibrillators), transient ventricular fibrillation (VF) is often induced at normothermia and without circulatory support. Duration of VF must be limited to less than 1 minute, and prompt hemodynamic resuscitation with at least 5 minutes of reperfusion should be maintained between episodes of VF to minimize cognitive injury [32].

4. **Intracerebral and extracerebral atherosclerosis.** Patient-related factors including intracerebral and extracerebral atherosclerosis compound the impact of perioperative hypotension. The incidence of neurologic injury after cardiac surgery is higher in patients with previous stroke, hypertension, advanced age, diabetes, and carotid bruit [3], all of which are factors related to more extensive cerebrovascular disease. In one series of 206 perioperative CAB patients, over 50% of patients exhibited concomitant cerebrovascular disease [33]. *Such patients are more prone to cerebral ischemia secondary to atheroemboli and perioperative hemodynamic instability.*

C. Inflammation

Ischemia can be defined as a critical decrease in tissue energy substrate (e.g., glucose, O_2), whether resulting from impaired bioavailability and/or decreased substrate delivery (perfusion/microcirculation), below which ion-pump failure triggers cytotoxic cascades and tissue necrosis. Whether precipitated by emboli or hypoperfusion, inflammatory cascades exacerbate and trigger various cytotoxic cascades, leading to cerebral damage and neuronal necrosis.

1. *Ischemic penumbra. A potentially viable brain region of unpredictable extent, variably responsive to resuscitative measures.* The ultimate size and histologic extent of the ischemic penumbra, which any of a diversity of ischemic insults will produce, is influenced by the duration of the ischemic insult, the affected vascular territory, the presence of collateral circulation, and factors that either ameliorate (e.g., hypothermia) or increase (e.g., proinflammatory mediators) the impact of ischemia on neuronal tissue [34]. This is the concept of the **"ischemic penumbra,"** and *salvage of the ischemic penumbra is the goal of neuroresuscitative efforts.*

   The correlations between markers of active systemic inflammation and perioperative stroke are manifold. These include perioperative elevations in C-reactive protein (and other biomarkers) and white blood cell count, which correlate with both the extent and incidence of end-organ injury in cardiac surgery and in nonoperated patients [35,36].

2. **"Panvascular inflammation"** is a term that has been used in patients presenting with unstable angina in reference to the correlation between markers of inflammation and the extent and magnitude of a *generalized heightened activity of systemic plaque*, as demonstrated in carotid and other major vessel groups [37], and which has been proposed as a mechanism for the significantly greater incidence of stroke in the SYNTAX trial of CAB versus PCI [37], despite other major cardiovascular and composite outcomes favoring CAB [1].

3. **Pathophysiology of neuronal ischemia**
   a. **Apoptosis, necrosis, and inflammation.** Two distinct phases of cellular death have been described after cerebral ischemia: apoptosis and necrosis. These are related to the intensity and duration of the ischemic insult. *Apoptosis is programmed cerebral cell death.* Its main features include cell shrinkage with preservation of cell membrane and mitochondrial integrity and lack of inflammation and injury to the surrounding tissue. There is some evidence that CPB may exacerbate apoptotic processes, thereby accelerating neuronal loss to manifest as delayed postoperative CNS injury. *Necrosis is a nonprogrammed event* leading to cellular swelling, disruption of cell membrane, and mitochondrial damage with inflammatory reaction, vascular damage, and edema formation [34]. The core of the ischemic tissue will show predominantly necrosis, and apoptosis will be found mostly in the periphery of the ischemic area. The sensitivity of neurons to ischemic insult varies by region, with hippocampal areas exhibiting marked vulnerability.
   b. **Lactic acidosis.** Glucose is essentially the sole substrate for energy production by the brain, being metabolized to produce 36 moles of adenosine triphosphate (ATP) per mole of glucose. Oxygen is essential for oxidative phosphorylation, and in the presence of ischemia, anaerobic glucose metabolism yields only 2 moles of ATP and results in lactate production with accumulation of hydrogen ion (H^+). *Anaerobic glycolysis is the primary cause of acidosis during ischemia,* and the severity of lactic acidosis is directly related to preischemic glucose concentrations. Hyperglycemia is associated with worsening of neurologic injury after cerebral ischemia and should be avoided in the perioperative period.
   c. **Ion gradients and role of calcium.** Neuronal function and structural integrity are dependent on ionic gradients, such that *up to 75% of ATP produced by resting neurons is utilized for extrusion of calcium by calcium-dependent ATPase.* With ischemia, decreased ATP production and evolving lactic acidosis impair transmembrane ionic pumps and consequently diminish cellular electrochemical gradients, leading to cell depolarization. Extraneuronal leakage of K^+ depolarizes adjacent neurons, thereby decreasing synaptic transmission and, along with extracellular calcium, promoting vasospasm in the adjacent vasculature.
   d. **Leukocytosis.** In a subanalysis of a trial randomizing 18,558 patients with symptomatic vascular disease to receive aspirin or clopidogrel, it was observed that in the week prior to a second vascular event, *the quartile with highest leukocyte counts had higher risks for ischemic stroke, MI, and vascular death* after adjustment for other risk factors [35]. In the week before a recurrent event, but not at earlier time points, the leukocyte count was significantly increased over baseline levels, suggesting that leukocyte counts (and mainly neutrophil counts) are independently associated with ischemic events in these high-risk populations. Consistent with this, in a prospective study of 7,483 patients who underwent CAB or valvular surgery or both, leukocyte count was compared with the occurrence of postoperative stroke [36]. There were a total of 125 postoperative strokes; leukocyte count was significantly higher preoperatively and immediately postoperatively in patients with stroke, and the magnitude of leukocyte count elevation correlated with stroke magnitude and extent. *These results strongly implicate inflammation and white cell activation as etiologic in both the extent and severity of perioperative cerebrovascular events.*
   e. **Excitotoxicity.** Glutamate is the most abundant excitatory amino acid (EAA) in the brain. It serves metabolic, neurotransmitter, and neurotropic functions and is normally compartmentalized in the neuron. Under normal conditions, brain cells quickly take up extracellular glutamate. Glutamate stimulates two kinds of receptors: ionophore-linked receptors and metabotropic receptors; the latter ones acting only as modifiers of the excitotoxic injury. The main excitotoxic role lies in the ionophore-linked receptors, and these include NMDA (*N*-methyl-D-aspartate), AMPA (alpha-amino-methylisoxazole-propionic acid), and kainate, responsible for mediating transmembrane Ca^{2+} and Na^+/K^+ passage.

Ischemia produces enhanced presynaptic EAA release and decreased reuptake, which causes activation of postsynaptic NMDA and AMPA receptors and produces massive efflux of K^+ and influx of Na^+ and Ca^+ and resultant osmolysis and calcium-related damage. EAAs also are increasingly implicated in free radical formation. ***Administration of ketamine, an NMDA-receptor antagonist, has shown variable efficacy to decrease neuronal ischemic injury.***

f. **Calcium.** With ischemia, ATP depletion causes loss of ionic gradients, resulting in cell membrane depolarization and influx of calcium ion (Ca^{2+}) through voltage-sensitive channels. Intracellular accumulation of Ca^{2+} is likely the final common pathway leading to neuronal death through enhanced protein and lipid catabolism. Elevated intracellular calcium activates both phospholipases, which leads to membrane cell breakdown and arachidonic acid and free radical formation, and endonucleases, which induces fragmentation of genomic DNA, mitochondrial dysfunction, and energy failure. The intensity of intracellular calcium overload is the key factor leading to irreversible cellular damage. Influx of Ca^{2+} can be minimized by calcium antagonists. Nimodipine has shown clinical benefit in decreasing vasospasm after subarachnoid hemorrhage, but has been associated with increased bleeding and mortality in cardiac surgical patients.

g. **Free fatty acids (FFAs).** Some of the earliest cell membrane changes with ischemia involve production of FFAs from membrane phospholipids. Intracellular Ca^{2+} activates calcium-dependent phospholipases C and A2, transforming membrane phospholipids into FFAs, which themselves are neurotoxic. FFAs are powerful uncouplers of oxidative phosphorylation and can undergo further oxidation from arachidonic acid, with resultant free radical formation. ***During cerebral ischemia, FFA production is decreased by administration of calcium antagonists and 21-aminosteroids (lazaroids), which are potent inhibitors of lipid peroxidation.*** Despite laboratory promise, clinical trials have so far been disappointing.

h. **Nitric oxide (NO).** NO is a free radical gas synthesized from L-arginine by NO synthase (NOS). NO functions as a neurotransmitter and has a role in regulating CBF and inflammation. In brain ischemia, the elevation of intracellular calcium markedly increases the activity of NOS. ***Increased NO combined with superoxide anion leads to the formation of other reactive oxygen species, hydroxyl free radicals, and nitrogen dioxide to produce proteolysis and cell damage.*** NO also mediates activation of ADP-polymerase leading to ATP and nicotinamide consumption and cell death [34]. Experimentally, lazaroids ameliorate neuronal ischemic damage when administered for ischemic stress, but results of clinical trials have not been positive.

IV. Intraoperative cerebral monitoring

A. Brain temperature

Accurate monitoring of brain temperature is essential, as temperature profoundly influences $CMRO_2$ and thus tolerance for ischemia. Mild hypothermia (less than 35°C) is disproportionately effective in decreasing ischemia-related injury due to inhibition of EAA release. During CPB, thermal gradients exist between various tissues; thus, brain temperature must be measured independent of other sites. Because of the small risk of trauma associated with placement of a tympanic thermistor, nasopharyngeal temperature (NPT) is the preferred site for clinical monitoring of brain temperature. Thermistor insertion should be through the nares to the level of the midpoint of the zygoma, a depth of 7 to 10 cm in an adult. Insertion of the thermistor before heparinization, using lubrication and exerting gentle pressure parallel to the floor of the nose, will minimize epistaxis—which can be problematic in a heparinized patient—and trauma to mucosa and turbinates. Esophageal temperature is a poor substitute for NPT because it variously reflects aortic inflow temperature, temperature of surrounding tissue, and the influence of residual ice or cooled fluid within the pericardial sac. For DHCA and high-risk patients, a thermistor/oximetric catheter can be placed retrograde into the jugular bulb, thus providing a sensitive clinical measure of global brain temperature and oxygenation. However, the invasivity, potential for wall artifact and other confounders have largely led to the use of cerebral NIRS in lieu of jugular oximetry.

TABLE 26.3 EEG confounders

- Anesthetic agents (e.g., propofol, sevoflurane, isoflurane, desflurane, thiopental, etomidate) producing EEG burst suppression (Fig. 26.10)
- High-dose narcotics or cerebral ischemia (similar EEG δ-wave activity)
- Biopotentials (e.g., cardiac depolarization [electrocardiogram], skeletal muscle [shivering], eye movement myopotentials, blood flow through aortic cannula)
- 60-Hz activity from electrical equipment (e.g., CPB pump motor, electrocautery, EEG)

CPB, cardiopulmonary bypass; EEG, electroencephalogram.

B. Electroencephalogram (EEG)

EEG represents the amplified, summated, and spontaneous electrical activity of the superficial cerebral cortex. Each electrode reflects microcurrent (10 to 200 μV) generated by electrical gradients across layers of neurons aligned at right angles to the monitored cortical surface in a 2- to 3-cm radius. EEG activity is commonly divided into four bands according to frequency: δ less than 4 Hz; θ 4 to 8 Hz; α 9 to 12 Hz; and β greater than 13 Hz. *In general, slower frequencies indicate a deeper level of anesthesia.* Several factors can confound interpretation of intraoperative EEG including the presence of various anesthetic agents, profound changes in body temperature, and the electrically hostile environment of an operating room (Table 26.3) which, along with its technical complexity, have limited its primary clinical use to postoperative monitoring for nonconvulsive seizures after suspected brain injury [28,38]. Although subtle EEG changes may be difficult to interpret, development of asymmetric EEG activity should be considered to represent hemispheric compromise (Table 26.4).

1. **Processed electroencephalogram (EEG).** Increasingly, processed EEG is employed intraoperatively (e.g., bispectral index [BIS] and others) for monitoring depth of anesthesia. Additionally, electrocortical "silence" or burst suppression can be readily identified with such devices and should be sought during cooling for DHCA to ensure adequacy of brain metabolic suppression. Most commercially available processed EEG monitors employ single- or two-channel adhesive pads that are fixed to frontotemporal areas. After initial electronic filtering, analog EEG voltages are rapidly digitized (150/sec) and analyzed over "epochs" (generally 2 to 4 seconds in duration) using analyses based on either frequency-domain or time-domain processing.

    a. **Compressed spectral array (CSA) and density-modulated display of power spectrum analysis (density spectral array, DSA).** For frequency-domain processing, some EEG applications use power spectral analysis. In this application, each EEG epoch is converted into a series of sine-wave components using Fourier transformation that treats the digitized EEG as a sum of sine waves of variable frequency and power. The amplitude (power) of each of the sine-wave components is indicated as a function of its frequency, and in the CSA, each EEG epoch is shown over time in a three-dimensional representation (frequency vs. power vs. time), with the most current epoch in the foreground. However, the vertical displacement, representing both power and time, hinders recognition of low-amplitude activity followed by high-amplitude activity in the same frequency band, reducing its efficacy. DSA is a representation in which each epoch is displayed using color-scale intensity or dot size proportional to the power of the individual frequency

TABLE 26.4 Causes of electroencephalographic asymmetry

- Unilateral carotid perfusion from aortic miscannulation
- Cerebral venous hypertension from asymmetric venous drainage (e.g., left superior vena cava)
- Cerebral hypoperfusion from low pump flow or systemic arterial hypotension, unmasking unilateral cerebrovascular disease
- Cerebral ischemia from embolus
- Unmasking of previous cerebrovascular accident (CVA)
- Artifact from proximity of arterial inflow cannula blood flow to ground electroencephalographic electrode

band. It can be difficult to recognize small changes in frequency using this display, but both CSA and DSA also calculate the *spectral edge frequency below which 95% of EEG power is located*.

    b. Spectral edge frequency (aperiodic analysis). Aperiodic analysis is a time-domain-based processing and does not use Fourier transformation. Instead, it is based on assessing voltage versus time of the raw EEG. Fast- and slow-wave components are analyzed separately and then combined for display. This model of analysis is also used to calculate the burst suppression ratio, which can be an indicator of anesthetic depth and cerebral metabolism depression. Epileptiform activity and artifact have been reported to be most readily identified by time-domain processing. EEG frequency carrying the median power (median frequency power) correlates with plasma levels of several narcotics. *The spectral edge frequency correlates with clinical assessment of anesthetic depth achieved with barbiturates or volatile anesthetics.*

  2. Bispectral index (BIS). Most frequency-domain processing (CSA, DSA) treats those component waveforms resulting from Fourier transformation as independent. BIS analysis measures potential interactions between the waves to determine the presence of interactive components (harmonics) indicative of phase coupling (biocoherence)—information that is not present in power spectral analysis. EEG slowing and synchrony often occur in relation to increasing depth of anesthesia. BIS measurement devices are the first ones specifically designed for the measurement of the hypnotic effects of drugs approved by the U.S. Food and Drug Administration (FDA).

  3. Evoked potentials (EPs). Metabolic and hemodynamic homeostasis determines the state of cerebral functional integrity. The latter can be inferred from EEG changes in response to repeated stimulation of intact afferent pathways. Separated from raw EEG and averaged, these EPs are described in terms of latency (time between the stimulus and respective EEG change) and amplitude (cortical microcurrent 1 to 5 µV). Reduction in CBF below 18 mL/100 g/min causes progressive decrease of the latter, which disappears at CBF below 15 mL/100 g/min. In clinical practice, only the response of sensory neurons of gray matter can be tested in this way. More commonly, EPs serve to monitor the function of sensory tracts as somatosensory-evoked potentials (SSEPs). Certain anesthetic agents complicate the recognition of specific effects of changing metabolic environment on cortical SSEPs (e.g., isoflurane increases latency and decreases amplitude of SSEPs) and have variable effects on different EPs (e.g., visual, somatosensory). Subcortical SSEP, which avoids anesthetic confounding, has recently been successfully introduced clinically [39]. Temperature alterations also affect the latency and amplitude of SSEP, confounding a primary use of SSEP for monitoring integrity of spinal cord during elephant trunk and other thoracic aortic procedures.

C. Transcranial Doppler (TCD)

Insonation of blood moving within a vessel produces a characteristic shift in signal frequency (Doppler shift) that is proportional to the flow velocity. Use of low-frequency sound waves (2 to 4 MHz) from depth-gated, direction-sensitive probes allows transmission through thin areas of skull (e.g., **the temporal window located above the zygomatic arch between the ear and orbit**). This transmission enables continuous assessment of blood flow velocity within the major intracerebral arteries (e.g., proximal MCA). Cerebral perfusion characteristics also can be assessed using TCD insonation for demonstration of laminar versus pulsatile flow or for detection of emboli. Because dissimilar acoustic echoes reflect inhomogeneities in the insonated substrate, microaggregate or microgaseous emboli can be detected within the bloodstream. Because TCD essentially functions as a microphone, artifactual noise transients can register as emboli. However, certain criteria have been employed to distinguish embolic signals from noise artifact (Table 26.5). Much greater acoustic resonance of gas emboli relative to formed elements creates *limits of TCD detection for formed elements greater than 100 µm wherein the amplitude of signal is proportional to the size of the embolus, whereas for bubble emboli, limits of resolution are 50 µm and the amplitude of the reflected signal is unrelated to the bubble size.*

TABLE 26.5 Transcranial Doppler (TCD) characteristics of emboli versus noise

	Emboli	Noise
Duration(s)	<0.1	0.5
Directionality	Unidirectional	Bidirectional
Frequency range (dB)	3–60	1–20
Sound	Chirpy	Noisy
Time delay (msec; bigate 10-mm distance)	11	0.08

Because of the ability to focus a pulsed ultrasound beam, however, by using a dual gating technique in which the vessel is insonated at two discrete sites, emboli can be discriminated from artifacts. This reflects the fact that emboli propagate with blood motion and artifact does not, and thus emboli (but not artifact) will be detected sequentially at different depths along the insonated cerebral artery.

One of the major goals in intraoperative TCD monitoring is discriminating solid versus gaseous cerebral emboli. Solid and gaseous microemboli may be differentiated with a new generation of multifrequency transducers, using both 2- and 2.5-MHz crystals, based on the principle *that solid microemboli reflect more ultrasound at the higher than at the lower frequency, whereas the opposite is the case for gaseous microemboli.* How robust this will prove in clinical practice remains to be seen and the results to date remain unconvincing.

D. Jugular oximetry

The characteristic attenuation of 650 to 1,100 nm of infrared light by a few specific light-absorbing chromophores (primarily oxyhemoglobin, deoxyhemoglobin, and oxidized cytochrome c oxidase) imparts wavelength (color) shift on the incident light. This spectral shift is proportionate to the degree of oxygenation, thereby enabling quantification of tissue oxygenation using optical spectroscopic devices. Placement of a fiberoptic oximetric catheter into the jugular bulb provides continuous monitoring of the hemoglobin saturation of effluent cerebral venous blood and reflects global cerebral O_2 supply and demand balance. **Jugular oximetry may provide an appropriate endpoint for termination of cooling before DHCA.** After jugular saturation has increased maximally and stabilized, $CMRO_2$ is at its lowest. Such monitoring has identified an association between rewarming after hypothermic CPB and significant cerebral venous blood desaturation. This indicates mismatching between cerebral O_2 supply and metabolic rate. Assuming adequate arterial oxygen saturation, increasing either hemoglobin concentration or depth of anesthesia (greater metabolic suppression) may be appropriate. However, the invasive nature and other confounders have led to cerebral NIRS largely supplanting jugular oximetry.

E. Near-infrared spectroscopy (NIRS)

Similar principles of light absorbance are used during noninvasive cerebral optical spectroscopy using scalp-attached probes. Most of the currently available commercial devices employ two-channel monitoring using adhesive pads, with one or more transmitting and two or more separately spaced receiving optodes. Differential spacing of the receiving optodes enables correction for extracerebral tissues to be made, allowing an assessment of regional oxygen saturation (rSO_2) of the cerebral cortex (Fig. 26.7). Current studies estimate that there is between 5% and 15% influence of extracerebral tissue on cerebral oximetry values as measured. Advantages and limitations of NIRS cerebral oximetry monitoring are shown in Table 26.6. This device enables indices of cerebral oxygenation to be determined in a continuous manner in a variety of clinical circumstances. There is no requirement for pulsatile blood flow, thus enabling continuous monitoring during CPB, and there are no temperature-related artifacts. A potential limitation is the fact that the cerebral sample volumes are on the order of 1 mL of frontal cortical tissue, thus rendering them highly localized. Since NIRS measures total tissue oxygenation, various factors including patient age, hemoglobin concentration at the measurement site, and sensor location can affect rSO_2 values. A prospective study demonstrated that avoidance of low intraoperative cerebral oximetry values decreases major organ morbidity and death in patients undergoing CABG surgery [40], and a recent multicenter study [41] has confirmed the

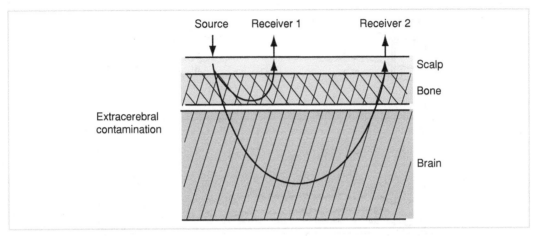

FIGURE 26.7 Schematic representation of tissue layers through which light must propagate to reach the brain. Light propagating from source to receiver 1 has a mean tissue path length such that it predominantly samples superficial tissue (scalp and skull), whereas light propagating to receiver 2 has a deeper mean path length into the brain. The signal from receiver 1 is used to correct the signal from receiver 2 for superficial tissue contamination. (From McCormick PW, Stewart M, Goetting MG, et al. Noninvasive cerebral optical spectroscopy for monitoring cerebral oxygen delivery and hemodynamics. *Crit Care Med.* 1991;19:89–97, with permission.)

successful treatment of cerebral desaturations using the original algorithm proposed [40]. While there is increasing clinical consensus that cerebral oximetry is beneficial in patients undergoing hypothermic circulatory arrest with direct cerebral perfusion [42], some clinicians remain skeptical [43]. Large-scale multicenter clinical outcomes studies will be required in order to make a solid recommendation for the widespread use of cerebral oximetry in cardiac surgical patients.

F. Cerebral perfusion pressure (CPP)

CPP represents the difference between driving pressure, or MAP, and downstream pressure, or intracranial pressure (ICP). During CPB, direct measure of ICP is not available; thus, CVP may be used as a surrogate. In the presence of impaired drainage from the SVC, which may occur during dislocation of the heart (particularly with use of a single two-stage cannula), cerebral venous hypertension may occur. Because atrial drainage is unimpaired, CVP measured from the atrium will be low; hence, this condition may be unrecognized unless proximal pressure is measured. If sustained, cerebral venous hypertension can lead to cerebral edema and substantially decreased CPP, despite apparently adequate MAP (Fig. 26.8). NIRS cerebral oximetry has been demonstrated to rapidly detect such events when cerebral desaturation occurs.

TABLE 26.6 Advantages and limitations of NIRS cerebral oximetry

▨ Advantages

No interference from electrocautery
Ease of use
Measures balance of O_2 delivery and demand
Does not require pulsatile blood flow
Monitors watershed zone at the border of anterior and middle
    cerebral arteries

▨ Limitations

Variable amount of extracerebral contamination (5–15%)
Approximately 70% venous weighted
Measures a small volume (1 mL) of cortical brain tissue

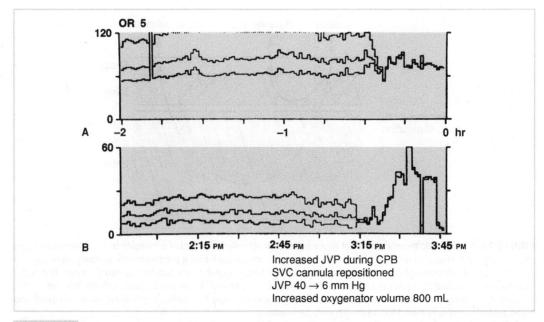

FIGURE 26.8 A: Systolic, mean, and diastolic arterial blood pressures (BPs), with commencement of cardiopulmonary bypass (CPB) indicated at 3:15 PM, after which mean arterial pressure (MAP) is shown. **B:** Pulmonary artery systolic, mean, and diastolic pressures with proximal jugular venous pressure (JVP) recorded at 3:15 PM, with commencement of CPB. A single two-stage venous cannula was used for CPB. With rotation of the heart, venous return to the oxygenator decreased and JVP approached MAP values. (Modified from Murkin JM. Intraoperative management. In: Estafanous FG, Barash PG, Reves JG, eds. *Cardiac Anesthesia: Principles and Clinical Practice.* Philadelphia, PA: J.B. Lippincott Company; 1994:326, with permission.)

CLINICAL PEARL During CPB, cerebral venous pressure should be monitored by a catheter placed proximally in the SVC (usually via introducer sheath of CVC or PA catheter) and by visual inspection of the face.

G. Lower limit of cerebral autoregulation

One of the most dynamic new developments in brain monitoring is the potential detection of individualized LLA intraoperatively. Based on studies initially conducted in head-injured patients, correlations were made between spontaneous fluctuations in MAP and corresponding changes in cerebral perfusion [44]. It has recently been determined that both TCD-monitored flow and cerebral NIRS velocity alterations correlate inconsistently with changes in MAP [44]. LLA is estimated by determining correlation coefficient (CC) between MAP and NIRS, which is taken to indicate pressure dependency of cerebral perfusion if greater than 0.35, or independence of pressure and flow (e.g., intact CA) if less than 0.35. The lowest MAP at which the CC exceeds 0.35 corresponds to the LLA as shown in Figure 26.3. Given its ease of use for data collection, cerebral NIRS is now utilized in clinical studies to detect LLA and has correlated with a variety of adverse outcomes [25–27,40]. Although individualized LLA currently is only used clinically as a research tool, ultimately it will become clinically available.

V. Prevention of central nervous system (CNS) injury

As discussed in detail below, Table 26.7 shows a series of evidence-based recommendations designed to limit the risk of perioperative cerebral injury in cardiac surgical patients [45]. Table 26.8 outlines specific interventions designed to limit or avoid particular risk factors.

TABLE 26.7 Evidence-based guidelines for best practice bypass

The clinical team should manage adult patients undergoing moderate hypothermic cardiopulmonary bypass (CPB) with α-stat pH management (class I, level A).
Limiting arterial line temperature to 37°C may be useful for avoiding cerebral hyperthermia (class IIa, level B).
The clinical team should maintain perioperative blood glucose concentration between 80 and 180 mg/dL in all patients including nondiabetics (class I, level B).
Direct reinfusion to the CPB circuit of unprocessed blood exposed to pericardial and mediastinal surfaces should be avoided (class I, level B).
Blood cell processing and filtration may be considered to decrease the deleterious effects of reinfused shed blood (class IIb, level B).
In patients undergoing CPB who are at increased risk of adverse neurologic events, strong consideration should be given to intraoperative TEE or epiaortic ultrasound scanning of the aorta: I. To detect nonpalpable plaque (class I, level A)   II. For reduction of cerebral emboli (class IIa, level B)
Arterial line filters should be incorporated in the CPB circuit to minimize the embolic load delivered to the patient (class I, level A).
Efforts should be made to reduce hemodilution including reduction of prime volume in order to avoid subsequent allogeneic blood transfusion (class I, level A).
Reduction of circuit surface area and the use of biocompatible surface-modified circuits may be useful/effective at attenuating the systemic inflammatory response to CPB and improving outcomes (class IIa, level B).

From Shann KG, Likosky DS, Murkin JM, et al. An evidence-based review of the practice of cardiopulmonary bypass in adults: a focus on neurologic injury, glycemic control, hemodilution, and the inflammatory response. *J Thorac Cardiovasc Surg*. 2006; 132(2):283–290.

TABLE 26.8 Perioperative strategies to minimize CNS brain injury

Mechanism of brain injury	Favorable intervention
Embolism	Epiaortic ultrasound No-touch technique in severe aortic atherosclerosis Dispersion aortic cannula Intra-aortic filters Cell Saver for shed blood Early postoperative DW-MRI in high-risk patients
Hypoperfusion	Preoperative carotid Doppler in high-risk patients High intraoperative arterial BP (emerging consensus to maintain MAP >70 mm Hg during normothermic and tepid CPB) Monitor SVP and MAP simultaneously (CPP) NIRS cerebral oximetry Early postoperative DW-MRI in high-risk patients
Inflammation	Minimal-volume CPB circuit Surface-modified CPB circuit Minimize allogeneic transfusion Perioperative statin administration
Aggravating factors	Labile perfusion pressures Rewarming and postoperative hyperthermia Hyperglycemia Postoperative atrial fibrillation

The interventions have been classified according to corresponding mechanisms of injury.
CNS, central nervous system; DW-MRI, diffusion-weighted magnetic resonance; SVP, superior vena cava pressure; BP, blood pressure; MAP, mean systemic arterial pressure; CPB, cardiopulmonary bypass; CPP, cerebral perfusion pressure; NIRS, near-infrared spectroscopy.

A. **Embolic load**
1. **Aortic instrumentation**
   a. Direct EAS of ascending aorta is the most sensitive technique for intraoperative assessment of atherosclerotic burden. Alternatively, initial TEE screening of descending aorta, followed by EAS if TEE detects descending aortic atherosclerosis, represents an acceptable screening strategy. Although it remains a standard of care, palpation of the aorta has not proven sensitive to detect noncalcific aortic atherosclerosis or to decrease stroke risk. Routine EAS is becoming standard of care in certain institutions [46]. With the identification of extensive aortic atherosclerosis, distal aortic arch or axillary artery cannulation and "no touch" anaortic techniques should be considered.
   b. Minimize the number of aortic clampings. Exclusive use of arterial grafts (e.g., mammary, gastroepiploic) or sutureless proximal anastomotic devices can avoid aortic partial clamping for proximal anastomoses. In cases of severe atheroscleroses, anaortic-technique OPCAB with zero manipulation of the ascending aorta significantly decreases stroke rate.

B. **Off-pump coronary artery bypass (OPCAB), coronary artery bypass (CAB), and minimally invasive extracorporeal circulation (MiECC)**
In a 2012 meta-analysis of risk of stroke in OPCAB versus conventional on-pump CAB surgery, analysis of 59 randomized clinical trials involving 8,961 randomly assigned patients, of whom 4,461 patients were assigned to OPCAB and 4,500 to CAB, found a composite stroke incidence of 1.4% in OPCAB versus 2.1% in CAB groups [47]. All studies to date have reported either no difference or a trend toward lower stroke incidence with OPCAB. A more recent meta-analysis of 13 studies with 37,720 patients compared outcomes between CAB and OPCAB both with and without aortic clamping, and found that anaortic OPCAB had the lowest rate of perioperative stroke. Avoidance of CPB reduced risk of short-term mortality, renal failure, atrial fibrillation, and bleeding [48].

CLINICAL PEARL   Anaortic OPCAB for patients at increased risk of stroke appears to be an effective strategy to minimize early stroke risk.

---

1. Current minimally invasive extracorporeal circulation (MiECC) systems have improved biocompatibility of CPB components. A meta-analysis including 22,778 patients favored CAB using MiECC over both OPCAB and non-MiECC-CAB for both morbidity (including renal failure and stroke) and mortality outcomes [49].

C. **Perfusion equipment and techniques**
1. Precirculation of CPB circuit for a minimum of 30 minutes with a 5-μm filter is recommended to remove plasticizers and other potential manufacturing microdebris.
2. Incorporation of a micropore (20 to 40 μm) filter into the cardiotomy return line keeps tissue and a variety of other particulate debris from the surgical field out of the CPB circuit, although lipid microemboli are not well removed.
3. Cell salvage processing prior to retransfusion of cardiotomy suction blood has been proposed to decrease lipid embolic load, but has not been shown to consistently improve early postoperative cognitive outcomes.
4. Use of a 40-μm filter on the arterial inflow line decreases delivery of emboli into the arterial circulation.
5. To minimize gas bubble formation due to decreased solubility with rewarming, the temperature gradient between the arterial inflow blood and the patient must be less than 10°C.
6. During rewarming, arterial blood inflow temperature must not exceed 37°C.
7. There is a possibility of air entrainment from cardiac vents in the surgical field. Meticulous de-airing of CPB venous cannulae and all syringes used for injection into the CPB circuitry are essential to minimize arterial gas embolization.

D. **Open-chamber de-airing techniques**
1. Before commencing ventricular ejection, needle aspiration of the LV and LA, combined with manual agitation of the heart, is required to dislodge air entrapped in the trabeculae. This process should be combined with concomitant manual ventilation of the lungs to mobilize residual air within the pulmonary veins.
2. TEE is used to detect residual intracavitary air and assist needle aspirations.
3. Steep Trendelenburg tilt is thought to divert cerebral emboli, though diffuse flow vortices within the atherosclerotic aorta can confound attempts at emboli diversion.
4. Transient bilateral carotid compression during defibrillation and initial filling and commencement of heart ejection should be reserved for instances where the risk of intracavitary air remains high and there is no suspicion of carotid atherosclerosis.
5. Insufflation of CO_2 into the surgical field decreases cerebral embolic load in open-chamber procedures, but to date has not been associated with improved neurologic or cognitive outcomes [29].

E. **Cerebral perfusion**
During moderate (28°C) hypothermic CPB, relative hypotension may be tolerated, as CA can be preserved to CPP 20 mm Hg during α-stat blood gas management [22]. However, in elderly patients or those with cerebrovascular disease, higher pressure should be maintained, because the lower autoregulatory threshold has been shown to vary markedly in such patients [23,24]. As assessed by NPT, the brain rewarms rapidly; therefore, hypotension (MAP less than 50 mm Hg) should be avoided after commencement of rewarming. Inadvertent compromise of CPP should also be avoided by monitoring proximal SVC pressure to detect cerebral venous hypertension. Diabetics and patients with previous CVA have impaired CA, and CBF is directly dependent on MAP. Such patients, as well as those with chronic hypertension, may benefit from close CNS monitoring and maintenance of higher perfusion pressures.

F. **Euglycemia**
There is considerable evidence from experimental models and from patients with CVA that hyperglycemia increases the magnitude and extent of neurologic injury during ischemia. Hyperglycemia should be avoided as a basic approach. *Glucose-free infusions and a glucose-free prime should be used for CPB circuits* because insulin resistance develops during CPB (partially as a result of increased endogenous catecholamines), producing glucose intolerance and increasing the tendency for refractory hyperglycemia. A structured approach to maintain normal values of blood glucose is considered favorable to patients' outcomes and is a recognized element of best practice CPB guidelines as shown in Table 26.7 [45]. However, the deleterious impact of hypoglycemia on mortality has tempered strict glycemic protocols in favor of permitting mild hyperglycemia, e.g., CPB glucose levels as high as 150–180 mg/dL.

G. **Mild hypothermia**
Increasing evidence shows EAAs as pivotal to the genesis of ischemic neurologic injury. Since EAA synthesis and release are critically temperature dependent and are significantly inhibited below 35°C [34], brain temperature (NPT) should be monitored continuously during rewarming, *hyperthermia (NPT greater than 37°C) must be avoided,* and brain temperature should be maintained less than 37°C after separating from CPB and up to 24 hours postoperatively [45].

H. **Best practice cardiopulmonary bypass (CPB)**
Recommendations from an evidence-based review for conducting safe, patient-centered CPB as based on a structured MEDLINE search coupled with a critical review of scientific literature and debates stemming from presentations at regional and national conferences are shown in Table 26.7 [45].

CLINICAL PEARL Hyperthermia during CPB must be avoided, especially during rewarming, because rewarming is associated with exacerbation of ischemic neurologic injury.

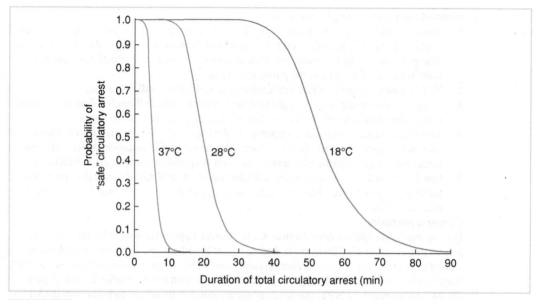

FIGURE 26.9 Nomogram of probability of "safe" total circulatory arrest according to duration of total arrest time at nasopharyngeal temperature (NPTs) of 37°C, 28°C, and 18°C, defined as the duration of total arrest after which no structural or functional damage has occurred. (From Kirklin JK, Kirklin JW, Pacifico AD. Deep hypothermia and total circulatory arrest. In: Arciniegas E, ed. *Pediatric Cardiac Surgery*. Chicago, IL: Year Book; 1985:79–85, with permission.)

VI. Pharmacologic cerebral protection

Despite a profound and ongoing increase in the understanding of the mechanisms involved in ischemic neuronal injury and the development of new subselective classes of drugs, currently none represent a standard of practice, but these or related compounds may become part of the therapeutic armamentarium.

A. Metabolic suppression

1. **Rationale and limitations.** Metabolic activity is temperature dependent, and hypothermia produces an exponential decrease in CMR. Unlike pharmacologic metabolic suppressants, hypothermia decreases metabolic activity related both to functional activity (e.g., EEG activity) and basal activity (e.g., ion pumps). Hypothermia prolongs the tolerance for global ischemia (Fig. 26.9) and is undertaken particularly for circulatory arrest. During cardiac surgery, however, the greatest risk for cerebral emboli occurs during normothermia with cannulation and decannulation; hence, pharmacologic metabolic suppressants have been investigated. While there was previously some interest in high-dose thiopental or propofol-induced burst suppression [50], no consistent clinical benefit was demonstrated.

2. **Agents.** As shown in Figure 26.10, various anesthetics have the ability to produce EEG burst suppression and decreases in CMR to approximately 70% of awake $CMRO_2$, averaging 2 to 2.5 mL/100 g/min.

   a. **Propofol.** Transient EEG burst suppression is obtained at dosages of 2 to 3 mg/kg with proportional decreases in CBF and $CMRO_2$. Infusion at 0.1 to 0.3 mg/kg/min produces sustained EEG suppression and is rapidly metabolized; therefore, it does not typically prolong recovery and extubation times. Hypotension from systemic vasodilation may require administration of phenylephrine or other such vasoconstrictors. Prolonged administration of propofol (>48 hours) has been associated with the rare occurrence of a severe metabolic syndrome characterized by metabolic acidosis, rhabdomyolysis of skeletal and cardiac muscle, renal failure, hepatomegaly, and death [51].

   b. **Isoflurane, sevoflurane, and desflurane.** At inspired concentrations of 1.5 to 2 MAC, burst suppression is produced. Unlike the intravenous agents, EEG suppression with

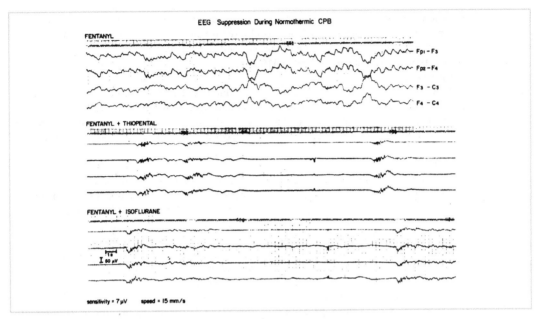

FIGURE 26.10 EEG tracings from three patients during normothermic cardiopulmonary bypass (CPB). The *top tracing* demonstrates characteristic low-voltage activity occurring during high-dose fentanyl anesthesia. The *middle tracing* shows the burst suppression pattern resulting from thiopental administration. The *lower pattern* demonstrates burst suppression occurring during isoflurane administration. (From Woodcock TE, Murkin JM, Farrar JK, et al. Pharmacologic EEG suppression during cardiopulmonary bypass: cerebral hemodynamic and metabolic effects of thiopental or isoflurane during hypothermia and normothermia. *Anesthesiology*. 1987;67:218–224, with permission.)

inhalational agents is not accompanied by any decrease in CBF, although $CMRO_2$ is reduced. Rapid elimination occurs upon discontinuation of volatile anesthetics. Of particular interest is the evidence of ischemic preconditioning and neuroprotection associated with administration of volatile anesthetics, which have been variously demonstrated to decrease glutamate release, modulate calcium flux, and inhibit generation of free radicals as well as modulate apoptosis [52]. Large-scale clinical studies are currently lacking but ***it does appear that volatile anesthetics do not increase and may decrease postoperative CNS dysfunction.***

B. Calcium channel blockers

Massive calcium influx is the final common pathway of ischemic neuronal injury. In clinical trials, calcium channel antagonists (nimodipine) have demonstrated efficacy in decreasing vasospasm after subarachnoid hemorrhage; however, nimodipine also has been associated with increased bleeding and higher mortality in cardiac surgical patients.

C. Glutamate antagonists

Since excitotoxicity is recognized as central to ischemic neuronal injury, EAA-receptor antagonists remain investigational. NMDA (e.g., ketamine) and AMPA-receptor antagonists have been found to be neuroprotective following cardiac arrest, but clinical studies in cardiac surgical patients remain inconclusive [53].

D. Lidocaine

Given its ability to decrease ischemia-mediated neuronal membrane depolarization and attendant excitotoxic cascades, two small clinical trials of lidocaine versus placebo have demonstrated lowered incidences of cognitive dysfunction in cardiac surgical patients. However, preliminary results from a larger clinical trial do not confirm these results.

E. Statins

An increasingly promising line of investigation is the role of perioperative statin therapy, either alone or in combination with other medications. Evidence is accruing that, when administered prior to CAB surgery, statins reduce the risk of perioperative mortality, stroke, and atrial fibrillation. When combined with chronic β-blocker usage, preliminary evidence suggests that statins may decrease risk for perioperative stroke in CAB patients [54].

VII. Deep hypothermic circulatory arrest (DHCA)

A. Clinical indications

DHCA sometimes is used for major surgical procedures because it provides a motionless, cannula-free, bloodless field. By allowing unobstructed surgical access, DHCA facilitates repair of complex congenital anomalies in neonates and infants. In adults, DHCA allows temporary interruption of cerebral perfusion, primarily for aortic arch reconstruction or for resection of giant cerebral aneurysms.

B. Technique

1. **Core and external cooling.** In most North American centers, active external cooling (e.g., ice baths) has been largely eliminated, but packing the head in ice is still recommended to inhibit secondary rewarming prior to onset of reperfusion. Core cooling using CPB allows efficient and controlled onset of hypothermia, and cooling persists until core temperature (bladder, rectal) is stable at 15° to 20°C in the absence of selective cerebral perfusion (SCP). Cooling must be continued until stable brain temperature (e.g., NPT, jugular thermistry) has been achieved. Some centers use development of isoelectric EEG, or plateau in cerebral NIRS (>90% saturation), as the endpoint for cooling.

2. **Decannulation.** Before circulatory arrest, administration of long-acting muscle relaxants is required to ensure profound motor block in order to minimize systemic O_2 consumption. With cessation of perfusion, venous cannulas are unclamped, allowing passive exsanguination into the CPB circuit and decreasing distention of the heart and bleeding into the surgical site. For pediatric surgery, venous cannulas are usually removed to facilitate surgical exposure. Often passive circulation of blood within the CPB circuit is continued ex vivo to avoid stasis.

C. Brain protection

1. **Temperature.** Hypothermia is the primary component of brain protection during circulatory arrest. The temperature coefficient (Q_{10}), which is the ratio of metabolic rates at temperatures 10°C apart, has been shown to be 2.3 for human brain such that CMR is still 17% of baseline at 15°C. A 20°C (37° to 17°C) decrease in brain temperature enhances cerebral tolerance for ischemia (see Fig. 26.9). Cooling the patient to a temperature of 10° to 15°C seems to offer the best protection to the brain. Minimizing rewarming of the brain is essential; therefore, external heat sources (e.g., overhead lights, ambient room temperature) should be minimized. Application of external ice packs to the head has been shown experimentally to delay brain rewarming and increase ischemic tolerance. Propofol and/or steroids are sometimes administered before circulatory arrest, although a beneficial effect is unproven.

2. **Anterograde and retrograde perfusion.** Because of CA with preferential shunting of blood to the brain, even low systemic perfusion rates (e.g., 10 to 25 mL/kg/min) during deep hypothermia have been shown to significantly improve cerebral ischemic tolerance in comparison to total circulatory arrest. A prospective randomized study has shown that continuous low-flow perfusion (0.71/min·m²) at 18°C for pediatric patients younger than 3 months old undergoing arterial switch operations results in significantly lower incidences of clinical seizures and brain creatinine kinase isoenzyme versus DHCA, and is now the standard of care.

   For aortic arch procedures in which arterial inflow is restricted, SCP via brachiocephalic or carotid perfusion is employed. Since these techniques assume adequacy of circle of Willis, there is increasing clinical interest in bihemispheric NIRS cerebral (and preoperative cerebral angiography) to assess adequacy of unilateral SCP. NIRS cerebral oximetry has been reported to detect catheter kinking or inadequacy of flow in a number of cases. Retrograde cerebral (CRP) perfusion does not provide sufficient substrate supply to continuously maintain brain metabolic demand, but may prevent rewarming

TABLE 26.9 Summary of deep hypothermic circulatory arrest (DHCA)

- Administer muscle relaxants prior to DHCA
- Cool until stable core (NPT) is achieved
- Eliminate glucose from solutions and pump prime
- Minimize ambient room temperature
- Place external ice packs around head
- Continuously monitor NPT during DHCA
- Use intermittent- or low-flow perfusion when possible
- Minimize duration of DHCA
- Ensure adequate anticoagulation prior to DHCA
- pH-stat during cooling, α-stat during rewarming
- Cerebral oximetry with use of RCP or SCP

and decrease cerebral embolization. In a recent case report, RCP with pressure-augmented perfusion guided by NIRS was felt to provide enhanced cerebral perfusion and was not associated with neurologic deficit despite prolonged duration of perfusion [55]. Consensus has emerged that cerebral oximetry monitoring is beneficial when SCP or retrograde cerebral perfusion (RCP) is employed.

3. **pH management.** In a large randomized clinical trial, use of either α-stat or pH-stat acid–base management strategy during reparative infant cardiac operations with DHCA was not consistently related to early neurodevelopmental outcomes, yet experimental and clinical studies have demonstrated more homogeneous brain cooling with pH-stat. Conversely, pH-stat impairs CA and potentially increases cerebral embolization; therefore, *a reasonable approach is to employ pH-stat during cooling and α-stat during SCP perfusion and rewarming* (Table 26.9).

CLINICAL PEARL One primary indication for pH-stat is during cooling for DHCA.

VIII. Cardiac surgery in patients with cerebrovascular disease
   A. Incidence
   Coronary atherosclerosis increases the likelihood of coexisting carotid arteriopathy. Presence or absence of carotid bruits is a poor predictor of carotid stenosis or the risk for perioperative stroke. In a survey of patients undergoing CABG, 5.5% showed significant unilateral carotid stenosis, 2.2% had bilateral stenoses, and 1.5% of patients had unilateral or bilateral carotid occlusion. Another study of over 200 CABG patients demonstrated a 54% incidence of significant cerebrovascular (carotid or intracranial) atherosclerosis preoperatively [33]. In general, however, noninvasive (ultrasonography) and invasive (contrast arteriography) investigations are usually reserved for patients who have had overt symptoms of cerebrovascular insufficiency (e.g., transient ischemic attacks or stroke) during the previous 3 to 6 months. In part, this reflects the clinical recognition that carotid endarterectomy (CEA) does not appreciably reduce risk of perioperative CVA in cardiac surgical patients [55].

   B. Morbidity
   Neurologic injury associated with cardiovascular surgery is a consequence of both cerebral emboli and hypoperfusion. Carotid disease is an important etiologic factor in the pathophysiology of post-CAB stroke but is probably only responsible for, at most, about 50% of all strokes [55,56]. Paradoxically, perioperative stroke is more frequent on the side contralateral to the stenosis and may reflect a relative diversion of flow and emboli to the nonstenotic side. Carotid stenosis is associated with a greater incidence of aortic atherosclerosis and concomitant intracerebral arterial disease. The presence of combined carotid and cardiac disease suggests more advanced and severe atherosclerosis and a higher risk of embolization and/or hypoperfusion

during cardiac surgery, and emphasizes the necessity for optimal intraoperative management (e.g., NIRS, EAS, and related best practices) [45].

C. **Combined carotid and cardiac procedures**

1. **Rationale.** Indications for CEA and CAB should be considered independently. There is no compelling evidence that, in the absence of significant symptomatology, CEA decreases perioperative stroke risk [55]. The role of carotid stenting is promising and is increasingly employed perioperatively for patients with symptomatic disease [56].

2. **Morbidity.** In asymptomatic patients, CEA does not decrease perioperative stroke risk. The reported combined risk of death, CVA, and MI for synchronous procedures (CEA + CAB) is 11.5%, and for staged procedures (CEA, then CAB), it is 10.2%, suggesting that institutional experience is of primary importance. Because of the paucity of natural history data, there is no systematic evidence that staged or synchronous operations confer any benefit over isolated CAB surgery [55].

As such, while there is a strong correlation between risk of perioperative stroke and presence of carotid stenosis, it is not clear that CEA mitigates this risk. In a meta-analysis of 11 studies in which 760 CAB patients underwent either staged or synchronous CAB plus CEA, it was noted that 87% of the patients were neurologically asymptomatic and 82% had unilateral carotid disease. Overall, the 30-day risk of death or stroke was 9.1%, and while it was observed that staged CAB and then CEA was considered less invasive, the authors concluded that *"it remains questionable whether the observed 9% risk of CEA can be justified in any asymptomatic patient with unilateral carotid disease"* [57].

IX. **Summary**

Strong evidence supports a number of procedural and technical modifications that have been shown to decrease perioperative CNS complications [45]. Avoidance of instrumentation of ascending aortic atheroma by enhanced screening techniques (e.g., preoperative MRI, intraoperative EAS) and selective use of OPCAB and anaortic techniques for patients with significant aortic atherosclerosis, more judicious use of NIRS for assessing adequacy of cerebral perfusion during CPB, avoidance of cerebral hyperthermia during rewarming on CPB and postoperatively, attenuation of perioperative and CPB-related inflammatory responses, enhanced usage of techniques to decrease postoperative atrial fibrillation, as well as administration of statins throughout the perioperative period have all been shown efficacious in decreasing perioperative CNS complications. *The challenge is not only to better understand which patients are at increased risk but to encourage more widespread assessment and adoption of cerebroprotective strategies.*

REFERENCES

1. **Serruys PW, Morice MC, Kappetein AP, et al; SYNTAX Investigators. Percutaneous coronary intervention versus coronary-artery bypass grafting for severe coronary artery disease. N Engl J Med. 2009;360(10):961–972.**
2. Bronster DJ. Neurologic complications of cardiac surgery: current concepts and recent advances. *Curr Cardiol Rep.* 2006; 8(1):9–16.
3. Messe SR, Acker MA, Kasner SE, et al. Stroke after aortic valve surgery: results from a prospective cohort. *Circulation.* 2014; 129(22):2253–2261.
4. **Leon MB, Smith CR, Mack MJ, et al; PARTNER 2 Investigators. Transcatheter or surgical aortic-valve replacement in intermediate-risk patients. N Engl J Med. 2016;374(17):1609–1620.**
5. Krasopoulos G, Falconieri F, Benedetto U, et al. European real world trans-catheter aortic valve implantation: systematic review and meta-analysis of European national registries. *J Cardiothorac Surg.* 2016;11(1):159–168.
6. Nishiyama K, Horiguchi M, Shizuta S, et al. Temporal pattern of strokes after on-pump and off-pump coronary artery bypass graft surgery. *Ann Thorac Surg.* 2009;87(6):1839–1844.
7. Hedberg M, Boivie P, Engström KG. Early and delayed stroke after coronary surgery—an analysis of risk factors and the impact on short- and long-term survival. *Eur J Cardiothorac Surg.* 2011;40(2):379–387.
8. Dacey LJ, Likosky DS, Leavitt BJ, et al. Perioperative stroke and long-term survival after coronary bypass graft surgery. *Ann Thorac Surg.* 2005;79(2):532–536.
9. Murkin JM, Martzke JS, Buchan AM, et al. A randomized study of the influence of perfusion technique and pH management strategy in 316 patients undergoing coronary artery bypass surgery. II. Neurologic and cognitive outcomes. *J Thorac Cardiovasc Surg.* 1995;110(2):349–362.
10. **Selnes OA, Grega MA, Bailey MM, et al. Do management strategies for coronary artery disease influence 6-year cognitive outcomes? Ann Thorac Surg. 2009;88(2):445–454.**

11. Sellke FW, DiMaio JM, Caplan LR, et al. Comparing on-pump and off-pump coronary artery bypass grafting: numerous studies but few conclusions: a scientific statement from the American Heart Association council on cardiovascular surgery and anesthesia in collaboration with the interdisciplinary working group on quality of care and outcomes research. *Circulation.* 2005;111(21):2858–2864.

12. Barber PA, Hach S, Tippett LJ, et al. Cerebral ischemic lesions on diffusion-weighted imaging are associated with neurocognitive decline after cardiac surgery. *Stroke.* 2008;39(5):1427–1433.

13. Kumar AK, Jayant A, Arya VK, et al. Delirium after cardiac surgery: a pilot study from a single tertiary referral center. *Ann Card Anaesth.* 2017;20(1):76–82.

14. **Lopez MG, Pandharipande P, Morse J, et al. Intraoperative cerebral oxygenation, oxidative injury, and delirium following cardiac surgery. *Free Radic Biol Med.* 2017;103:192–198.**

15. O'Neal JB, Shaw AD. Predicting, preventing, and identifying delirium after cardiac surgery. *Perioper Med (Lond).* 2016;5:7.

16. Rudiger A, Begdeda H, Babic D, et al. Intra-operative events during cardiac surgery are risk factors for the development of delirium in the ICU. *Crit Care.* 2016;20:264.

17. Barr J, Fraser GL, Puntillo K, et al. Clinical practice guidelines for the management of pain, agitation, and delirium in adult patients in the intensive care unit. *Crit Care Med.* 2013;41(1):263–306.

18. Bucerius J, Gummert JF, Borger MA, et al. Predictors of delirium after cardiac surgery delirium: effect of beating-heart (off-pump) surgery. *J Thorac Cardiovasc Surg.* 2004;127(1):57–64.

19. Tse L, Schwarz SK, Bowering JB, et al. Incidence of and risk factors for delirium after cardiac surgery at a quaternary care center: a retrospective cohort study. *J Cardiothorac Vasc Anesth.* 2015;29(6):1472–1479.

20. Maniar HS, Lindman BR, Escallier K, et al. Delirium after surgical and transcatheter aortic valve replacement is associated with increased mortality. *J Thorac Cardiovasc Surg.* 2016;151(3):815–823,e2.

21. Abawi M, Nijhoff F, Agostoni P, et al. Incidence, predictive factors, and effect of delirium after transcatheter aortic valve replacement. *JACC Cardiovasc Interv.* 2016;9(2):160–168.

22. Murkin JM, Farrar JK, Tweed WA, et al. Cerebral autoregulation and flow/metabolism coupling during cardiopulmonary bypass: the influence of $PaCO_2$. *Anesth Analg.* 1987;66(9):825–832.

23. Brady K, Joshi B, Zweifel C, et al. Real-time continuous monitoring of cerebral blood flow autoregulation using near-infrared spectroscopy in patients undergoing cardiopulmonary bypass. *Stroke.* 2010;41(9):1951–1956.

24. Murkin JM, Kamar M, Silman Z, et al. Intraoperative cerebral autoregulation assessment using ultrasound-tagged near-infrared-based cerebral blood flow in comparison to transcranial Doppler cerebral flow velocity: a pilot study. *J Cardiothorac Vasc Anesth.* 2015;29(5):1187–1193.

25. **Joshi B, Brady K, Lee J, et al. Impaired autoregulation of cerebral blood flow during rewarming from hypothermic cardiopulmonary bypass and its potential association with stroke. *Anesth Analg.* 2010;110(2):321–328.**

26. Ono M, Arnaoutakis GJ, Fine DM, et al. Blood pressure excursions below the cerebral autoregulation threshold during cardiac surgery are associated with acute kidney injury. *Crit Care Med.* 2013;41(2):464–471.

27. Hori D, Max L, Laflam A, et al. Blood pressure deviations from optimal mean arterial pressure during cardiac surgery measured with a novel monitor of cerebral blood flow and risk for perioperative delirium: a pilot study. *J Cardiothorac Vasc Anesth.* 2016;30(3):606–612.

28. **Murkin JM, Falter F, Granton J, et al. High-dose tranexamic acid is associated with nonischemic clinical seizures in cardiac surgical patients. *Anesth Analg.* 2010;110(2):350–353.**

29. Ryu KH, Hindman BJ, Reasoner DK, et al. Heparin reduces neurological impairment after cerebral arterial air embolism in the rabbit. *Stroke.* 1996;27(2):303–309.

30. **Ura M, Sakata R, Nakayama Y, et al. Ultrasonographic demonstration of manipulation-related aortic injuries after cardiac surgery. *J Am Coll Cardiol.* 2000;35(5):1303–1310.**

31. Johnson CE, Faulkner SC, Schmitz ML, et al. Management of potential gas embolus during closure of an atrial septal defect in a three-year-old. *Perfusion.* 2003;18(6):381–384.

32. Murkin JM, Baird DL, Martzke JS, et al. Cognitive dysfunction after ventricular fibrillation during implantable cardiovertor/defibrillator procedures is related to duration of the reperfusion interval. *Anesth Analg.* 1997;84(6):1186–1192.

33. Yoon BW, Bae HJ, Kang DW, et al. Intracranial cerebral artery disease as a risk factor for central nervous system complications of coronary artery bypass graft surgery. *Stroke.* 2001;32(1):94–99.

34. Auriel E, Bornstein NM. Neuroprotection in acute ischemic stroke—current status. *J Cell Mol Med.* 2010;14(9):2200–2202.

35. Grau AJ, Boddy AW, Dukovic DA, et al; CAPRIE Investigators. Leukocyte count as an independent predictor of recurrent ischemic events. *Stroke.* 2004;35(5):1147–1152.

36. Albert AA, Beller CJ, Walter JA, et al. Preoperative high leukocyte count: a novel risk factor for stroke after cardiac surgery. *Ann Thorac Surg.* 2003;75(5):1550–1557.

37. **Murkin JM. Panvascular inflammation and mechanisms of injury in perioperative CNS outcomes. *Semin Cardiothorac Vasc Anesth.* 2010;14(3):190–195.**

38. Gofton TE, Chu MW, Norton L, et al. A prospective observational study of seizures after cardiac surgery using continuous EEG monitoring. *Neurocrit Care.* 2014;21(2):220–227.

39. Chui J, Murkin JM, Turkstra T, et al. A novel automated somatosensory evoked potential (SSEP) monitoring device for detection of intraoperative peripheral nerve injury in cardiac surgery: a clinical feasibility study. *J Cardiothorac Vasc Anesth.* 2017;31(4):1174–1182.

40. Murkin JM, Adams SJ, Novick RJ, et al. Monitoring brain oxygen saturation during coronary bypass surgery: a randomized, prospective study. *Anesth Analg.* 2007;104(1):51–58.

41. Subramanian B, Nyman C, Fritock M, et al. A multicenter pilot study assessing regional cerebral oxygen desaturation frequency during cardiopulmonary bypass and responsiveness to an intervention algorithm. *Anesth Analg.* 2016;122(6):1786–1793.

42. Murkin JM, Arango M. Near-infrared spectroscopy as an index of brain and tissue oxygenation. *Br J Anaesth*. 2009;103 (suppl 1):i3–i13.
43. Murkin JM. Is it better to shine a light, or rather to curse the darkness? Cerebral near-infrared spectroscopy and cardiac surgery. *Eur J Cardiothorac Surg*. 2013;43(6):1081–1083.
44. Czosnyka M, Miller C; Participants in the International Multidisciplinary Consensus Conference on Multimodality Monitoring. Monitoring of cerebral autoregulation. *Neurocrit Care*. 2014;21(Suppl 2):S95–S102.
45. **Shann KG, Likosky DS, Murkin JM, et al. An evidence-based review of the practice of cardiopulmonary bypass in adults: a focus on neurologic injury, glycemic control, hemodilution, and the inflammatory response. *J Thorac Cardiovasc Surg*. 2006;132(2):283–290.**
46. Daniel WT 3rd, Kilgo P, Puskas JD, et al. Trends in aortic clamp use during coronary artery bypass surgery: effect of aortic clamping strategies on neurologic outcomes. *J Thorac Cardiovasc Surg*. 2014;147(2):652–657.
47. Afilalo J, Rasti M, Ohayon SM, et al. Off-pump vs. on-pump coronary artery bypass surgery: an updated meta-analysis and meta-regression of randomized trials. *Eur Heart J*. 2012;33(10):1257–1267.
48. Zhao DF, Edelman JJ, Seco M, et al. Coronary artery bypass grafting with and without manipulation of the ascending aorta: a network meta-analysis. *J Am Coll Cardiol*. 2017;69(8):924–936.
49. **Kowalewski M, Pawliszak W, Raffa GM, et al. Safety and efficacy of miniaturized extracorporeal circulation when compared with off-pump and conventional coronary artery bypass grafting: evidence synthesis from a comprehensive Bayesian-framework network meta-analysis of 134 randomized controlled trials involving 22778 patients. *Eur J Cardiothorac Surg*. 2016;49(5):1428–1440.**
50. Woodcock TE, Murkin JM, Farrar JK, et al. Pharmacologic EEG suppression during cardiopulmonary bypass: cerebral hemodynamic and metabolic effects of thiopental or isoflurane during hypothermia and normothermia. *Anesthesiology*. 1987;67(2):218–224.
51. Fodale V, La Monaca E. Propofol infusion syndrome: an overview of a perplexing disease. *Drug Saf*. 2008;31(4):293–303.
52. Yu Q, Wang H, Chen J, et al. Neuroprotections and mechanisms of inhalational anesthetics against brain ischemia. *Front Biosci (Elite Ed)*. 2010;2:1275–1298.
53. Bhutta AT, Schmitz ML, Swearingen C, et al. Ketamine as a neuroprotective and anti-inflammatory agent in children undergoing surgery on cardiopulmonary bypass: a pilot randomized, double-blind, placebo-controlled trial. *Pediatr Crit Care Med*. 2012;13(3):328–337.
54. Bouchard D, Carrier M, Demers P, et al. Statin in combination with β-blocker therapy reduces postoperative stroke after coronary artery bypass graft surgery. *Ann Thorac Surg*. 2011;91(3):654–659.
55. Kubota H, Tonari K, Endo H, et al. Total aortic arch replacement under intermittent pressure-augmented retrograde cerebral perfusion. *J Cardiothorac Surg*. 2010;5:97.
56. Naylor AR, Bown MJ. Stroke after cardiac surgery and its association with asymptomatic carotid disease: an updated systematic review and meta-analysis. *Eur J Vasc Endovasc Surg*. 2011;41(5):607–624.
57. Naylor AR, Mehta Z, Rothwell PM. A systematic review and meta-analysis of 30-day outcomes following staged carotid artery stenting and coronary bypass. *Eur J Vasc Endovasc Surg*. 2009;37(4):379–387.

27

Pain Management for Cardiothoracic Procedures

Brandi A. Bottiger, Rebecca Y. Klinger, Thomas M. McLoughlin, Jr.,
and Mark Stafford-Smith

I. Introduction

A. Incidence and severity of pain after cardiothoracic procedures

Pain is an unpleasant sensation occurring in varying degrees of severity as a consequence of injury or disease. Chest surgery, via sternotomy and especially via thoracotomy, is among the most debilitating for patients due to pain and consequent respiratory dysfunction. Important sources of postoperative discomfort after cardiothoracic surgery, in addition to incisional pain, include indwelling thoracostomy tubes, rib or sternal fractures, and costovertebral joint pain due to sternal retraction. Chronic pain due to intercostal nerve injury during thoracic surgery and persisting for >2 months, develops in approximately 50% of postthoracotomy patients, and in 5% this pain becomes severe and disabling. Persistent pain after cardiac surgery affects approximately 37% of patients in the first 6 months after cardiac surgery and remains present for more than 2 years in 17% [1]. Acute pain specifically attributed to median sternotomy is a frequent occurrence and is rated as severe by more patients [2] than expected. Poststernotomy pain also becomes chronic in up to 30% of patients [3], being rated as severe in 4% [4]. Furthermore, despite the hope that minimally invasive thoracic and cardiac surgical procedures involving smaller incisions would reduce the incidence and severity of postoperative pain compared to traditional approaches, clinical experience has not borne out this assumption for most patients. Recent trials demonstrate similar chronic pain incidences between open and minimally invasive approaches to thoracic surgery [5]. No single thoracotomy technique has been shown to reduce the incidence of chronic postthoracotomy pain, and patients should be warned in advance of this potential postoperative complication. Similarly, acute postoperative pain has been reported to be subjectively equivalent between conventional sternotomy and minimally invasive approaches to cardiac surgical procedures [6].

Psychosocial and genetic risk factors are associated with persistent pain states in various settings [7–9] including surgical populations [10]. However, this has yet to be proven in prospective trials involving thoracic surgical patients [5]. Notably, some evidence supports a protective effect from regional anesthesia techniques in the prevention of persistent postthoracotomy pain states [11].

B. **Transmission pathways for nociception**

An understanding of the anatomy and physiology of pain pathways underpins the logical choice of analgesic strategies during and after cardiothoracic surgery. Multimodal approaches take advantage of numerous therapeutic targets in the signaling chain to optimize pain control while minimizing side effects [12].

In the thoracic region, pain signals are relayed through myelinated Aδ and unmyelinated C fibers in peripheral intercostal nerves. The ventral, posterior, and visceral branches of each intercostal nerve innervate the anterior chest wall, posterior chest wall, and visceral aspects of the chest, respectively. These branches join together just before entering the paravertebral space and then pass through the intervertebral foramina in the spinal canal. Sensory intercostal nerve fibers form a dorsal root that fuses with the spinal cord dorsal horn to enter the central nervous system (CNS). Somatic pain is mediated predominantly through myelinated Aδ fibers in the ventral and posterior branches. Sympathetic (visceral) pain is mediated by unmyelinated C fibers in all three branches. Sympathetic afferent pain signals are directed from intercostal nerve branches through the sympathetic trunk (a paravertebral structure found just beneath the parietal pleura in the thorax) and then pass back into the peripheral nerves to enter the CNS from T1 to L2. In addition, the vagus nerve provides parasympathetic visceral innervation of the thorax. This cranial nerve enters the CNS through the medulla oblongata and, therefore, is not normally affected by epidural or intrathecal (IT) methods of pain control.

Spinal cord dermatomal segments typically lie cephalad to their respective vertebrae, since the spinal cord and spinal canal are different in length. Thus, knowledge of spinal anatomy is essential if regional analgesia techniques are to be successful. This is particularly important to remember when using lipid-soluble epidural opioids because the targeted dorsal horn often is significantly cephalad relative to the associated intervertebral foramen and nerve.

CLINICAL PEARL When using lipid-soluble epidural opioids in the neuraxial space, the targeted dorsal horn is often significantly cephalad relative to the associated intervertebral foramen and nerve.

Most spinal pain signals are transmitted to the brain after crossing from the dorsal horn to contralateral spinal cord structures (e.g., spinothalamic tract). Distribution of nociceptive messages occurs to numerous locations in the brain, resulting in cognitive, affective, and autonomic responses to noxious stimuli. Regional and neuraxial techniques involving local anesthetics target and block the afferent pathways from the peripheral nerve to the spinal cord.

Endogenous modification of pain signals begins at the site of tissue trauma and includes hyperalgesia related to inflammation and other CNS-mediated phenomena, such as "windup." The substantia gelatinosa of the dorsal horn is an important location for pain signal modulation, including effects that are mediated through opioid, adrenergic, and N-methyl-D-aspartate (NMDA) receptor systems.

C. **Analgesia considerations: the procedure, patient, and process**

The degree and location of surgical trauma, particularly in relation to the site of skin incision and route of bony access to the chest, are particularly important in anticipating analgesic requirements after cardiothoracic surgery. Notably, minimally invasive procedures that reduce total surgical tissue disruption but relocate it to more pain-sensitive regions may not translate into reduced postoperative pain or risk of chronic pain (e.g., minithoracotomy vs. sternotomy). Limited evidence in thoracic surgery suggests that enhanced recovery programs and decision support tools that guide therapies are important to consider in reducing length of stay and improving economic outcomes for select groups of patients [13,14]. However, specific analgesic choices should be reviewed for individual patients, in particular for high-risk patients in whom outcome benefits may be the greatest. This includes not only offering appropriate postoperative analgesia delivery but also preoperative education regarding pain reporting, procedures, devices to provide analgesia, and expectations for postoperative transition to oral medications and home administration.

CLINICAL PEARL Risks and benefits of specific analgesic choices should be reviewed for individual patients, in particular for high-risk patients in whom outcome benefits may be the greatest. Patient education and setting expectations prior to surgery are key elements for success.

D. **Adverse consequences of pain**

In addition to the unpleasant emotional aspects of pain, nociceptive signals have several other effects that can be harmful and delay patient recovery. These include activation of neuroendocrine reflexes constituting the surgical stress response (including inflammation and elevated circulating catecholamines), a catabolic state associated with high levels of several humoral substances (e.g., cortisol, vasopressin, renin, angiotensin), decreased vagal tone, and increased oxygen consumption. Spinal reflex responses to pain include localized muscle spasm and activation of the sympathetic nervous system.

Pathophysiologic consequences of the neuroendocrine local and systemic responses to pain include respiratory complications related to diaphragmatic dysfunction, myocardial ischemia, ileus, urinary retention and oliguria, thromboembolism, and immune impairment [15].

E. **Outcome benefits of good analgesia for cardiothoracic procedures**

A primary benefit of effective pain control is patient satisfaction and an improved recovery profile. Studies have documented additional advantages of optimizing analgesia, especially in recovery from thoracotomy. Belief that the pain of median sternotomy is less severe and inconsequential to outcomes leads many institutions to employ conventional analgesia protocols involving fixed dosing of analgesics on a timed schedule. However, after coronary bypass graft surgery, attention to profound analgesia in the early postoperative period may decrease the incidence and severity of myocardial ischemia.

Evidence supporting reductions in perioperative complications related to pain relief are reported for many different analgesic techniques and may be related to their effectiveness in blocking the surgical stress response and nociceptive spinal reflexes. In this regard, neuraxial and regional analgesia are most often reported as being effective. Nonetheless, beyond reduced pain, any outcome benefits related to the incidence of major morbidities and mortality of specific analgesia techniques remain difficult to prove, possibly due to the insufficient numbers of patients studied and the low frequency of these events, as is well summarized in a review by Liu et al. [16]. In general, reported benefits of good analgesia rely on reporting of surrogate markers that correlate with major adverse outcomes (e.g., arterial oxygen saturation) that imply attenuation of the adverse consequences of pain outlined in Section I.D. For example, in the setting of thoracic surgery, thoracic epidural analgesia provides superior pain relief compared to systemic opioids and decreases the incidence of atelectasis, pulmonary infections, hypoxemia, and other pulmonary complications [16]. In addition, effective analgesia established before surgery in some circumstances may provide preemptive protection against the development of chronic pain syndromes. Aggressive pain control in the early postoperative period was associated with a greater than 50% reduction in the number of patients continuing to experience chronic pain 1 year after thoracotomy in one study [17,18]. Unfortunately, in cardiac surgery, reports of neuraxial techniques generally involve small numbers and fail to demonstrate clinical outcome benefits, although benefits in hospital length of stay and cost avoidance have been commonly shown [19]. An outcome benefit following cardiac surgery with central neuraxial analgesia was not demonstrated in a meta-analysis published in 2004 or in a randomized trial published in 2011 [20,21].

II. **Pain management pharmacology**

Multimodal analgesia and regional techniques that spare opioids in the perioperative period are desirable, particularly in the context of the Centers for Disease Control and the World Health Organization's efforts to improve the communication between patients and providers regarding safety, efficacy, and the risks associated with long-term opioid therapy [22,23].

A. **Opioid analgesics**

1. **Mechanisms.** Opioid analgesics are a broad group of compounds that include naturally occurring extracts of opium (e.g., morphine, codeine), synthetic substances (e.g., fentanyl,

TABLE 27.1 Opioid receptors

Type	Mediated effects
μ_1	Analgesia
μ_2	Respiratory depression, euphoria, physical dependence, pruritus, nausea, and vomiting
K	Spinal analgesia, sedation, miosis, diuresis
Σ	Dysphoria, hypertonia
Δ	Spinal analgesia, μ-receptor modulation

hydromorphone), and endogenous peptides (e.g., endorphins, enkephalins). The analgesic effects of these drugs are all linked to their interaction with opioid receptors; however, individual agents may function as agonists, antagonists, or partial agonists at different receptor subtype populations. Opioid receptors are widely distributed throughout the body, but they are particularly concentrated within the substantia gelatinosa of the dorsal horn of the spinal cord and in regions of the brain including the rostral ventral medulla, locus coeruleus, and midbrain periaqueductal gray area. Stimulation of opioid receptors inhibits the enzyme adenyl cyclase, closes voltage-dependent calcium channels, and opens calcium-dependent inwardly rectifying potassium channels, resulting in inhibitory effects characterized by neuronal hyperpolarization and decreased excitability. Opioid receptor subtypes have been sequenced and cloned, and they belong to the growing list of G-protein–coupled receptors. The effects of agonist binding at different opioid receptor subtypes are summarized in Table 27.1.

2. **Perioperative use.** Opioids are commonly administered throughout the perioperative period for cardiothoracic procedures. Preoperatively, they can be given orally, intramuscularly (IM), or intravenously (IV) alone or as part of a sedative cocktail to provide anxiolysis and analgesia for transport and placement of intravascular catheters. Intraoperatively, they are given IV most commonly as part of a balanced anesthetic technique that includes potent inhaled anesthetics, benzodiazepines, and other agents. Finally, they can be injected directly into the thecal sac or included as a component of epidural infusions to provide intraoperative and postoperative analgesia. Opioids administered via the epidural route have varying spread and analgesic potency based in part on their water solubility. Matching analgesic requirements with knowledge of the position of the epidural catheter relative to the dermatomes affected requires understanding of the relative lipophilicity of the drug. Highly lipophilic drugs, such as fentanyl, may be best used with catheters placed near the involved dermatomes. Hydrophilic drugs, such as morphine, are generally useful even for remote catheters, such as those positioned in the lumbar region. Drugs with intermediate lipophilicity, such as hydromorphone, are considered ideal by most and can be used for more balanced dermatomal spread.

3. Side effects and cautions
   a. Respiratory depression (increased risk with higher dosing, coadministration of other sedatives, opioid-naïve patients, advanced age, central neuraxial administration of hydrophilic opioid agents)
   b. Sedation
   c. Pruritus
   d. Nausea
   e. Urinary retention, especially common in the elderly and in males receiving spinal opioids
   f. Inhibition of intestinal peristalsis/constipation
   g. CNS excitation/hypertonia, much more notable with rapid IV administration of lipophilic agents
   h. Miosis
   i. Biliary spasm

All of the above effects can be reversed with the administration of opioid antagonist drugs (e.g., naloxone). Opioid rotation, or changing the narcotic drug that a patient is receiving, may also be useful in reducing the incidence or severity of complicating side effects and also in enhancing the patient's experience of analgesia [24]. Notably, a new area of interest surrounds emerging evidence that choices as simple as the postoperative opioid analgesic selected (e.g., morphine vs. hydromorphone) may be associated with hospital lengths of stay and 30-day readmission rates [25].

B. **Nonsteroidal anti-inflammatory drugs (NSAIDs)**
   1. **Mechanisms.** NSAIDs act principally through both central and peripheral inhibition of cyclooxygenase, resulting in decreased synthesis of prostaglandins from arachidonic acid, including prostacyclin and thromboxane. Prostaglandins are involved in the physiology of numerous signaling pathways, including those influencing renal perfusion, bronchial smooth muscle tone, hemostasis, gastric mucosal secretions, and the inflammatory response. Prostaglandin E_2 is the eicosanoid produced in the greatest quantity at sites of trauma and inflammation and is an important mediator of pain. The full therapeutic effects of NSAIDs are complex and likely involve mechanisms that are independent of prostaglandin effects. For example, prostaglandin synthesis is effectively inhibited with low doses of most NSAIDs; however, much higher doses are required to produce anti-inflammatory effects.
   2. **Perioperative use.** NSAIDs are useful for postoperative analgesia. They are most commonly administered in cardiothoracic surgical patients as a complement to neuraxial techniques. Their principal advantage is the absence of respiratory depression and other opioid side effects. Many NSAIDs are available for oral or rectal administration. Ketorolac is a nonselective NSAID intended for short-term use (5 days or less) with preparations available for IV or IM injection, in addition to oral forms.
   3. **Side effects and cautions**
      a. Decreased renal blood flow/parenchymal ischemia
      b. Gastrointestinal mucosal irritation
      c. Impaired primary hemostasis
      d. Differential risk of myocardial and other ischemic events (in nonsurgical populations), of unknown importance in the perioperative period [26]
   4. **COX-2 inhibitors**
      The effects of cyclooxygenase are mediated by two distinct isoenzymes termed COX-1 and COX-2. COX-1 is the constitutive form responsible for the production of prostaglandins involved in homeostatic processes of the kidney, gut, endothelium, and platelets. COX-2 is predominantly an inducible isoform responsible for the production of prostaglandins during inflammation. Highly selective COX-2 inhibitors have potent analgesic properties and were previously popular for treating perioperative pain. Data from large randomized double-blind trials [27] revealed an increased incidence of cardiovascular complications, including myocardial infarction, with agents in this drug class. Celecoxib is the remaining COX-2 inhibitor widely available for prescription in the United States. The difference between celecoxib and the other agents may be due to its relatively modest COX-2 versus COX-1 subtype selectivity compared to the other agents (30:1 vs. >300:1). However, celecoxib is primarily recommended for the treatment of severe arthritis, rheumatoid arthritis, and ankylosing spondylitis in circumstances where treatment of these conditions with several other NSAIDs has failed.

C. **Acetaminophen (paracetamol)**
   1. **Mechanism**
      Acetaminophen is a synthetic, nonopiate, analgesic drug that is distinct from most other NSAIDs in that it is a weak inhibitor of the synthesis of prostaglandins and of COX-1 and COX-2. Its mechanisms appear to be primarily central, resulting in analgesia and antipyresis, with only minimal anti-inflammation. COX-3, a splice variant of COX-1, has been suggested to be the site of action. Other proposed mechanisms include the activation of descending serotonergic pathways and the inhibition of the nitric oxide pathway mediated

by a variety of neurotransmitter receptors including NMDA and substance P. Although the exact site and mechanism of analgesic action is not clearly defined, acetaminophen appears to produce analgesia by elevation of the pain threshold.

2. **Perioperative use and cautions**
    Although acetaminophen is primarily used for oral and rectal administration, in 2010, the FDA approved an IV form of the drug for relieving pain or fever in surgical patients in adults and children aged two and older. It is useful in the treatment of moderate to severe postsurgical pain, demonstrating an opioid-sparing effect with good patient acceptance and few adverse effects, especially in orthopedic surgical populations [28]. A modest opioid-sparing effect, with no reduction in the incidence of nausea and vomiting, was found when IV was compared to oral acetaminophen in a postoperative population of coronary artery bypass surgical patients [29].

    The primary risk of acetaminophen is hepatotoxicity secondary to overdose. Acetaminophen toxicity is the leading cause of acute liver failure in the United States. A typical IV adult dosing schedule involves the administration of 650 to 1,000 mg every 6 hours, with infusion of the drug timed to occur over at least 15 minutes.

D. **Local anesthetics**
    1. **Mechanisms.** Local anesthetics interrupt neural conduction, thus disrupting transmission of pain and other nerve impulses through the blockade of neuronal voltage-gated sodium channels. This blockade does not change the resting potential of the nerve. However, altered sodium ion channel permeability slows depolarization such that, in the presence of a sufficient concentration of local anesthetic, the threshold for the propagation of an action-potential cannot be reached.

    2. **Perioperative use.** Local anesthetics are used throughout the perioperative period for topical infiltration, for infiltration near peripheral nerves, or in the central neuraxial space. Their advantage lies in their capacity to provide profound analgesia without the undesired side effects seen with opioids or NSAIDs. Effective regional anesthesia is the best technique to most completely attenuate the neurohumoral stress response to pain. Thoracic epidural analgesia is particularly useful in treating pain, both somatic and visceral, for patients with occlusive coronary artery disease. Limited data support the use of systemic lidocaine to attenuate early postoperative pain after noncardiac surgery [30], but this has not yet been demonstrated in cardiac surgery [31].

    3. **Liposomal preparations.** Liposomal technology now allows for the extended-release delivery of local anesthetic medications using a single-injection technique. The purported advantage of liposomal delivery of local anesthetic is its prolonged analgesic effect.
        Currently the only commercially available preparation in the United States is liposomal bupivacaine (Exparel™; Pacira Pharmaceuticals, Inc., Parsippany, New Jersey), which demonstrates analgesic effects for up to 72 hours. However, infiltration of liposomal bupivacaine at the surgical site is not superior to bupivacaine hydrochloride [32]. There has been no international standard for the perioperative use of these preparations, and variability in practice exists as to whether liposomal bupivacaine is diluted with standard bupivacaine, or normal saline prior to injection. In some countries, legislative bodies have approved for use for subcutaneous (SC) infiltration, fascial plane blocks, and peripheral nerve blocks, but there has been no extensively studied or approved use for the neuraxial space [33–36]. Current cost/benefit assessment seems not in favor of the use of available liposomal preparations for cardiothoracic surgery patients.

    4. **Side effects and cautions**
        a. Not surprisingly, side effects from sodium channel blockade due to local anesthetic toxicity resemble those observed with severe extracellular hyponatremia. Excessive local anesthetic blood concentrations, achieved through absorption or inadvertent intravascular injection, predictably result in toxic effects on the CNS (seizures, coma) and the heart (negative inotropy, conduction disturbances, arrhythmias). Table 27.2 lists commonly accepted maximum local anesthetic dosing for infiltration anesthesia.

TABLE 27.2 Maximum recommended dosing of local anesthetic agents for local infiltration

Drug	Maximum dose (mg/kg)		Absolute maximum dose (mg)	
	Plain solution	Containing epinephrine (1:200,000)	Plain solution	Containing epinephrine (1:200,000)
Lidocaine	3	7	200	500
Mepivacaine	5	7	400	400
Bupivacaine	2.5	3	150	150
Ropivacaine	2–3	2–3	300	300

Dose may be increased modestly for use in compartments where absorption will be delayed (e.g., brachial plexus) and decreased for use in more vascular regions (e.g., epidural space, intercostal). Blood levels may be increased in the elderly and sick patient. Actual maximum dosage may be less than stated.

    b. Caution must be exercised in the performance of any invasive regional anesthesia procedure in the setting of ongoing or proposed anticoagulation or thrombolysis.

    c. Although regional anesthesia can be initiated without an apparent increase in the risk of bleeding in patients taking only aspirin or NSAIDs, the American Society of Regional Anesthesia and Pain Medicine (ASRA; www.ASRA.com) last published their consensus recommendations in 2010 for regional anesthesia in patients receiving antithrombotic therapy [37]. Recommendations include withholding antiplatelet agents clopidogrel (Plavix) for 7 days, ticlopidine (Ticlid) for 14 days, and GP IIb/IIIa antagonists for 4 to 48 hours prior to placement of a neuraxial block. ASRA also recommends holding warfarin for 4 to 5 days, low–molecular-weight heparins for 12 to 24 hours (depending on drug and dose), and unfractionated heparin for 8 to 12 hours (depending on dosing interval) before neuraxial block placement. Practice advisories regarding recommendations for time intervals for the new oral anticoagulants are being drafted in the United States, with some interim recommendations including holding dabigatran for 5 days, apixaban for 3 days, rivaroxaban for 3 days, prasugrel for 7 to 10 days, and ticagrelor for 5 to 7 days [37]. These guidelines recommend consideration of deep plexus or peripheral nerve blockade in the setting of drug-altered hemostasis.

    d. Allergic reactions are not uncommon, particularly to the para-aminobenzoic acid metabolites of ester local anesthetics or to the preservative materials found in commercial local anesthetic preparations. True allergic reactions to preservative-free amide local anesthetics (e.g., lidocaine) are rare, and suspected cases are often attributed in retrospect to inadvertent intravascular injection of epinephrine-containing solutions.

    e. Concentration-dependent neurotoxicity of local anesthetics (e.g., cauda equina syndrome following IT local anesthetic injection) is now well described [38].

    f. The liposomal bupivacaine (**Exparel™**) has specific cautions regarding its administration. The manufacturer (Pacira Pharmaceuticals, Inc., Parsippany, New Jersey) recommends that liposomal bupivacaine be administered 20 minutes after lidocaine. Furthermore, other formulations of bupivacaine should not be administered until 96 hours following the administration of liposomal bupivacaine. An additional caution is that liposomal bupivacaine should not be allowed to come into contact with antiseptic solutions (e.g., chlorhexidine, povidone iodine) as these solutions may cause disruption of the liposomes, leading to a sudden release of toxic amounts of bupivacaine into the plasma [39].

E. α_2-**Adrenergic agonists**

Clonidine is the prototypical drug in this class, although dexmedetomidine is also approved for clinical use. Both drugs produce analgesia through agonism at central α_2-receptors in the substantia gelatinosa of the spinal cord and sedation through receptors in the locus coeruleus in the brainstem. They may also act at peripheral α_2-receptors located on sympathetic nerve terminals to decrease norepinephrine output in sympathetically mediated pain. The analgesic effect of these drugs is distinct and complementary to that of opioids when used in combination. Clonidine may be administered orally to provide sedation and analgesia as a premedication. Preservative-free clonidine may be included as a component of epidural infusions or IT injections. Although these agents have limited respiratory depressant properties, hypotension, sedation, and dry mouth are common side effects from analgesic doses. Loss of standard cues for analgesia administration in unconscious patients (e.g., tachycardia, hypertension) due to the autonomic effects of α_2-adrenergic agonists may result in overestimation of the analgesic benefits of such agents.

F. Ketamine

Ketamine has complex interactions with a variety of receptors but is thought to act primarily through blockade of the excitatory effects of the neurotransmitter, glutamic acid, at the NMDA receptor in the CNS. It can be administered orally or parenterally to provide sedation, potent analgesia, and "dissociative anesthesia." The principal advantages of ketamine stem from its sympathomimetic properties and lack of respiratory depression. Cautions include increased secretions and dysphoric reactions. Ketamine administered by low-dose IV infusion as an adjunct to a poststernotomy and postthoracotomy analgesic regimen may increase patient satisfaction and provide an opioid-sparing effect [40]. Ketamine may also be added as an adjunctive medication to epidural infusions, including thoracic epidural infusions for acute postthoracotomy pain [41].

G. Gabapentinoids

Designed as analogs of GABA, the mechanism by which gabapentinoids affect neuropathy is through binding to the $\alpha_2\delta$-1 and $\alpha_2\delta$-2 subunits of calcium channels. Despite a meta-analysis of acute postoperative pain studies not finding a reduction of early perioperative pain scores or opioid consumption with a single dose of gabapentin or pregabalin, many general acute pain multimodal analgesic algorithms include gabapentinoid agents. Of importance are the known sedative and respiratory depressant side effects of these agents in a population such as cardiothoracic patients who are at high risk of serious postoperative respiratory complications. Although the short-term benefits of these agents are questionable in cardiothoracic patients, there may be longer-term value as an adjuvant analgesic strategy against chronic pain (e.g., postthoracotomy) [42,43].

H. Biologics

Presently, the genetic and molecular mechanism that may predict acute and chronic pain are being further elucidated [42]. This makes biologics (i.e., agents extracted or synthesized from biologic sources) an attractive potential future therapy. At the current time there are no biologics recommended for pain management in the cardiothoracic surgery setting; however, these agents may have promise as therapeutics for further research.

I. Nonpharmacologic analgesia

1. **Cryoablation.** A cryoprobe can be introduced into the intercostal space and used to produce transient (1 to 4 days) numbness in the distribution of the intercostal nerve. A cryoprobe circulates cold gas (approximately −80°C). When applied for two to three treatments of approximately 2 minutes each, this temporarily disrupts neural function. Cryoablation has been shown to reduce pain and the need for systemic analgesics after lateral thoracotomy for cardiac surgery [44].

2. **Nursing care.** Empathic nursing care and nursing-guided relaxation techniques are important components to patient comfort throughout the perioperative period and should not be overlooked [44].

III. Pain management strategies

A. Enteral

Gastrointestinal ileus is rarely a concern after routine cardiothoracic surgical procedures; therefore, transition to oral administration of analgesics should be considered as soon as pain management goals are likely to be effectively achieved by this route. This is particularly important because oral agents are currently the simplest, cheapest, and the most reliable way to continue effective analgesia after hospital discharge, and they should be used as the mainstay of any "fast-track" analgesia protocol.

B. Subcutaneous (SC)/intramuscular (IM)

SC and IM injections remain effective and inexpensive alternate parenteral routes to IV administration for the delivery of potent systemic analgesia using opioids (e.g., morphine, hydromorphone, meperidine). SC or IM injection results in slower onset of analgesia than the IV route and, therefore, is more suitable for scheduled dosing (e.g., every 3 to 6 hours) rather than "as needed." A notable disadvantage of the SC route is injection-related discomfort, which can largely be avoided by slow injection through an indwelling SC butterfly needle.

C. Intravenous

In the absence of neuraxial analgesia, IV opioid analgesia is generally the primary tool to provide effective pain relief for the early postoperative patient. The advantages of this route include rapid onset and ease of titration to effect. In addition, for the awake patient, patient-controlled IV delivery of opioids (i.e., patient-controlled analgesia [PCA]) has become widely available. PCA units combine options for baseline continuous infusion of drug with patient-administered bolus doses after programmed lockout periods to minimize the risk of overdose and maximize the patient's sense of "control" over their pain.

Patient satisfaction using PCA analgesia rivals that with neuraxial analgesia. Analgesic agents that have traditionally been available only for oral administration are becoming available for parenteral usage. IV ketorolac and acetaminophen have gained widespread acceptance as analgesic alternatives for thoracic surgical patients that are devoid of respiratory depressant effects.

D. Interpleural

Interpleural analgesia involves the placement of a catheter between the visceral and parietal pleura for the subsequent instillation of local anesthetic solution. The ensuing pain relief is believed to be the result of the blockade of intercostal nerves in addition to local actions on the pleura. Disadvantages of this technique include the requirement for relatively high doses of local anesthetic with relatively enhanced vascular uptake, poor effectiveness, and possible impairment of ipsilateral diaphragmatic function. For these reasons, interpleural analgesia has been largely abandoned as a strategy for pain control in cardiothoracic surgery patients.

E. Intercostal

Sequential intercostal blocks (e.g., T4 to T10) can contribute to unilateral postoperative chest wall analgesia for thoracic surgery. Bilateral intercostal nerve blocks (ICBs) may be used for pain relief after median sternotomy [45]. ICBs require depositing local anesthetic (e.g., 4 mL of 0.5% bupivacaine per nerve) at the inferior border of the associated rib near the proximal intercostal nerve. ICBs are generally performed through the skin before surgery or by the surgeon under direct vision within the chest. ICBs typically contribute to analgesia for up to 12 hours. However, they do not include blockade of the posterior and visceral rami of the intercostal nerve, thus they often require additional NSAID or parenteral analgesia to be effective.

F. Fascial plane blocks

The availability of ultrasound guidance to identify various thoracic fascial planes has facilitated the injection of local anesthetic to achieve ipsilateral chest wall analgesia with avoidance of the more invasive neuraxial and paravertebral approaches. Given the typically distant location from the neuraxis, fascial plane blocks are appealing since they may provide adequate analgesia for cardiothoracic surgical procedures while avoiding unwanted hypotension, urinary retention, and bleeding risk associated with neuraxial blockade. Single injection and catheter-based strategies in these fascial planes that may be applied to cardiac and thoracic surgery are described below.

1. **Pecs 1 and 2.** The so-called "Pecs" blocks are interfascial plane blocks of the anterior chest wall. Originally described [46] and primarily studied for use in breast surgery, when used in combination, these provide analgesia to the anterior and anterolateral chest wall. Pecs 1 is aimed to block the ipsilateral, lateral, and medial pectoral nerves, while Pecs 2 is aimed to block the lateral rami of the intercostal nerves and the long thoracic nerve. These blocks may be useful as part of a multimodal analgesia strategy for minimally invasive cardiac surgical procedures involving small anterior thoracotomies; such an approach has been described following minimally invasive mitral valve replacement [47].

2. **Serratus anterior plane block.** This chest wall block targets the thoracic intercostal nerves as well as the thoracodorsal and long thoracic nerves to provide analgesia to the anterolateral and a portion of the posterior hemithorax with a distribution from approximately T2 to T9 [48]. There are a few clinical reports of its efficacy for providing analgesia for rib fractures and for thoracic surgical procedures [49,50].

3. **Erector spinae plane block.** The erector spinae plane block involves depositing local anesthetic in the plane between the erector spinae musculature and the transverse process of the T5 vertebra [51]. Given its proximity to the midline relative to other fascial plane blocks, this approach may be more likely to achieve blockade of both the dorsal and ventral rami of the thoracic spinal nerves in a dermatomal distribution spanning approximately T2 to T9. Several case reports of this block have described its utility in thoracic surgery [51–53].

G. **Paravertebral blocks (PVBs)**
PVBs can provide unilateral chest wall analgesia for thoracic surgery. Sequential thoracic PVB injections (e.g., T4 to T10, 4 mL of 0.5% ropivacaine per level) may be combined with "light" general anesthesia for thoracotomy procedures and provide analgesia for several hours post-operatively. At some institutions, continuous PVB catheters are used interchangeably with epidural analgesia to provide pain relief with an apparent superior side-effect profile [54]. Anticipated chest tube insertion sites typically dictate the lowest PVB level required. Although the use of PVBs reduces intraoperative opioid requirement, NSAID and/or opioid supplementation is often required after thoracotomy to achieve adequate comfort. "Emergence" from PVB-mediated analgesia may occur on the day after surgery, often after transfer from an intensive care environment; therefore, it is important that other analgesia alternatives be immediately available at this time. Potential advantages of PVBs and ICBs relative to neur-axial techniques include the avoidance of opioid-related side effects, epidural hematoma, and hypotension related to bilateral sympathetic block. Nonetheless, ICB and PVB analgesia have the disadvantages that they may be less reliable than thoracic epidural analgesia and can them-selves be complicated by epidural spread of local anesthetic. Notably, compared to PVBs, ICBs do not affect the posterior and visceral rami of the intercostal nerves and tend to recede more rapidly. The paravertebral space, where peripheral nerves exit from the spinal canal, is limited superiorly and inferiorly by the heads of associated ribs, anteriorly by the parietal pleura, and posteriorly by the superior costotransverse ligament.

H. **Intrathecal (IT)**
IT opioid analgesia is a suitable strategy for major pain after median sternotomy or thoracotomy [55]. The benefits and risks of a spinal procedure should always be carefully weighed before using this technique, particularly with regard to the risk of spinal hematoma in patients receiv-ing anticoagulation or with abnormal hemostasis. Small-caliber noncutting spinal needles (e.g., 27-gauge Whitacre needle) are often selected for lumbar spinal injection of preservative-free morphine. Age rather than weight predicts proper IT opioid dosing in adults; 10 µg/kg IT morphine dosing is effective for cardiothoracic surgery in most adults and is usually adminis-tered before the induction of general anesthesia. Smaller doses (e.g., 0.3 to 0.5 mg, total dose) are required to reduce the likelihood of respiratory depression in elderly patients (older than 75 years of age). It is prudent to avoid the use of IT morphine in patients aged 85 years or older. Since rare patients will develop significant delayed respiratory depression, hourly monitoring of respiratory rate and consciousness for 18 to 24 hours is advisable with this technique. Reduced doses of sedative and hypnotic agents during general anesthesia may lower the likeli-hood of excessive postoperative somnolence. The onset of thoracic analgesia is approximately 1 to 2 hours after injection, lasting up to 24 hours. Postoperative NSAID therapy complements IT morphine analgesia without sedative effects. IT clonidine (1 µg/kg) combined with IT mor-phine produces superior analgesia compared to either drug administered alone [56]. IV or oral analgesia must be immediately available in anticipation of the resolution of IT morphine analgesia approximately 24 hours after injection because significant pain may develop rapidly. IT administration of other drugs for cardiac and thoracic surgeries, such as local anesthetic agents or short-acting opioids (e.g., sufentanil), is mainly limited to the intraoperative period.

I. **Epidural**
Epidural anesthesia is ideal for thoracic surgery and is the most widely studied and used form of regional analgesia for this purpose [18]. Although epidural catheter placement for use dur-ing and after cardiac surgery is reported to have benefits [57], this approach has not gained a similar level of acceptance. Of note, while many agree that thoracic epidural analgesia is the

gold standard for pain control after open thoracotomy, no regional anesthetic technique has yet emerged as superior for pain control after less-invasive video-assisted thoracoscopic surgical (VATS) approaches to lung resection [58]. The role of truncal and fascial plane blocks, some of which are described above, as viable options for pain relief following VATS procedures involving brief hospital stays has yet to be fully explored.

Thoracic epidural catheter placement (T4 to T10) is often preferred over lumbar for thoracic surgery. Proponents of thoracic catheter placement cite the reduced local anesthetic dosing requirements, closer proximity to the thoracic segment dorsal horns, and reduced likelihood of dislodgement postoperatively. Concern regarding increased risk of spinal cord injury using a thoracic compared to a lumbar approach for epidural catheter placement has not been borne out; however, some practitioners prefer that thoracic epidural catheter placement occur while the patient is sufficiently alert to reliably report paresthesias or other problems during the procedure. Selection of the thoracic interspace should be dictated by the surgical incision. The epidural catheter should be placed 4 to 6 cm into the epidural space and securely taped.

Intraoperative use of an epidural catheter enhances the value of regional anesthesia for thoracotomy surgery by permitting a "light general" anesthetic technique with reduced residual respiratory depressant effects. Epidural local anesthetic block should be preceded by a "test dose" of an epinephrine-containing local anesthetic to rule out intravascular or IT catheter placement. Epidural opioids should generally not be administered unless postoperative observation and monitoring for delayed respiratory depression is planned. To minimize postoperative somnolence and the risk of respiratory depression, the administration of potent IV sedatives and opioids should be reduced or avoided during surgery, and the agents used to maintain general anesthesia should be easily reversible (e.g., volatile anesthetic agents). A popular mixture for postoperative epidural analgesia is dilute local anesthetic (e.g., 0.125% bupivacaine) containing an opioid with intermediate lipid solubility (e.g., hydromorphone, 10 µg/mL); this is administered by continuous infusion at a starting rate of 4 to 7 mL/hr, ideally starting at least 15 minutes before the end of surgery and titrated to clinical effect. Since early titration of epidural analgesic infusions is often required, and pain is not effectively reported by the awakening patient, an initial analgesic dose of hydromorphone and local anesthetic agent should be administered (e.g., 200-µg hydromorphone bolus, 3-mL preservative-free 2% lidocaine) before emergence. IV ketorolac or acetaminophen can also be administered at this time when indicated. Ketorolac is often especially effective in helping to manage shoulder discomfort secondary to indwelling thoracostomy tubes, since this complaint often persists in the setting of good incisional pain control with epidural analgesia. Titration of epidural analgesia to comfort should be completed in the postoperative recovery area where transfer of care to the acute pain care team should occur.

CLINICAL PEARL   A primary benefit of effective pain control is patient satisfaction and improved recovery profile with avoidance of the negative consequences of pain; various analgesic strategies with or without neuraxial and regional techniques, can be considered. There is no "gold standard" recipe, as it is difficult to prove an outcome benefit with any single technique.

IV. Pain management regimens for specific cardiothoracic procedures
  A. Conventional coronary artery bypass grafting and open-chamber procedures
  The move away from standard high-dose opioid anesthesia and prolonged durations of postoperative ventilation has increased interest in different approaches to analgesia after cardiac surgery. Many procedures are suitable for early tracheal extubation and therefore require analgesia regimens compatible with a rapid recovery. Standard regimens for cardiac surgery now commonly involve modest intraoperative opioid dosing and the postoperative bedside availability of parenteral opioids as required in the first 12 to 24 hours, either patient controlled or administered by a nurse. Transition to oral agents is encouraged as soon as food is tolerated.

  Routine NSAID therapy for uncomplicated patients is a safe and cost-effective way to complement opioid analgesia. Preoperative IT morphine has gained popularity in some centers. In experienced hands, imaginative combinations, such as preoperative IT morphine and intraoperative IV remifentanil infusion, provide reproducible excellent analgesia with tracheal extubation often possible in the operating room [45].

B. Off-pump (sternotomy) cardiac procedures

One interpretation of "minimally invasive" cardiac surgery involves the avoidance of cardiopulmonary bypass (CPB). The more limited systemic inflammatory response–associated CPB avoidance oddly may *increase* the perception of pain. Additionally, off-pump cardiac surgery is often accompanied by a "fast-track" approach to pain relief, which further challenges traditional opioid-based analgesia regimens. Inadequate pain relief is an important addressable cause for delayed hospital discharge. Thus, interest in analgesic approaches other than parenteral opioids for off pump CABGs parallels the trend in traditional cardiac surgery on CPB, as outlined above (see Section IV.A).

C. Transcatheter and percutaneous procedures (transcatheter aortic valve replacement, mitral clip, electrophysiology procedures)

Percutaneous and transcatheter approaches to valvular disease and dysrythmias generally involve peripheral (e.g., groin) access and avoid the need for thoracic incisions. This can often be managed with local anesthetic infiltration at the site along with the use of nonopioid adjunct medications. Many European and American centers have moved to performing these procedures with sedation or local anesthesia only.

D. Minimally invasive (minithoracotomy/para- or partial sternotomy/robotic) cardiac procedures

In contrast to off-pump procedures, a second interpretation of "minimally invasive" cardiac surgery involves port-access catheter-based CPB employing very small incisions to achieve surgical goals. Although there were hopes that port-access procedures would be associated with less pain, this has not been proven to be true, most likely because of the relocation of the smaller incisions to more pain-sensitive areas (e.g., minithoracotomy). In addition to the alternate analgesic approaches outlined for patients undergoing traditional cardiac surgery with CPB (see Section IV.A), the possibility of using novel approaches to minithoracotomy analgesia, including ICBs, one-shot PVBs, continuous PVBs, and fascial plane blocks, exist but have not been sufficiently explored to recommend their routine use.

E. Thoracotomy/thoracoscopy procedures (noncardiac)

An increasing number of the patients presenting for lung surgery have end-stage lung disease and may not have been considered eligible for an operative procedure several years ago [59]. In part, these changes in eligibility for lung resection are due in part to the availability of less-invasive techniques, including minimally invasive VATS procedures. Patients with severe lung disease may have the most to gain from any improvements in outcome related to optimal postoperative analgesia (e.g., continuous thoracic epidural) [59]. Most physiologically invasive procedures (e.g., lobectomy) are now routinely performed using VATS approaches, although some procedures (e.g., pneumonectomy) typically still require the traditional and more painful thoracotomy incision. "Light" general anesthesia with regional blockade of the chest wall is a particularly suitable anesthetic approach for lung and other chest surgery. Sedatives (e.g., midazolam) should be used sparingly or completely avoided; often even a small dose of midazolam (e.g., 0.5 mg) will extend the action of shorter-acting agents, such as propofol (e.g., 10 mg), if sedation is absolutely necessary for line placement. Using this approach, residual sedative/hypnotic effects can be minimized, early tracheal extubation is more reliably achieved, and the transition to postoperative pain management is facilitated.

Analgesia for VATS and thoracotomy procedures in the intraoperative and postoperative period is often achieved through a multimodal approach including parenteral opioids, NSAIDs, and regional anesthesia; however, there is a large amount of variability between hospitals as to whether patients receive perioperative multimodal analgesia [60]. A spectrum of regional anesthesia procedures are available, including thoracic epidural, spinal, PVBs, intercostal blocks, interpleural blocks, and several potentially applicable thoracic fascial plane blocks. These can be performed transcutaneously under ultrasound needle guidance by the anesthesiologist or in some cases from within the rib cage during surgery by the surgeon. Selection of a regional analgesia approach should include a plan for transition to oral medication and match the anticipated hospital discharge timing; notably, neuraxial opioids may delay discharge if used inappropriately. Finally, many patients with normal pulmonary function having a minor surgical procedure will have good analgesia with IV PCA morphine or fentanyl alone.

Selection of a regional blockade technique is best made after evaluation of both the patient status and the demands of the surgery. American Society of Anesthesiologists class I to II patients anticipating postoperative hospital stays up to 48 hours may benefit from regional anesthetic blocks; however, anxious patients in this group should not be overly pressured to undergo a regional procedure. In contrast, patients who are deconditioned or undergoing more extensive procedures are more likely to benefit from regional anesthesia. Routine postoperative NSAID or acetaminophen therapy should be considered, since these agents are devoid of sedation and are particularly effective analgesics in combination with regional analgesia. Local anesthetic/opioid mixtures are popular analgesic regimens for use as continuous epidural infusions (see Section III.H). However, in high-risk cases (e.g., lung volume reduction or lung transplant surgery), where avoidance of all respiratory depressants is desirable, analgesia may be achieved using a dilute local anesthetic agent alone. Tachyphylaxis is a common problem with any local anesthetic–alone technique, requiring frequent rate readjustments. Removal of an epidural catheter subjects a patient to all the same risks as insertion. When transfer from epidural to oral analgesia is being considered, thromboprophylaxis protocols should be coordinated with epidural catheter removal to minimize the risk of epidural hematoma. If the patient is taking warfarin, the international normalized ratio at the time of catheter removal should be <1.5 to minimize the risk of bleeding.

F. **Open and closed (total endovascular aortic repair [TEVAR]) descending thoracic aortic procedures**

Major surgical procedures to treat diseases of the descending thoracic aorta often require both an extensive left thoracotomy incision and a long midline abdominal incision. Unfortunately, serious complications are common with these procedures and include high incidences of bleeding/coagulopathy due to the extensive surgery, paraplegia from spinal cord ischemia, and acute kidney injury. Despite the significant pain associated with these incisions, analgesia is often relegated to a secondary concern. In addition, increased risks of renal and spinal cord injury are relative contraindications to some of the most useful agents of a multimodal approach to severe postoperative pain. However, some creative approaches to analgesia are being considered. In addition to standard IV opioid techniques, a tunneled catheter under the left parietal pleura can be placed to extend cephalad over several dermatomes of the chest wall and deliver dilute local anesthetic. Unfortunately, there is little research in this area to guide clinicians. Some anesthesiologists and surgical teams even feel that the benefits of thoracic epidural analgesia merit placement of a thoracic epidural catheter either preoperatively or after surgery.

V. **Approach to specific complications and side effects of analgesic strategies**

A. **Complications of nonsteroidal anti-inflammatory drugs (NSAIDs)**

1. **Renal toxicity.** Normal patients exhibit a low rate of prostaglandin synthesis in the renal vasculature, such that cyclooxygenase inhibition has little effect. However, vasodilatory prostaglandins may play an important role in the preservation of renal perfusion in disease states. Nephrotoxicity, secondary to vasoconstriction of both afferent and efferent renal arterioles leading to reduced glomerular filtration rate, is commonly seen with NSAID administration in patients with dehydration, sepsis, congestive heart failure, or other causes of renal hypoperfusion. Avoiding NSAID-induced renal toxicity is best accomplished by limiting or avoiding their use in patients with decreased renal reserve and in those at risk for hypoperfusion. Risk appears to be low with perioperative ketorolac administration (1:1,000 to 1:10,000) [61]. NSAID-induced nephrotoxicity is usually reversible with discontinuation of the drug.

2. **Gastrointestinal mucosal irritation.** Gastrointestinal mucosal irritation is the most common NSAID side effect and can occur regardless of the route of administration. It may result in erosion and severe gastrointestinal bleeding. Prostaglandins are involved in multiple aspects of gastric mucosal protection, including mucosal blood flow, epithelial cell growth, and surface mucus and bicarbonate production. Prophylaxis may involve administration of histamine (H_2)-receptor antagonists, proton pump inhibitors (e.g., omeprazole), protective agents (e.g., sucralfate), or prostaglandin analogs (e.g., misoprostol). Each of these treatments appears to be effective in decreasing ulceration with NSAID treatment.

3. **Impaired primary hemostasis.** Nonspecific cyclooxygenase inhibition leads to impaired platelet aggregation that may increase intraoperative or postoperative bleeding. The duration of effect is highly variable depending on the individual drug (reversible vs. irreversible enzymatic inhibition). The only effective prophylaxis or treatment is to discontinue NSAIDs for a sufficient duration preoperatively (e.g., ibuprofen more than 3 days, aspirin more than 7 to 10 days).

B. **Nausea and vomiting**

Nausea and vomiting as a consequence of analgesia is most commonly associated with opioids. Opioids cause nausea primarily through activation of the chemoreceptor trigger zone of the brainstem in the floor of the fourth ventricle. A vestibular component is also postulated because it is clear that motion increases the incidence of nausea. Finally, the inhibitory effects of opioids on gastrointestinal motility may contribute. Nausea can accompany opioid therapy regardless of the route of administration. It occurs in roughly 25% to 35% of patients treated with spinal opioids and is more frequent with the spinal use of hydrophilic drugs (e.g., morphine) secondary to enhanced rostral spread of these agents [62]. The optimal pharmacologic treatment of nausea and vomiting involves such agents as ondansetron, prochlorperazine, chlorpromazine, promethazine, metoclopramide, and dexamethasone.

C. **Pruritus**

Pruritus is a common side effect of opioids administered by any route, but it can be particularly problematic after neuraxial administration. The mechanism is unclear and likely complex, but pruritus is not likely caused solely by either preservatives within the opioid preparation or histamine release. Pruritus often improves as the duration of opioid treatment lengthens. Pruritus is most effectively treated with antihistamines, mixed agonist–antagonist opioids (e.g., nalbuphine), or by naloxone infusion.

D. **Respiratory depression**

Hypoventilation is a potentially life-threatening complication of opioids. It can occur early after administration by any route, but it is particularly feared as a delayed complication of neuraxial opioid administration. Whatever the method of administration, opioid-related hypoventilation occurs secondary to elevated cerebrospinal fluid drug levels, either from systemic absorption or rostral spread of neuraxially administered drug, which then produce depression of the medullary respiratory center. Respiratory depression requiring naloxone administration is reported to occur in 0.2% to 1% of patients receiving epidural opioids [63], but the incidence is likely higher in opioid-naïve patients being treated for acute pain. Other factors that may increase the risk include advanced age, poor overall medical condition, higher opioid dosing (particularly of hydrophilic drugs), increased intrathoracic or intra-abdominal pressure (as may occur during mechanical ventilation), and coincident administration of other CNS depressants. Patients who have received spinal opioids in the prior 18 to 24 hours or in whom continuous infusions are being administered should have their ventilatory rate and level of alertness confirmed at least hourly. Caretakers should be aware that deteriorating levels of consciousness might portend severe respiratory depression even if ventilatory rates appear preserved. Arterial blood gas analysis should be used early in the investigation of decreased alertness. Modest doses of naloxone (0.04 to 0.1 mg IV) are usually sufficient to temporarily reverse respiratory depression if discovered before it has become severe.

E. **Neurologic complications**

Although neurologic complications from analgesic procedures are extremely rare, when these occur they can be catastrophic and appropriate management is key to minimizing adverse consequences. Nerve injury may be heralded by an acute discomfort with nerve trauma during a procedure but may only be apparent when local anesthetic effects recede. Therefore, it is essential that this diagnosis is not overlooked in the evaluation of a prolonged block. In particular, if a spinal cord hematoma is being considered, it should be remembered that the promptness of surgical decompression is the most important predictor of recovery of neurologic function [64].

Eighty-eight percent of neurologic deficits related to spinal hematoma will resolve if surgical decompression occurs within 12 hours of symptom onset, whereas only 40% will have improvement when surgery occurs beyond 24 hours. A key aspect in the evaluation of a possible nerve injury is the involvement of a neurologist in consultation. Most nerve injuries are transient and recover over several days, but the opinion of a specialist in this area will assure that effective acute treatments are not delayed.

F. Infectious complications

Infectious complications associated with neuraxial techniques are rare but potentially catastrophic, potentially requiring surgical intervention and drainage. Most recent practice advisories recommend looking for risk factors for infection and considering alternatives to neuraxial techniques for high-risk patients. A known epidural abscess is a contraindication to neuraxial blockade. According to this consensus document [65], if bacteremia is present, preprocedural antibiotics should be considered. Aseptic technique, with antiseptic skin preparation and use of sterile barriers and occlusive dressings, should be employed for placement of all neuraxial needles and catheters. Use of bacterial filters and avoidance of excessive catheter manipulation post placement is useful in preventing infection. Teams managing neuraxial or regional catheters should consider removal of accidentally disconnected or unnecessary catheters daily in the context of each patient's medical status, while balancing the benefits of good pain control.

VI. Risk versus benefit: epidural/intrathecal (IT) analgesia for cardiac surgical procedures requiring systemic anticoagulation

Controversy has surrounded the relative risks and benefits of neuraxial blockade for patients undergoing cardiac surgery requiring systemic anticoagulation. Clearly, extensive clinical experience and literature support the safety of neuraxial procedures in the setting of heparin anticoagulation accompanying major vascular surgery; but, in such cases, heparin dosing is generally lower than for cardiac surgery and is not accompanied by the added effects of CPB on impaired hemostasis. Established guidelines have been available to support decision making in this regard, including the avoidance of neuraxial interventions when patients have pre-existing hemostatic disorders, postponing surgery for 24 hours in the event of a traumatic ("bloody") tap at the time of needle or catheter insertion, and delaying heparin administration for at least 60 minutes after performance of an uncomplicated neuraxial procedure. These guidelines are largely based on the analysis of retrospective cohorts [66]. Current ASRA consensus guidelines indicate that "insufficient data and experience are available to determine if the risk of neuraxial hematoma is increased when combining neuraxial techniques with the full anticoagulation of cardiac surgery" [37].

Despite widespread belief in the salutatory effects of excellent analgesia, the principal patient-related benefit of central neuraxial analgesia for cardiac surgery is patient satisfaction. Importantly, a body of literature has assembled that does not support the belief that central neuraxial analgesia improves major clinical outcomes [20]. Epidural hematoma can complicate thoracic epidural placement for cardiac surgery, although to date there are no reports of spinal bleeding complicating single-shot IT drug placement prior to cardiac surgery, and the risk for epidural catheter insertion prior to cardiac surgery has been assessed to be equivalent to that for obstetric anesthesia [67,68]. Pending additional contributions to our understanding, the trend in expert opinion argues for caution, particularly regarding thoracic epidural catheter placement prior to "full" heparin anticoagulation for cardiac surgery.

CLINICAL PEARL Expert opinion leans toward caution in the setting of neuraxial blockade for cardiac surgery, with cognizance of holding systemic anticoagulation as appropriate per available practice guidelines.

VII. Considerations in facilitating transitions of care

A. Enhanced recovery after surgery (ERAS)

ERAS programs for thoracic surgery evolved from historical "fast-tracking" protocols to now include preoptimization, minimizing fasting time, thromboembolic prophylaxis, anesthetic and analgesic techniques, surgical approach, postoperative rehabilitation, and chest tube management. Such protocols demonstrate improvements in morbidity and length of stay for selected patient groups.

B. **Quality and safety considerations**

Reliable postoperative analgesia is a key component in facilitating prompt tracheal extubation (within 6 hours) after cardiac surgery. Such "fast tracking" of low-risk cardiac surgery patients appears to be safe and has been adopted by many centers as a process to shorten intensive care unit and hospital lengths of stay. Patients may receive additional benefits, such as improved cardiac function and reduced rates of respiratory infections and complications. Attention to reducing risk and to institutional resource utilization has expanded the focus on accelerating and improving transitions of care for all cardiothoracic surgical patients, not just those deemed "low risk" in advance. Similarly, the role of the anesthesiologist in care pathway design has expanded well beyond facilitating early extubation and early postoperative analgesia toward greater preoperative and postoperative integration as a key perioperative physician [69].

C. **Intrathecal (IT) morphine**

IT morphine is used in many centers for eligible cardiac surgery patients to provide analgesia and mild sedation in the early postoperative period. However, some studies have failed to demonstrate a beneficial effect of IT morphine either in improving early analgesia or in facilitating early extubation. NSAIDs complement opioid analgesia regardless of how the opioid is administered. Indomethacin, administered rectally as 100-mg suppositories, is a common component of fast-tracking protocols for cardiac surgery aimed at reducing pain and early postoperative narcotic use. Some NSAIDs may antagonize opioid-induced respiratory depression [70]. Intraoperative and postoperative continuous infusions of remifentanil or alfentanil (with or without supplemental propofol infusion) are used in some centers to allow for controlled analgesia and "scheduled extubation." Both a high-dose narcotic technique using the ultra–short-acting narcotic remifentanil [45] or an anesthetic incorporating high thoracic epidural conduction block [57] have been suggested as methods that may improve outcomes by inhibiting perioperative stress responses while facilitating early extubation and fast tracking.

Postoperative analgesia strategy for thoracic surgery patients often influences disposition when continuous epidural infusions are used, since the care team must be equipped and trained to intervene when potentially serious complications of postoperative analgesia occur, such as hypotension from local anesthetic–mediated reductions in sympathetic tone and delayed respiratory depression due to cephalad spread of neuraxial opioids. In formulating an analgesia plan for thoracic surgery, considerable respect must be paid to the failure to achieve tracheal extubation—a serious complication of emergence whose occurrence is partly under the influence of the anesthesiologist. This is particularly important since major pulmonary complications of lung resection surgery are more than twice as likely in the setting of postoperative respiratory failure and are highly associated with other markers of adverse outcome, including postoperative mortality. Contributors to the heightened risk of respiratory failure after lung resection include "variable" factors amenable to optimization, such as inadequate respiratory mechanics from pain-related chest wall splinting, poor positioning, and residual paralysis.

Since pain at emergence from anesthesia for lung resection is extremely difficult to treat without increasing the risk of acute respiratory depression and interfering with efforts to extubate the patient, the anesthesiologist must be confident that analgesia is established pre-emergence. If a thoracic epidural catheter has been placed, a common practice 10 to 15 minutes prior to emergence is to supplement existing analgesia with an additional 2-mL bolus of 2% preservative-free lidocaine for an average adult male; this represents a modest investment in protection from emergence pain that rarely causes block-mediated hypotension but allows for tracheal extubation before more pain management interventions are needed. Fortunately, difficult emergence sequences are relatively infrequent, but the patient with limited respiratory reserve likely has the most to gain from an experienced anesthesia team to avoid a prolonged episode of postoperative mechanical ventilation. Rarely, sequential blood gas determinations immediately following tracheal extubation (e.g., every 3 minutes) identify the marginal patient whose CO_2 levels are rising despite optimal analgesia, a concerning finding that requires further prompt intervention and optimization to avert respiratory failure and tracheal reintubation.

> **CLINICAL PEARL** Pain at emergence from anesthesia for lung resection is extremely difficult to treat without increasing the risk of acute respiratory depression in a patient with limited respiratory reserve, and can be optimized prior to extubation by modest dosing of neuraxial or regional catheters with local anesthetic prior to emergence.

REFERENCES

1. **Guimaraes-Pereira L, Reis P, Abelha F, et al. Persistent postoperative pain after cardiac surgery: a systematic review with meta-analysis regarding incidence and pain intensity. *Pain.* 2017;158(10):1869–1885.**
2. Lahtinen P, Kokki H, Hynynen M. Pain after cardiac surgery: a prospective cohort study of 1-year incidence and intensity. *Anesthesiology.* 2006;105(4):794–800.
3. Ho SC, Royse CF, Royse AG, et al. Persistent pain after cardiac surgery: an audit of high thoracic epidural and primary opioid analgesia therapies. *Anesth Analg.* 2002;95(4):820–823.
4. Meyerson J, Thelin S, Gordh T, et al. The incidence of chronic post-sternotomy pain after cardiac surgery—a prospective study. *Acta Anaesthesiol Scand.* 2001;45(8):940–944.
5. Bayman EO, Parekh KR, Keech J, et al. A prospective study of chronic pain after thoracic surgery. *Anesthesiology.* 2017; 126(5):938–951.
6. Glower DD, Landolfo KP, Clements F, et al. Mitral valve operation via port access versus median sternotomy. *Eur J Cardiothorac Surg.* 1998;14(1 Suppl):S143–S147.
7. Bayman EO, Brennan TJ. Incidence and severity of chronic pain at 3 and 6 months after thoracotomy: meta-analysis. *J Pain.* 2014;15(9):887–897.
8. **Kehlet H, Jensen TS, Woolf CJ. Persistent postsurgical pain: risk factors and prevention. *Lancet.* 2006;367(9522): 1618–1625.**
9. Bair E, Gaynor S, Slade GD, et al. Identification of clusters of individuals relevant to temporomandibular disorders and other chronic pain conditions: the OPPERA study. *Pain.* 2016;157(6):1266–1278.
10. Ip HY, Abrishami A, Peng PW, et al. Predictors of postoperative pain and analgesic consumption: a qualitative systematic review. *Anesthesiology.* 2009;111(3):657–677.
11. **Andreae MH, Andreae DA. Regional anaesthesia to prevent chronic pain after surgery: a Cochrane systematic review and meta-analysis. *Br J Anaesth.* 2013;111(5):711–720.**
12. Constantinides VA, Tekkis PP, Fazil A, et al. Fast-track failure after cardiac surgery: development of a prediction model. *Crit Care Med.* 2006;34(12):2875–2882.
13. **Jones NL, Edmonds L, Ghosh S, et al. A review of enhanced recovery for thoracic anaesthesia and surgery. *Anaesthesia.* 2013;68(2):179–189.**
14. Mehran RJ, Martin LW, Baker CM, et al. Pain management in an enhanced recovery pathway after thoracic surgical procedures. *Ann Thorac Surg.* 2016;102(6):e595–e596.
15. Brame AL, Singer M. Stressing the obvious? An allostatic look at critical illness. *Crit Care Med.* 2010;38(10 Suppl):S600–S607.
16. **Liu SS, Wu CL. Effect of postoperative analgesia on major postoperative complications: a systematic update of the evidence. *Anesth Analg.* 2007;104(3):689–702.**
17. Ochroch EA, Gottschalk A, Augostides J, et al. Long-term pain and activity during recovery from major thoracotomy using thoracic epidural analgesia. *Anesthesiology.* 2002;97:1234–1244.
18. **Gottschalk A, Cohen SP, Yang S, et al. Preventing and treating pain after thoracic surgery. *Anesthesiology.* 2006; 104(3):594–600.**
19. Fillinger MP, Yeager MP, Dodds TM, et al. Epidural anesthesia and analgesia: effects on recovery from cardiac surgery. *J Cardiothorac Vasc Anesth.* 2002;16(1):15–20.
20. Liu SS, Block BM, Wu CL. Effects of perioperative central neuraxial analgesia on outcome after coronary artery bypass surgery: a meta-analysis. *Anesthesiology.* 2004;101(1):153–161.
21. **Svircevic V, Nierich AP, Moons KG, et al. Thoracic epidural anesthesia for cardiac surgery: a randomized trial. *Anesthesiology.* 2011;114(2):262–270.**
22. United Nations Office on Drugs and Crime WHO. Opioid overdose: preventing and reducing opioid overdose mortality. Discussion paper UNODC/WHO 2013. 2013.
23. Dowell D, Haegerich TM, Chou R. CDC guideline for prescribing opioids for chronic pain—United States, 2016. *MMWR Recomm Rep.* 2016;65(1):1–49.
24. Inturrisi CE. Clinical pharmacology of opioids for pain. *Clin J Pain.* 2002;18(4 Suppl):S3–S13.
25. Gulur P, Koury K, Arnstein P, et al. Morphine versus hydromorphone: does choice of opioid influence outcomes? *Pain Res Treat.* 2015;2015:482081.
26. McGettigan P, Henry D. Cardiovascular risk and inhibition of cyclooxygenase: a systematic review of the observational studies of selective and nonselective inhibitors of cyclooxygenase 2. *JAMA.* 2006;296(13):1633–1644.
27. **Nussmeier NA, Whelton AA, Brown MT, et al. Complications of the COX-2 inhibitors parecoxib and valdecoxib after cardiac surgery. *N Engl J Med.* 2005;352(11):1081–1091.**
28. Sinatra RS, Jahr JS, Reynolds LW, et al. Efficacy and safety of single and repeated administration of 1 gram intravenous acetaminophen injection (paracetamol) for pain management after major orthopedic surgery. *Anesthesiology.* 2005;102(4):822–831.

29. Pettersson PH, Jakobsson J, Owall A. Intravenous acetaminophen reduced the use of opioids compared with oral administration after coronary artery bypass grafting. *J Cardiothorac Vasc Anesth.* 2005;19(3):306–309.

30. Dholakia U, Clark-Price SC, Keating SCJ, et al. Anesthetic effects and body weight changes associated with ketamine-xylazine-lidocaine administered to CD-1 mice. *PloS One.* 2017;12(9):e0184911.

31. Insler SR, O'Connor M, Samonte AF, et al. Lidocaine and the inhibition of postoperative pain in coronary artery bypass patients. *J Cardiothorac Vasc Anesth.* 1995;9(5):541–546.

32. Hamilton TW, Athanassoglou V, Mellon S, et al. Liposomal bupivacaine infiltration at the surgical site for the management of postoperative pain. *Cochrane Database Syst Rev.* 2017;2:Cd011419.

33. Boogaerts JG, Lafont ND, Declercq AG, et al. Epidural administration of liposome-associated bupivacaine for the management of postsurgical pain: a first study. *J Clin Anesth.* 1994;6(4):315–320.

34. Ilfeld BM. Liposome bupivacaine in peripheral nerve blocks and epidural injections to manage postoperative pain. *Expert Opin Pharmacother.* 2013;14(17):2421–2431.

35. Viscusi ER, Candiotti KA, Onel E, et al. The pharmacokinetics and pharmacodynamics of liposome bupivacaine administered via a single epidural injection to healthy volunteers. *Reg Anesth Pain Med.* 2012;37(6):616–622.

36. Ilfeld BM, Viscusi ER, Hadzic A, et al. Safety and side effect profile of liposome bupivacaine (exparel) in peripheral nerve blocks. *Reg Anesth Pain Med.* 2015;40(5):572–582.

37. **Horlocker TT, Wedel DJ, Rowlingson JC, et al. Regional anesthesia in the patient receiving antithrombotic or thrombolytic therapy: American Society of Regional Anesthesia and Pain Medicine evidence-based guidelines (third edition). *Reg Anesth Pain Med.* 2010;35(1):64–101.**

38. Neal JM, Kopp SL, Pasternak JJ, et al. Anatomy and pathophysiology of spinal cord injury associated with regional anesthesia and pain medicine: 2015 update. *Reg Anesth Pain Med.* 2015;40(5):506–525.

39. Pacira Pharmaceuticals, Inc. Exparel (bupivicaine liposomal injectable suspension) prescribing information. Available from https://www.exparel.com/sites/default/files/EXPAREL_Prescribing_Information.pdf. Accessed March 27, 2018.

40. Lahtinen P, Kokki H, Hakala T, et al. S(+)-ketamine as an analgesic adjunct reduces opioid consumption after cardiac surgery. *Anesth Analg.* 2004;99(5):1295–1301.

41. Ryu HG, Lee CJ, Kim YT, et al. Preemptive low-dose epidural ketamine for preventing chronic postthoracotomy pain: a prospective, double-blinded, randomized, clinical trial. *Clin J Pain.* 2011;27(4):304–308.

42. Cavalcante AN, Sprung J, Schroeder DR, et al. Multimodal analgesic therapy with gabapentin and its association with postoperative respiratory depression. *Anesth Analg.* 2017;125(1):141–146.

43. Zakkar M, Frazer S, Hunt I. Is there a role for gabapentin in preventing or treating pain following thoracic surgery? *Interact Cardiovasc Thorac Surg.* 2013;17(4):716–719.

44. Oates HB. Non-pharmacologic pain control for the CABG patient. *Dimens Crit Care Nurs.* 1993;12(6):296–304.

45. Zarate E, Latham P, White PF, et al. Fast-track cardiac anesthesia: use of remifentanil combined with intrathecal morphine as an alternative to sufentanil during desflurane anesthesia. *Anesth Analg.* 2000;91(2):283–287.

46. Blanco R. The "pecs block": a novel technique for providing analgesia after breast surgery. *Anaesthesia.* 2011;66(9):847–848.

47. Yalamuri S, Klinger RY, Bullock WM, et al. Pectoral fascial (PECS) I & II blocks as rescue analgesia in a patient undergoing minimally invasive cardiac surgery. *Reg Anesth Pain Med.* 2017;42(6):764–766.

48. Blanco R, Parras T, McDonnell JG, et al. Serratus plane block: a novel ultrasound-guided thoracic wall nerve block. *Anaesthesia.* 2013;68(11):1107–1113.

49. Kunhabdulla NP, Agarwal A, Gaur A, et al. Serratus anterior plane block for multiple rib fractures. *Pain Physician.* 2014;17(5):E651–E653.

50. Okmen K, Okmen BM. The efficacy of serratus anterior plane block in analgesia for thoracotomy: a retrospective study. *J Anesth.* 2017;31(4):579–585.

51. Forero M, Adhikary SD, Lopez H, et al. The erector spinae plane block: a novel analgesic technique in thoracic neuropathic pain. *Reg Anesth Pain Med.* 2016;41(5):621–627.

52. Forero M, Rajarathinam M, Adhikary S, et al. Continuous erector spinae plane block for rescue analgesia in thoracotomy after epidural failure: a case report. *A A Case Rep.* 2017;8(10):254–256.

53. Scimia P, Basso Ricci E, Droghetti A, et al. The ultrasound-guided continuous erector spinae plane block for postoperative analgesia in video-assisted thoracoscopic lobectomy. *Reg Anesth Pain Med.* 2017;42(4):537.

54. Davies RG, Myles PS, Graham JM. A comparison of the analgesic efficacy and side-effects of paravertebral vs epidural blockade for thoracotomy—a systematic review and meta-analysis of randomized trials. *Br J Anaesth.* 2006;96(4):418–426.

55. Rathmell JP, Lair TR, Nauman B. The role of intrathecal drugs in the treatment of acute pain. *Anesth Analg.* 2005;101(5 Suppl):S30–S43.

56. Lena P, Balarac N, Arnulf JJ, et al. Intrathecal morphine and clonidine for coronary artery bypass grafting. *Br J Anaesth.* 2003;90(3):300–303.

57. Scott NB, Turfrey DJ, Ray DA, et al. A prospective randomized study of the potential benefits of thoracic epidural anesthesia and analgesia in patients undergoing coronary artery bypass grafting. *Anesth Analg.* 2001;93(3):528–535.

58. Steinthorsdottir KJ, Wildgaard L, Hansen HJ, et al. Regional analgesia for video-assisted thoracic surgery: a systematic review. *Eur J Cardiothorac Surg.* 2014;45(6):959–966.

59. Licker MJ, Widikker I, Robert J, et al. Operative mortality and respiratory complications after lung resection for cancer: impact of chronic obstructive pulmonary disease and time trends. *Ann Thorac Surg.* 2006;81(5):1830–1837.

60. **Ladha KS, Patorno E, Huybrechts KF, et al. Variations in the use of perioperative multimodal analgesic therapy. *Anesthesiology.* 2016;124(4):837–845.**

61. Myles PS, Power I. Does ketorolac cause postoperative renal failure: how do we assess the evidence? *Br J Anaesth.* 1998;80(4):420–421.

62. Carr D, Cousins M. Spinal route of analgesia. In: Cousins M, Bridenbaugh P, eds. *Neural Blockade*. Philadelphia, PA: Lippincott-Raven Publishers; 1988:915–983.
63. Ready L. Regional anesthesia with intraspinal opioids. In: Loeser J, ed. *Bonica's Management of Pain*. Philadelphia, PA: Lippincott Williams & Wilkins; 2001:1953–1966.
64. Kunz U. Spinal hematoma: a literature survey with meta-analysis of 613 patients. *Neurosurg Rev*. 2003;26(1):52.
65. Practice advisory for the prevention, diagnosis, and management of infectious complications associated with neuraxial techniques: an updated report by the American Society of Anesthesiologists Task Force on Infectious Complications Associated with Neuraxial Techniques and the American Society of Regional Anesthesia and Pain Medicine. *Anesthesiology*. 2017;126(4):585–601.
66. Ho AM, Chung DC, Joynt GM. Neuraxial blockade and hematoma in cardiac surgery: estimating the risk of a rare adverse event that has not (yet) occurred. *Chest*. 2000;117(2):551–555.
67. Rosen DA, Hawkinberry DW 2nd, Rosen KR, et al. An epidural hematoma in an adolescent patient after cardiac surgery. *Anesth Analg*. 2004;98(4):966–969.
68. Bracco D, Hemmerling T. Epidural analgesia in cardiac surgery: an updated risk assessment. *Heart Surg Forum*. 2007;10(4): E334–E337.
69. **White PF, Kehlet H, Neal JM, et al. The role of the anesthesiologist in fast-track surgery: from multimodal analgesia to perioperative medical care. *Anesth Analg*. 2007;104(6):1380–1396.**
70. Moren J, Francois T, Blanloeil Y, et al. The effects of a nonsteroidal antiinflammatory drug (ketoprofen) on morphine respiratory depression: a double-blind, randomized study in volunteers. *Anesth Analg*. 1997;85(2):400–405.

Index

Note: Page number followed by f and t indicates figure and table only.